PRAISE FOR
THAT PARENTS AND
DOCTORS TRUST

❖ ❖ ❖ ❖ ❖

"Excellent. I recommend it to all my new patients. I have a 17 month old. This book was a bible even for me—a pediatrician."
—Claudia Somes, M.D.

❖

"**What to Expect When You're Expecting** has been my pregnancy bible."
—Cynthia Cravens Allen,
Kentucky

❖

"Wonderful. Well organized, readable."
—Catherine C. Wiley, M.D.

❖

"Your book . . . has been a godsend. I've faithfully read each chapter prior to beginning that month and have been reassured by your calm and compassionate writing."   —Carol Rozner, California

❖

"Contains useful information not available in other books."
—Jim Wiley, M.D.

❖

"Your calm and confident style fills me with courage for our transition to parenthood."   —Diane Wheeler, California

❖

"Very reassuring to the new mother."
                                   —Ralph Minear, M.D.

❖

"Your books have not left my night table for 18 months (except when they went to the hospital with me)! Your information is always *right on schedule,* clear, concise and unbiased."
                                   —Lori Slayton, New Jersey

❖

"Excellent—we used it as our bible during pregnancy."
                                   —Bruce Oran, M.D.

❖

"[It] has seen me through my first pregnancy... providing a concise, user-friendly source of information ... Thanks to your book, I feel our daughter had a head start on life."
                                   —Victoria Schei, Ontario

❖

"Extremely helpful. I've used this book as a valuable resource with my patients."   —Saundra Schoichet, Ph.D.
                                   Clinical Psychologist

❖

WHAT TO EXPECT WHEN YOU'RE EXPECTING

❖ ❖ ❖ ❖

Arlene Eisenberg

Heidi E. Murkoff

Sandee E. Hathaway, B.S.N.

With a foreword by Dr. Richard Aubry,
Assistant Chairman and Director of Obstetrics, Department of Ob-Gyn,
State University of New York Health Sciences Center at Syracuse

WORKMAN PUBLISHING, NEW YORK

To Emma, who inspired this book while still in the womb, who did her best to keep us from writing it once she was out, and who, we trust, will put it to good use one day.

To Howard, Erik, and Tim, without whom this book would not have been possible—in more ways than one.

To Rachel, Wyatt, and Ethan, who showed up a little late for our first edition, but whose gestations contributed plenty to this one.

Library of Congress Cataloging-in-Publication Data
Eisenberg, Arlene.
What to expect when you're expecting / by Arlene Eisenberg,
Heidi E. Murkoff, and Sandee E. Hathaway.—2nd ed.
p.   cm.
Includes index.
ISBN 0-89480-829-X
1. Pregnancy. 2. Childbirth. 3. Postnatal care.
I. Murkoff, Heidi Eisenberg. II. Hathaway, Sandee Eisenberg. III. Title.
RG525.E361991 618.2'4—dc20   90-50951
                                                   CIP

Book Design: Susan Aronson Stirling
Cover Illustration: Judith Cheng
Book Illustration: Carol Donner

Workman books are available at special discounts when purchased in
bulk for premiums and sales promotions as well as for fund-raising
or educational use. Special editions or book excerpts can also be
created to specification. For details, contact the Special Sales Director
at the address below.

Workman Publishing Company, Inc.
708 Broadway
New York, NY 10003

Manufactured in the United States of America
Second edition first printing, April 1991

85 84 83 82 81 80 79

A MILLION THANKS

Books and babies have a lot in common. Both take plenty of time, hard work, dedication, and care (not to mention a healthy dose of worry) to turn out the best possible product. Both also require the cooperation of a team of concerned people. We've been lucky to have a fine team involved in the creation of our book, all of whom we gratefully thank:

Elise and Arnold Goodman, our agents, for their confidence, advice, support, and friendship.

Suzanne Rafer, our terrific editor at Workman, for her perceptive suggestions, her patience, her sense of humor (she needed it), and her endless capacity for what sometimes seemed endless work.

Shannon Ryan, for a thousand and one things she's taken care of with efficiency, intelligence, and, incredibly, a smile. Kathie Ness, for her astute copy editing of this second edition.

Bert Snyder, Ina Stern, Saundra Pearson, Steve Garvan, Janet Harris, Andrea Glickson, Cindy Frank, Jill Bennett, Nicole Dawkins, Barbara McClain, Tom Starace, Anne Kostick, and everyone else at Workman who helped make our first edition a success and/or contributed to making this one come to fruition. And very special thanks to Peter Workman, for being a very special publisher.

Richard Aubrey, M.D., Professor of Obstetrics and Gynecology and Assistant Chairman and Director of Obstetrics, Department of Ob-Gyn, State University of New York Health Sciences Center at Syracuse, our invaluable medical advisor. Dick's wise, caring, perceptive, informed critique has added immeasurably to the quality of this book. We feel privileged to have worked with such a remarkable physician.

The American College of Obstetricians and Gynecologists (particularly Mort Lebow, Florence Foelak, and Kate Ruddon), the American Academy of Pediatrics (particularly Michelle Weber and Carolyn Kolbaba), and *Contemporary Pediatrics* (and editor Jim Swan) for supplying us with voluminous quantities of information and material, being available to answer our questions, and for helping us to keep our books up-to-date.

The many physicians who clarified points or answered our questions, including John Severs, Irving Selikoff, Michael Starr, Michelle Marcus, Roy Schoen, and the hundreds who answered questionnaires and have given us input at ACOG meetings.

Three men without whom this book (and those that followed) would literally not have been possible: Howard Eisenberg, Erik Murkoff, and Tim Hathaway. It's guys like these that give husbands and fathers a good name, and we thank them for their inspiration and support.

Those who were so instrumental in the success of the first edition, including designer Susan Aronson Stirling, cover illustrator Judith Cheng, and book illustrator Carol Donner; Henry Eisenberg M.D., Ann Appelbaum, and Beth Falk, and, of course, Mildred and Harry Scharaga, better known as Mimi and Gramps.

Friends like Sarah Jacobs who have offered ideas and insights.

The hundreds of readers who have written, phoned, or spoken to us over the years, for all their comments and suggestions.

CONTENTS

Foreword to the Second Edition: Another Word From the Doctor xvii

Foreword: A Word From the Doctor xviii

Introduction to the Second Edition: Why This Book Was Reborn xx

    What's in a Month?

Introduction: How This Book Was Born xxii

---------------------------------- *Part 1* ----------------------------------

IN THE BEGINNING

Chapter 1: Are You Pregnant?. 2

WHAT YOU MAY BE CONCERNED ABOUT .2

Signs of Pregnancy ♦ Pregnancy Tests ♦ *Possible Signs of Pregnancy* ♦ *Probable Signs of Pregnancy* ♦ *Positive Signs of Pregnancy* ♦ *Testing Smart* ♦ Due Date

WHAT IT'S IMPORTANT TO KNOW: CHOOSING (AND
WORKING WITH) YOUR PRACTITIONER 8

A Look Back ♦ What Kind of Patient Are You? ♦ Obstetrician? Family Practitioner? Nurse-Midwife? ♦ Type of Practice ♦ Finding a Candidate ♦ Birthing Alternatives ♦ Making Your Selection ♦ Making the Most of the Patient-Practitioner Partnership ♦ *Protecting Yourself Against Malpractice* ♦ *So You Won't Forget*

Chapter 2: Now That You Are Pregnant 18

WHAT YOU MAY BE CONCERNED ABOUT .18

Your Gynecological History ♦ Previous Abortions ♦ Fibroids ♦ Incompetent Cervix ♦ Your Obstetrical History Repeating Itself ♦ Repeat Cesareans ♦ Your Family History ♦ Pregnancies too Close Together ♦ Tempting Fate the Second Time Around ♦ Having a Big Family ♦ Being a Single Mother ♦ Having a Baby After 35 ♦ Age and Testing for Down Syndrome ♦ The Father's Age ♦ In-Vitro Fertilization (IVF) ♦ Living at a High Altitude ♦ Religious Objections to Medical

Care ♦ RH Incompatibility ♦ Obesity ♦ Herpes ♦ *Signs and Symptoms of Genital Herpes* ♦ Other STDs (Sexually Transmitted Diseases) ♦ Fear of Aids ♦ Hepatitis B ♦ An IUD Still in Place ♦ Birth Control Pills in Pregnancy ♦ Spermicides ♦ Provera ♦ DES ♦ Genetic Problems ♦ Your Opposition to Abortion

WHAT IT'S IMPORTANT TO KNOW: ABOUT PRENATAL
DIAGNOSIS 42

Amniocentesis ♦ *Amnio Complication* ♦ Ultrasound ♦ Fetoscopy ♦ Maternal-Serum Alpha-Fetoprotein Screening ♦ Chorionic Villus Sampling (CVS) ♦ *Reducing the Risk in Any Pregnancy* ♦ Other Types of Prenatal Diagnosis

Chapter 3: Throughout Your Pregnancy 52
WHAT YOU MAY BE CONCERNED ABOUT 52

Alcohol ♦ Cigarette Smoking ♦ *Breaking the Smoking Habit* ♦ When Other People Smoke ♦ Marijuana Use ♦ Cocaine and Other Drug Use ♦ *Perils in Perspective* ♦ Caffeine ♦ Sugar Substitutes ♦ *Your Pregnancy Lifestyle* ♦ The Family Cat ♦ Hot Tubs and Saunas ♦ Microwave Exposure ♦ Electric Blankets and Heating Pads ♦ X-Rays ♦ Household Hazards ♦ *Let Your House Breathe* ♦ *The Green Solution* ♦ Air Pollution ♦ Occupational Hazards ♦ *Getting all the Facts* ♦ *Quiet Please*

WHAT IT'S IMPORTANT TO KNOW: PLAYING BABY ROULETTE 76

Weighing Risk vs. Benefit

Chapter 4: The Best-Odds Diet 80

Nine Basic Principles for Nine Months of Healthy Eating ♦ The Best-Odds Daily Dozen ♦ *What's in a Pill?*

THE BEST-ODDS DIET FOOD SELECTION GROUPS 89

Protein Foods ♦ High-Protein Snacks ♦ Vitamin C Foods ♦ Calcium-Rich Foods ♦ Calcium-Rich Snacks ♦ Green Leafy and Yellow Vegetables and Yellow Fruits ♦ Other Fruits and Vegetables ♦ Whole Grains and Legumes ♦ Iron-Rich Foods ♦ High-Fat Foods

BEST-ODDS RECIPES 93

> Cream of Tomato Soup ♦ Best-Odds Fries ♦ Power-Packed
> Oatmeal ♦ Bran Muffins ♦ Whole-Wheat Buttermilk Pan-
> cakes ♦ Double-the-Milk Shake ♦ Fig Bars ♦ Fruity Oatmeal
> Cookies ♦ *Vegetarian Complete Protein Combinations* ♦
> *Dairy Complete Protein Combinations* ♦ Fruited Yogurt ♦
> Mock Strawberry Daiquiri ♦ Virgin Sangria

—————————— *Part 2* ——————————

NINE MONTHS AND COUNTING:
From Conception to Delivery

Chapter 5: The First Month 100
WHAT YOU CAN EXPECT AT YOUR FIRST PRENATAL VISIT 100

> *What You May Look Like*

WHAT YOU MAY BE FEELING 102

WHAT YOU MAY BE CONCERNED ABOUT 102

> Fatigue ♦ Depression ♦ Morning Sickness ♦ Excessive Saliva
> ♦ Frequent Urination ♦ Breast Changes ♦ Vitamin Supple-
> ments ♦ Ectopic Pregnancy ♦ The Condition of Your Baby ♦
> Miscarriage ♦ *Possible Signs of Miscarriage* ♦ Stress in Your
> Life ♦ *Relaxation Made Easy* ♦ Overwhelming Fear About
> Baby's Health ♦ Picking Up Other Children

WHAT IT'S IMPORTANT TO KNOW: GETTING REGULAR
  MEDICAL CARE 116

> A Schedule of Prenatal Visits ♦ *When to Call the Practi-
> tioner* ♦ Taking Care of the Rest of You

Chapter 6: The Second Month .119
WHAT YOU CAN EXPECT AT THIS MONTH'S CHECKUP 119

WHAT YOU MAY BE FEELING 119

WHAT YOU MAY BE CONCERNED ABOUT 120

Venous Changes ♦ *What You May Look Like* ♦ Complexion Problems ♦ Waistline Expansion ♦ Losing Your Figure ♦ Heartburn and Indigestion ♦ Food Aversions and Cravings ♦ Milk Aversion or Intolerance ♦ Cholesterol ♦ A Meatless Diet ♦ A Vegetarian Diet ♦ Junk-Food Junkie ♦ Eating Fast Food ♦ *Best-Odds Cheating* ♦ Chemicals in Food ♦ Reading Labels ♦ *Eating Safe*

WHAT IT'S IMPORTANT TO KNOW: PLAYING IT SAFE 133

Chapter 7: The Third Month 134

WHAT YOU CAN EXPECT AT THIS MONTH'S CHECKUP 134

WHAT YOU MAY BE FEELING 134

What You May Look Like

WHAT YOU MAY BE CONCERNED ABOUT 135

Constipation ♦ Flatulence (Gas) ♦ Weight Gain ♦ Headaches ♦ Trouble Sleeping ♦ Stretch Marks ♦ Baby's Heartbeat ♦ Sexual Desire ♦ Oral Sex ♦ Cramp After Orgasm ♦ Twins and More ♦ A Corpus Luteum Cyst

WHAT IT'S IMPORTANT TO KNOW: WEIGHT GAIN DURING
PREGNANCY 147

Breakdown of Your Weight Gain

Chapter 8: The Fourth Month 150

WHAT YOU CAN EXPECT AT THIS MONTH'S CHECKUP 150

WHAT YOU MAY BE FEELING 150

What You May Look Like

WHAT YOU MAY BE CONCERNED ABOUT 152

Elevated Blood Pressure ♦ Sugar in the Urine ♦ Anemia ♦ Breathlessness ♦ Forgetfulness ♦ Hair Dyes and Permanents ♦ Nosebleeds and Nasal Stuffiness ♦ Allergies ♦ Vaginal Discharge ♦ Fetal Movement ♦ Appearance ♦ Maternity Clothes ♦ Reality of Pregnancy ♦ Unwanted Advice

WHAT IT'S IMPORTANT TO KNOW: MAKING LOVE DURING
PREGNANCY 164

Understanding Sexuality During Pregnancy ♦ When Sexual
Relations May Be Limited ♦ Enjoying It More, Even if You're
Doing It Less

Chapter 9: The Fifth Month......................170
WHAT YOU CAN EXPECT AT THIS MONTH'S CHECKUP 170

WHAT YOU MAY BE FEELING................................170

What You May Look Like

WHAT YOU MAY BE CONCERNED ABOUT 171

Fatigue ♦ Faintness and Dizziness ♦ Hepatitis Testing ♦
Sleeping Position ♦ Backache ♦ Carrying Older Children ♦
Foot Problems ♦ Fast-Growing Hair and Nails ♦ Late Miscar-
riage ♦ Abdominal Pain ♦ Changes in Skin Pigmentation ♦
Other Strange Skin Symptoms ♦ Dental Problems ♦ Travel ♦
Eating Out ♦ *Eating Out, Best-Odds Style* ♦ Wearing a Seat
Belt ♦ Sports ♦ Vision ♦ A Low-Lying Placenta ♦ Outside
Influences in the Womb ♦ *Carrying Baby, Fifth Month* ♦
Motherhood

WHAT IT'S IMPORTANT TO KNOW: EXERCISE DURING
PREGNANCY 189

The Benefits of Exercise ♦ Developing a Good Exercise
Program ♦ *Don't Just Sit There...* ♦ Playing It Safe ♦
Choosing the Right Pregnancy Exercise ♦ If You Don't
Exercise

Chapter 10: The Sixth Month....................199
WHAT YOU CAN EXPECT AT THIS MONTH'S CHECKUP 199

WHAT YOU MAY BE FEELING................................199

What You May Look Like

WHAT YOU MAY BE CONCERNED ABOUT 200

Pain and Numbness in the Hand ♦ Pins and Needles ♦ Baby
Kicking ♦ Leg Cramps ♦ Rectal Bleeding and Hemorrhoids ♦

Itchy Abdomen ♦ Toxemia, or Preeclampsia ♦ Staying on the Job ♦ Clumsiness ♦ The Pain of Childbirth ♦ Labor and Delivery

WHAT IT'S IMPORTANT TO KNOW: CHILDBIRTH EDUCATION 209

Benefits of Taking a Childbirth Class ♦ Choosing a Childbirth Class ♦ *For Information on Childbirth Classes* ♦ The Most Common Schools of Thought

Chapter 11: The Seventh Month 214

WHAT YOU CAN EXPECT AT THIS MONTH'S CHECKUP 214

WHAT YOU MAY BE FEELING. 214

What You May Look Like

WHAT YOU MAY BE CONCERNED ABOUT 215

Increasing Fatigue ♦ Concern About the Baby's Well-Being ♦ Edema (Swelling) of the Ankles and Feet ♦ Overheating ♦ Orgasm and the Baby ♦ Premature Labor ♦ *Don't Hold It In* ♦ Approaching Responsibility ♦ Accidents ♦ Lower Back and Leg Pain (Sciatica) ♦ Skin Eruptions ♦ Fetal Hiccups ♦ Dreams and Fantasies ♦ A Low-Birthweight Baby ♦ A Birthing Plan

WHAT IT'S IMPORTANT TO KNOW: ALL ABOUT CHILDBIRTH
MEDICATION 226

What Kinds of Pain Relief Are Most Commonly Used? ♦ Making the Decision

Chapter 12: The Eighth Month. 233

WHAT YOU CAN EXPECT AT THIS MONTH'S CHECKUPS. 233

WHAT YOU MAY BE FEELING. 233

What You May Look Like

WHAT YOU MAY BE CONCERNED ABOUT 234

Shortness of Breath ♦ Not So Funny Rib Tickling ♦ Stress Incontinence ♦ Your Weight Gain and the Baby's Size ♦ How You're Carrying ♦ Presentation and Position of the Baby ♦

Carrying Baby, Eighth Month ♦ *How Does Your Baby Lie?* ♦ Your Safety During Childbirth ♦ Adequacy for Delivery ♦ Twin Labor and Delivery ♦ Banking Your Own Blood ♦ Having a Cesarean Section ♦ *Cesarean Questions to Discuss with Your Doctor* ♦ *Hospitals and Cesarean Rates* ♦ *Making the Cesarean Birth a Family Affair* ♦ Travel Safety ♦ Driving ♦ Braxton Hicks Contractions ♦ Bathing ♦ Relationship With Your Spouse ♦ Making Love Now

WHAT IT'S IMPORTANT TO KNOW: FACTS ABOUT
   BREASTFEEDING 251

Why Breast Is Best ♦ Why Some Prefer the Bottle ♦ Making the Choice ♦ When You Can't or Shouldn't Breastfeed ♦ Making Bottle-Feeding Work

Chapter 13: The Ninth Month 256
WHAT YOU CAN EXPECT AT THIS MONTH'S CHECKUPS. 256

WHAT YOU MAY BE FEELING. 257

What You May Look Like

WHAT YOU MAY BE CONCERNED ABOUT 258

Changes in Fetal Movements ♦ Fear of Another Long Labor ♦ Bleeding or Spotting ♦ Lightening and Engagement ♦ When You Will Deliver ♦ *Do-It-Yourself Labor Induction?* ♦ Labor and Delivery Rooms ♦ The Overdue Baby ♦ *How Is Baby Doing?* ♦ *What to Take to the Hospital* ♦ Membrane Rupturing in Public ♦ Breastfeeding ♦ Mothering

WHAT IT'S IMPORTANT TO KNOW: PRELABOR, FALSE LABOR,
   REAL LABOR 268

Prelabor Symptoms ♦ False Labor Symptoms ♦ Real Labor Symptoms ♦ When to Call the Doctor ♦ *Best Medicine for Labor?*

Chapter 14: Labor and Delivery. 271
WHAT YOU MAY BE CONCERNED ABOUT 271

Bloody Show ♦ Rupture of Membranes ♦ Darkened Amniotic Fluid (Meconium Staining) ♦ Induction of Labor ♦ Having a Short Labor ♦ Calling Your Practitioner During

Labor ♦ Back Labor ♦ Irregular Contractions ♦ Not Getting to the Hospital in Time ♦ *Emergency Delivery En Route to the Hospital* ♦ Enemas ♦ Shaving the Pubic Area ♦ *Emergency Delivery If You're Alone* ♦ Routine IVs ♦ Fetal Monitoring ♦ *Emergency Home (or Office) Delivery* ♦ The Sight of Blood ♦ Episiotomy ♦ Being Stretched by Childbirth ♦ Being Strapped to the Delivery Table ♦ The Use of Forceps ♦ *Apgar Table* ♦ The Baby's Condition

WHAT IT'S IMPORTANT TO KNOW: THE STAGES OF
CHILDBIRTH 288

Labor Positions

THE FIRST STAGE OF CHILDBIRTH: LABOR. 290

The First Phase: Early or Latent Labor ♦ *If You Aren't Making Progress* ♦ The Second Phase: Active Labor ♦ *On to the Hospital* ♦ The Third Phase: Advanced Active or Transitional Labor ♦ *Pain Risk Factors*

THE SECOND STAGE OF CHILDBIRTH: PUSHING AND
DELIVERY 299

A Baby Is Born ♦ *A First Look at Baby*

THE THIRD STAGE OF CHILDBIRTH: DELIVERY OF THE
PLACENTA, OR AFTERBIRTH 305

BREECH DELIVERY 306

CESAREAN SECTION: SURGICAL DELIVERY 307

--- *Part 3* ---

OF SPECIAL CONCERN

Chapter 15: If You Get Sick .310
WHAT YOU MAY BE CONCERNED ABOUT 310

Coming Down With a Cold or Flu ♦ Gastrointestinal Ills ♦ German Measles (Rubella) ♦ Toxoplasmosis ♦ Cytomegalovirus (CMV) ♦ Fifth Disease ♦ Group B Strep ♦ Lyme Disease ♦ Measles ♦ Urinary Tract Infection ♦ Hepatitis ♦

Mumps ♦ Chicken Pox (Varicella) ♦ Fever ♦ Taking Aspirin and Nonaspirin ♦ Taking Medications ♦ Herbal Cures

WHAT IT'S IMPORTANT TO KNOW: STAYING WELL 323

Chapter 16: Coping With a Chronic Condition 325

WHAT YOU MAY BE CONCERNED ABOUT 325

Diabetes ♦ *Safe Exercise Heart Rate for Diabetic Pregnancies* ♦ Asthma ♦ Chronic Hypertension ♦ Multiple Sclerosis (MS) ♦ An Eating Disorder ♦ Physical Disability ♦ Epilepsy ♦ Phenylketonuria (PKU) ♦ Coronary Artery Disease (CAD) ♦ Sickle-Cell Anemia ♦ Systemic Lupus Erythematosus (SLE)

WHAT IT'S IMPORTANT TO KNOW: LIVING WITH THE
HIGH-RISK OR PROBLEM PREGNANCY 339

Moms Helping Moms

Chapter 17: When Something Goes Wrong 342

CONDITIONS THAT MAY CAUSE CONCERN DURING PREGNANCY 343

Hyperemesis Gravidarum ♦ Ectopic Pregnancy ♦ *Bleeding in Early Pregnancy* ♦ *Bleeding in Mid- or Late Pregnancy* ♦ *If You've Had a Miscarriage* ♦ Early Miscarriage, or Spontaneous Abortion ♦ Late Miscarriage ♦ Trophoblastic Disease (Hydatidiform Mole) ♦ *When a Serious Fetal Defect Is Detected* ♦ Partial Molar Pregnancy ♦ Choriocarcinoma ♦ Gestational Diabetes ♦ Chorioamnionitis ♦ Preeclampsia (Pregnancy-Induced Hypertension) ♦ Eclampsia ♦ *Lowering the Risks for the Baby at Risk* ♦ Intrauterine Growth Retardation (IUGR) ♦ *Repeat Low-Birthweight Babies* ♦ Placenta Previa ♦ Placenta Accreta ♦ Abruptio Placenta ♦ Premature Rupture of the Membranes (PROM) ♦ Cord Prolapse ♦ Venous Thrombosis ♦ Preterm or Premature Labor

CONDITIONS THAT MAY CAUSE CONCERN DURING CHILDBIRTH 362

Uterine Inversion ♦ Uterine Rupture ♦ Shoulder Dystocia ♦ *First Aid for the Fetus* ♦ Fetal Distress ♦ Vaginal and Cervical Lacerations ♦ Postpartum Hemorrhage ♦ Postpartum Infection

COPING WITH PREGNANCY LOSS 366

When Multiple Fetuses Aren't Thriving ♦ *Loss of One Twin* ♦ *Why?*

—————— *Part 4* ——————
LAST BUT NOT LEAST:
Postpartum, Fathers, and the Next Baby

Chapter 18: Postpartum: The First Week 374

WHAT YOU MAY BE FEELING. 374

WHAT YOU MAY BE CONCERNED ABOUT 375

Bleeding ♦ Your Postpartum Condition ♦ Afterpains ♦ Pain in the Perineal Area ♦ Difficulty With Urination ♦ Having a Bowel Movement ♦ Excessive Perspiration ♦ Adequacy of Your Milk Supply ♦ Engorged Breasts ♦ *When to Call Your Practitioner* ♦ Engorgement If You're Not Breastfeeding ♦ Bonding ♦ Rooming-In ♦ Going Home ♦ Recovery From a Cesarean Section

WHAT IT'S IMPORTANT TO KNOW: GETTING STARTED
BREASTFEEDING 388

Breastfeeding Basics ♦ *Baby and Breast—A Perfect Feeding Team* ♦ When the Milk Comes In ♦ *Best-Odds Nursing Diet* ♦ Sore Nipples ♦ Occasional Complications ♦ *Medication and Breastfeeding* ♦ Breastfeeding After a Cesarean ♦ Breastfeeding Twins

Chapter 19: Postpartum: The First Six Weeks 396

WHAT YOU MAY BE FEELING. 396

WHAT YOU CAN EXPECT AT YOUR POSTPARTUM CHECKUP 397

WHAT YOU MAY BE CONCERNED ABOUT 397

Fever ♦ Depression ♦ Returning to Prepregnancy Weight and Shape ♦ Breast Milk ♦ Long-Term Cesarean Recovery ♦ Resuming Sexual Relations ♦ Lack of Interest in Making Love

♦ *Easing Back Into Sex* ♦ Becoming Pregnant Again ♦ Hair
Loss ♦ Taking Tub Baths ♦ Exhaustion

WHAT IT'S IMPORTANT TO KNOW: **GETTING BACK INTO
SHAPE** 408

Ground Rules ♦ Phase One: 24 Hours After Delivery ♦ Phase
Two: Three Days After Delivery ♦ Phase Three: After Your
Postpartum Checkup

Chapter 20: Fathers Are Expectant, Too 412
WHAT YOU MAY BE CONCERNED ABOUT 412

Feeling Left Out ♦ Fear of Sex ♦ Moodiness ♦ Impatience
With Your Wife's Mood Swings ♦ Sympathy Symptoms ♦
Anxiety Over Your Wife's Health ♦ Anxiety Over the Baby's
Health ♦ Anxiety Over Life Changes ♦ Your Wife's Looks ♦
Falling Apart During Labor ♦ Bonding ♦ Exclusion During
Breastfeeding ♦ Feeling Unsexy After Delivery

Chapter 21: Preparing for the Next Baby 424

Appendix 429

Common Tests During Pregnancy ♦ Non-Drug Treatments
During Pregnancy ♦ *Keeping Moist* ♦ Best-Odds Calorie and
Fat Requirements ♦ Sources and Resources

Pregnancy Notes 439

Index 462

Afterword 479

Another Word From the Doctor

Often, people who notice my name on the front cover of this book call to thank me for writing it. I thank them, in return, for their calls and compliments—and then explain that I *didn't* write it. My role, I tell them, was not author but medical advisor—in charge of the dotting of every anatomic "i" and the crossing of every biologic "t."

Like them, I'm pleased and excited about what these authors have done. What I wrote in my foreword in 1985 is every bit as true today. But with this complete revision, the book that I enthusiastically endorsed then is now even better.

It's even more up-to-date and more comprehensive, dealing in much greater depth with high-risk pregnancies, second pregnancies, and pregnancy loss. These topics are handled with sensitivity, clarity, and accuracy, avoiding the scare-on-every-page approach. The authors take the sensible view that, yes, there are things to be concerned about; any responsible mother-to-be would be concerned.

But then they add what is so often omitted elsewhere: "Here are some commonsense things you can do to avoid that complication."

That constructive approach, I am sure, is what has helped this book, written by non-physicians, win such wide acceptance among doctors and other health care providers in the first place. It's not only recommended (or given) to new patients by many ob/gyns, but used by those physicians and their spouses as well. My young residents read it to learn what patients are wondering and worrying about, so they'll be better prepared when they begin their own practice.

Clearly, expectant parents love this book. Physicians respect it. Those are two good reasons for the resounding success of *What to Expect When You're Expecting*. And if it didn't sound so appallingly unscientific, I'd hypothesize a third: babies appreciate it too.

Richard Aubry, M.D.,
M.P.H., F.A.C.O.G.

A Word From the Doctor

These are the best years in history to be expecting a baby. In recent decades, there has been a remarkable improvement in the outcome of human pregnancy—for mothers as well as for infants. Women enter pregnancy healthier; they get better, more complete prenatal care; and the hospital maternity wing has replaced the kitchen table and the four-poster as the place to have a baby.

Yet more can be done. To those of us in academic medicine it is becoming increasingly clear that superior doctors and superior equipment aren't enough. Further reductions in pregnancy and childbirth risks will require actively participating expectant couples as well. In order to participate more, couples will have to be more completely and accurately informed, not just about the climactic birth experience, but about the all-important nine months that precede it; not just about the risks that pregnancy presents, but about the steps parents can take to minimize and eliminate risks; not just about the medical aspects of pregnancy, but about psychosocial and lifestyle factors as well.

How can parents become so informed? High schools and colleges, have no time or place in their curricula for Babymaking 101. Professionals who provide obstetrical care have a time problem, too. And, they are sometimes overly scientific in their explanations and insufficiently sensitive to the psychological and emotional needs of expectant parents.

Consumer advocates have vaulted into the void with books, magazine articles, and classroom instruction. They are often tremendously helpful, but almost as often they're medically inaccurate, unnecessarily alarming, and/or disproportionately focused on the inadequacies of the health care profession, driving a wedge of suspicion and doubt between parents and their obstetrical caregivers.

The need for a book that provides accurate, up-to-date, and medically sound information with proper emphasis on nutrition, lifestyle, and the emotional aspects of pregnancy has long been apparent. Now, I believe, that need has been met in a highly readable and eminently practical month-by-month format.

The three authors—each an experienced "consumer" of maternity care—have given us that essential consumer perspective. They have wisely concentrated on giving expectant parents the information that will allow them to intelligently play their central role in the entire process, without threatening the doctors and nurse-midwives with whom they must work closely and congenially.

What to Expect When You're Expecting is lively in style, accurate, current, and well-balanced overall. But four aspects of its structure and content deserve special comment:

❖ The book's thoughtful family-centered approach to childbearing—with involvement of the husband throughout the pregnancy process and with a chapter responding to his special needs and problems—is excellent and important.

❖ Its practical chronological arrangement—sensibly answering all the big and little, trying and troubling questions that come up month after month—makes for timely reassurance and easy bedside-table reference.

❖ The book's emphasis on pre-

pregnancy and pregnancy nutrition and lifestyle, and its commonsense approaches to lactation and the psychosocial dimensions of motherhood, make it particularly valuable and unique.

❖ Its accurate and up-to-the-minute medical detail—particularly the clarity of its sections on genetics, teratology, preterm labor, delivery, cesarean section, and again, lactation—is outstanding.

All in all, I believe that this excellent book, should be *required reading* not only for expectant parents, but for doctors and nurses who are training to provide obstetrical care and for professionals already providing it. That is, I know, a long way out on a limb for a generally cautious medical school professor to go. But I say it out of strong conviction: the belief that only with properly informed and responsible consumers and providers working together can we draw near our common goal—healthy babies, mothers, and families. And, ultimately, society.

Richard Aubry, M.D.,
M.P.H., F.A.C.O.G.

Why This Book Was Reborn

Fourteen years ago, just hours before I delivered Emma, the baby who inspired it, my co-authors and I delivered the proposal for *What to Expect When You're Expecting*. In conceiving it, in researching it, in writing it, our goal was simple and single-minded: to bring reassurance to expectant parents.

Fourteen years later, our goal hasn't changed. But to help us meet the goal more fully, our book has.

The first copy of *What to Expect* was barely off the presses when we began to collect material in a folder marked "ADD." Though we managed to include the most significant new information, at least briefly, in subsequent printings, squeezing in a line here and a line there, the ADD file soon became a pile of files, then a boxful. When it started to become a roomful, we decided it was time to begin petitioning our publisher for the opportunity to begin a major revision, so that *all* our ADDs could finally be added.

Much of what we've revised reflects revisions in obstetrical practice. But many more of the changes reflect the input from a source we value as highly as any obstetrical journal or text: expectant parents. On a page at the end of the first edition of *What to Expect*, we asked readers to write and let us know if there was anything they worried about or experienced during pregnancy and postpartum that we didn't cover or didn't cover adequately. And though we received many letters from readers who said they felt we'd covered it all, we received others from readers who'd felt we hadn't.

Planning Ahead

If you aren't pregnant yet but are in the planning phase, turn to the last chapter of this book first. There you will find everything you need to know about getting a head start on a successful pregnancy and a healthy baby.

So, as requested, we've added more on second and subsequent pregnancies, more on chronic medical conditions that affect pregnancy, more on what to do if you get sick, more on coping with common (and not-so-common) pregnancy symptoms, and more on complications that may occur (but please, please, to spare yourself unnecessary worry, do not read this section unless a complication *does* occur).

More important than what we've changed, though, is what has stayed the same—namely, all that readers have told us they've appreciated about *What to Expect.* The practical step-by-step advice. The empathetic approach. The easy-to-read explanation of things medical. And, of course, the reassurance.

No book on pregnancy can anticipate and elaborate on every conceivable concern or situation and still fit comfortably on a single bookshelf. (After all, consider that no two pregnancies are identical and over 3½ million pregnancies take place each year in this country.) But we hope you'll find that this edition of *What to Expect When You're Expecting* comes close.

Thanks to you, our readers, for all the support and suggestions you've given us. And do keep those cards and letters coming. We'll do our best to keep responding.

Heidi E. Murkoff
New York City

What's in a Month?

There are several ways to count time in pregnancy: week by week for 40 weeks, month by month for ten four-week months, or month by month using the traditional nine months. We chose to divide *What to Expect When You're Expecting* into traditional months because so many women keep track of their pregnancies this way, because nine months are easily divided into trimesters, and because more women will have symptoms and experiences in common over the course of a month than in the limited span of a week.

So when using this book, remember that the first month begins seven days after the first day of your last menstrual period. If, for example, your last menstrual period began on March 5, your first month began on March 12. Your second month would then begin on April 12, your third on May 12 and so on. Your due date would be nine months later, on December 12.

When weeks are specified, however, for example in reference to first hearing the fetal heartbeat, we are talking about the number of weeks since the first day of the last menstrual period. If March 5 was a Sunday, 17 weeks into your pregnancy would be completed 17 Sundays from that day, or July 2. When counting 40 weeks to delivery, you would end up with a slightly earlier due date than when counting months, in this case December 10.

No matter which method your practitioner recommends for calculating your due date, keep in mind the nine-month format of this book when using it to follow your pregnancy's progress.

How This Book Was Born

I was pregnant, which about one day out of three made me the happiest woman in the world. And for the remaining two, the most worried.

Worried about the wine I'd sipped nightly with dinner, and the gin and tonics I'd downed more than a few times before dinner in my first six weeks of pregnancy—after two gynecologists and a blood test convinced me that I wasn't pregnant.

Worried about the seven doses of Provera one of the doctors had prescribed to bring on what she was certain was just a tardy period, but which proved two weeks later to be a nearly two-month gestation.

Worried about the coffee I'd drunk, and the milk I hadn't; the sugar I'd eaten, and the protein I hadn't.

Worried about the cramps in my third month, and the four days in my fifth month when I felt not even a flicker of fetal movement.

Worried about the time I fainted while touring the hospital I was to deliver in (I never did get to see the nursery), my middle-of-the-street belly-flop in the eighth month, and a bloody vaginal discharge in the ninth.

Worried, even, about feeling *good* ("But I'm not constipated. . . . I don't have morning sickness. . . . I'm not urinating more frequently—something must be wrong!").

Worried that I wouldn't be able to tolerate the pain during labor, or stand the sight of blood at delivery. And worried that because I couldn't squeeze out a drop of the colostrum all my books told me should fill my breasts by the ninth month, I wouldn't be able to breastfeed.

Where could I turn to find reassurance that all would be well? Not to the ever-growing stack of pregnancy books piled high on my bedside table. As common and normal as a few days of no fetal activity is in the fifth month, I couldn't find a single reference to it. As often as pregnant women take a tumble—almost always without harming their babies—I could find no mention of accidental falls.

When my symptoms, problems, or fears *were* discussed, it was usually in an alarming way which only compounded my concern. *Never* take Provera unless you would "absolutely abort," warned one volume—without adding that a woman who has taken the drug has so slight an increased risk of birth defects in her baby that an unwanted abortion need never be considered. "There is evidence that a single drinking 'binge' during pregnancy may affect some babies, depending on the stage of development they have reached," cautioned another book ominously—disregarding studies which show that a few drinking sprees in early pregnancy, when many women indulge unknowingly, appear to have no effect on a developing embryo.

I certainly couldn't find relief for my worries by opening a newspaper, flipping on the radio or television, or browsing through magazines. According to the media, threats to the pregnant lurked everywhere: in the air we breathed, in the food we ate, in the water we drank, at the dentist's office, in the drugstore, even at home.

My doctor offered some solace, of course, but only when I was able to summon up the courage to phone. (I was either afraid my worries would sound silly or afraid of what I would hear. Besides, how could I spend two days out of three on the phone badgering her?)

Was I (and my husband, Erik—who worried about everything I worried about, and then some) alone in my fears? Far from it. Worry, according to one study, is one of the most common complaints of pregnancy, affecting more expectant women than morning sickness and food cravings combined. Ninety-four out of every hundred women worry about whether their babies will be normal, and 93% worry about whether they and their babies will come through delivery safely. More women worry about their figures (91%) than their health (81%) during pregnancy. And most worry that they worry too much.

But though a little worry is normal for pregnant women and their mates, a lot of worry is an unnecessary waste of what should be a blissfully happy time. Despite all that we hear, read, and worry about, never before in the history of reproduction has it been safer to have a baby—as Erik and I discovered some seven and a half months of worrying later, when I gave birth to a healthier and more beautiful baby girl than I'd dared to dream possible.

Thus, out of our concerns, *What to Expect When You're Expecting* was born. It is dedicated to expectant couples everywhere (especially to my co-author and sister, Sandee, and her husband, Tim, whose first baby will be in a tight race with this book for publication), and written with the hope that it will help fathers- and mothers-to-be worry less and enjoy their pregnancies more.

Heidi E. Murkoff

Part 1

IN THE BEGINNING

1
Are You Pregnant?

A m I really pregnant? This is the first preoccupation of the hopeful expectant parent, and it arises the first moment one or another of the signs of pregnancy appears. Happily, it's a question that can very soon be answered, via the combination of a pregnancy test and a medical examination.

WHAT YOU MAY BE CONCERNED ABOUT

SIGNS OF PREGNANCY

'I only have some of the signs of pregnancy—can I still be pregnant?''

You can have all of the signs and symptoms of early pregnancy and not be pregnant. Or you can have only a few of them and be very definitely pregnant. The various signs and symptoms of pregnancy are only clues—important to pay attention to, but not to be relied upon for absolute confirmation.

Some of the pregnancy signs you may notice suggest the *possibility* you are pregnant, others the *probability*. *No* early signs are positive indications of pregnancy. In fact, the first sign that is proof positive of your pregnancy is your baby's heartbeat, which is audible at about 10, or more often 12, weeks with the sensitive ultrasound Doppler device, or with an or-

dinary stethoscope at 18 to 20 weeks.[1] Earlier signs only indicate the possibility or probability that you're carrying a child. Combined with a reliable pregnancy test and your doctor's examination, they can help provide an accurate diagnosis.

PREGNANCY TESTS

'My doctor said the exam and pregnancy test indicated I wasn't pregnant, but I really feel I am.''

As remarkable as modern medical science is, when it comes to pregnancy diagnosis, it still sometimes takes a backseat to a woman's intuition. The accuracy of the different

---

1. Verification of a pregnancy can be made earlier through ultrasound or via a blood test, but these are not routine procedures.

pregnancy tests varies, and none are accurate as early as some women begin to "feel" that they are pregnant—sometimes within a few days after conception. There are basically three kinds of pregnancy tests available today—and a rabbit needn't give its life for any of them.

POSSIBLE SIGNS OF PREGNANCY

SIGN	WHEN IT APPEARS	OTHER POSSIBLE CAUSES
Amenorrhea (absence of menstruation)	Usually entire pregnancy	Travel, fatigue, stress, fear of pregnancy, hormonal problems or illness, extreme weight gain or loss, going off the Pill, breastfeeding
Morning sickness (any time of day)	2–8 weeks after conception	Food poisoning, tension, infection, and a variety of diseases
Frequent urination	Usually 6–8 weeks after conception	Urinary tract infection, diuretics, tension, diabetes
Tingling, tender, swollen breasts	As early as a few days after conception	Birth control pills, impending menstruation
Changes in color of vaginal and cervical tissue*	First trimester	Impending menstruation
Darkening of areola (area around nipple) and elevation of tiny glands around nipple	First trimester	Hormonal imbalance or effect of prior pregnancy
Blue and pink lines under skin on breasts and later on abdomen	First trimester	Hormonal imbalance or effect of prior pregnancy
Food cravings	First trimester	Poor diet, stress, imagination, or impending menstruation
Darkening of line from navel to pubis	4th or 5th month	Hormonal imbalance or effect of prior pregnancy

*Signs of pregnancy looked for in medical examination.

The Home Pregnancy Test. This test is much more accurate than in the past, and a lot simpler to use. Like the urine test done in the lab or the doctor's office, it diagnoses pregnancy by detecting the presence of the hormone hCG (human Chorionic Gonadotropin) in the urine. Some tests can tell you if you're pregnant as early as the first day of your missed menstrual period (about 14 days after conception), and in as little as five minutes, with an any-time-of-the-day urine sample.

If it's done correctly—and this is increasingly possible as tests become less complicated to carry out and evaluate—an at-home test is now almost as accurate as a urine test done in a doctor's office or laboratory (the accuracy is close to 100%, according to the manufacturers), with a positive result much more likely to be correct than a negative one. Home tests offer the advantage of privacy and virtually

immediate results. And because they provide an accurate diagnosis very early in pregnancy—earlier than you would probably consider consulting a physician—they can give you the opportunity to start taking optimum care of yourself within days of conception, actually at about the same time as the pregnancy is implanting in your uterus. But they can be relatively expensive, and because you're less likely to feel confident in the results, you're more apt to want a retest, increasing the cost. (Some brands include a second test in the package.) Let your practitioner know which brand and type of test you used so that he or she can decide whether or not a retest is needed.

The major drawback with home pregnancy tests is that if a test produces a false-negative result and you actually are pregnant, you may postpone seeing a doctor and taking appropriate care of yourself. And even

PROBABLE SIGNS OF PREGNANCY

SIGN	WHEN IT APPEARS	OTHER POSSIBLE CAUSES
Softening of uterus and cervix*	2–8 weeks after conception	A delayed menstrual period
Enlarging uterus* and abdomen	8–12 weeks	Tumor, fibroids
Intermittent painless contractions	Early in pregnancy, increasing in frequency as pregnancy advances	Bowel contractions
Fetal movements	First noted at 16–22 weeks of pregnancy	Gas, bowel contractions

*Signs of pregnancy looked for in medical examination.

POSITIVE SIGNS OF PREGNANCY

SIGN	WHEN IT APPEARS	OTHER POSSIBLE CAUSES
Visualization of embryo or gestational sac through ultrasound*	As early as 4–6 weeks after conception	None
Fetal heartbeat*	At 10–20 weeks**	None
Fetal movements felt through abdomen*	After 16 weeks	None

*Signs of pregnancy looked for in medical examination.

**Depending on device used.

with a positive result, you may postpone the office visit because you assume that getting a diagnosis is the only reason to see your doctor at this point. So if you use such a test, keep in mind that it is not designed to take the place of a consultation with and examination by a medical professional. Medical follow-up to the test is essential. If the result is positive, you should have it confirmed by a physical exam and then get a complete prenatal checkup. If it is negative and your period still hasn't started, you and your doctor need to find out why.

The Lab or In-Office Urine Test. Like the at-home variety, this test can detect hCG in the urine with an accuracy of close to 100%—and as early as seven to ten days after conception. Unlike the home test, it is performed by a professional, who is, at least theoretically, more likely to do it correctly. If you plan on taking a urine test, call the doctor's office or lab the day before and ask if there are any instructions. The in-office test (which usually yields results in minutes) will probably not require first-morning urine; the lab version (you'll have to wait until they phone the news to the doctor's office) may. Urine tests are usually less expensive than blood tests, but they aren't used as often because they don't provide as much information; see below.

The Blood Test. The more sophisticated serum, or blood, pregnancy test can detect pregnancy with virtually 100% accuracy as early as one week after conception (barring lab error). It can also help to date a pregnancy by measuring the exact amount of hCG in the blood, since hCG values alter as pregnancy progresses. Occasionally a practitioner may order both a urine and a blood test to be doubly certain of the diagnosis.

No matter which test you use, the chances of the diagnosis being correct are enhanced when the test is followed by a medical examination. The physical signs of pregnancy—an enlarging and softening of the uterus, and a change in the texture of the cervix—may be apparent to your doc-

Testing Smart

To improve the chances that your home pregnancy test will be accurate, be sure to:

❖ Read test package directions carefully and thoroughly before use and follow them precisely. No matter how eager you are for results, if first-of-the-morning urine is required, wait until morning to perform the test.

❖ Have an easy-to-read clock or watch ready so that you can time the test precisely.

❖ Be sure containers, dipsticks, or any other equipment to be used with the test are clean and uncontaminated when you begin the test. Don't reuse containers if you want to try again.

❖ If a waiting period is required, place the sample away from the heat where it won't be disturbed.

❖ If the kit you've purchased contains a second test, or if you buy a second kit, wait a few days before trying a retest.

tor or midwife by the sixth week of pregnancy. But as with tests, a practitioner's diagnosis of "pregnant" is more likely to be correct than one of "not pregnant"—though false-negative results are fairly uncommon. False negatives are most likely to occur early in pregnancy, when a woman's body may not be producing enough hCG to test positive.

If you are experiencing the symptoms of early pregnancy (a missed period or two, breast fullness and tenderness, morning sickness, frequent urination, fatigue) and feel, test or no test, exam or no exam, that you are pregnant, act as though you are, taking all prenatal precautions, until you find out definitely otherwise. Neither tests nor medical practitioners are infallible. You know your own body—at least externally—better than your practitioner does. Ask for a retest (preferably a blood test) and another exam in a week or so; it may just be too early for an accurate diagnosis. More than one baby has arrived seven and a half or eight months after a pregnancy test and/or a doctor concluded that its mother wasn't pregnant.

If the tests continue to be negative but you still haven't begun to menstruate, be sure to check with your doctor to rule out an ectopic pregnancy, one that takes place outside of the uterus. (See page 109 for warning signs of this kind of pregnancy.)

It is possible, of course, to experience all the signs and symptoms of early pregnancy and not be pregnant at all. None of them alone or in combination is proof positive of pregnancy. After a second pregnancy test and physical exam determine that you are not pregnant, you must consider that the "pregnancy" may have psychological roots—possibly because you very strongly do, or don't, want to have a baby. In which case professional counseling is probably a good idea. Or it may be that the symptoms have some other biological cause that should be investigated by your doctor.

DUE DATE

"I am trying to plan my pregnancy leave. How do I know if my due date is really correct?"

Life would be a lot simpler if you could be certain that your due date is actually the day you will deliver. But life isn't that simple very often. According to some studies only 4 women in 100 give birth on their due date. Most, because a normal full-term pregnancy can last anywhere from 38 to 42 weeks, deliver within two weeks either way of that date.

That's why the medical term for "due date" is EDD, or the *estimated* date of delivery. The date your practitioner gives you is only an educated estimate. It is usually calculated this way: Take the date of the first day of your last normal menstrual period (LNMP) and add 7 to it. To that date, add nine months to get your due date. For example, say your last menstrual period began on April 11. Add 7 to 11, which brings you to April 18; then add nine months. Your due date would be January 18. Or, the date may be calculated based on a 40 week pregnancy, counting 40 weeks from your LNMP; in this case your EDD would be January 16.

If your periods come predictably every 28 days, you are more likely to deliver close to your estimated due date. If your cycles are longer than 28 days, you are more likely to deliver later than your EDD, and if they are shorter, earlier.

But if your cycle is irregular, this dating system may not work for you at all. Say you haven't had your period in three months and suddenly you're pregnant. When did you conceive? Because a reliable EDD is important, you and your practitioner will have to try to come up with one. Even if you can't pinpoint conception or are unaware of your most recent ovulation (some women recognize the release of an ovum by flank pain and cramping that lasts a few hours, clear stringy vaginal mucus, and if they're keeping track, the characteristic temperature drop just before and the rise afterward),

there are clues that can help.

The very first clue, the size of your uterus, will be noted when your initial internal pregnancy examination is performed. It should conform to your suspected stage of pregnancy. Later on there are other milestones that together can more accurately gauge just how pregnant you are: the first time the fetal heartbeat is heard (at about 10 to 12 weeks with a Doppler device, or at about 18 to 22 weeks with a stethoscope); when the first flutter of life is felt (at about 20 to 22 weeks with a first baby, or 16 to 18 with subsequent ones); the height of the fundus (the top of the uterus) at each visit (for example, it will reach the navel at about the 20th week). If all of these indications seem to correspond to the due date you and your practitioner have calculated, you can be pretty sure that it is close to accurate—that is, that you are quite likely to deliver within two weeks of that date. But if they don't correspond, the doctor may decide to do a sonogram sometime between the 12th and 20th weeks (the best information, some believe, can be garnered between weeks 16 and 20), which can more closely pinpoint the gestational age of your fetus. Some doctors will do a sonogram routinely, to obtain the most accurate date possible.

As delivery nears, there will be other clues to the date of the big event: painless contractions may become more frequent (and possibly uncomfortable), the fetus will drop into the pelvis (engagement), your cervix will begin to thin and shorten (effacement), and last of all, your cervix will begin to dilate. These clues will be helpful, but not definitive— only your baby knows for sure what his or her birthday will be. (For more information, see Lightening and Engagement, page 260; When You Will Deliver, page 261.)

WHAT IT'S IMPORTANT TO KNOW:
CHOOSING (AND WORKING WITH) YOUR PRACTITIONER

While it takes two to conceive a baby, it takes a minimum of three—mother, father, and at least one health care professional—to make that transition from fertilized egg to delivered infant a safe and successful one. Assuming you and your husband have already taken care of conception, the next challenge you face is selecting that third member of your pregnancy team. And making sure that it's a selection you can live with—and labor with.[2]

A LOOK BACK

The selection of a pregnancy caregiver wasn't a major consideration for mothers-to-be 30 years ago. Those were the days of no-questions-asked obstetrical care, when the few choices there were in childbirth were left up to the doctor. As far as selecting an obstetrician was concerned, one seemed pretty much like the next. And besides, since you were likely to be unconscious during delivery, it didn't ultimately matter much whether you had rapport with your doctor. Instead of being a participating team member, the mother-to-be was more or less a spectator, sitting obediently on the bench while her obstetrical captain called the plays.

Today there are almost as many choices in childbirth—yours for the choosing—as there are doctors in the Yellow Pages. The trick is in matching yourself up with a compatible practitioner.

2. Of course you can and ideally should make this selection even before you conceive.

WHAT KIND OF PATIENT ARE YOU?

Your first step in figuring out the kind of practitioner that is right for you is to give some thought to the kind of patient you are.

Do you believe that "doctor knows best" (after all, he or she's the one who went to medical school)? Would you prefer your physician to make all the decisions without consulting you, and do you feel safest when all the latest medical technology is being used in your care? In your medical fantasies, does the man in the white lab coat taking your pulse fit the description of Dr. Welby or Dr. Kildare? Then you may feel most comfortable with an obstetrician who has a traditional practice, a godlike aura, and an unswerving dedication to his or her own obstetrical philosophy.

Or do you believe that your body and your health are your business and no one else's? Do you have definite ideas about pregnancy and childbirth and feel you'd like to run the show, from conception to delivery, with minimal interference from your health professional? Then skip over the Welbys and Kildares, and look for a physician or midwife who's willing to relinquish the starring role and serve as your consultant on the production of your baby. Someone who will let you make as many of the childbirth decisions as is medically practical, who is dogmatic only when it comes to giving the patient a controlling vote. Don't assume, however, that a doctor who leans toward "New

Wave" obstetrics is going to be any less doctrinaire in his or her beliefs than a traditional physician.

Or perhaps you're somewhere in the middle and would prefer a practitioner who makes you a partner in your own care, one who makes decisions based on his or her experience and knowledge but always includes you in the process. If so, the practitioner for you is probably one who sees his or her role in your pregnancy as somewhere between star and consultant—who is neither a slave to medical gospel nor putty in your hands; who would like to give you the "natural" delivery you want but won't hesitate to do a cesarean if your baby's safety (or yours) requires it; who doesn't routinely either give or withhold medication; who sees nothing incongruous in using a fetal monitor and a birthing room at the same time; and who's more interested in a healthy mother and a healthy baby than in your personal preferences or his or her own. The practitioner for you sees the doctor-patient relationship as one in which each partner contributes what he or she does best.

Whatever your patienting style, if you believe that the father-to-be should have equal billing in the pregnancy-childbirth drama, you'll also need to determine if the caregiver you're considering does too. A practitioner's attitude is usually apparent at the first visit, sometimes even when you make the first appointment. Is the father invited to both the examination and the interview? Are his questions given full consideration? Does the practitioner direct comments to both the mother and father? Is it clear that, when the time comes, the father will be welcome to share in both labor and delivery?

OBSTETRICIAN? FAMILY PRACTITIONER? NURSE-MIDWIFE?

Narrowing your ideal practitioner down to one of three general personality types makes your job of finding him or her easier, but exam-tableside manner and philosophy aren't everything. You'll also have to give some thought to the kind of medical credentials that would best meet your requirements.

The Obstetrician. If yours is a high-risk pregnancy,[3] then you will very likely need and want a specialist who is trained to handle every conceivable complication of pregnancy, labor, and delivery: an obstetrician. You may even want to find a specialist's specialist, an obstetrician who specializes in high-risk pregnancies, or even a subspecialist in maternal-fetal medicine.

If your pregnancy looks pretty routine from an obstetrical point of view, you may still want to select an obstetrician (more than 8 out of 10 women do), or you can choose between a physician who is a family practice specialist (about 10% to 12% of women use one) and a certified nurse-midwife (selected by 1% to 2%).

The Family Physician. The family practitioner (FP), a relatively new specialist, is actually an updated version of the old-fashioned general practitioner (GP), who once provided one-stop medical service for the whole

---

3. Traditionally, a high-risk pregnancy is one in which the expectant mother has had a problem pregnancy before; has a medical problem, such as diabetes, hypertension, or heart disease; has an Rh or a genetic problem; or is under 17 or over 35 (though there is some question as to whether women in their 30s are really high risk).

family. The major difference between the GP and the family physician is training: the FP, unlike the GP, has had several years of specialty training in primary care, including obstetrics, after receiving an MD. If you decide on an FP, he or she can serve as your internist, obstetrician/gynecologist, and when the time comes, pediatrician. Ideally, an FP will become familiar with the dynamics of your family, will be interested in all aspects of your health, not just your pregnancy, and will view pregnancy as just a normal part of the life cycle, not an illness. If complications occur, your FP may call in a specialist for consultation, but may remain in charge of your case.

The Certified Nurse-Midwife.[4] If you are looking for a practitioner whose emphasis is on you the person and not you the patient, who will take extra time to talk with you about your feelings and problems, who will be oriented toward the "natural" in childbirth, then a certified nurse-midwife (CNM) may be right for you (though, of course, many physicians meet these requirements too). Although a nurse-midwife is a medical professional, thoroughly trained to care for women with low-risk pregnancies and to attend uncomplicated births (having received special education, training, and certification in midwifery), she is more likely to treat your pregnancy as a human, rather than a medical, condition. If you choose a midwife, be sure she's certified; a lay midwife cannot provide you and your baby with optimal care.

In recent years, the number of births attended by nurse-midwives has risen dramatically.

4. Today, some midwives are being trained and certified without first becoming nurses. So, in some parts of the country, you may find the Certified Midwife (CM) in addition to, or instead of, the CNM.

TYPE OF PRACTICE

You've decided on an obstetrician, a family practitioner, or a nurse-midwife. Next you've got to decide which kind of medical practice you would be most comfortable with. The most common kinds of practices, and their possible advantages and disadvantages, are:

Solo Medical Practice. In such a practice, a doctor works for him- or herself, using another doctor to cover when he or she is away or otherwise unavailable. An obstetrician or a family physician might be in solo practice; a nurse-midwife, in almost all states, must work in a collaborative practice with a physician. The major advantage of solo practice is that you see the same practitioner at each visit, one you can get to know and hopefully feel more comfortable with before delivery. The major disadvantage is that if your doctor is not available, a physician you don't know may deliver your baby.[5] A solo practice may also be a problem if, midway during your pregnancy, you find you're not really crazy about the doctor. You're stuck unless you can afford to pick up and change to another without worrying about the investment you've already made.

Partnership or Group Medical Practice. Two or more doctors in the same specialty care jointly for patients, seeing them on a rotating basis. Again, you can find both obstetricians and family doctors in this type of practice—sometimes both in one group. The advantage of this arrangement is that by seeing a different doctor each time, you will get to know them all, and when those labor pains

5. You can remedy this by asking to meet the covering physician in advance.

are coming strong and fast there will be a familiar face in the room with you. The disadvantage is that you may not like all of the doctors in the practice equally, and you usually won't be able to choose the one who attends your birthing. Also, depending on whether you find it reassuring or unsettling, hearing different points of view from the various partners may be an advantage or a disadvantage.

Combination Practice. A group practice that includes one or more obstetricians and one or more nurse-midwives. The advantages and disadvantages are similar to those of any group practice. In addition, there is the advantage of having at some of your visits the extra time and attention a midwife may offer and at others the security of a physician's expertise. You may have the option of a midwife-coached delivery, assured that if a problem develops, a physician you know is in the wings.

Maternity or Birth Center–Based Practice. In these facilities, certified nurse-midwives provide the bulk of the care, and physicians are on call as needed. Some maternity centers are based in hospitals with special birthing rooms, and others are separate units. All maternity centers provide care for low-risk patients only.

The obvious advantage of this type of practice is to those women who prefer certified midwives as their primary practitioners. The major disadvantage is the fact that if a complication arises during pregnancy (as it does 20% to 30% of the time), you may have to switch to a physician and start developing a relationship all over again; if one arises during labor or delivery (as occurs 10% to 15% of the time), you may need to be delivered by the doctor on call, who may be a perfect stranger. If complications arise at a free-standing maternity center,

you may have to be transported to the nearest hospital for emergency care.

Independent Certified Nurse-Midwife Practice. In the states in which they are permitted to practice independently, CNMs offer women with low-risk pregnancies the advantage of personalized pregnancy care and a low-tech natural delivery (sometimes at home, but more often in birthing centers or hospitals). An independent CNM should have a physician available for consultation as needed and on call in case of emergency—during pregnancy, childbirth, or postpartum. Care by a certified nurse midwife is covered by most insurers and health plans.

FINDING A CANDIDATE

When you have a good idea of the kind of practitioner you want and the type of practice you'd prefer, where can you find some likely candidates? The following are all good sources:

❖ Your gynecologist or family doctor (if he or she doesn't do deliveries) or your internist, assuming you're happy with his or her style of practice. (Doctors tend to recommend others with philosophies similar to their own.)

❖ Friends who have recently had babies and whose childbearing philosophies are similar to yours.

❖ An obstetrical nurse, if you're lucky enough to know one.

❖ The county medical society, which can give you a list of names of physicians who deliver babies, along with information on their medical training, specialties, special interests, type of practice, and board certification. The society may also be able to tell you whether or not a specialist will be helpful in your situation, and if so, what kind of specialist.

❖ The *Directory of the American Medical Association* or the *Directory of Medical Specialties,* often available at your public library or doctor's office.

❖ The local La Leche League, if you're strongly interested in breastfeeding.

❖ A nearby hospital with facilities that appeal to you; for example, a neonatal intensive care unit, birthing rooms, rooming-in, father participation. They can give you the names of attending physicians.

❖ The International Childbirth Education Association, P.O. Box 20852, Milwaukee, WI 53220, or the American Society for Prophylaxis in Obstetrics (ASPO) / Lamaze, 1411 K Street NW, Suite 200, Washington, DC 20005, if you are interested in a practitioner who emphasizes prepared childbirth.

❖ A local maternity or birth center, or the American College of Nurse-Midwives, 818 Connecticut Avenue NW, Washington, DC 20006, if you are looking for a CNM.

❖ The Yellow Pages, if all else fails, under Physicians—Obstetrics and Gynecology, Maternal-Fetal Medicine, or Family Physicians.

BIRTHING ALTERNATIVES

Never before have women had so much control over the process of having a baby. For millennia it was largely nature's whims that decided a woman's obstetrical fate; then early in this century it became the physician who decided how she was to deliver. Now, at last, though nature still holds a few cards and physicians still have a

say, more and more of the decisions are falling to women and their spouses. It is becoming increasingly possible for a woman to choose the best time to conceive (thanks to better birth control methods and ovulation prediction kits) and often, barring complications, how she will give birth. Among birthing options the array is dizzying, even in a hospital setting. Leave the hospital, and there's yet more to select from.

Though your preliminary preferences for delivery shouldn't be your only criteria in choosing a practitioner, they should certainly come into play. (Keep in mind, however, that no firm decisions can be made until further into your pregnancy, and many can't be finalized until the delivery itself.) The following birthing options are among those that expectant mothers today can consider and might want to ask about before making a final decision on a practitioner and hospital:

Family-Centered Care. What many feel is the ideal in hospital maternity care, complete family-centered care is not yet a reality in many hospitals, though there's definitely a trend in that direction. ASPO/Lamaze has set criteria for this ideal, which include an official hospital policy of family-centered maternity care; childbirth education programs that reflect such a policy; management of labor without unnecessary technological interference and with attention to psychosocial needs; an atmosphere in which questions, self-help, and self-knowledge are encouraged, in which adaptations are made for cultural differences, and in which breastfeeding is encouraged within one hour of birth unless medically contraindicated; and a program that assesses a mother's basic infant care skills and determines satisfactory initiation of breastfeeding, if applicable, prior to discharge. Patient rooms should have a door (for privacy), comfortable furnishings, private toilet and bath/shower facilities, as well as sufficient space to accommodate family (siblings included) and other support persons, professional personnel and medical equipment, personal possessions, a newborn crib and supplies, and a sofa bed for family members staying overnight. There should also be an area nearby for support persons to take relaxation breaks away from the scene of the labor.

Birthing Rooms. At one time, every woman about to have a baby labored in a labor room, delivered in a delivery room, and recovered in a postpartum room. Her newborn was immediately whisked from her after birth and tucked away in a nursery to be cared for behind glass windows. Today, the availability of birthing rooms in many hospitals makes it possible for women to stay in the same bed from labor through recovery, sometimes even for their entire hospital stay, and for their babies to remain by their sides from birth on. Birthing rooms are fully equipped for uncomplicated deliveries and for unexpected emergencies (in most hospitals, cesareans and other complications must be handled in a delivery or operating room), but they look much like a cozy bedroom or hotel room (with soft lighting, pictures on the wall, curtains on the windows, an arm or rocking chair, and a comfortable bed—which usually converts to a birthing bed).

In most hospitals, a newly delivered mother (and her baby, if she's rooming in) is moved from the birthing room to a postpartum room after an hour or so of largely uninterrupted family togetherness. In a few more progressive hospitals, she can plan to stay in the birthing room straight through to check-out—sometimes with daddy, and even siblings, sharing the room.

Birthing rooms are usually available only for women who are at low risk for childbirth complications. Since the supply of birthing rooms at some hospitals is far exceeded by the demand, and they are often assigned on a first-come, first-served basis, there's the possibility that you won't get one. Fortunately, you may be able to experience unrushed, family-oriented, noninterventionist labor and delivery in some more traditional hospital settings, too.

Birthing Bed. The hard, flat delivery table on which your mother probably delivered you is losing out to a soft, roomy bed that is comfortable for labor and then, with a flip of a lever, becomes ideal for delivery. Usually the back can be raised to support the mom in a squatting or semi-squatting position and the foot of the bed can snap off to make way for the birthing attendant. After delivery, a change of linens, a few switches flipped, and presto, you're back in bed.

Birthing Chairs. Advocates of squatting deliveries prefer the birthing chair over the birthing bed. This chair is designed to support a woman in a sitting position during delivery. Since this position allows for an assist from gravity, theoretically speeding labor, it is appealing to some mothers and their birth attendants. Occasionally, however, the increased pressure of the baby's head against the pelvis when the mother is squatting in a birthing chair can lead to excessive tearing of the perineum. Though such tears can be repaired, they can prolong postpartum recuperation and discomfort.

Leboyer Births. When the French obstetrician Frederick Leboyer first propounded his theory of childbirth without violence, the medical community scoffed. Today many of the procedures he proposed, aimed at making a newborn's arrival in the world more tranquil, are common practice. Many babies are delivered in birthing rooms, without the aid of the bright lights once deemed necessary, on the theory that gentle lighting can make the transition from the dark uterus to the bright outside world more gradual and less jolting. Upending and slapping the newborn is no longer routine anywhere, and less violent procedures are preferred for establishing breathing when it doesn't start on its own. In some hospitals, the umbilical cord isn't cut immediately; instead, this last physical bond between mother and baby remains intact while they get to know each other for the first time. And though the warm bath Leboyer recommended for soothing the new arrival (and smoothing the transition from a watery home to a dry one) isn't common, being put immediately into mother's arms is.

In spite of the growing acceptance of many Leboyer theories, a full-blown Leboyer birth—with soft music, soft lights, and a warm bath for baby—isn't widely available. If you're interested in one, ask about it when you're interviewing practitioners.

Underwater Births. The concept of delivering underwater to simulate the environment in the womb is one that is not widely accepted in the medical community. Though many women who have experienced such a birth report that it was exhilarating, most physicians and hospitals feel that the risk of the fetus drowning, though probably remote, is still too great to make the procedure an acceptable one.

Home Births. For some women, the idea of being hospitalized when they aren't sick isn't appealing, but delivering at home is. And sometimes such a birth is very successful. The newborn arrives amid family and friends in a warm and loving atmosphere. The

risk, of course, is that if something goes wrong, the facilities for an emergency cesarean or resuscitation of the newborn will not be close at hand. For many women a maternity center or a hospital birthing room is an ideal compromise, combining homey atmosphere with the security of high-tech backup. Those low-risk women who insist on a home birth need to be certain they will be attended by a qualified physician or certified nurse-midwife, and that emergency transportation to a nearby hospital will be available at a moment's notice. In Great Britain home births are not uncommon, but a fully equipped ambulance or "flying squad" is usually standing by, ready to transport the mother and, if delivery has already taken place, her baby to the hospital in case of emergency.

MAKING YOUR SELECTION

Once you've secured your prospective practitioner's name, call and make an appointment for an interview. Go armed with questions that will enable you to sense if your philosophies are in sync and if your personalities mesh comfortably. But don't expect that you will agree on everything—that doesn't happen even in the happiest of marriages. If it's important that your doctor be a good listener or a careful explainer, does this one seem to fulfill those requirements? If you're concerned with the emotional aspects of pregnancy, will this practitioner take your concerns seriously? Ask about his or her positions on any of the following issues that you feel strongly about: natural childbirth vs. anesthetized childbirth vs. pain relief as needed in childbirth; breastfeeding; induction of labor; use of fetal monitoring; enemas; forceps; cesarean sections; or anything else that concerns you. That way there won't be any unpleasant last-minute surprises.

Perhaps the most important thing you can do at this first meeting is to let the practitioner know what kind of patient you are. You can judge from the response whether he or she will be comfortable with you.

You will probably also want to know something about the hospital the doctor is affiliated with. Does it have features that are important to you, such as birthing rooms, birthing chairs, facilities for Leboyer birth, rooming-in, a neonatal intensive care unit, the latest fetal monitoring equipment? Are they flexible about routines that concern you, such as shaving and enemas? Do they allow fathers in the labor, delivery, and operating rooms even during a cesarean? Will you have to keep your legs in stirrups during delivery?

Before you make a final decision, think about whether the practitioner inspires a feeling of trust. Pregnancy is one of the most important voyages you'll ever make—you'll want a skipper (or first mate) in whom you have complete faith.

MAKING THE MOST OF THE PATIENT-PRACTITIONER PARTNERSHIP

Choosing the right practitioner is only the first step. For the vast majority of women, those who are ready neither to cede all responsibility to the physician nor to take over entirely themselves, the next step is nurturing a good working partnership with that professional. Here's how:

❖ When a question or concern you think is worth mentioning crops up between visits, write it down on a list that you will take to your next appointment. (It helps to keep a few notepads in convenient places—the refrigerator door, your purse, your desk at work, your bedside table—so that you'll always be within jotting distance of one; consolidate the lists before each doctor's visit.) That's the only way you can be sure that you won't forget to ask all your questions and report all your symptoms. And that you won't be wasting your time, or your practitioner's, while you try to remember what it was you wanted to ask.

❖ Along with your list of questions, bring a pen and pad to each office visit so you can make a note of your practitioner's recommendations. Many people are too nervous in a medical setting to remember directions accurately. If your practitioner doesn't volunteer adequate information, make inquiries before you leave, so there's no confusion once you get home. Ask about such things as side effects of treatments, when to stop taking a medication if one is prescribed, when to check back about a problem situation.

❖ Though you don't want to call your physician at every pelvic twinge, you shouldn't hesitate to call about worries that you can't resolve by checking in a book such as this one, and that you feel can't wait until the next visit. Don't be afraid that your concerns will sound silly. Unless your practitioner is just out of training, he or she's heard them all before. Be prepared to be very specific about your symptoms. If you are experiencing pain, be precise about its location, duration, quantity (is it sharp, dull, crampy?), and severity. If possible, explain what makes it worse or better—changing positions, for example. If you have a

Protecting Yourself Against Malpractice

Recognizing that the modern obstetrical practitioner-patient relationship is a partnership, and that when there is a less than perfect outcome it isn't always the physician who's at fault, doctors are no longer allowing themselves to be sitting ducks while patients take malpractice pot shots at them. They're fighting back and even in rare instances turning the tables and charging with malpractice the very same patients who are hurling malpractice charges at them. Still, though a few doctor vs. patient countersuits are actually coming to trial, you needn't worry that you will have to pay your doctor a million dollars if you don't take the vitamins he or she prescribes. What you do need to worry about, however, if you are guilty of malpractice, is that you and your baby will pay the price in possibly more devastating ways—with health and even life being the cost.

If you want to be a patient whom no one can charge with malpractice, take the following precautions:

❖ Tell the whole truth, and nothing but the truth. Don't give your practitioner a false or incomplete medical history. Make sure he or she knows about any drugs—prescription or non-, legal or illegal, medicinal or recreational, including alcohol and tobacco—that you are currently taking as well as about any past or present illnesses or operations.

❖ Don't reject necessary x-rays, tests, or medications unless you have an authoritative second opinion that backs up your decision.

❖ Follow instructions carefully when undergoing a medical procedure. You can't blame the radiologist for a blurred x-ray if you moved when you were told to stand still.

❖ Follow your practitioner's recommendations as to appointment schedule, weight gain, bed rest, exercise, medication, vitamins, and so on—unless, again, you have respected medical opinion that advises you otherwise.

❖ Do not allow anyone who is clearly under the influence of drugs or alcohol to treat you. Doing so makes you an accomplice to his or her crime.

❖ Always alert a practitioner to an obvious adverse effect of a medication or treatment, as well as to any other worrisome symptoms that you experience in your pregnancy. Also speak up if you believe your practitioner's instructions may be incorrect (see page 15).

❖ Never threaten or otherwise alarm a physician in a manner that could interfere with the treatment you are receiving.

❖ Take good care of yourself, following the Best-Odds Diet (see page 80), getting adequate rest and exercise, and absolutely avoiding alcohol, tobacco, and other nonprescribed drugs and medications, once you find out you're pregnant, or better still, once you start trying to conceive.

If you feel you can't follow your practitioner's instructions or go along with his or her recommended course of treatment, right or wrong, you clearly have little faith in the person you've chosen to care for you and your baby during your pregnancy, labor, and delivery. In such a case, all sides will be better served if you find a replacement.

vaginal discharge, describe its color (bright red, dark red, brownish, pinkish, yellowish), when it started, and how heavy it is. Also report accompanying symptoms (such as fever, nausea, vomiting, chills, diarrhea). (See When to Call the Practitioner, page 117.)

❖ When you read about something new in obstetrics, don't brandish the clipping in front of the practitioner at your next visit saying, "I must have this." Instead ask if he or she feels there is any value to this new procedure or validity to that new theory. Often the media report medical advances prematurely, before they are proven safe and effective through controlled studies. If indeed it is a legitimate advance, your practitioner may already be aware of it or may want to find out more about it. Whether it is or not, you may both learn something through the exchange.

❖ When you hear something that doesn't correspond with what your practitioner has told you, ask for an opinion on what you've heard. Not in a challenging way, just in order to get more information.

❖ If you suspect that the practitioner may be mistaken about something (for example, okaying intercourse when you have a history of miscarriage), speak up. You can't assume that he or she, even with your chart in hand, will always remember every aspect of your medical and personal history—and you share the responsibility of making sure errors are not made. The best approach in such a situation is to lay out your understanding of the situation and your concerns in a non-combative way. Almost invariably you will find that your provider really cares and will be glad for your candid input.

❖ If you have a gripe about anything (from being kept waiting to not getting answers to your questions), air it. Letting it fester will jeopardize the practitioner-patient relationship.

❖ If your relationship with your practitioner breaks down irreparably, think about changing doctors. He or she probably doesn't enjoy the bad feelings any more than you do. Don't, however, expect to get good obstetrical care if you regularly switch from doctor to doctor, trying to find one who will follow *your* orders. Consider, instead, that the problem with the care you've been receiving may originate with you.

So You Won't Forget

Because there'll be times when you'll want to do a little writing with your reading—jot down a symptom so you can share it with your doctor, make a note of this week's weight so you can compare it to next week's, record what needs recording so you'll remember what needs remembering—we've added note pages to *What to Expect*, starting on page 439.

If You're Not Pregnant ...

If your pregnancy test is negative this time, but you'd very much like to become pregnant soon, start making the most of the preconception period by taking the steps in Chapter 21. Such preconception preparation will help ensure the best possible pregnancy outcome when you do conceive.

2
Now That You Are Pregnant

WHAT YOU MAY BE CONCERNED ABOUT

Now that you no longer have to worry about what the result of the pregnancy test will be, you're sure to come up with a whole new set of concerns: What effect will my age or my husband's age have on my pregnancy and on our baby? How will chronic medical problems or family genetic problems affect him or her? Will our past lifestyles make a difference? Can my previous obstetrical history repeat? What can I do to lower any risks my history may present?

YOUR GYNECOLOGICAL HISTORY

"I haven't mentioned a previous pregnancy to my obstetrician because it occurred before I was married. Is there any reason I should?"

Your past gynecological history can be as important to your practitioner as the information he or she gains at each checkup during this pregnancy. Previous pregnancies, miscarriages, abortions, surgery, or infections may or may not have an impact on what happens in this pregnancy, but any information you have about them should be passed on to your practitioner. It will be handled with confidentiality. And don't worry about what your doctor will think. It's the job of the physician to help mothers and babies, not to judge them.

PREVIOUS ABORTIONS

"I've had two abortions. Will they affect this pregnancy?"

Probably not, if they were done in recent years and during the first trimester. Though abortions performed before 1973 have been linked to an increased risk of midtrimester miscarriage (because of damage in the course of the procedure that weakened the cervix, making it "incompetent"), improved techniques in first-trimester abortions since that time appear to have eliminated the risk of this type of cervical injury.

Multiple second-trimester abortions (14 to 26 weeks), however, do appear to increase the risk of premature delivery. If you had your abortions after the third month, see page 218 for reducing the risks of premature birth.

In either case, be sure your practitioner knows about the abortions. The more familiar he or she is with your gynecological history, the better care you will receive.

FIBROIDS

"I've had fibroids for several years, and they've never caused me any problem. But now that I'm pregnant, I'm worried that they will."

Fibroids occur most commonly in women over 35, and since the ranks of women in that age group who are having babies are swelling, fibroids are becoming relatively common in pregnancy (estimates range from 1 to 2 women in 100). The vast majority of pregnant women with fibroids can expect to go to term without added complications related to this condition. Occasionally, however, these small nonmalignant growths in the inner walls of the uterus do cause problems, increasing slightly the risk of ectopic pregnancy, miscarriage, placenta previa (a low-lying placenta), abruptio placenta (a premature separation of the placenta from the uterine wall), premature labor, premature rupture of membranes, stalled labor, fetal malformation, and breech and other more-difficult-to-deliver fetal posi-

tions. To minimize these risks, you should: be under the care of a physician; discuss the fibroids with your physician so that you become better informed on the condition in general and the risks in your particular case; reduce other pregnancy risks (see page 50); and be particularly attentive to symptoms that could signal impending trouble (see page 117).

Sometimes a woman with fibroids notices pressure or pain in the abdomen. And though it should be reported to the doctor, it usually isn't anything to worry about. Bed rest and safe pain relievers (see page 320) for four or five days usually bring relief. Sometimes the fibroids degenerate or twist, causing abdominal pain often accompanied by fever. Rarely, surgery may be needed to remove such a degenerating fibroid or one that is otherwise causing problems. If doctors suspect that the fibroids could interfere with a safe vaginal delivery, they may opt to deliver by cesarean section.

"I had a couple of fibroids removed a few years ago. Will this cause problems now that I'm pregnant?"

In most cases, surgery for the removal of small uterine fibroid tumors doesn't affect a subsequent pregnancy. Extensive surgery for large fibroids could, however, weaken the uterus enough so that it would be unable to tolerate labor. If, on reviewing your surgical records, your physician decides this might be true of your uterus, a cesarean delivery will be planned. You should become familiar with the signs of early labor in case contractions begin before the planned surgery (see page 221). And you should have an emergency plan for getting to the hospital immediately if you do go into labor.

INCOMPETENT CERVIX

"I had a miscarriage in my fifth month in my first pregnancy. The doctor said it was caused by an incompetent cervix. I just had a positive home pregnancy test and I'm terrified that I will have the same problem again."

Now that your incompetent cervix has been diagnosed, your physician should be able to take steps to prevent it from causing you to miscarry again. An incompetent cervix, one that opens prematurely under the pressure of the growing uterus and fetus, is estimated to occur in 1 or 2 of every 100 pregnancies; it is believed responsible for 20% to 25% of all second-trimester miscarriages. An incompetent cervix can be the result of genetic weakness of the cervix (the neck of the uterus); exposure of the mother to DES (diethylstilbestrol; see page 40) when she was in her mother's womb; extreme stretching of or severe lacerations to the cervix during one or more previous deliveries; cervical surgery or laser therapy; or traumatic D and Cs or abortions (particularly those performed before 1973). Carrying more than one fetus can also lead to incompetent cervix, but if it does, the problem will not usually recur in subsequent single-fetus pregnancies.

Incompetent cervix is usually diagnosed when a woman miscarries in the second trimester after experiencing progressive painless effacement (thinning) and dilatation of the cervix without apparent uterine contractions or vaginal bleeding. Ideally, doctors would like to be able to diagnose the problem before the miscarriage occurs so that steps can be taken to save the pregnancy. Recent attempts at diagnosing an opening cervix early on with ultrasound look promising.

If you lost a prior pregnancy because of an incompetent cervix, tell your obstetrician about it immediately if he or she is not already familiar with that fact. It is likely that cerclage (suturing, or stitching closed, the opening of the cervix) can be performed early in the second trimester (12 to 16 weeks) to prevent a repeat of this tragedy. The simple procedure is performed in the hospital after a normal pregnancy has been confirmed by ultrasound. After surgery and 12 hours of bed rest, the patient is usually allowed to get up to go to the bathroom and 12 hours later can resume normal activities. Sexual intercourse may be prohibited for the duration of the pregnancy, and frequent exams by the doctor may be necessary. Rarely, complete bed rest and the use of a specially designed appliance called a pessary to support the uterus may be substituted for cerclage. Treatment may also be initiated when ultrasound or a vaginal examination shows the cervix is opening, even if there was no previous late miscarriage.

When or whether the sutures will be removed will depend partly on the doctor's preference and partly on the type of sutures. Usually they are removed a few weeks before the estimated due date; in some cases they may not be removed until labor begins unless there is infection, bleeding, or premature rupture of the membranes.

Regardless of which course of treatment is taken, your chances of carrying to term are good. Still, you will have to be alert for signs of an impending problem in the second or early third trimester: pressure in the lower abdomen, vaginal discharge with or without blood, unusual urinary frequency, or the sensation of a lump in the vagina. If you experience any of these, go immediately to the doctor's office or the emergency room. (For more on midtrimester miscarriage, see page 177.)

YOUR OBSTETRICAL HISTORY REPEATING ITSELF

"My first pregnancy was very uncomfortable—I must have had every symptom in the book. Will I be that unlucky again?"

In general, your first pregnancy is a pretty good predictor of future pregnancies, all things being equal. So you are a little less likely to breeze comfortably through pregnancy than someone who already has. Still, there's always the hope that your luck will change for the better. All pregnancies, like all babies, are different. If, for example, morning sickness or food cravings plagued you in your first pregnancy, they may be barely noticeable in the second (or vice versa, of course). While luck, genetic predisposition, and the fact that you've experienced certain symptoms before have a lot to do with how comfortable or uncomfortable this pregnancy will be, other factors—including some that are within your control—can alter the prognosis to some extent. The factors include:

General Health. Being in good all-round physical condition gives you a better shot at having a comfortable pregnancy. Ideally, attend to chronic conditions (allergies, asthma, back problems) and clear up lingering infections (such as urinary tract infections or vaginitis) before conception (see Chapter 15). Once you become pregnant, continue to take good care of yourself as well as your pregnancy.

Diet. While it can't offer any guarantees, following the Best-Odds Diet gives every pregnant woman the best odds of having a comfortable pregnancy. Not only can it better your chances of avoiding or minimizing the miseries of morning sickness and indigestion, it can help fight excessive fatigue, combat constipation and hemorrhoids, prevent urinary tract infections and iron-deficiency anemia, and give you a leg up against leg cramps. (And even if your pregnancy turns out to be uncomfortable anyway, you'll have bestowed on your baby the best odds of developing well and being born healthy.)

Weight Gain. Gaining weight at a steady rate and keeping the gain within the recommended boundaries (between 25 and 35 pounds) can improve your chances of escaping or minimizing such pregnancy miseries as hemorrhoids, varicose veins, stretch marks, backache, fatigue, indigestion, and shortness of breath.

Fitness. Getting enough and the right kind of exercise (see page 189 for guidelines) can help improve your general well-being. Exercise is especially important in second and subsequent pregnancies because abdominal muscles tend to be laxer, making you more susceptible to a variety of aches and pains, most notably backache.

Lifestyle Pace. Leading a harried and frenetic life, as so many women do today, can aggravate or sometimes even trigger one of the most uncomfortable of pregnancy symptoms—morning sickness—and exacerbate others such as fatigue, backache, and indigestion. Getting some help around the house, taking more breaks away from whatever frazzles your nerves (including older children, if any), cutting back on job responsibilities, or letting low-priority tasks go undone for the time being can bring some relief (see page 102 for more tips).

Other Children. Some pregnant women with other children at home find that keeping up with their off-spring keeps them so busy that they barely have time to notice pregnancy discomforts, major or minor. But for many others, having one or more older children tends to aggravate pregnancy symptoms. For example, morning sickness can increase during times of stress (the getting-to-school or the getting-dinner-on-the-table rush, for instance); fatigue can be heightened because there doesn't seem to be any time to rest; backaches can be aggravated if you're doing a lot of child toting; even constipation becomes more likely if you never have a chance to use the bathroom when the urge strikes. The key to lessening the toll that caring for your other children can take on your pregnant body is sometimes elusive, but worth seeking: more time to take care of yourself. Take advantage of any potential helper you can find (paid or volunteer) to lighten your load and to help free up personal time.

"My first pregnancy was rough, with several serious complications. I'm very nervous now that I'm pregnant again."

One complicated pregnancy doesn't necessarily predict another. Often a woman who weathered high seas the first time around is rewarded with smooth sailing the next. If it was a one-time event, such as an infection or an accident, that caused the complications, then they aren't likely to recur. Nor will they recur if they were caused by lifestyle habits that you've now changed (like smoking, drinking, or using drugs), an exposure to an environmental hazard (such as lead) to which you are no longer exposed, or by failure to seek medical care early in pregnancy (assuming you've sought such care early on this time).

If the cause was a chronic health problem, such as diabetes or high blood pressure, correcting or controlling the condition prior to conception or very early in pregnancy can greatly reduce the risk of repeat complications.

If you had a specific complication during your first pregnancy that you would like to avoid the second time around, it's a good idea to discuss it with your practitioner now to see if anything can be done to prevent a repeat. No matter what the problem or its cause (even if it's been labeled "cause unknown"), the tips in the response to the previous question can help make your pregnancy more comfortable and safer for both you and your baby.

"With my first child, I had a very comfortable and uneventful pregnancy. That's why the 42-hour labor with 5 hours of pushing I had came as such a shock. I'm glad I'm pregnant again, but I dread another labor like the first one."

Relax, enjoy your pregnancy, and put thoughts of another difficult labor out of your mind. Second and subsequent deliveries are, barring a less than ideal fetal position or some other unforeseen complication, almost always easier than first ones, thanks to a more experienced uterus and a laxer birth canal. All phases of labor tend to be shorter, and the amount of pushing necessary to deliver generally decreases dramatically.

REPEAT CESAREANS

"When I had my first baby by cesarean I was told I could never deliver vaginally because of my abnormal pelvis. I want to have six kids just like my mother did, but I understand three cesareans is the limit."

Tell that to Ethel Kennedy, the indomitable wife of Robert F. Kennedy, who is reported to have had 11 cesareans in an era when the procedure was neither as safe nor as easy as it is today. Of course, sometimes having numerous cesareans isn't possible. Much depends upon the kind of incision that was made and the kind of scar that formed. Talk to your obstetrician about your concern, because only someone fully familiar with your clinical history can predict whether or not you can do an "Ethel Kennedy" (or even half an "Ethel Kennedy"). You may be pleasantly surprised.

If you do have multiple cesareans, however, you may, because of numerous scars, be at increased risk for uterine rupture caused by labor contractions. For this reason, you should be particularly alert for the signs of oncoming labor (contractions, bloody show, ruptured membranes; see page 269) in the final months of pregnancy. Should they occur, notify your doctor and go to the hospital immediately. You should also notify him or her at *any* time in your pregnancy if you have bleeding or unexplained, persistent abdominal pain.

"I had my last baby by cesarean. I'm pregnant again and I'm wondering what the chances are of my having a vaginal delivery."

"Once a cesarean always a cesarean" was, until very recently, an obstetrical edict engraved in stone, or rather in the uteruses of women who'd had one or more surgical deliveries. Today the American College of Obstetricians and Gynecologists has turned that theory upside-down. The new position: Repeat cesareans should not be considered routine; Vaginal Birth After Cesarean (VBAC) should be the norm. Experience shows that between 50% and 80% of women who

have had cesareans are able to go through a normal labor and a vaginal delivery in subsequent deliveries. Even women who have had more than one cesarean or are carrying twins have a good chance of being able to successfully deliver vaginally.

Whether or not you will be able to try VBAC will depend on the type of uterine incision (which may be different from your abdominal incision) made in your previous c-section and on the reason your baby was delivered surgically. If you had a low-transverse incision (across the lower part of the uterus), as 95% of women do today, your chances of succeeding at VBAC are good; if you had a classic vertical incision (down the middle of your uterus), as was popular in the past and is still occasionally needed, you will not be allowed to attempt a vaginal delivery because of the risk of uterine rupture. If the reason for your c-section was one that isn't likely to repeat (fetal distress, premature separation of the placenta, faulty placement of the placenta, infection, breech, toxemia), it's very possible you can have a vaginal delivery this time. If it was a chronic disease (diabetes, high blood pressure, heart disease) or an uncorrectable problem (a badly contracted pelvis, for example), you will probably require a repeat cesarean. Don't rely on your recollection of the type of uterine incision you had or the reason you needed a cesarean last time—check, or have your physician check, the medical records of your prior delivery.

If you feel strongly about wanting a vaginal delivery this time, then discuss the possibility with your physician now. Some doctors still cling to the old adage and will not permit a woman with a cesarean-scarred uterus to go through a trial of labor. If you are to succeed at VBAC, you will need to find an amenable doctor who is willing to be with you from the very beginning of labor through delivery. And for safety's sake, you must plan on delivering in a hospital fully equipped and staffed for emergency cesarean sections, should one become necessary.

Your role in ensuring a safe vaginal delivery is as important as your doctor's. You should:

❖ Take childbirth education classes, and take them seriously, so that you will be able to labor as efficiently as possible to minimize the stress on your body.

❖ Notify your doctor when the first signs of labor (see page 269) occur.

❖ Tell your doctor immediately if *between* contractions you notice any unusual abdominal pain or tenderness.

You may also be asked to limit medication, to avoid masking signs of an impending rupture. But some doctors, who believe continuous monitoring will warn of a rupture, will okay epidurals.

Though your chances of having a normal vaginal delivery are good, even the woman who has never had a cesarean has a 20% or better chance of needing one. So don't be disappointed if you end up with a repeat. After all, the safest possible birth of that wonderful baby of yours is what this is all about.

"I had a cesarean my first time after an agonizing, long labor. My doctor said I should try to have a vaginal delivery this time, but I would rather have a cesarean and avoid another ordeal."

To read what staunch cesarean opponents have to say about it, one would quickly conclude that the medical establishment is solely responsible for the high rate of cesareans in this country. But there's another side of the story that isn't often told, and that

is that many repeat cesareans (and repeats make up at least one-third of the total performed each year) are performed at the request of the expectant mother. And the most common reason these mothers give for opting for the planned surgical delivery over VBAC is the desire to avoid another prolonged and painful labor.

It's normal for the human being not to want to suffer—it's an automatic reflex designed to protect against injury. Your eyelid blinks when a sharp object approaches; you pull your hand away from a flame. Those actions make sense. But though it might seem that choosing a cesarean just to avoid the pain of labor also makes sense, it doesn't. It's true that labor may cause more pain than a cesarean, but it isn't as likely to inflict injury. Your risks actually increase with a surgical delivery, and though the risks remain minute (with the chances of dying during a vaginal delivery at 1 in 10,000 and the chances of dying during a surgical delivery at 4 in 10,000), increasing risk without reason never makes sense.

Remember, too, that your labor this time is likely to be much easier and shorter. And if the VBAC is successful, you'll avoid the two or three days of abdominal pains that often follow a c-section. You owe it to yourself to give it a try.

YOUR FAMILY HISTORY

"I recently discovered that my mother and one of her sisters both lost babies shortly after delivery. No one knows why. Could that happen to me?"

It used to be that family histories of infant illness or death were often concealed, as though losing a baby or a child were somehow sinful or something to be ashamed of. But now we realize that exposing the history of past generations can help keep today's generation healthy. Though the deaths of the two babies under similar circumstances may just be coincidental, it would certainly make sense to see a genetic counselor or maternal-fetal subspecialist to get some advice. Your practitioner can recommend one.

Any couple that does not have information on possible hereditary defects in their families might be wise to make an effort to learn more, possibly by questioning older family members. Because prenatal diagnosis is possible for many hereditary disorders, being armed with such information beforehand may make it possible to prevent problems before they occur or to treat them when they do.

"There are several stories in our family about babies who seemed fine at birth but then started to get sicker and sicker. Eventually they died in early infancy. Should I be concerned?"

A mong the major causes of infant illness and death in the first few days and weeks of life are what are known as inborn errors of metabolism. Babies born with this type of genetic defect are missing an enzyme or other chemical substance, making it impossible for them to metabolize a particular dietary element; which element depends on which enzyme is missing. Ironically, the baby's life is in jeopardy as soon as feeding begins.

Fortunately most such disorders can be diagnosed prenatally, and many can be treated. So consider yourself lucky if you turn out to have this information available to you in advance, and be sure to act on it. Discuss this information with your practitioner and, if it's recommended, with a genetic counselor.

PREGNANCIES TOO CLOSE TOGETHER

"I became pregnant again just ten weeks after I delivered my first child. I'm worried about what effect this might have on my health and on the baby I'm now carrying."

C onceiving again before you've fully recovered from a recent pregnancy and delivery puts enough strain on your body without adding the debilitating effects of worry. So first of all, *relax*. Though conception in the first three postpartum months is rare (almost a miracle if the new baby is exclusively breastfed), it's taken other women by surprise too. And most have delivered normal, healthy infants, little the worse for wear themselves.

However, it's essential to be aware of the toll two quickly consecutive pregnancies can take, and to do everything possible to compensate. Conception within three months of delivery puts the new pregnancy in a high-risk category, which in this case isn't as ominous as it sounds, particularly with the proper care and precautions, including:

❖ The best prenatal care, starting as soon as you think you're pregnant. As with any high-risk pregnancy, you're probably best off with an obstetrician, or with a nurse-midwife who practices with one. You should be scrupulous about following doctor's orders and not missing office visits.

❖ The Best-Odds Diet (see page 80), adhered to, if not religiously, at least faithfully. It's possible your body has not had a chance to rebuild its stores and you may still, even some time after delivery and particularly if you are nursing, be at a nutritional disadvantage. That means you may need to overcompensate nutritionally to be sure both you and the baby you are carrying will not be deprived. Pay particular attention to protein (have at least 100 grams or four Best-Odds servings daily) and iron (you should take a supplement).

❖ **Adequate weight gain.** Your new fetus doesn't care whether or not you've had time to shed the extra pounds his or her sibling put on you. The two of you need the same 25-to-35-pound gain this pregnancy. So don't even think about losing weight, not even early on. A carefully monitored gradual weight gain will be relatively easy to take off afterward, particularly if it was gained on the highest-quality diet, and especially once you have two children to keep up with.

Be certain, too, that you don't let lack of time or energy keep you from eating enough. Feeding and caring for the child you already have shouldn't keep you from feeding and caring for your child-to-be. Watch your weight gain carefully, and if you're not progressing as you should (see page 147), monitor your calorie intake more closely and follow the suggestions given on page 81 for aid in increasing weight gain.

❖ **Weaning your older baby immediately if you're nursing.** He or she's already reaped many of the benefits of breastfeeding, and weaning at this stage should be neither difficult nor traumatic for your baby, though it may be uncomfortable for you. Some women do continue nursing, but trying to rally the nutritional forces for both nursing and pregnancy can be a losing battle for all concerned. For tips on weaning at any age, see *What to Expect the First Year*.

❖ **Rest**—more than is humanly (and new-motherly) possible. This will require not only your own determination but help from your husband and possibly others as well. Set priorities: let less important chores or work go undone, and force yourself to lie down when your baby is napping. Have Daddy take over as many nighttime feedings as he can rise to the occasion for, as well as much of the cooking, housework, and baby care (particularly tasks that involve a lot of heavy lifting or carrying).

❖ **Exercise**—just enough to keep you in shape and relax you, but not enough to overtax your system. If you can't seem to find the time for a regular pregnancy exercise routine, build physical activity into your day with your baby. Take him or her for a brisk walk in the stroller or in a baby carrier. Or enroll in a pregnancy exercise class (see page 194 for tips on choosing one) or swim at a club or Y that offers baby-sitting services. But avoid jogging or other strenuous exercise.

❖ **Eliminating or minimizing all other pregnancy risk factors,** such as smoking and drinking (see page 50). Your body and your baby shouldn't be subjected to any additional stress.

TEMPTING FATE THE SECOND TIME AROUND

"I had a perfect first baby. Now that I'm pregnant again, I can't get rid of the fear that I won't be so lucky this time."

A million-dollar lottery winner isn't likely to hit the jackpot again, though his or her odds remain as good as any other player's. A mother who has had a "perfect" baby, however, is not only likely to win again, her odds are better than they were before she had a successful pregnancy under her belt. In addition, with each subsequent pregnancy, she has the chance to improve her odds a little—by eliminating any existing negatives (smoking, drinking, drug use) and accentuating all positives (proper diet, exercise, and medical care).

HAVING A BIG FAMILY

"I'm pregnant for the sixth time. Does this pose any additional risk for my baby or for me?"

Time-honored medical theory has it that not only does practice in childbearing not make perfect, it may make imperfect. It has long been believed in medical circles that women who have five or more children are putting both themselves and their babies at increased risk with each additional pregnancy. This may have been true before the advances in modern obstetrical care—and it is probably true today for women who receive inadequate care—but the fact is that women getting good prenatal care have an excellent chance of having healthy, normal babies even in fifth or later pregnancies. In a recent study the only increased risk discovered for fifth and subsequent pregnancies was a small jump in the incidence of multiple births (twins, triplets, and so on) and in babies born with trisomy 21, a chromosomal disorder.[1] So enjoy your pregnancy *and* your large family. But do take a few precautions:

---

1. Though according to this study having a large family doesn't seem to be particularly risky for the babies, another study has shown that with each baby the mother's risk of developing noninsulin-dependent diabetes later in life increases.

❖ Consider prenatal testing if you are 30 years old or older (rather than waiting until you're 35), since the incidence of offspring with chromosomal problems appears to increase earlier in women with many pregnancies.

❖ Be sure to get all the help you can solicit or pay for. And drop nonessential chores for the duration. Teach your older children to be more self-sufficient (even toddlers can dress and undress themselves, put away toys, and so on). Exhaustion isn't good for any pregnant woman, particularly not one with a large brood to look after.

❖ Watch your weight. It's not uncommon for women who've had several pregnancies to put on a few extra pounds with each baby. If that's been the case with you, be particularly careful to eat efficiently and not gain too much (see page 147). Overweight does increase some risks, particularly that of having a difficult labor, and it can complicate cesarean delivery and recovery. On the other hand, make sure you're not so busy you don't eat enough to gain adequate weight.

❖ Keep all other pregnancy risks to a minimum—see page 50.

❖ Be particularly aware of signs that something may be wrong during pregnancy, labor, or postpartum (see pages 117 and 381). One study showed that, although there was no increased risk of either the many-time mother or her baby dying during pregnancy or delivery, there was an increased risk of such complications as breech or other unusual presentations, premature separation of the placenta, rupture of the uterus, and postpartum hemorrhage, and of the need for forceps and cesarean deliveries.

BEING A SINGLE MOTHER

"I'm single, I'm pregnant, and I'm happy about it—but I'm also a little nervous about going through this alone."

Just because you don't have a husband doesn't mean you'll have to go through pregnancy alone. The kind of support you'll need can come from other sources besides a spouse. A good friend or a relative you feel close to and comfortable with (a mother, aunt, sibling, or cousin) can step in to hold your hand, emotionally and physically, throughout pregnancy. That person can, in many ways, play the role of the father during the nine months and beyond—accompanying you to prenatal visits and childbirth education classes, lending an ear when you need to talk about your concerns and fears as well as your joyous anticipation, helping you get both your home and life ready for the new arrival, and acting as coach, supporter, and advocate during labor and delivery.

Something you might want to keep in mind when reading this book: the many references to "husband" and "father-to-be" aren't meant to exclude you. Since the majority of our readers are in traditional families, it's just simpler to use these terms consistently than try to include all the other possibilities that exist. We hope that you'll understand, and that as you read this book you'll find that it's meant as much for you as for married mothers-to-be.

HAVING A BABY AFTER 35

"I'm 38 and pregnant with my first—and probably last—baby. It's so important that it be healthy, but I've read so much about the risks of pregnancy after 35."

Becoming pregnant after 35 puts you in good—and growing—company. While the pregnancy rate has been dropping among women in their 20s, it has been zooming among women over 35. Nowadays, it isn't unheard of for a woman to have her first child, or start a second family, after 40 or even 45.

If you've lived for more than 35 years, however, you know that nothing one does in life is completely risk-free. Pregnancy, at any age, certainly isn't. And though these days the risks are very small to begin with, they do increase slightly as age advances. Most older mothers, however, feel that the benefits of starting a family at the time that is right for them far outweigh any risks. And they are buoyed by the fact that new medical discoveries are rapidly reducing these risks.

The major reproductive risk faced by a woman in your age group is not becoming pregnant at all because of decreased fertility. Once she's overcome that and become pregnant, she also faces a greater chance of having a baby with Down syndrome. The incidence increases with the mother's age: 1 in 10,000 for 20-year-old mothers, about 3 in 1,000 for 35-year-old mothers, and 1 in 100 for 40-year-old mothers. It's speculated that this and other chromosomal abnormalities, though still relatively rare, are more common in older women because their ova are older too (every woman is born with a lifetime supply of eggs) and have had more exposure to x-rays, drugs, infections, and so on. (It is now known, however, that the egg is not always responsible for such chromosomal abnormalities. An estimated minimum of 25% of Down syndrome cases have been linked to a defect in the father's sperm. See page 30.)

While Down syndrome (characterized by varying degrees of mental retardation, certain facial characteristics, loose muscle tone, and sometimes other health problems) isn't preventable at this time, it can be diagnosed in utero, through prenatal diagnosis (see page 42). Such diagnostic testing is now routine for mothers over 35 and others in high-risk categories, including those who have low MSAFP readings (see page 47). Should an abnormality be discovered, the parents then must decide, with input from genetic counselors, pediatricians, maternal-fetal subspecialists, and other professionals, whether to terminate or continue the pregnancy. In making the decision, it is important for expectant parents to keep in mind that only 10 percent of children with Down syndrome are severely retarded and many have the potential for living fulfilling lives. They are exceptionally loving and lovable, and most can, with early intervention[2] learn to read and write (sometimes even to go to college) and to become self-reliant.

Mothers who are 35-plus also are slightly more likely to develop high blood pressure (especially if they are overweight), diabetes, and cardiovascular disease—all of which are more common in older groups in general and are usually controllable. Older mothers are also somewhat more subject to miscarriage (often due to a blighted embryo), preterm labor, and postpartum hemorrhage. Because studies are contradictory, it isn't clear whether or not labor and delivery are on the average longer, more difficult, or more complicated in older mothers than in younger ones. But if they are, the differences are probably small. In some older women, a decrease in muscle tone and joint flexibility may contribute to labor difficulties, but in many

others, thanks to excellent physical condition resulting from healthy lifestyles, this is not a problem.

In spite of the increased risks—which, as you can see, are far less threatening than many women fear—today's older mothers have a lot going for them. Medical science, for example. Screening for birth defects can be done in utero through amniocentesis, chorionic villous sampling, ultrasound, and other newer procedures (see About Prenatal Diagnosis, page 42) and can potentially reduce the risk of bearing an infant with a severe birth defect to a level comparable to that of younger women. Drugs and close medical supervision can sometimes forestall preterm labor. Electronic fetal monitoring during labor can warn of fetal distress, allowing speedy measures to be taken to protect the fetus from further trauma.

As successful as these advances have been in reducing the risks of pregnancy after 35, they pale next to the strides older mothers have taken—and can take—to improve the odds for themselves and their babies through exercise, diet, and quality prenatal care. Advanced reproductive age alone does not necessarily put a mother in a high-risk category. But an accumulation of many individual risks can. When the older mother makes a concerted effort to eliminate or minimize as many risk factors as possible, she can take years off her pregnancy profile—making her chances of delivering a healthy baby virtually as good as those of a younger mother. (See Reducing Risk in Any Pregnancy, page 50.)

And there may be some additional pluses. It's been theorized that this new breed of woman—better educated (more than half of older mothers have gone to college), career-oriented, and more settled—make better parents, thanks to their maturity and stability. Because they are

---

2. Such intervention, which includes training of parents as well as daily exposure of the infant to a specially designed program, can have a remarkable effect on children with Down syndrome.

older and have probably had their share of the fast lane, they are now less likely to resent being tied down by a baby. One study showed that these mothers were generally more accepting of parenting and displayed more patience and other strengths that were beneficial to the development of their children. And though they may have less physical stamina than when they were younger, are separated by a wide generation gap from their children, and often find the lifestyle change more stressful because they're more set in their ways, few regret having become parents. Most, in fact, are thrilled about it.

AGE AND TESTING FOR DOWN SYNDROME

"I'm 34, and I'm due to deliver just two months before my 35th birthday. Should I consider testing for Down syndrome?"

The chances of having a baby with Down syndrome don't escalate suddenly on a woman's 35th birthday. The risk increases gradually from the early 20s on, with the greatest jump coming as a woman passes 40. So there is no clear scientific answer to whether or not it makes sense to resort to prenatal diagnosis when you are just shy of 35. The 35 cutoff is simply an arbitrary age, selected by doctors trying to detect as many fetuses with Down syndrome as possible without exposing more mothers and babies than necessary to the slight risk of some types of prenatal diagnosis. Some practitioners do advise women who will turn 35 during pregnancy to consider prenatal diagnosis; others don't.

In many cases, the practitioner will suggest that an MSAFP test (see page 47) be evaluated first, before a woman under 35 undergoes amniocentesis. A low reading on this simple blood test indicates the possibility, but not the probability, of Down syndrome in the fetus and suggests that a follow-up amniocentesis is a good idea. And though the test doesn't catch all cases of the syndrome, it is a useful screening tool. If the MSAFP reading is normal, on the other hand, amniocentesis becomes somewhat less essential— assuming there are no indications for it other than advanced age. Discuss the options, and your concerns, with your practitioner or genetic counselor.

THE FATHER'S AGE

"I'm only 31, but my husband is over 50. Does advanced paternal age pose risks to a baby?"

Throughout most of history, it was believed that a father's responsibility in the reproductive process was limited to fertilization. Only during this century (too late to help those queens who'd lost their heads for failing to produce a male heir) was it discovered that a father's sperm held the deciding genetic vote in determining his child's sex. And only in the last few years has it begun to be postulated that an older father's sperm might contribute to birth defects such as Down syndrome. Like the older mother's ova, the older father's primary oocytes (undeveloped sperm) have had longer exposure to environmental hazards and might conceivably contain altered or damaged genes or chromosomes. And from the isolated studies that have been done, there is some evidence that in about 25% or 30% of Down syndrome cases, the faulty chromosome can be traced to the father. It also appears that there is an increase in the incidence of Down syndrome when the father is over 50 (or 55, depending on the study), though the association is weaker than in the case of maternal age.

But the evidence remains inconclusive—mostly because of the inadequacy of the existing research. Setting up the kind of large-scale studies required to obtain conclusive results has been difficult so far, for two reasons. First of all, Down syndrome is relatively rare (about 1 or 2 in 1,000 live births). Second, in the majority of cases, older fathers are married to older mothers, making it tricky to clarify the independent role of paternal age.

So the question of whether or not Down syndrome and other birth defects can be linked to advanced paternal age remains largely unanswered. Experts believe that there probably is some connection (although it's not clear at what age it begins), but that the risk is almost certainly very small. At this time, genetic counselors do not recommend amniocentesis on the basis of paternal age alone. If, however, you're going to spend the rest of your pregnancy worrying about the possible—though unlikely—effects of your husband's age on your baby, you might discuss your fears with your practitioner to see if amniocentesis is at all warranted.

IN-VITRO FERTILIZATION (IVF)

"I conceived my baby through in-vitro fertilization. Are my chances of having a healthy baby as good as anyone else's?"

The fact that you conceived in a laboratory rather than in bed apparently doesn't affect your chances of having a healthy baby.[3] Recent studies have shown that all other factors

being equal (age, DES exposure, the condition of the uterus, the number of fetuses, for example), there is no significant increase in such complications as prematurity, pregnancy-induced hypertension, prolonged labor, delivery complications, or the need for c-sections in IVF mothers. Nor does there appear to be more risk of a baby being born with abnormalities. There is a slightly higher miscarriage rate, but this is probably due to the fact that women who have IVF are so closely monitored that every pregnancy is diagnosed and therefore every miscarriage noted. This, of course, is not the case in the general population, in which many miscarriages occur before diagnosis and go unobserved or unreported.

There will, however, be some differences between your pregnancy and others, at least in the beginning. Because a positive test doesn't necessarily mean a pregnancy, because trying again can be so emotionally and financially draining, and because it's not known right off how many of the test-tube embryos are going to develop into fetuses, the first six weeks of an IVF pregnancy are usually more nerve-wracking than most. In addition, if an IVF mother has miscarried in previous tries, intercourse and other physical activities may be restricted, or complete bed rest may even be ordered. And the hormone progesterone may be prescribed to help support the developing pregnancy during the first two months. But once this period is past, you can expect that your pregnancy will be pretty much like everyone else's—unless you're carrying more than one fetus, as 5% to 25% of

3. Although less information is available on GIFT (gamete intrafallopian transfer) and intratubal insemination, it is assumed that the picture is pretty much the same for babies conceived through these newer methods.

IVF mothers do. If you are, see page 143.

And as with everyone else, your odds of having a healthy baby can be improved significantly by good medical care, excellent diet, moderate weight gain, a healthy balance of rest and exercise, and avoidance of alcohol, tobacco, and unprescribed drugs. See page 50 for tips on reducing pregnancy risk.

LIVING AT A HIGH ALTITUDE

"I'm concerned because we live at a high altitude, and I've heard that this can cause problems in pregnancy."

Since you're accustomed to breathing the thinner air where you live, you're far less likely to encounter an altitude-induced problem in your pregnancy than if you'd just moved there after thirty years at sea level. Though women who live at high altitudes run a *very slightly* increased chance of developing such pregnancy complications as hypertension and water retention, and of giving birth to a somewhat smaller than average baby, good prenatal care coupled with sensible self-care (eating a top-notch diet, gaining adequate weight, abstaining from alcohol and other drugs) can greatly minimize these risks. So can avoiding tobacco smoke—yours and/ or anybody else's. Smoking, which deprives babies of oxygen and optimum development at any altitude, appears to do still further damage at higher elevations, more than doubling the decrease in average birthweight. Strenuous exercise can also rob your baby of oxygen in high altitudes, so choose brisk walking over jogging, for example, and (of course this goes for all pregnant women) quit before you reach exhaustion.

Though you should be able to handle the high altitude without any trouble, women accustomed to living at low altitudes may have difficulty handling pregnancy high above sea level. Some doctors suggest postponing a contemplated move or visit (see page 180) from low altitude to high until after delivery. And of course attempting Mt. Rainier is definitely out.

RELIGIOUS OBJECTIONS TO MEDICAL CARE

"Because of my religious beliefs, I am opposed to seeking medical care. That holds especially for pregnancy, which after all is a natural process. My in-laws insist this is dangerous."

They're right. One study shows that women who refuse prenatal care on religious grounds are 100 times more likely to die in childbirth than women who get prenatal care, and that their babies are 3 times as likely to die at birth. You have to decide if these are risks you want to take for yourself and your child-to-be. And beyond the personal risk, are you willing to subject yourself to the legal risk if any injury that you might have prevented befalls your baby? Some courts are holding mothers responsible for behavior potentially damaging to the fetus they are carrying.

It's not likely that your in-laws are saying that your religious principles aren't important, rather that human life, not religious principle, is what is at stake here. Not only yours, but that of your precious baby.

Finally, it may help you to know that almost all religious convictions are fully compatible with good and safe obstetrical care. Discuss your convictions with two or three prospective practitioners. It's very possible that you can find a physician or nurse-midwife who will be able to find ways to safely adapt your pregnancy care to your religious rules.

RH INCOMPATIBILITY

"My doctor said my blood tests show I am Rh negative and my husband is Rh positive. He said not to worry, but my mother lost her second child because of Rh disease."

Every human being inherits a blood type that is either Rh positive (has the dominant Rh factor) or negative (lacks the factor). All pregnant women are tested for the Rh factor early in pregnancy. If a woman turns out to be Rh positive (85% are), or if both she and her husband are negative, there is no cause for concern. If, however, she is Rh negative and her husband Rh positive, she is a candidate for Rh incompatibility problems and her pregnancy must be kept under careful obstetrical surveillance.

When your mother had children, the problem of Rh incompatibility was indeed an ominous one. But thanks to several medical advances, your worry about losing a child to this condition is now largely unnecessary.

First of all, if this is your first pregnancy, there is very little threat to the baby. Trouble doesn't start brewing until the Rh factor enters the Rh-negative mother's circulatory system during the delivery (or abortion or miscarriage) of a child who has inherited the Rh factor from his or her father. The mother's body, in a natural protective immune response to the "foreign" substance, produces antibodies against it. The antibodies themselves are harmless—until she becomes pregnant again with another Rh-positive baby. Then the antibodies cross the placenta and attack the fetal red blood cells, causing very mild (if maternal antibody levels are low) to very serious (if they are high) anemia in the fetus. Only very rarely do these antibodies form in first pregnancies, in reaction to fetal blood leaking back through the placenta into the mother's circulatory system.

Today, prevention of the development of Rh antibodies is the key to protecting the fetus when there is Rh incompatibility. Most doctors use a two-pronged attack. At 28 weeks, an expectant Rh-negative woman who shows no antibodies in her blood is given a dose of Rh-immune globulin. Another dose is administered within 72 hours after delivery, if the baby is Rh positive. (A dose of vaccine is also administered after a miscarriage, an abortion, an amniocentesis, or bleeding during pregnancy.) Giving immune-globulin as required now can head off serious problems in future pregnancies.

If tests determine that a woman has developed Rh antibodies previously, amniocentesis (see page 44) can be used to check the blood type of the fetus. If it is Rh positive, and thus incompatible with the mother's, the maternal antibody levels are monitored regularly. If the levels become dangerously high tests will be done to assess the condition of the fetus. If at any point the safety of the fetus is threatened, indicating the development of erythroblastosis fetalis (also known as hemolytic or Rh disease), a transfusion of Rh negative blood may be necessary. When the incompatibility is severe, which is rare, the fetal transfusion can take place while the fetus is still in the uterus. More often it can wait until immediately after delivery. In mild cases, when antibody levels are low, a transfusion may not be needed. But doctors will be ready to do one at delivery if necessary.

The use of Rh vaccines has reduced the need for transfusions in Rh-incompatible pregnancies to less than

1%, and in the future may make this lifesaving procedure a medical miracle of the past.

OBESITY

"I'm about 60 pounds overweight. Does this put me and my baby at higher risk during pregnancy?"

Most overweight mothers and their babies come through pregnancy and delivery safe and sound. Still, health risks do multiply as the pounds do, in pregnancy as well as out of it. The risk of both hypertension and diabetes, for example, is increased when you are overweight, and both of these conditions can complicate pregnancy (in the form of preeclampsia and gestational diabetes). In addition, there appears to be an increased risk of spina bifida and other neural tube defects. And accurate dating of a pregnancy may be tricky because ovulation is often erratic in obese women and because some of the yardsticks doctors traditionally use to estimate the date (the height of the fundus, the size of the uterus) may be made indecipherable by layers of fat. An overly padded abdomen can also make it impossible for the doctor to determine a fetus's size and position manually, so that technological assistance might be necessary to avoid surprises during delivery. And delivery difficulties can result if the fetus is much larger than average, which is often the case in obese mothers (even those who don't overeat during pregnancy). Finally, if a cesarean delivery is necessary, the ample abdomen can complicate both the surgery and recovery from it.

As with other high-risk pregnancies, top-notch medical care can greatly increase the odds in favor of mother and baby. Right from the start you will probably undergo more tests than the typical low-risk pregnant woman: ultrasound early on to more accurately date your pregnancy, and later to determine the baby's size and position; at least one glucose tolerance test or screening for gestational diabetes, probably late in the second trimester, to determine if you are showing any signs of developing diabetes; and toward the end of your pregnancy, nonstress and other diagnostic tests to monitor your baby's condition.

Self-care will also be important. Your doctor will probably warn you not to smoke and to reduce all the other pregnancy risks that are within your control (see page 50).You will be cautioned against dieting, but also warned not to gain excessive weight. Most of the time, obese women can gain less than the recommended 25 to 35 pounds during pregnancy without adversely affecting the weight or health of their fetus.[4] But their lower-calorie diets must contain at least 1,800 calories and be packed with foods that are dense with vitamins, minerals, and protein (see Best-Odds Diet, page 80). Making every bite count is especially important for you, as is taking a pregnancy vitamin and mineral supplement. Getting regular exercise, within the guidelines recommended by your doctor, will also help keep your weight gain in check without your having to reduce food intake drastically.

For your next pregnancy, if you are planning on one, try to get as close as possible to your ideal weight *prior* to conception. It will make the course of your pregnancy easier.

---

4. Definitions vary, but usually a woman is considered obese if her weight is 120% of her ideal weight, very obese if it measures 150%. Thus a woman who should weigh 100 pounds is obese at 120 and very obese at 150 pounds.

HERPES

"I was anxious for a positive pregnancy test; but now that I am definitely pregnant, I'm terrified because I have genital herpes."

With the notable exception of AIDS (acquired immune deficiency syndrome), herpes has had the dubious distinction of generating more frightening headlines in recent years than any other sexually transmitted disease (STD). And many of the accompanying stories have emphasized that not only can adults contract the disease through sexual intercourse, but babies can contract it by passing through an infected birth canal. Though the disease is merely annoying in adults, it can be serious in newborns, whose immune systems are immature.

Certainly concern is warranted, but hysteria, in spite of alarmist headlines, isn't. First of all, neonatal infection is quite rare—occurring in an estimated 1 in 3,000 to 1 in 20,000 deliveries. Second, though still very serious, the disease seems to be somewhat milder in newborns than it was in the past.

Third, a baby has only a 2% to 3% chance of infection if its mother has a recurrent herpes infection during pregnancy—and recurrent infections are much more common than primary ones. Even among those babies at greatest risk, those whose mothers have their first herpes outbreak as delivery nears, 60% to 75% will escape infection. And though a primary infection earlier in pregnancy increases the risk of miscarriage and premature delivery, such infection is relatively rare.

So if you picked up your herpes infection before pregnancy, which is most likely, the risk to your baby is low. And with good medical care it can be lowered still further. For moms who test negative, taking steps to prevent a first time infection, especially in the third trimester, is important.

When a woman has an active (new or recurrent) herpes infection near delivery, a cesarean delivery will greatly reduce the chances of infection being passed on to the baby. Women previously positive or who are at high risk should be screened for active infection prior to delivery; if they test positive, they should be delivered by C-section.

Signs and Symptoms of Genital Herpes

Since it is during a primary, or first, episode that genital herpes is most likely to be passed on to the fetus, your doctor should be informed if you experience the following symptoms of the disease: fever, headache, malaise, achiness for two or more days, accompanied by genital pain, itching, pain with urination, vaginal and urethral discharge, and tenderness in the groin (inguinal adenopathy), as well as lesions that blister and then crust over. Healing generally takes place within two to three weeks, during which time the disease can be transmitted.

If you have genital herpes, be careful not to pass it to your partner (and he should likewise be careful if he's infected). Avoid intercourse when either of you has lesions; wash hands thoroughly with mild soap and water after using the toilet or having sexual relations; shower or bathe daily; keep lesions clean, dry, and dusted with cornstarch; and wear cotton underpants and avoid wearing clothes that are constricting in the crotch area.

Presently a cesarean for a woman with a history of herpes is performed only when the infection is active as she goes into labor. Some doctors test weekly for active infection when a woman develops lesions close to her due date[5] and continue doing cultures into labor; others simply check for active lesions (or signs that an active infection is about to erupt) as labor begins. Both approaches reduce the rate of c-sections. Because of the slight risk of fetal infection when the protection of the amniotic sac is gone, cesarean delivery is usually carried out within four to six hours after the membranes rupture, unless the fetus is not mature enough for immediate delivery.

Newborns at risk for herpes infection are usually isolated from other newborns at birth to prevent the possible spread of infection. In the unlikely event that infection does occur, treatment with an antiviral drug will reduce the risk of permanent damage. If the mother has an active infection, she can still care for her baby and even breastfeed if she takes special precautions to avoid transmitting the virus.

OTHER STDs (SEXUALLY TRANSMITTED DISEASES)

'I've heard that herpes can harm the fetus. Is this also true of other sexually transmitted diseases?''

The bad news: Yes, there are other STDs that present a hazard to the fetus. The good news: Most are easily diagnosed and treated.

---

5. Since antiviral drugs haven't yet been approved for use in pregnancy, their use is reserved for life-threatening situations.

Gonorrhea. Gonorrhea has long been known to cause conjunctivitis, blindness, and serious generalized infection in the fetus delivered through an infected birth canal. For this reason, pregnant women are routinely tested for the disease, usually at their first prenatal visit (see page 101). Sometimes, particularly in women at high risk for STDs, the test is repeated late in pregnancy. If infection with gonorrhea is found, it is treated immediately with antibiotics. Treatment is followed by another culture, to be sure the woman is infection-free. As an added precaution, drops of silver nitrate or an antibiotic ointment are squeezed into the eyes of every newborn at birth. (This treatment can be delayed for as long as an hour—but no longer—if you want to have some eye-to-eye contact with your baby first.)

Syphilis. The fetal bone and tooth deformities, the progressive nervous system damage, the stillbirths, and the eventual brain damage caused by syphilis have long been recognized too. And testing for this disease is also routine at the first prenatal visit. Antibiotic treatment of infected pregnant women before the fourth month, when the infection usually begins to cross the placental barrier, will almost always prevent damage to the fetus.

Chlamydia. More recently recognized as a potential danger to the fetus, chlamydia is now reported to the Center for Disease Control more often than gonorrhea. It is the most common infection passed from mother to fetus—which is why chlamydia screening in pregnancy is a good idea, particularly if you have had multiple sexual partners in the past (which increases your chance of infection). Since about half the women with chlamydial infection experience no symptoms, it often goes undiagnosed when not tested for.

Prompt treatment of chlamydia prior to or during pregnancy can prevent chlamydial illness (pneumonia, which fortunately is most often mild, and eye infections, which are occasionally severe) from being transmitted by the mother to the baby during delivery. Though the best time for treatment is prior to conception, administering antibiotics to the pregnant infected mother can also effectively prevent infant infection. Antibiotic ointment used at birth protects the newborn from chlamydial eye infection.

Nonspecific vaginitis (NSV).

NSV, also known as bacterial vaginosis or Gardnerella vaginitis, can cause such pregnancy complications as premature rupture of the membranes and intra-amniotic infection, which may lead to premature labor. Some experts believe pregnant women should be screened for NSV, so it may be among the infections you are tested for at your first visit.

Venereal, or genital, warts.

These sexually transmitted warts may appear anywhere in the genital area and are caused by the human papilloma virus. Their appearance can vary from a barely visible lesion to a soft, velvety, flat bump or a cauliflower-like growth. The warts range in color from pale to dark pink. Highly contagious, venereal warts are particularly important to treat not only because they can be transmitted to the baby or even block delivery, but because 5% to 15% of cases go on to produce inflammation of the cervix, which can progress to cervical cancer. Treatment may include a prescribed topical medication safe for use in pregnancy—*do not* use OTC wart remedies. If necessary, large warts may be removed late in pregnancy by freezing, electrical heat, or laser therapy.

Acquired Immune Deficiency Syndrome (AIDS).

Infection in pregnancy by the HIV virus, which causes AIDS, is a threat not just to the expectant mother but to her baby as well. A large proportion (estimates range from 20% to 65%) of babies born to mothers who are HIV positive develop the infection within six months, and it is suspected that pregnancy itself could speed up the progress of the disease in the mother. For these reasons, some infected women choose to terminate their pregnancies. Before taking any action, anyone who tests HIV positive should consider retesting (tests are not always accurate and can sometimes be positive in someone who does not have the virus).[6] If a second test is positive, then formal counseling about AIDS and the treatment options is absolutely imperative. Treating the HIV positive mother with AZT can dramatically reduce the chance of her passing the infection on to her child. Combined with a planned cesarean section, AZT treatment can reduce the risk of transmission to almost zero—apparently without damaging side effects.

If you suspect that you may have been infected with any sexually transmitted disease, be sure you have been tested; if you haven't, ask to be. If a test turns out to be positive, be sure that you—and your partner, if necessary—are treated. Treatment will protect not only your health, but that of your baby.

FEAR OF AIDS

"Both my husband and I had a number of partners before we met. Since I heard that AIDS sometimes doesn't show up for

---

6. Occasionally, a woman who has had several children will test false-positive for HIV. If you have a large family and test positive, discuss this possibility with your physician.

years, I can't get rid of the fear that I might have it and give it to my baby."

The chance that you or your husband contracted the human immunodeficiency virus (HIV) that causes AIDS, before you met is slight if neither one of you is in a high risk group (hemophiliacs, IV drug users, those who've had sex with bisexual or homosexual males or with IV drug users), even if you've had multiple partners. A test for HIV will probably relieve your worry. If, however, the test turns out positive, you can be treated immediately, which could help not just you but your baby as well (see page 37).

"I was surprised when my doctor asked if I wanted to be tested for HIV—I don't think I'm in a high-risk category."

It is becoming increasingly common for all pregnant women to be tested for HIV, whether or not they have a prior history of high-risk behavior. So don't be offended; be glad your practitioner cares enough to recommend the test. (For more on HIV, see page 37.)

HEPATITIS B

"I'm a carrier of hepatitis B, and just found out that I'm pregnant. Will my being a carrier hurt my baby?"

Knowing you're a carrier for hepatitis B is the first step in making sure that your condition won't hurt your baby. Though babies born to some carriers (those with a certain antigen) are at high risk for infection, treating them within 12 hours of birth with hepatitis B vaccine and immune globulin can almost always prevent such infection. So be sure that your practitioner knows that you're a carrier, that a titer is taken to determine how contagious you are, and that your baby is treated as needed. For more information on hepatitis infections, see page 318.

AN IUD STILL IN PLACE

"I've been wearing an IUD for two years and just discovered that I'm pregnant. We want to be able to keep the baby; is it possible?"

Getting pregnant while using birth control is always a little unsettling, but it does happen. The odds of it happening with an IUD are 1 to 5 in 100, depending on the type of device used and whether or not it has been properly inserted. A woman who conceives with an IUD in place and doesn't want to terminate her pregnancy has two choices—which she should discuss as soon as possible with her doctor: leaving the IUD in place or having the IUD withdrawn. Which is preferable usually depends on whether or not the removal cord is found, on examination, to be visibly protruding from the cervix. If it isn't visible, the pregnancy has a very good chance of proceeding uneventfully with the IUD in place. The IUD will simply be pushed up against the wall of the uterus by the expanding amniotic sac surrounding the baby, and during childbirth, will usually deliver with the placenta. If, however, the IUD string is visible early in pregnancy, the chances of a safe and successful pregnancy are greater if the IUD is removed as soon as feasible, once conception is confirmed. If it isn't, there is a significant chance that the fetus will spontaneously miscarry; when it's removed, the risk is only 20%. If that doesn't sound reassuring, keep in mind that the rate of miscarriage in all known pregnancies is estimated to be about 15% to 20%.

If you do continue your pregnancy with the IUD left in, you should, during the first trimester, be especially alert for bleeding, cramps, or fever, because the IUD puts you at higher risk for early pregnancy complications (see Ectopic Pregnancy, page 109, and Miscarriage, page 111.) Notify your doctor of such symptoms promptly.

BIRTH CONTROL PILLS IN PREGNANCY

"I got pregnant while using birth control pills. I kept taking them for over a month because I had no idea I was pregnant. Now I'm worried about the effect this may have on my baby."

Ideally, you should stop using oral contraceptives three months, or for at least two normally occurring menstrual cycles, before you want to become pregnant. But conception doesn't always wait for ideal conditions, and occasionally a woman becomes pregnant while taking the Pill. In spite of warnings you might have read on drug inserts, there's no reason for alarm. Statistically, there is no good evidence of an increased risk of fetal malformation when the mother has conceived while on oral contraceptives. A discussion of the subject with your practitioner should further relieve your concern.

SPERMICIDES

"I conceived while using a spermicide with my diaphragm, and used it several times again before I knew I was pregnant. Could the chemicals have damaged the sperm before conception, or the embryo after it?"

It is estimated that between 300,000 and 600,000 women who become pregnant each year used spermicides around the time of conception and in the early weeks of pregnancy before finding out that they'd conceived. So the question of what effects spermicides may have during conception and pregnancy is of great significance to a great many expectant couples—and to those choosing a method of birth control.

Fortunately, the answers so far have been reassuring. No more than a tentative link has ever been suggested between the use of spermicides and the incidence of certain birth defects, specifically Down syndrome and limb deformities. And the most recent and most convincing studies have found no increase in the incidence of such defects even with the repeated use of spermicides in early pregnancy. So according to the best information available, you and the other 299,999 to 599,999 mothers-to-be can relax—there appears to be nothing to worry about.

You may, however, be more comfortable with a different, and perhaps more reliable, method of birth control in the future. And because any chemical exposure of embryo or fetus is suspect, if you do continue to use a spermicide, you should plan on discontinuing its use before you decide to become pregnant again—assuming your next pregnancy is planned.

PROVERA

"Last month my doctor gave me Provera to bring on a late period. It turns out that I was pregnant. The package insert warns that pregnant women should never take this drug. Could my baby be malformed? Should I consider an abortion?"

Having taken the progesterone drug Provera during pregnancy, though it isn't recommended, is no reason to consider an abortion—as your obstetrician will probably tell you. It's not even a reason to worry. The drug company's warnings are not only for your protection but for theirs: in case of a lawsuit. It's true that some studies show a 1 in 1,000 risk of certain birth defects when an embryo or fetus has been exposed to Provera, but that risk is only minimally higher than for the risk of the same defects occurring in any pregnancy.

Whether Provera actually does cause birth defects or not isn't even certain. Some physicians who prescribe Provera to prevent miscarriage believe that it only *appears* to cause defects—by occasionally enabling a woman to sustain a blighted pregnancy that would have otherwise miscarried. It will probably take years more study on hundreds of thousands of pregnant women to definitely determine the effects—if any—of progesterone drugs on the fetus. But from what is presently known, it is believed that if Provera is actually a teratogen (a substance that can harm an embryo or fetus), it is a very weak one (see Playing Baby Roulette, page 76). Cross this one off your worry list.

DES

"My mother took DES when she was pregnant with me. Can this affect my pregnancy or my baby in any way?"

Before the dangers of using the synthetic estrogen drug diethylstilbestrol (DES) to prevent miscarriage were known, more than a million pregnant women took it. Now that their daughters, many of whom were born with structural abnormalities of the reproductive tract (the majority so minor that they are of no gynecological or obstetrical signifi-

cance), are of childbearing age, they are concerned about the effects DES exposure will have on their own pregnancies. Happily, these effects appear to be minimal for most women—it is estimated that at least 80% of DES-exposed women have been able to have children.

The women with the most severe abnormalities, however, do appear to have an increased risk of certain pregnancy problems: ectopic pregnancy (probably because of malformed fallopian tubes), and midtrimester miscarriage and preterm birth (usually because of a weakened, or incompetent, cervix, which under the weight of a growing fetus can open prematurely). Because of the risks involved with all of these complications, it's important that you advise your physician of your DES exposure.[7] It is also important for you to be aware of the symptoms of these pregnancy mishaps and, should they occur, to report them to your doctor at once. If an incompetent cervix is suspected, one of two courses will probably be taken. Either a preventive stitch will be placed around the cervix between the 12th and 16th weeks of your pregnancy or your cervix will be examined regularly for signs of premature opening; if such signs are noted, steps will be taken to prevent further progression toward premature delivery.

GENETIC PROBLEMS

"I keep worrying that I might have a genetic problem and not know it. Should I get genetic counseling?"

---

7. Because of the slightly increased risk of pregnancy complications, DES-exposed women are probably better off with an obstetrician overseeing their pregnancy care.

Probably all of us carry one or more deleterious gene for mild or serious genetic disorders. But fortunately, because most disorders (Tay-Sachs or cystic fibrosis, for example) require a matching one-from-mom, one-from-dad pair of genes, they rarely manifest themselves in our children. One or both parents can be tested for some of these disorders before or during pregnancy. But testing makes sense only if there is a better-than-average possibility that both parents are carriers of a particular disorder. The clue is often ethnic or geographic. For example, Jewish couples whose forebears came originally from Eastern Europe should be tested for Tay-Sachs. (In most cases, a practitioner will recommend a test for one parent; testing the second parent becomes necessary only if the first test is positive.) Similarly, black couples should be tested for the sickle-cell anemia trait.

Diseases that can be passed on via a single gene from one carrier parent (hemophilia, for example) or by one affected parent (Huntington's chorea) have usually turned up in the family before, but this may not be common knowledge. That's why it's important to keep records of family health histories.

Most expectant parents, happily, are at low risk for transmitting genetic problems and need never see a genetic counselor. In many cases an obstetrician will talk to a couple about the most common genetic issues, referring to a genetic counselor or a maternal-fetal subspecialist those with a need for more expertise:

❖ Couples whose blood tests show them both to be carriers of a genetic disorder.

❖ Parents who have already borne one or more children with genetic birth defects.

❖ Couples who know of a hereditary disorder on any branch of either of their family trees. In some cases, as with certain thalassemias (hereditary anemias common among Mediterranean peoples), doing DNA testing of the parents before pregnancy makes interpreting later testing of the fetus much easier.

❖ Couples in which one partner has a congenital defect (such as congenital heart disease).

❖ Pregnant women who have had positive screening tests for the presence of a fetal defect.

❖ Closely related couples, because the risk of inherited disease in offspring is greatest when parents are related (for example, 1 in 8 for first cousins).

❖ Women over 35.

A genetic counselor is a sort of heredity bookmaker, trained to give such couples the odds of their having a healthy child and to guide them in deciding whether or not to have children. If they are already pregnant, the counselor can suggest appropriate prenatal testing.

Genetic counseling has saved hundreds of thousands of high-risk couples from the heartbreak of bearing children with serious problems. The best time to see a genetic counselor is before getting pregnant, or in the case of close relatives, before getting married. But it's not too late even after pregnancy is confirmed.

If testing uncovers a serious defect in a fetus, the expectant parents are faced with the decision of whether or not to continue with the pregnancy. Though the decision is theirs, a genetic counselor can provide important input.

YOUR OPPOSITION TO ABORTION

"My husband and I don't believe in abortion. Why should I have to go through amniocentesis?"

Amniocentesis isn't only appropriate for those couples who would consider abortion should a serious fetal defect be detected via the procedure. For the vast majority of expectant parents the best reason for prenatal diagnosis is the reassurance it almost always brings.

And although many couples opt for terminating the pregnancy when the news is bad, testing can also be valuable when abortion is not an option. When the defect discovered is a fatal one, it gives the parents time to grieve before the birth and eliminates the sense of shock later. When other kinds of defects are present, it provides parents a head start on preparing for life with a special-needs child.

They can also begin working through the inevitable reactions (denial, resentment, guilt) that come with discovering their baby has a defect rather than waiting until after delivery, when such feelings can compromise parent-child bonding. They can learn about the particular problem in advance and prepare to ensure the best possible life for their child. They may even discover that the defect is treatable in the uterus or that special precautions at or after birth will increase the odds that the baby will be okay. For parents who feel unable to cope, knowing in advance will allow them to consider a special-needs adoption.

So, if prenatal diagnosis is indicated, don't reject it out-of-hand. Talk to your practitioner, a genetic counselor, or a maternal-fetal subspecialist to help you clarify your options before you make your decision. And don't let your opposition to abortion deprive you and your doctors of potentially valuable information.

WHAT IT'S IMPORTANT TO KNOW: ABOUT PRENATAL DIAGNOSIS

Is it a boy—or a girl? Will it have blond hair like Grandma, green eyes like Grandpa? Daddy's voice and Mommy's flair for figures or—heaven forbid!—the other way around? The questions of pregnancy far outnumber the answers, providing lively material for nine months of dinner table debate, neighborhood speculation, and office pools.

But there's one question that isn't a topic for casual wagering. It's one most parents hesitate to talk about at all: "Is my baby okay?"

Until recently, that question could be answered only at birth. Today it can to some extent be answered as

early as six weeks after conception, through prenatal diagnosis.

Because of inherent risks, small as they are, prenatal diagnosis isn't for everyone. Most parents will continue to play the waiting game, with the happy assurance that the odds are overwhelming that their babies are indeed "okay." But for those whose concerns represent more than normal expectant-parent jitters, the benefits of prenatal diagnosis can far outweigh the risks. Women who are good candidates for prenatal diagnosis include those who:

❖ Are over 35.

❖ Have a family history of genetic disease and/or have been shown to be carriers of such a disease.

❖ Have been exposed to infection (such as rubella or toxoplasmosis) that could cause a birth defect.

❖ Have been exposed since conception to a substance or substances that they fear might have been harmful to their developing baby. (Consultation with a physician can help determine whether prenatal diagnosis is warranted in a particular case.)

❖ Have had unsuccessful pregnancies previously, or have had babies with birth defects.

In more than 95% of cases, prenatal diagnosis turns up no apparent abnormalities. In the remainder, the expectant couple's discovery that something is wrong with their baby isn't comforting. But, teamed with expert genetic counseling, the information can be used to make vital decisions about this and future pregnancies. Possible options include:

Continuing the Pregnancy. This option is often chosen when the defect uncovered is one the family feels that both they and the baby they are awaiting can live with, or when the parents are opposed to abortion under any condition. Having some idea of what is to come allows parents to make preparations (both emotional and practical) for receiving a child with special needs into the family, for coping with the inevitable loss of a child, or for considering a special-needs adoption.

Terminating the Pregnancy. If testing suggests a defect that will be fatal or extremely disabling, and retesting and/or interpretation by a genetic counselor confirms the diagnosis, many parents opt for terminating the pregnancy. In such a case, careful examination of the products of the pregnancy for abnormalities is a must, and may be helpful in determining the chances of a repeat in future pregnancies. Most couples, armed with this information and the guidance of a physician or genetic counselor, do try again, with the hope that the tests and the pregnancy will turn out better next time around. And most often they do.

Prenatal Treatment of the Fetus. This option is available in only a few instances, though in the future it can be expected to become more and more common. Treatment may consist of blood transfusion (as in Rh disease), surgery (to drain an obstructed bladder, for instance), or administration of enzymes or medication (such as steroids to accelerate lung development in the fetus who must be delivered before term). As technology advances, more kinds of prenatal surgery, genetic manipulation, and other fetal treatments may also become commonplace.

Donating the Organs. If diagnosis indicates that the fetal defects are not compatible with life, as when all or most of the brain is missing, it may be possible to donate one or more of the other organs to an infant in need. Some parents find that this provides at least some small consolation for their own loss. A neonatologist at a local medical center may be able to provide helpful information in such a situation.

Of course it's important to remember that nothing is perfect, not even high-tech prenatal diagnosis. For that reason, all results that indicate there is something wrong with the fetus should be confirmed by further testing or consultation with additional professionals. Acting too quickly to terminate a pregnancy has on occasion resulted in the aborting of a normal fetus.

The most commonly used methods of prenatal diagnosis follow.

AMNIOCENTESIS

The fetal cells, chemicals, and microorganisms in the amniotic fluid surrounding the fetus provide a wide range of information—genetic makeup, present condition, level of maturity—about the new human being. Thus being able to extract and examine some of the fluid through amniocentesis has been one of the most important advances in prenatal diagnosis. It is recommended when:

❖ The mother is over age 35. Between 80% and 90% of all amniocentesis is performed solely on the basis of advanced maternal age, primarily to determine if the fetus has Down syndrome, which is most prevalent among children of older mothers.

❖ The couple has already had a child with a chromosomal abnormality, such as Down syndrome, or with a metabolic disorder, such as Hunter's syndrome.

❖ The couple has already had a child or has a close relative with a neural tube defect. (A test to determine maternal-serum alpha-fetoprotein, or MSAFP, levels in the mother's blood will probably be performed first.)

❖ The mother is a carrier of an x-linked genetic disorder, such as hemophilia (which she has a 50-50 chance of passing on to any son she bears). Amniocentesis can identify the sex of the fetus, although not whether the baby has inherited the gene.

❖ Both parents are carriers of an au-tosomal recessive inherited disorder, such as Tay-Sachs disease or sickle-cell anemia, and thus have a 1 in 4 chance of bearing an affected child.

❖ It is necessary to assess the maturity of the fetal lungs (among the last organs ready to function on their own).

❖ A parent is known to have a condition such as Huntington's chorea, which is passed on by autosomal dominant inheritance, giving the baby a 1 in 2 chance of inheriting the disease.

❖ Results of screening test (usually MSAFP, sonogram, estriol, and/or hCG) turn out to be abnormal, and evaluation of the amniotic fluid is necessary to determine whether or not there actually is a fetal abnormality.

When Is It Done? Diagnostic second-trimester amniocentesis is usually performed between the 16th and 18th weeks of pregnancy, though occasionally as early as the 14th or as late as the 20th week. Studies on earlier amniocentesis (between the 11th and 14th weeks) have shown a significant increase in complications. Most tests, because cells must be cultured in the laboratory, take from 24 to 35 days to be completed, though a few, such as those for Tay-Sachs disease, Hunter's syndrome, and neural tube defects, can be performed immediately.

Amniocentesis can also be performed in the last trimester to assess the maturity of fetal lungs.

How Is It Done? After changing into an examination gown and emptying her bladder, the expectant mother is positioned on the examining table on her back, her body draped so that only her abdomen is exposed. The fetus and placenta are then located via ultrasound, so that the doctor will be able to steer clear of them during the procedure. (A more detailed ultrasound will have previously been done to identify any easily visible fetal abnormalities.) The abdomen is swabbed with antiseptic solution, and in some cases, numbed with an injection of a local anesthetic, similar to the novocaine used by dentists. (Because this injection is as painful as the passage of the amniocentesis needle itself, some practitioners omit it.) Then a long, hollow needle is inserted through the abdominal wall into the uterus and a small amount of fluid is withdrawn. The slight risk of accidentally pricking the fetus during this part of the procedure is further reduced by the use of simultaneous ultrasound guidance. The mother's vital signs and the fetal heart tones are checked before and after the procedure, which, from start to finish, shouldn't take more than 30 minutes. Rh-negative women are usually given an injection of Rh-immune globulin after an amniocentesis to be sure the procedure does not result in Rh problems.

Unless it is a necessary part of the diagnosis, parents have the option not to be told their baby's sex when the report comes back, but to find out the old-fashioned way, in the delivery room. (Keep in mind that mix-ups, though rare, do happen.)

How Safe Is It? Most women experience no more than a few hours of mild cramping after the procedure; rarely there is slight vaginal bleeding or amniotic fluid leak. Although fewer than 1 in 200 women experience an infection or other complication that may lead to miscarriage, amniocentesis, like most other prenatal diagnostic tests, should be performed only when the benefits outweigh the risks.

ULTRASOUND

The advent of ultrasonography has made obstetrics a much more precise science and pregnancy a much less worrisome experience for many expectant parents. Through the use of sound waves that bounce off internal structures, it allows visualization of the fetus without the hazards of x-ray. If the apparatus used has a TV-like viewing screen, it provides a unique opportunity to "see" your baby—and maybe even get a sonogram photo to show to friends and family—though it may take an expert to make out a head or buttocks in the blurry image.

A level 1 ultrasound is usually done to date a pregnancy. A more detailed, or level 2, ultrasound is used for more sophisticated diagnostic purposes. Ultrasound may be recommended when the mother has a poor obstetrical history; for example, when she's had an ectopic (tubal) pregnancy, a hydatidiform mole (the placenta develops into a bunch of grapelike cysts that can't support a developing embryo); a ce-

Amnio Complication

Although complications with amniocentesis are rare, it is estimated that following about 1 in 100 procedures there is some leakage of amniotic fluid. If you should notice such leakage from your vagina, report it to your practitioner at once. The odds are very good that the leakage will stop after a few days, but bed rest and careful observation are usually recommended until it does.

sarean section; or a baby with a birth defect or genetic disease. It may also be used to:

❖ Verify a due date by checking to see if it correlates with the baby's size.[8]

❖ Determine the condition of the fetus when there is a greater than average risk of an abnormality, or when there is greater than average concern. This can be done earlier and often more accurately with transvaginal ultrasound.

❖ Rule out pregnancy by the seventh week if there's been a suspected false-positive pregnancy test.

❖ Determine the cause of bleeding or spotting in early pregnancy, such as a tubal pregnancy or a blighted ovum (an embryo that has stopped developing and is no longer viable).

❖ Locate an IUD that was in place at the time of conception.

❖ Locate the fetus prior to amniocentesis and during chorionic villus sampling biopsy.

❖ Determine the condition of the fetus if no heartbeat has been detected by the 14th week with a Doppler device, or if there has been no fetal movement by the 22nd week.

❖ Diagnose the existence of multiple fetuses, usually when the mother has taken fertility drugs and/or the uterus is larger than expected for the date.

❖ Determine if abnormally rapid uterine growth is being caused by an excess of amniotic fluid.

---

8. Some physicians believe this should be done routinely because verifying the date early on reduces the possibility of unnecessarily inducing labor when a baby is (incorrectly) believed to be late; this in turn reduces the need for cesareans for failed induction.

❖ Determine the condition of the placenta, when deterioration might be responsible for fetal growth retardation or distress. Detect cervical changes that predict preterm labor.

❖ Visualize the placenta to determine if bleeding late in pregnancy is due to the placenta being located low in the uterus (placenta previa) or to its separating prematurely (abruptio placenta). Blood clots behind the placenta can also be visualized.

❖ Determine the size of the fetus when preterm delivery is being contemplated or when the baby is believed to be late.

❖ Evaluate the condition of the fetus through observation of fetal activity, breathing movements, amniotic fluid volume (see Biophysical Profile, page 263).

❖ Verify breech presentation or other uncommon fetal or cord position prior to delivery.

When Is It Done? Depending on the reason for it, ultrasound can be used any time from the fifth week of gestation through delivery. Transvaginal ultrasound may be used earlier than the transabdominal (through the abdomen) procedure to determine whether there is a multiple gestation or abnormal fetal development.

How Is It Done? Ultrasound examination may be through the abdomen or through the vagina; sometimes, when there's a special need, the doctor may have a look both ways. The procedures are quick (five to ten minutes) and painless, except for the discomfort of the full bladder necessary for the transabdominal exam (which is probably why most women appear to prefer the transvaginal). During either exam, the expectant mother lies on her back. For the transabdominal, her bare abdomen is spread with a film of oil or gel that will improve the conduction of sound. A transducer is then moved slowly over the abdomen. For the transvaginal, a probe is inserted into the vagina. The instruments record echoes of sound waves as they bounce off parts of the baby. With the help of a technician or doctor, you may be able to differentiate the beating heart; the curve of the spine; the head, arms, and legs. You may even catch sight of your baby sucking its thumb. Sometimes even the genital organs are distinguishable and the sex can be surmised, although with less than 100% reliability. (If you don't want to know your baby's sex yet, inform the doctor in advance.)

How Safe Is It? In 25 years of clinical use and study, no known risks and a great many benefits have been associated with the use of ultrasound photography. Still, because of the slim possibility that side effects may show up in the future, it's generally recommended by U.S. experts that ultrasound be used in pregnancy only when valid indications exist. Although British studies have tended to support the use of routine ultrasound, U.S. studies have found that the outcome is not improved when ultrasound is used routinely in normal pregnancies.

FETOSCOPY

Fetoscopy is science fiction turning fast into medical fact. In a voyage as fantastic as any penned by Isaac Asimov, a miniaturized telescope-like instrument, complete with lights and lenses, is inserted through tiny incisions in the abdomen and uterus into the amniotic sac, where it can view and photograph the fetus. At the same time, fetoscopy makes it possible to diagnose, through blood and tissue sampling, several blood and skin diseases that amniocentesis can't detect. Because it's a relatively high-risk procedure, however, and because other safer techniques are becoming available to detect the same disorders, fetoscopy is not widely used.

When Is It Done? Usually after the 16th week.

How Is It Done? After the abdomen is swabbed with antiseptic and numbed with a local anesthetic, tiny incisions are made in the abdomen and uterus. With ultrasound monitoring to guide the instrument, a fiber-optic endoscope is passed through the incisions and into the uterus. With this miniature telescope, the fetus, placenta, and amniotic fluid can be observed, blood samples can be taken from the junction of the umbilical cord and the placenta, and/or a tiny bit of fetal or placental tissue can be removed for examination.

How Safe Is It? Fetoscopy is, at this point, still a relatively risky procedure, carrying between a 3% and 5% chance of fetal loss. Though this risk is greater than that of other diagnostic tests, it is outweighed for the occasional woman who needs it by the benefit of discovering, and possibly treating or correcting, a defect in her fetus.

MATERNAL-SERUM ALPHA-FETOPROTEIN SCREENING

Elevated levels in the mother's blood, or serum, of alpha-fetoprotein (MSAFP), a substance produced by the fetus, can indicate a neural tube defect such as spina bifida (a deformity of the spinal column) or anencephaly (the absence of all or part of the brain). Abnormally low levels suggest an increased risk of Down syndrome or other chromosomal defect. This is only a screening test, and any abnormal result requires further testing to confirm the existence of a problem.

When Is It Done? Between the 16th and 18th weeks.

How Is It Done? This simple test requires only a maternal blood sample. If MSAFP levels are found to be abnormally high, a second test is run. If the second test duplicates the initial results, then a variety of other procedures—including genetic counseling; ultrasound to date the pregnancy, check for multiple fetuses, or look for abnormalities in the fetus; and/or amniocentesis to determine MSAFP and acetylcholinesterase levels in the amniotic fluid—are performed to confirm or rule out the presence of a neural tube defect. Only 1 or 2 out of 50 women with high initial readings will eventually be shown to have an affected fetus. In the other 48, further testing will reveal that the reason MSAFP levels are elevated is that there is more than one fetus, or that the pregnancy is further along than at first believed, or that the original readings were inaccurate. Still, though elevated MSAFP levels are not usually a cause for alarm, practitioners may recommend extra rest and vigilance for women with high readings because they may be at a slightly increased risk of having low-birthweight or preterm babies.

If MSAFP levels are abnormally low, ultrasound, genetic counseling, and/or amniocentesis will be offered to determine whether or not the fetus actually does suffer from Down syndrome or another chromosomal defect.

How Safe Is It? The initial screening test itself poses no more risk to mother or baby than does any other standard blood test. The major risk of the test is that a false-positive result may lead to follow-up procedures that present greater risk—and in rare cases, to therapeutic or accidental abortion of perfectly normal fetuses. Before you consider taking any action on the basis of prenatal testing, be sure the results have been evaluated by an experienced physician or genetic counselor. Get a second opinion if you have any doubts. A maternal-fetal medicine subspecialist may be particularly helpful.

CHORIONIC VILLUS SAMPLING (CVS)

Chorionic villus sampling can give results (and most often, reassurance) earlier in pregnancy than amniocentesis. The earlier diagnosis is particularly helpful for those who might consider a therapeutic pregnancy termination if something is seriously wrong since an earlier abortion is less complicated and traumatic. CVS may also be valuable when amniocentesis is not possible, as when there is very little amniotic fluid (oligohydramnios).

It is believed that chorionic villus sampling will eventually be able to detect virtually all of the 3,800 or so disorders for which defective genes or chromosomes are responsible. And in the future it may make possible the treatment or correction in utero of many of these conditions. At present, CVS is useful only to detect disorders for which the technology exists, such as Tay-Sachs, sickle-cell anemia, most types of cystic fibrosis, the thalassemias, and Down syndrome. Testing for specific diseases (other than Down syndrome) is usually done only when there is a family history of the disease or the parents are known to be carriers. The indications for doing the test are the same as those for amniocentesis, though CVS is not used to assess fetal lung maturity. Occasionally, both CVS and amniocentesis may be needed.

When Is It Done? For genetic determinations, generally between the 10th and 13th weeks of pregnancy. The procedure may be used later in pregnancy (when villi are no longer present) to obtain cells for a placental biopsy.

How Is It Done? CVS may someday be an office procedure, but at the moment it is performed in medical centers only. Though originally the sampling of cells was always taken via the vagina and cervix (transcervical CVS), it is now often taken via a needle inserted in the abdominal wall (transabdominal CVS). Neither procedure is entirely pain-free; the discomfort can range from very mild to severe.

In the transcervical procedure, the expectant mother lies on an examining table and a long thin tube is inserted through the vagina into the uterus. Guided by ultrasound imaging, the doctor positions the tube between the uterine lining and the chorion, the fetal membrane that will eventually form the fetal side of the placenta. A sampling of the chorionic villi (finger-like projections of the chorion) is then snipped or suctioned off for diagnostic study.

In the transabdominal procedure, the patient also lies on an examining table, tummy up. Ultrasound is used to determine the location of the pla-

9. Women who have a placenta that is located deep in the back of the uterus or who have fibroids in the uterine walls are not good candidates for this type of ultrasound.

centa and to view the uterine walls.[9] It also helps the physician to find a safe spot in which to insert the needle. This area is washed and disinfected, then injected with a local anesthetic to numb it. Still under ultrasound guidance, a guide needle is inserted through the abdomen and the uterine wall to the edge of the placenta. then a narrower needle, which will draw up the cells, is inserted through the guide needle. The narrow needle is rotated and pushed in and out 15 or 20 times per sampling, then withdrawn with the sample of cells to be studied.

Since the chorionic villi are of fetal origin, examining them can give a complete picture of the genetic makeup of the developing fetus. Though results are possible from the rapidly dividing cells of the outer layer of cells (the cytotrophoblast) in as little as three days, more reliable results can be obtained by culturing cells from the inner layer of fibroblasts for seven to ten days. For this reason, CVS procedures now routinely use the inner layer of cells.

How Safe Is It? Though most studies so far conclude CVS is safe and reliable, there have been reports from at least one testing center linking it to limb deformities in the fetus. The procedure also increases the risk of miscarriage slightly (more so than amniocentesis). And there is a slim risk that a pregnancy could be terminated on the basis of incorrect information, since an abnormality called mosaicism may be detected in the villi when it doesn't exist in the fetus. This problem can be eliminated by rechecking such a diagnosis with amniocentesis. These risks have to be weighed against the benefit of earlier diagnosis with CVS. Risks can be reduced by choosing a testing center with a good safety record and waiting until after the 10th week.

Some vaginal bleeding can occur af-

Reducing the Risk in Any Pregnancy

Good Medical Care. Even a low-risk pregnancy is put at high risk if prenatal care is absent or poor. Seeing a qualified practitioner regularly, beginning as soon as pregnancy is suspected, is vital for all expectant mothers. (Choose an obstetrician experienced in your particular condition if you are in a high-risk category.) But just as important as having a good doctor is being a good patient. Be an active participant in your medical care—ask questions, report symptoms—but don't try to be your own doctor. (See page 15.)

Good Diet. The Best-Odds Diet (see page 80) gives every pregnant woman the best odds of having a successful and comfortable pregnancy and a healthy baby.

Fitness. It's best to begin pregnancy with a well-toned, fit body, but it's never too late to start deriving the benefits of exercise. Regular exercise can prevent constipation and improve respiration, circulation, muscle tone, and skin elasticity, contributing to a more comfortable pregnancy and an easier, safer delivery. (See page 189).

Sensible Weight Gain. A gradual, steady, and moderate weight gain may help prevent a variety of complications, including diabetes, hypertension, varicose veins, hemorrhoids, low birth weight, and difficult delivery due to an overly large fetus. (See page 147.)

No Smoking. Or quitting as early in pregnancy as possible to reduce its many risks to mother and baby, including prematurity and low birth weight. (See page 54.)

Abstinence from Alcohol. Drinking very rarely or not at all will reduce the risk of birth defects, particularly fetal alcohol syndrome (the result of heavy drinking) and fetal alcohol effect (the result of moderate drinking). See page 52.)

Avoidance of Drugs. All illicit drugs are dangerous to the fetus and should be avoided during pregnancy. Medication should be used only when its benefits outweigh its risks, and only when it has been approved or prescribed by a physician who is aware that you are pregnant. (See page 58.)

Avoidance of Environmental and Occupational Toxins. Though everything we touch, breathe, eat, and drink isn't as hazardous as newspaper headlines would have us believe, avoiding known hazards (such as excessive x-rays, lead, and so on; see individual topics) is prudent.

Prevention of and Prompt Treatment for Infection. All infections—from the common cold to urinary tract and vaginal infections to the increasingly common sexually transmitted diseases—should be avoided whenever possible. When contracted, however, infection should be treated promptly by a physician who knows you are pregnant.

Being Wary of the Superwoman Syndrome. Often well established in their careers and highly motivated in everything they do, today's mothers tend to be overachievers and overdoers. Getting enough rest during pregnancy is far more important than getting everything done, especially in high-risk pregnancies. Don't wait until your body starts pleading for relief before you slow down. If your doctor recommends that you begin your maternity leave earlier than you'd planned, take the advice. Some studies have suggested a higher incidence of premature delivery among women who work up until term, if their job entails physical labor or long periods of standing.

ter CVS and should not be a cause for concern, though it should be reported to your doctor. Your doctor should also be informed if the bleeding lasts for three days or longer. Since there is also a very slight risk of infection, be sure to report any fever in the first few days following the procedure.[10]

Since many women feel physically and emotionally drained following CVS (it's not unusual to fall into bed and sleep around the clock), it's generally recommended that those undergoing the procedure arrange to have someone drive them home afterward and that they make no other plans for the rest of the day.

OTHER TYPES OF PRENATAL DIAGNOSIS

The field of prenatal diagnosis is expanding so rapidly that new methods are constantly being evaluated. In addition to the standard methods listed above, there are others that are being used experimentally or only occasionally. These include:

❖ **Maternal blood screening for hCG** (human chorionic gonadotropin), which may eventually turn out to surpass age as the most important criterion for determining who should have amniocentesis to detect Down syndrome. Researchers have found that a high level of hCG in a pregnant woman's blood means she is at greater than normal risk for having a baby with Down syndrome. She then becomes a good candidate for amniocentesis.

❖ **Maternal serum markers.** Combining MSAFP and hCG tests with a test for low levels of unconjugated estriol in the blood may be used to routinely screen mothers of any age for the possibility of a fetus with Down syndrome. Amniocentesis is done if screening tests are abnormal. This testing can eliminate the need for routine amniocentesis in women over 35 while allowing for a prenatal diagnosis that might otherwise be missed in younger women (who don't have routine amnios).

❖ **Percutaneous umbilical cord sampling (PUBS),** in which blood is drawn from the umbilical cord for study. It is somewhat safer than fetoscopy when done under ultrasound guidance, and can detect the same conditions. Blood may also be drawn from the fetal hepatic vein for study.

❖ **Fetal skin sampling,** in which a tiny sample of fetal skin is taken and studied. This method is particularly useful in detecting certain skin disorders.

❖ **Magnetic resonance imaging,** a method that is still investigational but offers some promise of being able to give a clearer picture than ultrasound of what the newborn will be like, inside and out.

❖ **Radiography (x-ray),** once the predominant way of visualizing an infant prenatally, has been almost entirely replaced by ultrasound.

❖ **Echocardiography,** with which defects in the fetal heart can be detected.

❖ **Maternal blood testing to determine the gender** of a fetus, though still experimental, could be valuable in screening for certain hereditary diseases that affect male offspring only.

10. Since there is the potential for leakage of fetal red blood cells into the mother's circulatory system, some doctors believe all Rh-negative women should be given an immune globulin called anti-D-globulin prior to CVS.

3
Throughout Your Pregnancy

WHAT YOU MAY BE CONCERNED ABOUT

Pregnant women have always worried. What they worry about, however, has changed considerably over the generations, as obstetrical medicine—and expectant parents—have learned more and more about what does and does not affect the health and well-being of the unborn. Our grandmothers, vulnerable to a variety of old wives' tales, feared that seeing a monkey while pregnant would result in monkey-like offspring, or that slapping their bellies in fright would leave their babies with hand-shaped birthmarks. We, vulnerable instead to a daily deluge of modern media tales (usually as frightening, sometimes as unfounded), have other fears: Is the air I'm breathing polluted? Is my drinking water safe? Is my job, or my husband's smoking, or that cup of coffee I had this morning hazardous to my baby's health? What about that x-ray I had at the dentist's? As a basis for worry, these concerns can make pregnancy unnecessarily nervewracking. As a basis for action,

they can give you an enhanced sense of control and greatly improve the odds of your having a healthy baby.

ALCOHOL

"I had a few drinks on several occasions before I knew I was pregnant. I'm afraid that the alcohol may have harmed my baby."

"Behold, thou shalt conceive, and bear a son; now beware, drink no wine or strong drink," an angel tells Samson's mother in the Book of Judges. Lucky lady. She was able to start ordering Evian when her son was just a gleam in his father's eye. Not many of us receive such advance notice of our pregnancies. And because we're often unaware that we're pregnant until we are into our second month, we're apt to have done things we wouldn't have done if only we had known. Like having a few, a few times too often. Which is why your concern is one of the most common brought to the first prenatal visit.

Fortunately, it's also one of the concerns that can most easily be put aside. There's no evidence that a few drinks on a couple of occasions early in pregnancy will prove harmful to a developing embryo. In fact, one recent study showed that women who'd had two or three such drinking episodes early in pregnancy weren't any more likely to have babies with structural defects or growth retardation than were teetotalers.

Continuing to drink heavily throughout pregnancy, however, is associated with a wide variety of problems in the offspring. That's not surprising when you consider that alcohol enters the fetal bloodstream in approximately the same concentrations present in the mother's blood; each drink a pregnant woman takes is shared with her baby. Since it takes the fetus twice as long as its mother to eliminate the alcohol from its system, the baby can be at the point of passing out when the mother is just pleasantly high.

Heavy drinking (generally considered to be the consumption of five or six drinks of wine, beer, or distilled spirits a day) throughout pregnancy can result, in addition to many serious obstetrical complications, in what is known as fetal alcohol syndrome (FAS). Described as the hangover that lasts a lifetime, this condition produces infants who are born undersized, usually mentally deficient, with multiple deformities (particularly of the head and face, limbs, heart, and central nervous system), and a high neonatal mortality rate. Later, children with FAS display learning, behavioral, and social problems, and generally lack judgment.

The risks of continued drinking are certainly dose-related: the more you drink, the more potential danger to your baby. But even moderate consumption (one to two drinks daily or occasional heavy binging on five or more drinks) throughout pregnancy is related to a variety of serious problems, including the increased risk of miscarriage, prematurity, low birthweight, and complications during labor and delivery. It has also been linked to the somewhat more subtle fetal alcohol effect (FAE), which is characterized by numerous developmental and behavioral problems. Even one or two drinks daily apparently increases the risk of miscarriage, stillbirth, abnormal growth, and developmental problems. Drinking in the last six months of pregnancy may increase the risk of leukemia in the infant.

Although some women drink lightly during pregnancy—one glass of wine nightly, for instance—and still manage to deliver an apparently healthy baby, there is no assurance that this is a wise practice. The safe daily alcohol dose in pregnancy, if there is one, is not known.

All that is known about alcohol and pregnancy leads us to suggest that although you shouldn't worry about what you drank before you knew you were pregnant, it would be prudent to abstain for the rest of your pregnancy —except perhaps for a celebratory half glass of wine on a birthday or anniversary (taken *with* a meal, since food reduces the absorption of alcohol).

That's as easily done as said for some women—especially those who develop a distaste for alcohol in early pregnancy, which may linger through delivery. For others, particularly those who are accustomed to "unwinding" with cocktails at the end of the day or to taking wine with dinner, abstinence may require a concerted effort, possibly including a lifestyle change. If you drink to relax, for example, try substituting other methods of relaxation: music, warm baths, massage, exercise, reading. If drinking is part of a daily ritual that you don't want to give up, try a Virgin Mary (a Bloody Mary without the vodka) at brunch, sparkling cider or grape juice or nonalcoholic malt beer at dinner, juice spritzer (half juice, half seltzer, with a twist) or a Mock Strawberry Daiquiri or Virgin Sangria (see page 98) at cocktail hour—served at the accustomed time, in the accustomed glasses, with the accustomed ceremony.[1] If your husband joins you on the wagon (at least while in your company), the ride will be considerably smoother.

In the United States, alcohol use during pregnancy is the major cause of mental retardation and a leading cause of birth defects generally; but these defects are preventable. The sooner a heavy drinker stops drinking during pregnancy, the less risk to her baby. The heavy drinker who refuses to abstain or to seek help from Alcoholics Anonymous, a certified alcohol counselor or physician, or an alcohol treatment program may want to consider terminating her pregnancy and postponing childbearing until her illness is under control.

CIGARETTE SMOKING

"I've been smoking for ten years. Will this hurt my baby?"

There's no clear evidence that smoking *prior* to conception will harm a developing fetus—though parental smoking *can* interfere with conception. But it's well documented that smoking during pregnancy is hazardous. It has been linked to some

---

1. Though substituting nonalcoholic look-alikes for favorite alcoholic beverages during pregnancy can work for the occasional drinker, the heavy drinker may find that these beverages serve to trigger a desire for alcohol. If they do in you, avoid any drink, or even setting, that reminds you of alcohol.

115,000 miscarriages and 5,600 infant deaths a year as well as to ectopic pregnancy. It can also increase the risk of a wide variety of pregnancy complications. Among the more serious of these are vaginal bleeding, abnormal placental implantation, premature placental detachment, premature rupture of the membranes, and early delivery. It has been suggested that as many as 14% of preterm births in the United States are related to maternal cigarette smoking.

There is also strong evidence that an expectant mother's smoking adversely and very directly affects her baby's development in utero. The most widespread risk is low birthweight. In industrialized nations, such as the United States and Britain, smoking is blamed for as many as a third of all the babies who are born too small. And being born too small is the major cause of infant illness and perinatal death (those that occur just before, during, or after birth).

But there are other potential risks as well. Babies of smoking moms are more likely to suffer from apnea (breathing lapses) and are twice as likely to die of SIDS (sudden infant death syndrome, or crib death) as babies of nonsmokers. In general, babies of smokers aren't as healthy at birth as babies of nonsmokers, with three-pack-a-day maternal smoking associated with a quadrupled risk of low Apgar scores (the standard scale used to evaluate an infant's condition at birth). And there's evidence that, on the average, they may never catch up to the children of nonsmokers, that they may have long-term physical and intellectual deficits, and that they may also be hyperactive. At age 14, one study showed, children of smokers tended to be more prone to respiratory disease, to be shorter than children of nonsmokers, and to be less successful in school.

It was once believed that the reason

Breaking the Smoking Habit

Identify Your Motivation for Smoking. For example, do you smoke for pleasure, stimulation, or relaxation? To reduce tension or frustration, to have something in your hand or mouth, to satisfy a craving? Perhaps you smoke out of habit, lighting up without thinking about it. Once you understand your motivations, you should be able to find substitutes.

Identify Your Motivation for Quitting. When you're pregnant, that's easy.

Choose Your Method of Withdrawal. Do you want to go cold turkey or to taper off? Either way, pick a "last day" that isn't far off. Plan a full day of activities for that date—those you don't associate with smoking.

Try to Sublimate Your Urge to Smoke. Use any and all of the following that you think will help:

❖ If you smoke mainly to keep your hands busy, try playing with a pencil, beads, a straw; knit, polish silver, create a new nutritious recipe, write a letter, play the piano, learn to paint, make rag dolls, do jigsaw or crossword puzzles, challenge someone to a game of chess or Scrabble—anything that might make you forget to reach for a cigarette.

❖ If you smoke for oral gratification, try a substitute: sorbitol- or aspartame-sweetened gum, raw vegetables, popcorn, a whole-wheat breadstick, a toothpick, an empty cigarette holder. Do avoid empty-calorie nibbles.

❖ If you smoke for stimulation, try to get your lift from a brisk walk, an absorbing book, good conversation. Be sure your diet contains all essential nutrients and that you eat frequently, to avoid feeling draggy because of low blood sugar.

❖ If you smoke to reduce tension and relax, try exercise instead. Or relaxation techniques. Or listening to soothing music. Or a long walk. Or a massage. Or making love.

❖ If you smoke for pleasure, seek pleasure in other pursuits, preferably in no-smoke situations. Go to a movie, visit baby boutiques, tour a favorite museum, attend a concert or a play, have dinner with a friend who is allergic to smoke. Or try something more active, like tennis doubles.

❖ If you smoke out of habit, avoid the settings in which you habitually smoke and friends who smoke; frequent places with no-smoking rules instead.

❖ If you associate smoking with a particular beverage, food, or meal, avoid the food or beverage, eat the meal in a different location. (Say you smoke with breakfast but you never smoke in bed. Have breakfast in bed for a few days.)

❖ When you feel the urge to smoke, take several deep breaths with a pause between each. Hold the last breath while you strike a match. Exhale slowly, blowing out the match. Pretend it was a cigarette and crush it out.

If You Do Slip Up and Have a Cigarette, Don't Despair. Just get right back on your program, knowing that every cigarette you *don't* smoke is going to help your baby.

Look at Smoking as a Non-Negotiable Issue. When you were a smoker, you couldn't smoke in a theater, subway, or department store, even in some restaurants. That was that. Now you have to tell yourself that you can't smoke, period. That is that.

for the difficulties these children display was poor prenatal nutrition: their mothers smoked rather than ate during their pregnancies. But recent studies disprove this theory; smoking mothers who eat as much and gain as much weight as nonsmoking mothers still give birth to smaller babies. This seems to be the result of carbon monoxide poisoning and a reduction of oxygen to the fetus through the placenta. Gaining weight in excess of 40 pounds may somewhat reduce the risk of a smoking mother having an undersized baby, but that kind of weight gain poses other risks to the mother and child.

In effect, when you smoke, your baby is confined in a smoke-filled womb. His heartbeat speeds, he coughs and sputters, and worst of all, due to insufficient oxygen, he can't grow and thrive as he should.

Studies show that the effects of tobacco use, like those of alcohol use, are dose-related: tobacco use reduces the birthweight of babies in direct proportion to the number of cigarettes smoked, with a pack-a-day smoker 130% more likely to give birth to a low-birthweight child than a nonsmoker. So cutting down on the number of cigarettes you smoke may help some. But cutting down can be illusory because the smoker often compensates by taking more frequent and deeper puffs and smoking more of each cigarette. This can also happen when she tries to reduce the risk by using low-tar or low-nicotine cigarettes.

The news, however, isn't all bad. Some studies show that women who quit smoking early in pregnancy—no later than the fourth month—can reduce the risk of damage to the fetus to the level of the nonsmoker. Sooner is better, but quitting even in the last month can help preserve oxygen flow to the baby during delivery. For some smoking women, quitting will never be easier than in early pregnancy, when they develop a sudden distaste for cigarettes—probably the warning of an intuitive body. If you're not lucky enough to develop such a natural aversion, try quitting with the help of Smoke Enders or another smoking-cessation group. Or ask your practitioner to recommend other local resources. You may even want to try hypnosis.

Most people experience withdrawal symptoms when they quit smoking, though the symptoms and their intensity vary from person to person. Some of the most common include a craving for tobacco, irritability, anxiety, restlessness, tingling or numbness in the extremities, lightheadedness, fatigue, and sleep and gastrointestinal disturbances. Some people also find that both physical and mental performance are impaired at first. Most find that for a while they are coughing more, rather than less, because their bodies are suddenly better able to bring up all the secretions that have accumulated in the lungs.

To try to slow the release of nicotine and the nervousness that may result, increase your intake of fruit, fruit juice, milk, and mixed greens and temporarily cut back on meat, poultry, fish, and cheese; avoid caffeine, which can add to the jitters. Get plenty of rest (to counter fatigue) and exercise (to replace the kick you used to get from nicotine). Let your mind go fallow for a few days, if necessary and if possible, doing mindless tasks or going to the movies or other places where smoking is prohibited.

The worst effects of withdrawal will last a few days to a few weeks. The benefits, however, will last a lifetime—for you and your baby. (For more tips on improving your pregnancy lifestyle, see page 63.)

"My sister-in-law smoked two packs a day through three pregnancies, and had no

complications and big healthy babies. Why should I quit?"

Everyone has heard inspiring stories of someone beating the odds—a cancer patient given a 10% chance of survival living to a ripe age, or a quake victim found alive after being trapped under rubble without food or drink for days. But there's something much less inspiring about an expectant mother who consciously stacks the odds against her unborn babies by choosing to smoke, yet manages to beat the odds and produce healthy offspring anyway.

There are no sure things when it comes to making a baby, but there are many ways of bettering the odds. And giving up smoking is one of the most tangible ways you can improve the odds of your having an uncomplicated pregnancy and delivery and a healthy baby. Though there's the chance that you, too, can have a vigorous full-term baby even if you smoke your way through your pregnancy, there's also a significant risk that your baby would suffer some or all of the effects detailed on page 54. Your sister-in-law was lucky (and to a certain extent, this luck could have gotten a boost from heredity or other factors that might not hold for you)[2]; but do you really want to take the gamble that you will be lucky too? And then again that luck may not be all that it seems to be. Some of the deficits—physical and intellectual—that afflict babies of smokers aren't apparent immediately. The seemingly

---

2. It's possible that the reason her babies were not undersized is that she gained an excessive amount of weight by consuming an excessive number of calories. Taking in more calories than are usually required can, in some cases, reduce the risk of a smoker's baby being born smaller than average—but can present other problems.

healthy infant can grow into a child who is often sick, who is hyperactive, or who has trouble learning.

In addition to the effect smoking could have on your baby while you're still pregnant, there is the effect it would have once he or she has moved from your smoke-filled womb to your smoke-filled rooms. Babies of parents (mothers and/or dads) who smoke are sick more often than the babies of nonsmokers and are more likely to be hospitalized through infancy and childhood.

So as you can see, quitting is your best bet.

WHEN OTHER PEOPLE SMOKE

"I quit smoking, but my husband still goes through two packs a day, and a couple of my co-workers smoke like chimneys. I keep worrying that somehow this may hurt our baby."

Smoking, it is becoming more and more apparent, doesn't just affect the person who is puffing away—it affects everyone around him. Including a developing fetus whose mother happens to be nearby. So if your husband (or anyone else who lives in your home or works at the next desk) smokes, your baby's body is going to pick up nearly as much contamination from tobacco smoke by-products as if *you* were lighting up.

If your husband says he can't quit smoking, ask him to at least do all his smoking out of the house or in a different room, away from you and the baby. Quitting, of course, would be better, not just for his own health but for the baby's long-term well-being. Studies show that parental smoking—mother's or father's—can cause respiratory problems in their children, impairing lung development even into adulthood. It can also increase the odds that the children themselves will end up becoming smokers.

You probably won't be able to get your friends and co-workers to kick the habit, but you may be able to get them to curtail smoking around you. If there are laws protecting non-smokers where you live or work, then it will be relatively easy to do this. If there are no such laws, try tactful persuasion—show them the material in this book on the danger of tobacco smoke to a fetus. If that fails, try to get a regulation passed where you work that limits smoking to certain areas, such as a lounge, and prohibits smoking in the vicinity of nonsmokers. If all else fails, then try to move your office for the duration of your pregnancy.

MARIJUANA USE

"I've been a social smoker of marijuana —indulging only at parties—for about ten years. Could this have caused harm to the baby I'm now carrying? And is smoking pot during pregnancy dangerous?"

As it was with cigarette smoking over 20 years ago, all the evidence on the effects of marijuana use is not yet in. Consequently, those who choose to smoke it today are guinea pigs testing a substance whose dangers may not be fully documented for some time to come. And since marijuana crosses the placenta, mothers who smoke it during pregnancy make guinea pigs out of their unborn children as well.

It is usually recommended that couples trying to conceive abstain from marijuana use, since it can interfere with conception. But if you are already pregnant, you needn't worry about your past smoking—there is no

present evidence that it will harm your fetus.

Continuing to smoke marijuana now that you've found out you're pregnant, however, might well be a story with a less happy ending. Some, though not all, studies show that women who use marijuana even as infrequently as once a month throughout pregnancy are more likely to: gain inadequate weight; suffer from hyperemesis (severe and chronic vomiting), which can interfere seriously with prenatal nutrition if not treated; have dangerously rapid labor, prolonged or arrested labor, or a cesarean section; have a low-birthweight baby (though the increased risk is small); show meconium staining of the amniotic fluid during labor (a complication that can indicate fetal distress); and have a baby that needs resuscitation after delivery. Although there is no clear-cut evidence of an increased incidence of malformations in the babies of marijuana users, there have been reports of Fetal Alcohol Syndrome–like characteristics (see page 53) as well as tremors, vision abnormalities, and a withdrawal-like cry during the newborn period. Marijuana has also been shown to adversely affect placental function and the fetal endocrine system, potentially interfering with the successful completion of pregnancy. Based on the available evidence, the United States surgeon general has warned that marijuana use by a pregnant woman may be hazardous to the health of the fetus she is carrying.

So treat marijuana as you would any other drug during pregnancy: Don't take it unless it is medically required and prescribed. If you have already smoked early in your pregnancy, don't worry. Since most of the negative effects of marijuana appear to occur as pregnancy progresses, it's very unlikely any harm was done. Any pregnant woman who can't seem to break her marijuana habit should tell her practitioner or seek other professional help as soon as pregnancy is confirmed.

COCAINE AND OTHER DRUG USE

"I did some cocaine a week before I found out I was pregnant. Now I'm worried about what that could have done to my baby."

D on't worry about past cocaine use; just make sure it was your last. While the good news is that using the drug before you found out you were pregnant isn't likely to have had any effect, the bad news is that continuing to use it during pregnancy could be catastrophic. Cocaine not only crosses the placenta, it can damage it, reducing blood flow to the fetus and retarding fetal growth. It can also result in a variety of serious pregnancy complications, including miscarriage, premature labor, and stillbirth. In the baby who survives, there's the risk of stroke at birth and numerous long-term effects. Among them are chronic diarrhea, irritability, excessive crying and other behavioral problems, and abnormal breathing patterns and brain waves. It's also suspected, though not yet confirmed, that babies born to cocaine users are at an increased risk of SIDS.

Certainly, the more often the expectant mother uses cocaine, the greater the risk to her baby. But even very occasional use later on in pregnancy can be hazardous. For instance,

Perils in Perspective

Open a newspaper or turn on the television or radio, and chances are you'll encounter yet another report on the hazards of being pregnant in modern times. To hear the media tell it, an expectant mother can't eat, drink, breathe, or work without exposing her fetus to potential harm. Yet the reassuring truth is that pregnancy has never been so safe; never before in the history of reproduction have babies had a better chance of being born alive and well. Most environmental risks are theoretical, and those that are substantiated account for only a tiny fraction of all birth defects and pregnancy complications.

What's a mother-to-be to do? Read about the environmental risks listed in this chapter, eliminate some of them, minimize some of them, learn to live with some of them, and most important, put all of them in sensible perspective. The fact is that all of the environmental factors that are not within your control when you're pregnant—a job that has you sitting in front of a video display terminal, a hometown that's polluted with carbon monoxide, incidental brief exposures to paint fumes, hair dyes, insecticides—have far less impact on the outcome of your pregnancy than the factors you have complete control over, such as getting good, regular medical care, eating an excellent diet, and not drinking, smoking, or taking nonprescribed drugs once you find out you're pregnant. The woman who worries about the permanent she had before she found out she was pregnant but continues to smoke a pack a day is misdirecting her concern. She'd be much wiser to concentrate on those factors that will almost definitely have an effect on her baby's well-being instead of worrying about those that almost certainly will not.

a single use in the third trimester can trigger contractions and an abnormal fetal heartbeat.

Tell your practitioner about any cocaine use since you've conceived. As with every aspect of your medical history, the more your doctor knows, the better care you and your baby will receive. If you have any difficulty giving cocaine up entirely, seek professional help immediately.

Pregnant women who use drugs of any kind—other than those that have been prescribed by a physician who knows they are pregnant—are also putting their babies in jeopardy. Every known illicit drug (including heroin, methadone, crack, "ice," LSD, and PCP), and every prescription drug of abuse (including narcotics, tranquilizers, sedatives, and diet pills) can cause serious harm to a developing fetus and/or to the pregnancy with continued use. Check with your practitioner or another knowledgeable doctor about any drugs you've used during pregnancy, or call one of the hotlines listed in the Appendix to see what effect they could have had. Then, if you are still using drugs, get professional support (from a certified addiction counselor, an addictionologist, or a treatment center) to help you quit now.

CAFFEINE

"I find it difficult to start the day without my two cups of coffee. Is caffeine risky during pregnancy?"

Possibly. Caffeine (found in coffee, tea, colas and other soft drinks) does cross the placenta and enter the fetal circulation. Animal studies have shown numerous harmful effects from caffeine on developing fetuses, but human studies are less clear. One found as little as one and a half to two cups of coffee a day could double the risk of miscarriage.

Others found four or more cups a day caused withdrawal in the newborn (with heartbeat abnormalities, tremors, and rapid breathing) and increased the risk of SIDS. Though some have found no problem, until more is known, it makes sense to try to avoid caffeine.

Here are some additional reasons to give up caffeinated coffee (and tea and colas) during pregnancy. First of all, caffeine has a diuretic effect, drawing fluid and calcium—both vital to maternal and fetal health—from the body. If you're having a problem with frequent urination anyway, caffeine intake will compound it. Second, coffee and tea, especially when taken with cream and sugar, are filling and satisfying without being nutritious and can spoil your appetite for the nutritious food you need. Colas are not only filling but may contain questionable chemicals in addition to unneeded sugar. Third, caffeine can exacerbate your normal pregnancy mood swings and also interfere with adequate rest. Fourth, caffeine may interfere with the absorption of the iron both you and your baby need. Fifth, research suggests excessive caffeine use could result in temporary abnormal heartbeat, rapid respiration, and tremors in the newborn and the development of diabetes[3] later in life. Finally, the fact that many women lose their taste for coffee early in pregnancy suggests that mother nature herself considers the substance to be unsuitable for pregnant women.

How Do You Break the Caffeine Habit?
The first step, finding your motivation, is easy in pregnancy: giving your

3. In countries where caffeine consumption is highest, the incidence of diabetes is highest too; it is suspected that caffeine builds up in the fetal pancreas and eventually damages the cells that produce insulin.

baby the healthiest possible start in life. Next you need to determine why you indulge, and which beverages you can safely substitute to satisfy this need. If it's the taste of coffee or tea, or the comfort of a warm drink, that appeals to you, then switch to a naturally decaffeinated replacement (but don't let it take the place of your milk, orange juice, or other nutritious beverages).[4] If you drink cola for the taste, you can substitute caffeine-free soft drinks occasionally, but soft drinks have no regular place in a pregnancy diet; instead explore the varied flavors of unsweetened 100% fruit juices (papaya, passion fruit, mango, cherry, berry, cran-apple, and so on, in the countless combinations available) and flavored seltzers. If it's refreshment you're thirsting for, you'll find that juices and plain or carbonated water are better thirst quenchers than colas, anyway. If it's the caffeine lift you crave, you'll get a more natural, longer-lasting boost from exercise and good food, especially complex carbohydrates and protein, or from doing something that exhilarates you: dancing, jogging, making love. Though you'll doubtless sag for a few days after giving up caffeine, you'll soon feel better than ever. (Of course, you will still experience the normal fatigue of early pregnancy.)

If you drink coffee, tea, or cola for something to do, do something else—something good for your baby. Knit him or her a sweater, go for a walk or shop for a crib, scrub a bunch of vegetables for dinner. If you drink your caffeinated beverage as part of a daily ritual (the coffee break, reading the paper, watching TV), change the location of that ritual, and change the beverage that accompanies it.

---

4. Though decaffeinated teas are okay, beware of medicinal or heavy use of herbal teas; see page 323.

Minimizing Caffeine Withdrawal Symptoms. As any coffee, tea, or cola addict is well aware, it is one thing to want to give up caffeine and another thing to do it. Caffeine is an addictive drug; heavy imbibers who quit cold turkey can expect to experience withdrawal symptoms, including headache, irritability, fatigue, and lethargy. Which is why it's probably a better idea to ease off the caffeine gradually—starting by cutting down to an almost certainly safe level of two cups (taken with food to buffer the effect on your system) for a few days. Then, once you've adjusted to two cups, gradually reduce your daily intake, a quarter of a cup at a time, down to one cup, and finally, as the need for the drug lessens, to none. Or switch temporarily to a half caffeinated–half decaffeinated brew during the withdrawal period, gradually increasing the proportion of decaffeinated until your mug is completely caffeine-free. (If your taste buds miss the flavor of coffee, continue to satisfy them by using a brewed decaffeinated coffee. It isn't necessary to spring for the costlier water-processed varieties—the chemically processed coffees appear to pose no health risks. Even espresso lovers can be appeased with decaffeinated espressos, which are nearly as rich and flavorful as the caffeinated ones.)

Withdrawal will be less uncomfortable and easier to handle if you heed these energizing suggestions:

❖ Keep your blood sugar, and thus your energy level, up. Eat frequent small meals that are rich in protein and complex-carbohydrate foods. And be sure to take your pregnancy vitamin-mineral supplement.

❖ Get some outdoor exercise every day.

❖ Be sure to get enough sleep—

which will probably be easier without caffeine.

If you decide that a completely caffeine-free life isn't for you, don't despair. Based on the evidence, a cup or two of caffeinated beverage daily should pose no problem.

SUGAR SUBSTITUTES

"I'm trying not to gain too much weight. Can I use sugar substitutes?"

It usually comes as an unpleasant surprise to hopeful dieters, but the use of sugar substitutes rarely helps control weight. Maybe it's because the person who uses a substitute in her tea figures she's saved enough calories to have a few cookies with it. Even if sugar substitutes could guarantee weight control, however, caution would be recommended concerning their use by expectant mothers.

Unfortunately, not much human research has been done on saccharin use in pregnancy. Animal studies, however, show an increase in cancer in the offspring when pregnant mothers ingest the chemical. Added to evidence that the sweetener crosses the placenta in humans and is eliminated very slowly from fetal tissues, these studies suggest that it is sensible not to use saccharin while preparing for pregnancy, around the time of conception, or during pregnancy itself. Don't worry, however, about saccharin you've had before finding out that you're pregnant, since the risks, if any, are certainly extremely slight.

On the other hand, studies have shown no harmful effects from the use of typical amounts of the sweetener aspartame (Equal, NutraSweet) by most women during pregnancy.[5] Aspartame is composed of two common amino acids (phenylalanine and aspartic acid) plus methanol, and most doctors will okay *moderate* use of this sweetener for pregnant women. But because so many products sweetened with aspartame are nutritionally unworthy of a Best-Odds dieter—they're often overloaded with artificial additives and underloaded with nutrients—pregnant women should be selective in choosing among them. Adding a packet of Equal to your homemade ice cream or hot chocolate or using NutraSweet-sweetened yogurt should be fine. Filling up on diet sodas in place of more nourishing fare wouldn't be.

During pregnancy, the best sweeteners to rely on are natural and nutritious fruits and fruit juices. In the past few years, products sweetened entirely with fruit and fruit juice concentrates have proliferated in health food stores and supermarkets. Besides the Best-Odds treats you can bake (see the recipes on page 96 and in *What to Eat When You're Expecting,* or modify your own favorites), there are dozens that you can buy, including jams and jellies, cookies and muffins, ice creams and sorbets, candy bars and granola bars—even pop-up toaster pastries and sparkling natural "sodas." And unlike most products sweetened with sugar or sugar substitutes, the majority are nourishing, combining whole-grain flours with a host of other wholesome ingredients. Avoid those that, like most sugar-sweetened products, are made with refined flours, "bad" fats, or a long list of chemicals.

5. Women with PKU (phenylketonuria), however, must limit their intake of phenylalanine and are generally advised not to use aspartame. The suggestion has been made that some women—estimates vary from 1 in 10 to 1 in 50—may not metabolize phenylalanine properly, yet exhibit no symptoms of PKU. The theory that these women may damage their babies' brains by ingesting large amounts of aspartame remains unproven.

Your Pregnancy Lifestyle

Whereas most of your lifestyle habits used to affect only your body, many now have the potential of affecting your baby's body too. Old habits may now be bad habits, ones you'd like to break in a hurry.

Fortunately, there are some strategies that can help.

Eliminate Temptation. That means keeping everything that you shouldn't have out of sight. No wine in the fridge; no liquor on top of the bar. No cake mixes in the kitchen cupboard; no white bread in the bread box.

Stock Up on Substitutes. Sparkling cider in your wineglass at dinner, a Mock Strawberry Daiquiri (page 98) at cocktail time (unless imitations make you yearn for the real thing). Fruit-sweetened cookies and cakes in the cupboard; delicious whole-grain breads and muffins in the freezer.

Use Cues. One of the major obstacles to changing habits is forgetting what your goals are; they can easily slip from your mind when temptation is near. So tape pictures of babies (cute, healthy-looking babies) on the refrigerator, inside kitchen cupboards, on the outside of the liquor cabinet, on your desk at work. If skipping breakfast is your vice, put a sign inside your front door that asks, "Have you fed your baby breakfast today?"

Forgive Yourself. If you slip up and eat something that's less than good for your baby, or even if you have a glass of wine or a beer, don't throw in the towel and go back to your old ways. Get right back on the healthy-living wagon. Try to analyze what it was that caused you to fall off, and try to avoid such situations for the duration.

Identify, Then Squelch, Feelings That Weaken Your Resolve. Many people find it difficult to stay on a diet, avoid alcohol, tobacco, or drugs, or shun other negative habits in the face of hunger, anger, boredom, fatigue, or loneliness. So get a jump on these saboteurs. Eat frequent small meals to keep hunger in check. Diffuse feelings of annoyance or resentment immediately, before they get the best of you. Get plenty of rest—when your body says "slow down," listen. And if you feel isolated or bored a good deal of the time, join a prenatal group, do some volunteer work, or take some stimulating courses. Make sure your spouse knows that you're craving extra attention—and the important reasons why you need it now more than ever.

Rely on Relaxation. It's often tension that makes us susceptible to forgetting our good intentions, so take spare moments during the day to do relaxation exercises (see page 114).

Learn to Say No... to that second cup of coffee, that social cigarette, that glass of bubbly being passed your way, one too many fudge brownies. Be polite but firm: "You know I love your brownies, Grandma, but my baby's too young for them" or "Thanks, but I'll toast your birthday with orange juice—my baby's underage."

Enlist an Ally. Your husband is the most logical one, but it can also be a friend at work, a sister, or someone else you spend a lot of time with. Your ally should be willing to stick to the rules with you when you're together; this will help strengthen your resolve and remove a good deal of temptation.

If You Can't Do It Alone, Get Help. Some habits are harder to break than others. If you're having difficulty kicking a potentially dangerous habit, whether it's smoking, drinking, or taking drugs, then talk to your practitioner or seek other professional help.

THE FAMILY CAT

"I have two cats at home. I've heard that cats carry a disease that can harm a fetus. Do I have to get rid of my pets?"

Probably not. Since you've lived with cats for a while, the odds are pretty good that you've already contracted the disease, toxoplasmosis (see page 313), and developed an immunity to it. It's estimated that about half of the American population has been infected (the estimates in some countries—France, for example—are as high as 90%), and the rates of infection are much higher among people who have cats or who frequently eat raw meat or drink unpasteurized milk (both of which can also harbor and transmit the infection). If you weren't tested prenatally to see if you were immune, it's not likely you will be tested now—unless you show symptoms of the disease (although some doctors will run regular tests on pregnant women who live with a lot of cats).

If you were tested prenatally and were not immune, or if you're not sure whether you are or not, you should take the following precautions to avoid infection:

❖ Have your cats tested by a veterinarian to see if they have an active infection. If one or both of them does, board them at a kennel or ask a friend to care for them for at least six weeks—the period during which the infection is transmissible. If they are free of infection, keep them that way by not allowing them to eat raw meat, roam outdoors, hunt mice or birds (which can transmit toxoplasmosis to cats), or fraternize with other cats. Have someone else handle the litter box. If you must do it yourself, use

gloves when handling the litter box and wash your hands when you've finished. The litter should be changed daily since the oocytes that transmit the disease become more infectious with time.

❖ Wear gloves when gardening. Don't garden in soil, or let your children play in sand, in which cats may have deposited feces. Wash fruits and vegetables, especially those grown in home gardens, with dish detergent (rinsing very thoroughly), and/or peel or cook them.

❖ Don't eat raw or undercooked meat or unpasteurized milk; a thermometer inserted in the center of the meat when it comes from the oven should register at least 140°F. In restaurants, order meat well done.

Some doctors are urging routine testing before conception or in very early pregnancy for all women, so that those who test positive can relax, knowing they are immune, and those who test negative can take the necessary precautions to prevent infection. Other doctors believe the costs of such testing may outweigh the benefits it may provide.

HOT TUBS AND SAUNAS

"We have a hot tub. Is it safe for me to use it while I'm pregnant?"

You won't have to switch to cold showers, but it's probably a good idea to refrain from long stays in the hot tub. Anything that raises the body temperature over 102°F (38.9°C) and keeps it there for a while—whether it's a dip in a hot tub or an extremely hot bath, too long a session in the sauna or steam room, an overzealous workout in hot weather, or a virus—is potentially hazardous to the developing embryo or fetus, particularly in the early months. Some studies have shown that a hot tub doesn't raise a woman's temperature to dangerous levels immediately—it takes at least 10 minutes (longer if the shoulders and arms are not submerged or if the water is 102°F or less)—but because individual responses and circumstances vary, play it safe by keeping your belly out of the hot tub. But feel free to soak your feet.

If you've already had some brief sojourns in the hot tub, there is probably no cause for alarm. Studies show that most women spontaneously get out of a hot tub before their body temperatures reach 102°F, because they've become uncomfortable. It's likely you did too. If you are concerned, however, speak to your doctor about the possibility of having an ultrasound exam or other prenatal test to help put your mind at ease.

Lengthy stays in the sauna may also be unwise, though the evidence is not clear. The weekly sauna is customary in Finland, even for pregnant women, and yet the kind of central nervous system defects believed to be caused by hyperthermia (a dangerous rise in body temperature) aren't common in babies there. Still, most U.S. experts recommend avoiding the sauna.

MICROWAVE EXPOSURE

"I've read that exposure to microwave ovens is dangerous to a developing fetus. Should I unplug ours until after the baby's born?"

A microwave oven can be a working mother-to-be's best friend, helping to make nutritious eating-on-the-run possible. But like so many of our modern miracles, there's talk that it may also be a modern menace. Whether or not we can be zapped by exposure to microwaves is still very controversial. Much more research needs to be done before the answer is definitively known. It is believed, however, that two types of human tissue—the developing fetus and the eye—are particularly vulnerable to the effects of microwaves because they have a poor capacity to dissipate the heat the waves generate. However, rather than unplugging your microwave oven, you should take some precautions.

First of all, be sure your oven doesn't leak. Don't operate it if seals around the door are damaged, if the oven doesn't close properly, or if something is caught in the door. Since inexpensive home devices for measuring radiation are unreliable, don't attempt to test for leaks yourself. Consult an appliance service center, the city or state consumer protection office, or your local health department. They may be able to do the testing for you, or recommend someone who can. Second, don't stand in front of the oven when it is in operation. Finally, follow the manufacturer's directions to the letter.

ELECTRIC BLANKETS AND HEATING PADS

'We use an electric blanket all winter long. Is this safe for the baby we're expecting?''

Cuddle up to your sweetie instead, or if his toes are as cold as yours, invest in a down comforter, push up the thermostat, or heat the bed with the blanket and then turn it off before you get in. Electric blankets can raise body temperature excessively, and although their use hasn't been clearly associated with fetal damage, the theory is there. Furthermore, although studies have been contradictory, some researchers have suggested that there is also some potential risk from the electromagnetic field created by electric blankets. So it would be prudent to try alternative routes to warmth. Don't, however, worry about nights you've already spent beneath an electric blanket—the chance that your baby was harmed is extremely remote, even in theory.

Be cautious, too, when using a heating pad. If treatment with one has been recommended by the doctor, wrap it in a towel to reduce the heat it passes along, limit applications to 15 minutes, and don't sleep with it.

Electrically heated water beds have also been linked to pregnancy problems, specifically miscarriage. Scientists believe this may be due to the electromagnetic fields the heaters emit. New super-low EMF water-bed heaters, however, emit EMF levels equivalent to background radiation and are probably safe. If you have an older heater, you can warm the bed, then turn the heater off when you are ready to retire.

X-RAYS

"I had an x-ray series at the dentist before I found out I was pregnant. Could this have hurt my baby?"

Don't worry. First of all, dental x-rays are directed far away from your uterus. Second, a lead apron shields your uterus and your baby effectively from any radiation.

Determining the safety of other types of x-rays during pregnancy is more complicated, but it is clear that diagnostic x-rays rarely pose a threat to the embryo or fetus. Three factors affect whether or not radiation from x-rays might be harmful:

❖ **The Amount of Radiation.** Severe damage to the embryo or fetus occurs only at very high doses (50 to 250 rads). No damage appears to occur at doses lower than 10 rads. Since modern x-ray equipment rarely delivers more than 5 rads during a typical diagnostic exam, such exams should not present a problem in pregnancy.

❖ **When the Exposure Occurs.** Even at high doses, there appears to be no teratogenic risk to the embryo before implantation (the sixth to eighth day postconception). There is a somewhat greater risk of damage during the period of early development of a baby's organs (the third and fourth weeks after conception), and some continued risk of damage to the central nervous system throughout pregnancy. But again, only at high doses.

❖ **Whether There Is Actual Exposure of the Uterus.** Today's x-ray equipment is able to precisely pinpoint the area that needs to be viewed, which protects the rest of the body from radiation exposure. Most x-rays can be done with the mother's abdomen and pelvis, and thus the uterus, shielded by a lead apron. But even an abdominal x-ray is unlikely to be hazardous, since it practically never delivers more than 10 rads.

Of course it still isn't wise to take unnecessary risks, no matter how small, so it's usually recommended that elective x-rays be postponed until after delivery. Necessary risks are another matter. Since the likelihood of damage to the fetus from x-ray exposure is slight, the health of the expectant mother shouldn't be endangered by putting off an x-ray that is genuinely needed. And the already minimal hazards of an x-ray during pregnancy can be minimized still further by observing the following guidelines:

❖ Always inform the doctor ordering the x-ray and the technician performing it that you are pregnant.

❖ Never have an x-ray, even a dental x-ray, during pregnancy if the benefit does not outweigh the risk. (Read Weighing Risk vs. Benefit, page 77.)

❖ Do not have an x-ray if a safer diagnostic procedure can be used instead.

❖ If an x-ray is necessary, be certain that it is taken in a licensed or regularly inspected facility. Equipment should be up-to-date, in good condition, and operated by well-trained, conscientious technicians under the supervision of a full-time radiologist. The x-ray equipment should, when possible, be directed so that only the minimum area necessary is exposed to radiation; the uterus should be shielded with a lead apron.

❖ Follow the technician's directions precisely, being especially careful not to move during the shot, so that retakes won't be needed.

❖ Most important, if you've had an x-ray, or need an x-ray, don't waste your time worrying about the possible consequences. Your baby is in more danger when you forget to buckle your seat belt.

HOUSEHOLD HAZARDS

"The more I read, the more I'm convinced that the only way to protect my baby in this day and age is to spend the next nine months locked up in a sterile room. Even my home isn't safe."

T he threats you and your baby face from the increasing number of environmental hazards, including those in your own backyard, quickly pale when compared to those faced by your great-grandmothers, when modern obstetrical medicine was in its infancy. All of today's environmental perils combined (alcohol, tobacco, and other drugs excepted) are far less of a threat to you and your baby than one untrained midwife with unwashed hands was to your ancestresses. So in spite of all the trumpeting about the perils around us, we repeat: Pregnancy and childbirth have never been so safe.

But while you won't have to trade in your home for a sterile room, a little caution is certainly warranted when dealing with hazards around the house:

Household Cleaning Products. Since many cleaning products have been in common use for the better part of the century and no correlation has ever been noted between clean homes and birth defects, it's unlikely that disinfecting your toilet bowl or polishing your dining-room table will in any way compromise the well-being of your baby. In fact, much the opposite is probably true: The elimination of bacteria and other germs by chlorine, ammonia, and other cleaning agents can protect your baby by preventing infection.

No studies have proven that the occasional incidental inhalation of ordinary household cleansers has any detrimental effect on the developing fetus; on the other hand, no studies have proven frequent inhalation completely safe. If you've already been "exposed" to cleaning products, there's no reason for concern. But for the rest of your pregnancy, clean with prudence. Let your nose, and the following tips, be your guide in screening out potentially hazardous chemicals:

❖ If the product has a strong odor or

fumes, don't breathe it in directly. Use it in an area with plenty of ventilation, or don't use it at all.

❖ Use pump sprays instead of aerosols.

❖ Never (even when you're not pregnant) mix ammonia with chlorine-based products; the combination produces deadly fumes.

❖ Try to avoid using products such as oven cleaners and dry-cleaning fluids whose labels are plastered with warnings about toxicity.

❖ Wear rubber gloves when you're cleaning. Not only will they spare your hands a lot of wear and tear, they'll prevent the absorption through the skin of potentially toxic chemicals.

Lead. Not that expectant mothers need something else to worry about, but in recent years it's been discovered that lead—long known to reduce the IQ of children who ingest it from crumbling paint—can also affect pregnant women and their fetuses. Heavy exposure to the mineral can put a woman at increased risk of developing pregnancy-induced hypertension, and even of pregnancy loss. It puts her baby at risk for a variety of problems, ranging from serious behavioral and neurological problems to relatively minor birth defects. The risks multiply when a baby is exposed to lead in the uterus and then continues to be exposed after birth.

Fortunately, it's fairly easy to avoid lead exposure, along with all the problems it can cause. Here's how: Since drinking water is a common source of lead, be sure that yours is lead-free (see below). If your home dates back to 1955 or earlier and layers of paint are to be removed for any reason, stay away from the house while the work is being done. Still another common source of lead is food or drink contaminated by lead leached from earthenware, pottery, or china. If you have pitchers or dishes that are home-crafted, imported, antique, just plain old (the FDA did not set limits on lead in dishes until 1971), or of otherwise questionable safety, don't use them for serving or storing, particularly of acidic food or beverages (citrus, vinegar, tomatoes, wine, soft drinks).

Tap Water. Water ranks second only to oxygen on the list of substances essential to life. Humans can survive for at least a week without food (though starvation isn't medically recommended), but for only a few days without water. In other words, you've got more to worry about if you *don't* drink the water than if you do.

It's true that water once posed a serious threat to the lives it sustained, carrying deadly typhoid and other diseases. But modern water treatment has eliminated such threats, at least in developed areas of the world. Though there are some who suspect that a new threat to the unborn now exists in the very chemicals that are used to purify water, there is no conclusive evidence that this is true. Any possible hazard is eliminated in systems that use filters instead of chemicals in the water purification process.

Most tap water in the United States is safe and drinkable. But there are exceptions. Some water is contaminated with lead as it passes through old lead pipes or through newer pipes that were soldered with lead. And in a few areas, seepage of sewer wastes and chemicals from factories, toxic waste sites, dumping grounds, underground storage tanks, and farms has also led to potentially hazardous contamination. Water that comes from an underground well is at least as subject to such contamination as water from rivers, lakes, and streams. To be sure that when you fill a glass of water you will be drinking to your—and your baby's—health, do the following:

❖ Check with your local Environmental Protection Agency (EPA) or health department about the purity and safety of community drinking water. If you lack confidence in the answers, you can also consult a local environmental group (contact the Environmental Defense Fund for a referral). If there is a possibility that the quality of your water (because of pipe deterioration, because your home borders on a waste disposal area, or because of odd taste or color) might differ from the rest of the community's, arrange to have it tested (your local EPA or health department can tell you where).

❖ If your tap water looks suspicious or has an "off" taste, invest in a carbon filter for your kitchen sink. (It will last longer if it is used only for cooking and drinking water and not for the dishwasher and other purposes.) Or use bottled water for drinking and cooking.

Be aware, however, that no water that is bottled and advertised as "pure" is automatically free of impurities. Some bottled waters are as contaminated as contaminated tap water, and most do not contain fluorides, which could be important for your bones and teeth, and later for your baby's.

❖ If you suspect lead in your water, or if testing reveals high levels, changing the plumbing would be the ideal solution, but this is not always feasible. To reduce the levels of lead in the water you drink, use only cold water for drinking and cooking (hot leaches more lead from the pipes), and run the cold-water tap for about five minutes in the morning (as well as any time the water has been off for six hours or more) before using it. You can tell that fresh water from the street pipes has reached your faucet when the water has gone from cold to warmer to cold again.

❖ If your water smells and/or tastes like chlorine, boiling it or letting it stand for 24 hours will evaporate much of the chemical.

Insecticides. Though some insects, such as gypsy moths, pose a considerable threat to trees and plants, and others, such as roaches and ants, to your esthetic sensibilities, they rarely pose a health risk to human beings—even pregnant ones. And it's generally safer to live with them than to eliminate them through the use of chemical insecticides, some of which have been linked to birth defects.

Of course, your neighbors and/or your super (if they don't happen to be pregnant or have small children) may not agree. If your neighborhood is currently being sprayed, avoid being outdoors as much as possible until the chemical odors have dissipated—about two to three days. When indoors, keep the windows closed. If your super is spraying apartments for roaches or other insects, ask him to skip yours if possible. If not, be sure that all closets and kitchen cabinets are tightly closed to prevent contamination of their contents, and that all food preparation surfaces are covered. Stay out of the apartment for a day or two if that's possible, and ventilate with open windows for as long as practical. The chemicals are potentially dangerous only as long as the fumes linger. Once the spray has settled, have someone else scrub all the food preparation surfaces in or near the sprayed area.

Whenever possible, try to take the natural approach to pest control. Pull weeds instead of spraying them. Have someone remove gypsy moth larvae or other insect pests manually from trees and plants, then drop them in a jar of kerosene. Some pests can be eliminated from garden and house plants by spraying with a forceful stream from the garden hose or with a biodegradable insecticidal soap mixture, though the procedure may need to be repeated several times to be effective. Investing in an infantry of ladybugs or other beneficial predators (available from some garden supply houses) can also wipe out some unfriendly pests.

Inside the house, use "motel" or Combat-type traps, strategically placed in heavy bug traffic areas, to get rid of roaches and ants; use cedar blocks instead of mothballs in clothes closets; and use other nontoxic types of pest control. If you have young children or pets, avoid boric acid, which can be toxic when ingested. For more information on natural pest control, contact your regional Cooperative Extension Service or a local environmental group.

If you have been accidentally exposed to insecticides or herbicides, don't be alarmed. Brief, indirect exposure isn't likely to have done any harm to your baby. What does increase the risk is frequent, long-term exposure, the kind that working daily around such chemicals (as in a factory or heavily sprayed field) would involve.

Paint Fumes. In the entire animal kingdom, the period before birth (or egg laying) is passed in hectic preparation for the arrival of the new offspring. Birds feather their nests, squirrels line their tree-trunk homes with leaves and twigs, and human mothers and fathers sift madly through volumes of wallpaper and fabric samples.

And almost invariably, painting the baby's room is involved—which, in the days of arsenic- or lead-based paints, might have posed some threat to the health of the unborn. For a long while it was believed modern latex paints were much safer, but it was recently reported that they contain unsafe amounts of mercury. Federal regulations now require that paints be reformulated so they don't contain mercury. But because you don't know what hazard may turn up in paint next, it's a good idea to consider painting an inappropriate avocation for an expectant mother—even one who's trying desperately to keep busy in those last weeks of waiting. In addition, balancing on ladder tops is precarious, to say the least, and paint odors can bring on an attack of nausea. Try, instead, to get the expectant father, or someone else, to handle this aspect of the preparations.

While the painting is being done, try to arrange to be out of the house. Whether you're there or not, be sure to keep windows open for ventilation (for this reason human nest renovations are best accomplished, as they are for much of the animal kingdom, during the mild days of spring.) Avoid

Let Your House Breathe

Though making your house as airtight as possible will cut your fuel bills, it will also increase the risk of indoor air pollution. So don't caulk every crack and weatherstrip every door. Allow some fresh air to leak in and some indoor air to leak out. Weather permitting, keep some windows open.

The Green Solution

There is no way to totally eliminate indoor air pollution. Furniture, paints, carpets, paneling, all can give off invisible fumes and pollute the air you breathe at home. Though there's no evidence that at typical levels such pollution is harmful to you or your baby, you may be more comfortable if you know you are doing something to reduce it. You can accomplish this very easily and effectively by filling your home with house plants. Plants have the ability to absorb noxious fumes in the air while adding oxygen, and of course beauty, to the indoor environment.

entirely exposure to paint removers, which are highly toxic, and steer clear of the paint removing process (whether chemicals or sanders are used), particularly if the paint that's being removed might be mercury- or lead-based.

AIR POLLUTION

"It seems it isn't even safe to breathe when you're pregnant. Will city air pollution hurt my baby?"

Living in a bus terminal or sleeping nightly in a tollbooth on a congested highway might, of course, expose your fetus to excessive pollutants while depriving it of essential oxygen. Ordinary breathing in the big city, however, isn't as risky as you might think, particularly when you consider the alternative. Millions of women live and breathe in major cities across the nation and give birth to millions of healthy babies. Even in the 1960s, when pollution was at its worst levels in such smoggy places as Los Angeles and New York, no damage to the unborn was documented.

Day-to-day breathing, then, will have no detrimental effect on your baby. Even enough carbon monoxide to cause illness in the mother appears not to have deleterious effects on the fetus early in pregnancy (although carbon monoxide poisoning later in pregnancy might). It's common sense, however, to avoid extraordinarily high doses of most air pollutants. Here's how:

❖ Avoid smoke-filled rooms for extended, repeated periods. Keep in mind that cigars and pipes, because they aren't inhaled, release even more smoke into the air than cigarettes do. Ask family, guests in your home, and co-workers not to smoke in your presence.

❖ Have the exhaust system on your car checked to be sure there is no leakage of noxious fumes and that the exhaust pipe isn't rusting away. Never start your car in the garage with the garage door closed; keep the tailgate on a station wagon closed when the engine is running; avoid waiting in gas lines with other cars spewing out carbon monoxide; keep your car's air vent closed when driving in heavy traffic.

❖ If a pollution alert is called in your city, stay indoors as much as you can, with the windows closed and the air conditioner, if you have one, running. Follow any other instructions given by the city for residents who are at special risk.

❖ Don't run, walk, or bicycle along congested highways, or exercise outdoors when there's a pollution alert, since you breathe in more air—and pollution—when you're active.

❖ Make sure gas stoves, fireplaces, and wood-burning stoves in your home are vented properly. If they aren't, they can fill the air with carbon monoxide and other possibly hazardous gases.

❖ Keep the air around you cleaner with greenery. Living plants improve air quality in and around your home.

❖ If you *do* work in a bus terminal or in a tollbooth on a busy highway, consider asking for a temporary transfer to a desk job to eliminate even the hypothetical risk that the pollution might pose to your baby.

OCCUPATIONAL HAZARDS

"You hear a lot about dangers on the job, but how do you know if your workplace is safe?"

The hazards of the workplace, and the threats they may pose to the reproductive capabilities of both male and female workers and to the well-being of their unborn children, have only just begun to be explored and identified. Conclusive answers have been elusive, as they are whenever cause-and-effect connections between environmental factors and poor pregnancy outcomes are sought. First of all, it's hard to separate out all the various possible contributing risk factors in a woman's life, or to prove that an unfavorable outcome wasn't caused by a genetic accident. Second, though animal studies often yield interesting results, there's no way to ascertain whether the results apply to humans, since experiments on humans aren't, of course, feasible.

Therefore, effects on humans can be determined only through epidemiological studies. These studies can be done in two ways: Large groups of women who are exposed to certain substances can be looked at to see if they show an increase in one or more types of poor pregnancy outcome (miscarriages, birth defects, etc.). Or small groups of women who have poor outcomes can be studied to see if there is a common risk factor shared by all of them. Either way, such studies give us clues but not definitive answers.

From what we presently know, it is clear that some workplaces do present hazards for the pregnant woman (e.g., chemical factories, operating rooms, x-ray departments). Other workplaces so far have fallen into gray areas because not enough research has been done to establish their safety—or lack of it. In the majority of workplaces, much of the concern about potential risks on the job is unwarranted.

The following is a brief rundown on what's known (and what's not) about the safety of certain jobs during pregnancy:

Office Work. Far and away the most controversial potential occupational hazard sits on the desks of over 10 million American women of childbearing age: the video display terminal. VDTs have become the intensely scrutinized focus of media and public attention since the early 1980s, when reports began to link them with pregnancy problems. Several studies have been done since then, and very little solid incriminating evidence has been uncovered. No study has been able to prove a definite link between the low-level radiation (actually lower than that of sunshine) emitted by VDTs and miscarriages, though the link had been suggested. And the most recent government study (sponsored by NIOSH) has shown no greater miscarriage rate among women who use

VDTs than those who don't. One study did show an increase in miscarriages among clerical workers (but not executives) who worked 20 or more hours in front of a VDT, but experts suggest that other factors might have been responsible. Isolated reports of birth defects in babies of VDT users have not been consistent with the kinds of defects that would be expected from radiation exposure; researchers therefore considered it unlikely that the defects are related to VDT use.

Unquestionably, more large-scale study needs to be done—and it's very possible that when it is, VDTs will be vindicated. In the meantime, panic is certainly not justified, nor, according to researchers, is a change of career, even if you spend the better part of your work week in front of a terminal. If all the reassurances in the world won't make you comfortable sitting at your VDT, however, and you feel as though you would like to take some concrete steps to minimize any possible risks, consider the following:

❖ No pregnancy-related problems have been reported among pregnant women who used a VDT for 20 hours a week or less. A temporary decrease in hours spent in front of the screen to under this number would seem to wipe out even a theoretical risk.

❖ If the radiation is responsible for any negative effects, some theorize, then it would be more dangerous to sit *behind* someone else's terminal (more radiation is emitted from the back of a unit) than in front of your own. If your desk is in a less than ideal position relative to other VDTs, see if you can change its location or change desks temporarily, or if barriers can be erected between units.

❖ Some experts have suggested that wearing a protective apron or using a grounded electrically conductive filter over the screen may protect against nonionizing radiation; others have termed these precautions ineffective. Discuss this option with your practitioner.

Though there isn't any hard evidence that working with a VDT can cause miscarriage, there is evidence that it can cause a multitude of physical discomforts, including neck, eye, wrist, arm, and back strain, dizziness, and headaches, all of which can compound the normal discomforts of pregnancy. To reduce these symptoms, try the following:

❖ Take frequent breaks from the sitting position during the day—even a brisk walk to the rest room or to deliver a memo will help.

❖ Do stretching and/or relaxation exercises (see page 194) periodically while sitting at the terminal.

❖ Use a height-adjustable chair with a backrest that supports your lower back. And be sure the keyboard and monitor are at comfortable heights.

❖ Make sure that your eyeglasses are appropriate for use at a VDT.

Health Care Work. Ever since the first doctor cared for the first patient, health care workers (physicians, dentists, veterinarians, nurses, laboratory and x-ray technicians) have taken risks with their own lives in order to save or improve the quality of the lives of others. And while some such risks are an inevitable part of the job, it makes sense for the health care worker, particularly the pregnant one, to protect herself from as many as possible. Potential risks include exposure to waste anesthesia gases (either through leakage in the operating room or the exhaled breath of recovery room patients), to chemicals (such as ethylene

Getting all the Facts

By law, you have the right to know what chemicals you are exposed to on the job; your employer is obliged to tell you. Information on workplace hazards can also be obtained by contacting the National Institute of Occupational Safety and Health, Clearing House for Occupational Safety and Health Information, 4676 Columbia Parkway, Cincinnati, OH 45226; or the Occupational Safety and Health Administration, 200 Constitution Avenue NW, Washington, DC 20210. NIOSH also makes available a booklet titled *Technical Guidelines for Protecting the Safety and Health of Hospital Workers.* Information about the safety of machinery or other equipment that you operate on the job can often be secured by writing directly to the manufacturer's corporate medical director.

If your job does expose you to hazards, either ask to be transferred temporarily to a safer post or, finances permitting, begin your maternity leave early.

oxide and formaldehyde) used for sterilization of equipment, to ionizing radiation (such as that used in diagnosis or treatment of disease),[6] to anti-cancer drugs, and to infections, such as hepatitis B and AIDS. Depending upon the particular risk you are exposed to, you might want to either take safety precautions as recommended by the National Institute of Occupational Safety and Health (NIOSH; see box above) or switch to safer work for the time being.

Manufacturing Work. How safe conditions are in a factory depends on what's being made in it and, to a certain extent, on how principled the people who run it are. The Occupational Safety and Health Administration (OSHA) lists a number of substances that a pregnant woman should avoid on the job. They include such chemicals as alkylating agents, arsenic, benzene, carbon monoxide, chlorinated hydrocarbons, dimethyl sulfoxide, organic mercury compounds, lead, lithium, aluminum, arsenic, ethylene oxide, dioxin, and polychlorinated biphenyls. Where proper safety protocols are implemented, exposure to such toxins can be avoided. Your union or other labor organization may be able to help you determine if you are protected. You can also get useful information from OSHA (see box above).

In-Flight Work. It has recently been suggested that flight attendants and airline pilots (possibly along with very frequent flyers) may run the risk of excessive exposure to radiation from the sun if their flights often bring them to very high altitudes. Radiation is more intense nearer the poles and less so near the equator, so flights across the southern United States pose less potential risk than those across the northern states. Though at this

---

6. Most technicians working with low-dose diagnostic x-ray will not be exposed to dangerous levels of radiation. It is recommended, however, that women of childbearing age working with higher-dose radiation wear a special device that keeps track of daily exposure, to ensure that cumulative annual exposure does not exceed safe levels.

time the risk appears to be very small, those who ordinarily spend a lot of time flying long distances, particularly at closer proximity to the poles, might want to consider a switch during pregnancy to shorter routes that fly at lower altitudes, or to ground work. If you're concerned about the flying you did before you found out you were pregnant, discuss this with your practitioner—you're more than likely to find reassurance.

Physically Strenuous Work. Work that involves heavy lifting, physical exertion, long hours, rotating shifts, or continuous standing may somewhat increase a woman's risk for early and late miscarriage as well as preterm deliveries and stillbirth. If you have such a job, you should request a transfer to a less strenuous position until after delivery and postpartum recovery. (See page 204 for recommendations on how long it is safe for you to stay at various strenuous jobs during your pregnancy.)

Other Work. Teachers and social workers who deal with young children may come into contact with potentially dangerous infections, such as rubella. Animal handlers, meat cutters, and meat inspectors may be exposed to toxoplasmosis (but may well have developed immunity already, in which case their babies would not be at risk), and laundry workers to a variety of infections. If you work where infection is a risk, be sure you're immunized as needed and take appropriate precautions, such as using gloves, masks, and so on. (See individual infections.)

Artists, photographers, chemists, cosmeticians, dry cleaners, agricultural and horticultural workers, and others may be exposed to a variety of possibly hazardous chemicals in the course of their work. If you work with any suspect substances, you should take appropriate precautions, which in some cases may mean avoiding that part of your work that involves the use of chemicals. Don't be overly concerned about exposure that's already occurred, since in most cases exposure to toxins that isn't massive enough to cause illness in the mother rarely results in damage to the fetus.

Quiet Please

Noise is probably the most prevalent of all occupational hazards, and has long been known to cause hearing loss in those exposed to it on a regular basis. Recent studies suggest that it may also cause high-frequency hearing loss in the unborn and that it may be associated with prematurity and intrauterine growth retardation as well. More research needs to be done, but in the meantime expectant mothers who work in an extremely noisy environment where protective hearing devices are required or who are exposed to heavy vibration on the job should play it safe and ask for a temporary transfer. All expectant mothers should avoid listening to loud music (especially in an enclosed place like a car) and going to rock concerts.

WHAT IT'S IMPORTANT TO KNOW:
PLAYING BABY ROULETTE

When a gambler playing roulette puts down a bet on his lucky number, the odds are very high against the wheel coming to a stop there. It's the same when a pregnant woman plays baby roulette (intentionally or inadvertently), exposing her baby to teratogens, substances potentially harmful to the fetus. Almost all of the time the baby roulette wheel will pass innocuously by, and the baby won't be affected.

Although the gambler will call it luck, where the roulette wheel stops depends on the weight of the wheel, the friction it encounters, and the force with which it is spun. And though baby roulette may also appear to be a game of chance, its outcome, too, is actually dependent on a variety of factors:

How Strong Is the Teratogen? A very few drugs are powerful teratogens. For example, thalidomide, a drug used in the early 1960s, caused severe deformities in all fetuses who were exposed in utero at a particular time in their development (1 in 5 of all babies exposed at any time prenatally), and the acne medicine Accutane, a more recently recognized teratogen, caused defects in almost 1 in 5 exposures. At the other extreme are drugs such as the hormone Provera—a progestin—that are believed to cause defects only rarely (an estimated 1 in 1,000 exposed fetuses for Provera). Most drugs fall somewhere in between, and fortunately, few are as potent as thalidomide and Accutane (and Accutane-like compounds).

Often it's very difficult to tell whether a drug is teratogenic at all, even when its use appears to be related to the occurrence of certain birth defects. Say, for example, a defect shows up in babies whose mothers took a particular antibiotic for infection with high fever when they were pregnant; the cause of the defect could turn out to be the fever or the infection, not the medication. Or, as some surmise may be the case with Provera, which has been used to prevent miscarriage, the malformations associated with its use may have nothing to do with the drug, but may show up only because the drug averted the miscarriage of an embryo that was blighted to begin with.

Is the Fetus Genetically Susceptible to the Teratogen? Just as not everybody exposed to cold germs succumbs, not every fetus who is exposed to a teratogen is affected by it.

When Was the Fetus Exposed to the Teratogen? The period of gestation during which most teratogens are capable of doing harm is very brief. For example, thalidomide caused no damage at all when taken after the 52nd day. Likewise, the rubella virus causes damage in less than 1% of fetuses if exposure takes place after the third month.

During the six to eight days after conception (before a woman has even missed her period), the fertilized egg, or conceptus, which expands into a ball of cells and travels down the fallopian tubes to the uterus, is largely insensitive to assault from what passes through its mother's system, and rarely suffers malformation. In fact, if it does sustain a minor injury, it has the ability to repair itself. The only risk at this point is that the conceptus will fail to survive because of a genetic mistake or that it will be destroyed by certain external factors, such as a very powerful dose of radiation.

The period during which the organs are being formed—from implantation of the conceptus in the uterus around days six to eight through the end of the first trimester—is the interval when the risk of malformation is greatest. After the third month, the risk of this kind of injury is greatly reduced; any damage that does occur usually affects the rate of growth of the fetus or its central nervous system.

How Much Exposure Was There? Most teratogenic effects are dose-related. One brief diagnostic x-ray will be unlikely to cause a problem. A series of heavy-dose radiation treatments could. Smoking lightly for the first few months is not likely to harm a fetus; heavy smoking for the entire pregnancy increases certain risks very significantly.

What Is the Mother's General Nutritional Status? Animal experiments show that defects apparently caused by a drug were, in some cases, actually caused by poor nutrition; the drug only reduced appetite, and thus water and food intake. Just as you will resist a cold virus more effectively if you are well nourished and not run-down, so will your fetus resist teratogens better if he or she is well nourished—through you, of course.

Was the Mother Affected by the Exposure? It's reassuring to know that chemical exposure that isn't toxic enough to cause symptoms in the mother usually is not toxic enough to cause problems in the fetus.

Are Several Factors Combining to Increase Risk? The trio of poor diet, smoking, and alcohol abuse, the duet of smoking and tranquilizers, and other "losing combinations" can greatly increase risk.

Is Some Unknown Protective Factor in Play? Even when all factors appear identical, not all fetuses are affected in the same way. In experiments with mouse fetuses of identical genetic strains who were exposed to the same teratogens at identical stages in development and at identical dosages, only 1 in 9 was born malformed. No one knows exactly why, though perhaps someday medical science will come up with the solution to this mystery.

WEIGHING RISK VS. BENEFIT

Should today's pregnant woman fear for her baby's life and well-being because he or she is developing in a world filled with environmental threats? Absolutely not—and for several reasons. First of all, drugs and other environmental factors account for less than 1% of all birth defects—and birth defects affect only 3% to 4% of all newborns. The general risk is extremely slight, even if you have already been exposed to a specific teratogen. Second, if you haven't, knowing what the risks are can help you to avoid them, improving your baby's odds still more. Third, in spite of the dire warnings making headlines and highlighting news programs daily, never have the chances of having a healthy, normal baby been better.

Of course, no decision is totally without risk. But when making choices, we need to learn to weigh risks against benefits. This is never more important than during pregnancy, when each decision potentially affects the safety and well-being of not one but two lives. When you're faced with the decision of whether or not to smoke, to have a before-dinner cocktail, to nibble on a chocolate bar instead of an apple while watching TV, you should weigh risk against benefit. Are the benefits, if any, you are going to derive from smoking, drinking, or junk-food snacking worth the risks to your baby?

Well, most of the time your answer will probably be no. But once in a while you may decide that a little risk will be worth it. One small glass of wine, for example, to toast your anniversary: the risk to your baby is practically nil, and the benefit (a more festive anniversary) is really important. Or a big chunk of sugar- and butter-rich cake for your birthday—a lot of empty calories, true. But they won't really deprive baby of necessary nutrients over the long run, and after all, it *is* your birthday.

Some risk vs. benefit decisions are easy. For instance, regular heavy alcohol consumption throughout pregnancy can handicap your child for life (see page 52). Giving up the pleasure you derive from drinking may take considerable effort, but the risks if you don't are clear.

Or say you have the flu and you are running a fever that's high enough to pose a threat to your baby. Your doctor won't hesitate to prescribe a safe medication to bring down the fever. In this case, the benefit of using the drug far outweighs its possible harm. On the other hand, if your temperature is only slightly elevated, it poses no threat to your baby and will actually help your body fight the flu virus. So before resorting to medication, your doctor will feel secure in giving your body a chance to cure itself, on the grounds that the possible risk of taking the drug outweighs its potential benefits.

Other decisions are not so clear-cut. What if you have a terrible cold with sinus headaches that have been keeping you up at night? Should you take a cold tablet to help you get some rest? Or should you suffer through sleepless nights, which won't do you or the baby any good? The best way to approach such decisions is:

❖ Determine if there are alternative lower-risk ways of obtaining the benefits you are seeking—perhaps through non-drug approaches (see Appendix). Try them. If they don't work, continue to evaluate your original option—in this case, cold tablets.

❖ Ask your physician about risks and benefits. It's important to remember that not all drugs are known to cause birth defects, and that many have been used safely in pregnancy. New studies are turning up more information on drug safety, or lack of it, daily. Your practitioner has access to this information.

❖ Do some research on your own. For the latest information on the safety of a particular drug during pregnancy, check with the Federal Drug Administration or the March of Dimes. (See Appendix.)

❖ Determine if there are ways of increasing the benefits and/or decreasing the risks (taking the safest, most effective pain reliever in the smallest effective doses for the shortest possible time), and try to ensure that if you do take the risk, you will receive the benefit (take your cold tablet before you go to bed, when you are most likely to get that needed rest).

❖ In consultation with your practitioner and, if necessary, a genetic counselor or maternal-fetal subspecialist, review all the information you've gathered—weighing risks against benefits—and make your decision.

During pregnancy you will be challenged to make intelligent decisions in dozens of situations, weighing risk against benefit. Almost every decision you make will impact on your chance of having a healthy baby. But an occasional wrong choice isn't likely to be catastrophic—it will change the odds only very slightly. If you've already made a few not-so-terrific choices and there's no way to undo them, forget them. Just try to make better decisions for the rest of your pregnancy. And remember, the odds are very much in your baby's favor!

4
The Best-Odds Diet

There's a tiny new being developing inside you. The odds are already fairly good that he or she will be born healthy. But you have the chance to improve those odds significantly—to come as close as possible to guaranteeing your baby not just good health, but excellent health—with every bite of food you put in your mouth.

That's not just idle theory. A study done at the Harvard School of Public Health dramatically illustrates how closely the state of a baby's health at birth is tied to its mother's diet during pregnancy. Of the women in the study whose diets were good to excellent, fully 95% had babies in good or excellent health. On the other hand, only 8% of women whose diets were really awful (composed largely of junk foods) had babies in good or excellent health, and 65% of them had infants who were stillborn, premature, functionally immature, or who had congenital defects.

Of course, the diets of most of the women in the study (like those of most pregnant women) were neither excellent nor extremely poor. They were average, and so was the health of their children. Eighty-eight percent had babies in good or fair health. But only 6% had infants in really excellent health—which is, after all, what most of us want for our children.

Other studies, too, have shown that what a pregnant woman eats or does not eat can have an effect on her developing fetus. For example, lack of folic acid just before conception and early in pregnancy can increase the risk of spinal tube defects and possibly lip and palate deformities; lack of protein and calories in the last trimester can interfere with brain development. Inadequate food intake or the wrong kinds of food can retard fetal growth.

Research also shows that her eating habits can have an effect on the course of her pregnancy (some complications, such as anemia and pre-eclampsia, are more common among poorly nourished women); her comfort (fatigue, morning sickness, constipation, leg cramps, and a host of other pregnancy symptoms can be minimized or avoided altogether with good diet); her labor and delivery (in general, women on excellent diets are less likely than women on poor diets to deliver too early; specifically, deficiency in zinc has been linked to an increased risk of premature labor); her emotional state (good diet can help to moderate mood swings); and her postpartum recovery (a well-nourished body can bounce back faster and more easily, and weight that's been gained at a sensible rate and on nutritious foods can be shed more quickly).

If your eating habits aren't that disciplined or virtuous to begin with, following the Best-Odds Diet will probably present you with quite a challenge. But when you consider the result of your extra efforts—better odds that your baby will be born in excellent health and better odds that you'll recover faster from pregnancy and delivery—we think you'll agree that it's a challenge worth accepting.

NINE BASIC PRINCIPLES FOR NINE MONTHS OF HEALTHY EATING

Every Bite Counts. You've got only nine months of meals and snacks with which to give your baby the best possible start in life. Make every one of them count. Before you close your mouth on a forkful of food, consider, "Is this the best bite I can give my baby?" If it will benefit your baby, chew away. If it'll only benefit your sweet tooth or appease your appetite, put your fork down.

All Calories Are Not Created Equal. For example, the 150 calories in a doughnut are not equal to the 150 calories in a whole-grain, juice-sweetened bran muffin. Nor are the 100 calories in ten potato chips equal to the 100 in a baked potato served in its skin (or in a batch of Best-Odds Fries; see page 93). So choose your calories with care, selecting quality over quantity. Your baby will benefit a lot more from 2,000 nutrient-rich calories daily than from 4,000 mostly empty ones.

Starve Yourself, Starve Your Baby. Just as you wouldn't consider starving your baby after it's born, you shouldn't consider starving it in utero. The fetus can't thrive living off your flesh, no matter how ample. It needs regular nourishment at regular inter-

vals. Never, never skip a meal.[1] Even if you're not hungry, the baby is. If persistent heartburn or a constant bloated feeling is spoiling your appetite, spread your daily requirements out over six small meals instead of three large ones.

Efficiency Is Effective. Fill your daily nutritional requirements in the most efficient way possible within your caloric needs. Eating 6 tablespoons of peanut butter (if you can get it down) at 600 calories, or about 25% of your daily allotment, is a considerably less efficient way of getting 25 grams of protein than eating 3½ ounces of water-packed tuna at 125 calories. And eating a cup and a half of ice cream (about 450 calories) is a far less efficient way of getting 300 milligrams of calcium than drinking a glass of skim milk (90 calories) or eating a cup of nonfat yogurt (100 calories). Fat, because it has more than twice as many calories per gram as either proteins or carbohydrates, is a particularly inefficient source of calories. Choose lean meats over fatty ones, low-fat milk and dairy products over full-fat, broiled foods over fried; spread butter lightly; sauté in a teaspoon of fat, not a quarter of a cup.

Efficiency is important, too, if you're having trouble gaining enough weight. To start tipping the scale toward a healthier weight gain, choose foods that are dense in nutrients and calories—avocados, nuts, and dried fruits, for instance—that can fill you and your baby out without filling you up too much. And avoid such calorie bargains as popcorn and large salads, which will do just the opposite.

---

1. Never fast during pregnancy, either. An Israeli study shows a jump in deliveries just after Yom Kippur, the Day of Atonement, suggesting that fasting late in pregnancy could trigger labor.

Whether you are trying to gain less or gain more, or just trying to squeeze your Daily Dozen into a queasy, upset, or too-full tummy, whenever possible opt for foods that efficiently fulfill two or more requirements with one serving—for example, broccoli (Vitamin C, Green Leafy, and Calcium); yogurt or canned salmon (Protein and Calcium); dried apricots (Yellow Fruits and Iron). (The Daily Dozen requirements are described beginning on page 83.)

Carbohydrates Are a Complex Issue. Some women concerned about gaining too much weight during pregnancy mistakenly drop carbohydrates from their diets like so many hot potatoes. True, refined and/or simple carbohydrates (like white bread, white rice, refined cereals, cakes, cookies, pretzels, sugars, syrups) are nutritionally weak —supplying little but calories. But unrefined and/or complex carbohydrates (whole-grain breads and cereals, brown rice, vegetables, dried beans and peas, and, of course, hot potatoes—especially in their skins) and fresh fruit supply essential B vitamins, trace minerals, protein, and important fiber. Good not only for your baby, but for you. They'll help keep nausea and constipation in check, and because they are filling and fiber-rich but not fattening (as long as they're not bathed in buttery sauces or slathered with rich toppings), they'll help keep your weight gain in check, too. Recent research suggests yet another bonus for complex carbohydrate eaters: consuming plenty of fiber may reduce the risk of developing gestational diabetes. *Note:* Move from a low-fiber to a high-fiber diet slowly.

Sweet Nothings: Nothing But Trouble. No calorie is as empty, and therefore as wasted, as a calorie of sugar. In addition, researchers are finding that sugar may be not only void of value, but harmful. Research suggests that, in addition to causing tooth decay, it may be implicated in diabetes, heart disease, depression, and in some cases of hyperactivity. Perhaps the worst thing about sugar is that it is most often found in foods that are on the whole nutritionally bankrupt: sweets and baked goods made with bleached white flour and excessive quantities of unhealthy fats. Sugar substitutes (even aspartame, which is believed to be safe for use in pregnancy; see page 62) are a questionable replacement for all the sugar the average pregnant woman is used to consuming, partly because these sweeteners, too, are often found in less-than-best foods.

For delicious *and* nutritious sweetness, substitute fruit and fruit juice concentrates (undiluted frozen juices) for sugar. They are about as sweet as sugar but contain more vitamins and trace minerals. Products sweetened with them are almost invariably made with whole grains and healthy fats and without questionable chemical additives. Make your own at home, using recipes such as those found in this chapter, or choose from the increasingly abundant selection available in health food stores and supermarkets. But read labels to be sure that the fruit sweeteners have not simply replaced the sugar in what is otherwise a poor food choice.

The Best-Odds Diet recommends limiting refined sugars (brown, white, turbinado, honey, maple syrup, corn syrup, fructose, and so on) during pregnancy to an occasional special-occasion fling. Every sugar calorie can better come from foods that yield a higher nutritional return for baby.

Good Foods Remember Where They Came From. If your green beans haven't seen their native fields for months (having been boiled, processed, preserved, and canned since harvesting), they probably don't have much of their natural goodness left to offer you or your baby. Choose fresh vegetables and fruits when they're in season, or fresh-frozen when fresh are unavailable or you don't have time to prepare them (they're as nutritious as fresh because they're frozen immediately after harvesting). Try to eat some raw vegetables and/or fruit every day. When cooking vegetables, steam or stir-fry them lightly, so they'll retain their vitamins and minerals. Poach fruits in juice with no sugar added. Avoid prepared foods that have picked up a lot of chemicals, sugar, and salt on the assembly line; they're frequently low in nutrition. Choose a fresh chicken breast over processed chicken roll; a casserole made from fresh ingredients rather than a dehydrated mix of overprocessed ingredients and chemicals; fresh oatmeal made from rolled oats (you can flavor it with cinnamon and chopped dried fruit) rather than the sugared instant varieties.

Healthful Eating Should Be a Family Affair. If there are subversive elements at home, urging you to bake chocolate chip cookies or to add potato chips to your shopping list, it's a sure bet that the Best-Odds Diet won't stand a chance. So make other family members your allies by putting the whole household on the diet with you. Bake naturally sweet Fruity Oatmeal Cookies (page 96) instead of chocolate chip; bring home whole-wheat pretzels or toasted sunflower seeds instead of potato chips. In addition to a healthier baby and a relatively slimmer you, there will be the postpartum bonus of a fitter, trimmer husband and older children (if you have them) with better eating habits. Continue the Best-Odds Diet for the whole family after delivery and you will be giving each member—particularly that important newest member—the best odds for a longer and healthier life.

Bad Habits Can Sabotage a Good Diet. The best prenatal diet in the world is easily undermined if the expectant mother fails to heed the advice to eliminate alcohol, tobacco, and other unsafe drugs from her life. Read about these saboteurs in Chapter 3, and if you haven't done so already, change your habits accordingly.

THE BEST-ODDS DAILY DOZEN

Calories. The old adage that a pregnant woman is eating for two is true. But it's important to remember that one of the two is a tiny developing fetus whose caloric needs are significantly lower than yours—a mere 300 a day, more or less. So, if you're of average weight, you need only about 300 calories more than was necessary to maintain your prepregnancy weight.[2] During the first trimester you may need fewer than 300 extra calories daily, unless you're trying to compensate for starting out underweight. As your metabolism speeds up later in pregnancy, you may need somewhat more than 300 extra calories daily. In spite of the numerous pregnancy diets you may see that seem to recommend you eat enough food to feed a family of four, consuming calories beyond what your baby needs for growth and what you need for baby-making is not only unnecessary but unwise. Eating fewer calories, on the other hand, is

2. To determine roughly how many calories you need to maintain your prepregnancy weight, multiply that weight by 12 if you're sedentary, 15 if you're moderately active, and up to 22 if you're very active. Because the rate at which calories are burned varies from person to person even during pregnancy, calorie requirements vary too, so the figure you arrive at is just an estimate.

not only unwise but potentially dangerous; women who don't take in sufficient calories during pregnancy—particularly in the second and third trimesters—can seriously hamper the development of their babies.

There are four exceptions to this basic formula. In each of these cases the expectant mother should discuss her caloric needs with her practitioner: the overweight woman, who, with proper nutritional guidance, can possibly do with fewer calories; the seriously underweight woman, who certainly needs more; the adolescent, who is still growing herself and has special nutritional needs; and the woman carrying multiple fetuses, who will have to add 300 calories for each of them.

Having to eat 300 extra calories a day sounds like a food lover's fantasy, but sad to say, it isn't. By the time you've guzzled your four glasses of milk (total of 380 calories for skim) or the equivalent in calcium-rich foods and taken your required extra servings of protein, you've exceeded your allowance. Which means that instead of adding tantalizing frills, you'll probably have to cut out those you're accustomed to in order to nourish your baby adequately and keep your weight gain reasonable. To make sure you get the maximum nutritional punch out of your calories, become a dietary efficiency expert (see page 81).

But while calories count during pregnancy, they don't have to be counted. Instead of concerning yourself with complicated computations at every meal, step on a reliable scale once a week to check your progress. Weigh yourself at the same time of day, naked or wearing the same clothing (or clothing that weighs about the same), so that your calculations won't be thrown off by a heavy meal one week or a heavy sweater the next. If your weight gain is going according to schedule (an average of about 1 pound a week in the second and third trimesters; see page 147), you're getting the right number of calories. If it's less than that, you're getting too few; if it's more than that, you're getting too many. Maintain or adjust your food energy intake as necessary, but be certain you never cut out required nutrients along with calories. And continue to weigh yourself weekly to make sure you stay on track.

Protein: four servings daily. Protein is composed of substances called amino acids, which are the building blocks of human cells; they are particularly important in building the cells of a new baby. Research has shown that inadequate protein intake in expectant mothers, like inadequate calorie intake, can result in babies being smaller than normal at birth. Therefore, the pregnant woman should aim to have at least 60 to 75 grams of protein every day. It's possible that 100 grams, the amount often recommended in high-risk pregnancies, may be a better goal since the increased intake may help prevent a pregnancy from becoming high risk in the first place.[3] Though a goal of 100 grams of protein may seem like a lot, most Americans consume that much or more per day. To get your 100 grams, all you have to do is eat a total of four servings of Protein Foods from the Best-Odds Food Selection Groups (see page 89). When tallying your protein servings, don't forget to count the protein found in many high-calcium foods: a glass of milk and an ounce of cheese each provide a third of a protein serving; a cup of yogurt equals

3. Women who are not taking in an adequate amount of calories (perhaps because of nausea and vomiting) need a greater protein intake so that there is enough both for energy and for baby-building purposes. They should be sure to get at least four servings daily.

half a serving; 4 ounces of canned salmon, a whole serving.

If at the end of the day you come up a half or even a whole serving short, you can meet your quota quickly with a high-protein bedtime snack. For example, try egg salad (half a protein serving when made with 1 egg and 2 egg whites) with whole-wheat crackers; a Double-the-Milk Shake (two-thirds of a protein serving; see page 95); or ¾ cup of low-fat cottage cheese (a full protein serving) garnished either with fresh fruit, raisins, and cinnamon or chopped tomato and basil. *Do not,* however, use liquid or powdered high-protein supplements to help fill your protein requirement—they could be harmful.

Vitamin C Foods: two servings daily.

You and baby both need vitamin C for tissue repair, wound healing, and various other metabolic (nutrient-utilizing) processes. Your baby also needs it for proper growth and for the development of strong bones and teeth. Vitamin C is a nutrient the body can't store, so a fresh supply is needed every day. Vitamin C–rich foods are best eaten fresh and uncooked, as exposure to light, heat, and air destroys the vitamin over time. As you can see from the list of Vitamin C Foods on page 90, the old standby orange juice is far from the only, or even the best, source of this essential vitamin.

Calcium Foods: four servings daily.

Back in elementary school you probably learned that growing children need plenty of calcium for strong bones and teeth. Well, so do growing fetuses on their way to becoming growing children. Calcium is also vital for muscle, heart, and nerve development, blood clotting, and enzyme activity. But it's not only your baby who stands to lose when you don't get enough calcium. If incoming supplies are inadequate, your baby-making fac-tory will draw upon the calcium in your own bones to help meet its quota, setting you up for osteoporosis later in life. Still another reason to drink your milk (or take your calcium in other forms) is the recent research indicating that a high calcium intake may help prevent pregnancy-induced hypertension (preeclampsia).

So be diligent about getting your four servings of calcium-rich foods a day. And don't worry if the idea of four glasses of milk doesn't appeal to you. Calcium doesn't have to be served in glasses at all. It can be served up as a cup of yogurt, a piece of cheese, or a large portion of cottage cheese. It can be disguised in soups, casseroles, breads, cereals, desserts; this is especially easy when it's in the form of nonfat dry milk or evaporated skim milk (⅓ cup and ½ cup, respectively, measure up to a full glass of liquid milk, or one Calcium serving). And if you do opt for the glass, you can double the calcium power in each one by stirring in ⅓ cup of nonfat dry milk (see Double-the-Milk Shake, page 95). For those who can't tolerate or don't eat milk products at all, calcium can also come in nondairy form. The Calcium-Rich Foods listing on page 90 provides a variety of nondairy equivalents.

For those who cannot be sure of getting enough calcium from their diets (such as vegetarians or the lactose-intolerant), a calcium supplement may be recommended.

Green Leafy and Yellow Vegetables and Yellow Fruits: three servings daily, or more.

These bunny-set favorites supply the vitamin A, in the form of beta-carotene, that is vital for cell growth (your baby's cells are multiplying at a fantastic rate), healthy skin, bones, and eyes, and may even reduce the risk of some types of cancer. The green leafies and yellows also deliver doses of essential vitamins (vitamin E, riboflavin, folic acid, B₆), numerous minerals (many green leafies provide a good deal of calcium as well as trace minerals), and constipation-fighting fiber. A bountiful selection of nature's most efficient sources of vitamin A can be found in the Green Leafy and Yellow Vegetables and Yellow Fruits list on page 91. Those with an anti-vegetable bent may be surprised to discover that carrots and spinach are not the only sources of vitamin A and, in fact, that the vitamin comes packaged in some of nature's most tempting sweet offerings—dried apricots, yellow peaches, cantaloupe, and mangoes, for example. And those who like to drink their vegetables may be happy to know that they can occasionally count a glass of vegetable juice cocktail toward their Green Leafy and Yellow allowance.

Other Fruits and Vegetables: two servings daily, or more. In addition to produce rich in beta-carotene-vitamin A and vitamin C, you need at least two other types of fruit or vegetable daily—for extra fiber, vitamins, and minerals. Many of these are rich in potassium and/or magnesium, both of which are important to good pregnancy health, and in boron, the importance of which is only beginning to be understood. A variety of these fruits and vegetables are suggested on page 91.

Whole Grains and Legumes: six to eleven servings a day. Whole grains (whole wheat, oats, rye, barley, corn, rice, millet, triticale, soy, and so on) and legumes (dried peas and beans) are packed with nutrients, particularly the B vitamins that are needed for just about every part of your developing baby's body. These concentrated complex carbohydrates are also rich in trace minerals, such as zinc, selenium, and magnesium, which have been shown to be very significant in preg-

nancy. Starchy foods may also help reduce morning sickness.

Though these staff-of-life foods have many nutrients in common, each has its own strengths. To get the maximum benefit, include a variety of complex carbohydrates in your diet. Be adventurous: Bread your fish with oat bran seasoned with herbs and Parmesan cheese. Add triticale to your rice pilaf. Use rolled barley in your favorite oatmeal cookie recipe. Substitute navy beans for limas in your soup.

Don't count refined grains (breads or cereals made with white flour, for example) as meeting this requirement on a regular basis. Even if they are "enriched," they are still lacking in the fiber and in more than a dozen vitamins and trace minerals that are found in the originals.

Iron-Rich Foods: some daily. Since large amounts of iron are essential for the developing blood supply of the fetus and for your own expanding blood supply, you'll need more during these nine months than at any other time in your life. Get as much of your iron as you can from your diet (see the list on page 92). Eating foods rich in vitamin C at the same sitting as iron-rich foods will increase the absorption of the mineral by the body.

Because it's often difficult to fill the pregnancy iron requirement through diet alone, it is recommended that, from about the 12th week on, pregnant women take a daily supplement of 30 milligrams of ferrous iron. To enhance the absorption of the iron in the supplement, it should be taken between meals with a fruit juice rich in vitamin C or with water (but not with milk, tea, or coffee). If a pregnant woman's iron stores are low, 60 to 120 milligrams may be prescribed by her practitioner.

High-Fat Foods: four full or eight half servings, or an equivalent combina-

tion daily. According to generally accepted nutritional guidelines, no more than 30% of an adult's calories should come from fat (in the average American diet, 40% of calories come from fat). The same guidelines apply to pregnant adults. That means that if you weigh about 125 pounds and need about 2,100 calories a day (see page 83 and the Appendix if you weigh more or less), no more than 630 of these should come from fat. Since it takes only 70 grams of fat (as much as you would find in a hefty slice of quiche) to reach 630 calories, this requirement is definitely the easiest to fill—and the easiest to overfill. And though there's no harm in having a couple of extra Green Leafies or Vitamin C foods, or even additional Whole Grains or Calcium foods, excess fat servings could spell excess pounds. Still, while keeping fat intake moderate is a good idea, eliminating all fat from your diet is a potentially dangerous one. Fat is vital to your developing baby; the essential fatty acids in them are just that—essential. Crucial in the ninth month are omega-3 fatty acids (in salmon, flax seed, sardines).

Keep track of your fat intake; fill your daily quota but don't exceed it. Don't forget that the fat used in cooking and preparing foods counts, too. If you've fried your eggs in ½ tablespoon of margarine (½ a serving) and mashed your tuna with a tablespoon of mayonnaise (1 serving), include these amounts in your daily tally.

If you're not gaining enough weight, and increasing your intake of other nutritious foods is not effective, try adding one extra fat serving each day (but no more); the concentrated calories it provides may help you hit your optimum weight gain stride.

For information on cholesterol in pregnancy, see page 126.

Salty Foods: in moderation. At one time, the medical establishment pre- scribed limiting salt (sodium chloride) during pregnancy because it contributed to water retention and bloating. Now it is believed that some increase in body fluids in pregnancy is necessary and normal, and that a moderate amount of sodium is needed to maintain adequate fluid levels. Still, very large quantities of salt and very salty foods (such as pickles, soy sauce, and potato chips) aren't good for anyone, pregnant or not. High sodium intake is closely linked to high blood pressure, a condition that can cause a variety of potentially dangerous complications in pregnancy, labor, and delivery. Though iodine deficiency is not a problem in the United States, you may want to use iodized salt to be sure that you meet the increased need for iodine in pregnancy. As a general rule, rather than adding salt during cooking, salt your food to taste at the table.

Fluids: at least eight 8-ounce glasses daily. You're not only eating for two, you're drinking for two. If you've always been one of those people who goes through the day with barely a sip of anything, now's the time to change. As body fluids increase during pregnancy, so does your need for fluid intake. Your fetus, too, needs fluids. Most of its body, like yours, is composed of water. Extra fluids also help keep your skin soft, lessen the likelihood of constipation, rid your body of toxins and waste products, and reduce excessive swelling and the risk of urinary tract infection. Be sure to get at least 8 cups (2 quarts) a day—more if you're retaining a lot of fluid (paradoxically, a plentiful fluid intake can flush out excess fluids) or it's very hot (dehydration may increase preterm labor risk). Of course, all your water doesn't have to come from the tap. You can count milk (which is two-thirds water), fruit and vegetable juices, soups, caffeine- and sugar-free soft drinks, and bottled plain and sparkling water. Limit caloric fluids, however, or you may end up with too many calories each day.

Using 12-ounce glasses or mugs each time you take a drink will give you 1½ cups of fluid at a shot and mean fewer refills. Spread your fluid intake out over the day, and don't try to drink more than two glassfuls at a sitting—which could dilute your blood excessively, causing a chemical imbalance.

Nutritional Supplements: a pregnancy formula taken daily. Vitamin supplements have always generated controversy in the scientific community. The controversy surrounding prenatal vitamin supplements has now intensified with a statement from the National Academy of Sciences, which concluded that there is currently insufficient evidence to encourage routine use of supplements (except for 30

What's in a Pill?

There are no standards set either by the FDA or by the American College of Obstetricians and Gynecologists specifying exactly what must be in a pill for it to be called a prenatal supplement. So selecting the right formula can be complicated. Often a practitioner will prescribe a supplement, and in general prescribed formulas are superior to those bought over the counter.

If you are selecting a vitamin/mineral supplement yourself, look for a formula that contains:

❖ No more than 4,000 or 5,000 IU of vitamin A; amounts over 10,000 IU can be toxic. Beta-carotene form is safer.

❖ 800 to 1,000 mcg (1 mg) of folic acid.

❖ No more than 400 IU of vitamin D.

❖ 200 to 300 mg calcium. If you're not getting high calcium foods, you will need additional supplementation to reach the 1,200 mg RDA. Do not take more than 250 mg of calcium (or more than 25 mg of magnesium) *along with* supplementary iron since these minerals interfere with iron absorption. Take any larger doses at least two hours before or after your iron supplement.

❖ Approximately the RDA for vitamin C (70 mg); thiamine (1.5 mg); riboflavin (1.6 mg); pyridoxine (B_6; 2.6 mg); niacinamide (17 mg); vitamin B_{12} (2.2); vitamin E (10 mg). Most formulas contain 2 to 3 times the RDA of these; there are no known harmful effects from such doses.

❖ Approximately the RDA for zinc (15 mg) and iron (30 mg elemental).* More iron may be prescribed if you are anemic.

❖ Some preparations may also contain magnesium, copper, biotin, and/or pantothenic acid. Such trace minerals as chromium, manganese, and molybdenum are rarely found in pregnancy supplements.

---

*Copper is necessary in any supplement containing zinc, since zinc can interfere with the body's absorption of copper, increasing the need for this mineral. Zinc and copper are both necessary in a supplement containing iron, since the iron may interfere with their absorption. Zinc is also necessary if you are taking large doses (1,200 to 1,500 mg) of calcium.

milligrams of iron) for all pregnant women. The Academy urged more research to see if supplementation with certain vitamins and minerals could indeed be valuable for everyone. But for the present, they recommend that physicians carefully evaluate the diet of each patient and prescribe supplements only when they determine that the diet is lacking—with routine supplementation limited to those at nutritional high risk, including vegetarians, women carrying more than one fetus, heavy smokers, and alcohol and drug abusers.

The theory that a healthy pregnant woman can get virtually all of her nutritional requirements at the kitchen table is a common one. And, indeed, she could—if she lived in a laboratory where her food was prepared to ensure retention of vitamins and minerals and measured to ensure an adequate daily intake, if she never ate on the run or felt too sick to eat, if she always knew for sure that she was carrying only one baby and that her pregnancy wouldn't turn out to be high-risk. But in the real world, a nutritional supplement provides extra health insurance—and women who like to play it safe may feel safer with such insurance.

Still, a supplement is just a *supplement*. No pill, no matter how complete, can replace a good diet. It's very important that most of your vitamins and minerals come from foods, because that is the way nutrients can be most effectively utilized. Fresh foods (not processed) contain not only nutrients that we know about, and that can be synthesized in a pill, but probably a great many others that are as yet undiscovered. Thirty years ago, a prenatal supplement didn't contain zinc and the other trace minerals we now know to be necessary to good health. But whole-wheat bread has always contained it. Likewise, food supplies fiber and water (fruits and vegetables are loaded with both) and important calories and protein—none of which come packaged in a pill. (Incidentally, beware of those pills claiming to be equivalent to daily vegetable requirements—those claims are totally fraudulent.)

And don't think that because a little is good, a lot is better. Vitamins and minerals at high doses act as drugs in the body and should be treated as drugs, especially by expectant moms; a few, such as vitamins A and D, are toxic at levels not much beyond the RDA (recommended daily allowance).[4] Any supplementation beyond the RDA should be taken only under medical supervision, when benefits outweigh risks.

THE BEST-ODDS DIET FOOD SELECTION GROUPS

Many foods fill more than one nutritional requirement, so Food Selection Groups may overlap. The same three glasses of milk, for example, will give you three Calcium and one Protein serving.

PROTEIN FOODS

Every day have four of the following, or a combination equivalent to four servings. Servings contain between 18 and 25 grams of protein, and you should consume 75 to 100 grams a day.

3 8-ounce glasses of skim or low-fat milk or low-fat buttermilk

4. Getting more than the RDA of such vitamins from your daily diet, however, is not considered dangerous.

¾ cup low-fat cottage cheese
1¾ cups low-fat yogurt
1¾ ounces (½ cup) Parmesan cheese
2½ ounces Edam cheese
3 ounces Swiss or Cheddar cheese or low-fat cheese
5 large egg whites
2 large whole eggs, plus 2 egg whites
3½ ounces tuna
2½ ounces white meat chicken or turkey, without skin
3½ ounces fish or shrimp
5 ounces clams, crab, or lobster meat
3 ounces lean beef, lamb, or pork, or dark meat chicken
3 ounces veal
4 ounces fatty beef or lamb
3 ounces liver (use infrequently)
5 or 6 ounces tofu (bean curd)
Texturized vegetable protein[5]
1 serving of a complete protein combination (see box, page 97)

HIGH-PROTEIN SNACKS

Nuts and seeds
Whole-grain baked goods
Soy baked goods
Yogurt
Hard cheese
Hard-cooked eggs
Wheat germ

VITAMIN C FOODS

Have at least two Vitamin C foods, or a combination equal to two, every day. Your body can't store this vitamin, so don't skip a day.

½ grapefruit

½ cup grapefruit juice
2 small oranges
½ cup orange juice
2 tablespoons orange juice concentrate
½ medium mango
½ cup cubed papaya
¼ small cantaloupe
½ cup strawberries
1⅓ cup blackberries or raspberries
1½ large tomatoes
1 cup tomato juice
¾ cups vegetable juice (V-8)
1½ cups shredded raw cabbage or coleslaw
½ small red or green pepper
⅔ cup cooked broccoli
¾ cup cooked cauliflower
¾ cup cooked fresh kale
1 cup collard greens, frozen chopped
¾ cup cooked kohlrabi
3 cups raw spinach

CALCIUM-RICH FOODS

Take four servings of these foods daily, or any combination that is equivalent to four servings. You need 1,280 to 1,300 milligrams of calcium daily. Each serving contains about 300 milligrams of calcium.

8 ounces skim or 1% milk or low-fat buttermilk[6]
½ cup evaporated skim or low-fat milk
1¾ cups low-fat cottage cheese
1½ ounces Cheddar or American cheese
1¼ ounces Swiss cheese
1 cup low-fat or nonfat plain yogurt
⅓ cup nonfat dry milk
6 ounces calcium-added mild

---

5. Recipes vary; some have a high protein/calorie ratio, others low, so read nutrition labels, remembering that 20 to 25 grams of protein equals 1 Protein serving.

6. Stick to non-fat or 1% milk; drinking 3 or more glasses of *whole* milk daily may be linked to preeclampsia (see page 351). Use lactose-reduced milk if you are lactose intolerant.

6 ounces calcium-added orange juice
4 ounces canned salmon with bones
3 ounces canned sardines with bones
3½ ounces canned Pacific mackerel
  with bones
2 to 3 tablespoons ground sesame
  seeds
Soy milk and soy protein[7]
1 cup collard greens
1½ cups cooked kale
1½ cups cooked mustard or turnip
  greens
1¾ cups broccoli
2½ tablespoons blackstrap molasses
2 corn tortillas
10 dried figs
3 cups cooked dried beans (Great
  Northern, navy, pinto)

CALCIUM-RICH SNACKS

Almonds, filberts, peanuts
Dried fruit
Baked goods made with sesame seeds,
  soy flour, or carob

GREEN LEAFY AND YELLOW VEGETABLES AND YELLOW FRUITS

You need three or more servings a day, one of which should be raw. Try to choose some yellow and some green daily.

⅛ cantaloupe (about 5 inches long)
2 large fresh or dried apricots
½ medium mango
1 large nectarine or yellow peach

1 cup cubed papaya
½ medium persimmon
1 tablespoon canned unsweetened
  pumpkin
⅓ cup cooked beet greens
¾ cup cooked broccoli or turnip
  greens
½ raw carrot, or ⅓ cup cooked
½ cup cooked collard greens
1½ cups endive or escarole
⅓ cup cooked kale or mustard greens
8 to 10 large leaves dark green leafy
  lettuce
½ cup raw spinach, or ¼ cup cooked
¼ cup cooked winter squash
¼ small sweet potato or yam
⅓ cup cooked Swiss chard

OTHER FRUITS AND VEGETABLES

Have at least two of the following daily.

1 apple or ½ cup unsweetened applesauce
6 to 7 asparagus spears
1 small banana
1 cup bean sprouts
¾ cup green beans
⅔ cup blueberries or lingonberries
⅔ cup Brussels sprouts
⅔ cup pitted fresh cherries
⅔ cup grapes
1 cup fresh mushrooms
1 medium white peach
9 pods okra
½ cup parsley
1 medium pear
1 medium slice fresh or unsweetened
  canned pineapple
1 medium potato
⅔ cup zucchini

WHOLE GRAINS AND LEGUMES

Have six to eleven of the following every day, closer to six if you are

7. Soy formulas vary; check the nutrition label to determine calcium equivalents, keeping in mind that 1 Calcium serving is equal to about 300 milligrams.

gaining quickly, closer to eleven if you are gaining slowly:

1 slice whole-wheat, whole-rye, other whole-grain or soy bread
½ cup cooked brown rice
½ cup cooked wild rice
½ cup cooked whole-grain cereal (oatmeal, Wheatena, Ralston)
1 ounce whole-grain ready-to-eat cereal with no added sugar (shredded wheat, some health food brands)
2 tablespoons wheat germ
½ cup cooked millet, bulgur, triticale, or kasha (buckwheat groats)
½ cup cooked whole-grain, soy, or high-protein-type pasta
2 x 2 x 1-inch cornbread (made with nondegerminated meal)
½ cup cooked beans or peas
1 corn or whole-wheat tortilla

IRON-RICH FOODS

Small amounts of iron are found in most of the fruits, vegetables, grains, and meats you eat every day. But try to have some of the following higher-iron-content foods daily, along with your supplement.

Duck
Beef
Liver and other organ meats (choose infrequently)
Oysters (cooked; don't eat raw)
Sardines
Collards, kale, and turnip greens
Jerusalem artichokes
Pumpkin
Potatoes in their skin
Spinach
Spirulina (seaweed)
Legumes (green peas, chick-peas, lentils, kidney and lima beans, for example)
Soybeans and soy products
Carob flour and carob powder
Blackstrap molasses
Dried fruits

HIGH-FAT FOODS

Have four full or eight half servings, or a combination, daily, if you weigh about 125 pounds (see Appendix if you weigh more or less). Do not exceed this quantity unless you are gaining weight too slowly (see page 147); do not reduce this quantity unless you are gaining weight too quickly. Prefer healthy fats over unhealthy fats (see page 126). On most days, no more than two servings should come from pure fats, such as butter, margarine, or oil.

Half Servings

1 ounce cheese (Swiss, Cheddar, provolone, mozzarella, blue, Camembert)
1½ ounces skim-milk mozzarella
2 tablespoons grated Parmesan cheese
1½ tablespoons light cream
1 tablespoon heavy, or whipping, cream
2 tablespoons whipped cream
2 rounded tablespoons sour cream
1 tablespoon cream cheese
1 cup whole milk
1½ cups 2% milk
⅔ cup whole evaporated milk
½ cup regular ice cream
1 cup whole-milk yogurt
1 tablespoon "light" margarine
1 tablespoon peanut butter
½ cup white sauce
⅓ cup hollandaise sauce
1 egg or 1 egg yolk
¼ small avocado
2 servings Best-Odds cake, cookies, or muffins
6 ounces tofu
7 ounces light-meat turkey or chicken, no skin
3½ ounces dark-meat turkey or chicken, no skin
4 ounces fresh or canned salmon
3 ounces canned tuna in oil

Full Servings[8]

1 tablespoon vegetable oil
1 tablespoon regular margarine or
butter

1 tablespoon regular mayonnaise
2 tablespoons regular salad dressing[9]
3 to 6 ounces lean meat (varies with
cut)
¾ cup tuna salad

BEST-ODDS RECIPES

Here are some recipes to pacify your sweet or snacking tooth and to give you a few cocktail or breakfast ideas. For more, see *What to Eat When You're Expecting.*

CREAM OF TOMATO SOUP

Makes 3 servings

> **1 tablespoon margarine or butter**
> **2 tablespoons whole-wheat flour**
> **1 ¾ cups evaporated skim milk**
> **3 cups tomato or vegetable juice**
> **¼ cup tomato paste**
> **Salt and pepper to taste**
> **Fresh or dried oregano and basil to taste (optional)**

Optional Garnishes
> **6 tablespoons cottage cheese (½ Protein serving) *or***
> **2 tablespoons grated Parmesan cheese (¼ Protein serving; ½ Calcium serv-**

ing) *or* 1 tablespoon wheat germ (½ Whole Grains serving)

1. In a saucepan, melt the margarine over low heat. Add the flour, and blend over very low heat for 2 minutes. Gradually blend in the milk and continue cooking over low heat, stirring occasionally, until thickened.

2. Stir in the juice, tomato paste, and seasonings until smooth. Continue cooking over low heat, stirring frequently, for 5 minutes.

3. Serve soup warm, topped with cottage cheese, Parmesan cheese, or wheat germ if desired.

1 serving = 1+ Calcium serving; 1 Vitamin C serving; 1 Green Leafy serving if vegetable juice is used.

BEST-ODDS FRIES

Makes 2 servings

> **1 ½ teaspoons vegetable oil**
> **2 large baking potatoes**
> **2 egg whites**
> **Kosher (coarse) salt and pepper to taste**

1. Preheat the oven to 425°F. Grease a nonstick baking sheet with the vegetable oil.

---

8. There are a great many other sources of fat in the diet, most of which add up very quickly and most of which do not fit into the Best-Odds mold. For example, you can get 1 Fat serving and very little nutrition from: 1 typical croissant, doughnut, brownie, or Danish pastry; 1 slice of apple or ½ slice of pecan pie; ½ of a fast-food burger or a small fried chicken drumstick; ¼ cup premium ice cream (16% butterfat); 4 small biscuits. Be wary.

---

9. Since the fat content of salad dressings varies, read the labels; each 14 grams of fat is 1 Fat serving. In homemade dressings, each tablespoon of oil is equal to 1 Fat serving.

2. Scrub the potatoes thoroughly under running water; pat dry. Slice them lengthwise into ¼-inch-thick slices, then cut into fries of the desired size. Pat the fries dry.

3. In a medium-size bowl, beat the egg whites with a whisk until foamy. Add the potatoes and toss until coated with the egg whites.

4. Arrange the fries in a single layer on the prepared baking sheet. Leave some space between them so they don't stick together. Bake until crisp and lightly brown and tender, 30 to 35 minutes. Sprinkle with salt and pepper, and serve immediately.

1 serving = 1 Other Vegetable serving

POWER-PACKED OATMEAL

Makes 1 serving

> 1 ¼ cups water
> ½ cup rolled oats
> 2 tablespoons wheat germ (if constipation is a problem, substitute unprocessed bran for all or part of wheat germ)
> Salt to taste (optional)
> ⅓ cup instant nonfat dry milk

1. Bring the water to a boil in a small saucepan. Add the oats, wheat germ, and salt, if desired, stirring to mix thoroughly. Lower the heat and cook 5 minutes or longer, according to desired texture, adding more water if necessary.

2. Remove the pan from the heat and stir in the dry milk. Serve immediately.

SWEET VARIATION: Add 2 tablespoons raisins and 1 tablespoon apple juice concentrate (or to taste) when you add the oats, or during the last minute of cooking if you like firmer raisins; add ground cinnamon and/or salt to taste

(both optional) when you add the milk.

SAVORY VARIATION: Add pepper, grated Parmesan or Cheddar cheese (½ ounce = ½ Calcium serving) when you add the milk.

1 serving = 1 Protein serving; 1 Whole Grains serving; 1 Calcium serving; high fiber.

BRAN MUFFINS

Makes 12 to 16 muffins

> Vegetable cooking spray
> ⅔ cup raisins
> 1 cup apple juice concentrate
> ¼ cup orange juice concentrate
> 1 ½ cups whole-wheat flour
> ½ cup wheat germ
> 1 ½ cups unprocessed bran
> 1 ¼ teaspoons baking soda
> ½ cup chopped nuts
> 1 teaspoon ground cinnamon (optional)
> 1 ½ cups low-fat buttermilk
> 2 egg whites, slightly beaten
> ⅓ cup instant nonfat dry milk
> 2 tablespoons margarine or butter, melted and cooled

1. Preheat the oven to 350°F. Lightly grease nonstick muffin tins with vegetable cooking spray.

2. In a small saucepan, combine the raisins, ¼ cup of the apple juice concentrate, and the orange juice concentrate. Simmer, stirring occasionally, for 5 minutes.

3. Blend in a mixing bowl the flour, wheat germ, bran, baking soda, chopped nuts, and cinnamon.

4. In a separate bowl, beat together the buttermilk, egg whites, dry milk, margarine, and remaining apple juice concentrate.

5. Combine the dry and liquid ingredients, blending thoroughly in a few strokes. Fold in the raisins with their cooking juice. Fill the prepared muffin tins, or paper muffin cups placed in regular tins, two-thirds full.

6. Bake until a toothpick inserted in the center of a muffin comes out clean, about 20 minutes.

VARIATION: Add 2 medium apples or pears, diced, along with the nuts. If constipation is no problem, substitute 1 cup oats, oat bran, or barley flakes for the unprocessed bran.

1 large muffin (12 in a recipe) = 1½ Whole Grains servings; ½ Protein serving; very high fiber. Fruit Variation adds 1 Other Fruit serving.

WHOLE-WHEAT BUTTERMILK PANCAKES

Makes approximately 12 pancakes (3 servings)

Note: Allow 1 hour preparation time for batter to settle.

> 1 cup low-fat buttermilk
> 1 teaspoon apple juice concentrate
> ¾ cup whole-wheat flour
> 5 tablespoons wheat germ
> ⅓ cup nonfat dry milk
> Dash of salt, or to taste (optional)
> Ground cinnamon to taste (optional)
> 2 teaspoons baking powder
> 2 large egg whites
> Margarine or butter

Optional Garnishes
> Unsweetened applesauce (1 Other Fruit serving)
> Unsweetened (fruit only) preserves or apple butter
> ½ cup low-fat yogurt (½ Calcium serving)

1. Purée in a blender all the ingredients except the egg whites, margarine, and the garnishes.

2. In a mixing bowl, beat the egg whites until stiff. Quickly beat the buttermilk-flour mixture into the egg whites. Let the batter stand for 1 hour.

3. Heat a nonstick skillet, and when it is hot, lightly brush it with margarine or butter. Stir the batter, and spoon it onto the skillet to make 3-inch pancakes. When the surface of the pancakes begins to bubble and the undersides are lightly browned, turn and brown the other side. Continue making pancakes, brushing on additional margarine between batches, until the batter is used up. Serve the pancakes with any or all of the garnishes.

VARIATIONS: Add to the batter any of the following: ¼ cup raisins (½ Other Fruit serving); 6 whole dried apricots, diced (some Iron; 1 Yellow Fruit serving); ½ banana, pear, or apple, sliced (½ Other Fruit serving); ¼ cup chopped nuts (¼ Fat serving; some Protein).

⅓ recipe = 1 Whole Grains serving; 1 Protein serving; ½ Calcium serving; high fiber.

DOUBLE-THE-MILK SHAKE

Makes 1 serving

Note: Freeze an overripe banana, peeled and wrapped, 12 to 24 hours before making this shake.

> 1 cup skim or low-fat milk
> ⅓ cup nonfat dry milk
> 1 frozen overripe banana, cut into chunks
> 1 teaspoon vanilla extract
> Dash of ground cinnamon, or to taste (optional)

Purée all the ingredients in a blender. Serve immediately.

BERRY VARIATION: Add ½ cup berries, fresh or unsweetened frozen, and 1 tablespoon frozen apple juice concentrate (thawed) before blending; omit the cinnamon, if desired.

"CREAMSICLE" VARIATION: Add 2 tablespoons frozen orange juice concentrate (thawed); omit the cinnamon.

1 shake = 2 Calcium servings; ⅔ Protein serving; 1 Other Fruit serving. Berry Variation adds 1 Other Fruit serving, 1 Vitamin C serving if strawberries are used. "Creamsicle" Variation adds ½ Vitamin C serving.

FIG BARS

Makes about 36 cookie bars

> Vegetable oil or vegetable
>   cooking spray
> 1 tablespoon fructose
> 4 tablespoons (½ stick) margarine or butter
> 1 cup plus 2 tablespoons
>   apple juice concentrate,
>   heated until warm
> 1½ cups whole-wheat flour
> 1 cup wheat germ
> 1½ teaspoons vanilla extract
> 1 pound dried figs, chopped
> 2 tablespoons ground almonds or other nuts

1. Preheat the oven to 350°F. Lightly grease a nonstick baking sheet with oil or vegetable cooking spray.

2. Cream the fructose and margarine together in a bowl. Add ½ cup plus 2 tablespoons of the apple juice concentrate, and continue to cream.

3. Add the flour, wheat germ, and vanilla, and mix to form a dough. Divide the dough in half, forming each half into a rectangular bar. Wrap them, separately, in waxed paper and chill for 1 hour.

4. Combine the figs and remaining apple juice concentrate in a saucepan, and cook over low heat until soft. Remove from the heat, and stir in the ground nuts until smooth.

5. Roll out one rectangular bar of dough on the prepared baking sheet until it is very thin, evening out the edges as much as possible. Spread the fig mixture evenly over the dough. Roll out the second rectangle of dough between two sheets of waxed paper to the same size as the first rectangle. Remove one sheet of waxed paper, and flip the dough as evenly as possible over the fig mixture. Press down lightly, and trim the ends as needed with a sharp knife.

6. Bake until lightly browned, 15 to 30 minutes. Cut into squares or diamond shapes while still hot.

3 cookies = 1 Whole Grains serving; 1 Other Fruit serving; some Iron; high fiber.

FRUITY OATMEAL COOKIES

Makes 24 2-inch cookies

> Vegetable oil or vegetable
>   cooking spray
> 10 dates, pitted
> 6 tablespoons apple juice
>   concentrate
> 2 tablespoons vegetable oil
> 1½ cups rolled oats (or a
>   mixture of oats and raw
>   wheat flakes)
> 1 cup raisins
> ¼ to ½ cup chopped nuts
> Ground cinnamon to taste
> 1 egg white

1. Preheat the oven to 350°F. Lightly grease a nonstick baking sheet with the oil or vegetable cooking spray.

2. Combine the dates and the apple juice concentrate in a saucepan, and simmer until the fruit has softened. Purée the mixture in a blender or food

VEGETARIAN COMPLETE PROTEIN COMBINATIONS

The following selections are nutritious foods for all pregnant women; however, non-vegetarians should count only one serving a day as part of their protein allowance. Additional servings can count toward the Whole Grains and Legumes requirement. Strict vegetarians should have five of these protein servings daily.

Choose one serving (10 to 13 grams protein) from the legumes list plus one serving (10 to 13 grams protein) from the grains list for a complete protein combination.

LEGUMES

1 cup broad beans or black-eyed peas
¾ cup mung, black, Great Northern, lima, navy, pinto, or kidney beans
¾ cup soybeans or soy grits
1 cup chick-peas
⅔ cup lentils or split peas

GRAINS

1½ cups brown rice, groats, barley, millet, bulgur*
1⅓ cups wild rice
2 ounces (before cooking) soy pasta

2 to 4 ounces (before cooking; weight depending on protein content) whole-wheat pasta
2 ounces (before cooking) Superoni or soy pasta
⅔ cup (before cooking) oats
¾ cup seeds: sesame, sunflower, pumpkin
½ cup Brazil nuts or peanuts
2 ounces cashews, walnuts, or pistachios
⅓ cup wheat germ
2½ to 3 tablespoons peanut butter

DAIRY COMPLETE PROTEIN COMBINATIONS

Choose one serving (about 10 grams protein) from the legumes and grains list and one serving (about 12 grams protein) from the dairy foods list for a complete protein.

LEGUMES AND GRAINS

1 portion beans, peas, lentils, grains, pasta, noodles (see above)
4 slices whole-grain bread
⅔ cup cooked oatmeal
1½ ounces whole-grain ready-to-eat cereal

DAIRY FOODS

1¼ cups skim milk
1½ ounces Cheddar, American, Swiss, low-fat cheese
½ cup cottage cheese
¼ cup Parmesan cheese
⅓ cup nonfat dry milk plus 2 tablespoons wheat germ
1¼ cups yogurt
1 egg plus 2 egg whites

---

*These grains are low in protein; enrich with 2 tablespoons of wheat germ per serving.

processor, then pour it into a bowl. Add the 2 tablespoons oil and the oats, raisins, nuts, and cinnamon.

3. In a separate bowl, beat the egg white lightly. Fold it gently into the cookie mixture. Drop the batter in tablespoonsful onto the prepared sheet.

4. Bake until lightly browned, 10 to 12 minutes.

3 cookies = 1 Other Fruit serving; ½ Whole Grains serving; some Iron; high fiber.

FRUITED YOGURT

Makes about 1 cup

- ¾ cup plain low-fat yogurt
- ½ teaspoon freshly grated orange zest
- ½ cup fresh or frozen (thawed) unsweetened strawberries
- 1 tablespoon orange juice concentrate
- 5 teaspoons apple juice concentrate
- ½ teaspoon ground cinnamon, or to taste (optional)

Purée all the ingredients in a blender or food processor. Serve plain, or as a sauce for fruit, cake, or pancakes.

1 cup = 1 Vitamin C serving; ¾ Calcium serving.

MOCK STRAWBERRY DAIQUIRI

Makes 4 servings

- 2 cups washed, hulled fresh or frozen (unsweetened) strawberries (or substitute 2 very ripe bananas, cut into small pieces)

- 1 cup ice cubes, cracked (½ cup if using frozen berries)
- ¼ cup apple juice concentrate, or to taste
- 1 tablespoon fresh lime juice
- 1 teaspoon pure rum extract

Purée all the ingredients in a blender. Serve cold in tall glasses.

1 serving = 1 Other Fruit serving; 1 Vitamin C serving. Or 2 Other Fruit servings if bananas used.

VIRGIN SANGRIA

Makes 5 to 6 servings

- 3 cups unsweetened grape juice
- ¾ cup apple juice concentrate
- 1 tablespoon fresh lime juice
- 1 tablespoon fresh lemon juice
- 1 small unpeeled lemon, sliced and seeded
- 1 small unpeeled orange, sliced and seeded
- 1 small unpeeled McIntosh apple, cored, cut into eighths
- ¾ cup seltzer (unsalted club soda)

Combine all the ingredients except the seltzer in a large pitcher. Stir well, and chill. Add seltzer just before serving. Serve over ice in wineglasses.

1 serving = 1 Other Fruit serving.

Part 2

NINE MONTHS AND COUNTING:

From Conception to Delivery

5
The First Month

WHAT YOU CAN EXPECT AT YOUR FIRST PRENATAL VISIT

The first is the most comprehensive of all the prenatal visits.[1] A complete medical history will be taken, and certain tests and procedures will be performed only at this exam. One practitioner's routine may vary slightly from another's. In general, the examination will include:

Confirmation of Your Pregnancy. Your practitioner will want to check the following: the pregnancy symptoms you are experiencing; the date of your last normal menstrual period, to determine your estimated date of delivery (EDD), or due date (see page 6); your cervix and uterus, for signs and approximate age of the pregnancy. If there's any question, a pregnancy test may be ordered if you haven't already had one.

A Complete History. To give you the

best care possible, your practitioner will want to know a great deal about you. Come prepared by checking home records and refreshing your memory, as necessary, on the following: your personal medical history (chronic illness, previous major illness or surgery, medications you are presently taking or have taken since conception, known allergies, including drug allergies); your family medical history (genetic disorders and chronic diseases); your social history (age, occupation, and habits, such as smoking, drinking, exercise, diet); your gynecological and obstetrical history (age at first menstrual period, usual length of menstrual cycle, duration and regularity of menstrual periods; past abortions, miscarriages, and live births; course of past pregnancies, labors, and deliveries); and factors in your personal life that might affect your pregnancy.

A Complete Physical Examination. This may include: assessment of your

---

1. See the Appendix for an explanation of the procedures and tests performed.

WHAT YOU MAY LOOK LIKE

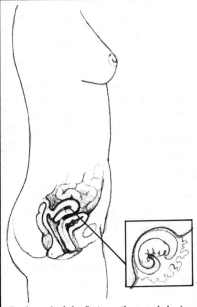

By the end of the first month, your baby is a tiny, tadpole-like embryo, smaller than a grain of rice. In the next two weeks, the neural tube (which becomes the brain and spinal cord), heart, digestive tract, sensory organs, and arm and leg buds will begin to form.

general health through examination of heart, lungs, breasts, abdomen; measurement of your blood pressure to serve as a baseline reading for comparison at subsequent visits; notation of your height and weight, usual and present; inspection of extremities for varicose veins and edema (swelling from excess fluid in tissues), to serve as a baseline for comparison at subsequent visits; inspection and palpation of external genitalia; internal examination of your vagina and cervix (with a speculum in place); examination of your pelvic organs bimanually (with one hand in the vagina and one on the abdomen) and also through the rectum and vagina; assessment of the size and shape of your bony pelvis.

A Battery of Tests. Some tests are routine for every pregnant woman; some are routine in some areas of the country or with some practitioners, and not others; some are performed only when circumstances warrant. The most common prenatal tests include:

❖ A blood test to determine blood type and check for anemia.

❖ Urinalysis to screen for sugar, protein, white blood cells, blood, and bacteria.

❖ Blood screens to determine immunity to such diseases as rubella.

❖ Tests to disclose the presence of such infections as syphilis, gonorrhea, hepatitis, chlamydia, and in some cases, AIDS.

❖ Genetic tests for sickle-cell anemia or Tay-Sachs disease.

❖ A Pap smear for the detection of cervical cancer.

❖ A gestational diabetic screening test to check for any tendency toward diabetes, particularly for women who have previously had an excessively large baby or gained excessive weight with an earlier pregnancy.

An Opportunity for Discussion. Come prepared with a list of questions, problems, and symptoms you would like to talk about. This is also a good time to bring up any special concerns that weren't addressed at an earlier consultation.

WHAT YOU MAY BE FEELING

You may experience all of these symptoms at one time or another, or only one or two.

PHYSICALLY:

❖ Absence of menstruation (though you may stain slightly when your period would have been expected or when the fertilized egg implants in the uterus)

❖ Fatigue and sleepiness

❖ Frequent urination

❖ Nausea, with or without vomiting, and/or excessive salivation (ptyalism)

❖ Heartburn, indigestion, flatulence, bloating

❖ Food aversions and cravings

❖ Breast changes (most pronounced in women who have breast changes prior to menstruation): fullness, heaviness, tenderness, tingling; darkening of the areola (the pigmented area surrounding the nipple). Sweat glands in the areola become prominent (Montgomery's tubercles), looking like large goose bumps; a network of bluish lines appear under the skin as blood supply to the breasts increases (though these lines may not appear until later)

EMOTIONALLY:

❖ Instability comparable to premenstrual syndrome, which may include irritability, mood swings, irrationality, weepiness

❖ Misgivings, fear, joy, elation—any or all of these

WHAT YOU MAY BE CONCERNED ABOUT

FATIGUE

"I'm tired all the time. I'm worried that I won't be able to continue working."

It would be surprising if you weren't tired. In some ways, your pregnant body is working harder even when you're resting than a nonpregnant body is when mountain-climbing; you just can't see its efforts. For one thing, it's manufacturing your baby's life-support system, the placenta, which won't be completed until the end of the first trimester. For another, it's adjusting to the many other physical and emotional demands of pregnancy, which are considerable. Once your body has adjusted and the placenta is complete (around the fourth month), you should have more energy. Until then, you may need to work fewer hours or take a few days off if you're really dragging. But if your pregnancy continues normally, there is absolutely no reason why you shouldn't stay at your job (assuming your doctor hasn't restricted your activity and/or the work isn't overly strenuous or hazardous; see page 72). Most pregnant women are happier and less anxious if they keep busy.

Since your fatigue is legitimate, don't fight it. Consider it a signal from your body that you need more rest. That, of course, is more easily suggested than done. But it is worth a try.

Baby Yourself. If you're a first-time expectant mother, enjoy what will probably be your last chance for a long while to focus on taking care of yourself without feeling guilty. If you already have one or more children at home, you will have to divide your focus. But either way, this is not a time to strive for Super-Mom-to-Be status. Getting adequate rest is more important than keeping your house white-glove-test clean or serving dinners worthy of four-star ratings. Keep evenings free of unessential activities. Spend them off your feet when you can, reading, watching TV, scouring baby-name books. If you have older children, read to them, play quiet games with them, or watch classic kiddie videos with them rather than traipsing off to the playground. (Fatigue may be more pronounced when there are older children at home, simply because there are so many more physical demands and so much less time to rest. On the other hand, it may be less noticed, since a mother of young children is usually accustomed to exhaustion and/or too busy to mind.)

And don't wait until nightfall to take it easy—if you can afford the luxury of an afternoon nap, by all means indulge. If you can't sleep, lie down with a good book. A nap at the office isn't a reasonable goal, of course, unless you have a flexible schedule and access to a comfortable sofa, but putting your feet up at your desk or in the ladies' lounge during breaks and lunch hours may be. (If you choose lunch hour to rest, don't forget to eat too.) Napping when you're mothering may also be difficult, but if you can time your rest with the children's nap-time, you may be able to get away with it—assuming you can tolerate the unwashed dishes and the dust balls under the bed.

Let Others Baby You. Accept your mother-in-law's offer to vacuum and dust the house when she's visiting. Let your dad take the older kids to the zoo on Sunday. Enlist your husband for chores like laundry and marketing.

Get an Hour or Two More Sleep Each Night. Skip the 11 o'clock news and turn in earlier; ask your husband to fix breakfast so you can turn out later.

Be Sure That Your Diet Isn't Deficient. First-trimester fatigue is often aggravated by a deficiency in iron, protein, or just plain calories. Double-check to make certain you're filling all of your requirements (see the Best-Odds Diet, page 80). And no matter how tired you're feeling, don't be tempted to rev up your body with caffeine, candy bars, and cake. It won't be fooled for long, and after the temporary lift, your blood sugar will plummet, leaving you more fatigued than ever.

Check Your Environment. Inadequate lighting, poor air quality (sick building syndrome), or excessive noise in your home or workplace can contribute to fatigue. Be alert to these problems and try to get them corrected.

Take a Hike. Or a slow jog. Or a stroll to the grocery store. Or the time to do a pregnancy exercise routine. Paradoxically, fatigue can be heightened by too much rest and not enough activity. But don't overdo the exercise. Stop before that exercise high dissolves into a low, and be sure to follow the precautionary guidelines on page 195.

Though fatigue will probably ease up by month four, you can expect it to return in the last trimester—probably as nature's way of preparing you for those long sleepless nights once the baby has arrived.

When fatigue is severe, especially if it is accompanied by fainting, pallor, breathlessness, and/or palpitations, it's wise to report it to your practitioner (see Anemia, page 154).

DEPRESSION

"I know I should feel happy about my pregnancy, but I seem to be suffering from postpartum depression prematurely."

First of all, you may be mistaking depression for the very normal mood swings of pregnancy. These swings may be more pronounced in the first trimester and, in general, in women who ordinarily suffer from emotional instability premenstrually. Feelings of ambivalence about the pregnancy once it's confirmed, which are common even when a pregnancy is planned, may exaggerate the swings still more. Though there's no cure for mood swings, avoiding sugar, chocolate, and caffeine (all of which can push a low even lower), following the Best-Odds Diet, getting a good balance of rest and exercise, and talking your feelings out can help to keep them from swinging too far.

If your lows are consistent or frequent, you may be one of the 10% of pregnant women who battle mild to moderate depression during pregnancy. Some of the factors that can put a woman at risk for such depression are:

❖ A personal or family history of mood disorder.

❖ Socioeconomic stress.

❖ Lack of emotional suppport from the baby's father.

❖ Hospitalization or bed rest because of pregnancy complications.

❖ Anxiety about her own health, especially if she experiences pregnancy complications or illness during pregnancy.

❖ Anxiety about her baby's health.

The most common symptoms of depression, in addition to feeling down, empty, and flat, include sleep disturbances; changed eating habits (not eating at all or eating endlessly); prolonged or unusual fatigue; extended loss of interest in work, play, and other activities or pleasures; and exaggerated mood swings. If that sounds like what you're experiencing, try those tips for dealing with postpartum depression that seem applicable to your life now (see page 398).

If the symptoms continue for longer than two weeks, speak to your practitioner about your depression or ask for a referral to a therapist. Except in extreme cases, antidepressant medication, the safety of which in pregnancy is not certain, will be bypassed in favor of supportive therapy, which can often be just as effective. Getting help is important, because your depression can lead to your not taking optimum care of your baby.

MORNING SICKNESS

"I haven't had any morning sickness. Can I still be pregnant?"

Morning sickness, like a craving for pickles and ice cream, is one of those truisms about pregnancy that ain't necessarily so. Studies show that only about one-half of all expectant women ever experience the nausea and vomiting associated with morning sickness. If you're among those who never, or rarely, suffer from it, you can consider yourself not only pregnant but lucky.

If you have no pregnancy symptoms at all, or suddenly lose those you've had, however, check with your doctor.

"My morning sickness lasts all day. I'm afraid I'm not able to keep down enough food to nourish my baby."

Fortunately, morning sickness (a misnamed malady, because it can strike morning, noon, or night—or even all day long) rarely interferes with proper nutrition enough to harm the developing fetus. And for most women, it doesn't last past the third month—though an occasional expectant mother won't experience it until well into the second trimester and a few, particularly those expecting twins, may enjoy its dubious pleasures for a full nine months. The major plus: these symptoms, like other pregnancy symptoms, are a sign that your hormones are doing their job.

What causes morning sickness? No one knows for sure, but there's no shortage of theories. It is known that the command post for nausea and vomiting is located in the brain stem. A myriad of physical reasons why this area may be overstimulated during pregnancy have been suggested, including the high level of the pregnancy hormone hCG in the blood in the first trimester, the rapid stretching of the uterine muscles, the relative relaxation of the muscle tissue in the digestive tract (which makes digestion less efficient), the excess acid in the stomach, and an enhanced sense of smell.

Not all pregnant women experience morning sickness, and among those who do, not all experience it to the same degree. Some have a few queasy moments, others feel nauseated round the clock, and still others vomit several times a day. There are probably several reasons for these variations: *Hormone levels.* Excessive levels (as when a woman is carrying multiple fetuses) can increase morning sickness; lower levels may eliminate it. *The response of the brain's nausea and vomiting command post to pregnancy hormones and other triggers.* This response can affect whether or not a woman experiences morning sickness and to what degree. A woman whose command center is particularly sensitive (for example, she gets seasick out in a boat) is likely to have more severe nausea and vomiting in pregnancy. *Stress levels.* It's well known that stress of various kinds can cause stomach upset so it's not surprising that stress can trigger gastrointestinal symptoms or increase their severity in pregnancy. *Fatigue.* Physical or mental fatigue can also increase the risk of morning sickness (severe morning sickness can conversely increase fatigue).

The fact that morning sickness is more common and tends to be more severe in first pregnancies supports the concept that both physical and psychological factors are involved. Physically, the novice pregnant body is less prepared for the onslaught of hormones and other changes than one that has been through it all before. Emotionally, those pregnant for the first time are more likely to be subject to the anxieties and fears that can turn a stomach, whereas women in subsequent pregnancies may be distracted from their nausea by the demands of caring for older children.

No matter the cause, morning sickness is no fun for the woman who is experiencing it and she needs all the support she can get—from her spouse, her family, and her practitioner. Unfortunately, medical experts are even less certain of the cure for the morning sickness than they are of its cause. They do, however, agree that there are many ways of alleviating its symptoms and minimizing its effects. See which work best for you:

❖ Eat a diet high in protein and complex carbohydrates (see the Best-Odds Diet, page 80)—both of which fight nausea. So does good nutrition, so eat as well as you can under the circumstances.

❖ Take plenty of fluids—especially if you're losing them through vomiting. If they are easier to get down than solids when your stomach is upset, use them to get your nutrients. Concentrate on any of the following you can handle: Double-the-Milk Shakes (see page 95); fruit or vegetable juices; soups, broths, and bouillons. If you find fluids make you queasier, eat solids with a high water content, such as fresh fruits and vegetables—particularly lettuce, melons, and citrus fruits. Some women find that drinking and eating at the same sitting puts too much strain on their digestive tract; if this is true for you, try taking your fluids between meals.

❖ Take a prenatal vitamin supplement (see page 88) to compensate for nutrients you may not be getting. But take it at a time of day when you are least likely to chuck it back up—possibly before you go to bed. Your doctor may recommend an additional 50-milligram ration of B$_6$, which seems to help relieve nausea in some women. *Do not take any medication for morning sickness unless it is prescribed by your physician.* Such a prescription will almost certainly be written only when morning sickness is severe enough to be debilitating (see hyperemesis, page 343) and threatens to compromise your nutritional status and your baby's.

❖ Avoid the sight, smell, and taste of foods that make you queasy. Avoid food smells entirely if they trigger nausea. Don't be a martyr and prepare a sausage and onion hero for your spouse if it sends you rushing to the bathroom. And don't force yourself to eat foods that don't appeal, or worse, make you sick. Instead, with a little nutritional guidance from your conscience, let your eyes, nose, and tongue be your guides in menu planning. Choose only sweet foods if they're all you can abide (get your vitamin A and

protein from peaches and pancakes at dinner instead of from broccoli and chicken). Or only savories if they're your ticket to a less tumultuous tummy (have a grilled cheese and tomato sandwich for breakfast instead of cereal and orange juice.)

❖ Avoid tobacco smoke which appears to increase morning sickness.

❖ Eat often—and before you feel hungry. When your stomach is empty, its acids have nothing to digest but its own lining. This can trigger nausea. So can the low blood sugar caused by long stretches between meals. Six small meals are better than three large. Carry nutritious snacks (dried fruit, whole-grain crackers) with you for snacking.

❖ Eat before nausea strikes. Food will be easier to get down and may prevent an attack.

❖ Eat in bed—for the same reasons you should eat often: to avoid an empty stomach and keep your blood sugar at an even keel. Before you go to sleep at night, have a snack that is high in protein and complex carbohydrates: a glass of milk and a bran muffin, for example. Twenty minutes before you plan to get out of bed in the morning, have a high-carbohydrate snack: a few whole-wheat crackers or rice cakes, or a handful of raisins. Keep them next to the bed so you don't have to get up for them, and in case you wake up hungry in the middle of the night.[2]

❖ Get some extra sleep and relaxation. Both emotional and physical fatigue can exacerbate nausea.

❖ Greet the morning in slow motion—rushing tends to aggra-

---

2. If you start to associate a particular carbohydrate snack (crackers, for instance) with your nausea, switch to a different snack.

vate nausea. Don't jump out of bed and dash out the door. Stay in bed digesting your crackers for 20 minutes, then rise slowly to a leisurely breakfast. This may seem impossible if you have other children, but try to wake up before they do to get some quiet time, or let your spouse handle their early morning needs.

❖ Brush your teeth (with a toothpaste that doesn't increase queasiness) or rinse your mouth (ask your dentist to recommend a good rinse, check with your practitioner to make sure it's okay to use) after each bout of vomiting, as well as after each meal. Not only will this help keep your mouth fresh and reduce nausea, it will decrease the risk of damage to teeth or gums that can occur when bacteria work on regurgitated residue in your mouth.

❖ Minimize stress. Morning sickness is more common among women who are under a great deal of stress, either at work or at home. See page 113 for tips on dealing with stress during pregnancy.

❖ Try Sea-Bands. The 1-inch bands, worn on both wrists, put pressure on the inner wrist and often relieve nausea. They cause no side effects and are widely available.

❖ Try acupuncture. It often works to lessen nausea.

In an estimated 7 of every 2,000 pregnancies, nausea and vomiting become so severe that medical treatment is needed. If this seems to be the case with you, see page 343.

EXCESSIVE SALIVA

"My mouth seems to fill up with saliva all the time—and swallowing it makes me queasy. What's going on?"

An excess of saliva, also called ptyalism, is another common symptom of pregnancy. It's unpleasant but harmless. Happily, it usually disappears after the first few months. It's more common in women who are also experiencing morning sickness, and it seems to compound the queasiness. There's no sure cure, but brushing your teeth frequently with a minty toothpaste, rinsing with a minty mouthwash, or chewing gum can help dry things up a bit.

FREQUENT URINATION

"I'm in the bathroom every half hour. Is it normal to be urinating this often?"

Most—though by no means all—pregnant women do make frequent detours to the toilet in both the first and last trimesters. One of the reasons for an initial increase in urinary frequency is the increased volume of body fluids and the improved efficiency of the kidneys, which helps rid the body more quickly of waste products. Another is the pressure of the growing uterus, which is still in the pelvis next to the bladder. This pressure on the bladder is often relieved once the uterus rises into the abdominal cavity, around the fourth month. It probably won't return until the baby "drops" back down into the pelvis in the ninth month. But because the arrangement of internal organs varies slightly from woman to woman, the degree of urinary frequency in pregnancy may also vary.

Leaning forward when you urinate will help ensure that you empty your bladder completely and may reduce trips to the bathroom. If you find you go frequently during the night, try limiting fluids after 4 P.M. Don't, however, limit fluids otherwise.

*"How come I'm not urinating fre-
quently?"*

No noticeable increase in the frequency of urination may be perfectly normal for you, especially if
you ordinarily urinate often. You
should, however, be certain you're
getting enough fluids (at least eight
glasses a day). Not only can insufficient fluid intake be the cause of infrequent urination, it could also lead to
urinary tract infection.

BREAST CHANGES

*"I hardly recognize my breasts anymore—
they're so huge. And they're tender too.
Will they stay that way, and will they sag
after I give birth?"*

Get used to the chesty look for
now. Although it may not always
be in fashion, it's one of the hallmarks
of pregnancy. Your breasts are swollen
and tender because of the increased
amounts of estrogen and progesterone
your body is producing. (The same
mechanism operates premenstrually,
when many women experience breast
changes—but the changes are more
pronounced in pregnancy.) These
changes are not random; they are
aimed at preparing you to feed your
baby when it arrives. If, however, they
are less marked in a second or subsequent pregnancy (as they often are), it
doesn't mean that you will be less
capable of breastfeeding.

In addition to their enlarging, you
will probably notice other changes in
your breasts. The areola (the pigmented area around the nipple) will
darken, spread, and may be spotted
with even darker areas. This darkening may fade but not disappear entirely after birth. The little bumps you
may notice on the areola are seba-
ceous (sweat) glands, which become
more prominent during pregnancy

and return to normal afterward. The
complex road map of blue veins that
traverses the breasts—often quite
vivid on a fair-skinned woman—
represents a mother-to-baby delivery
system for nutrients and fluids. After
delivery or sometime after nursing is
discontinued, the appearance of the
skin will return to normal.

What you won't have to get used to,
fortunately, is the sometimes agonizing sensitivity of your breasts. Though
they will continue to grow throughout your pregnancy—possibly increasing as much as three cup sizes—
they are not likely to remain tender to
the touch past the third or fourth
month. As for whether or not they
will sag after the baby is born, that is
at least partly up to you. Stretching
and sagging of the breast tissue result
from a lack of support during
pregnancy—not from pregnancy
itself—though the tendency to sag
may be genetic. No matter how firm
your breasts are now, protect them for
the future by wearing a good support
bra. If your breasts are particularly
large or have a tendency to sag, it's a
good idea to wear a bra even at night.

If your breasts enlarge early in pregnancy and then suddenly diminish in
size (and especially if other pregnancy
symptoms also disappear without explanation), contact your practitioner.

*"My breasts became very large in my first
pregnancy, but they haven't seemed to
change at all now that I'm in my second.
Could something be wrong?"*

Small-chested women who look
forward to having their cups running over in pregnancy are sometimes
in for a disappointment, at least temporarily, the second or third time
around. Though some experience as
much enlargement early on as they
did in the first pregnancy, others do
not—perhaps because the breasts,

thanks to their previous experience, don't need as much preparation and respond to the pregnancy hormones less dramatically. In these women, the breasts may gradually enlarge during pregnancy, or may hold off their expansion until after delivery, when milk production begins.

VITAMIN SUPPLEMENTS

"Should I be taking vitamins?"

Virtually no one gets a nutritionally perfect diet every day, especially early in pregnancy, when morning sickness is a common appetite suppressant and when what little nutrition some women manage to get down often comes right back up. A daily vitamin supplement, while it does not take the place of a good prenatal diet, can serve as your dietary insurance, guaranteeing that should your body not cooperate or should you slip up occasionally, your baby won't be cheated. In addition, some studies have shown that women who take vitamin supplements prior to pregnancy and during the first month significantly reduce the risk of neural tube defects (such as spina bifida) in their babies. Good formulations designed especially for expectant mothers are available by prescription or over the counter. (See page 88 for what the supplement should contain.) Do not take any kind of dietary supplements other than such a prenatal formula without your doctor's recommendation.

Many women find that taking a vitamin supplement increases nausea in early pregnancy, and sometimes beyond. Switching formulas may help, as may taking your pill after meals (unless that's when you usually throw up). If swallowing a standard-size pill is difficult for you, consider switching to a child-size formula, a chewable supplement, or a capsule that can be opened and sprinkled on food or drink. But be sure the formula you select approximates the requirements for supplements designed for pregnancy (see page 88). If your supplement was prescribed by your practitioner, check with him or her before switching.

In some women, the iron in a prenatal vitamin can cause constipation or diarrhea. Again, switching formulas may bring relief. Taking a pregnancy supplement without iron and a separate iron preparation (your doctor can prescribe one that dissolves in the intestines rather than in the more sensitive stomach) may also reduce irritation and relieve symptoms. Ask your practitioner for advice.

ECTOPIC PREGNANCY

"I've been having occasional cramping. Could I have an ectopic pregnancy without knowing it?"

The fear of ectopic, or tubal, pregnancy lurks somewhere in the mind of nearly every newly pregnant woman who has heard of this abnormal type of implantation. Fortunately, for the vast majority it's an unfounded fear—a fear that can be dismissed completely by the eighth week of pregnancy, by which time most tubal pregnancies have been diagnosed and terminated.

Only about 2 in 100 pregnancies are ectopic, that is, implanted outside the uterus, usually in the fallopian tubes.[3] A good many of these are diagnosed before a woman even realizes she is

---

3. This usually occurs because some irregularity in the tube blocks the passage of the egg down to the uterus. Rarely, the fertilized egg implants in the ovary, the abdominal cavity, or the cervix.

pregnant. So chances are that if your doctor has confirmed your pregnancy through a blood test and a physical exam and you've had no signs of ectopic pregnancy, then you can cross this worry off your list.

There are several factors that can make women more susceptible to ectopic pregnancy. They include:

❖ A previous ectopic pregnancy.

❖ Previous pelvic inflammatory disease.

❖ Previous abdominal or tubal surgery with postoperative scarring.

❖ Tubal ligation (surgical sterilization), unsuccessful tubal ligation, or tubal ligation reversal.

❖ An IUD in place when conception occurs (an IUD is more likely to prevent conception in the uterus than outside it—increasing the risk of ectopics in IUD users).[4]

❖ Maternal smoking—the more cigarettes smoked daily, the more risk.

❖ Possibly, multiple induced abortions (the evidence isn't clear).

❖ Possibly, exposure to diethylstilbestrol (DES) in the womb, especially if it resulted in significant structural abnormalities of the reproductive tract.

Rare as ectopic pregnancies are, every pregnant woman—particularly those at high risk—should be familiar with the symptoms. Occasional cramping, probably the result of ligaments stretching as the uterus grows, is not one of them. But any or all of the following might be, and do require immediate evaluation by a physician. If you can't reach your physician, go at once to the hospital emergency room.

4. But having worn an IUD in the past does not appear to increase risk.

❖ Colicky, crampy pain with tenderness, usually in the lower abdomen —on one side initially, though the pain can radiate throughout the abdomen. Pain may worsen on straining of bowels, coughing, or moving. If tubal rupture occurs, pain becomes very sharp and steady for a short time before diffusing throughout the pelvic region.

❖ Brown vaginal spotting or light bleeding (intermittent or continuous), which may precede pain by several days or weeks, though sometimes there is no bleeding unless the tube ruptures.

❖ Heavy bleeding if the tube ruptures.

❖ Nausea and vomiting—in about 25% to 50% of women—though this may be difficult to distinguish from morning sickness.

❖ Dizziness or weakness, in some women. If the tube ruptures, weak pulse, clammy skin, and fainting are common.

❖ Shoulder pain, in some women.

❖ Feeling of rectal pressure, in some women.

If an ectopic pregnancy is present, quick medical attention can often save the fallopian tube and the woman's fertility (see page 343 for the treatment of ectopic pregnancies).

THE CONDITION OF YOUR BABY

"I'm very nervous because I can't really feel my baby. Could it die without my knowing it?"

At this stage, with no noticeable enlargement of the abdomen or obvious fetal activity, it's hard to imagine that there's really a living, growing baby inside you. But the death of a fetus or embryo that isn't expelled from the uterus in a miscarriage is very rare. When it does happen, a woman eventually loses all signs of pregnancy, including breast tenderness and enlargement, and may develop a brownish discharge, though no actual bleeding. Upon examination, the physician will find that the uterus has diminished in size.

If at any time all of your pregnancy symptoms disappear or you feel as though your uterus isn't growing, call your doctor. That's a more positive approach than sitting around worrying.

MISCARRIAGE

"Between what I read and what my mother tells me, I'm afraid everything I've done, am doing, and will do might cause a miscarriage."

For many expectant women, the fear of miscarriage keeps their joy guarded in the first trimester. Some even refrain from spreading their happy news until the fourth month, when they begin to feel secure that the pregnancy will indeed continue. And for most of them—probably 90%—it will.[5]

There is still much to be learned about the reasons behind early miscarriage, but several factors are believed *not* to cause the problem. They include:

❖ Previous trouble with an IUD. Scarring of the endometrium (the lining of the uterus) caused by IUD-triggered infection could prevent a pregnancy from implanting in the uterus, but should not cause miscarriage once implantation is well established. Nor should previous difficulty holding an IUD in place affect a pregnancy.

❖ History of multiple abortions.[6] Scarring of the endometrium from multiple abortions, as from IUD-caused infections, could prevent implantation but should not otherwise be responsible for early miscarriage.

❖ Emotional upset—resulting from an argument, stress at work, or family problems.

❖ A fall or other minor accidental injury to the mother. But serious injury could result in miscarriage, so safety precautions—such as wearing a seat belt and not climbing on rickety chairs or ladders—should always be observed.

❖ Usual and accustomed physical activity, such as housework; lifting children, groceries, or other moderately heavy objects (see page 204); hanging curtains; moving light furniture; and moderate and safe exercise (see page 189).[7]

❖ Sexual intercourse—unless a woman has a history of miscarriage or is otherwise at high risk for pregnancy loss.

There are several factors, however, that *are* believed to increase the risk of spontaneous abortion. Some are not likely to recur and should not

---

5. Roughly 10% of diagnosed pregnancies end in clinically apparent miscarriage. Another 20% to 40% of pregnancies end before a pregnancy diagnosis is made; these are the miscarriages that usually go unnoticed.

6. Though not a direct cause of early miscarriage, repeated abortions or other procedures requiring dilation of the cervix may result in a weakened or incompetent cervix—often a cause of late miscarriage. (See page 177.)

7. In a high-risk pregnancy, the physician may limit these activities or even prescribe strict bed rest. But you need limit activity only on direction of your doctor.

Possible Signs of Miscarriage

**When to Call Your Doctor
Immediately, Just in Case**

❖ When you experience bleeding with cramps or pain in the center of your lower abdomen. (Pain on one side in early pregnancy could be triggered by an ectopic pregnancy, and also warrants a call to the doctor.)

❖ When pain is severe or continues unabated for more than one day, even if it isn't accompanied by staining or bleeding.

❖ When bleeding is as heavy as a menstrual period, or light staining continues for more than three days.

**When to Get Emergency
Medical Attention**

❖ When you have a history of miscarriage, and experience either bleeding or cramping or both.

❖ When bleeding is heavy enough to soak several pads in an hour, or when pain is so severe you can't bear it.

❖ When you pass clots or grayish or pink material—which may mean a miscarriage has already begun. If you can't reach your doctor, go to the nearest emergency room or to the one recommended by his or her office. The doctor may want you to save the material you pass (in a jar, plastic bag, or other clean container) so he or she can try to determine whether or not the miscarriage is simply threatening, is complete, or is incomplete and requires a D and C (dilation and curettage) to complete it.

affect future pregnancies. For example, exposure to rubella or other teratogenic disease, to radiation, or to drugs harmful to the fetus; a high fever; or an IUD in place at conception. Other risk factors, once identified, can be controlled or eliminated in future pregnancies (poor nutrition; smoking; hormonal insufficiency; and certain maternal medical problems). A few miscarriage risk factors are not easily overcome, such as a malformed uterus (though it can sometimes be surgically corrected) and certain chronic maternal illnesses.

Rarely, repeated miscarriages are traced to the mother's immune cells attacking cells in the embryo—her own (an autoimmune reaction) or the father's. Immunotherapy may be helpful in such instances.

When Not to Worry. It's important to recognize that each cramp, ache, or bit of spotting isn't necessarily a warning of an impending miscarriage. Just about every normal pregnancy will include at least one of these usually innocuous symptoms at one time or another:[8]

❖ Mild cramps, achiness, or a pulling sensation on one or both sides of the abdomen. This is probably caused by the stretching of ligaments that support the uterus. Unless cramping is severe, constant, or accompanied by bleeding, there's no need to worry.

❖ Staining a bit around the time you

---

8. You should routinely tell your practitioner about *any* pains, cramping, or bleeding. In most cases his or her response will put your worries to rest.

would have expected your period, about seven to ten days after conception, when the little ball of cells that is going to develop into your baby attaches itself to the uterine wall. Slight bleeding at this time is common and doesn't necessarily indicate a problem with your pregnancy—as long as it isn't accompanied by lower abdominal pain.

If You Suspect Miscarriage. If you experience any of the symptoms listed in the box on page 112, put a call in to your practitioner. If your symptoms are listed under "When to Get Emergency Medical Attention" and your practitioner is not available, leave a message for him or her, and either call 911 or your local EMS (emergency medical service) or go straight to the nearest emergency room.

While waiting for help, lie down if you can, or rest in a chair with your feet up. This may not prevent a miscarriage if it's about to happen, but it should help you to relax. It should also help you to relax to know that most women who have episodes of bleeding in early pregnancy carry to term and deliver healthy babies.

If miscarriage is suspected or diagnosed, see page 346.

"I don't really feel pregnant. Could I have miscarried without knowing it?"

Fear of miscarrying without realizing it, though common, is unwarranted. Once a pregnancy is established, the signs that it is aborting are not easily overlooked. Simply "not feeling pregnant" is not usually a reason for concern—many women with normal pregnancies don't feel pregnant, at least until they begin to notice fetal movement. You will likely be reassured by your practitioner at your next prenatal visit.

Occasionally, an embryo dies and is not spontaneously expelled. In such a "missed miscarriage," signs of pregnancy usually diminish or vanish[9] suddenly and there may be a brownish discharge. A call to the practitioner is important under such circumstances.

STRESS IN YOUR LIFE

"My job is a high-stress one. I wasn't planning to have a baby now, but I got pregnant. Should I quit work?"

Stress has, over the past couple of decades, become an important area for study because of the effect it can have on our lives. Depending on how we handle and respond to it, stress can be good for us (by sparking us to perform better, to function more effectively) or it can be bad for us (when it gets out of control, overwhelming and debilitating us). If the stress at work has you working at top efficiency, has you excited and challenged, then it shouldn't be harmful to your pregnancy. But if the stress makes you anxious, sleepless, or depressed, or if it is causing you to experience physical symptoms (such as headache, backache, or loss of appetite), then it could be. It could also be detrimental if it is exhausting you (see page 102 for tips on handling fatigue).

Negative reactions to stress can be compounded by the normal mood swings in pregnancy. And since such reactions as appetite loss, bingeing on the wrong foods, and sleeplessness can take a toll on you—and, if allowed

---

9. Don't forget, however, that by the end of the first trimester, morning sickness is usually gone, urinary frequency has lessened, and breast tenderness is less pronounced—all of which is normal.

Relaxation Made Easy

There are many routes to relaxation, including yoga. Here are a couple of relaxation techniques that are easy to learn and to do anywhere, anytime. If you find them helpful, you can do them when anxiety strikes, or regularly several times a day to try to ward it off.

1. Sit with your eyes closed. Relax your muscles, starting with those in your feet and working up slowly through the legs, torso, neck, and face. Breathe only through the nose (unless it's too stuffy, of course). As you breathe out, repeat the word "one" (or "peace," or any other simple word) to yourself. Continue the repetitions for 10 to 20 minutes.

2. Inhale slowly and deeply through your nose, pushing your abdomen out as you do. Count to four. Then, letting your shoulders and neck muscles relax, exhale slowly and comfortably to the count of six. Repeat this sequence four or five times to banish tension.

to continue into the second and third trimesters, on your baby—learning to handle the stress constructively should become a priority now. The following should help:

Talk About It. Allowing your anxieties to surface is the best way of making sure they don't get you down. Maintain open lines of communication with your spouse, spending some time at the end of each day airing concerns and frustrations. (Of course he, too, is probably in need of a friendly ear, so be prepared to do your fair share of listening.) Together you may be able to find some relief, even some humor, in your respective situations. If you find instead that you get on each other's nerves, talk to another family member, your practitioner, a friend, or a member of the clergy. If nothing seems to help, consider professional counseling.

Do Something About It. Identify sources of stress in your job and in other areas of your life, and determine how they can be modified to reduce the stress. If you're clearly trying to do too much, cut back in some areas.

If you've taken on too many responsibilities at home or at work, set priorities and then decide which can be postponed or passed to someone else. Learn to say no to new projects or activities before you're overloaded.

Sometimes sitting down with a notepad and making lists of the hundreds of things you need to get done (at home or at work), and the order you're planning to do them in, can help you feel more in control of the chaos in your life. Cross them off your list as they're taken care of for a rewarding sense of accomplishment.

Sleep It Off. Sleep is the ticket to regeneration—for mind and body. Often feelings of tension and anxiety are prompted by our not getting enough shut-eye. If you're having trouble sleeping, see the tips on page 140.

Nourish It. Hectic lifestyles can lead to hectic eating styles. Inadequate nutrition during pregnancy can be a double whammy: it can hamper your ability to handle stress as well as affect your baby's growth and development. So be sure to get three squares a day plus adequate snacks, within the Best-

Odds framework (see page 80).

Wash It Away. A warm bath (but not a hot tub) is an excellent way to relieve tension. Try one after a hectic day; it will also help you to sleep better.

Get Away from It Temporarily. Combat stress with any activity you find relaxing—sports (check first with your practitioner, and observe the guidelines on page 195); reading; moviegoing; listening to music (consider taking a cassette player with headphones to work, so you can listen to relaxing music during coffee breaks and lunch, or even while you work if that's feasible); long walks (or short ones during breaks or lunch—but be sure to leave time for eating); meditation (just close your eyes and picture a bucolic scene, or keep them open and gaze at a soothing picture or photo placed strategically in your office). Practice relaxation techniques (see page 114), not just because they'll come in handy during childbirth, but because they can help drain the strain anytime.

Get Away from It Permanently. Maybe the problem isn't worth the stress and anxiety it's generating. If it's your job, consider taking early maternity leave, cutting back to part-time, or switching positions for the time being to reduce stress to a manageable level.

Remember, your stress quotient is only going to increase once the baby is born; it makes sense to try to learn how to handle it now.

OVERWHELMING FEAR ABOUT BABY'S HEALTH

"I know it's probably irrational, but I can't sleep or eat or concentrate at work because I'm afraid my baby won't be normal."

Every expectant mother worries about whether her baby will be normal. But while even a moderate dose of worry that doesn't respond to reassurance (such as is found in this book) is an unavoidable side effect of pregnancy, worry that is so all-consuming that it interferes with functioning needs professional attention. Talk to your practitioner. Perhaps an ultrasound evaluation of the fetus can be arranged to help calm your fears. Many physicians are willing to order such an exam when a patient is extremely anxious, particularly if she feels she has a specific reason to fear for her baby's health (perhaps she spent a lot of time in a hot tub or had a few too many a few too many times before she found out she was pregnant), and even if her concerns seem unfounded or exaggerated. This is because the possible risks of the procedure to mother and fetus (research has yet to reveal any) are outweighed by the risks of such overwhelming anxiety (especially if it is keeping the mother-to-be from eating and sleeping).

Though ultrasound can't detect every potential problem, it can, once significant fetal development has taken place, show a great deal. Even the outline, as blurry as it is, of a normal baby—with all its limbs and organs in place—can offer enormous comfort. That, teamed with verbal reassurance from her own practitioner, and perhaps from the specialist who has evaluated the ultrasound, can help an expectant mother get on with the vital business at hand: caring for herself and nourishing her baby. If it doesn't, professional counseling may be necessary.

Other kinds of prenatal diagnosis, such as amniocentesis and chorionic villus sampling, which can also offer some reassurance, are usually recommended only when there is a valid medical reason (see pages 44 and 48), since the procedures themselves carry some risk.

PICKING UP OTHER CHILDREN

"I'm afraid to pick up my two-year-old daughter, who is pretty heavy, because I've heard physical strain can cause miscarriage."

You'll have to come up with a better excuse to get her to walk on her own two feet. Unless your physician has instructed you otherwise, carrying moderately heavy loads (even a strapping preschooler) is okay, though you should avoid exerting yourself to the point of exhaustion (see page 174 for tips on avoiding back strain when lifting). And in fact, blaming your child's as yet unborn sibling for your reluctance to carry her can needlessly set up feelings of rivalry and resentment toward the baby even before the pint-size competition arrives on the scene.

As your pregnancy progresses, however, your back may not be amenable to the strain of toting both a fetus and a toddler, and in that case, you should keep lifting of the latter to a minimum. But be sure you blame your back, and not the baby, for this slowdown in pickups, and that you compensate for it with plenty of holding and hugging in the sitting position.

WHAT IT'S IMPORTANT TO KNOW: GETTING REGULAR MEDICAL CARE

In the past decade, the self-care health movement has instructed Americans in everything from taking their own blood pressure and pulse to home-treating muscle strains and self-evaluating a scratchy throat or an aching ear. The impact this has had on the effectiveness of our health care has been unquestionably positive—cutting down on the number of trips we have to make to our doctors and making us better patients when we do go. Best of all, it's made us aware of the responsibility we each have for our own health, and it has the potential of making us a lot healthier in the years to come.

Even in pregnancy, as you can see throughout this book, there are countless steps you can take to make your own nine months safer and more comfortable, your labor and delivery easier, and your expected end product healthier. But to try to go it alone, even for a few months, is to abuse the concept of self-care—which is built on the foundation of a cooperative partnership between patient and health professional. Regular professional input in pregnancy is crucial. One major study found that women who had many prenatal visits (an average of 12.7) had bigger babies with better survival rates than those who had only a few prenatal visits (an average of 1.4).

A SCHEDULE OF PRENATAL VISITS

Ideally, your first visit to a physician or nurse-midwife should take place while that baby is still in the planning stages. That's an ideal many of us, especially those whose pregnancies are unplanned, can't always manage.

When to Call the Practitioner

It's best to set up an emergency protocol with your practitioner before an emergency strikes. If you haven't, and you are experiencing a symptom that requires immediate medical attention, try the following: First call the practitioner's office. If he or she isn't available and doesn't call back within a few minutes, call again and leave a message saying what your problem is and where you are headed. Then go directly to the nearest emergency room or call the emergency medical squad.

When you report any of the following, be sure to mention any other symptoms you may be experiencing, no matter how remote they may seem from the immediate problem. Also be specific, mentioning how long the symptom has existed, how frequently it recurs, what seems to relieve or exacerbate it, and how severe it is. Call immediately for any of the following, except as noted.

❖ Severe lower abdominal pain, on one or both sides, that doesn't subside: call your practitioner the same day. If it is accompanied by bleeding, or nausea and vomiting: call immediately.

❖ Severe upper mid-abdominal pain, with or without nausea and swelling hands and face.

❖ Slight vaginal spotting: call your practitioner the same day.

❖ Heavy vaginal bleeding (especially when combined with abdominal or back pain).

❖ Bleeding from nipples, rectum, bladder: call your practitioner the same day.

❖ Coughing up of blood.

❖ A gush or steady leaking of fluid from the vagina.

❖ A sudden increase in thirst, accompanied by a paucity of urination, or no urination at all for an entire day.

❖ Swelling or puffiness of hands, face, eyes: call your practitioner the same day. If very sudden and severe, or accompanied by headache or vision difficulties: call immediately.

❖ Severe headache that persists for more than two or three hours: call your practitioner the same day. If accompanied by vision disturbances or puffiness of eyes, face, hands: call immediately.

❖ Painful or burning urination: call your practitioner the same day. If accompanied by chills and fever over 102 degrees and/or backache: call immediately.

❖ Vision disturbances (blurring, dimming, double vision) that persist for two hours.

❖ Fainting or dizziness: call your practitioner the same day.

❖ Chills and fever over 100 degrees (in the absence of cold or flu symptoms): call your practitioner the same day. Fever over 102 degrees: call immediately.

❖ Severe nausea and vomiting, vomiting more often than two or three times a day in the first trimester, vomiting later in pregnancy when you haven't earlier: call your practitioner the same day. If vomiting is accompanied by pain and/or fever: call immediately.

❖ Sudden weight gain of more than two pounds not related to overeating: call your practitioner the same day. If accompanied by swelling of the hands and face and/or headache or visual disturbance: call immediately.

❖ Absence of noticeable fetal movement for more than 24 hours after the 20th week: call your practitioner the same day. Fewer than ten movements per hour (see page 201) after 28 weeks: call immediately.

❖ All-over itching, with or without dark urine, pale stools, jaundice; call your practitioner the same day.

When in Doubt

Sometimes the body's signals that something is wrong aren't clear. You feel unusually exhausted, achy, not quite right. But there are none of the clear-cut symptoms listed on page 117. If a good night's sleep and some extra rest don't team up to make you feel better in a day or two, don't be embarrassed to check with your physician. It's likely that you only need more rest than you're getting. But it is also possible that you are anemic or harboring an infection of some kind. Certain infections—cystitis, for one— can do their dirty work without showing any obvious symptoms.

Second best, and still very good, is a visit as soon as you suspect you have conceived. An internal exam will help to confirm your pregnancy, and a physical will uncover potential problems that may need monitoring. After that, the schedule of visits will vary depending on the practitioner you are seeing and whether or not yours is a high-risk pregnancy. In an uneventful low-risk pregnancy you can probably expect to see your practitioner monthly, or occasionally even less often, until the end of the 32nd week. After that you may begin going every two weeks until the last month, when weekly visits are customary.[10]

For what you can expect at each prenatal visit, see the monthly chapters.

TAKING CARE OF THE REST OF YOU

You're understandably preoccupied with prenatal matters during pregnancy. But though your health care should begin with your belly, it shouldn't end there. And don't just wait for problems to drop into your lap. Pay a visit to your dentist; most dental work, particularly the preventive kind, can be done safely during pregnancy (see page 179). See your allergist, if necessary. You probably won't begin a course of allergy shots now, but if your allergies are severe, he or she may want to monitor your condition. Your family doctor or a specialist should also be monitoring any chronic illnesses or other medical problems that don't fall under the purview of the obstetrician; if you're seeing a nurse-midwife for pregnancy, you should see an obstetrician or your family physician for *all* medical problems.

If new medical problems come up while you're pregnant, don't ignore them. Even if you've noticed symptoms that seem relatively innocuous, it's more important now than ever to consult with your physician promptly. Your baby needs a *wholly* healthy mother.

---

10. A recent study suggests that healthy, well-educated women do well with as few as 9 scheduled pregnancy visits.

6
The Second Month

WHAT YOU CAN EXPECT AT THIS MONTH'S CHECKUP

If this is your first prenatal visit, see What You Can Expect at Your First Prenatal Visit (page 100). If this is your second exam, you can expect your practitioner to check the following, though there may be variations depending upon your particular needs and your practitioner's style of practice:[1]

❖ Weight and blood pressure

❖ Urine, for sugar and protein

❖ Hands and feet for edema (swelling), and legs for varicose veins

❖ Symptoms you have been experiencing, especially unusual ones

❖ Questions or problems you want to discuss—have a list ready

WHAT YOU MAY BE FEELING

You may experience all of these symptoms at one time or another, or only one or two. Some may have continued from last month, others may be new. Don't be surprised, no matter what your symptoms, if you don't feel pregnant yet.

PHYSICALLY:

❖ Fatigue and sleepiness

❖ A need to urinate frequently

---
1. See Appendix for an explanation of the procedures and tests performed.

❖ Nausea, with or without vomiting, and/or excessive salivation (ptyalism)

❖ Constipation

❖ Heartburn, indigestion, flatulence, bloating

❖ Food aversions and cravings

❖ Breast changes: fullness, heaviness, tenderness, tingling; darkening of areola (the pigmented area around the nipple); sweat glands in the areola become prominent (Montgomery's tubercles), like large goose bumps; a network of bluish lines appear under the skin as blood supply to the breasts increases

❖ Occasional headaches (similar to headaches in women taking birth control pills)

❖ Occasional faintness or dizziness

❖ Tightness of clothing around waist and bust; abdomen may appear en-

larged, probably due to bowel distention rather than uterine growth

EMOTIONALLY:

❖ Instability comparable to premenstrual syndrome, which may include irritability, mood swings, irrationality, weepiness

❖ Misgivings, fear, joy, elation—any or all of these

WHAT YOU MAY BE CONCERNED ABOUT

VENOUS CHANGES

"I have unsightly blue lines under the skin, on my breasts and abdomen. Is that normal?"

Very normal. What you see is part of the network of veins that has expanded to carry the increased blood supply of pregnancy. Not only are the veins nothing to worry about, they are a sign that your body is doing what it should. They may show up earliest in very slim or light-complexioned women. In some women this venous network may be less visible or not noticeable at all, or may not become obvious until later in pregnancy.

"Since I became pregnant I've got awful-looking spidery purplish-red lines on my thighs. Are they varicose veins?"

They aren't pretty, but they aren't varicose veins. They are probably spider nevi, or telangiectases, which can result from the hormone changes of pregnancy. They may fade and disappear after delivery; if they don't, they can be removed.

"My mother and grandmother both had varicose veins during pregnancy and had trouble with them ever after. Is there anything I can do to prevent the problem in my own pregnancy?"

Because varicosities often run in families, you're wise to think about prevention now—especially since varicose veins tend to worsen with subsequent pregnancies.

Normal, healthy veins carry blood from the extremities back to the heart. Because they must work against gravity, they are designed with a series of valves that prevent back flow. When these valves are missing or faulty, as they are in some people, blood tends to pool in the veins where the pressure of gravity is greatest (usually the legs, but sometimes the rectum or the vulva), resulting in the bulging of varicosities. Veins that are easily distended, or distensible, can further contribute to the condition. The problem is more common in people who are obese, and occurs four times more often in women than in men. In women who are susceptible, the condition often surfaces for the first time during pregnancy. There are several reasons for this: increased pressure from the uterus on the pelvic veins;

WHAT YOU MAY LOOK LIKE

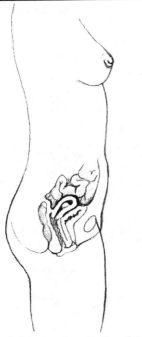

By the end of the second month, the embryo is more human-looking, about 1¼ inches long from head to buttocks (one-third of it is the head), and weighs about ⅓ ounce. It has a beating heart, and arms and legs with the beginnings of fingers and toes. Bone starts to replace cartilage.

increasing pressure on leg veins; expanded blood volume; and pregnancy-hormone-induced relaxation of the muscle tissue in the veins.

The symptoms of varicose veins aren't difficult to recognize, but they vary a great deal in severity. There may be severe pain, mild achiness, a sensation of heaviness, or none of these symptoms in the legs. A faint outline of bluish veins may be visible, or serpentine veins may bulge from ankle to upper thigh or vulva. In severe cases the skin overlying the veins

becomes swollen, dry, and irritated. Occasionally, thrombophlebitis (the inflammation of a vein due to a blood clot) may develop at the site of a varicosity (see page 360).

Fortunately, varicose veins during pregnancy can often be prevented, or the symptoms minimized, by taking measures to eliminate unnecessary pressure on the leg veins.

❖ Avoid excessive weight gain.

❖ Avoid long periods of standing or sitting. When sitting, elevate your legs above the level of the hips when possible. When lying down, raise your legs by placing a pillow under your feet or lie on your side.

❖ Avoid heavy lifting.

❖ Avoid straining during bowel movements.

❖ Wear support pantyhose (light support hose seem to work well without being uncomfortable) or elastic stockings, putting them on before getting out of bed in the morning (before blood pools in your legs) and removing them at night before getting into bed.

❖ Don't wear restrictive clothing. Avoid tight belts or girdles, especially panty-leg girdles (even those designed for pregnancy); stockings and socks with elastic tops; garters; and snug shoes.

❖ Don't smoke. A possible correlation has been found between smoking and varicose veins (and of course a host of other health problems, including pregnancy complications; see page 54).

❖ Get some exercise—such as a brisk 20- to 30-minute walk—every day.

❖ Be sure to get enough vitamin C, which some physicians believe helps to keep veins healthy and elastic.

Surgical removal of varicose veins isn't recommended during pregnancy, although it can certainly be considered a few months after delivery. In most cases, however, the problem will clear up or improve spontaneously after delivery, usually by the time pre-pregnancy weight is reached.

COMPLEXION PROBLEMS

"My skin is breaking out the way it did when I was a teenager."

The glow of pregnancy that some women are lucky enough to radiate is caused not simply by joy over impending motherhood, but by an increased secretion of oils brought about by hormonal changes. And so, alas, are the less-than-glowing break-outs of pregnancy that some not-so-lucky women experience (particularly those whose skin ordinarily breaks out before their periods). Though such eruptions are hard to eliminate entirely, the following suggestions may help keep them to a minimum:

❖ Be faithful to the Best-Odds Diet— it's good for your skin as well as for your baby.

❖ Don't pass a tap without filling your glass. Water is one of the most effective pore-purifiers around.

❖ Wash your face two or three times a day with a gentle cleanser. Avoid skin-clogging creams and makeup.

❖ If your practitioner approves, take a vitamin B_6 supplement (no more than 25 to 50 milligrams). This vitamin is used in treating hormonally induced skin problems, though the evidence that it helps is not clear.

❖ If your skin problems are severe enough to warrant your seeing your internist and/or consulting a dermatologist, be sure to let him or her know you are expecting. Some drugs used for acne, particularly Accutane and possibly Retin-A, should not be used by pregnant women because they can be harmful to the fetus.

For some pregnant women, dry, often itchy, skin is a problem. Moisturizers may be helpful. (For optimum absorption, they should be applied while the skin is still damp after bath or shower.) So may drinking plenty of fluids and keeping rooms well humidified in the heating season. Too-frequent bathing, particularly with soap, tends to increase dryness. So cut down on bathing, and try using a mild soapless cleanser.

WAISTLINE EXPANSION

"Why does my waist seem to be expanding already? I thought I wouldn't 'show' until the third month at least."

Your expanding waistline may very well be a legitimate by-product of pregnancy, especially if you started out slender, with little excess flesh for your growing uterus to hide behind. Or it may be the result of bowel distention, very common in early pregnancy. On the other hand, it's also quite possible that your "show" may be an indication that you're gaining weight too quickly. If you've gained more than 3 pounds so far, analyze your diet—you are very likely taking in too many calories, possibly empty ones. Review the Best-Odds Diet, and read about weight gain on page 147.

LOSING YOUR FIGURE

"I'm worried that my figure will never be the same after I have a baby."

The 2 to 4 permanent pounds the average woman puts on with each pregnancy, and the flab that usually accompanies them, are not the inevitable result of being pregnant. They're the result of gaining too much weight, eating the wrong foods, and/or not getting enough exercise during those nine months.

The weight gain of pregnancy has just two legitimate purposes: to nourish the developing fetus now, and to store up reserves for breastfeeding to nourish the baby after delivery. If only enough weight to serve those purposes is gained and a woman keeps physically fit, her figure will generally return to prepregnancy form within a few months after her baby is born, especially if she is using up fat stores by breastfeeding.[2] So stop worrying and start taking action. Follow the Best-Odds Diet, and observe the recommendations about weight gain on page 147 and exercise on page 189.

With attention to diet and exercise now, you can look better than ever after pregnancy, because you will have learned how to take optimum care of your body. If your husband joins you in your healthier lifestyle, he can look better after your pregnancy too.

HEARTBURN AND INDIGESTION

"I have indigestion and heartburn all the time. Will this affect my baby?"

While you are painfully aware of your gastrointestinal discomfort, your baby is blissfully oblivious to and unaffected by it—as long as it isn't interfering with your eating the right foods.

Though indigestion can have the same cause (usually overindulgence) during pregnancy as when you're not pregnant, there are additional reasons

why it may be plaguing you now. Early in pregnancy, your body produces large amounts of progesterone and estrogen, which tend to relax smooth muscle tissue everywhere, including the gastrointestinal (GI) tract. As a result, food sometimes moves more slowly through your system, resulting in bloating and indigestion. This may be uncomfortable for you, but it is beneficial for your baby because this alimentary slowdown allows better absorption of nutrients into your bloodstream and subsequently through the placenta, into your baby's system.

Heartburn results when the ring of muscle that separates the esophagus from the stomach relaxes, allowing food and harsh digestive juices to back up from the stomach to the esophagus. These stomach acids irritate the sensitive esophageal lining, causing a burning sensation right about where the heart is; thus the term heartburn—which has nothing to do with your heart. During the last two trimesters the problem can be compounded by your blossoming uterus as it presses up on your stomach.

It's nearly impossible to have an indigestion-free nine months; it's just one of the less pleasant facts of pregnancy. There are, however, some pretty effective ways of avoiding heartburn and indigestion most of the time, and of minimizing the discomfort when it strikes:

❖ Avoid gaining too much weight; ex-

2. A few nursing mothers find they can shed very little weight while breastfeeding; they are usually able to return to prepregnancy weight soon after weaning their babies. If they don't, it is because they are consuming too many calories and burning too few. Bottle-feeding mothers will have to lose weight postpartum through diet and exercise.

cess weight puts excess pressure on the stomach.

❖ Don't wear clothing that is tight around your abdomen and waist.

❖ Eat many small meals rather than three big ones.

❖ Eat slowly, taking small mouthfuls and chewing thoroughly.

❖ Eliminate from your diet any food that causes GI discomfort. The most common offenders are hot and highly seasoned foods; fried or fatty foods; processed meats (hot dogs, bologna, sausage, bacon); chocolate, coffee, alcohol, carbonated beverages; spearmint and peppermint (even in gum).

❖ Don't smoke.

❖ Avoid bending over at the waist; bend instead with your knees.

❖ Sleep with your head elevated about 6 inches.

❖ Relax.

❖ If all else fails to relieve your symptoms, ask your doctor to recommend a low-sodium antacid or other over-the-counter medication that is safe for use in pregnancy. Avoid preparations containing sodium or sodium bicarbonate.

FOOD AVERSIONS AND CRAVINGS

"Certain foods—particularly green vegetables—that I've always liked taste funny now. Instead, I have cravings for foods that are less nutritious."

T he pregnancy cliché of a harried husband running out in the middle of the night, raincoat over his pajamas, for a pint of ice cream and a jar of pickles to satisfy his wife's cravings is probably played out more often in the heads of cartoonists than in real life. Not many pregnant women's cravings carry them—or their husbands—that far.

But most of us do find that our tastes in food change somewhat in pregnancy. Studies show that between 66% and 90% of expectant mothers experience a craving for at least one food (most often ice cream or fruit), and between 50% and 85% have at least one food aversion. To a certain extent, these sudden gastronomic eccentricities can be blamed on hormonal havoc—which probably explains why food aversions and cravings are most common in the first trimester of first pregnancies, when that havoc is at its height.

Hormones, however, don't offer the only explanation for pregnancy food aversions and cravings. The long-favored theory that these are sensible signals from our bodies—that when we develop a distaste for something, it's usually bad for us, and that when we crave something, it's usually something we need—has some merit. Such a signal comes when the black coffee that used to be the mainstay of your workday becomes totally unappealing. Or the cocktail before dinner seems too strong even when it's weak. Or you suddenly can't get enough citrus fruit. On the other hand, when you can't stand the sight of fish, or broccoli suddenly tastes bitter, or you crave ice-cream sundaes, you can't credit your body with sending accurate signals.

The fact is that body signals relating to food are notoriously unreliable, probably because we've departed so significantly from the food chain in nature that we can no longer interpret these signals correctly. Before ice-cream sundaes were invented, when food came from nature, a craving for carbohydrates and calcium would have steered us toward fruits or berries and milk or cheese. With the wide variety of tempting (but often unwholesome) foods available today, it's no wonder our bodies are confused.

You can't totally ignore cravings and aversions. But you can respond to them without putting your baby's nutritional needs in jeopardy. If you crave something that's good for you and baby, by all means go ahead and enjoy it. If you crave something that you really shouldn't have, then seek a substitute that satisfies the craving without sabotaging your baby's nutritional interests: raisins, dried apricots, or a fruit-juice-sweetened muffin, cookie, or chocolate bar instead of sugary candies; lightly salted whole-wheat pretzels instead of the usually oversalted, nutritionally vacant variety. When substitutes don't satisfy, sublimation may be helpful—try exercise, knitting, reading, a leisurely bath, or other distractions when unwholesome urges strike. And, of course, occasionally give in to your cravings and cheat (see page 129).

If you experience a sudden aversion to coffee or alcohol or chocolate ice cream, great. It will make giving them up for the duration all the easier. If it's fish or broccoli or milk you can't tolerate, you don't have to force-feed yourself, but you do have to find compensating sources of the nutrients they supply. (See the Best-Odds Diet for appropriate substitutions.)

Most cravings and aversions disappear or weaken by the fourth month. Cravings that hang in there longer may be triggered by emotional needs—the need for a little extra attention, for example. If both you and your spouse are aware of this need, it should be easy to satisfy. You might, instead of requesting a middle-of-the-night pint of Rocky Road, settle for some quiet cuddling or a romantic bath-for-two.

Some women find themselves craving, even eating, such peculiar sub-

stances as clay, ashes, and laundry starch. Since this habit, known as pica, can be a sign of nutritional deficiency, particularly of iron, it should be reported to your practitioner.

MILK AVERSION OR INTOLERANCE

"I can't tolerate milk, and drinking four cups a day would make me ill. Will my baby suffer if I don't drink milk?"

First of all, it's not milk your baby needs, it's calcium. Since milk is the most convenient source of calcium in the American diet, it's the one most often recommended for filling the greatly increased requirement during pregnancy. But there are many substitutes that fill the nutritional bill just as well. Many people who are lactose-intolerant (can't digest the milk sugar, lactose) can tolerate some kinds of dairy products, such as hard cheeses, fully processed yogurts, and the new lactose-reduced milk, in which 70% of the lactose has been converted to a more easily digested form. If you can't tolerate any dairy products, you can still get all the calcium your baby requires by eating the nondairy foods listed under Calcium-Rich Foods on page 90.

You may find, however, that even though you have been lactose-intolerant for years, you are able to handle some dairy products during the second and third trimesters, when fetal needs for calcium are the greatest. Even if that's so, don't overdo it; try to stick primarily to those products that are less likely to provoke a reaction.

If your problem with milk isn't physiological but just a matter of distaste, there are many sources of calcium that should not offend your taste buds. You'll find them all in the

Calcium-Rich Foods list. Or you can try to fool your taste buds with non-fat dry milk that comes to your table incognito (in oatmeal, soups, muffins, sauces, shakes, frozen desserts, puddings, and so on).

If, in spite of all your best efforts, you can't seem to get enough calcium into your diet, ask your practitioner about prescribing a calcium supplement.

CHOLESTEROL

"My husband and I are very careful about our diets, and we limit our cholesterol and fat intake. Should I continue to do this while I'm pregnant?"

Pregnant women, and to a lesser extent nonpregnant women of childbearing age, are in an enviable position: they do not have to limit their cholesterol intake as drastically as do men and older women. In fact, cholesterol is necessary for fetal development, so much so that the mother's body automatically increases its production, raising blood cholesterol levels by anywhere from 25% to 40%.[3] Though you don't have to eat a high-cholesterol diet to help your body step up production, you can feel free to indulge a bit. Have an egg every day[4] if you like, use cheese to meet your calcium requirement, and enjoy an occasional steak—all without guilt. But don't overdo, because many high-cholesterol foods are high in fat and

calories, and an excess of them could send the numbers on your scale soaring. Too much fat could also put you over your fat quota (see page 87). And remember that many foods high in cholesterol are also high in animal fats that may be contaminated by undesirable chemicals (see page 131).

But while you don't necessarily have to hold the mayo (and the butter, and the egg yolks, and the lamb chops), everyone else in your household (except for under-two-year-olds)[5] should, most of the time. That goes most emphatically for adult men, both those with borderline-to-high cholesterol counts and those who just want to avoid developing a problem. Because serving two sets of breakfasts, lunches, and dinners—one cholesterol-lenient and one cholesterol-trimmed—is not only a strain on the cook but also unfair to those being denied, it's wise to continue, or to institute, a healthy heart regimen for family meals. Lean toward lean meats, poultry without the skin, low-fat dairy products, cholesterol-combating oils (such as olive and canola), and the white of the egg rather than the yolk. Enjoy your cholesterol on the sly, when no one else is around to drool.

A MEATLESS DIET

"I eat chicken and fish but no red meat. Can I supply my baby with all the nutrients he needs without meat?"

Your baby can be just as happy and healthy as any beef-eating mother's offspring. Fish and poultry, in fact, give you more protein and less fat

---

3. Women who have hypercholesteremia, a familial type of high blood cholesterol, are exceptions to the loosening of the cholesterol reins in pregnancy. These women should continue to follow their doctors' advice about diet.

4. Not raw, however, or even undercooked, because of the risk of salmonella poisoning.

5. Babies under two need fat and cholesterol for proper growth and brain development, and should never be placed on a fat- and cholesterol-restricted diet except under medical supervision.

for your calories than beef, pork, lamb, and organ meats. A red-meatless diet also contains less cholesterol, which may not make a big difference to you while you're pregnant, but represents a plus for your spouse and perhaps other family members.

A VEGETARIAN DIET

"I'm a vegetarian and in perfect health. But everyone—including my doctor—says that I have to eat meat and fish, eggs, and milk products to have a healthy baby. Is this true?"

Vegetarians of every variety can have healthy babies without compromising their dietary principles. But they have to be even more careful in planning their diets than meat-eating mothers-to-be, being particularly sure to get all of the following:

Adequate Protein. For the ovo-lacto vegetarian, who eats eggs and milk products, adequate protein intake can be ensured by taking ample quantities of both. A vegan (a strict vegetarian who eats neither milk nor eggs) has to depend on combinations of vegetable proteins to meet her five-serving protein allowance (see Vegetarian Complete Protein Combinations, page 97). Some meat substitutes are good protein sources; others are low in protein and high in fat and calories. Read the labels.

Adequate Calcium. This is no problem for the vegetarian who eats dairy products, but adroit maneuvering is needed for those who don't. Many soy products are fairly high in calcium, but beware of soy milks loaded with sucrose (sugar, corn syrup, honey); look for a pure soybean product instead. For tofu to be counted as a calcium food, it must have been coagulated with calcium; otherwise it

will contain little or none of that mineral. Some brands of stone-ground corn tortillas are good nondairy sources of calcium, providing as much as half a calcium serving per piece (check the labels). Another easy-to-take nondairy source of calcium is calcium-added orange juice. For yet others, see the Calcium-Rich Foods list on page 91. For added insurance, it is recommended that vegans also take a prescribed calcium supplement (vegetarian formulas are available).

Vitamin B$_{12}$. Vegetarians, particularly vegans, often don't get enough of this vitamin because it is found primarily in animal foods. So they should be certain to take a vitamin supplement that includes B$_{12}$ as well as folic acid and iron.

Vitamin D. This important vitamin occurs naturally only in fish liver oils. It is also produced by our skin when we are exposed to sunlight, though because of the vagaries of weather, cover-up clothing, and the dangers of spending too much time in the sun, this is an unreliable source of the vitamin for most women. To ensure adequate intake of vitamin D, particularly for children and pregnant women, U.S. law requires that milk be fortified with 400 mg of vitamin D per quart. If you don't drink milk, be sure that there is vitamin D in the supplement you are taking (see page 88). Be careful, however, not to take vitamin D in doses beyond pregnancy requirements, since it can be toxic in excessive amounts.

JUNK-FOOD JUNKIE

"I'm addicted to junk foods—doughnuts for breakfast; fast-food burgers, fries, and Cokes for lunch. I'm afraid that if I can't break these bad habits, my baby will be undernourished."

Y ou're right to worry. Before you became pregnant, your dietary indiscretions could hurt only you; now they can hurt your baby as well. Make a daily diet of doughnuts, fast-food burgers, and Cokes, and you'll be denying your baby adequate nourishment during the most important nine months of his or her life. Eat the junk food on top of a balanced diet, and your baby won't be the only one growing.

Happily, addictions can be broken. Heroin. Tobacco. Even junk food. Here are several ways to make your withdrawal almost as painless as it is worthwhile:

Change the Locale of Your Meals. If breakfast usually consists of a danish at your desk, have a better breakfast before you leave for work. If you can't resist a burger at lunch, go to a restaurant that doesn't serve burgers, or order in a nutritious sandwich from the local deli or bring one from home.

Stop Thinking of Eating as a Catch-as-Catch-Can Proposition. Rather than settling for what's easiest, select what's best for your baby. Plan meals and snacks ahead of time to be sure you get all of your Daily Dozen.

Don't Give Temptation a Tumble. Keep candy, chips, sugary cookies made with refined flours, and sugar-sweetened soft drinks out of the house (other family members will survive without them, and in fact will benefit from their absence). When the coffee wagon bell chimes at work, don't answer it. Stock home and workplace with such wholesome snacks as fresh and dried fruit, nuts, fruit-juice-sweetened baked goods, whole-wheat breadsticks and crackers, juices, hard-cooked eggs, and string cheese (the last two will need refrigeration at work, or the company of an ice pack in your lunch box).

Don't Use Lack of Time as an Excuse for Sloppy Eating. It takes no more time to make a tuna sandwich to take to work than to stand on line at Burger King. Or to slice a fresh peach into a container of yogurt than to cut a slab of peach pie. If the prospect of preparing a real dinner every night seems overwhelming, cook enough for two or three dinners at one time and give yourself alternate nights off. And keep it simple: fancy sauces aren't nutritious, only high in fat and calories. Utilize frozen vegetables or the fresh, prewashed, cut-up vegetables at salad bars or in supermarket produce sections when you don't have the time to do it yourself (raw vegetables can be quickly steamed or stir-fried at home).

Don't Use a Tight Budget as an Excuse for Eating Junk Foods. A glass of orange juice or milk is cheaper than a can of Coke. A homemade broiled chicken breast and baked potato cost a lot less than a Big Mac and fries.

Quit Cold Turkey. Don't tell yourself you can have just one cola today or just one doughnut. That approach almost never works when you're trying to break an addiction. Just tell yourself that junk food is out—at least until you deliver. You may be surprised to find, once the baby's born, that your new good eating habits are as hard to break as your old bad ones—which will make setting a good example for your child all the easier.

Study the Best-Odds Diet. Make it part of your life.

EATING FAST FOOD

"I go out with friends for fast food after a movie about once a month. Do I have to skip this for the rest of my pregnancy?"

Best-Odds Cheating

Unless you have a food allergy or sensitivity, no food need be completely off limits, even during pregnancy. The Best-Odds Diet recognizes that all of us slip up—really *need* to slip up—every once in a while. To eliminate guilt, the diet allows for cheating. So once a week give in to something that is not quite perfect but not totally terrible: a bagel, some bread, or pancakes made with refined flour; frozen yogurt or ice milk made with sugar; french fries or fried chicken; a fast-food burger; a bran or whole-grain muffin made with sugar or honey. Once a month, treat yourself to something terribly wicked: a slice of cake or pie; an ice-cream sundae; a candy bar. Always try to cheat selectively—choose carrot cake or cheesecake over butter-cream-frosted yellow cake; ice cream over milkless frozen desserts (unless you can't tolerate milk); cookies made with oats, raisins, or nuts rather than chocolate chips. Cheat only on something you really want and love. And don't cheat at all if you find that you can't stop once you get started.

Though fast food still can't be called health food, the major chains have gone a long way recently to improve the nutritive quality of the fare they offer. Still, you have to pick and choose to be sure you get the best of the offerings. At some fast-food establishments you can get help from the nutrition information posted or available on request. Look for grilled chicken, broiled or baked fish, baked potatoes (without the fat-rich toppings), a taco, a slice of pizza, occasionally a plain burger, salads that aren't swimming in oily dressings (select fresh vegetables instead, and lightly dress them and sprinkle with cheese), or other main-course items that are not excessively high in fat and sodium. Avoid the fries (though they may no longer be made with beef fat, they're still high in fat and calories), double burgers, processed cheese toppings for potatoes (use some fresh cheese from the salad bar instead), sugary canned fruits and puddings, sodas, and fruit pies. If the shakes or frozen desserts are made with real milk, treat yourself occasionally—but avoid those that are primarily sugar, saturated fat, and chemicals. Drink juice, milk, soda water, or plain water, and bring along your own dessert (a couple of fruit-juice-sweetened cookies or a piece of fruit) if you fear your sweet tooth may get the better of you if it isn't appeased. If you come away without having had a single green leafy or yellow vegetable, munch a carrot or enjoy a slice of cantaloupe when you get home.

CHEMICALS IN FOODS

"With additives in packaged foods, insecticides on vegetables, PCBs in fish, DES in meat, and nitrates in hot dogs, is there anything I can safely eat during pregnancy?"

Reports of hazardous chemicals in just about every item in the American diet are enough to scare the appetite out of anyone—and especially a pregnant woman afraid not only for her own health but for that of her unborn child. Thanks to the media, "chemical" has become synonymous with "dangerous," and "natural" with "safe." But neither generalization is true. Everything we eat is made up of chemicals. Some chemicals are harmful, some are not; some are even beneficial. And although "natural" is often better than artificial or unnatural, it can also be deadly. A "natural" mushroom can be poisonous; "natural" eggs, butter, and animal fats are associated with heart disease; and "natural" sugar and honey cause cavities.

That's not to say that you have to give up eating altogether in order to protect your baby from danger at the table. In spite of anything you might have heard, no food or additive presently in use has been shown to cause birth defects. And in fact, most American women fill their shopping carts without giving safety a second thought and have perfectly normal babies. Clearly, the danger that exists from the chemical additives in food is remote.

If you want to do your best to eliminate even this remote risk, use the following as a guide to help you decide what to drop into your shopping cart and what to pass up.

❖ Use the Best-Odds Diet as the foundation for food selection; it steers you clear of most potential perils. It also supplies Green Leafies and Yellows that are rich in protective beta-carotene, which may counteract the negative effects of toxins in our food.

❖ Use sweeteners wisely. Entirely avoid foods sweetened with saccharin; it crosses the placenta and its long-term effects on the fetus are unknown. If you do not have difficulty handling the amino acid phenylalanine, you can, however, use aspartame (Equal, NutraSweet). The components of this sweetener do not appear to cross the placenta in any significant amounts, and studies show no harm to the fetus with moderate maternal use in nor-

mal women. (But there are reasons why foods made with aspartame may not be the best ones for you; see page 62.) Sweeteners made of slowly absorbed carbohydrates, such as sorbitol and mannitol, are also believed safe, but be aware that they are not low in calories and that even moderate doses can cause diarrhea.

❖ Whenever possible, cook from scratch with fresh ingredients. You'll avoid many questionable additives found in processed foods, and your meals will be more nutritious too.

❖ Contact your local Environmental Protection Agency (EPA) or health department for a list of fish in your area that have not been contaminated with PCBs or other chemicals. If the fish you are planning to enjoy is the bounty of a family fishing expedition, be especially careful to check on its safety since such fish is more suspect than most commercially caught seafood.

Because chemicals in the mother's body can be passed on to and damage the fetus (PCBs, for example can lower IQ), pregnant women should play it safe. They should avoid bluefish and striped bass, believed to pose the greatest risk. As a general rule, they should also skip freshwater fish caught in polluted lakes and rivers (most are). It's also recommended that they limit intake of swordfish, fresh tuna, and shark (all high in mercury) to no more than one serving a month (though because levels are lower in canned tuna, a couple of cans a week are okay). Beware, too, of eating fish from waters that are grossly contaminated—with sewage for example—or tropical fish, such as grouper, amberjack, mahimahi, which can cause poisoning.

Since unwanted chemicals collect in fatty tissue, you'll be safest.

sticking to lean seafood, such as sole, flounder, haddock, Pacific halibut, ocean perch, pollack, and cod. Also okay are most salmon (especially farm raised) and cooked shellfish. (*All* seafood should be well cooked.)[6]

❖ Generally avoid foods preserved with nitrates and nitrites: frankfurters, salami, luncheon meats, smoked fish and meats.

❖ Whenever you have a choice between a product with artificial colorings, flavorings, preservatives, and other additives and one without, opt for the one that's additive-free.

❖ In cooking, don't use MSG or flavor enhancers that contain it. In Chinese restaurants, request no MSG when ordering.

❖ Choose lean cuts of meat and poultry and remove visible fat and skin before cooking, since chemicals that are fed to livestock tend to concentrate in these parts of the animal. Don't eat organ meats (liver, kidneys, etc.) very often, for the same reason. When possible, buy poultry and meat that has been raised organically, without hormones or antibiotics. Free-range chickens, for example, are not only less likely to be contaminated with these chemicals, they are also less likely to carry such infections as salmonella because the birds are not kept in cramped disease-breeding quarters.

❖ As a precaution, give all nonorganic vegetables and fruits a bath (in wa-ter, a produce wash product, or dish detergent) just before using them; rinse thoroughly. Scrub skins when possible, and be sure to rinse thoroughly. Peel when practical, to remove surface chemical residues, especially when a vegetable has a waxy coating (as cucumbers, and sometimes tomatoes, apples, and peppers, often do).

❖ Beware of picture-perfect produce. Fruits and vegetables that appear to have been embalmed, so unblemished are they, may very well have been heavily protected by pesticides in the fields. The less pretty produce may be the healthier bet.

❖ Buy organic produce when possible and practical. Produce that is certified organic usually is as close as possible to being free of all chemical residues. Transitional produce may still contain some residues from soil contamination, but should be safer than conventionally grown produce. If organic produce is available locally and you can afford the premium price, make it your choice. If it isn't available, ask the produce manager at your favorite market to order it.

❖ Favor domestic produce. Imported produce (and foods made from such produce) may contain higher levels of pesticides than that grown in the U.S., since pesticide regulation in other countries is often lax or nonexistent. Bananas, all of which are imported, are apparently safe, however; government monitoring sources have found them virtually free of pesticides.

❖ Vary your diet. Variety ensures not only a more interesting gastronomic experience and better nutrition, but also better odds of avoiding excessive exposure to any one potentially toxic substance. Switch between broccoli, kale, and car-

---

6. For the latest information on fish safety call the FDA, 1-800-FDA-4010, or The American Seafood Institute (an industry source), 1-800-EAT-FISH (in Rhode Island, dial 401-783-4200), between 9 A.M. and 5 P.M. Monday through Friday.

rots, for instance; melon, peaches, and strawberries; salmon, tuna, and sole; wheat, oats, and rice.

❖ Don't be fanatic. Though trying to avoid theoretical hazards in food is a commendable goal, making your life stressful in order to do so is not.

READING LABELS

"I'm eager to eat well, but it's difficult to figure out what's in the products I buy."

L abels aren't designed to help you as much as to sell you. Keep this in mind when food shopping, and learn to read the small print, especially the ingredients list and the nutrition label.

The ingredients listing will tell you, in order of predominance (with the first ingredient the most plentiful and the last the least), exactly what is in the product. A quick perusal will tell you whether the major ingredient in a cereal is sugar or a wholegrain. It will also tell you when a product is high in salt, fat, or additives.

Nutritional labels appear on more than half the products on your grocer's shelves, and these are particu- larly valuable for a pregnant woman counting her protein and watching her calories, as they provide the grams of the former and the number of the latter in each serving. The listing of percentages of the government's rec- ommended daily allowance, however, is less useful, because the RDA for pregnant women is different from the RDA used on package labels. Still, a food high in a wide variety of nutri- ents is a good product to purchase.

While it's important to pay atten- tion to the small print, it's sometimes just as important to ignore the large print. When a box of English muffins trumpets boldly, "Made with whole wheat, bran, and honey," reading the small print may reveal that that the major ingredient (first on the list) is *white,* not whole-wheat, flour, that the muffins contain precious little bran (it's near the bottom of the ingre- dients list), and that there's a lot more sugar (it's high on the list) than honey (it's low).

"Enriched" and "fortified" are also banners to be wary of. Adding a few vitamins to a poor food doesn't make it a good food. You'd be much better off with a bowl of oatmeal, which comes by its vitamins honestly, than with a refined cereal that is 50% sugar

---

Eating Safe

A more immediate threat than the chemicals in your food are the little organisms—bacteria and parasites— that can contaminate it. These villains can cause anything from mild stom- ach upset to severe illness, and in very rare instances even death. So beware of dishes that have been prepared un- der less than sanitary conditions; cooked food that has been left stand- ing unrefrigerated for more than a couple of hours; food from cans that are swollen or jars that don't pop when you open them; unpasteurized juices, milk, or cheese; undercooked or raw eggs and any kind of raw, or even undercooked, meat, fish, or poul- try. To be sure that you don't conta- minate food yourself, carefully wash your hands with soap and water be- fore cooking or eating.*

---

*For more on safe food preparation, see *What to Eat When You're Expecting.*

(the nutrition label usually lists the percentage of sugar) but has a few pennies' worth of vitamins and minerals added.

A "TILTED" UTERUS

"My doctor said my uterus is tilted. Is this a problem?"

Probably not. About one in five women has a tilted (or retroverted) uterus, in which the fundus (or top) of the uterus is tilted toward the back instead of the front. In most cases, the uterus rights itself by the end of the first trimester. In the rare cases where it doesn't, and where it becomes lodged in the pelvis, putting pressure on the bladder, a catheter may be inserted to drain urine and the uterus gently pushed back into the proper position.

WHAT IT'S IMPORTANT TO KNOW: PLAYING IT SAFE

The home. The highway. The backyard. The most significant risks faced by pregnant women are not from pregnancy complications, but from accidental injuries.

Accidents often seem "accidental," that is, to happen by chance. Yet most are the direct result of carelessness—often on the part of the victim herself—and many can be avoided with a little extra caution and common sense. There are a wide variety of steps you can take to prevent injuries and accidents:

❖ Recognize that you're not as graceful as you were prepregnancy. As your abdomen grows, your center of gravity will shift, making it easier for you to lose your balance. You will also find it increasingly difficult to see your feet. These changes can contribute to your becoming accident-prone.

❖ Always fasten your seat belt—and keep it fastened—in autos and on airplanes. If you are sitting in the front passenger seat in a car with an airbag, be sure your seat is as far back as possible. If you are driving a car with an airbag in the steering wheel, tilt the wheel toward your chest, away from your tummy and, sit at least 10 inches from the steering wheel. Keep objects off your lap and off the dashboard, since they can become projectiles. When you can, ride in the back seat.

❖ Never climb on a shaky chair or ladder, or better still, don't climb at all.

❖ Don't wear high spiky heels, sloppy slippers, or thongs that can snap, all of which encourage falls and twisted ankles. Don't walk on slippery floors in your stocking feet or in smooth-soled shoes.

❖ Be careful getting in and out of the tub; be sure your tub and shower are equipped with nonskid surfaces and sturdy grab bars.

❖ Check your house and backyard for hazards: rugs without skidproof bottoms, especially at the top of stairs; toys or junk on stairways; poorly lit stairs and hallways; wires strung across the floor; overwaxed floors; icy sidewalks and steps.

❖ Observe the safety rules of whatever sport you play; follow all the tips for safe exercise and activity on page 195.

❖ Don't overdo. Fatigue is a major contributor to accidents.

7
The Third Month

WHAT YOU CAN EXPECT AT THIS MONTH'S CHECKUP

This month you can expect your practitioner to check the following, though there may be variations depending upon your particular needs and your practitioner's style of practice:[1]

❖ Weight and blood pressure

❖ Urine, for sugar and protein

❖ Fetal heartbeat

❖ Size of uterus, by external palpa-

tion, to see how it correlates to estimated date of delivery (EDD), or due date

❖ Height of fundus (the top of the uterus)

❖ Hands and feet for edema (swelling), and legs for varicose veins

❖ Questions or problems you want to discuss—have a list ready

WHAT YOU MAY BE FEELING

You may experience all of these symptoms at one time or another, or only a few of them. Some may have continued from last month, others may be new. You may also have additional, less common, symptoms.

PHYSICALLY:

❖ Fatigue and sleepiness

---

1. See Appendix for an explanation of the procedures and tests performed.

❖ A need to urinate frequently

❖ Nausea, with or without vomiting, and/or excessive salivation

❖ Constipation

❖ Heartburn, indigestion, flatulence, bloating

❖ Food aversions and cravings

❖ Breast changes: fullness, heaviness, tenderness, tingling; darkening of the areola (the pigmented area surrounding the nipple); sweat glands

WHAT YOU MAY LOOK LIKE

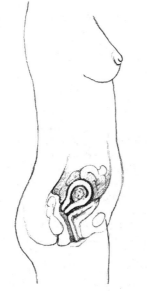

By the end of the third month, this tiny human, now a fetus, is 2½ to 3 inches long and weighs about ½ ounce. More organs are developing; circulatory and urinary systems are operating; the liver produces bile. Reproductive organs are developed, but the gender of the fetus is difficult to distinguish externally.

in the areola become prominent (Montgomery's tubercles), like large goose bumps; network of bluish lines under the skin expands

❖ Additional veins visible elsewhere, as blood supply to abdomen and legs also increases

❖ Occasional headaches

❖ Occasional faintness or dizziness

❖ Tightness of clothing around waist and bust, if it wasn't tight already; abdomen may appear enlarged by end of month

❖ Increasing appetite

EMOTIONALLY:

❖ Instability comparable to premenstrual syndrome, which may include irritability, mood swings, irrationality, weepiness

❖ Misgivings, fear, joy, elation—any or all

❖ A new sense of calmness

WHAT YOU MAY BE CONCERNED ABOUT

CONSTIPATION

"I've been terribly constipated for the past few weeks. Is this common?"

Very common. And there are sound reasons why. For one, increased relaxation of the musculature of the bowel, due to the high levels of certain hormones circulating during pregnancy, makes elimination sluggish. For another, the pressure from the growing uterus on the bowels inhibits their normal activity.

But there's no sound reason for accepting constipation as inevitable with every pregnancy. Irregularity can be overcome by taking the following measures, which can also head off a common result of irregularity, hemorrhoids (see page 203):

Fight Back with Fiber. Avoid constipating refined foods and focus on such fiber-rich items as fresh fruit and vegetables (raw or lightly cooked, with skin left on when possible); whole-grain cereals, breads, and other baked goods; legumes (dried beans and peas); and dried fruit (raisins, prunes, apricots, figs). If you normally eat little fiber, add these high-fiber foods to your diet gradually or you may find your stomach unsettled. (You may find it unsettled for a while anyway, since flatulence is a frequent but usually temporary side effect of a fiber-infused diet, as well as a common complaint of pregnancy.) Spreading your daily fare out over six small meals rather than trying to squeeze everything into three overly filling ones may make you less uncomfortable.

If your case is a desperate one that doesn't seem to respond to such dietary manipulation or to the tactics below, add some wheat bran to your diet, starting with a sprinkle and working up to a couple of tablespoons. But avoid larger quantities of wheat bran; as it moves speedily through your system, it can carry away important nutrients before they've had a chance to be absorbed.

Drown Your Opponent. Constipation doesn't stand a chance against an ample fluid intake. Most fluids—particularly water and fruit and vegetable juices—are effective in softening stool and keeping food moving along the digestive tract. Some people find cups of hot water flavored with lemon (but no sugar) especially helpful. If constipation is severe, prune juice may do the trick.

Start an Exercise Campaign. Fit a brisk walk of at least half an hour into your daily routine; supplement it with any exercise you enjoy that is safe during pregnancy (see Exercise During Pregnancy, page 189).

If your efforts don't seem to be productive, consult with your practitioner. He or she may prescribe a bulk-forming stool softener for occasional use.

"All my pregnant friends seem to have problems with constipation. I don't; in fact, I've been more regular than ever. Is my system working right?"

Pregnant women are so programmed by mothers, friends, books, even doctors, to expect constipation that those who do become constipated accept it as normal and inevitable, and those who don't worry that there's something wrong.

But from the sound of things, your system couldn't be working better. Chances are your new digestive efficiency is attributable to a change in your diet—almost undoubtedly a change for the better.[2] Stepping up your consumption of fruits, vegetables, whole grains and other complex carbohydrates, and fluids, as recommended by the Best-Odds Diet, is bound to counteract the natural digestive slowdown of pregnancy and keep things moving smoothly. As your system gets used to the rough stuff, its productivity may decrease a little (and flatulence, which often temporarily accompanies such dietary changes, may ease up), but you will probably continue to be "regular."

If your stools are either very frequent (more than twice a day), or loose, watery, bloody, or mucousy, however, consult with your practitioner. Diarrhea during pregnancy requires prompt intervention.

---

2. Iron supplements may contribute to diarrhea *or* to constipation. If your supplement seems to unsettle your system, ask your practitioner to suggest a different formula.

FLATULENCE (GAS)

"I'm very bloated from gas and worry that the pressure, which is so uncomfortable for me, might also be hurting the baby."

Snug and safe in a uterine cocoon, protected on all sides by impact-absorbing amniotic fluid, your baby is impervious to your intestinal distress. If anything, he or she probably is soothed by the bubbling and gurgling of your gastric Muzak.

The only possible threat to your baby's well-being is if bloating—which often worsens late in the day—is preventing you from eating regularly and properly. To avoid this risk (and to minimize your own discomfort), take the following measures:

Stay Regular. Constipation is a common cause of gas and bloating.

Don't Gorge. Large meals just add to the bloated feeling. They also overload your digestive system, which isn't at its most efficient to begin with during pregnancy. Instead of three large meals a day, eat six small ones.

Don't Gulp. When you rush through meals or eat on the run, you're bound to swallow as much air as food. This captured air forms painful pockets of gas in your gut.

Keep Calm. Particularly during meals: Tension and anxiety can cause you to swallow air.

Steer Clear of Gas-Producers. Your stomach knows what they are—possibly onions, cabbage and cabbage-family members such as Brussels sprouts and broccoli, fried foods and sugary sweets (which you shouldn't be having now anyway), and of course the notorious beans.

WEIGHT GAIN

"I'm concerned that I didn't gain any weight in my first trimester."

Many women have trouble putting on an ounce in the early weeks; some even lose a few, usually courtesy of morning sickness. Fortunately, nature offers some protection for the babies of mothers who are too queasy to eat well during the first trimester: the fetus's need for calories and certain nutrients during this time is not as great as it will be later, so not gaining early on isn't likely to have an effect. But not gaining weight from here on in *can* have an effect—a significant one—because calories and nutrients will be more and more in demand as your baby-making factory picks up steam.

So don't worry, but do eat. And start watching your weight carefully to make sure it begins to move upward at a satisfactory rate (about 1 pound a week through the eighth month). If you continue to have trouble gaining weight, try packing more of a nutritional wallop with the calories you take in, through efficient eating (see page 81). Try, too, to eat a little more food each day, by adding more frequent snacks. But don't try to add pounds by adding junk food to your diet—that kind of weight gain will round out your hips and thighs, not your baby.

"I was shocked to find out that I'd already gained 13 pounds in the first trimester. What should I do now?"

You can't turn back the scales—that weight is there to stay for now, at least until some time after delivery. And you can't apply the extra pounds toward next trimester's gain, either. Your fetus needs a steady supply of calories and nutrients, particularly during the months to come. You can't cut back on calories now, expecting it to get sufficient nourishment from the excess weight you've already accumulated. Dieting to lose or maintain weight is never appropriate during pregnancy, and it is an especially dangerous game during the second and third trimesters, when fetal growth is dramatically swift and significant.

But while you can't do anything about the weight you've gained so far, there's plenty you can do to ensure that you don't continue putting on pounds at an excessive rate. Some women experience an early weight gain blitz because they overindulge in the kinds of starchy sweets they find comforting to their morning-sick tummies. If that was your problem, it should be less and less of one as queasiness tapers off and an appetite for a more varied diet returns. Other women gain too much in the first trimester because they've bought into the misconception that no-holds-barred eating is a pregnant woman's right and responsibility. Review the Best-Odds Diet (see page 80 and *What to Eat When You're Expecting*) to find out why it isn't, and to learn how you can eat for your baby's health without munching your way to a 60-pound weight gain. Gaining efficiently, on the highest-quality foods possible, will not only accomplish that goal but will make the weight you do gain easier to shed in the postpartum period.

HEADACHES

"I find that I'm getting a lot more headaches than ever before. Do I have to suffer with them because I can't take pain relievers?"

That women are more susceptible to headaches during the time they're supposed to stay away from pain relievers is one of the ironies of pregnancy. Although it may be one you'll have to live with, it's not necessarily one you'll have to suffer excessively with. While it's true that you can't turn to your medicine cabinet for a quick cure (see Appendix), prevention, teamed with home remedies, can offer some relief from the recurrent headaches of pregnancy. The best way of preventing and treating the headache depends on the cause or causes. Pregnancy headaches are most commonly the result of hormonal changes (which are responsible for the increased frequency and severity of many types of headaches, including sinus headaches), fatigue, tension, hunger, physical or emotional stress, or any combination of these.

With many of the following ways of overcoming and preventing headaches, you can fit the cure to the cause:

Relax. Pregnancy can be a time of high anxiety, with tension headaches a common result. Some women find relief through meditation and yoga. You can take a course or read a book on these or other relaxation techniques, or try those on page 114.

Of course, relaxation exercises don't work for everyone—some women find that they increase tension instead of alleviating it. For them, lying down in a dark, quiet room, or stretching out on the sofa or with their feet up at their desk for 10 or 15 minutes is a better foil for tension and tension headaches.

See the other tips for stress reduction on page 113.

Get Enough Rest. Pregnancy can also be a time of high fatigue, particularly in the first and last trimesters, and often for the full nine months for women who work long hours at a job or caring for their other children.

Sleep can be elusive once the belly starts burgeoning (how will I ever get comfortable?) and the mind starts racing (how will I ever get everything done before the baby comes?), compounding fatigue. Making a conscious effort to get more rest, day *and* night, can help keep headaches at bay. But be careful not to sleep *too much,* as excess sleep can also give you a headache.

Eat Regularly. To avoid hunger headaches triggered by low blood sugar, be sure not to miss meals. Carry high-energy snacks (complex carbohydrates and protein will work most effectively) with you in your purse, stash them in the glove compartment of your car and in your office desk drawer, and always keep a supply on hand at home.

Seek Some Peace and Quiet. If you're "allergic" to noise, stay away from it whenever possible. Avoid loud music, noisy restaurants, roaring parties, and crowded department stores. At home, lower the volume on the telephone's ring, the TV, and the radio.

Don't Get Stuffy. If an overheated, smoke-filled, unventilated room touches off headaches, leave it for a stroll outdoors now and then—or better still, avoid such locations entirely. Dress in layers when you know you're going somewhere stuffy, and keep comfortable by removing layers as needed. If your workplace is poorly ventilated, move to a better-ventilated office or area if that's possible; take frequent breaks if it isn't.

Go Hot and Cold. For relief of sinus headaches, apply hot and cold compresses to the aching area, alternating 30 seconds of each for a total of 10 minutes, four times a day. For tension headaches, try ice applied to the back of the neck for 20 minutes while you close your eyes and relax. (Use an ordinary ice pack or a special neck pillow that holds a gel-based cold pack.)

Straighten Up. Slouching or looking down to read, sew, or do other close work for long stretches of time can also cause headaches, so watch your posture.

If an unexplained headache persists for more than a few hours, returns very often, is the result of fever, or is accompanied by visual disturbances or puffiness of the hands and face, notify your practitioner at once.

"I suffer from migraine headaches. I heard they are more common in pregnancy. Is this true?"

Some women find their migraines strike more frequently during pregnancy. Others find they are less frequent. It isn't known why this should be so, or even why some people have recurrent migraines and others never have a single one.

Migraines are headaches that are in a class by themselves. Their development is related to constriction, or narrowing, of the blood vessels in the head, followed by their sudden dilation, or opening. This interferes with blood flow and causes pain and other symptoms. Though symptoms vary from person to person, a migraine is usually preceded by fatigue. The fatigue may then be followed by nausea with or without vomiting and diarrhea, sensitivity to light, and possibly a misting or zigzagging over one or, occasionally, both eyes. When the headache finally arrives, anywhere from minutes to hours after the first warning symptom, the pain, which is intense and throbbing, is usually localized on one side, but it can spread to the other side. Some people also experience tingling or numbness in one arm or side of the body, dizziness, ringing in the ears, runny nose, runny and/or bloodshot eyes, and temporary mental confusion.

If you've had migraines in the past, be prepared for dealing with them during pregnancy, preferably through prevention. If you know what brings on an attack, you can try to avoid the culprit. Stress is a common one (see page 113 for tips on handling it), as are chocolate, cheese, coffee, and red wine (not an approved pregnancy beverage, anyway). Try to determine what, if anything, can stave off a full-blown attack once the warning signs appear. For some people, splashing the face with cold water helps, or lying down in a darkened room for two or three hours, eyes covered (napping, meditating, or listening to music, but not reading or watching TV). Discuss with your physician which migraine medications are safe to take during pregnancy, and which might be most effective.

If you experience for the first time what seems like a migraine, call your doctor immediately. The same symptoms could also be indicative of a pregnancy complication. If an unexplained headache persists for more than a few hours, returns very often, is the result of fever, or is accompanied by visual disturbances or puffiness of the hands and face, also notify your practitioner at once.

TROUBLE SLEEPING

"I've never had a sleep problem in my life—until now. I can't seem to settle in at night."

Your mind is racing, your belly burgeoning—it's no wonder you can't settle in for a good night's sleep. You could write this insomnia off as good preparation for the sleepless nights that likely lie ahead in the first

months of your baby's life, or you could try the following tips:

❖ Get enough exercise. A body that gets a workout by day (see page 189 for guidelines) will be a sleepier body at night. But don't exercise too close to bedtime, since the exercise-induced high could keep you from crashing when your head hits the pillow.

❖ Set a leisurely pace at dinner. Don't gobble your meals on a television tray; partake at the table, with your spouse and a healthy helping of relaxing conversation.

❖ Develop a bedtime routine and stick with it. After dinner, maintain the easy pace, focusing on activities that relax you. Indulge in light reading (but nothing you can't put down) or television (no violent or emotionally wrenching dramas), soothing music, relaxation exercises (see page 114), a warm bath, a backrub, some lovemaking.

❖ Have a light snack to keep your blood sugar level up. Too much food or none at all before bedtime can interfere with sleep. Good soporific snacks include whole-grain fruit-sweetened cookies and milk; fruit and cheese; cottage cheese and unsweetened applesauce.

❖ Get comfortable. Be sure your bedroom is neither too hot nor too cold, that your mattress is firm and your pillow supportive. See page 173 for comfortable sleep positions; the sooner in pregnancy you learn to sleep comfortably on your side, the easier it will be for you to do it later on.

❖ Get some air. A stuffy environment is not a good sleeping environment. So open a window in all but the coldest or hottest weather (when a fan or air conditioning can help circulate the air). And don't sleep with the covers over your head. This will decrease the oxygen and increase the carbon dioxide you breathe in, which can cause headaches and even abnormal heart rhythms.

❖ Stay out of your bedroom except to sleep.

❖ If frequent trips to the bathroom are interfering with your sleep, limit fluids after 4 P.M. and stand as little as possible during the day, since standing increases night-time urination.

❖ Clear your mind. If you've been losing sleep over problems at work or at home, try to solve them during the day, or at least talk about them with your spouse early in the evening. But put any worries out of your mind in the hours just before bedtime. (See other tension relief tips on page 113.)

❖ Don't use such crutches as medications or alcohol to assist you in falling asleep. These could be harmful in pregnancy, and they don't help in the long run anyway. Avoid caffeine (in tea, coffee, colas) and/or large quantities of chocolate (not very Best-Odds anyway) after noontime. These can interfere with sleep in the short run.

❖ Stay up later. You may need less sleep than you think you do. Putting off your bedtime may, paradoxically, help you sleep better. Avoiding daytime napping may help, too.

❖ Judge the adequacy of your sleep by how you feel, not by how many hours you stay in bed. Remember that most people with sleep problems actually get more sleep than they think. You're getting enough rest if you're not chronically tired (beyond the normal fatigue of pregnancy).

❖ Don't worry about your insomnia —it won't hurt you or your baby. When you can't sleep, get up and read, knit, or watch TV until you get drowsy. Worrying about not sleeping will certainly be more stressful than lack of sleep itself.

STRETCH MARKS

"I'm afraid I'm going to get stretch marks. Can they be prevented?"

For many women—especially those who favor bikinis—stretch marks are more to be dreaded than flabby thighs. Nevertheless, 90% of all women will develop these pink or reddish, slightly indented, sometimes itchy streaks on their breasts, hips, and/or abdomen sometime during pregnancy.

As their name implies, stretch marks are caused by the skin stretching, generally due to a large and/or rapid increase in weight. Expectant mothers who have good, elastic skin tone (because they either inherited it or earned it through years of excellent nutrition and exercise) may slip through several pregnancies without a single telltale striation. Others may be able to minimize, if not prevent, stretch marks by keeping weight gain steady, gradual, and moderate. Promoting elasticity in your skin by nourishing it with the Best-Odds Diet (page 80) may help, but no cream, lotion, or oil, no matter how expensive, will prevent or alleviate stretch marks—although they may be fun for your husband to rub on your tummy, and will prevent your skin from drying.

If you do develop stretch marks during pregnancy, you can console yourself with the knowledge that they will gradually fade to a silvery sheen some months after delivery. If positive thinking doesn't work, later on you can consider laser treatment that will make them even less noticeable.

BABY'S HEARTBEAT

"My friend heard her baby's heartbeat at 2½ months. I'm a week ahead of her and my doctor hasn't picked up my baby's yet."

It's possible to pick up the fetal heartbeat as early as the 10th or 12th week with a highly sensitive instrument called a Doppler (a hand-held ultrasound device that amplifies the sound). But an ordinary stethoscope isn't powerful enough to detect the heartbeat until the 17th or 18th week at the earliest. Even with sophisticated instruments, the heartbeat may not be audible this early because of the baby's position or other interfering factors, such as excess layers of maternal fat. It's also possible that a slightly miscalculated due date may be causing the delay. Wait until next month. By your 18th week, the miraculous sound of your baby's heartbeat is certain to be available for your listening pleasure. If it isn't, or if you are very anxious, your doctor may order an ultrasound, which will pick up a heartbeat that, for some reason, is difficult to hear with a stethoscope.

SEXUAL DESIRE

"All of my pregnant friends say that they had an increased desire for sex early in pregnancy—some had orgasms and multiple orgasms for the first time. How come I feel so unsexy?"

Pregnancy is a time of change in many aspects of your life, not the least of them sexual. Some women who have never had either orgasm or much of a taste for sex suddenly experience both for the first time when pregnant. Other women, accustomed to having a voracious appetite for sex and to being easily orgasmic, suddenly find that they are completely lacking in desire and are difficult to arouse. These changes in sexuality can be disconcerting, guilt-provoking, wonderful, or a confusing combination of all three. And they are perfectly normal.

As you will see by reading Making Love During Pregnancy (page 164), there are many logical explanations for such changes and for the feelings that they may provoke. Some of these factors may be strongest early in pregnancy, when nausea and fatigue make you feel understandably unsexy, when being able to make love without worrying about trying to get (or trying not to get) pregnant frees you of inhibitions and makes you sexier than ever, when guilt results because you're feeling sexy and you think you should be feeling motherly instead. Other factors, such as physical alterations that may make orgasm easier to achieve, more powerful, or more elusive, continue throughout gestation.

Most important is recognizing that your sexual feelings—and your husband's as well—during pregnancy may be more erratic than erotic; you may feel sexy one day and not the next. Mutual understanding and open communication will see you through.

ORAL SEX

"I've heard that oral sex is dangerous during pregnancy. Is this true?"

Cunnilingus is safe throughout pregnancy as long as your mate is careful not to blow any air into your vagina. Doing this could force air into your bloodstream and cause an air embolism (obstructing a blood vessel), which might prove deadly to both mother and baby.

Fellatio, because it doesn't involve the female genitalia, is always safe during pregnancy and for some couples is a very satisfactory substitute when intercourse isn't permitted.

CRAMP AFTER ORGASM

"I get an abdominal cramp after orgasm. Is this a sign that sex is hurting my baby? Will it cause a miscarriage?"

Cramping—both during and after orgasm, and sometimes accompanied by backache—is very common and harmless during a normal, low-risk pregnancy. Its cause can be physical: a combination of the normal venous congestion in the pelvic area during pregnancy and the equally normal congestion of the sexual organs during arousal and orgasm. Or it can be psychological: a result of the common fear of hurting the baby during intercourse.

The cramping is not a sign that sex is hurting the fetus. Most experts agree that sexual relations and orgasm during a normal, low-risk pregnancy are perfectly safe and are not a cause of miscarriage. If the cramps bother you, ask your husband for a gentle low back rub. It may relieve not only the cramps but any tension that might be triggering them, too.[3] (see Making Love During Pregnancy, page 164.)

TWINS AND MORE

"I'm already very big. Could I be carrying twins?"

It's more likely that you're just carrying a little extra weight because you gained more than your share in the first trimester. Or that you're small-boned to begin with and on you, uterine expansion is noticeable earlier than it would be on a larger frame. A relatively large abdomen in and of itself is not generally considered a sign that an expectant mother is carrying multiple fetuses; in making the diagnosis, a practitioner will look at other factors, including:

❖ A large-for-date uterus. The size of the uterus, not of the abdomen, is what counts in the diagnosis of multiple fetuses. If your uterus seems to be growing more rapidly than expected for your due date, a multiple pregnancy would be suspected. Other possible explanations for a large-for-date uterus include a miscalculated due date or an excessive amount of amniotic fluid (polyhydramnios).

❖ Exaggerated pregnancy symptoms. When twins are being carried, the troubles of pregnancy (morning sickness, indigestion, edema, and so on) can be doubled, or seem that way. But all of these can also be exaggerated in a singleton pregnancy.

❖ More than one heartbeat. Depending on the position the babies are in, a practitioner may be able to hear two (or more) distinctly separate heartbeats. But because the heartbeat of a single fetus may be heard at several locations, the locating of two (or more) confirms twins (or more) only if the heartbeats are different in rate. So twins aren't often diagnosed this way.

❖ Predisposition. Though there are no factors that increase the chances of having identical twins, there are several that make a woman more likely to have nonidentical twins. These include nonidentical twins in the mother's family, advanced

---

3. Some women also experience crampiness in the legs after intercourse. See page 202 for tips on relieving such discomfort.

age (women over 35 more frequently release more than one egg), the use of drugs to stimulate ovulation (fertility drugs), and in-vitro fertilization. Twins are also more common among black women than white, and less common among Asians.

If one or more of these factors lead the practitioner to the conclusion that there's a possibility of more than one fetus, an ultrasound exam will be ordered. In virtually every case (except in the rare instance where one camera-shy fetus remains stubbornly hidden behind the other), this technique will accurately diagnose a multiple pregnancy.

"We'd barely adjusted to the fact that I was pregnant when we found out I'm carrying twins. I'm worried about the risks involved for them—and for me."

Multiple births are multiplying at a fantastic rate; 2 in 100 sets of parents can expect to see double (or triple, or more) in the delivery room, up from 1 in 100 a generation ago. And although some multiple births are still conceived the old-fashioned way—as a result of random throws of nature's dice or because of an inherited predisposition—scientists point to several new factors in explaining the current baby-baby boom. One is the increase in older mothers: women over 35, because their ovulation tends to be erratic (with greater chances of more than one egg being released at a time), are more likely to conceive a multiple birth. Another is the use of such fertility drugs as Pergonal and Clomiphene (again, more often by older women, since fertility decreases with age), which increase the likelihood of multiple birth. Still another is the use of in-vitro fertilization, a procedure wherein eggs fertilized in a test tube are implanted into the uterus,

which, since several ova are involved, also yields an increased risk of multiple birth.

But if today's mother is more likely to conceive twins, she is also more likely to deliver those twins in good condition. Better than 90% of twin pregnancies, studies show, have happy endings. Much of this success is attributable to the advance-warning capabilities of ultrasound; rare is the couple nowadays who is taken by surprise by twins in the delivery room. Advance warning makes not only for fewer practical and logistical complications after birth (having to go back to the store at the last minute for an extra crib and layette), but also for fewer medical complications during pregnancy and at delivery. Armed with the knowledge that she is carrying more than one baby, an expectant mother and her practitioner can take many precautions that can reduce her risk of certain pregnancy complications (hypertension, anemia, and abruptio placenta are more common in multiple pregnancies) and improve her chances of carrying the babies to term and delivering them in top-notch condition:

Extra Medical Care. Much of the higher risk a multiple pregnancy carries can be reduced with expert medical monitoring by an obstetrician (high-risk pregnancies should not be overseen by a midwife). You will be scheduled for more frequent appointments than will the woman carrying a single fetus—often seeing the doctor every other week after the 20th week and weekly after the 30th. And you will be watched more closely for signs of complications so that if one develops, it can be treated quickly.

Extra Nutrition. Eating for three (or more) is at least double the responsibility of eating for two. On top of all the other good things it can do for all babies (see page 80), excellent nutrition can have a dramatic impact on one of the most common problems of multiple pregnancies: low birthweight. Instead of being born at 5 pounds and less (once the standard in multiple births), twins who are nourished on a superior diet can weigh in at a much healthier 6 to 7 pounds or more.

Many of the Best-Odds dietary requirements are multiplied with each fetus you're carrying. Specifically, that translates to approximately 300 additional calories, one additional Protein serving, one additional Calcium serving, and one additional Whole Grain serving. Because that's a lot of food to fit into a stomach cramped by a rapidly growing uterus, and because prenatal gastrointestinal discomforts, such as morning sickness and indigestion, are often multiplied in multiple pregnancies, the quality of the food you eat will be particularly important. Avoiding nutritionless frills will help ensure that you'll have room for the good stuff. Eating efficiently (see page 81) and spreading your requirements out over at least six small meals and many snacks, rather than trying to get your Daily Dozen and then some in at three sittings, should help too.

Extra Weight Gain. An additional baby means additional weight gain—not just because of the baby itself, but because of the extra baby by-products (often including an extra placenta and additional amniotic fluid). Your physician will probably advise a carefully monitored weight gain of at least 35 to 45 pounds above your prepregnancy weight (unless you're very overweight), or about 50% more than is recommended in a singleton pregnancy. That means about 1½ pounds a week after the 12th week. Particularly if this weight is gained on an excellent diet, it will go a long way toward producing healthier babies.

Extra Vitamins and Minerals. An additional fetus also means an increased need for such nutrients as iron and folic acid (needed to prevent anemia; see page 154), zinc, copper, calcium, B_6, vitamin C, and vitamin D. Because of this increased need, it's been stated by the Food and Nutrition Board of the American Academy of Sciences that women carrying more than one fetus are in the high-risk group that should take a prenatal vitamin-mineral supplement daily. So be sure you do. *Do not,* however, take any supplements beyond that, unless recommended by your physician.

Extra Rest. Your body will be working twice as hard at baby building, so it's going to need twice as much rest for its efforts. It's your job to make sure it gets it whenever it needs it. Make time for a nap or a rest with your feet up by depending more on others for help around the house and with errands, and by relying more on modern conveniences (use frozen vegetables, which are just as nutritious as fresh, or precut ones from a salad bar or supermarket produce section). And, if at all possible, work fewer hours at your job, or even stop work early if fatigue is severe.

Extra Caution. Depending on how your pregnancy is going, the doctor may prescribe taking an early leave from work (as early as the 24th week in some cases), getting help with the housework, and, sometimes, complete bed rest at home. Hospital bed rest during the last months of pregnancy is usually reserved for complicated multiple pregnancies; most studies show that for normal twin pregnancies, routine hospital admission at this time does not prevent preterm labor. Following doctor's orders to the letter, no matter how difficult that might be, is one of the best ways you can help your babies go to term.

Extra Help for the Extra Symptoms of Multiple Pregnancies. Since the common discomforts of pregnancy (including morning sickness, indigestion, backache, constipation, hemorrhoids, edema, varicose veins, shortness of breath, and fatigue) are likely to be exaggerated in a mom carrying more than one fetus, she needs to be aware of the various routes to relief. Though relief may be more elusive in a twin pregnancy, the suggestions in this book for dealing with these complaints apply to all mothers, whether they are expecting one baby or more than one (refer to the complaints individually; see the index). Consult with your doctor for additional advice, or if symptoms seem particularly severe.

An extremely uncommon complaint that occasionally complicates a multiple pregnancy is separation of the symphysis pubis, or the lower joint of the pelvic bone. This separation can cause limited mobility and severe localized pain in the pelvic area; contact your obstetrician if you experience either of these symptoms.

"Everybody thinks it's so exciting that we're going to have twins—except us. We're disappointed and scared. What's wrong with us?"

Nothing. Our prenatal daydreams rarely involve two cribs, two diaper pails, two high chairs, two strollers, or two babies. We prepare ourselves psychologically, as well as physically, for the arrival of one baby; when we hear that we're going to have two, feelings of disappointment are not unusual. Nor is fear. The impending responsibilities of caring for one new infant are daunting enough without having them doubled.

So accept the fact that you are ambivalent about the dual arrivals, and don't burden yourself with guilt. Instead, use this time before delivery to get used to the idea of twins. Talk to each other and to anyone you know who has twins. Your practitioner may also be able to provide the name of a local parents-of-twins support group or the name of a mother of twins in your area. Sharing your feelings, and recognizing that you're not the first expectant parents to experience them, will help you feel more accepting of, and in time even excited about, this pregnancy.

A CORPUS LUTEUM CYST

"My doctor said that I have a corpus luteum cyst on my ovary. She said that it won't be a problem, but I'm concerned."

Every month of a woman's reproductive life, a small yellowish body of cells forms after ovulation. Called a corpus luteum (literally "yellow body"), it occupies the space in the Graafian follicle formerly occupied by the ovum, or egg. The corpus luteum produces progesterone and estrogen, and is programmed by nature to disintegrate in about 14 days. When it does, diminishing hormone levels trigger menstruation. In pregnancy the corpus luteum, sustained by the hormone hCG (human Chorionic Gonadotropin) that is generated by the trophoblast (the cells that develop into the placenta), continues to grow and produce progesterone and estrogen to nourish and support the new pregnancy until the placenta takes over. In most cases, the corpus luteum starts to shrink about six or seven weeks after the last menstrual period and ceases to function at about 10 weeks, when its work of providing bed and board for the baby is done.

In an estimated 1 in 10 pregnancies, however, the corpus luteum fails to regress at the expected time and develops into a corpus luteum cyst. Usually, as your doctor has already assured you, the cyst won't present a problem. But just as a precaution, the physician will monitor its size and condition regularly via ultrasound, and if it becomes unusually large or if it threatens to twist or rupture, will consider removing it surgically. Such intervention is necessary with only about 1% of all corpus luteum cysts, and after the 12th week the surgery rarely threatens the pregnancy.

INABILITY TO URINATE

"The last few nights I've been unable to urinate, even though my bladder seems very full."

In about 15 to 20% of women the uterus lies in what is called "a retroverted position." In most of these women the postion changes by the end of the first trimester and there are no problems. Occasionally, however, the uterus remains retroverted and presses on the urethra, the tube leading from the bladder, making urination impossible.[4] There may also be urinary leakage when the bladder becomes very overloaded.

Sometimes the problem can be solved by actually manipulating the uterus off the urethra and into the proper position by hand. Other times catheterization (removing the urine through a tube) is necessary in addition. Speak to your practitioner about what would be best in your case.

WHAT IT'S IMPORTANT TO KNOW:
WEIGHT GAIN DURING PREGNANCY

Put two pregnant women together anywhere—in a doctor's waiting room, on a bus, at a business meeting—and the questions are certain to start flying. "When are you due?" "Have you felt the baby kicking yet?" "Have you been feeling sick?" And perhaps the favorite query of all: "How much weight have you gained?"

The comparisons are inevitable, and sometimes a little disturbing. Women who started off with a bang, enthusiastically eating their way to 10-pound first-trimester gains, wonder "how much is too much?" Others who, appetites daunted by bouts with morn-

ing sickness, ended up with net gains that barely registered on the practioner's scale (perhaps even with a slight weight loss), wonder "what's too little?" All wonder "how much is just right?"

Total Increase. Though it was once in medical vogue to limit a woman's pregnancy weight gain to 15 pounds, it is now recognized that this kind of weight gain was insufficient. Babies whose mothers gain under 20 pounds are more likely to be premature, small for their gestational age, and to suffer growth retardation in the uterus.

Almost as hazardous, however, was the next vogue, which urged women to eat to their hearts' and souls' content and gain any amount of weight. There are serious risks in gaining too much weight: assessment and mea-

4. Rarely the inability to urinate may be caused by over use of antihistamines or even garlic pills. If your uterus does not seem retroverted, this may be the root of your problem.

surement of the fetus become more difficult; excess weight overworks muscles and results in backache, leg pain, increased fatigue, and varicose veins; the baby may become so large that a vaginal delivery becomes difficult or impossible; if surgery, such as cesarean section, is needed, it becomes more difficult, and postoperative complications more common; and after pregnancy the excess weight may be hard to shed.

Though there's a good chance that a woman with an enormous weight gain may have an oversized baby, the mother's weight gain and the weight of her infant don't always correlate. It's possible to gain 40 pounds and deliver a 6-pound baby, and to gain 20 and have an 8-pounder. The quality of the food that contributes to the weight gain is more important than the quantity.

The sensible and safe pregnancy weight gain for the average woman is between 25 and 35 pounds, with a petite, small-boned woman's gain likely to fall at the lower end of the range and a larger, big-boned woman's gain likely to fall on the high end. That gain allows about 6 to 8 pounds for baby and 14 to 24 pounds for pla-

centa, breasts, fluids, and other by-products (see page 148). It also ensures a speedier return to prepregnancy weight for mom.

The formula changes for women with special needs. Women who begin pregnancy extremely underweight should try to gain enough weight during the first trimester so that they start the second trimester at or close to their ideal weight; then they should aim to gain the requisite 25 to 35 pounds on top of that. Women who start pregnancy 10% to 20% or more overweight can safely gain somewhat less weight, though not less than fifteen pounds and only on the best-quality food and under careful medical supervision. Pregnancy is never a time for weight loss or maintenance, because a fetus can't survive on a mother's fat stores alone since they provide calories but no nutrients.

Women who are carrying more than one fetus also need to have their weight gain goal adjusted by their physicians. Though it doesn't double for twins or triple for triplets, it does increase significantly—to 35 to 45 pounds for twins, and more when there are more than two fetuses.

Breakdown of Your Weight Gain
(All weights are approximate)

Baby	7 ½ pounds
Placenta	1 ½ pounds
Amniotic fluid	2 pounds
Uterine enlargement	2 pounds
Maternal breast tissue	2 pounds
Maternal blood volume	4 pounds
Fluids in maternal tissue	4 pounds
Maternal fat stores	7 pounds
Total average	30-pound overall weight gain

• **Rate of Increase.** The average-weight woman should gain approximately 3 to 4 pounds during the first trimester, and about a pound a week, 12 to 14 pounds in all, during the second trimester. Weight gain should continue at a rate of about 1 pound a week during the seventh and eighth months, and in the ninth month drop off to a pound or 2—or even none at all—for a total of 8 to 10 pounds during the third trimester.

Rare is the woman who can tailor her weight gain precisely to the ideal formula. And it's fine to fluctuate a little—a ½ pound gain one week, 1½ pounds the next. But the goal of every pregnant woman should be to keep weight gain as steady as possible, without any sudden jumps or drops. If you don't gain any weight for two weeks or more during the fourth to eighth months, if you gain more than 3 pounds in any one week in the second trimester, or if you gain more than 2 pounds in any week in the third

trimester, especially if it doesn't seem to be related to overeating or excessive intake of sodium, check with your doctor. Check, too, if you gain no weight for more than two weeks in a row.

If you find that your weight gain has strayed significantly from what you planned (for instance, that you gained 14 pounds in the first trimester instead of 3 or 4, or that you gained 20 pounds in the second trimester instead of 12), take action to see that it gets back on a sensible track, but don't try to stop it in its tracks. With your practitioner, readjust your goal to include the excess you've already gained (which your baby can't thrive on) and the weight you still have to gain (which your baby needs). Keep in mind that your baby requires a steady daily shipment of nutrients throughout the pregnancy. Watch your diet carefully, but never diet. Monitor your weight from the beginning, and you'll never have to put your baby on a diet to keep yourself from getting fat.

Weight Insurance

A recent study found that underweight women can improve the weight of their babies by taking a nutritional supplement formulated for pregnancy that contains 25 milligrams of zinc. Especially if you're 5 feet 4 inches tall or less and weigh less than 110 pounds, make sure your supplement includes that amount of zinc.

8
The Fourth Month

WHAT YOU CAN EXPECT AT THIS MONTH'S CHECKUP

This month you can expect your practitioner to check the following, though there may be variations depending upon your particular needs and upon your practitioner's style of practice:[1]

❖ Weight and blood pressure

❖ Urine, for sugar and protein

❖ Fetal heartbeat

❖ Size of uterus, by external palpation

❖ Height of fundus (top of the uterus)

❖ Hands and feet for edema (swelling), and legs for varicose veins

❖ Symptoms you've been experiencing, especially unusual ones

❖ Questions or problems you want to discuss—have a list ready

WHAT YOU MAY BE FEELING

You may experience all of these symptoms at one time or another, or only a few of them. Some may have continued from last month, others may be new. You may

also have other, less common, symptoms.

PHYSICALLY:

❖ Fatigue

❖ Decreased urinary frequency

❖ An end to, or a decrease in, nausea

---

1. See Appendix for an explanation of the procedures and tests performed.

and vomiting (in a few women, "morning sickness" will continue; in a very few it is just beginning)

❖ Constipation

❖ Heartburn, indigestion, flatulence, bloating

❖ Continued breast enlargement, but usually decreased tenderness and swelling

❖ Occasional headaches

❖ Occasional faintness or dizziness, particularly with sudden change of position

❖ Nasal congestion and occasional nosebleeds; ear stuffiness

❖ "Pink toothbrush" from bleeding gums

❖ Increase in appetite

❖ Mild swelling of ankles and feet, and occasionally of hands and face

❖ Varicose veins of legs and/or hemorrhoids

❖ Slight whitish vaginal discharge (leukorrhea)

❖ Fetal movement near the end of the month (but usually this early only if you are very slender or if this is not your first pregnancy)

EMOTIONALLY:

❖ Instability comparable to premenstrual syndrome, which may include irritability, mood swings, irrationality, weepiness

❖ Joy and/or apprehension—if you have started to feel pregnant at last

❖ Frustration—if you don't really feel pregnant yet but are too big for

WHAT YOU MAY LOOK LIKE

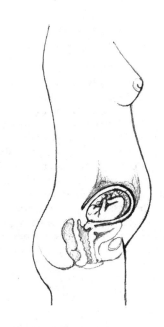

By the end of the fourth month, the 4-inch fetus, now nourished by the placenta, is developing reflexes, such as sucking and swallowing. Body growth begins to outstrip that of the head; tooth buds appear; fingers and toes are well defined. Though human-looking, it cannot survive outside the uterus.

your regular wardrobe and too small for maternity clothes

❖ A feeling you're not quite together. You're a scatterbrain, you forget things, drop things, have trouble concentrating

WHAT YOU MAY BE CONCERNED ABOUT

ELEVATED BLOOD PRESSURE

"I'm worried because at my last visit my blood pressure was up a little bit."

Worrying about your blood pressure will only send the readings higher, and a slight increase at one visit probably doesn't mean much of anything. Perhaps you were just nervous, or were late for your appointment and ran all the way, or were worrying about a report you had to finish at work. An hour later your pressure might very well have been normal. But because it is often difficult to determine the cause of an isolated elevated reading, your practitioner may advise you to take it easy and possibly to limit sodium and fat intake and increase your servings of fruits and vegetables to 8 to 10 per day.

If your blood pressure remains slightly elevated, however, you may be among the 1% to 2% of pregnant women who develop transient high blood pressure during pregnancy. This type of hypertension is perfectly harmless, as far as is known, and disappears after delivery.

What is considered normal blood pressure in pregnancy varies somewhat over the course of nine months. A baseline reading (what is normal for you) is obtained at the first prenatal visit. Generally blood pressure drops a little over the next several months. But somewhere around the seventh month, it usually begins to rise a bit.

During the first or second trimester, if systolic pressure (the upper number) rises 30 mmHg or the diastolic pressure (the lower number) rises 15 mmHg over the baseline reading, and stays up for at least two readings taken at least six hours apart, close observation, and possibly treatment, is warranted. In the third trimester, treatment is usually begun only if the rise is greater than that.

If such an increase in blood pressure is accompanied by sudden weight gain (more than 3 pounds in one week in the second trimester, or more than 2 pounds in one week in the third), severe edema (swelling due to water retention), particularly of hands and face, as well an ankles, and/or protein in the urine,[2] the problem may turn out to be preeclampsia (also called pregnancy-induced hypertension—PIH; see page 351). In women who receive regular medical care, this condition is generally diagnosed before it progresses to more serious symptoms, which include blurred vision, headaches, irritability, and gastric pain. If you should experience any of the symptoms of preeclampsia, call your doctor immediately (see page 204).

SUGAR IN THE URINE

"At my last office visit the doctor said that there was sugar in my urine. She said not to worry, but I'm convinced I have diabetes."

Take your doctor's advice—don't worry. A small amount of sugar in the urine on one occasion during pregnancy does not a diabetic make. Your body is probably doing just what it's supposed to do: making sure that your fetus, which depends on you for its fuel supply, is getting enough glucose (sugar).

---

2. See Appendix for an explanation of protein in the urine.

Since it is insulin that regulates the level of glucose in your blood and ensures that enough is taken in by your body cells for nourishment, pregnancy triggers *anti*-insulin mechanisms to make sure enough sugar remains circulating in your bloodstream to nourish your fetus. It's a perfect idea that doesn't always work perfectly. Sometimes the anti-insulin effect is so strong that it leaves more than enough sugar in the blood to meet the needs of both mother and child—more than can be handled by the kidneys. The excess is "spilled" into the urine. Thus your "sugar in the urine"—a not uncommon occurrence in pregnancy, especially in the second trimester, when the anti-insulin effect increases. In fact, roughly half of all pregnant women show some sugar in the urine at some point in their pregnancies.

In most women, the body responds to an increase in blood sugar with an increased production of insulin, which will usually eliminate the excess sugar by the next office visit. This may well be the case with you. But some women, especially those who are diabetic or have tendencies toward diabetes, may be unable to produce enough insulin at one time to handle the increase in blood sugar, or they may be unable to use the insulin they do produce efficiently. Either way, these women continue to show high levels of sugar in both blood and urine. In those who were not previously diabetic, this is known as gestational diabetes.

If sugar appears in your urine at your next visit, your doctor may test your blood for sugar and may order a glucose-tolerance test, a procedure that accurately reflects the body's response to sugar in the bloodstream and identifies individuals with diabetes. Symptoms that may suggest gestational diabetes include excessive hunger and thirst; frequent urination; even in the second trimester; recurrent vaginal monilial infections; and an increase in blood pressure.

About 1% to 2% (some estimates are as high as 10%) of pregnant women develop this condition—which probably could more appropriately be called "carbohydrate intolerance of pregnancy" rather than the alarming "gestational diabetes"—making it the most common pregnancy complication. Because it is so common, most doctors now screen for it routinely with a blood sugar test between the 24th and 28th weeks of pregnancy. Higher-risk mothers-to-be are screened earlier and more often. Those at higher risk include older mothers (since the tendency toward diabetes increases as we get older) and women with a family history of diabetes mellitus; women with a history of sugar in the urine during pregnancy or of glucose intolerance outside of pregnancy; women who are obese, were large babies themselves (over 9 pounds), or have had one or more large babies previously; and women who have a poor obstetrical history (including previous gestational diabetes, toxemia, repeated urinary tract infection, excessive amniotic fluid, recurrent miscarriage, unexplained stillbirth, or a baby with a congenital anomaly).

Though diabetic mothers-to-be and their fetuses were once at great risk, thanks to modern medicine this is no longer the case. When blood sugar is closely controlled through diet and, if needed, medication, women with diabetes can have normal pregnancies and healthy babies. If you should de-

---

3. Women with abnormal blood glucose but normal glucose-tolerance tests may still be at risk for having large babies and may need to control their diets carefully. If you have an abnormal blood sugar screening, consult your physician.

velop gestational diabetes, see pages 325 and page 350.

Blood sugar abnormalities disappear after delivery in about 97% to 98% of women with gestational diabetes, but some of these women, particularly those who are obese, may develop diabetes later in life. To reduce this risk, those with gestational diabetes should take the following preventive measures: have regular medical checkups, maintain ideal weight, cultivate good diet and exercise habits, and learn the symptoms of the disease so they can be reported promptly to the physician.

ANEMIA

"A friend of mine became anemic during pregnancy. How can I tell if I am, and can I prevent it?"

As blood volume builds during pregnancy, the amount of iron needed for producing red blood cells gradually increases. Because not all pregnant women get the iron they need, nearly 20% become iron-deficient. Fortunately iron-deficiency anemia is easily corrected—in most cases by eating a varied and nutritious diet and taking an iron supplement. Note: Taking caffeine at the same time as high iron foods or supplements will reduce iron absorption.

A blood test for anemia is administered at the first prenatal visit, but few women turn out to be iron-deficient at this time. Some may have come into pregnancy with the condition (common during the childbearing years because of monthly menstrual blood loss). But with conception and the cessation of menstruation, iron stores —if dietary intake is adequate—are replenished. It isn't until the 20th week (when expanding maternal blood volume and a growing fetus increases the need for iron significantly)

that most cases of iron-deficiency anemia develop.

When the iron deficiency is mild, there may be no symptoms; but as oxygen-carrying red blood cells are further depleted, the mother begins to exhibit such symptoms as pallor, extreme fatigue, weakness, palpitations, breathlessness, and even fainting spells. This may be one of the few instances where the fetus's nutritional needs are met before the mother's, since the baby of an anemic mother is rarely iron-deficient at birth. However, there is some evidence, not yet conclusive, that babies of anemic mothers who don't take iron supplements may be at a slightly increased risk of being small or premature.

While all pregnant women are susceptible to iron-deficiency anemia, certain groups are at particularly high risk: those who have had several babies in quick succession, those who are carrying more than one fetus, those who have been vomiting a lot or eating little because of morning sickness, and those who came to pregnancy undernourished and/or have been eating poorly since they conceived. Not surprisingly, low-income women often fall into this last category, putting them at higher risk.

To prevent iron-deficiency anemia, it is generally recommended that expectant mothers eat a diet rich in iron (see the Iron-Rich Food Selection list, page 92). But because it is difficult to impossible to get adequate iron from dietary sources alone, daily iron supplementation of 30 mg is also usually prescribed (see page 86). Additional supplementation, usually another 30 mg, is recommended when iron-deficiency anemia is diagnosed.

Sometimes, when iron deficiency is ruled out as a cause of anemia in pregnancy, testing may be needed to check for the presence of one of the other types of anemia, such as folic acid deficiency, sickle-cell, or thalassemia.

BREATHLESSNESS

"Sometimes I feel like I am having trouble breathing. Is this because of my pregnancy?"

Probably. Many pregnant women experience a mild breathlessness beginning in the second trimester. Once again, pregnancy hormones are at work. The hormones swell the capillaries of the respiratory tract as they do other capillaries in the body and relax the muscles of the lungs and bronchial tubes as they do other muscles. As pregnancy progresses, another factor comes into play and it becomes more of an effort to take a deep breath because the growing uterus pushes up against the diaphragm, crowding the lungs and making it difficult for them to expand fully. Such breathlessness is normal.

Severe breathlessness, on the other hand, especially when breathing is rapid, lips or fingertips seem to be turning bluish, and/or there is chest pain and rapid pulse, could be a sign of trouble and requires an immediate call to the doctor or trip to the emergency room.

FORGETFULNESS

"Last week I left the house without my wallet; this morning I completely forgot an important business meeting. I can't focus on anything, and I'm beginning to think I'm losing my mind."

You're not alone. Many pregnant women begin to feel that as they're gaining pounds, they're losing brain cells. Even women who pride themselves on their organizational skills, their capacity to deal with complicated issues, and their ability to maintain their composure suddenly find themselves forgetting appoint-ments, having trouble concentrating, and losing their cool. Fortunately the scatterbrain syndrome (similar to one that many women experience premenstrually) is only temporary. Like numerous other symptoms, it's caused by the hormonal changes wrought by pregnancy.

Feeling tense about this intellectual fogginess will only compound it. Recognizing that it is normal, even accepting it with a sense of humor, may help to ease it. Reducing the stresses in your life as much as possible will also help (see page 113). It just may not be feasible to do as much as efficiently as you did before you took on the added job of baby-making. Taking informal inventory or keeping written checklists at home and at work (and referring to them before leaving home or work) can help contain the mental chaos as well as keep you from making potentially dangerous mistakes (such as forgetting to lock the door or turn off the burner under the tea kettle before leaving the house).

And you might as well get used to working at a little below peak efficiency. The fog may well continue through the early weeks after your baby's arrival (due to fatigue, not hormones) and perhaps may not lift completely until baby is sleeping through the night.

HAIR DYES AND PERMANENTS

"As if the weight I've been putting on hasn't been depressing enough, my hair has started to lose all its body. Is it safe to get a permanent?"

Though the pregnant belly is the most obvious physical effect a gestating fetus has on its mother, it's by no means the only one. The changes are evident everywhere—

from the palms of the hands (which may temporarily turn a ruddy red) to the inside of the mouth (gums may swell and bleed). The hair is no exception. It can take a turn for the better (as when lackluster hair suddenly takes on a brilliant shine) or for the worse (as when once bouncy hair goes limp).

Ordinarily, a permanent or a body wave would be the obvious answer to hair that has taken a wrong turn, but it isn't during pregnancy. For one thing, hair responds unpredictably under the influence of pregnancy hormones; a permanent might not take at all, or might result in an unflattering frizz instead of bouncy waves. For another thing, the chemical solutions used in permanents are absorbed through the scalp into the bloodstream, raising questions about the safety of their use during pregnancy. So far, studies of the effects of such chemicals on the fetus have been extremely reassuring: no link has been found between the use of permanents and the development of birth defects. But since more study will be necessary before these substances are completely exonerated, the very cautious may wish to stay "straight" until after delivery. Don't be concerned, however, about a permanent you've already had—the risk is only theoretical, and certainly not worth worrying about. (The same can be said for hair relaxers and prescription dandruff shampoos. Avoid using them from now on, but don't worry about any previous use.)

Excellent nutrition may help revive some of your hair's luster; "extra body" shampoos and curling irons may help restore the bounce. But by and large, your hair will probably continue to limp its way through your pregnancy. So, it might make sense to switch to a style that doesn't depend on fullness, such as a very short cut, or one that builds fullness in, such as a blunt cut.

"After I went for my three-month coloring appointment last week, I was horrified to hear from a friend that hair dyes can cause birth defects. What should I do?"

Relax. As with permanents, there has been no solid evidence that hair dyes cause birth defects. Since the risk is only theoretical, there's no point in worrying about applications you've already had. But since it's wise to be extra prudent during pregnancy, at least when that's possible and practical, you might not want to schedule any more appointments until after delivery.

If you're determined to "hide that gray" or those pesty roots and want to be totally cautious at the same time, ask your hairdresser about using pure vegetable colorings.

NOSEBLEEDS AND NASAL STUFFINESS

"My nose has been congested a lot, and sometimes it bleeds for no apparent reason. I'm worried because I know bleeding can be a sign of illness."

Nasal congestion, often with associated nosebleeds, is a common complaint in pregnancy, probably because the high levels of estrogen and progesterone circulating in the body bring increased blood flow to the mucous membranes of the nose, causing them to soften and swell—much as the cervix does in preparation for childbirth.

You can expect the stuffiness to get worse before it gets better—which won't be until after delivery. You may also develop a postnasal drip, which can occasionally lead to nocturnal coughing or gagging. Don't use medication or nasal sprays (unless prescribed by your doctor) to deal with the problem.

The congestion and bleeding are more common in winter, when heating systems force hot, dry air into the house, drying delicate nasal passages. Using a humidifier may help overcome this dryness. You might also try lubricating each nostril with a dab of petroleum jelly.

Taking an extra 250 mg of vitamin C (with your practitioner's approval), in addition to your required vitamin C foods, may help to strengthen your capillaries and reduce the chance of bleeding. (But don't take megadoses of the vitamin.)

Sometimes a nosebleed will follow overly energetic nose-blowing. Correct nose-blowing is an art, which you would do well to master: First gently close one nostril with the thumb, and then carefully blow the mucus out the opposite side. Repeat with the other nostril, continuing to alternate until you can breathe through your nose.

To stem a nosebleed, sit or stand leaning slightly forward, rather than lying down or leaning backward. Press your nostrils together with your thumb and forefinger and hold for five minutes; repeat if the bleeding continues. If the bleeding isn't controlled after three tries, or if the bleeding is frequent and heavy, call your doctor.

ALLERGIES

"My allergies seem to have worsened since my pregnancy began. My nose is runny and my eyes tear all the time."

You may be mistaking the normal nasal stuffiness of pregnancy for allergies. Or, though some fortunate women find temporary relief during this time, pregnancy may have indeed aggravated your allergies. If this is the case, check with your physician to see what you can safely use to relieve any severe symptoms. Some antihista-

mines and other medications appear to be relatively safe for use in pregnancy (your usual medication may not be one of these). But, because no tests for safety are absolutely conclusive, drugs should be used only when all else fails. If your nose is very runny, the secretions are thick, or you're sneezing a lot, increase your fluid intake to compensate for any loss and to thin the secretions.

In general, however, the best approach to dealing with allergies in pregnancy is preventive—avoiding the offending substance or substances, assuming you know what they are:

❖ If pollens or other outdoor allergens trouble you, stay indoors in an air-conditioned and air-filtered environment as much as you can during your susceptible season. Wash your hands and face if you've been outdoors, and wear large curved sunglasses to keep pollens from floating into your eyes.

❖ If dust is a culprit, try to have someone do the dusting and sweeping for you. A vacuum cleaner, damp mop, or a damp cloth-covered broom kicks up less dust than an ordinary broom, and an absorbent cloth will do better than a feather duster. Stay away from musty places like attics and libraries full of old books. Have someone pack away dust collectors in your home, such as draperies and rugs.

❖ If you're allergic to certain foods, stay away from them, even if they are good foods for pregnancy. Consult the Best-Odds Diet (page 80) for substitutes.

❖ If animals bring on allergy attacks, let friends know of the problem in advance so that they can rid a room of both pets and their dander before you visit. And of course, if your own pet is suddenly triggering an allergic response, try to keep one or more areas in your home (particularly your bedroom) pet-free.

❖ Tobacco-smoke allergy is easier to control these days, since fewer people smoke and more smokers oblige if they are asked to refrain. To ease your allergy, as well as for the benefit of your baby, you should avoid exposure to cigarette, pipe, and cigar smoke. Don't be embarrassed to say, "Yes, I mind very much if you smoke."

VAGINAL DISCHARGE

"I've noticed a slight vaginal discharge that is thin and whitish. I'm afraid I have an infection."

A thin, milky, mild-smelling discharge (leukorrhea) is normal throughout pregnancy. It's much like the discharge many women have prior to their menstrual periods. Since it increases until term and may become quite heavy, some women are more comfortable wearing sanitary pads during the last months of pregnancy. Do not use tampons, which could introduce unwanted germs into the vagina.

Aside from offending your esthetic sensibilities (and possibly your husband's—who may be turned off oral sex by the unusual taste and odor), the discharge should be of no concern. It is important to keep the genital area clean and dry; cotton, or cotton-crotched, underwear may help to do this. Avoid tight pants, jeans, leotards, and spandex exercise suits. Rinse the vaginal area thoroughly after soaping during a bath or shower, and avoid exposing it to such irritants as deodorant soaps, bubble baths, and perfumes.

Do *not* use a douche unless it is prescribed by your doctor. (Even then, *do not use a bulb syringe,* such as the disposable variety. Use a douche bag or can, and hold it *no higher than 2 feet above the nozzle* to keep the water pressure low. The tip should not be inserted more than 1 inch past the entrance of the vagina, and the labia should be held open, allowing the fluid to run freely out. These precautions should be followed to reduce the risk of introducing air and causing a life-threatening air embolism.)

If you develop a vaginal discharge that is yellowish, greenish, or thick and cheesy, has a foul odor, or is accompanied by burning, itching, redness, or soreness, infection is likely. Notify your doctor or nurse-midwife so that the infection can be treated (probably with vaginal suppositories or gels, ointments, or creams inserted with an applicator). Unfortunately, though medication may banish the infection temporarily, it often returns off and on until after delivery. Though it may require retreatment, simple vaginitis is not cause for worry and does not pose a risk to your baby.

If your vaginitis is caused by a yeast called monilia, your doctor will be careful to treat it with medication so you won't pass the infection on to your baby during delivery (in the form of thrush, a yeast infection of the mouth)—although the infection is not hazardous to the newborn and is easily treated.

You may be able to hasten your recovery and prevent reinfection by maintaining scrupulous cleanliness, especially after going to the bathroom (always wipe from front to back), and by following the Best-Odds Diet—being especially careful to avoid refined sugars, which may help to create a breeding ground for infectious organisms. Recent research indicates that eating 1 cup of yogurt containing live lactobacillus acidophilus cultures (check the label) daily can reduce the risk of vaginal infections dramatically.

If the infection is a sexually transmittable one, avoiding intercourse and any other sexual contact until both you and your spouse are infection-free is generally recommended. Condoms may be suggested for six months after the condition has cleared. To prevent reinfection, care should be exercised to avoid transferring germs from anus to vagina (with fingers, penis, or tongue).

FETAL MOVEMENT

"I haven't felt the baby moving yet; could something be wrong? Or could I just not be recognizing the kicking?"

Fetal movement may be the greatest source of joy in your pregnancy, and lack of it the greatest cause of anxiety. More than a positive pregnancy test, an expanding belly, or even the sound of the fetal heartbeat, the presence of fetal movement affirms that you've got a new life growing inside you. Its absence breeds terror that the new life is not thriving.

Though the embryo begins to make spontaneous movements by the seventh week, these movements do not become apparent to the mother until much later. That first momentous sensation of life, or "quickening," can occur anywhere between the 14th and 26th weeks, but generally closer to the average of the 18th to 22nd week. Variations on that average are common. A woman who's had a baby before is likely to recognize movement earlier (because she knows what to expect and because her uterine muscles are laxer, making it easier to feel a kick) than one who is expecting her first child. A very slender woman may notice very early, weak movements,

whereas an overweight woman may not be aware of movements until they've become more vigorous.

Sometimes the first perception of movement is delayed slightly because of a miscalculated due date. Or sometimes it's delayed because a woman has failed to recognize fetal movement when she felt it.

Nobody can tell a first-time mother-to-be exactly what she can expect to feel; a hundred pregnant women may describe that first movement in a hundred different ways. Perhaps the most common descriptions are "a fluttering in the abdomen" and "butterflies in the stomach." But early fetal movements have also been described as "a bumping or nudging," "a twitch," "a growling stomach," "someone hitting my stomach," "a bubble bursting," "the squirmies," "like being turned upside down on an amusement park ride." Often the first noticeable movements are mistaken for gas or hunger pains. And one woman recalls, "I thought a bug was on my shirt, but when I went to brush it off, I realized it was the baby moving."

Although it isn't unusual to be unaware of fetal movements until the 20th week or later, your practitioner may order a sonogram to check on the baby's condition if you haven't felt anything—and he or she hasn't been able to elicit fetal response by prodding—by the 22nd week. If the fetal heartbeat is strong, however, and everything else seems to be progressing normally, the practitioner may hold off even longer on testing.

"I felt little movements every day last week, but I haven't felt anything at all today. What's wrong?"

Anxiety over when the first movement will be felt is often replaced by anxiety that fetal movements don't seem frequent enough, or that they haven't been noticed for a while. At this stage of pregnancy, however, these anxieties, while understandable, are usually unnecessary. The frequency of noticeable movements at this point may vary a great deal; patterns of movement are erratic at best. Though the fetus is stirring almost continuously, only some of these movements are strong enough for you to feel. Others may be missed because of the fetal position (facing and kicking inward, for instance, instead of outward). Or because of your own activity (when you're walking or moving about a lot, your fetus may be rocked to sleep; or it may be awake, but you may be too busy to notice its movements). It's also possible that you're sleeping right through your baby's most active period—which for many babies is in the middle of the night.

One way to elicit fetal movement if you haven't noticed any all day is to lie down for an hour or two in the evening, preferably after a glass of milk or other snack; the combination of your inactivity and the jolt of food energy may be able to get the fetus going. If that doesn't work, try again in a few hours, but don't worry. Many mothers find they don't notice movement for a day or two at a time, or even three or four, before the 20th week. After that time, though there's still no need to panic, it's probably a good idea to call your practitioner for reassurance if 24 hours go by without perceptible fetal activity (assuming, of course, that you've already started feeling movement).

After the 28th week fetal movements become more consistent, and studies show that it's a good idea for mothers to get into the habit of checking fetal activity daily (see page 202).

APPEARANCE

"I get depressed when I look in the mirror or step on a scale—I'm so fat."

In a society as obsessed with slenderness as ours, where those who can "pinch an inch" despair, the weight gain of pregnancy can easily become a source of depression. It shouldn't. There's an important difference between pounds added for no good reason (willpower gone astray) and pounds gained for the best and most beautiful of reasons: your child and its support system growing inside you.

Yet in the eyes of many beholders, a pregnant woman isn't just beautiful inside but outside as well. Many women and their husbands consider the rounded pregnant reflection to be the most lovely—and sensuous—of feminine shapes.

As long as you're eating right and not exceeding the recommended limits for pregnancy weight gain (see page 147), you needn't feel "fat"—just pregnant. The added inches you're seeing are all legitimate byproducts of pregnancy and will disappear soon after the baby is born. If you *are* exceeding the limits, self-defeating depression won't keep you from getting fatter (and may even fuel your appetite), but careful scrutiny of your eating habits might. Remember, however, that dieting to lose or keep from gaining weight during pregnancy is extremely unsafe. Never cut back on the Best-Odds Diet requirements because you're afraid of putting on too much weight.

Watching your weight gain isn't the only way to give your appearance an edge. Wearing clothes that flatter your changing figure will also help; choose from the growing selection of creative maternity styles available instead of trying to squeeze into outfits in your prepregnancy wardrobe (see below).

You'll like your mirror image better, too, if you get an easy-care hairstyle (one that doesn't require a permanent; see page 155), take care of your complexion, and take the time to apply makeup if you ordinarily wear it.

MATERNITY CLOTHES

"I can't squeeze into my baggy jeans anymore, but I dread buying maternity clothes."

There's never been a more fashionable time to be pregnant. Gone are the days when pregnancy wardrobes were limited to dowdy smocks and overblouses. Not only are today's maternity clothes a lot more interesting to look at and practical to wear, but pregnant women can supplement and mix-and-match these specialized purchases with a variety of other items that they can continue to wear even after they get their shape back.

Consider the following when preparing to make your pregnancy fashion statement:

❖ **You've still got a way to grow.** Don't go on a whirlwind spending spree at the local maternity boutique on the first day you can't button your jeans. Maternity clothes can be costly, especially when you consider the relatively short period of time they can be worn. So buy as you grow, and then buy only as much as you need (once you've checked what you can use that's already in your closet, you may end up needing a lot less than you'd figured). Though the pregnancy pillows available in try-on rooms in maternity stores can give a good indication of how things will fit later, they can't predict how you will carry (high, low, big, small) and which outfits will end up being the most comfortable when you need comfort most.

❖ **You're not limited to maternity clothes.** If it fits, wear it, even if it isn't from the maternity department. Buying nonmaternity clothing for maternity use (or using items you already own) is, of course, the best way of getting your money's worth. And depending on what the designers are showing in a particular season, anywhere from a few to many of the fashions on the regular racks may be suitable for pregnant shapes. But be wary of spending a lot on such purchases. Though you may love the clothes now, you may love them considerably less after you've worn them throughout your pregnancy; postpartum, the impulse may be great to pack them away like so many maternity clothes.

❖ **Your personal sense of style counts when you're pregnant too.** If you normally dress in tailored clothes, or casual clothes, don't try to talk yourself into a wardrobe of frilly smocked maternity dresses. Though the novelty of looking the part of the lady-in-waiting may carry you contentedly through a month or two, it's doomed to fizzle out long before you're able to relinquish the maternity clothes, leaving you to face the rest of your pregnancy in clothes you despise.

❖ **Accessories deserve a starring role.** When you're not pregnant, accessories are a nice touch. When you are pregnant, they're essential. The boost you get from an interesting scarf, an exotic pair of earrings, an electric shade of hosiery, even a bright-colored pair of sneakers, will compensate for a lot of the inevitable fashion compromises expectant mothers have to make.

❖ **Among your most important accessories are the ones the public never** sees. A well-fitting, supportive bra is vital during pregnancy, when breast expansion generally makes your old bras useless. Bypass the sale racks and put yourself in the hands of an experienced fitter at a well-stocked lingerie department or shop. With any luck, she will be able to tell you approximately how much extra room and support you need and which kind of bra will provide it. But don't stock up. Buy just a couple (one to wear and one to wash), and then go back for another fitting when you start growing out of them.

Special maternity underwear isn't usually necessary and, unless you're used to high-waisted briefs, won't be terribly comfortable. A nice alternative is bikini underwear, bought in a larger than usual size, that you can wear *under* your belly. Buy them in favorite colors and/or sexy fabrics to give your spirits a lift (but make sure crotches are cotton).

❖ A pregnant woman's best friend can be her husband's closet. It's all there for the taking (though it's probably a good idea to ask first): oversized T-shirts and regular shirts that look great over pants or under jumpers (try belting them under the belly for an interesting silhouette), sweatpants that will accommodate more inches than yours will, running shorts that will keep up with your waistline for at least a couple more months, belts with the few extra notches you need.

❖ Both a borrower and a lender be. Accept all offers of used maternity clothes, even if the offerings don't suit your usual style. In a pinch, any extra dress, jumper, or pair of slacks may do—you can make any borrowed item more "yours" with accessories. When your term is over, offer to lend those maternity

outfits you can't or don't want to wear postpartum to newly pregnant friends; between you and your friends, you'll be getting your money's worth from your maternity clothes.

❖ Cool is in. Hot stuff (fabrics that don't breathe, such as nylon and other synthetics) isn't so hot when you're pregnant. Since your metabolic rate is higher than usual, making you warmer, you'll feel more comfortable in cottons. Light colors, mesh weaves, and loose garments will also help to keep you cool. Knee-highs are more comfortable than pantyhose, but avoid those that have a narrow constrictive band at the top. When the weather turns cold, dressing in layers is ideal, since you can selectively peel off as you heat up or when you go indoors.

REALITY OF PREGNANCY

"Now that my abdomen is swelling, the fact that I'm really pregnant has finally sunk in. Even though we planned this pregnancy, I suddenly feel scared, trapped by the baby—even antagonistic toward it."

Even the most eager of expectant parents may be surprised (and guilt-ridden) to find themselves with second thoughts as their pregnancy starts to become a reality. An unseen little intruder has suddenly come between them, turning their lives upside down, depriving them of freedoms they'd always taken for granted, making more demands on them—both physically and emotionally—than anyone ever has before. Every aspect of the lifestyle they had become accustomed to—from how they spent their evenings, to what they ate and drank, to how often they made love—is being altered by this child even before its birth. And the knowledge that these changes will become still more imposing after delivery compounds their mixed feelings, deepens their apprehension.

Studies show that not only is a little ambivalence, a little fear, even a little antagonism, normal, it's healthy—as long as these feelings are acknowledged and confronted. And now is the best time to do that. Work out any resentments now (over not being free to stay out late on Saturday nights, to pick up and go on a weekend trip when the spirit moves you, to work full time, or to spend your money any way you please), and you won't find yourself venting them at your baby after he or she's arrived. Sharing your feelings with your partner is the best way to do this—and encourage him to do likewise.

Although the lifestyle changes may be greater or lesser, depending on how you and your spouse decide to order your priorities, it's true that your life is never going to be the same again once your "two" becomes "three." But as some parts of your world become more constricted, others will open up. You may find yourself reborn with your baby's birth. And this new life may turn out to be the best yet.

UNWANTED ADVICE

"Now that it's obvious I'm expecting, everyone—from my mother-in-law to strangers on the elevator—has advice for me. It drives me crazy."

Short of taking up a reclusive existence on a desert island, there's no way for a pregnant woman to escape the unsolicited advice of those around her. There's just something about a bulging belly that brings out the "expert" in all of us. Take your morning jog around the park and someone is sure to chide: "You shouldn't be running in your condition!" Lug home two bags of groceries from the supermarket and you're bound to hear: "Do you think you ought to be carrying such heavy bundles?" Or reach up for a subway strap and you may even be warned: "If you stretch that way the cord will wrap around your baby's neck and strangle it."

Between such gratuitous advice and the inevitable predictions about the sex of the baby, what's an expectant mother to do? First of all, keep in mind that most of what you hear is probably nonsense. Old wives' tales that *do* have foundation in fact have been scientifically substantiated and have become part of standard medical practice. Those that do not, though still tightly woven into the tapestry of pregnancy mythology, can be confidently dismissed. Those recommendations that leave you with a nagging doubt—"What if they are right?"—and are therefore impossible to dismiss are best checked with your doctor, nurse-midwife, or childbirth educator.

Whether it's possibly plausible or obviously ridiculous, however, don't let unwanted advice get your dander up. Neither you nor your baby will profit from the added tension. Instead, keeping your sense of humor handy, you can take one of two approaches: Politely inform the well-meaning stranger, friend, or relative that you have a trusted physician who counsels you on your pregnancy and that you can't accept advice from anyone else. Or, just as politely, smile, say thank you, and go on your way, letting their comments go in one ear and out the other—without making any stops in between.

But no matter how you choose to handle unwanted advice, you'd also do well to get used to it. If there's anyone who attracts a crowd of advice-givers faster than a pregnant woman, it's a woman with a new baby.

WHAT IT'S IMPORTANT TO KNOW:
MAKING LOVE DURING PREGNANCY

Religious and medical miracles aside, every pregnancy begins with the sexual act. So why is it that what got you into this situation in the first place may now have become one of your biggest problems?

Whether sex becomes virtually non-existent, just a little uncomfortable, or better than ever, almost every expectant couple finds that their sexual relationship undergoes some kind of change during the nine months of pregnancy.

Variations in sexual appetite and response before conception are wide to begin with. What constitutes a satisfying sex life to one couple—"obligatory" relations once a week, for instance—would be completely unsatisfactory for another, for whom once a day might not always be enough. After conception, such variations may be even more exaggerated. And to further complicate matters sexual, physical and emotional upheaval sometimes leaves the once-a-day couple less in the mood for love than the once-a-week couple, and vice versa.

Though there are variations from couple to couple, a general down-up-down pattern of sexual interest during the three trimesters of pregnancy is common. It's not surprising that a diminution of sexual interest may occur early in pregnancy (in one survey, 54% of women reported reduced libido in the first trimester). After all, fatigue, nausea, vomiting, and painfully tender breasts do make less than ideal bedfellows. In women with comfortable first trimesters, however, sexual desire often remains more or less the same. And a sizable minority of expectant women find it increases

significantly—often because the hormonal changes of early pregnancy leave the vulva engorged and ultrasensitive, and/or because the heightened breast sensitivity that is painful for other women is pleasurable for them. These women may experience orgasms or multiple orgasms for the first time.

Interest often—but not always—picks up during the midtrimester, when a couple is physically and psychologically better adjusted to the pregnancy. It usually wanes again as delivery nears, even more drastically than in the first trimester—for obvious reasons: first, the bulk of the abdomen is more and more difficult to get around; second, the aches and discomforts of advancing pregnancy are capable of cooling the hottest passion; and third, late in the trimester it's hard to concentrate on anything but that eagerly and anxiously awaited event.

Sexual pleasure, like sexual interest, seems to diminish in some—but certainly not all—couples. In one group of women, only 21% received little or no pleasure from sex before conception. The percentage of these women finding sex not pleasurable rose to 41% at 12 weeks of gestation, and to 59% going into the ninth month. The same study found that at 12 weeks, about 1 in 10 couples were not having sex at all; by the ninth month, more than a third were abstaining. But encouragingly, the study also found that more than 4 in 10 women were still enjoying sex at this point—more than half of these with *no* problems.

So you may find that sex during pregnancy is the best you've ever had. Or something you wish you could enjoy but can't. Or it may become an uncomfortable obligation. You may even abandon it altogether. Normalcy in pregnancy lovemaking, as in so many other aspects of pregnancy, is what is right for you.

UNDERSTANDING SEXUALITY DURING PREGNANCY

U nfortunately, some practitioners are as inhibited about sexuality as the rest of us. Often they don't tell expectant couples what to expect, or not to expect, in the intimate part of their relationship. And that leaves many couples uncertain how to proceed.

Understanding why making love during pregnancy is different than it is at other times can help ease fears and worries, and can make having intercourse (or not having it) more acceptable and more pleasurable.

First of all, there are many physical changes that affect desire and actual sexual pleasure both positively and negatively. Some negative factors can be dealt with to minimize their interference in your sex life; others you may just have to learn to live with—and love with.

Nausea and Vomiting. If your morning sickness stays with you day and night, you may just have to wait its symptoms out. (In most cases, queasiness will start letting up by the end of the first trimester.) If it strikes just at certain hours, keep your schedules flexible, and put the good times to good use. Don't pressure yourself to feel sexy when you're feeling lousy; morning sickness can be aggravated by emotional stress. (See page 104 for tips on minimizing morning sickness.)

Fatigue. This, too, should pass by the fourth month. Until then, make love while the sun shines (when the opportunity presents itself), instead of trying to force yourself to stay up late for romance. If your weekend afternoons are free, cap off a nap with a lovemaking session. (See page 102 for more on easing fatigue.)

The Changing Shape. Making love can be both awkward and uncomfortable when a bulging belly seems to loom as large and forbidding as a Himalayan mountain. As pregnancy progresses, the gymnastics required to scale that growing abdomen may not seem, to some couples, worth the effort. (But there are ways to get around the mountain; see page 169.) In addition, the woman's full-figured silhouette may actually turn off one or both partners. You may be able to psych yourself out of this socially conditioned reflex by thinking: big (in pregnancy) is beautiful.

The Engorgement of Genitals. Increased blood flow to the pelvic area, caused by the hormonal changes of pregnancy, can heighten sexual response in some women. But it can also make sex less satisfying (especially later in pregnancy) if a residual fullness persists after orgasm, leaving a woman feeling as though she didn't quite make it. For the male, too, the engorgement of the pregnant woman's genitalia may increase pleasure (if he feels pleasantly and snugly caressed) or decrease it (if the fit is so tight he loses his erection).

Leakage of Colostrum. Late in pregnancy, some women begin producing the premilk called colostrum. Colostrum can leak from the breasts during sexual stimulation, and it can be disconcerting in the middle of foreplay. It's nothing to worry about, of course, but if it bothers you or your partner, it can easily be avoided by refraining from breast play.

Breast Tenderness. Some fortunate couples revel throughout pregnancy in the fun of full-and-firm-for-the-first-time breasts. But many find that in early pregnancy, the breasts may have to be neglected during love play because they are painfully tender. (Be certain to communicate your discomfort to your partner, rather than suffering, and resenting, his touch in silence.) However, as the tenderness diminishes toward the end of the first trimester, the extreme sensitivity of the breasts enhances sex for some couples.

Alterations in Vaginal Secretions. These secretions increase in volume and change in consistency, odor, and taste. The increased lubrication may make intercourse more enjoyable for a couple if the woman's vagina has always been dry and/or uncomfortably narrow. Or it might make the vaginal canal so wet and slippery that a man may have trouble holding an erection. The heavier scent and taste of the secretions may also make oral sex unpleasant to some men. Massaging scented oils into the pubic area or the inner thighs may help to disguise the problem.

Bleeding Caused by the Sensitivity of the Cervix. The mouth of the uterus also becomes engorged during pregnancy—crisscrossed with many additional blood vessels to accommodate increased blood flow to the uterus—and much softer than before pregnancy. This means that deep penetration can occasionally cause bleeding, particularly late in pregnancy when the cervix begins to ripen for delivery. If this occurs (and threatened miscarriage or any other complications that require abstinence from intercourse are ruled out by your practitioner), simply avoid deep penetration.

There is a full complement of psychological hangups that can interfere with sexual enjoyment during pregnancy. These, too, can be minimized.

Fear of Hurting the Fetus or Causing a Miscarriage. In normal pregnancies sexual intercourse will do neither. The fetus is well cushioned and protected inside the amniotic sac and uterus, and the uterus is securely sealed off from the outside world with a mucous plug in the mouth of the cervix.

Fear That Having an Orgasm Will Stimulate Miscarriage or Early Labor. Although the uterus does contract following orgasm—and these contractions can be quite pronounced in some women, lasting as long as half an hour after intercourse—such contractions are not a sign of labor and pose no danger in a normal pregnancy. However, orgasm, particularly the more intense kind triggered by masturbation, may be prohibited in pregnancies at high risk for miscarriage or premature labor.

Fear That the Fetus Is "Watching" or "Aware." Though a fetus may enjoy the gentle rocking of uterine contractions during orgasm, neither can it see what you're doing nor has it any idea what is happening during intercourse, and your baby will certainly have no memory of it. Fetal reactions (slowed movement during intercourse, then furious kicking and squirming and speeded-up heartbeat after orgasm) are responses solely to hormonal and uterine activity.

Fear That the Introduction of the Penis into the Vagina Will Cause Infection. As long as the male does not have a sexually transmittable disease, there appears to be no danger of infection to either mother or fetus through intercourse during the first seven or eight months—in the amniotic sac, the baby is safe from both semen and infectious organisms. Most physicians believe this is true even during the ninth month—as long as the sac remains intact (the membranes haven't ruptured). But because they could rupture at any time, some suggest that a condom be worn during intercourse in the last four to eight weeks of pregnancy, as added insurance against infection.

Anxiety Over the Coming Attraction. Both the mother- and father-to-be are subject to mixed feelings over the upcoming blessed event; thoughts about the responsibilities and lifestyle changes and the financial and emotional cost of bringing up a baby can inhibit relaxed lovemaking. This ambivalence, which many expectant parents experience, should be confronted and talked through openly rather than being brought to bed.

The Changing Relationship Between Husband and Wife. A couple may have trouble adjusting to the idea that they will no longer be just lovers, or husband and wife, but mother and father as well. After all, many of us still avoid associating our own parents with sex, though we are living proof that such an association exists. On the other hand, some couples may discover that the new dimension in their relationship brings a new intimacy into bed with them—and with it, a new excitement.

Subconscious Hostility. Of the expectant father toward the expectant mother, because he is jealous that she has become the center of attention. Or of mom-to-be toward dad-to-be because she feels she is doing all the suffering (particularly if the pregnancy has been a rough one) for the baby they both want and will both enjoy. Such feelings are important to talk out, but not in bed.

Belief That Intercourse During the Last Six Weeks of Pregnancy Will Cause Labor to Begin. It *is* true that the uterine contractions triggered by orgasm become stronger as pregnancy proceeds. But unless the cervix is "ripe," these contractions do not appear to bring on labor—as many hopeful and eager overdue couples can attest. However, since no one knows exactly what mechanism initiates labor, and because some studies do show an increase in premature births among couples having intercourse in the last weeks of pregnancy, abstinence is often prescribed for women with a tendency toward preterm delivery.

Fear of "Hitting" the Baby Once the Head Is Engaged in the Pelvis. Even couples who were relaxed about having intercourse earlier can tighten up now because the baby is too close for comfort. Many doctors suggest that though you can't hurt the baby, deep penetration won't be comfortable at this time and should be avoided.

Psychological factors can also affect sexual relations for the better:

Switching from Procreational to Recreational Sex. Some couples who worked hard at becoming pregnant may be delighted at being able to have sex for its own sake—free from thermometers, charts, calendars, and anxiety. For them, sex becomes really enjoyable for the first time in months, or even years.

Though sexual intercourse during pregnancy may be different from what you've experienced before, it is in most cases perfectly safe. In fact, it can be good for you, both physically and emotionally: it can keep you and your spouse close; it can help you get in shape, preparing your pelvic muscles for delivery; and it's relaxing—which is beneficial for everyone concerned, baby included.

WHEN SEXUAL RELATIONS MAY BE LIMITED

Since lovemaking has so much to offer the expectant couple, it would be ideal if every couple could take advantage of it throughout pregnancy. Alas, for some this isn't possible. In high-risk pregnancies, intercourse may be restricted at certain times, or even for nine months. Or, intercourse may be permitted without orgasm for the wife, or petting may be allowed as long as penetration is avoided. Knowing precisely *what* is safe and *when* is essential; if your doctor instructs you to abstain, ask why and whether he or she is referring to intercourse, orgasm, or both, and whether the restrictions are temporary or apply for the entire gestation.

Intercourse will probably be restricted under the following circumstances:

❖ Any time unexplained bleeding occurs.

❖ During the first trimester if a woman has a history of miscarriages or threatened miscarriage, or shows signs of a threatened miscarriage.

❖ During the last 8 to 12 weeks if a woman has a history of premature or threatened premature labor, or is experiencing signs of early labor.

❖ If amniotic membranes (the bag of waters) have ruptured.

❖ When placenta previa is known to exist (the placenta is located near or over the cervix, where it could be prematurely dislodged during intercourse, causing bleeding and threatening mother and baby).

❖ In the last trimester if multiple fetuses are being carried.

ENJOYING IT MORE, EVEN IF YOU'RE DOING IT LESS

Good, lasting sexual relationships—like good, lasting marriages—are rarely built in a day (or even a really terrific night). They grow with practice, patience, understanding, and love. This is true, too, of an already established sexual relationship that undergoes the emotional and physical assaults of pregnancy. Here are a few ways to "stay on top":

❖ Never allow how frequently or infrequently you have intercourse to interfere with other aspects of your relationship. The quality of lovemaking is always more important than the quantity—and never more so than during pregnancy.

❖ Keep the emphasis on love, rather than lovemaking. If one or both of you don't feel like having intercourse, or if intercourse is frustrating because it isn't fully satisfying, find alternative routes to intimacy. The possibilities are far more numerous than positions in a sex manual. For example: old-fashioned kissing and necking, hand holding, back rubs, foot massage, sharing a milkshake in bed (see page 95 for a recipe), reading love poems, watching television while cuddling under the blanket, taking a shower together, going out (or staying in) for a romantic dinner by candlelight, meeting for a quiet lunch—or whatever else makes the lovebird in you coo.

❖ Recognize the possible strains that expectant parenthood may have placed on your relationship, and acknowledge any changes in the intensity of sexual desire that either or both of you may be feeling. Discuss any problems openly; don't sweep them under the bedcovers. If any problems seem too big to handle by yourselves, seek professional help.

❖ Think positive: Making love is good physical preparation for labor and delivery. (Not many athletes have this much fun in training.)

❖ Think of having to try new positions during pregnancy as an adventure. But give yourselves time to adjust to each position you try. (You might even consider a "dry run"—trying out a new position fully clothed first, so that it'll be more familiar when you try it for real.) Usually comfortable positions include: male on top, but off to one side or supported by his arms (to keep his weight off the woman); woman on top (but avoid deep penetration); both partners on their side—front-to-front or front-to-back.

❖ Keep your expectations within reality's reach. Though some women achieve orgasm for the first time during pregnancy, at least one study showed that most women are less likely to achieve orgasm *regularly* during pregnancy than before conception—particularly in the last trimester, when only 1 out of 4 women reach climax consistently. Your goal doesn't always have to be orgasm; sometimes just physical closeness can satisfy.

❖ If the doctor has ruled out sexual intercourse during any period of your pregnancy, ask if orgasm is okay—via mutual masturbation. If it's taboo for you, you might still get pleasure out of pleasuring your husband in this way.

❖ If the doctor has prohibited orgasm for you but not coitus, you might still be able to enjoy lovemaking without your reaching climax. Though this may not be completely satisfying, it can provide a sense of intimacy. Another possibility: intercourse between the thighs.

Even if the quality, or quantity, of your sexual relations isn't quite what it once was, understanding the dynamics of sexuality during pregnancy can keep the relationship strong— even strengthen it—without spectacular or frequent intercourse.

A Scary Ultrasound

In about 1 to 4% of second trimester ultrasounds a choroid plexus cyst is detected in the fetal brain. Though this sounds very scary, the vast majority resolve before birth and don't result in any developmental problems later. If there are no other signs of abnormalities in the fetus, the prognosis is very good.

9
The Fifth Month

WHAT YOU CAN EXPECT AT THIS MONTH'S CHECKUP

This month, you can expect your practitioner to check the following, though there may be variations depending upon your particular needs and upon your practitioner's style of practice:[1]

❖ Weight and blood pressure

❖ Urine, for sugar and protein

❖ Fetal heartbeat

❖ Size and shape of uterus, by external palpation

❖ Height of fundus (top of uterus)

❖ Feet and hands, for edema (swelling), and legs for varicose veins

❖ Symptoms you have been experiencing, especially unusual ones

❖ Questions and problems you want to discuss—have a list ready

---

WHAT YOU MAY BE FEELING

You may experience all of these symptoms at one time or another, or only a few of them. Some may have continued from last month, others may be new. Still others may hardly be noticed because you've become so used to them. You may also have other, less common, symptoms.

1. See Appendix for an explanation of the procedures and tests performed.

PHYSICALLY:

❖ Fetal movement

❖ Increasing whitish vaginal discharge (leukorrhea)

❖ Lower abdominal achiness (from stretching of the ligaments supporting the uterus)

❖ Constipation

❖ Heartburn, indigestion, flatulence, bloating

WHAT YOU MAY LOOK LIKE

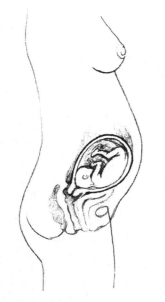

By the end of the fifth month, the activity of this 8- to 10-inch fetus is strong enough to be felt by its mother. Soft downy lanugo covers its body; hair begins to grow on its head; brows and white eyelashes appear. A protective vernix coating covers the fetus.

- ❖ Occasional headaches, faintness or dizziness
- ❖ Nasal congestion and occasional nosebleeds; ear stuffiness
- ❖ "Pink toothbrush" from bleeding gums
- ❖ Hearty appetite
- ❖ Leg cramps
- ❖ Mild swelling of ankles and feet, and occasionally of hands and face
- ❖ Varicose veins of legs and/or hemorrhoids
- ❖ Increased pulse (heart rate)
- ❖ Easier—or more difficult—orgasm
- ❖ Backache
- ❖ Skin pigmentation changes on abdomen and/or face

EMOTIONALLY:

- ❖ An acceptance of the reality of pregnancy
- ❖ Fewer mood swings, but irritability still occasionally occurs; continued absentmindedness

WHAT YOU MAY BE CONCERNED ABOUT

FATIGUE

"I get tired when I am exercising or doing heavy cleaning; should I stop?"

Not only should you stop when you get tired, you should, whenever possible, stop before then. Exerting yourself to the point of exhaustion is never a good idea. During pregnancy it's a particularly bad one, since overwork takes its toll not only on

you but on the baby as well. Pay careful attention to your body's signals. If you become breathless when you're jogging, or find the vacuum suddenly feels as if it weighs a ton, take a break.

Instead of marathon activity sessions, pace yourself. Work or exercise a bit, rest a bit. Most of the time the work, or the workout, will get done, and you won't feel drained afterward. If occasionally something doesn't get done, you're getting good training for the days when the demands of parent-hood will often keep you from finish-ing what you start. See page 102 for tips on dealing with fatigue.

FAINTNESS AND DIZZINESS

"I feel dizzy when I get up from a sitting or lying-down position. And yesterday I nearly fainted while I was shopping. Am I okay? Can this hurt my baby?"

On late-show movies, a fainting spell is a more reliable indicator of pregnancy than a dead rabbit. Screenwriters in the '40s were, how-ever, off the mark. Though dizziness is fairly common in pregnancy, fainting, also called syncope, is less so. There are a variety of reasons, known or suspected, for a pregnant woman feel-ing lightheaded or dizzy.

In the first trimester, dizziness may be related to a blood supply that is inadequate to fill the rapidly expand-ing circulatory system; in the second trimester, it may be caused by the pressure of the expanding uterus on maternal blood vessels. Dizziness can occur anytime you rise from a sitting or prone position. This is called pos-tural hypotension. It's caused by a sudden shifting of blood away from the brain when blood pressure drops rapidly. The cure is simple: Always get up very gradually. Jumping up quickly to answer the phone is likely to land you right back on the sofa.

You might also feel dizzy because your blood sugar is low. Generally this is caused by going too long without food and can be avoided by getting some protein (which helps keep blood sugar level) at every meal and by tak-ing more frequent, smaller meals or eating snacks between your usual mealtimes. Carry a box of raisins, a piece of fruit, or some whole-wheat crackers or breadsticks in your bag for quick blood-sugar lifts.

Dizziness can strike, too, in an over-heated store, office, or bus, especially if you are overdressed. The best way to handle such dizziness is to get some fresh air by going outside or opening a window. Taking off your coat and loosening your clothes—especially around the neck and waist—should help, too.

If you feel lightheaded and/or think you are going to faint, try to increase circulation to your brain by lying down, if possible, with your feet (not your head) elevated, or by sitting down with your head between your knees, until the dizziness subsides. If there's no place to lie or sit, kneel on one knee and bend forward as though you were trying to tie your shoelace. Actual fainting is rare, but if you do faint, there is no need for worry or concern—although the flow of blood to your brain is temporarily being re-duced, this will not affect your baby.[2]

Tell your practitioner about any diz-ziness or faintness you experience when you see him or her next. Report actual fainting promptly. Frequent fainting—occasionally a sign of severe anemia or other illness—needs to be evaluated by a physician.

HEPATITIS TESTING

"I'm in my fifth month and my obstetri-cian just tested me for hepatitis B. Why?"

As a routine precaution, it's now recommended that all women be tested for hepatitis B at least once during their pregnancy, usually late in the second trimester. That's because hepatitis B, unlike hepatitis A, can be passed on to the fetus, almost always during childbirth, though very occa-

---

2. First aid for mothers-to-be who've actually fainted is the same as the preventive mea-sures.

sionally during pregnancy itself. Nearly 9 in 10 infected babies, if untreated, will become chronic carriers of hepatitis B, and are at risk of later developing liver inflammation or more serious liver disease. Routine testing allows doctors to diagnose the disease in infected mothers so that their babies can be treated at birth (see page 318), which almost always prevents the infection from taking hold.

SLEEPING POSITION

"I've always slept on my stomach. Now I'm afraid to. And I just can't seem to get comfortable any other way."

G iving up your favorite sleeping position during pregnancy can be as traumatic as giving up your teddy bear was when you were six. You're bound to lose some sleep over it—but only until you get used to the new position. And the time to get used to it is now, before your expanding belly makes getting comfortable even more difficult.

Two common favorite sleeping positions—on the belly and on the back—are not the best choices during pregnancy. The belly position, for obvious reasons: as your stomach grows, sleeping on it would be about as

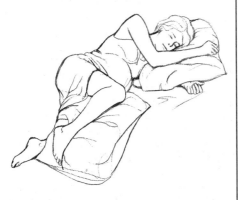

Sleep on your left side.

comfy as sleeping on a watermelon. The back position, though more comfortable, rests the entire weight of your pregnant uterus on your back, your intestines, and the inferior vena cava (the vein responsible for returning blood from the lower body to the heart). This can aggravate backaches and hemorrhoids, inhibit digestive function, interfere with breathing and circulation, and possibly cause hypotension, or low blood pressure.

This doesn't mean you have to sleep standing up. Curling up or stretching out on your side—preferably the left side—with one leg crossed over the other and with a pillow between them, is best for both you and your fetus. It not only allows maximum flow of blood and nutrients to the placenta but also enhances efficient kidney function, which means better elimination of waste products and fluids and less edema (swelling) of ankles, feet, and hands.

Very few people, however, manage to stay in one position through the night. Don't be alarmed if you wake up and find yourself on your back or abdomen. No harm done—just turn back to your side. You may feel uncomfortable for a few nights, but your body will soon adjust to the new position.

BACKACHE

"I'm having a lot of backaches. I'm afraid I won't be able to stand up at all by the ninth month."

T he aches and discomforts of pregnancy are not designed to make you miserable. They are the side effects of the preparations your body is making for that momentous moment when your baby is born. Backache is no exception. During pregnancy, the usually stable joints of the pelvis begin to loosen up to allow easier passage for the baby at delivery. This, along with your oversized abdomen, throws your body off balance. To compensate, you tend to bring your shoulders back and arch your neck. Standing with your belly thrust forward—to be sure that no one who passes fails to notice you're pregnant—compounds the problem. The result: a deeply curved lower back, strained back muscles, and pain.

Even pain with a purpose hurts. But without defeating the purpose, you can conquer (or at least subdue) the pain. The best approach, as usual, is prevention: coming into pregnancy with strong abdominal muscles, good posture, and graceful body mechanics. But it's not too late to learn body mechanics that will minimize pregnancy backache. To align your body properly, practice the pelvic tilt, as shown on page 191. The following should also help:

❖ Try to keep weight gain within the recommended parameters (see

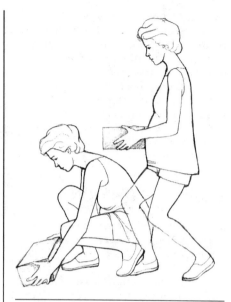

Bend at the knees.

page 147). Excess poundage will only add to the load your back is struggling under.

❖ Don't wear very high heels, or even very flat ones without proper support. Some doctors recommend wide 2-inch heels to help keep the body properly aligned. There are shoes and shoe inserts especially designed to help alleviate leg and back problems during pregnancy; ask your practitioner or a salesperson at a good shoe store.

❖ Learn the proper way to lift heavy loads (packages, children, laundry, books, etc.). Don't lift abruptly. Stabilize your body first by assuming a wide stance (feet shoulder-width apart) and tucking your buttocks in. Bend at the knees, not at the waist, and lift with your arms and legs rather than your back. (See illustration, above.) If backache is a problem, try to limit the carrying you do. If you're forced to carry a heavy load of groceries, divide them between two shopping bags

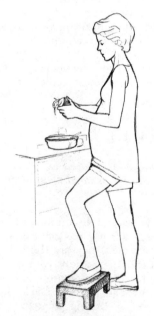

Take an anti-backache position.

and carry one in each arm, rather than carrying the lot in front of you.

❖ Try not to stand for long periods. If you must, keep one foot up on a stool with your knee bent to prevent strain on your lower back. (See illustration, facing page.) When standing on a hard-surfaced floor, as when cooking or washing dishes, put a small skid-proof rug underfoot.

❖ Sit smart. Sitting puts more stress on your spine than almost any other activity, so it pays to do it right. That means sitting, when possible, in a chair that offers adequate support, preferably one with a straight back, arms (use them for assistance when you rise from the chair), and a firm cushion that doesn't allow you to sink down into it. Avoid backless stools and benches. And wherever you're sitting, never cross your legs. Not only can leg crossing promote circulation problems, it can cause you to tilt your pelvis too far forward, aggravating backache. Whenever possible, sit with your legs slightly elevated (see illustration, right); when driving, keep your seat forward so you can keep one knee higher and bent.

Sitting too long can be as bad as sitting the wrong way. Try not to sit for more than an hour without taking a walking/stretching break; setting a half-hour limit would be even better.

❖ Sleep on a firm mattress, or put a board under an overly soft one. A comfortable sleeping position (see page 173) will help minimize aches and pains when you're awake. When getting out of bed in the morning, swing your legs over the side of the bed to the floor, rather than twisting to get up.

❖ Ask your practitioner if a pregnancy girdle or a crisscross support sling for your belly will be helpful in lessening the strain on your lower back.

❖ Don't stretch to put dishes back into the cupboard or to hang a painting. Instead, use a low, steady footstool. Reaching above your head puts a strain on the back muscles.

❖ Use a heating pad (wrapped in a towel) or warm (but not hot) baths to temporarily relieve sore muscles.

❖ Learn to relax. Many back problems are aggravated by stress. If you think yours might be, try some relaxation exercises when pain strikes. Also follow the suggestions beginning on page 113 for dealing with stress in your life.

❖ Do simple exercises that strengthen your abdominal muscles, such as the Dromedary Droop (page 192) and the Pelvic Tilt (page 191).

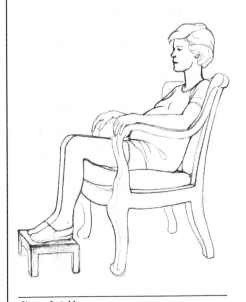

Sit comfortably.

CARRYING OLDER CHILDREN

"I have a 3½-year-old who always wants to be carried up the stairs. But my back is breaking from her weight."

It would be a good idea to break her habit rather than continue breaking your back; the strain of carrying a growing fetus is enough without adding some 30 or 40 pounds of preschooler. Be careful not to blame her sibling-to-be for the change in parental policy, however—blame your back instead. And make much ado about her efforts when she does agree to walk on her own.

Of course there will be times when your child won't take "walk" for an answer. So learn the proper way to lift (see page 174), and be assured that such lifting in no way compromises your unborn baby, unless your practitioner has restricted such strenuous activities.

FOOT PROBLEMS

"My shoes are all beginning to feel uncomfortably tight. Could my feet be growing along with my belly?"

Not growing in the usual sense, but they may indeed be getting larger. First of all there is the swelling, or edema, caused by the normal fluid retention of pregnancy. There may also be extra fat on the feet if your weight gain is excessive. Then there is the spreading of your foot joints (along with all your other joints) as the hormone relaxin sets about its job of loosening up your pelvis for delivery. The swelling in your feet will go down after delivery and the weight will probably be lost. But though the joints will tighten up, it's possible that your feet will be permanently larger—

by as much as a full shoe size.

In the meantime, try the tips for reducing excessive swelling (see page 217) if that seems to be your problem, and get a couple of pairs of shoes that fit you comfortably now—one for walking and working, and one for dress wear. Both should have heels no more than 2 inches high, nonskid soles, and plenty of space for your feet to spread out in (try them on at the end of the day, when your feet are the most swollen); and both should be made of leather or canvas so your feet can breathe. If you choose carefully, you can find not just walking shoes, but dress shoes too, that meet these requirements.

Shoes, or orthotic inserts, that are designed to correct the distorted center of gravity of pregnancy can not only make your feet more comfortable but reduce back and leg pain as well. They are available in two different designs, one to take you through the first six months of pregnancy and the other to take you through the final trimester. Ask your practitioner for a recommendation.

Elasticized slippers worn for several hours a day have also been useful in reducing fatigue and achiness in feet and lower legs, though they don't seem to reduce swelling. If your legs are aching and tired at the end of the day, wearing such slippers while you are at home—or even at work, if that's feasible—may help.

FAST-GROWING HAIR AND NAILS

"It seems to me that my hair and nails have never grown so fast before."

The bounteous circulation and increased metabolism caused by pregnancy hormones is nourishing your skin cells well. Happy effects of this increased nourishment are nails that grow faster than you can manicure them, and hair that grows faster (and if you're really lucky, is thicker and more lustrous) than you can secure appointments with your stylist.

The extra nourishment can, however, also have less happy effects. It can cause hair to grow in places women would rather it didn't. Facial areas (lips, chin, and cheeks) are most commonly plagued with this pregnancy-induced hirsutism, but arms, legs, back, and belly can be affected too. Much of the excess hair disappears within six months postpartum, though some may linger longer.

Though there's no known risk, it's probably not a good idea to use depilatories or bleach cream once you find out you're pregnant. Your skin may not react well to the chemicals, and it's even possible that they may be absorbed into your bloodstream. Plucking facial hair and shaving legs and underarms present no problem.

LATE MISCARRIAGE

"I know they say that once you pass the third month, you don't have to worry about miscarriage. But I know someone who lost her baby in the fifth month."

While it's essentially true that there's little reason to worry about miscarriage after the first trimester, it does occasionally happen that a fetus is lost between the 12th and 20th weeks. This is known as a *late* miscarriage, and accounts for fewer than 25% of all spontaneous abortions; it is rare in an uneventful, low-risk pregnancy. After the 20th week, when the fetus usually weighs over 500 grams (17½ ounces) and there is the possibility that it can survive with specialized care, its delivery is considered a premature birth and not a miscarriage.

Unlike the causes of early miscarriages, which are frequently related to the fetus, the causes of second-trimester miscarriages are usually related to either the placenta or the mother.[3] The placenta may separate prematurely from the uterus, be implanted abnormally, or fail to produce adequate hormones to maintain the pregnancy. The mother may have taken certain drugs, or may have undergone surgery that affected her pelvic organs. Or she may suffer from serious infection, uncontrolled chronic illness, severe malnutrition, endocrine dysfunction, myomas (tumors of the uterus), an abnormally shaped uterus, or an incompetent cervix that opens prematurely. Serious physical trauma, such as that sustained in an accident, appears to play only a small role in miscarriage at any stage in pregnancy.

Early symptoms of a midtrimester miscarriage include a pink vaginal discharge for several days, or a scant brown discharge for several weeks. Should you experience such a discharge, don't panic—it could be nothing serious. But do call your practitioner the day you first notice it. If you have heavy bleeding with or without cramping, call your practitioner immediately or go to the hospital. See page 348 for treatment of threatened miscarriage and prevention of future miscarriages.

ABDOMINAL PAIN

"I'm very worried about the pains I've been getting on the sides of my pelvis."

What you are probably feeling is the stretching of muscles and ligaments supporting the uterus—

---

3. Many maternal causes of late miscarriage can be prevented by good medical care.

something most pregnant women experience. The discomfort may be crampy or sharp and stabbing, and often is most noticeable when you are getting up from a bed or chair, or when you cough. It may be brief, or may last for several hours. As long as the pain is occasional and not persistent—and is not accompanied by fever, chills, bleeding, increased vaginal discharge, faintness, or other unusual symptoms—there's no cause for concern. Getting off your feet and resting in a comfortable position should bring some relief. You should, of course, mention the pain to your practitioner at your next visit.

CHANGES IN SKIN PIGMENTATION

"I have a dark line down the center of my abdomen and dark spots on my face. Is this discoloration normal, and will it remain after pregnancy?"

Once again those pregnancy hormones are at work. Just as they caused the darkening of the areolas around your nipples, they are now responsible for the darkening of the *linea alba*—the white line you probably never noticed—which runs down the center of your abdomen to the top of your pubic bone. During pregnancy, it's renamed the *linea nigra,* or black line.

Some women, usually those with darker complexions, also develop discolorations in a mask-like configuration on foreheads, noses, and cheeks. The patches are dark in light-skinned women and light in dark-skinned women. This mask of pregnancy, or chloasma, will gradually fade after delivery. In the meantime, bleaching probably won't lighten chloasma (and is not a good idea anyway), though cover-up makeups may camouflage it.

Sun can intensify the coloration, so use a sun block with a sun protection factor (SPF) of 15 or more when outdoors in sunny weather, or wear a hat that completely shades your face. Since there is some evidence that the excess pigmentation may be related to folic acid deficiency, be sure that your vitamin supplement contains folic acid and that you are eating green leafy vegetables, oranges, and whole-wheat bread or cereal daily.

Hyperpigmentation (darkening of the skin) may occur in high-friction areas, such as between the thighs. This, too, will fade after delivery.

OTHER STRANGE SKIN SYMPTOMS

"My palms seem to be red all the time. Is it my imagination?"

No, and it isn't your dishwashing liquid, either. It's your hormones. Increased levels of pregnancy hormones cause red, itchy palms (and sometimes red, itchy soles of the feet) in two-thirds of white and one-third of black pregnant women. The dishpan look will disappear soon after delivery.

Your nails may not escape pregnancy unscathed either. You may find they are more brittle or soft, and have developed grooves. Nail polish may make them worse. If they show signs of infection, ask your practitioner about treatment.

"My legs and feet turn bluish and blotchy sometimes. Is something wrong with my circulation?"

Due to stepped-up estrogen production, many women experience this kind of transitory, mottled discoloration when they're chilly. It is insignificant, and will disappear post-partum.

"I've developed a tiny, floppy growth of skin under my arm at the bra line. I'm worried that it could be skin cancer."

What you're describing is proba-bly a skin tag, another benign skin problem common in pregnant women and often found in high-friction areas, such as under the arms. Skin tags frequently develop in the second and third trimesters and may regress after delivery. If they don't, they can be easily removed by your physician.

To be sure of the diagnosis, show it to your practitioner at your next visit.

"I seem to have broken out in a heat rash. I thought only babies got that."

Actually, anyone can develop a heat rash. But it is particularly common in pregnant women because of the increase in eccrine perspiration, the kind that comes from sweat glands that are distributed over the entire body surface and that are involved in heat regulation. Patting on some corn-starch after your shower and trying to keep as cool as possible will help min-imize discomfort and recurrence.

On the plus side, apocrine perspira-tion, the kind produced by glands un-der the arms, under the breasts, and in the genital area, diminishes in preg-nancy—so though you may have heat rash you are less likely to have body odor. If you itch all over but have no rash, call your practitioner.

DENTAL PROBLEMS

"My mouth has suddenly become a disas-ter area. My gums bleed every time I brush, and I think I have a cavity. But

I'm afraid to go to the dentist because of the anesthesia."

With so much of your attention centered on your abdomen during pregnancy, it's easy to over-look your mouth—until it begins to scream for equal time, which it fre-quently does because of the heavy toll a normal pregnancy can take on the gums. The gums, like the mucous membranes of the nose, become swol-len, inflamed, and tend to bleed easily because of pregnancy hormones.

It's best not to wait until your mouth is hollering for help. If you suspect a cavity or other incipient trouble, make an appointment right away. Sometimes there's actually more risk to the fetus in putting off neces-sary dental work than there is in hav-ing it done. For example, badly de-cayed teeth that are not taken care of can be a source of infection that spreads throughout the system, put-ting both mother and fetus in danger. Impacted wisdom teeth that are either infected or causing severe pain should also be attended to promptly.

However, special precautions must be taken when dental work is done during pregnancy to ensure that the supply of oxygen to the fetus is not compromised through the use of gen-eral anesthetics, and that no anes-thetic is used that is known to cause harm to a fetus. In most cases a local anesthetic will suffice. If a general an-esthetic is absolutely required, then it should be administered by an experi-enced anesthesiologist. Discuss the anesthesia with both your dentist and your physician beforehand to ensure safety. Check with your physician to see if an antibiotic will be needed prior to or at the time of dental work.

If after the dental work you're left with chipmunk cheeks and can't chew solids, you're going to have to make some dietary alterations. On a fluid-only diet you can obtain adequate nutrients temporarily by sipping milkshakes (see Double-the-Milk Shake, page 95). Supplement the shakes with citrus juices (if they don't burn your gums) and homemade "creamed" soups made from cooked vegetables puréed with cottage cheese, yogurt, or skim milk. Once you can manage soft foods, add puréed vegetables and meats, scrambled eggs, unsweetened yogurt, apple sauce, mashed bananas, mashed potatoes, and creamy cooked cereals enriched with nonfat dry milk.

Of course, for all dental difficulties the best treatment is prevention. Following a program of preventive dental care throughout pregnancy—and preferably throughout life—will avert most dental problems:

❖ Make an appointment with your dentist at least once during the nine months for a checkup and cleaning—once each trimester may be even better. The cleaning is important to remove plaque, which can not only increase the risk of cavities but also make your gum problems worse. Avoid x-rays unless they are absolutely necessary, and then take the special precautions suggested on page 66. Routine repair work requiring anesthesia should be postponed, because even a local anesthetic can enter your bloodstream and reach the fetus. If you've had gum problems in the past, you should also see your periodontist during your pregnancy.

❖ Follow the Best-Odds Diet, eating little or no refined sugar, particularly between meals (also avoid dried fruit between meals), and plenty of foods high in vitamin C. Sugar contributes to both decay and gum disease; vitamin C strengthens gums, reducing the possibility of bleeding. Also be sure to fill your calcium requirements

daily (see page 85). Calcium is needed throughout life to keep teeth and bones strong and healthy.

❖ Floss and brush regularly, according to your dentist's prescription. (If your dentist does not instruct you in such preventive measures, you are probably going to the wrong dentist.)

❖ To further reduce bacteria in the mouth, brush your tongue when you brush your teeth. This will also help keep your breath fresh.

❖ When you can't brush after eating, chewing a stick of sugarless gum (preferably sweetened with xylitol) or nibbling on a chunk of cheese or a handful of peanuts (all seem to have antibacterial cleansing capabilities) can stand in temporarily for a thorough brushing.

"I found a nodule on the side of my gum that bleeds every time I brush my teeth."

What you discovered is probably a pyogenic granuloma, which can appear on the gum or elsewhere on the body. Though it bleeds easily and is also known by the ominous-sounding term "pregnancy tumor," it is perfectly harmless. It usually regresses on its own after delivery. If it becomes very annoying before that, it can be removed surgically.

TRAVEL

"Is it safe for me to go ahead with the vacation my husband and I had planned for this month?"

For most women, travel during the midtrimester is not only safe but the perfect chance to get away with their husbands for a last fling (at least for a while) as a twosome. And with no diapers, no bottles, no jars of messy baby food to worry about, it'll certainly never be as easy to vacation with your baby again.

Of course you will need your doctor's permission; if you have high blood pressure, diabetes, or other medical or obstetrical problems, you may not get the green light. (That doesn't mean you can't vacation at all. If you can't travel, pick a hotel or resort within an hour's drive of your doctor's office—and enjoy!) Even in a low-risk pregnancy, traveling a great distance isn't a terrific idea in the first trimester, when the possibility of miscarriage is greatest and when your body is still making its initial physical and emotional adjustment to pregnancy. Likewise, long-distance travel is not recommended in the last trimester because, should labor begin early, you would be far from your practitioner.

Travel to a hot climate may be uncomfortable because of your increased metabolism (see page 217). Travel to areas at high altitude may be dangerous, since adjusting to the decrease in oxygen may be too taxing for both mother and fetus. If you must make such a trip, you should plan on limiting exertion for several days after arrival to minimize the risk of developing acute mountain sickness (AMS).[4] If you are in your last trimester, your doctor may recommend you have a nonstress test on arrival at your destination and then daily for the next two days, then semi-weekly. Any signs of fetal distress will probably warrant the administration of oxygen and a return to a lower altitude.

Other inappropriate destinations are developing regions of the world for which vaccinations would be nec-

essary, since some vaccines may be hazardous during pregnancy. Not insignificantly, these same locales may be hotbeds of certain potentially dangerous infections for which there are no vaccines—another reason to avoid them.

Once you have your doctor's permission, you will only need to do a little planning and take a few precautions to ensure a safe and *bon* voyage for you and your baby:

Plan a Trip That's Relaxing. A single destination is preferable to a Grand Tour that takes you to nine cities in six days. A trip on which you set the pace is a lot better than a group tour that sets it for you. A few hours of sightseeing or shopping should be alternated with time spent sitting reading, relaxing, or napping.

Take Your Best-Odds Diet with You. You may be on vacation, but your baby is working as hard as ever at growing and developing, and has the same nutritional requirements he or she always has. Total self-sacrifice isn't required at mealtimes, but prudence is. Order thoughtfully and you will be able to savor the local cuisine while also fulfilling your baby's requirements. (See Eating Out Best-Odds Style, page 184.) Don't skip breakfast or lunch in order to save up for a lavish dinner.

Don't Drink the Water if you're traveling to a foreign country, unless you're certain it's safe. (But do substitute fruit juices and bottled water to get your daily fluids.) In some regions, it may not be safe to eat raw unpeeled fruits or vegetables. For complete information on such restrictions, on other foreign health hazards, and on immunizations for travel, contact the American College of Obstetricians and Gynecologists, 409 12th Street, S.W. Washington, DC 20024-2188; (202) 484-3321.

---

4. Symptoms of AMS includes: lack of appetite, nausea, vomiting, flatulence, restlessness, headache, lassitude, shortness of breath, scanty urine, and psychological changes.

Pack a Pregnancy Survival Kit. Make sure you take enough vitamins to last the trip; packets of dry skimmed milk if you think you won't be able to find fresh milk; a small jar of wheat germ to enrich white bread or cereal in case whole-grain versions aren't available; medication for traveler's stomach *prescribed by your doctor;* your favorite pregnancy book for reference; comfortable shoes roomy enough to accommodate feet swelled by long hours of sightseeing; and a spray disinfectant in case you have to sanitize a public toilet.

Have the Name of a Local Obstetrician Handy, just in case. Your doctor may be able to provide you with one. If not, contact the local medical association in the city you're traveling to or the International Association for Medical Assistance to Travelers, Suite 5620, Empire State Building, 350 Fifth Avenue, New York, NY 10001—which will, for a small donation, provide you with a directory of English-speaking physicians throughout the world. Some major hotel chains can also provide you with this kind of information. If for any reason you find yourself in need of a doctor in a hurry and can't find one, call the nearest hospital or head for its emergency room.

Carry a Medical History. It is always wise, but particularly when you're pregnant, to travel with a medical information card listing your blood type, medications you're taking and/or are allergic to, and any other pertinent medical data, along with your doctor's name, address, and telephone number. Tuck an extra prescription for each medication you are taking into your passport folder, in case your bags and medication are lost—temporarily or permanently—en route. You may have to have a prescription you've brought from home cosigned by a local doctor; often a doctor at a hospital emergency room will agree to do the honors.

Head Off Traveler's Irregularity. Changes in schedule and diet can compound constipation problems. To avoid this, make sure you get plenty of the three most effective constipation-combators: fiber, fluids, and exercise. (See Constipation, page 135.) It may also help to eat breakfast a little early, so you'll have time to use the bathroom before you set out for the day.

When You've Got to Go, Go. Don't encourage urinary tract infection or constipation by postponing trips to the bathroom. Go as soon as you feel the urge.

Get the Support You Need. Support hose, that is. Particularly if you already suffer from varicose veins—but even if you only suspect you may be predisposed to them—wear support hose when you'll be doing a lot of sitting (in cars, planes, trains, for example) and when you'll be doing a lot of standing (in museums, on lines).

Don't Be Stationary While on the Move. Sitting for long periods can restrict the circulation in your legs, so be sure to get up and walk at least every hour or two when you are on a plane or train. When traveling by automobile, don't go for more than two hours without stopping for a stretch. While you're sitting, do the simple exercises described on page 194.

If You're Traveling by Plane: Check with the airline in advance to see if it has special regulations concerning pregnant women (many airlines do). Arrange ahead of time for a seat in the front of the plane (preferably on the aisle, so you can get up and stretch or use the restroom as needed), or if seating is not reserved, ask for pre-boarding. *Do not fly in an unpressur-*

ized cabin. All commercial jets are pressurized; but small private or feeder airline planes may not be, and pressure changes at high altitudes may rob you—and your baby—of oxygen.

When booking your flight, ask about the special meals available and order one that provides a good protein serving along with a whole-grain bread, if it's available. On some airlines, low-cholesterol, ovo-lacto vegetarian, or seafood meals provide more of the Daily Dozen than do the regular menu selections. Drink plenty of water, milk, and fruit juice to counter the dehydration caused by air travel, and bring along whole-grain crackers or bread sticks, individually wrapped packets of cheese, raw vegetables, fresh fruit, and other healthful snacks to supplement the airline meal.

Wear your seat belt comfortably fastened below your abdomen. If you're traveling to a different time zone, take jet lag into account. Rest up in advance, and plan on taking it easy for a few days once you arrive. It may also help to try to gradually switch yourself to the time zone you're headed for by moving meal- and bedtimes forward or back, and once you've arrived, by exposing yourself to bright outdoor-like light during the time you would ordinarily be asleep at home.

If You're Traveling by Car: Keep a bagful of nutritious snacks and a thermos of juice or milk handy for when hunger strikes. For long trips, be sure the seat you will occupy is comfortable; if it isn't, consider buying or borrowing a special back-supporting cushion, available in auto supply stores and through some catalogs. A neck support pillow may also add to your comfort. If you aren't behind the wheel, set your seat as far back as possible to give your legs maximum stretching space. And of course keep your seat belt fastened at all times (see page 186).

If You're Traveling by Train: Check to be sure there's a dining car with a full menu. If not, bring adequate meals and snacks along. If you're traveling overnight, arrange for a sleeper. You don't want to start your vacation exhausted.

EATING OUT

"I try hard to stay on a proper diet, but with a business lunch nearly every day, it seems impossible."

For most pregnant women it isn't substituting mineral water for martinis that poses a challenge at business lunches (or when dining out after hours); it's trying to put together a meal that's nutritionally sound from a menu of cream sauces, elegant but empty starches, and tempting sweets. But with the following suggestions, it is possible to take the Best-Odds Diet out to lunch or dinner:

❖ Push away the breadbasket unless it's filled with whole-grain choices (make an exception if you're unhealthily hungry and no other sustenance is on the near horizon). Be aware that "dark" breads, such as pumpernickel or dark rye, may get their wholesome-looking color from caramel color or molasses rather than from whole grains.[5] Be sure that you tally the butter or margarine you spread on your bread into your daily fat allowance;

---

5. The occasional serving of white pasta, white rice, or white bread won't diminish the odds in your Best-Odds Diet, but frequent servings of such foods will. If that's all you can get when eating out, and you éat out frequently, carry a small flask of toasted wheat germ (you *can* develop a taste for it) and sprinkle some on these depleted foods to bring them closer to the way they were meant to be. Or bring along your own whole-grain roll or bread.

Eating Out, Best-Odds Style

❖ **Best** restaurants are seafood, American, continental, and steak houses where broiled, grilled, or poached fish, poultry, and lean cuts of meat are served, along with simply prepared fresh vegetables, salads, and potatoes.

Another excellent choice, if your stomach isn't too out of sorts for spices, is an Indian restaurant, where wholesome, protein-rich baked and roasted entrées (often marinated in yogurt) are served alongside vegetables and salads (also often made with yogurt), whole-grain Indian breads, which are sometimes stuffed with vegetables, and vegetable curries. (Vegetarians can easily make a high-protein meal out of the lentil, pea, chickpea, and cheese vegetarian selections.)

A new entry in the Best category are health food establishments and restaurants of any stripe that, heeding currently accepted dietary guidelines, limit fat, sugar, and excess sodium in some or all of their dishes (or at least are willing to do so on request); offer whole-grain breads, rice, and pasta; use olive oil or polyunsaturated vegetable oil rather than other less healthful shortenings; and emphasize fresh salads and vegetables.

❖ **Next Best** are ethnic restaurants where meats, fish, and poultry are featured. Included in this group are Italian eateries, if cream-based pasta sauces are eschewed for lighter ones (such as marinara or a tomato primavera), or fish, chicken, and veal entrées and fresh vegetables (arugula, spinach, kale, broccoli rabe) are chosen; French nouvelle (lighter than classic French), though sauces should still be ordered on the side; Cajun, or Louisiana-style, if you stick with boiled, steamed, broiled, and grilled fish or seafood and hearty seafood/poultry/vegetable stews such as jambalayas (but easy on the white rice); Jewish, if you avoid fatty meats (and those deli specials laced with nitrates), gravies, superfluous starches, rye bread, and salty pickles; and Greek or Middle Eastern, if you order baked or grilled fish, meats, and poultry accompanied by bulgur wheat or brown rice.

Chinese restaurants are fast securing a Next Best rating, as more and

when spreading, keep in mind that there may be other fats in your meal (for example, salad dressing and buttered vegetables).

❖ Order salad as a first course, and ask for the dressing (or plain oil and vinegar) on the side so you can stay within the Best-Odds Diet guidelines for fat intake. Other good first-course choices include fresh mozzarella and tomatoes, shrimp cocktail, and grilled or marinated vegetables.

❖ If you're ordering soup, opt for a clear consommé or broth, or a vegetable-, milk-, or yogurt-based soup. Generally steer clear of cream soups (unless you know they're made with milk).

❖ Select a high-protein, low-fat main course. Fish, chicken, and veal are usually the best bets, as long as they're broiled, grilled, or poached and not fried or bathed in butter or rich sauces. If everything comes with a sauce, ask for yours on the

more offer brown rice, "light" or steamed preparations that don't contain whopping amounts of soy sauce, and the option of ordering dishes without MSG (but steer clear of deep-fried and high-sugar sweet-and-sour dishes). An abundance of tofu dishes makes Chinese restaurants a "Best" bet for vegetarians.

Mexican and Spanish restaurants that feature lighter cuisine, prepare foods with vegetable oil rather than lard, and include vegetables on their menus (a bowl of gazpacho can do it all) can also provide a Next-Best meal; they're in the Best category for vegetarians, who can get plenty of protein and calcium from corn enchiladas stuffed with cheese and beans.

Also Next Best, particularly for lunches, are delis (if you avoid cold cuts and stick with a tuna, egg, chicken, or chef's salad, or a tuna, egg, chicken, turkey, or roast beef sandwich on whole-wheat bread with lettuce and tomato and a side of cole slaw); coffee shops, where you can get everything from broiled fish to salads to poached eggs to sandwiches on whole-wheat bread; some fast-food restaurants, specifically those that offer salad bars or other healthier menu selections; and traditional health food and vegetarian restaurants (these are "Best" for vegetarians, of course, and many of the more modern ones fall into the "Best" category for everyone), where you can get a wholesome meal as long as you're careful not to overdose on fat or fall short on protein.

❖ **Least Best** restaurants to frequent during pregnancy include: Japanese, since sushi, like all uncooked fish and meat, is completely taboo, tempura is deep-fried, and sukiyaki and teriyaki dishes are heavy on the soy sauce (which is extremely high in sodium); German, Russian, and Middle European, where empty calories lurk in breading, deep-frying fat, dumplings, and gravies, and excesses of fat and nitrates are found in sausages and wursts; Southern, where vats of deep-frying fat dominate the kitchens, vegetables are overcooked, usually in pork fat, and whole grains are unheard of; and fast-food restaurants that don't offer salad bars or other healthy options (see page 128).

A very occasional dining-out indiscretion won't upset the odds of the Best-Odds Diet. But frequent ones may—so diner beware.

side. Often chefs will accommodate a request for fish broiled with little or no fat. If you're a vegetarian, scan the menu for tofu, beans and peas, cheeses, and combinations of these. A vegetable lasagne, for example, might be a good choice in an Italian restaurant, bean curd and vegetables in a Chinese one.

❖ As side dishes, white or sweet potatoes (in any form but fried, heavily buttered, or candied), brown rice, kasha or groats, pasta, legumes (dried beans and peas), and lightly cooked fresh vegetables are all appropriate.

❖ Desserts should, except on special occasions, be limited to unsweetened and unliqueured fresh or cooked fruits and berries (with a dollop of whipped cream, if you like). An occasional swirl of frozen yogurt or scoop of ice cream is okay, too. If you crave something more, take a couple of bites of a dining companion's desert. Indulge in juice-sweetened treats when you get home; see pages 93 to 98 for recipes, or try some of the numerous commercially available varieties.

WEARING A SEAT BELT

"Is it safe to fasten my seat belt in the car or on an airplane?"

What's the major cause of death among women of childbearing age? Toxemia? Childbirth? Postpartum infection? Actually, none of the above. The most common way for a young woman to lose her life is in an auto crash. And the best way to avoid such a fatality—as well as serious injury to you and your unborn child—is to always buckle up. Statistics prove conclusively it is a lot safer to fasten your seat belt than not to fasten it.

For maximum safety and minimum discomfort, fasten the belt below your belly, across your pelvis and upper thighs. If there is a shoulder harness, wear it over your shoulder (not under your arm), diagonally, between your breasts and to the side of your belly. And don't worry that the pressure of an abrupt stop will hurt the baby—it is well cushioned by amniotic fluid. Since airbags could be a problem, ride in the rear seat when possible, or put the front seat as far back as you can. When driving, tilt the wheel up and away from the fetus (see page 133).

SPORTS

"I like to play tennis and swim. Is it safe to continue?"

Keeping fit is certainly recommended for anyone; the pregnant woman is no exception. And in most cases, pregnancy doesn't mean giving up the sporting life—just remembering you are carrying a new life and practicing a little extra common sense and moderation. Most practitioners permit patients whose pregnancies are progressing normally to continue participating in sports they are proficient at for as long as is practical—but with several caveats. Among the most important: "Never exercise to the point of fatigue." (See Exercise During Pregnancy, page 189 for more information.)

VISION

"My eyesight seems to be deteriorating since I got pregnant. And my contacts don't seem to fit anymore. Am I imagining it?"

No, chances are you really aren't seeing as well as you were pre-pregnancy. Your eyes are just another of the seemingly unrelated body parts that can fall prey to pregnancy hormones. Not only can your vision seem less sharp, but hard contact lenses, if your wear them, may suddenly no longer feel comfortable. And though these eye effects, which are probably related to fluid retention, are temporary, they can be annoying.

Your vision should clear up after delivery, and your eyes return to normal. Since being refitted for new hard lenses during pregnancy doesn't make financial sense, you might consider switching to glasses or soft contacts, if that's possible, until you deliver.

Though a slight deterioration in visual acuity is not unusual in pregnancy, other symptoms could signal a problem. If you experience blurring, dimming, spots or floaters, or double vision that persists for more than two or three hours, don't wait further for it to pass; call your doctor at once.

A LOW-LYING PLACENTA

"The doctor said my sonogram showed that the placenta was down near the cervix. He said that it was too early to worry about it now; when should I start worrying?"

Like a fetus, a placenta can do a lot of moving around during pregnancy. It doesn't actually pick up and relocate, but it does appear to migrate upward as the lower segment of the uterus stretches and grows. Though an estimated 20% to 30% of placentas are in the lower segment in the second trimester (and an even larger percentage before 20 weeks), the vast majority move into the upper segment by the time delivery nears. If this doesn't happen and the placenta remains low in the uterus, a diagnosis of "placenta previa" is made. This complication occurs in only about 1%, or less, of full-term pregnancies. And in only 1 out of 4 of these cases is the placenta located low enough—partially or completely covering the os, or mouth of the uterus—to cause a serious problem.

So as you can see, your doctor is right. It's too early to worry—and statistically speaking, the chances are slim that you'll ever have to worry. If a sonogram still shows a low-lying placenta once you're well into your eighth month, read about placenta previa on page 356.

OUTSIDE INFLUENCES IN THE WOMB

"I have a friend who insists that taking her unborn baby to concerts will make him a music lover, and another one whose husband reads to her tummy every night to give their baby a love of literature. Isn't this all nonsense?"

In the study of the unborn, it's getting harder and harder to distinguish between nonsense and fact. And while there's plenty of pure nonsense out there, scientists are coming to believe that some of these apparently outlandish theories may turn out to have a basis in fact. Still, much more research needs to be done before anyone can answer your question with certainty.

Because the ability to hear is quite well developed in the fetus by the end of the second trimester or the beginning of the third, it's true that your friends' babies are hearing the music and the readings. What that will mean in the long run isn't really clear. Some researchers in the field believe that it is actually possible to stimulate the fetus prior to birth to produce, in a sense, a "super baby." At least one has claimed to turn out babies who can speak at six months and read at a year and a half, by exposing the fetus to increasingly complex rhythmic imitations of a mother's heartbeat. Others question the wisdom of tampering with nature in this way, believing that it could, in the long run, be harmful.

Certainly, anyone who understands child development should be very wary of trying to create a super baby, either before birth or after it. It's much more important for a baby to be taught that he or she is loved and wanted than to be taught how to speak and read.

That isn't to say that attempting to make contact with your baby before birth, and even reading to it or playing music for it, is either harmful or a waste of time. Any kind of prenatal communication may give you a head start on the long process of parent-baby bonding. This may not necessarily translate into more closeness as your baby gets older, but it may make those earliest days easier.

Of course, if you feel silly talking to your bloated abdomen, you needn't

Carrying Baby, Fifth Month

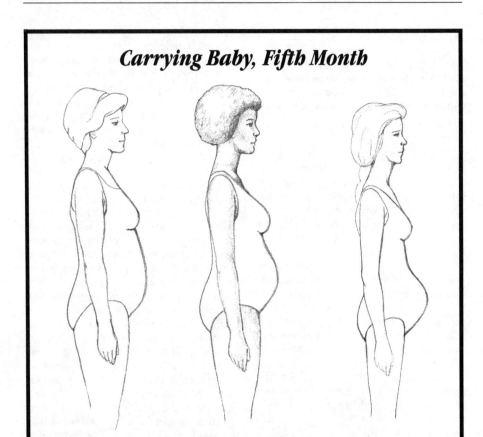

Here are just three of the very different ways that a woman may carry near the end of her fifth month. The variations on these are endless. Depending on your size, your shape, the amount of weight you've gained, and the position of your uterus, you may be carrying higher, lower, bigger, smaller, wider, or more compactly.

worry that your baby will miss out on getting to know you. He or she is getting used to the sound of your voice—and probably that of your spouse's, too—every time you talk to each other or someone else. That's why so many newborns seem to recognize their parent's voices. They may even be familiar with other sounds that are common in their mother's surroundings. Whereas a newborn who had little prenatal exposure to a barking dog may startle at hearing the sound, one who's heard a lot of barking won't even blink.

Exposure to music, too, may have some impact on the fetus. There have been reports that some fetuses have shown a preference (by a change in their movements) for certain types of music—usually the gentler kind. And reports that playing a certain piece (in the study, it was one by Debussy) over and over for the fetus at times when both mother and fetus were tranquil has resulted in the baby later seeming to like the piece, and to quiet down and be soothed upon hearing it. Of course, most experts would agree that exposing a baby to good music after he or she is born is probably a lot more significant in the creation of a music lover than exposing a fetus in utero.

It's also been suggested that, since the sense of touch is also already developed in the uterus, stroking your abdomen and "playing" with a little knee or bottom when it's pushed up may also help parent-child bonding—and whether this is true or not, there's certainly no harm in trying. Of course, it's unlikely that you'll need to make a conscious effort to touch your baby more; even strangers can hardly keep their hands off a pregnant belly.

So enjoy making baby contact now, but don't worry about teaching facts or imparting information—there'll be plenty of time for that later. As you'll soon discover, children grow up all too soon anyway. There's no need to rush the process, particularly before birth.

MOTHERHOOD

"Will I be happy with the baby once I have it?"

Most people approach any major change in their lives—marriage, a new career, or an impending birth—wondering whether it will be a change they'll be happy with. And if they start out with unrealistic expectations, they may very well end up disappointed. If your visions of motherhood consist of nothing but leisurely morning walks through the park, sunny days at the zoo, and hours coordinating a wardrobe of miniature, sparkling clean clothes, you're in for a heavy dose of reality shock. There'll be many mornings that will turn into evenings before you and your baby ever have the time to see the light of day, many sunny days that will be spent largely in the laundry room, and few tiny outfits that will escape unstained by spit-up puréed bananas and baby vitamins. And if you have images of bringing a cooing, enchanting Gerber baby home from the hospital, you are headed for certain postpartum disillusionment. Not only won't your newborn be smiling or cooing for many weeks, he or she may hardly communicate with you at all, except to cry—most notably when you're sitting down to dinner or starting to make love, have to go to the bathroom, or are so tired you can't move.

What you *can* expect realistically, however, are some of the most wondrous, miraculous experiences of your life. The fulfillment you will feel when cuddling a warm, sleeping bundle of baby (even if that cherub was a colicky devil moments before) is incomparable. That—along with that first toothless smile meant just for you—will be well worth all the sleepless nights, delayed dinners, mountains of laundry, and frustrated romance.

Can you expect to be happy with your baby? Yes, as long as you expect a real baby and not a fantasy.

WHAT IT'S IMPORTANT TO KNOW: EXERCISE DURING PREGNANCY

Executives do it. Senior citizens do it. Doctors, lawyers, and construction workers do it. If they do it, pregnant women wonder, shouldn't we?

"It," of course, is exercise. And the answer for most women with normal pregnancies seems to be: yes. The

Basic Position and Kegel Exercises

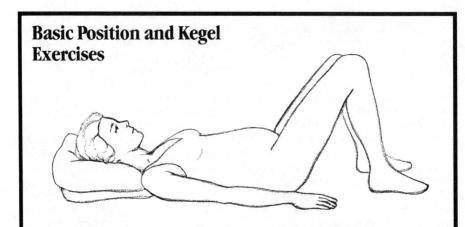

Lie on your back, knees bent, feet about 12 inches apart, soles flat on the floor. Your head and shoulders should be supported by cushions, and your arms resting flat at your sides. To do Kegels, firmly tense the muscles around your vagina and anus. Hold for as long as you can (working up to 8 to 10 seconds), then slowly release the muscles and relax. These also can be done, and after the fourth month should be done, in a standing or sitting position. Do at least 25 repetitions at various times during the day. Note: The Basic Position should be used only through the fourth month. After that time exercising flat on one's back is not recommended, since the growing uterus could put excessive weight on major blood vessels.

concept of pregnancy as an illness, and of the pregnant woman as an invalid too delicate to climb a flight of stairs or carry a bag of groceries, is as dated as general anesthesia in routine deliveries. Though there still isn't a vast body of research on the subject of exercise during pregnancy, moderate physical activity is now considered not only thoroughly safe, but extremely beneficial for most expectant mothers and their babies.

As anxious as you might be to hit the jogging trail, however, there is one vitally important stop you must make first—at your doctor's office. Even if you're feeling terrific, you must obtain medical clearance before suiting up in your husband's sweatpants. Pregnant women who are in a high-risk category may have to curb exercise or even eliminate it entirely for now. But if yours is among the great majority of normal pregnancies, and your doctor has given you the go-ahead, suit up and read on.

THE BENEFITS OF EXERCISE

It appears that women who don't get any exercise during pregnancy become progressively less fit as the months pass by—particularly because they are becoming heavier and heavier. A good exercise program (which can be built right into your daily lifestyle) can counteract this trend toward decreasing fitness.

There are four kinds of exercise that can be useful during pregnancy: aerobics, calisthenics specifically designed for pregnancy, relaxation techniques, and Kegel exercises.

Aerobics. These are rhythmic, repetitive activities strenuous enough to demand increased oxygen to the muscles, but not so strenuous that demand exceeds supply (walking, jogging, bicycling, swimming, tennis singles). Aerobic exercises stimulate the heart and lungs, and muscle and joint activity—producing beneficial overall body changes, especially an increase in the ability to process and utilize oxygen, which is a plus for you and your baby. Exercise too strenuous to be sustained for the 20 to 30 minutes necessary to reach this "training effect" (such as sprinting), or not strenuous enough (tennis doubles), is not considered aerobic.

Aerobic exercise improves circulation (enhancing the transport of oxygen and nutrients to your fetus while decreasing the risk of varicose veins, hemorrhoids, and fluid retention); increases muscle tone and strength (often preventing or relieving backache and constipation, making it easier to carry the extra weight of pregnancy, and facilitating delivery); builds endurance (making you better able to cope with a lengthy labor); may help control blood sugar; burns calories (allowing you to eat more of the good food you and your baby need without gaining excessive weight, and promis-

ing a better postpartum figure); lessens fatigue and promotes good sleep; imparts a feeling of well-being and confidence; and in general heightens your ability to cope with the physical and emotional challenges of childbearing.

Calisthenics. These are rhythmic, light gymnastic movements that tone and develop muscles and can improve posture. Calisthenics especially designed for pregnant women can be very useful in relieving backache, in improving physical and mental well-being, and in preparing your body for the arduous task of childbirth. Calisthenics designed for the general population, however, may be unsafe.

Relaxation Techniques. Breathing and concentration exercises relax mind and body, help conserve energy for when it's needed, assist the mind to focus on a task, and increase body awareness—all of which can help a woman better meet the challenges of childbirth. Relaxation techniques are

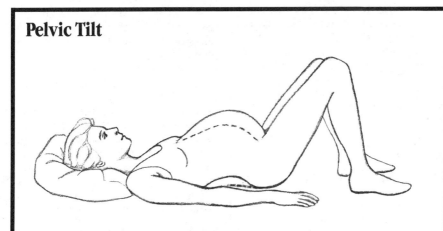

Pelvic Tilt

Assume the basic position (see Note at the end of the Basic Position and Kegel Exercises on the facing page). Exhale as you press the small of your back against the floor. Then inhale and relax your spine. Repeat this several times. The tilt can also be done standing up straight, with your back against a wall (inhale while pressing the small of your back into the wall). The standing version is an excellent way to improve your posture and should be used after the fourth month.

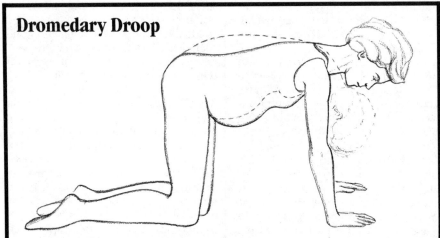

Dromedary Droop

This exercise is useful throughout pregnancy and into labor, to relieve the pressure of the enlarged uterus on your spine. Get down on your hands and knees, with your back in a naturally relaxed position (don't let your spine sag). Keep your head straight, your neck aligned with your spine. Then hump your back, tightening your abdomen and buttocks, and allow your head to drop all the way down. Gradually release your back and raise your head to the original position. Repeat several times.

valuable in combination with more physical routines, or alone—especially in pregnancies when more active exercise is prohibited.

Pelvic Toning. Kegel exercises are simple techniques for toning the muscles in the vaginal and perineal area, strengthening them in preparation for delivery. This will also aid recovery postpartum. This exercise is one virtually every pregnant woman can perform and benefit from, any time, any place.

DEVELOPING A GOOD EXERCISE PROGRAM

Get Started. The best time to get fit is before you get pregnant. But it's never too late to start exercising—even if you're already pushing nine months.

Get Off to a Slow Start. Once you've decided to begin a fitness program, it's tempting to start off with a bang, running 3 miles the first morning or

working out twice the first afternoon. But such enthusiastic beginnings lead not to fitness but to sore muscles, sagging resolve, and abrupt endings. They can also be dangerous.

Of course, if you followed an exercise program before pregnancy, you can probably continue it—though possibly in a modified form (see Playing It Safe, page 195). If you're a fledgling athlete, however, build up slowly. Start with 10 minutes of warm-ups followed by 5 minutes of more strenuous workout and a 5-minute cool-down. Stop strenuous exercise sooner if you begin to tire. After a few days, if your body has adjusted well, increase the period of strenuous activity by a couple of minutes a day up to 20 to 30 minutes or more, if you feel comfortable.

Get Off to a Slow Start Every Time You Start. Warm-ups can be tedious when you're eager to get your workout started (and over with). But as every athlete knows, they're an essential part of any exercise program. They ensure that the heart and circulation aren't taxed suddenly, and reduce the chances of injury to muscles and joints, which are more vulnerable when cold" —and particularly vulnerable during pregnancy. Walk before you run, stretch lightly before you begin calisthenics, swim slowly before you start your laps.

Finish as Slowly as You Start. Collapse seems like the logical conclusion to a workout, but it isn't physiologically sound. Stopping abruptly traps blood in the muscles, reducing blood supply to other parts of your body and to your baby. Dizziness, faintness, extra heartbeats, or nausea may result. So finish your exercise with exercise: about 5 minutes of walking after running, paddling after a vigorous swim, light stretching exercises after almost any activity. Top off your cool-down with a few minutes of relaxation.

You can also help avoid dizziness (and a possible fall) if you get up slowly when you've been exercising on the floor. Do your stretches after aerobics, and be sure not to stretch to your limit, since this can damage joints that have been loosened by pregnancy.

Watch the Clock. Too little exercise won't be effective; too much can be debilitating. A full workout, from warm-up to cool-down, can take anywhere from 30 minutes to an hour or even more. If you have been working out prepregnancy and you have your practitioner's okay, you can continue the same schedule—as long as the exercises you choose are safe (see page 197). But keep the level of exertion mild to moderate. If you haven't exercised regularly in the past, working up to a half an hour three times a week, including warming up and cooling down is a realistic and safe goal. If time is limited, try brisk walking for ten minute stretches three times a day.

Keep It Up. Exercising erratically (four

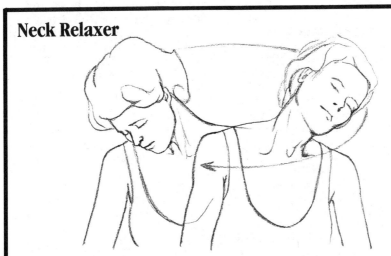

Neck Relaxer

The neck is often a focus of tension, tightening under stress. This exercise can help to relax both your neck and the rest of you: Sit in a comfortable position (Tailor Sit, page 195, might be best) with your eyes closed. Gently roll your head around, making a full circle, and inhaling as you do. Exhale and relax, letting your head drop forward comfortably. Repeat 4 or 5 times, alternating the direction of the roll and relaxing between rolls. Do this exercise several times a day.

Don't Just Sit There . . .

Sitting for an extended period without a break is not a good idea for anyone, but it is particularly unwise when you're pregnant. It causes blood to pool in your leg veins, can cause your feet to swell, and could lead to other problems. If your work entails a lot of sitting, or if you watch TV for hours at a time or travel long distances frequently, be sure to break up every hour or so of sitting with five or ten minutes of walking. And at your seat, periodically do some exercises that enhance circulation, such as taking a few deep breaths; extending your lower legs, flexing your feet, and wiggling your toes; and contracting the muscles in your abdomen and buttocks (a sort of sitting pelvic tilt). If your hands tend to swell, also try stretching your arms above your head and opening and closing your fists.

---

times one week and none the next) won't get you in shape. Exercising regularly (three or four times a week, every week) will. If you're too tired for a strenuous workout, don't push yourself; but do try to do the warm-ups so that your muscles will stay limber and your discipline won't dissolve. Many women find they feel better if they do some exercise every day.

Work Exercise into Your Schedule. The best way to be sure of doing your exercise is to allot a specific time for it: first thing in the morning; before going off to work; during a coffee break; or before dinner. If you have no regular block of free time for an exercise session, you can build exercise into your existing schedule. Walk to work, if you can, or park your car or get off the bus a distance from the job and walk part of the way. Or walk an older child to school (or to a friend's) instead of driving. Do your vacuuming in a steady, 20-minute stretch after a few warm-ups, and you will exercise your body and clean the carpets at the same time. Instead of flopping down in front of the TV with your spouse after the dinner dishes are done, ask him to join you for a walk. No matter how busy your day, if there's the will, there's always a way to fit in some form of exercise.

Compensate for the Calories You Burn. Probably the best part of a pregnancy exercise program is the extra eating you'll have to do. As always, make those calories count. Take this opportunity to add even *more* good-for-baby nutrients to your diet. You'll have to consume about 100 to 200 additional calories for every half hour of strenuous exercising. If you believe you're consuming enough calories but you still are not gaining weight, you may be exercising too much.

Replace the Fluids You Use Up. For every half hour of strenuous activity, you will need at least a full glass of extra liquid to compensate for fluids lost through perspiration. You will need more in warm weather, or when you are perspiring profusely: drink before, during, and after exercising. The scale can give you a clue to how much extra fluid you need to drink: 2 cups for each pound lost during exercise.

If You Choose the Group Approach: take an exercise class that is specifically designed for pregnant women. Since not everyone who claims to be an expert is one, ask for the instructor's credentials before enrolling. Classes are better for some women than solo exercising (particularly when self-discipline is lacking) and provide support and feedback. The best programs maintain moderate intensity; meet at least three times weekly; individualize to each woman's capabilities; don't use fast-tempoed music, which may push participants into working too hard; and have a network of medical specialists available for questions.

PLAYING IT SAFE

Don't Work Out on an Empty Stomach. Mother's rule about not swimming after a meal had some validity. But exercising on an empty stomach can be hazardous too. If you haven't eaten for hours, it's a good idea to have a light snack and a drink—choose items high in potassium, such as a banana or oj— 15 to 30 minutes before beginning your warm-ups. If you're uncomfortable eating that close to exercising, have your snack an hour before.

Dress for the Occasion. Wear clothes that are loose or that stretch when you move. Fabrics should let your body breathe—right down to your underwear, which should be cotton. Well-fitting athletic shoes, designed for the appropriate activity, will protect your feet and joints.

Select the Right Surface. Indoors, wood floors or a tightly carpeted surface is better than tile or concrete for your workouts. (If a surface is slippery, don't exercise in socks or footed tights.) Outdoors, soft running tracks and level grassy or dirt trails are better than hard-surfaced roads or sidewalks; avoid surfaces that are uneven.

Do Everything in Moderation. *Never* exercise to the point of exhaustion when you're pregnant; the chemical

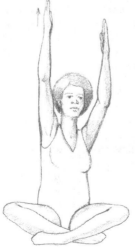

Tailor Sit, Tailor Stretch

Sitting cross-legged is particularly comfortable during pregnancy. Sit this way often and do arm stretches: Place your hands on your shoulders, then lift both arms above your head. Stretch one arm higher than the other, reaching for the ceiling, then relax it and repeat with the other arm. Repeat 10 times on each side. Do not bounce.

Leg Lifts

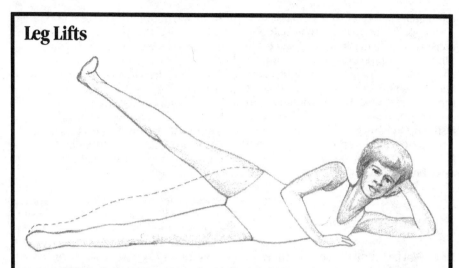

Lie on your left side, with your shoulders, hips, and knees in a straight line. Place your right hand on the floor in front of your chest and support your head with your left. Relax and inhale; then exhale while slowly raising your right leg as high as you can, keeping your foot flexed (pointing up toward your belly) and your inner ankle facing directly down. Inhale while slowly lowering your leg. Repeat 10 times on each side. This exercise can be done with the leg either straight or bent at the knee.

by-products of overexertion are not good for the fetus. (If you're a trained athlete, you still shouldn't exercise to your fullest capacity, whether it exhausts you or not.) There are several ways of checking to see whether you're overdoing it. First, if it feels good, it's probably okay. If there's any pain or strain, it's not. A little perspiration is fine; a drenching sweat is a sign to slow down. So is being unable to carry on a conversation as you go. A pulse that is still over 100 beats per minute five minutes after completing a workout means you've worked too hard. So does needing a nap when you're finished. You should feel exhilarated, not drained.

Know When to Stop. Your body will signal when it's time. Signals include: pain anywhere (hip, back, pelvis, chest, head, and so on); a cramp or stitch; lightheadedness or dizziness; tachycardia, or palpitations; severe breathlessness; difficulty walking or loss of muscle control; headache; increased swelling of your hands, feet, ankles, face; amniotic fluid leakage or vaginal bleeding; or after the 28th week, a slowing down or cessation of fetal movement. If any of these symptoms aren't relieved by a short rest, check with your doctor (but call immediately if you have any bleeding or amniotic fluid leakage). In the second and third trimesters, you may notice a gradual decrease in your performance and efficiency. It's best to slow down.

Stay Cool. Don't exercise in very hot or humid weather; don't use saunas, steam rooms, or hot tubs. Until research shows otherwise, exercise or environments that raise a pregnant woman's temperature more than 1½ to 2 degrees Fahrenheit should be considered dangerous (blood is shunted away from the uterus to the skin as the body attempts to cool off). So don't exercise in the heat of the day or in a warm or stuffy room. And

Choosing the Right Pregnancy Exercise

Select the type of exercise that's right for you. Though you can probably continue a sport or activity you are already proficient at, it's not advisable to take up a new one during pregnancy. Exercises that even a novice can do during pregnancy include:

❖ Walking at a brisk pace

❖ Swimming in shallow water that is neither too hot nor too cold*

❖ Cycling on a stationary bike at a comfortable tension and speed*

❖ Land and water** workouts designed especially for pregnancy

❖ Pelvic toning (Kegel exercises)

❖ Pregnancy yoga or relaxation routines

Exercises that only a well-trained, experienced athlete should engage in during pregnancy:

❖ Jogging, up to 2 miles per day**

❖ Doubles tennis (but not singles, which can be too strenuous)

❖ Cross-country skiing below 10,000 feet

❖ *Light* weight lifting (breathe out on lifting; avoid Valsalva maneuver—holding your breath and straining)

❖ Cycling (with extreme caution)

❖ Ice skating (with extreme caution)

Exercises that even an athlete should avoid, because of their greater risks, include:

❖ Jogging more than 2 miles per day**

❖ Horseback riding

❖ Waterskiing

❖ Diving and jumping into pools

❖ Sprinting (too much oxygen is demanded too quickly)

❖ Scuba diving (diving gear may restrict circulation; decompression sickness is hazardous to the fetus)

❖ Downhill skiing (risky because of the possibility of a serious fall)

❖ Cross-country skiing above 10,000 feet (the high altitude deprives both mother and fetus of oxygen)

❖ Bicycling on wet pavement or winding paths (where falls are likely), and cycling leaning forward in racing posture (can cause backache)

❖ Contact sports, such as football (they carry a high risk of injury)

❖ Workouts not designed for pregnancy. Avoid exercises that pull on the abdomen (such as full sit-ups or double leg lifts); that might force air into the vagina (such as upside-down "bicycling," shoulder stands, or exercises where you bring your knee to your chest while kneeling on all fours); that stretch the inner thigh muscles (such as sitting on the floor with the soles of the feet together and pressing down on or bouncing your knees); that cause the small of the back to curve inward; that require "bridging" (bending over backward) or other contortions; or that involve deep flexion or extension of joints (such as deep knee bends), jumping, bouncing, sudden changes in direction, or jerky motions.

*These non-weight-bearing exercises are okay for all 9 months of pregnancy.

**Water workouts are ideal because of minimal impact on maternal and fetal heart rates and mom's joints.

***A few very fit women continue more rigorous exercise programs with no apparent ill effects, though their babies may weigh less than average. Check with your doctor before doing so yourself.

don't overdress. Wear light clothes in summer, and under-dress in winter. You should feel slightly chilly when you go out—the exercise will warm you quickly. Or wear layers, so you can remove one or two as you heat up. And don't wait for your body to tell you when you're overheated—stop before you reach that point.

Proceed with Caution. Even the most skilled sportswoman can lack grace when she's pregnant. As the center of gravity shifts forward with the uterus, a fall becomes an ever-increasing possibility. Be aware, and be careful. Late in pregnancy, avoid sports that require sudden moves or a good sense of balance, such as tennis.

Be Aware of the Added Risk of Injury. For a variety of reasons (an altered center of balance, lax joints, absent-mindedness), women are more subject to injury when they are expecting.

Stay Off Your Back, and Don't Point Your Toes. After the fourth month, don't exercise flat on your back, as the weight of your enlarging uterus could compress major blood vessels, restricting circulation. Pointing, or extending, your toes—at any time in pregnancy—could lead to cramping in your calves. Flex your feet instead, turning them up toward your face.

Taper Off in the Last Trimester. Though everyone has heard stories of pregnant athletes who have stayed in the pool or on the jogging trails right up until delivery, it is wise for most women to slack off during the last three months. And, in fact, in one study, only 10% of trained athletes maintained their performance at or near prepregnancy levels until delivery. Cutting back is particularly wise the ninth month, when stretching routines and brisk walking should provide adequate exer-cise. Serious athletic pursuits can be resumed at about six weeks postpartum.

IF YOU DON'T EXERCISE

Exercising during pregnancy can certainly do you a lot of good. It can relieve backache, prevent constipation and varicose veins, give you a general sense of well-being, make childbirth a little quicker and easier, and leave you in better physical shape postpartum. But sitting it out (whether by choice or on doctor's orders), getting most of your exercise from opening and closing your car door, won't do you or your baby any harm. In fact, if you're abstaining from exercise on doctor's orders, you're helping your baby and yourself. Your doctor will almost certainly restrict exercise if you have a history of three or more spontaneous abortions or of premature labor, or if you have an incompetent cervix, bleeding or persistent spotting in the second or third trimester, heart disease, or a diagnosis of placenta previa, pregnancy-induced hypertension (toxemia), or, intrauterine growth retardation. Your activity may also be limited if you have high blood pressure, diabetes, thyroid disease, anemia or other blood disorders; or a fetus that isn't thriving; are seriously over- or underweight; or have had an extremely sedentary lifestyle up until now. A history of precipitous (very brief) labor or of a fetus that didn't thrive in a previous pregnancy might also be a reason for a red light on exercise.

In some cases arm-only exercises may be okayed when other exercises are taboo. Check with your doctor.

10
The Sixth Month

WHAT YOU CAN EXPECT AT THIS MONTH'S CHECKUP

This month you can expect your practitioner to check the following, though there may be variations depending upon your particular needs and upon your practitioner's style of practice:[1]

❖ Weight and blood pressure

❖ Urine, for sugar and protein

❖ Fetal heartbeat

❖ Height of fundus (top of uterus)

❖ Size of uterus and position of fetus, by external palpation

❖ Feet and hands for edema (swelling), and legs for varicose veins

❖ Symptoms you may have been experiencing, especially unusual ones

❖ Questions and problems you want to discuss—have a list ready

WHAT YOU MAY BE FEELING

You may experience all of these symptoms at one time or another, or only a few of them. Some may have continued from last month, others may be new. Still others may hardly be noticed because you've become so used to them. You may also have other, less common, symptoms.

1. See Appendix for an explanation of the procedures and tests performed.

PHYSICALLY:

❖ More definite fetal activity

❖ Whitish vaginal discharge (leukorrhea)

❖ Lower abdominal achiness (from stretching of ligaments supporting the uterus)

❖ Constipation

❖ Heartburn, indigestion, flatulence, bloating

❖ Occasional headaches, faintness or dizziness

❖ Nasal congestion and occasional nosebleeds; ear stuffiness

❖ "Pink toothbrush" from bleeding gums

❖ Hearty appetite

❖ Leg cramps

❖ Mild swelling of ankles and feet, and occasionally of hands and face

❖ Varicose veins of legs and/or hemorrhoids

❖ Itchy abdomen

❖ Backache

❖ Skin pigmentation changes on abdomen and/or face

❖ Enlarged breasts

EMOTIONALLY:

❖ Fewer mood swings; continued absentmindedness

❖ A beginning of boredom with the pregnancy ("Can't anyone think about anything else?")

❖ Some anxiety about the future

WHAT YOU MAY LOOK LIKE

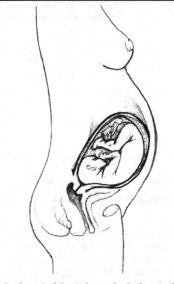

By the end of the sixth month, the fetus is about 13 inches long and weighs about 1 ¾ pounds. Its skin is thin and shiny, with no underlying fat; its finger and toe prints are visible. Eyelids begin to part, and the eyes open. With intensive care, the fetus may survive if born now.

WHAT YOU MAY BE CONCERNED ABOUT

PAIN AND NUMBNESS IN THE HAND

"I keep waking up in the middle of the night because some of the fingers on my right hand are numb; sometimes they even hurt. Is that related to my pregnancy?"

If the numbness and pain are confined to your thumb, index finger, middle finger, and half of your ring finger, you probably have carpal tunnel syndrome. Though this condition is most common in people who regularly perform tasks that require repetitive motions of the hand (such as meat cutting, piano playing, typing), it is also common in pregnant women. That's because the carpal tunnel in the wrist, through which the nerve to the affected fingers runs, becomes swollen during pregnancy (as do so many other tissues in the body), with the resultant pressure causing numbness, tingling, burning, and/or pain. The symptoms can also affect the hand

and wrist, and can radiate up the arm. Because fluids accumulate in your hands all day thanks to gravity, the swelling and accompanying symptoms may be more severe at night. Try to avoid sleeping on your hands, which can aggravate the problem. When numbness occurs, hanging the affected hand over the side of the bed and shaking it vigorously may relieve it. If it doesn't, and the numbness (with or without pain) is interfering with your sleep, discuss the problem with your doctor. Often wearing a wrist splint and taking vitamin B_6 daily is helpful. Some people have gotten relief from acupuncture. The nonsteroidal anti-inflammatory drugs and steroids usually prescribed for carpal tunnel syndrome may not be recommended during pregnancy. If other treatments fail and the condition persists after delivery, simple surgery may be indicated.

PINS AND NEEDLES

"I frequently get a tingling sensation in my hands and feet. Does this indicate a problem with my circulation?"

As if it weren't enough to be on tenterhooks during pregnancy, some women occasionally experience the disconcerting tingling sensation of pins and needles in their extremities. Although it may feel as if your circulation is being cut off, this isn't the case. No one knows why this phenomenon occurs or how to eliminate it, but it is known that it doesn't indicate anything serious. Changing your position may help. If the tingling interferes in any way with your functioning, report it to your practitioner.

BABY KICKING

"Some days the baby is kicking all the time; other days he seems very quiet. Is this normal?"

Fetuses are only human. Just like us, they have "up" days, when they feel like kicking up their heels (and elbows and knees), and "down" days, when they'd rather lie back and take it easy. Most often, their activity is related to what you've been doing. Like babies out of the womb, fetuses are lulled by rocking. So when you're on the go all day, your baby is likely to be pacified by the rhythm of your routine, and you're likely not to notice much kicking—partly because baby's slowed down, partly because you're so busy. As soon as you slow down, he or she is bound to start acting up. That's why most expectant mothers feel fetal movement more often in bed at night or in the morning. Activity may also increase after the mother has had a meal or snack, perhaps in reaction to the surge of glucose (sugar) in her blood. Some pregnant women also report increased fetal activity when they are excited or nervous; the baby may be stimulated by the mother's adrenalin response.

Babies are actually most active between weeks 24 and 28. But their movements are erratic and usually brief, so though they are visible on ultrasound, they aren't always felt by the busy mother-to-be. Fetal activity usually becomes more organized and consistent, with more clearly defined periods of rest and activity, between 28 and 32 weeks.

Don't be tempted to compare baby-movement notes with other pregnant women. Each fetus, like each newborn, has an individual pattern of activity and development. Some seem always active; others mostly quiet. The kicking of some is regular; that of others may exhibit no discernible pattern. As long as there is no radical slowdown or cessation of activity, all variations are normal.

Recent research suggests that from the 28th week on it may be a good idea for mothers to test for fetal movements twice a day—once in the morning, when activity tends to be sparser, and once in the more active evening hours. Your doctor may recommend a test or you can use this one:

Check the clock when you start counting. Count movements of any kind (kicks, flutters, swishes, rolls). Stop counting when you reach ten, and note the time. Often, you will feel ten movements within ten minutes or so. Sometimes it will take longer.

If you haven't counted ten movements by the end of an hour, have some milk or another snack; then lie down, relax, and continue counting. If the two hours go by without ten movements, call your practitioner without delay. Though such an absence of activity doesn't necessarily mean there's a problem, it can occasionally indicate fetal distress. In such cases, quick action may be needed.

The closer you are to your due date, the more important regular checking of fetal movements becomes.

"Sometimes the baby pushes so hard it hurts."

A s your baby matures in the uterus, he or she becomes stronger and stronger, and those once butterfly-like fetal movements pack more and more power. Don't be surprised if you get kicked in the ribs or poked in the abdomen or cervix with such force it hurts. When you seem to be under a particularly fierce attack, try changing your position. It may knock your little linebacker off balance and temporarily stem the assault.

"The baby seems to be kicking all over. Could I be carrying twins?"

A t some point in her pregnancy, just about every woman begins to think that she's carrying either twins or a human octopus. For most, of course, neither is true. Until a fetus grows to the point that his movements are restricted by the confines of his uterine home (usually at about 34 weeks), he's able to perform numerous acrobatics. So, while it may sometimes feel as if you're being pummeled by a dozen fists, it's more likely to be two fists that really get around—along with tiny knees, elbows, and feet.

For more on twins and how they are diagnosed, see page 143.

LEG CRAMPS

"I have leg cramps at night that interfere with my sleep."

B etween your racing mind and your bulging belly, you probably have enough trouble sleeping without having to suffer from leg cramps. Unfortunately, these painful spasms, which occur most often at night, are very common among pregnant women in the second and third trimesters. Fortunately, however, there are ways of both preventing and alleviating them.

Since some leg cramps are believed to be caused by an excess of phosphorus and a shortage of calcium circulating in the blood, taking calcium supplements that do not contain phosphorus may be effective in alleviating them. If not, it may be necessary—but only on your practitioner's advice—to reduce phosphorus intake by cutting down on milk and meat. (But be certain that you are getting your calcium and protein elsewhere. See the Best-Odds Diet, page 80, for substitutes.) Because fatigue and pressure of the enlarging uterus on certain nerves are also thought to be possible contributing factors, wearing support hose during the day and alternating periods of rest (with your feet up) with periods of physical activity may also be helpful in eliminating the problem of leg cramps.

If you do get a cramp in your calf, straighten your leg and flex your ankle and toes slowly up toward your nose. This should soon lessen the pain. (Doing this several times with each leg before retiring at night may even help ward off the cramps.) Standing on a cold surface sometimes works, too. If either technique reduces the pain, massage or local heat can then be used for added relief. If neither reduces it, don't massage your calves or apply heat. Do contact your doctor if the pain continues, as there is a slight possibility that a blood clot may have developed in a vein, making medical treatment necessary (see Venous Thrombosis, page 360).

RECTAL BLEEDING AND HEMORRHOIDS

"I'm concerned about the rectal bleeding I've been having."

Bleeding is always a frightening symptom, especially during pregnancy—and particularly in an area so close to your birth canal. But unlike vaginal bleeding, rectal bleeding is not a sign of a possible threat to your pregnancy. During pregnancy it's frequently caused by external and, less often, internal hemorrhoids. Hemorrhoids, which are varicose veins of the rectum, afflict between 20% and 50% of all pregnant women. Just as the veins of the legs are more susceptible to varicosities at this time, so are the veins of the rectum. Constipation often causes or compounds the problem.

Hemorrhoids (also called piles because of the resemblance these swollen veins sometimes bear to a pile of grapes or marbles) can cause itching and pain as well as bleeding. Rectal bleeding may also stem from fissures—cracks in the anus caused by constipation, which can accompany hemorrhoids or appear independently. Fissures are generally extremely painful.

Don't try to self-diagnose hemorrhoids. Rectal bleeding is occasionally a sign of serious disease and should always be evaluated by a physician. But if you do have hemorrhoids and/or fissures, your role will be the most crucial in treating them. Good self-care can often eliminate the need for more radical medical therapy.

❖ Avoid constipation. It is *not* a necessary component of pregnancy; see page 135. (Preventing constipation from the start is, incidentally, frequently an excellent way to prevent hemorrhoids completely.)

❖ Avoid pressure on rectal veins: Sleep on your side, not your back; avoid long hours of standing or sitting; don't strain when having a bowel movement or linger on the toilet (reading is not recommended). Sitting with your feet on a step stool may make evacuation easier.

❖ Do Kegel exercises regularly: they improve circulation to the area (see page 190).

❖ Take warm sitz baths twice a day (see page 434).

❖ Apply witch hazel soaks or ice packs (whichever is more soothing) to the hemorrhoids.

❖ Use topical medications, suppositories, laxatives, or stool softeners only if prescribed by a doctor who knows you're pregnant. Do not take mineral oil.

❖ Keep the perineal area (from vagina to rectum) scrupulously clean. Wash the area with warm water after bowel movements, always wiping from front to back. Use only white toilet paper.

❖ Lie down several times a day—if possible, on your side. Watch TV, read, and talk to your husband in this position.

With good care, hemorrhoids can be kept from becoming chronic. They may be made worse by delivery, especially if the pushing phase is long, but usually disappear postpartum if preventive measures are continued.

ITCHY ABDOMEN

"My belly itches constantly. It's driving me crazy."

Join the club. Pregnant bellies are itchy bellies, and they can become progressively itchier as the months pass and the skin is stretched taut across the abdomen. The result is dryness, causing more pronounced itching in some women. Try not to scratch. Lubricating lotion may ease the itch, but probably won't cure it. An anti-itching lotion (such as calamine) may provide more relief. If you itch all over, check with your practitioner.

TOXEMIA, OR PREECLAMPSIA

"Recently a friend of mine was hospitalized for toxemia. How can you tell if you have it?"

Fortunately toxemia, also known as preeclampsia/eclampsia or pregnancy-induced hypertension (PIH), is uncommon. Even in its mildest form it occurs in only 5% to 10%

of pregnancies—and most of these cases are among women who came into pregnancy with chronic high blood pressure. Toxemia is most common in first pregnancies and beyond the 20th week of gestation. In women who are receiving regular prenatal care, it is diagnosed and treated early, preventing needless complications. Though routine office visits sometimes seem a waste of time in a healthy pregnancy, it is at such visits that the earliest signs of preeclampsia can be picked up.

If you have had a sudden weight gain apparently unrelated to excess food intake, severe swelling of your hands and face, unexplained headaches or itching, and/or vision disturbances, call your practitioner. Otherwise, assuming regular medical care, you needn't worry about toxemia. See page 152 for tips on preventing and dealing with high blood pressure in pregnancy, and page 351 for more information on toxemia.

STAYING ON THE JOB

"I stand a lot on my job. I was planning to work up until I deliver, but is that safe?"

The question of how a mother-to-be's job affects an unborn fetus is an important one, especially these days, when so many expectant mothers are working. The answer at this point, however, isn't all that clear. We all know women who went from the office or the studio or the shop right to the hospital and delivered perfectly healthy babies. And, in fact, one study of pregnant doctors in arduous residency training programs found that although these women were on their feet for 65 hours a week, they didn't seem to have any more pregnancy complications than the male residents' pregnant wives, who worked many fewer usually less stressful hours. Other studies, however, suggest that steady strenuous or stressful activity or long hours of standing during the last half of pregnancy may increase the risk of the mother developing high blood pressure, as well as the risk of a damaged placenta and a low-birthweight baby. Some studies show the risk of complications from standing on the job after 28 weeks increases if the expectant mother has other children at home to care for.

Should women who stand on the job—salespeople, cooks, police officers, waitresses, doctors, nurses, and so on—work past the 28th week? Clearly, more study will need to be done before definitive answers to that question will be available. The American Medical Association, in fact, recommends that women who work at jobs requiring more than four hours a day on their feet should quit by the 24th week, and that those who must stand for 30 minutes out of each hour should quit by the 32nd. But many practitioners feel this recommendation is too strict, and will permit women who feel fine to work longer. Standing on the job all the way to term, however, may not be a good idea, less because of the theoretical risk to the fetus than the real risk that such pregnancy discomforts as backache, varicose veins, and hemorrhoids will be aggravated.

Research shows that underweight women who gain little weight during, pregnancy are at a greater risk of having small babies when they have outside employment than when they don't, so it may be wise for such women—if they are really unable to gain adequate weight (gaining should be their first approach to the problem; see page 81)—to temporarily give up employment if they can, or at least to reduce their hours.

Some experts recommend that a woman not stay past the 20th week at a job that requires heavy lifting,[2] pulling, pushing, climbing (stairs, poles, or ladders), or bending below the waist, if this kind of work is intensive, and past the 28th week if it is moderate. It's probably also a good idea to take early leave from a job that requires frequent shift changes (which can upset appetite and sleep routines, and worsen fatigue); one that seems to exacerbate any pregnancy problems, such as headache, backache, or fatigue; or one that increases the risk of falls or other accidental injuries.

On the other hand, you can probably plan on going straight from a desk job to the delivery room without any threat to you or your baby. A sedentary job that isn't particularly stressful may actually be less of a strain on you both than staying at home with a vacuum cleaner and mop. And doing a small amount of walking—up to an hour or two daily—on the job or off, is not only harmless but may be beneficial (assuming you aren't carrying heavy loads as you go).

No matter how long you keep working, there are ways of reducing physical on-the-job stress during pregnancy:

❖ Wear support hose.

❖ If you are standing for long stretches, keep one foot on a low stool, knee bent, to take some of the pressure off your back. (See illustration, page 174.)

2. Lifting weights of 25 pounds or less, even repetitively, is usually not a problem, nor is lifting weights of up to 50 pounds intermittently (which should be reassuring to pregnant mothers of babies and preschoolers). But women in jobs requiring repetitive lifting of weights of 25 to 50 pounds should probably quit by the 34th week, by the 20th week if the weights are over 50 pounds. Those in jobs requiring only intermittent lifting of weights over 50 pounds should quit by the 30th week.

❖ Take frequent breaks. Stand up and walk around if you've been sitting; sit down with your feet up if you've been standing. Do some stretching exercises, especially for your back and legs.

❖ Rest a lot when you are not working; cut down on strenuous activities such as running, tennis, climbing, and so on. The more strenuous your job, the more you need to cut down on other strenuous activities.

❖ Rest on your left side during your lunch hour, if possible. Sleep on your left side at night.

❖ At your desk, keep your legs elevated (on a stool or carton) when possible.

❖ Listen to your body. Slow down your pace if you're feeling tired; go home early if you're exhausted.

❖ Stay out of smoke-filled areas; they are not only bad for the baby but can increase your fatigue.

❖ Avoid extremes in temperature.

❖ Avoid noxious fumes and chemicals (see page 67).

❖ Do any necessary lifting properly to avoid strain on your back (see page 174), and reduce the weight you ordinarily lift by at least 25%.

❖ Empty your bladder at least every two hours.

❖ If you must stand or walk on the job, cut down on your hours, if possible, and increase the time you spend napping or resting with your feet up.

❖ Remember that no job is as important as that of nourishing your baby. Don't let your other work interfere with your getting breakfast, lunch, and dinner every day, supplemented by nutritious snacks (keep a plentiful supply at your workplace or bring them in daily.)

CLUMSINESS

"Lately I've been dropping everything I pick up. Why am I so clumsy suddenly?"

Like the extra inches on your belly, the extra thumbs on your hands are part and parcel of being pregnant. As with so many pregnancy side effects, this temporary clumsiness is caused by the loosening of joints and the retention of water, both of which can make your grasp on objects less firm and sure. Another factor may be a lack of concentration as a result of the scatterbrain syndrome (see page 155).

Besides making a conscious effort to pick up things more carefully, there isn't much you can do about pregnancy "dropsies"—so it might be a good idea to let your husband handle the good china for the next few months.

THE PAIN OF CHILDBIRTH

"Now that pregnancy has become an inescapable reality, I'm worrying about whether I will be able to tolerate the pain of childbirth."

Though almost every expectant mother eagerly awaits the birth of her child, very few look forward to the labor and delivery that precede it. Especially for those who've never experienced significant discomfort, the fear of this unknown is very real—and very normal. Unhappily, it's often compounded for these women by the horror tales of mothers, aunts, and friends in whose footsteps to the labor room they dread to follow.

There's no point in dreading the pain—which may end up being worse than you bargained for or not so bad after all—but there's a lot to be said for being prepared for it. When women who anticipate that labor will be an incomparably exhilarating and ultimately fulfilling experience end up with 24 hours of excruciating back labor, they suffer as much from disappointment as from pain. And because the pain is unexpected, they have trouble dealing with it.

In general, both women who fear pain the most and those who expect it the least have a harder time during labor and delivery than women who are realistic in their expectations and are prepared for any eventuality.

If you prepare both your mind and your body, you should be able to reduce your anxiety now, and at the same time help make your actual labor more comfortable and tolerable.

Get Educated. One reason earlier generations of women found labor so unbearable was that they didn't understand what was happening to their bodies. Take a good childbirth education class with your husband if at all possible (see Childbirth Education, page 209); otherwise, read as much on the subject of labor and delivery as you can (try to touch on all the major schools of thought), including the descriptions beginning on page 212. What you don't know can hurt you more than it should.

Get Moving. You wouldn't think of running a marathon without the proper physical training. Neither should you consider going into labor (which is a no less Herculean feat) untrained. Work out faithfully with all the breathing and toning-up exercises your practitioner and/or childbirth educator recommends. (If they have not recommended any, see page 189 for several basic exercises.)

Put Pain in Perspective. There are at least two good things to be said about the pain of childbirth, no matter how intense. First, it has a definite time limit. Though it may be difficult to believe at the time, you will not be in labor forever. Average labor with a first child is between 12 and 14 hours—and only a few of those hours are likely to be very uncomfortable. (Many doctors will not allow labor to continue much beyond 24 hours, and will perform a cesarean at that point if adequate progress has not been made.) Second, it's a pain with a very definite positive purpose: Contractions progressively thin and open your cervix, each contraction bringing you closer to the birth of your baby. Don't feel guilty, however, if you lose sight of that purpose during very hard labor and care very little about anything but getting it over with. Your tolerance for pain does not reflect on the depth of your maternal love.

Don't Plan on Going It Alone. Even if you don't feel like holding hands with your mate during labor, it will be comforting to know he (or a close friend or relative) is there to mop your brow, to feed you ice chips, to massage your back or neck, to coach you through contractions, or just for you to curse at. Your coach should go through childbirth classes with you if possible, or if it's not, should read up on the coach's role, starting on page 288.

Be Ready to Accept Pain Relief If It's Needed. Asking for or accepting medication is a sign neither of failure nor of weakness (you don't have to be a martyr to be a mother), and some kind of pain relief is sometimes absolutely necessary to keep a laboring woman at her most effective. See page 226 for more on pain relief during labor and delivery.

LABOR AND DELIVERY

"I'm getting very anxious about labor and delivery. What if I fail?"

The advent of childbirth education probably did as much as any of the miraculous medical advancements in the past decades to improve the experience of women in labor. However, by creating a mystique of the perfect labor and delivery, it sometimes left parents-to-be feeling pressured to achieve that ideal. Couples prepared themselves for childbirth as if for a final exam. It's not surprising that many worried about failing, and of thereby letting down not only themselves and each other but also their doctors, nurse-midwives, and especially their childbirth educators.

But fortunately most childbirth educators have now come to recognize that there isn't just one way to experience childbirth, and that the only goal—which all parents share—is a healthy mother and a healthy baby. They are letting parents know that labor and delivery aren't a test that a mother passes (if she does her breathing exercises, has a vaginal delivery, and takes no medication) or fails (if she neglects her breathing exercises, has a cesarean, or accepts pain relief). That's something you need to recognize, too. Even forgetting, because of pain and excitement, everything you're "supposed" to do won't change the outcome of the delivery or make you a failure.

Learn everything you can in your classes and from your reading, but don't become so obsessed that you forget that childbirth is a natural process—one that women managed to stumble through successfully for thousands of years before Mrs. Lamaze gave birth to her son, the doctor.

"I'm afraid I'll do something embarrassing during labor."

The prospect of screaming or crying out, or of involuntarily emptying your bladder or bowel, might seem embarrassing now. During labor, however, avoiding humiliation will be the farthest thing from your mind. Besides, nothing you can do or say during labor will shock or disgust your birth attendants, who've doubtless seen and heard it all before. The important thing is to be yourself, to do what makes you feel most comfortable. If you are ordinarily a vocal, emotive person, don't try to hold in your moans or hold back your grunts and groans. On the other hand, if you're normally very inhibited and would rather whimper quietly into your pillow, don't feel obligated to out-yell the woman in the next room.

"I dread losing control during labor and delivery."

To members of the take-charge-of-your-life generation, the thought of relinquishing control of your labor and delivery to the medical staff can be a little unnerving. Of course you want the doctors and nurses to take the best possible care of you and your baby. But you'd still like to maintain a modicum of control. And you can—by working hard now at your childbirth preparation exercises, becoming familiar with the birth process (see page 288), and by developing rapport with a practitioner who respects your opinions. Setting up a birthing plan (see page 225) with your practitioner, specifying what you would like and would not like during labor and delivery, also increases your control.

But with that said and done, it's important to understand that you won't necessarily be able to stay in complete control of your labor and to have everything go your way. The best-laid plans of obstetrical patients and their practitioners can give way to a variety of unforeseen circumstances. It's only sensible to be mentally prepared for the more common scenarios that can unfold at a birth, and for the possibility that procedures and interventions that you'd hoped to avoid may become unavoidable at the last minute. For instance, you'd hoped to deliver without an episiotomy but your perineum refuses to budge after three hours of pushing. Or you'd planned to go through labor completely unmedicated, but an extremely long and trying active phase has zapped you of your strength. Learning when relinquishing the reins will be in the best interest of you and your baby is an important part of your childbirth education.

WHAT IT'S IMPORTANT TO KNOW: CHILDBIRTH EDUCATION

When your parents were expecting you, being prepared for childbirth meant that the baby's room was painted, the layette was ordered, and a suitcase packed with pretty nightgowns for the hospital stay was waiting at the door. It was the arrival of the child—not the childbirth experience—that was anticipated, planned for, and looked forward to. Women knew little of what to expect from labor and delivery; husbands knew even less. And since mother was likely to be unconscious during the birth and father was likely to be absently thumbing through *Time* magazines in the waiting room, their ignorance was of little consequence.

Now that general anesthesia is reserved mainly for emergency cesareans, waiting rooms are for nervous grandparents, and mom and dad can go through childbirth together, ignorance is neither wise nor acceptable. Preparing for childbirth has come to mean preparing for the labor and delivery experience as much as for the new baby. Expectant couples devour stacks of books, magazine articles, and pamphlets. They participate fully in their prenatal visits, seeking answers to all their questions, reassurance for all their worries. And more and more often, they attend childbirth education classes.

Just what are these classes about, and why are they proliferating faster than stretch marks in the sixth month? The original, pioneering classes were intended to explain a new approach to childbirth—without medication and without fear—and were commonly known as "natural childbirth" classes. Since then, there has been a shift in emphasis from natural childbirth (though it's still considered the ideal) to education and preparation for many of the possible eventualities of labor and delivery—so that whether the birth turns out to be medicated or unmedicated, vaginal or surgical, with an episiotomy or without one, parents will have an understanding of what is happening and will be able to participate as fully as possible.

Most curricula are based on the following:

❖ The imparting of accurate information, intended to reduce fears, improve the ability to cope with pain, and enhance decision-making skills.

❖ The teaching of specially designed techniques of relaxation, distraction, muscular control, and breathing—all of which can increase a couple's sense of being in control while contributing to the woman's endurance and a reduction in her perception of pain.

❖ The development of a productive working relationship between the laboring mother and her coach, which, if maintained during labor and delivery, may serve to provide a supportive environment that can, in turn, help the mother to minimize her anxieties and maximize her efforts during labor.

BENEFITS OF TAKING A CHILDBIRTH CLASS

J ust how much a couple benefits from childbirth education depends on the course they take, on the teacher, and on their own attitudes. These classes work better for some couples than for others. Some thrive in group situations and find sharing feelings natural and helpful; others are uncomfortable in groups and find sharing difficult and unproductive. Some enjoy learning the relaxation and breathing techniques, while others feel that the repetition of such exercises is forced and intrusive, tension-producing rather than tension-alleviating. Some ultimately find these exercises effective in the control of pain during labor; others end up not using them at all. Just about every couple, however, stands to gain something from taking a *good* childbirth class—and certainly has nothing to lose. Some benefits include:

❖ The opportunity to spend time with other expectant couples: to share pregnancy experiences, compare progress, and swap tales of woes, worries, aches and pains. It's also a chance to make friends-with-babies, for later. Many classes hold "reunions" once everyone has delivered.

❖ Increased involvement of the father in the pregnancy, particularly important if he isn't able to attend prenatal visits. Classes will familiarize him with the process of labor and delivery so that he can be a more effective coach, and will allow him to meet other expectant fathers. Some courses even include a special session for fathers only, which gives them the chance to express and find relief for the anxieties they're reluctant to burden their partners with.

❖ A weekly chance to ask questions that come up between prenatal visits, or that you don't feel comfortable asking your practitioner.

❖ An opportunity to get hands-on instruction in breathing, relaxation, and coaching techniques, and to get feedback from an expert.

❖ An opportunity to develop confidence in your ability to meet the strenuous demands of labor and delivery, through increased knowledge (which helps banish fear of the unknown) and the acquisition of coping skills, which may enable you to feel more in control.

❖ A chance to learn coping strategies that may help to decrease your perception of pain and, hopefully, increase your ability to tolerate it during labor and delivery—which may translate into less need for medication.

❖ The possibility of an improved, less stressful labor, thanks to a better understanding of the birthing process and the development of coping skills. Couples who've had childbirth preparation generally rate their childbirth experiences as more satisfying overall than those who haven't.

❖ Possibly, a slightly shorter labor. Studies show that the average labor of women who have had childbirth education is somewhat shorter than that of women who haven't, probably because the training and preparation better enable them to work with, instead of against, the work of the uterus. (There is no guarantee of a short labor, only the possibility of a *shorter* one.)

CHOOSING A CHILDBIRTH CLASS

In some communities where childbirth classes are few and far between, the choice is a relatively simple one. In others, the variety of offerings can be overwhelming and confusing. There are courses run by hospitals, by private instructors, by practitioners through their offices. There are "earlybird" prenatal classes—taken in the first or second trimester—which cover such concerns of pregnancy as nutrition, exercise, fetal development, hygiene, sexuality, dreams and fantasies; and there are down-to-the-wire six- to ten-week childbirth classes, usually begun in the seventh or eighth month, which concentrate on labor, delivery, and postpartum mother and baby care.

If the pickings are slim, taking any childbirth class is probably better than taking none at all—as long as you keep your perspective and don't accept every word spoken in class as gospel. If there is a selection of courses where you live, it may help to consider the following when making your decision:

❖ Taking a class that is run either by your practitioner or under the auspices of your practitioner, or is recommended by him or her, often works out best. If the laboring and delivering philosophies of your childbirth education teacher vary greatly from those of the person who'll be assisting you during labor and delivery, you're bound to run into contradictions and conflicts. If differences of opinion do arise, make sure you address them with your practitioner well before your delivery date.

❖ Small is best. Five or six couples to a class is ideal; more than ten isn't recommended. Not only can a teacher give more time and individual attention to couples in an intimate group—particularly important during the breathing and relaxation technique practice sessions—but the camaraderie in a small group tends to be stronger.

❖ Classes that set up unrealistic expectations can work against you. (If you're guaranteed that taking the class will make labor short or painless or glorious, for instance, beware.) There's no way to know for sure what a teacher's philosophy of childbirth is until you take the class—but sitting in on one or talking to her before signing up can give you some idea.

❖ What is the rate of drug-free labors among class "graduates?" This may be helpful information, but it can also be misleading. Does a low rate indicate that students were so well prepared in the various natural pain-reducing strategies that they rarely needed medication? Or were they so convinced that asking for medication was a sign of failure that they stoically withstood severe pain? Perhaps the best way to find the answer is to talk to some of the graduates.

❖ What is the curriculum like? Ask for a course outline, and if you can,

For Information on Childbirth Classes

Ask your practitioner for information on classes in your area, or call the hospital where you plan to deliver. If you are interested in pregnancy classes, ask at one of your early visits; otherwise the question can wait until the third trimester. You can also obtain referrals on local classes from:

❖ *Gamper Method:* Midwest Parentcraft Center, 627 Beaver Rd., Glenview, IL 60025; 312-248-8100.

❖ The Read Natural Childbirth Foundation, P.O. Box 956, San Rafael, CA 94915; 415-456-3143 (for general information only).

❖ *Lamaze:* American Society for Psychoprophylaxis in Obstetrics, 1840 Wilson Blvd., Suite 204, Arlington, VA 22201; 800-368-4404.

❖ International Childbirth Education Association, P.O. Box 20038, Minneapolis, MN 55420; 612-854-8660 (ICEA provides referrals from other groups as well).

❖ *Bradley:* American Academy of Husband-Coached Childbirth, P.O. Box 5224, Sherman Oaks, CA 91413; 800-4ABIRTH.

sit in on a class. A good course will include a discussion of cesarean section (recognizing that 15% to 25% of students may end up having one) and of medication (recognizing, too, that some will need this). It will deal with the psychological and emotional as well as the technical aspects of childbirth.

❖ How is the class taught? Are films of actual childbirths shown? Will you hear from mothers and fathers who've recently delivered? Is there discussion, or just lecture? Will there be an opportunity for parents-to-be to ask questions? Is adequate time provided during class for practicing the various techniques that are taught? Is one particular philosophy espoused—Lamaze or Bradley, for example?

THE MOST COMMON SCHOOLS OF THOUGHT

There are three major childbirth education philosophies, though many instructors combine elements of each in their classes.

Grantly Dick-Read. Combining relaxation techniques and prenatal education to break the fear-tension-pain cycle of labor and delivery, this psychophysical childbirth philosophy dates back to the '40s and '50s and represents the first organized approach to childbirth preparation in the United States. It was the first to include fathers in the education process and to bring them into the labor room. Programs begin in the fourth month and are conducted by instructors trained and certified in the Gamper method, named for Margaret Gamper, the nurse who inspired Dr. Dick-Read.

Lamaze. Also called the psychoprophylactic method, this approach, pioneered by Dr. Ferdinand Lamaze, is similar in some ways to the psychophysical approach in that its major weapons against pain are knowledge and relaxation techniques. In addition, Dr. Lamaze's approach depends on conditioning, à la Dr. Pavlov, who conditioned dogs to salivate at the sound of a bell. The expectant mother is conditioned, through intensive training and practice, to substitute useful responses to the stimulus of labor contractions in place of counterproductive ones. The father or other coach trains with the mother to assist her during both labor and delivery.

Bradley. This approach, which originated the husband-coached delivery, emphasizes good diet and uses exercise to ease the discomforts of pregnancy and to prepare muscles for birth and breasts for nursing. Women learn to imitate their sleeping position and breathing (which is deep and slow) and to use relaxation to make the first stage of labor more comfortable. Rather than the usual panting and Lamaze breathing patterns, the Bradley method employs deep abdominal breathing; instead of using distraction and a focus of concentration outside the body to take the mind off discomfort, Bradley recommends that the laboring woman concentrate within and work with her body. Medi-

cation is reserved for complications and cesareans, and about 94% of Bradley graduates go without it. "Early bird" Bradley classes are offered, as are classes that continue into the postpartum period, but they aren't mandatory. The typical Bradley course runs 12 weeks, beginning in the 5th or 6th month.

Other Childbirth Classes. Childbirth educators certified by the International Childbirth Education Association support family-centered maternity care and a minimum of medical intervention. There are also childbirth education classes designed to prepare parents to deliver in a particular hospital, and classes sponsored by a medical group, health maintenance organization (HMO), or other health-care provider group. Many childbirth classes take no particular party line, selecting the best from what is known about childbirth preparation and changing their curricula as new information becomes available. In some cities, education for pregnancy as well as childbirth is offered, in classes that usually begin in the first trimester.

When Something Just Doesn't Feel Right

Maybe it's a twinge of abdominal pain that feels too much like a cramp to ignore, a sudden change in your vaginal discharge (a leaking of fluid, a thick and albuminous discharge, with or without blood), an aching in your lower back or in your pelvic floor—or maybe it's something so vague, you can't even put your finger on it. Chances are nothing's wrong—but to play it safe, check the symptoms on page 221 and page 361. Early detection of premature labor (as well as of other complications of pregnancy) can often make a big difference in successful outcome.

11
The Seventh Month

What You Can Expect at This Month's Checkup

This month you can expect your practitioner to check the following, though there may be variations depending upon your particular needs and upon your practitioner's style of practice:[1]

❖ Weight and blood pressure

❖ Urine, for sugar and protein

❖ Fetal heartbeat

❖ Height of fundus (top of uterus)

❖ Size and position of fetus, by external palpation

❖ Feet and hands for edema (swelling), and legs for varicose veins

❖ Symptoms you have been experiencing, especially unusual ones

❖ Questions and problems you want to discuss—have a list ready

What You May Be Feeling

You may experience all of these symptoms at one time or another, or only a few of them. Some may have continued from last month, others may be new. Still others may hardly be noticed because you've become so used to them. You may also have other, less common, symptoms.

PHYSICALLY:

❖ Stronger and more frequent fetal activity

❖ Increasingly heavy whitish vaginal discharge (leukorrhea)

❖ Lower abdominal achiness

❖ Constipation

❖ Heartburn, indigestion, flatulence, bloating

❖ Occasional headaches, faintness, or dizziness

---

1. See Appendix for an explanation of the procedures and tests performed during office visits.

- Nasal congestion and occasional nosebleeds; ear stuffiness
- Pink toothbrush from bleeding gums
- Leg cramps
- Backache
- Mild swelling of ankles and feet, and occasionally of hands and face
- Varicose veins of the legs
- Hemorrhoids
- Itchy abdomen
- Shortness of breath
- Difficulty sleeping
- Scattered Braxton Hicks contractions, usually painless (the uterus hardens for a minute, then returns to normal)
- Clumsiness (which increases the risk of falling)
- Colostrum, either leaking or expressed, from enlarged breasts

EMOTIONALLY:

- Increasing apprehension about motherhood, baby's health, and about labor and delivery
- Continued absentmindedness
- Increased dreaming and fantasizing about the baby
- Increased boredom and weariness with the pregnancy, the beginning of anxiousness for it to be over

WHAT YOU MAY LOOK LIKE

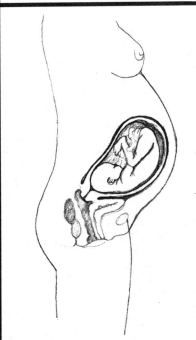

By the end of the seventh month, fat begins to be deposited on the fetus. It may suck its thumb, hiccup, cry; can taste sweet or sour; responds to stimuli, including pain, light, and sound. Placental function begins to diminish, as does the volume of amniotic fluid, as the 3-pounder fills the uterus. Good chance of survival if born now.

WHAT YOU MAY BE CONCERNED ABOUT

INCREASING FATIGUE

'I've heard women are supposed to feel terrific in the last trimester. I feel tired all the time."

"Supposed to" is a phrase that ought to be stricken from a pregnant woman's vocabulary. There's no one way you're supposed to feel at any time in pregnancy. Though some women feel less tired in the third trimester than in the first and second, it can be perfectly normal to continue feeling fatigued or to feel even more fatigued. Actually, there are probably more reasons to feel tired than to feel terrific in the last trimester. First of all, you're carrying around a lot more weight than you were earlier. Second, because of your bulk, you may be having trouble sleeping. You may also be losing sleep because your mind is overloaded with baby concerns, plans, and fantasies. Taking care of other children, a job, or both may be taking a toll on you—and so may preparing for the new baby.

Just because fatigue is a normal part of pregnancy doesn't mean you should ignore it. As always, it's a signal from your body that you should slow down. Take the hint: Rest and relax as much as you can. You'll need every bit of strength you can save up for labor, delivery, and—more important—what follows them.

Extreme fatigue that doesn't ease up when you get more rest should be reported to your doctor. Anemia (see page 154) sometimes strikes at the beginning of the third trimester, which is why many practitioners do a routine blood test for it in the seventh month.

CONCERN ABOUT THE BABY'S WELL-BEING

"I worry all the time that something is wrong with my baby."

There probably isn't an expectant mother (or father) who hasn't been haunted by this same fear. Some will even put off buying baby clothes and furniture, or choosing the baby's name, until toes and fingers have been counted, the Apgars have been calculated, and the doctor has congratulated them on their healthy baby.

But the odds of having a completely normal baby have never been better. The U.S. infant mortality rate is the lowest in history, down to a little over 9 per 1,000 births (and lower than that for middle-class women).[2] Most of these perinatal (around the time of birth) deaths occur in the newborns of women who receive medical care late or not at all and who are inadequately nourished. A majority of the remainder, occur in infants of high-risk women: those with a family history of genetic disease; with uncontrolled chronic illnesses; who drink heavily and/or smoke or take drugs; or who are carrying multiple fetuses. Even for these women, close medical supervision and improved prenatal care have recently greatly increased the chances of having healthy babies.

Some experts had forecast that as the death rate fell—because more babies with birth defects would be saved by medical miracles—the rate of children with handicaps would rise. This hasn't happened; the percentage of birth defects, in fact, appears to be declining. And when a child *is* born with a birth defect, he or she isn't necessarily permanently handicapped. Most minor, and many serious, defects are now correctable. If diagnosed in utero, some can be treated even before birth through surgery or medication. Shortly after birth, many heart defects and other internal abnormalities can be repaired with surgery, as can cleft palates and bone or limb abnormalities later on. Children who are intellectually disabled can, with early intervention, make remarkable strides.

So when worry strikes, strike

---

2. Estimated by government sources for 1990. Though this is an improvement over the past, it is still much higher than the rates in many other countries. The reason: inadequate health care for the poor.

back—with the knowledge that your baby couldn't have picked a better time to be born (and to grow up) healthy. And, of course, continue to do all you can to give your baby the best odds possible.

EDEMA (SWELLING) OF THE ANKLES AND FEET

"My ankles seem to be swollen, especially when the weather is warm. Is this a bad sign?"

Any degree of edema (swelling due to excessive accumulation of fluids in the tissues) was once considered a potential danger sign in pregnancy. Now doctors recognize that mild edema is related to the normal and necessary increase in body fluids in pregnancy. Some swelling of the ankles and legs, without accompanying symptoms to suggest the development of preeclampsia (see below), is considered completely normal. In fact, 75% of women develop such edema at some point in their pregnancies.[3] It's particularly common late in the day, in warm weather, or after standing or sitting for a period of time. Most women find that much of the swelling disappears overnight—after several hours spent lying down.

Generally, edema is nothing but a little uncomfortable. To ease the discomfort, elevate your legs or lie down when you can, preferably on your left side; wear comfortable shoes or slippers; avoid elastic-top socks or stockings.

If you find the swelling very bothersome, try support hose. Several types are available for pregnancy wear—including full pantyhose (with roomy tummy space) and knee highs—so check with your practitioner to see if he or she has a recommendation for you. When shopping, select the size based on your prepregnancy weight. Put the support hose on before you get up in the morning, while the swelling is down.

Help your system to flush out waste products by drinking at least eight to ten 8-ounce glasses of liquid a day. Paradoxically, drinking even greater amounts of liquids—up to a gallon a day—helps many women avoid excess water retention. But don't drink more than 16 ounces (2 glassfuls) at once, and don't fill up with so much liquid that you have no room for the other 11 components of your Daily Dozen. Though it's no longer believed that salt restriction is wise during a normal pregnancy (salt may be restricted for some women with high blood pressure), excessive salt intake isn't any smarter and could increase excess fluid retention.

If your hands and/or face become puffy, or if edema persists for more than 24 hours at a time, you should notify your doctor. Such swelling may be insignificant, or—if accompanied by rapid weight gain, a rise in blood pressure, and protein in the urine—it could signal the beginning of preeclampsia (pregnancy-induced hypertension; see page 204).

OVERHEATING

"I feel so warm most of the time, and I sweat a lot. Is this normal?"

With your basal metabolic rate (the rate at which your body expends energy at total rest) up about 20% during pregnancy, the heat's on. Not only are you likely to feel too warm in warm weather, you may even

---

3. One in 4 pregnant women never experience edema, and this can be completely normal, too. Others may not notice swelling.

feel overheated in the winter—when everyone else is shivering. You will also probably perspire more, especially at night. This is a mixed blessing. While it helps to cool you off and rids your body of waste products, it is admittedly unpleasant.

To minimize discomfort, bathe often; use a good antiperspirant; and dress in layers—especially in the winter—so you can peel down to shirtsleeves when you start heating up. And don't forget to take in extra fluids to replace those lost through your pores.

ORGASM AND THE BABY

"After I have an orgasm my baby usually stops kicking for about half an hour. Is sex harmful to him or her at this stage of pregnancy?"

Babies are individuals, even in the womb. And their responses to their parents' lovemaking vary. Some, perhaps like your baby, are rocked to sleep by the rhythmic motion of coitus and the uterine contractions that follow orgasm. Others, stimulated by the activity, may become more lively. Both responses are normal; neither indicates any awareness of the proceedings on the part of the fetus or that the fetus has been harmed in any way.

Whether sexual intercourse is totally safe during the last two months of pregnancy, even in a normal pregnancy, is a matter of increasing controversy in the obstetrical community. Acquitted several years ago as an accessory to premature labor and perinatal infection, coitus in the final weeks of gestation is once again being implicated in such complications by researchers. To learn what is believed safe in sexual relations for expectant parents, see Making Love During Pregnancy, page 164.

PREMATURE LABOR

"Is there anything I can do to ensure that my baby won't be born prematurely?"

Far more babies are born late than early. In the U.S., only 7 to 10 in every 100 deliveries are premature or preterm—that is, take place before the 37th week of pregnancy. One-third of preterm births occur because labor begins early; one-third because the membranes rupture prematurely; and one-third because of a maternal or fetal problem. About 3 in 4 occur in women who are known to be at high risk for premature delivery. The rate of premature deliveries is lower for white women (fewer than 6 in 100) and higher for black women (nearly 13 in 100), only partly for socio-economic reasons. In spite of efforts aimed at preventing preterm births, there has been little progress made, and, in fact, the number of babies born early has increased in recent years.

There are a wide variety of factors that are believed to be related to increased risk of preterm delivery. The more risk factors in a woman's history, the greater the chance that she will deliver prematurely. Altering the risk factors that follow may help increase the odds of carrying a pregnancy to term:

Smoking. Quit before conception or as early as possible in pregnancy.

Alcohol Use. Avoid regular consumption of beer, wine, and liquor (no one yet knows how much is too much, so it's safer to abstain).

Drug Abuse. Don't take any medication without the approval of a physician who knows you are pregnant; don't take any other drugs at all.

Inadequate Weight Gain. If your pre-pregnant weight was normal, gain a minimum of 25 pounds; if you were significantly underweight before conceiving, gain closer to 35 pounds. (Overweight women, with excellent nutrition and their doctor's permission, may safely be able to gain less.)

Inadequate Nutrition. Follow a well-balanced diet (See the Best-Odds Diet, page 80) throughout pregnancy. Be sure that your vitamin supplement contains zinc; some recent studies have linked zinc deficiency with preterm labor.

Standing, or Heavy Physical Labor. If your job alone or your job plus housework require you to stand for several hours each day, stop working or cut back.

Sexual Intercourse (for Some Women). Expectant mothers who are at high risk for premature delivery are generally advised to abstain from intercourse and/or orgasm during the final two or three months of pregnancy because, in these women, orgasm might activate uterine contractions.

Hormonal Imbalance. Just as it can trigger late miscarriage, an imbalance of hormones can sometimes trigger premature delivery; hormone replacement may prevent both.

Other risk factors are not always possible to eliminate, but their effects can sometimes be modified:

Infections (such as rubella; certain venereal diseases; and urinary tract, vaginal, and amniotic fluid infections). When there is an infection that could harm the fetus, early labor seems to be the body's way of trying to get the baby out of a dangerous environment. In the case of amniotic fluid infection (chorioamnionitis), which may be a major cause of preterm labor, the body's immune response apparently triggers production of prostaglandins, which can initiate labor, as well as of substances that can damage the fetal membranes, leading to their premature rupture.

To reduce the risk that you will contract an infection, stay away from people who are ill and make sure you get adequate rest and exercise, optimum nutrition, and regular prenatal care. Some doctors also recommend using a condom during the last months of pregnancy to reduce the risk of amniotic fluid infection.

Incompetent Cervix. This condition, in which a weak cervix opens prematurely, often goes undiagnosed until after at least one instance of late miscarriage or premature labor. Once the condition is diagnosed, premature delivery can be avoided by suturing the cervix closed at about the 14th week. It is also suspected that in some women, for reasons unknown and apparently not related to incompetent cervix, the cervix begins to efface and dilate early, leading to early delivery. Routine examination of the cervix to uncover such changes in the last months of pregnancy in high-risk women is a common and probably useful procedure.

Uterine Irritability. Research suggests that in some women the uterus is particularly irritable, and that this irritability makes it susceptible to untimely contractions. If these women could be identified and monitored in the third trimester, it's possible, some believe, that their premature labor could be prevented by full or partial bed rest and/or the use of medication to quiet the contractions.

Placenta Previa (a low-lying placenta located near or over the cervix). This condition may be discovered in an ultrasound exam, or may not be suspected until bleeding is noted in mid- or late pregnancy. Premature labor may be headed off by complete bed rest.

Chronic Maternal Illness (high blood pressure; heart, liver, or kidney disease; diabetes). Good medical care, sometimes including bed rest, can often prevent premature delivery.

Stress. Sometimes the cause of stress can be eliminated or minimized (by quitting a high-pressure job or getting counseling for a floundering marriage, for example); sometimes eliminating the cause is more difficult (when you lose your job or are pregnant and alone). But all kinds of stress can be reduced through education, relaxation techniques, good nutrition, a balance of exercise and rest, and by talking out the problem—often in a self-help group (see page 113).

Age Under 17. Optimal nutrition and prenatal care can help compensate for the fact that the mother, like her fetus, is still growing.

Age Over 35. Optimal nutrition, good prenatal care, reduction of stress, and prenatal screening for genetic and obstetrical problems specific to older women all reduce risk.

Low Educational or Socioeconomic Level. Again, good nutrition and early access to, and participation in, culturally sensitive prenatal care, as well as the elimination of as many risk factors as possible, can decrease the risk.

Structural Abnormalities of the Uterus. Once the problem has been diagnosed, prepregnancy surgical repair can frequently prevent future preterm births.

Multiple Gestations. Women carrying more than one fetus deliver an average of three weeks early. Meticulous prenatal care, optimal nutrition, the elimination of other risk factors, along with more time spent lying down and resting, and restrictions on activity as needed in the last trimester, may prevent a too-early birth.

Fetal Abnormality. In some instances, prenatal diagnosis may pick up a defect that can be treated while the fetus is still in the uterus; sometimes correcting the problem can allow the pregnancy to continue to term.

History of Premature Deliveries. A diagnosed cause can be corrected; topnotch prenatal care, reduction of other risk factors, and limitations on activities may help to prevent a repeat. Testing for and treating vaginal infection in the second trimester can reduce risk.

Occasionally none of the above risk factors is present. A healthy woman with a perfectly normal pregnancy suddenly goes into labor early, for no apparent reason. Perhaps someday a cause will be identified for such premature births, but presently they are labeled "cause unknown."

It's been suggested that when risk factors are present, the use of home uterine monitoring could help reduce the incidence of premature deliver. From studies so far, it isn't clear whether or not the technique works. There is some indication, however, that education about the symptoms of preterm labor and regular contact with a medical professional may be helpful.

If preterm labor does begin, the delivery can often be held off until the baby is more mature. Even a brief delay can be beneficial; each additional day the baby remains in the uterus until term improves its chances of survival. So you can see that it's important to be familiar with the signs of early labor, and to alert your practitioner if you've the slightest suspicion that labor is beginning. *Don't worry about bothering your doctor*—no matter what the day or hour.

❖ Menstrual-like cramps, with or without diarrhea, nausea, or indigestion.

❖ Lower back pain or pressure, or a change in the nature of lower backache.

❖ An achiness or feeling of pressure in the pelvic floor, the thighs, or the groin.

❖ A change in vaginal discharge, particularly if it is watery or tinged or streaked pinkish or brownish with blood. The passage of a thick, gelatinous mucous plug may or may not precede this "bloody show."

❖ Rupture of membranes (a trickle or rush of fluid from your vagina).

You can have all these symptoms and not be in labor, but only your practitioner can tell you for sure. If he or she suspects you're in labor, you will probably be examined promptly. For information about how premature labor is treated, see page 361.

If premature labor does occur—despite steps taken to prevent or postpone it—your chances of bringing a healthy, normal baby home from the hospital are excellent. (Of course, that trip home with the baby may have to be delayed days, weeks, or even months to increase those chances.)

APPROACHING RESPONSIBILITY

"I'm beginning to worry that I won't be able to manage my job, my house, my marriage—and the baby too."

You probably won't be able to manage if you attempt to be a full-time career woman, housekeeper, wife, and mother—expecting perfection in each role. Many new mothers have tried to be "superwoman"; few have succeeded without sacrificing their health and sanity.

But it will be possible to survive if you reconcile yourself to the reality that you can't do it all—at least in the beginning. If job, husband, and baby are top priorities, perhaps keeping the house immaculate will have to take a backseat for now. If full-time motherhood appeals to you and you can afford to stay home for a while, maybe you can shelve your career temporarily. Or work part-time, as a compromise. It's just a matter of deciding what your priorities are.

Whatever decision you make, your new life will be easier if you don't have to go it alone. Behind most successful moms there's a cooperative dad, willing to share the workload. Don't feel guilty about asking your husband to change diapers and bathe the baby after a long day at the office. There's probably no better way for him to unwind and at the same time to get to know his child. If Dad isn't available (all or part of the time), then

---

Don't Hold It In

Making a habit of not urinating when you feel the need increases the risk that your inflamed bladder may irritate the uterus and set off contractions, so *don't hold it in.*

you are going to need to consider other sources of assistance: the baby's grandparents or other relatives, child-care or household workers, play-groups, day care centers.

ACCIDENTS

"I missed the curb today when I was out walking and fell belly-first on the pavement. I'm not worried about my skinned knees and elbows, but I'm terrified that I've hurt the baby."

A woman in the last trimester of pregnancy isn't exactly the most graceful creature on earth. A poor sense of balance (because her center of gravity keeps shifting forward) and looser, less stable joints contribute to her awkwardness and make her prone to minor falls—particularly belly-flops. So do her tendency to tire easily, her predisposition to preoccupation and daydreaming, and the difficulty she may be having seeing past her belly to her feet.

But while a curbside spill may leave you with multiple scrapes and bruises (particularly to your ego), it's extremely rare for a fetus to suffer the consequences of its mother's clumsiness. Your baby is protected by the world's most sophisticated shock-absorption system, comprised of amniotic fluid, tough membranes, the elastic, muscular uterus, and the sturdy abdominal cavity girded with muscles and bones. For it to be penetrated, and for your baby to be hurt, you'd have to sustain very serious injuries—the kind that would very likely land you in the hospital.

Even though there's probably no harm done, you should let your practitioner know if you have a fall. You may be asked to come in so that your baby's heartbeat can be checked—mostly to set your mind at ease.

On the rare occasion when damage to a pregnancy does occur as a result of an accident, it's most likely to involve separation (abruption) of the placenta, partially or completely, from the uterine wall—an injury that requires swift action on the part of the physician. If you notice vaginal bleeding, leakage of amniotic fluid, abdominal tenderness, or uterine contractions, or if your baby seems unusually inactive, seek medical attention *immediately*. Have someone take you to the emergency room if you can't reach your doctor.

LOWER BACK AND LEG PAIN (SCIATICA)

"I've been having pain on the right side of my back, running right down my hip and leg. What's happening?"

T his sounds like another of the occupational hazards of expectant motherhood. The pressure of the enlarging uterus, which has been responsible for so many other discomforts, can also affect the sciatic nerve—causing lower back, buttock, and leg pain. Rest, and a heating pad applied locally, may help. The pain may pass as your baby's position changes, or it may linger until you've delivered. In severe cases, a few days of bed rest or special exercises may be recommended.

SKIN ERUPTIONS

"It's not bad enough that I have stretch marks, now I seem to have some kind of itchy pimples breaking out in them."

Cheer up. You have less than three months left until delivery, when you'll be able to bid a grateful good-bye to most of the unpleasant side effects of pregnancy—among them, these new eruptions. Until then, it may help to know that although they may be uncomfortable, the lesions aren't dangerous to you or your baby. Known medically, and unpronounceably, as pruritic urticarial papules and plaques of pregnancy, or PUPPP, the condition generally disappears after delivery and doesn't recur in subsequent pregnancies. Though PUPPP most often develops in abdominal stretch marks, it sometimes also appears on the thighs, buttocks, or arms of the expectant mother. Show your rash to your practitioner, who may prescribe topical medication, an antihistamine, or a cortico steroid shot to ease any discomfort.

There are a variety of other skin conditions and rashes that can develop during pregnancy. Though they should always be shown to your practitioner, they are rarely serious. Some will need to be treated; others will run a mild course and disappear after delivery.

FETAL HICCUPS

"I sometimes feel regular little spasms in my abdomen. Is this kicking, or a twitch, or what?"

Believe it or not, your baby's probably got hiccups. This phenomenon is not uncommon in fetuses in the last half of pregnancy. Some get hiccups several times a day, every day. Others never get them at all. The same pattern may continue after birth.

But before you start holding a paper bag over your belly, you should know that hiccups don't cause the same discomfort in babies (in or out of the uterus) as they do in adults—even when they last as long as 20 minutes or more. So just relax and enjoy this little entertainment from within.

DREAMS AND FANTASIES

"I've been having so many vivid dreams about the baby that I'm beginning to think I'm going mad."

Though the many night- and day-dreams (both horrifying and pleasant) a pregnant woman can experience in the last trimester may make her feel as though she's losing her sanity, they're actually helping to keep her sane. Dreams and fantasies are both healthy and normal, and help expectant women to sort out worries and fears in a nonthreatening way.

Each of the dream and fantasy themes commonly reported by pregnant women expresses one or more of the deep-seated feelings and concerns that might otherwise be suppressed:

❖ Being unprepared, losing things, forgetting to feed the baby; missing a doctor's appointment; going out to shop and forgetting the baby; being unprepared for the baby when it arrives; losing car keys, or even the baby—can express the fear of not being adequate to the task of motherhood.

❖ Being attacked or hurt—by intruders, burglars, animals; falling down the stairs after a push or a slip—may represent a sense of vulnerability.

❖ Being enclosed or unable to escape—trapped in a tunnel, a car, a small room; drowning in a pool, a lake of snowy slush, a car wash—can signify the fear of being tied down and deprived of freedom by the baby.

❖ Going off your pregnancy diet—gaining too much weight, or gaining a lot of weight overnight; overeating; eating or drinking the wrong things (two hot fudge sundaes or a bottle of wine) or not eating the right things (forgetting to drink milk for a week)—is a theme common among those trying to adjust to a restricted dietary regimen.

❖ Losing appeal—becoming unattractive or repulsive to her husband; her husband finding another woman—expresses nearly every woman's fear that pregnancy will destroy her looks forever and drive her husband away.

❖ Sexual encounters—either positive or negative, pleasure- or guilt-provoking—may reflect the sexual confusion and ambivalence often experienced during pregnancy.

❖ Death and resurrection—lost parents or other relatives reappearing—may be the subconscious mind's way of linking old and new generations.

❖ Family life with the new baby—getting ready for the baby; loving and playing with the baby—is practice parenting, bonding mother with the baby prior to birth.

❖ What the baby will be like—can represent a wide variety of concerns. Dreams about the baby being deformed or unusual in size express anxiety about its health. Fantasies about the infant having unusual skills (like talking or walking at birth) may indicate concern about the baby's intelligence and ambition for his or her future. Premonitions that the baby will be a boy or a girl could mean your heart's too set on one or the other. So could dreams about the baby's hair or eye color or resemblance to one parent

or the other. Nightmares of the baby being born fully grown could signify another problem—your fear of having to handle a tiny baby.

Though dreams and fantasies can be more anxiety-provoking in pregnancy than they are at other times, they can also be more useful. If you listen to what your motherhood fantasies are telling you about your feelings and deal with them now, you can make the transition into real-life motherhood more easily.

A LOW-BIRTHWEIGHT BABY

"I've been reading a lot about the high incidence of low-birthweight babies. Is there anything I can do to be sure I won't have one?"

Since most cases of low birthweight are preventable, you can do a lot—and inasmuch as you're reading this book, chances are you already are. Nationally, nearly 7 of every 100 newborns are categorized as low birthweight (under 5 pounds 8 ounces, or 2,500 grams), and slightly more than 1 in 100 babies as *very* low birthweight (3 pounds 5 ounces, or 1,500 grams, or less). But among informed women who are conscientious about both medical and self care as well as their lifestyle habits, the rate is much lower. Most of the common causes of low birthweight are preventable (tobacco, alcohol, or drug use by the mother, poor nutrition, inadequate prenatal care, for example); many others (such as chronic maternal illness) can be controlled by a good working partnership between the mother and her practitioner. A major cause—premature labor—can in some instances also be prevented (see page 218).

Of course, sometimes a baby is small at birth for reasons that no one can control—the mother's own low weight when she was born, for example, or an inadequate placenta, or a genetic disorder (see page 354 for more on causes of growth retardation in the fetus). But even in these cases, excellent diet and prenatal care can often compensate. And when a baby does turn out to be small, the top-notch medical care currently available gives even the very smallest an increasingly good chance of surviving and growing up healthy.

If you think you have reason to worry about the possibility of having a low-birthweight baby, you should share your concern with your practitioner. A sonogram will probably be able to determine right now whether or not your fetus is growing at a normal pace. If it isn't, then steps can be taken to uncover the cause of the slow growth and, if possible, correct it (see page 355).

A BIRTHING PLAN

"A friend who recently delivered said she worked out a birthing plan with her doctor before delivery. Is this common?"

Birthing plans are becoming increasingly common as practitioners recognize that more and more women—and their partners—would like to be involved in making as many of the childbirth decisions as they possibly can. Some practitioners routinely ask expectant parents to fill out a birthing plan; most others are willing to discuss such a plan if a patient requests it. The typical plan combines the parents' wishes and preferences with what the practitioner and hospital find acceptable—and what is feasible from a practical point of view. It's not a contract but a written understanding between practitioner and/or hospital and patient with the goal of bringing childbirth as close as possible to the patient's ideal while heading off unrealistic expectations, minimizing disappointment, and avoiding major conflict during labor and delivery.

A birthing plan may deal with a wide variety of topics; the precise content of each will depend on the parents, practitioner, and hospital involved, as well as on the particular situation. Some of the issues that you may want to express your preferences about include the following (refer to the appropriate pages before making your decision):

❖ How far into your labor you would like to remain at home (see page 270).

❖ Eating and/or drinking during active labor (page 291).

❖ Being out of bed (walking about or sitting up) during labor (page 289).

❖ Wearing contact lenses during labor and delivery (usually not permitted if general anesthesia is required).

❖ The locale of your labor and delivery—birthing room, labor room, delivery room (page 261).

❖ Personalizing the atmosphere (with music, lighting, items from home).

❖ The use of a still camera or videotape.

❖ Administration of enemas (page 277).

❖ Shaving of the pubic area (page 278).

❖ The use of an IV (intravenous fluid administration; page 279).

❖ Routine catheterization (page 378).

❖ The use of pain medication (page 226).

❖ External fetal monitoring (continuous or intermittent); internal fetal monitoring (page 280).

❖ The use of oxytocin (to induce or augment contractions; page 273).

❖ Delivery positions (page 300).

❖ Episiotomy; the use of steps to reduce the need for an episiotomy (page 283).

❖ Forceps use (page 286).

❖ Cesarean section (page 242).

❖ Suctioning of the newborn; suctioning by the father.

❖ The presence of significant others (besides your spouse) during labor and/or at delivery.

❖ The presence of older children at delivery or immediately after.

❖ Holding the baby immediately after birth; breastfeeding immediately.

❖ Postponing weighing the baby and administering eye drops until after you and your baby greet each other.

❖ Cord blood banking (see page 255).

You may also want to include some postpartum items on your birthing plan, such as:

❖ Your presence at the weighing of the baby, the administration of eye drops, the pediatric exam, and baby's first bath.

❖ Baby feeding in the hospital (whether it will be controlled by the nursery's schedule or your baby's hunger; whether breastfeeding will be supported; whether supplementary bottles can be avoided).

❖ Management of breast engorgement if you're not breastfeeding (page 382).

❖ Circumcision.

❖ Rooming in.

❖ Other children visiting with you and/or with the new baby.

❖ Postpartum medication or treatments for you or your baby.

❖ The length of the hospital stay, barring complications.

Of course with some of these items, your practitioner's judgment or hospital rules will affect the final plan. And remember that while it is ideal if your plans can be carried through the way you drew them up, it isn't always possible. Since there is no way to predict in advance precisely how labor and delivery will progress, childbirth plans you make before the process begins may not end up being in the best interests of you and your baby, and may have to be changed at the last minute. If this happens, try to keep in mind that the priorities in any birth should be the health and safety of mother and child—and that all other considerations must be secondary.

WHAT IT'S IMPORTANT TO KNOW:
ALL ABOUT CHILDBIRTH MEDICATION

On January 19, 1847, Scottish physician James Young Simpson splashed a half teaspoonful of chloroform on a handkerchief and held it over the nose of a laboring woman. Less than half an hour later, she became the first woman to deliver while under anesthesia. (There was only one complication: When the

4. For more information on these postpartum issues, see *What to Expect the First Year*.

woman—whose first baby had been born after three days of painful labor—awoke, Dr. Simpson was unable to convince her that she'd actually given birth.)

This revolution in obstetrical practice was welcomed by women but fought by both the clergy and some members of the medical profession, who believed that pain in childbirth (woman's punishment for Eve's indiscretions in Eden) was a burden that women were born to carry. Relief of the pain would be immoral.

But opponents didn't stand a chance at halting the revolution. Once word got around that childbirth didn't have to hurt, obstetrical patients wouldn't take "no pain relief" for an answer. No longer was it a question of whether anesthesia had a place in obstetrics, but what kind of anesthesia would fill that place best.

The search for the perfect pain reliever—a drug that would eliminate pain without harming mother or child—was on. Enormous progress was made (and is still being made); analgesics and anesthetics became safer and more effective every year.

And then, during the 1950s and '60s, the love affair between childbirth medication and obstetrical patients began to get shaky. Women wanted to be awake for their deliveries and to experience every sensation, in spite of the discomfort. And they wanted their babies to arrive as alert as they were—not drugged from the effects of anesthesia.

Through the 1970s and into the 1980s, singleminded women waged war against recalcitrant physicians, the battle cry being "natural childbirth for all." Today enlightened practitioners and patients alike recognize that wanting relief from excruciating pain is natural, and that therefore pain relief medication can play a role in natural childbirth. Though an unmedicated birth is still considered the

ideal, it's understood that there are times when it's not in the best interests of mother and/or child. Medication is recommended when:

❖ Labor is long and complicated—since pain stress can lead to chemical imbalances that can interfere with contractions, compromise blood flow to the fetus, and exhaust the mother, reducing her ability to push effectively.

❖ The pain is more than the mother can tolerate, or is interfering with her ability to push.

❖ Outlet forceps (to ease the baby out once its head is visible at the vaginal outlet) are required.

❖ It's necessary to slow down a precipitous (dangerously rapid) labor.

❖ A mother is so agitated that she is hindering the progress of labor.

Prudent use of any type of medication always requires a careful weighing of risk against benefit. In the case of obstetrical drugs used during labor and delivery, risks and benefits must be examined for both mother and baby, making the equation a more complicated one. In some instances, the risks of medications clearly outweigh the benefits they offer—such as when the fetus, because of prematurity or other factors, doesn't appear strong enough to cope with the combined stress of labor *and* drugs.

Most experts agree that when childbirth medication is used, benefits can be increased and risks reduced by:

❖ Selecting a drug that has minimal side effects and presents the least risk to mother and baby while still providing pain relief; giving it in the smallest dose that will be effective; and administering it at the optimum time in the course of labor. Exposure to general anesthetic agents is usually minimized in cesarean deliveries by extracting the fetus within minutes of administering the drug to the mother, before it has a chance to cross the placenta in significant amounts.

❖ Having an expert anesthesiologist or anesthetist administer anesthesia. (You have the right to insist on this if you are having general or regional—spinal, epidural, etc.— anesthesia.)

A major concern of careful medicating in obstetrics is not only the safety of the direct recipient (the mother), but that of the indirect recipient and innocent bystander (the baby). A baby whose mother has been given medication during delivery may be born drowsy, sluggish, unresponsive, and, less often, with breathing and sucking difficulties and an irregular heartbeat. Studies show, however, that when drugs have been properly used, these adverse effects largely disappear soon after birth. A fetus can handle a certain degree of the depression or arrested activity that sometimes results from too much medication in labor or too much anesthesia during delivery; only extreme depression is hazardous. If a baby is so drugged that he doesn't breathe spontaneously at birth, quick resuscitation (a simple procedure) will prevent long-term damage.

Yet another concern in administering pain relief is how it will affect the progress of labor; given at the wrong time, it could slow or even stop it.

WHAT KINDS OF PAIN RELIEF ARE MOST COMMONLY USED?

A variety of analgesics (pain relievers), anesthetics (substances that produce loss of sensation), and ataraxics (tranquilizers) may be given during labor and delivery. Which drug, if any, will be administered will depend on the stage of labor, the patient's preference (except in an emergency), the past health history of the mother, and her present condition as well as that of her baby, as well as upon the obstetrician's and/or anesthesiologist's preference and expertise. The efficacy will depend upon the woman, the dosage, and other factors. (Very rarely, a drug won't produce the desired effect, and will give little or no pain relief.) Obstetrical pain relief is most commonly accomplished with the following drugs:

Analgesics. Meperidine hydrochloride, a powerful pain reliever commonly known under the trade name Demerol, is one of the most frequently used obstetrical analgesics. It is most effectively administered intravenously (injected slowly into an IV apparatus, so that its effects can be gauged) or intramuscularly (one shot, usually in the buttocks, though the medication may be repeated every two to four hours as needed). Demerol does not usually interfere with the contractions or their work, though with larger doses the contractions may become less frequent or weaker. It may actually help normalize contractions in a dysfunctional uterus (one that is functioning abnormally). Like other analgesics, Demerol is not generally administered until labor is well established and false labor has been ruled out, but at least two to three hours before delivery is expected. A mother's reaction to the drug and the degree of pain relief achieved vary widely. Some women find it relaxes them and makes them better able to cope with contractions. Others very much dislike the drowsy feeling and find they are less able to cope. Side effects may, depending on a woman's sensitivity, include nausea, vomiting, depression, and a drop in blood pressure. The effect Demerol will have on the newborn depends on the total dose and how close to delivery it has been administered. If it has been given too close to delivery, the baby may be sleepy and unable to suck; less frequently, respiration may be depressed and supplemental oxygen may be required. These effects are generally short-term and, if necessary, can be counteracted. Demerol may also be given postpartum to relieve the pain of an episiotomy repair or a cesarean.

Tranquilizers. These drugs (such as Phenergan or Vistaril) are used to calm and relax an anxious woman so that she can participate more fully in childbirth. Tranquilizers can also enhance the effectiveness of analgesics, such as Demerol. Like analgesics, tranquilizers are usually administered once labor is well established, and considerably before delivery. But they are occasionally used in early labor if a first-time mother is extremely nervous. Women's reactions to the effects of tranquilizers vary. Some welcome the gentle drowsiness; others find it interferes with their control. A small dose may serve to relieve anxiety without impairing alertness. A larger dose may cause slurring of speech and dozing between contraction peaks—making use of prepared childbirth techniques difficult. Though the risks to a fetus or newborn from tranquilizers are minimal (except in cases of fetal distress), it's a good idea for you and your coach to try nondrug relaxation techniques before asking for medication.

Inhalants. Nitrous oxide is rarely used today, except in combination with other drugs to induce general anesthesia.

Regional Nerve Blocks. Anesthetics injected along the course of a nerve or nerves may be used to deaden sensation in that region. In childbirth, anesthetics may completely numb the area from the waist down for surgical delivery, or numb a smaller area partially or totally for a vaginal one. Regional blocks have an advantage over general anesthesia for surgical delivery, in that the mother is awake during the birth and is alert afterward. In a vaginal delivery, they have the possible disadvantage of inhibiting the urge to push. Occasionally, oxytocin may be administered to rev up contractions that have become sluggish because of the anesthetic effect. Sometimes a catheter (tube) is inserted into the bladder to drain urine (because the urge to urinate is also suppressed). The most frequently used blocks are: pudendal, epidural, spinal, and caudal.

A pudendal block, occasionally used to relieve early second-stage pain, is usually reserved for the vaginal delivery itself. Administered through a needle inserted into the perineal or vaginal area (while the mother lies on her back with her feet in stirrups), it reduces pain in the region, but not uterine discomfort. It is useful when outlet forceps are used, and its effect can last through episiotomy and repair. It is frequently used in combination with Demerol or a tranquilizer to provide excellent pain relief with relative safety—even when an anesthesiologist is not available.

The epidural block (or lumbar epidural) is becoming increasingly popular for both vaginal and cesarean deliveries, as well as for the relief of severe labor pain. The major reason is its relative safety (less drug is needed to achieve the desired effect) and its ease of administration. The drug (usually bupivacaine, lidocaine, or chloroprocaine) is administered as needed during labor and/or delivery, through a fine tube that has been inserted through a needle in the back (after a local anesthetic numbs the area), into the epidural space between the spinal cord and the outer membrane, usually while the mother lies on her left side or sits up and leans over a table to steady herself. The medication can be stopped in time to allow the mother to have full control over pushing and then be restarted after delivery, during the repair of any episiotomy. Blood pressure is checked frequently because the procedure can cause it to drop suddenly. Intravenous fluids, and possibly medication, may be given to counteract this reaction. Leaning the uterus to the left may also help. Because of the risk of a blood pressure drop, an epidural is generally not used when there is a bleeding complication, such as placenta previa, severe preeclampsia or eclampsia, or fetal distress. Because an epidural is sometimes associated with slowing of the fetal heartbeat, continuous fetal monitoring is usually required.

Epidurals have been associated with an increased need for cesarean, forceps, and vacuum deliveries. But recent studies have shown that when it is administered after the cervix has dilated to 4 cm and active labor has begun, there is no increase in c-sections. Nor is there an increase with a "walking epidural" (used with growing frequency), which uses a lower dose and a different mix of drugs than the traditional epidural. Although it diminishes pain, the walking epidural does not diminish sensation or motor function, allowing the laboring woman to sense the contractions and to get up and walk around if she wishes.

If you feel the need for an epidural, be sure it is given after labor begins and dilation reaches 4 cm; ask, too, that the level of medication not be so high as to totally block your motor function. Or ask for a walking epidural.

[5] It's been suggested that women with pain severe enough to require an epidural may be destined for a difficult labor, which may explain some of the increased need for interventions.

Spinal blocks (for cesarean) and low spinal, or saddle, blocks (for forcepsassisted vaginal delivery) are administered in a single dose just prior to delivery. The mother lies on her side (back arched, neck and knees flexed) and an anesthetic is injected into the fluid surrounding the spinal cord. There may be some nausea and vomiting while the drug is in effect, about 1 to 1½ hours. As with an epidural, there is a risk of a drop in blood pressure. Elevation of the legs, leaning the uterus to the left, intravenous fluids, and, occasionally, medication may be used to prevent or counteract this complication. After delivery, spinal-block patients must usually remain flat on their backs for about eight hours, and a few may experience post-spinal headache. As with epidurals, spinals are not usually used when there is placenta previa, preeclampsia or eclampsia, or fetal distress.

The caudal block blocks sensation in a more limited area than the epidural, is more difficult to administer and takes a larger dose to be effective. It also inhibits labor. For these reasons, it is used infrequently.

General Anesthesia. Once the most popular pain relief for delivery, general anesthesia—which puts the patient to sleep—is used today almost exclusively for surgical births, and occasionally for delivering the head in a vaginal breech. Because of its rapid effect, it is more likely to be used in emergency cesareans, when there is no time for a regional anesthetic to be administered.

Inhalants, such as those used for analgesic effect, are used to induce general anesthesia—often in conjunction with other agents. This is done by an anesthesiologist in an operating/delivery room. The mother is awake during the preparations and unconscious for however long it takes to complete the delivery (usually a matter of minutes). When she comes to she may be groggy, disoriented, and restless. She may also have a cough and sore throat (due to the endotracheal tube), experience nausea and vomiting, and find her bowels and bladder sluggish. A temporary drop in blood pressure is another possible side effect.

The major problem with general anesthesia is that as the mother is sedated, so is the fetus. Sedation of the fetus can be minimized, however, by administering the anesthesia as close to the actual birth as possible. That way the baby can be delivered before the anesthetic has reached him or her in meaningful amount. Administering oxygen to the mother and tilting her to the side (usually the left side), can also help get oxygen to the fetus.

The other major risk of general anesthesia is that the mother may vomit and aspirate (inhale) the vomited material, which can cause complications, such as aspiration pneumonia. That's why you are asked not to eat or drink a lot of liquids when in active labor and why, if you do have general anesthesia, an endotracheal tube will be inserted through your mouth into your throat to prevent aspiration. You may be given oral antacids just prior to the procedure to neutralize the acids in your stomach in case you do aspirate.

Hypnosis. Despite the somewhat disreputable image it's developed on the nightclub circuit, hypnosis, in qualified hands, provides a legitimate, medically acceptable route to pain relief. There's really nothing mysterious about hypnosis. Suggestion and the power of mind over matter are taught in every good childbirth preparation class. With hypnosis a very high level of suggestibility is achieved, which (depending on an individual's susceptibility and the type of hypnosis used) can do anything from making the patient more relaxed and comfortable to completely eliminating awareness of pain. Only about 1 in 4 adults is hypnotizable to some degree. (A very small percentage can even go through an unmedicated cesarean section without feeling any pain.)

Training of a subject in hypnosis for childbirth should start weeks or months in advance, under a physician certified in the subject or another practitioner recommended by your physician. You may use auto- or self-hypnosis, or you may depend upon the practitioner to make the suggestions. Either way, use caution—hypnosis can be misused.

Other Methods of Pain Relief. There are several techniques aimed at reducing the perception of pain that do not require the use of drugs, and that are sometimes effective. They are particularly good choices for women who are in drug or alcohol recovery and those who do not want to use drugs for other reasons.

TENS (Transcutaneous Electrical Nerve Stimulation). TENS uses electrodes to stimulate nerve pathways to the uterus and cervix. It's theorized that this stimulation jams other sensory inputs along those pathways, such as pain. The intensity of stimulation is controlled by the patient, allowing her to increase it during a contraction, reduce it in between. More hospitals are making TENS available and it may be worthwhile checking to see if yours is one of them.

Acupuncture. Long popular in China and sometimes used in the U.S., acupuncture probably works according to the same principles as TENS. But the stimulation is supplied by needles inserted and manipulated through the skin.

Alteration of the risk factors for increased pain perception. A number of factors, emotional and physical, can affect how a woman perceives the pain of childbirth. Altering them can often increase comfort during labor (see page 298).

Physical therapy. Massage, heat, pressure, or counterpressure administered by a health professional or a loving spouse or friend often lessens the perception of pain.

Distraction. Anything—watching TV, listening to music, meditating. practicing breathing exercises—that takes your mind off the pain can decrease your perception of it. Visualization exercises (create your own) can also help.

MAKING THE DECISION

Women have more options in childbirth today than ever before. And with the exception of certain emergency situations, the decision of whether or not to have medication during labor and delivery will be largely yours. To try to make the best possible decision, for you and your baby:

❖ Discuss the topic of pain relief and anesthesia with your practitioner long before labor begins. Your practitioner's expertise and experience make him or her an invaluable partner in your decision-making process. Well before your first contraction, find out what kinds of drugs or procedures he or she uses most often, what side effects may be experienced, when he or she considers medication absolutely necessary and when the option is yours.

❖ Recognize that, although childbirth is a natural experience that many women can go through without medication, it is not supposed to be a trial by ordeal or a test of bravery, strength, or endurance. The pain of childbirth has been described as the most intense in the human experience. Medical technology has given women the option of relief through medication or other techniques. Not only is such relief acceptable, it is, sometimes, preferable.

❖ Keep in mind that taking childbirth medication (or any medication) en-

tails both risks and benefits, and it should be used only when the benefits outweigh the risks.

❖ Don't make up and close your mind in advance. Though it's okay to theorize what might be best for you under certain circumstances, it's impossible to predict what kind of labor and delivery you'll have, how you will respond to the contractions, and whether or not you'll want, need, or have to have medication. Even if you're scheduled for a cesarean, you can plan only tentatively on an epidural; last-minute complications could necessitate general anesthesia.

❖ If during labor you feel you need medication, discuss it with your coach and the nurse or doctor. But don't insist on it immediately. Try holding out 15 minutes or so and putting that time to the best possible use—concentrating extra-hard on your relaxation or breathing techniques and taking in all the comfort your coach can give you. You may find that with a little more support you can handle the pain, or that the progress you make in those 15 minutes gives you the will to go on without help. If after waiting you find that you need the relief as much or even more, ask for it—and don't feel guilty. If, of course, your physician decides that you need medication immediately, for your sake or your baby's, waiting may not be advisable.

❖ Remember that your well-being and that of your baby are your number one priority (as they have been all through pregnancy), not some preconceived, idealized childbirth scenario. All decisions should be made with that priority in mind.

12
The Eighth Month

WHAT YOU CAN EXPECT AT THIS MONTH'S CHECKUPS

After the 32nd week, your practitioner may ask you to come in every two weeks so you and your baby can be more closely monitored. You can expect the following to be checked, depending upon your particular needs and upon your practitioner's style of practice:[1]

❖ Weight and blood pressure

❖ Urine, for sugar and protein

❖ Fetal heartbeat

❖ Height of fundus (top of uterus)

❖ Size (you may get a rough weight estimate) and position of fetus, by palpation

❖ Feet and hands for edema (swelling), and legs for varicose veins

❖ Symptoms you have been experiencing, especially unusual ones

❖ Questions and problems you want to discuss—have a list ready

WHAT YOU MAY BE FEELING

You may experience all of these symptoms at one time or another, or only a few of them. Some may have continued from last month, others may be new or hardly noticeable. You may also have other, less common, symptoms.

1. See Appendix for an explanation of the procedures and tests performed during office visits.

PHYSICALLY:

❖ Strong, regular fetal activity

❖ Increasingly heavy whitish vaginal discharge (leukorrhea)

❖ Increased constipation

❖ Heartburn, indigestion, flatulence, bloating

❖ Occasional headaches, faintness or dizziness

❖ Nasal congestion and occasional nosebleeds; ear stuffiness

❖ Bleeding gums

❖ Leg cramps

❖ Backache

❖ Mild swelling of ankles and feet, and occasionally of hands and face

❖ Varicose veins of legs

❖ Hemorrhoids

❖ Itchy abdomen, protruding navel

❖ Increasing shortness of breath as uterus crowds the lungs, which eases when the baby drops

❖ Difficulty sleeping

❖ Increasing Braxton Hicks contractions

❖ Increasing clumsiness

❖ Colostrum, either leaking or expressed, from breasts (though this premilk substance may not appear until after delivery)

EMOTIONALLY:

❖ Increasing eagerness for the pregnancy to be over

❖ Apprehension about the baby's health, about labor and delivery

❖ Increasing absentmindedness

❖ Excitement at the realization that *it* won't be long now

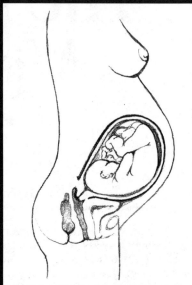

WHAT YOU MAY LOOK LIKE

By the end of the eighth month, the baby is about 18 inches long and weighs 5 pounds. Growth, especially of the brain, is great in this period, and the fetus can see and hear. Most systems are well developed, but the lungs may still be immature. Baby has an excellent chance of survival if born now.

WHAT YOU MAY BE CONCERNED ABOUT

SHORTNESS OF BREATH

"Sometimes I have trouble breathing. Could this mean that my baby isn't getting enough oxygen?"

Shortness of breath doesn't mean you—or your baby—are short of oxygen. Changes in the respiratory system during pregnancy actually allow women to take in *more* oxygen and to use it more efficiently. Still, most women experience varying degrees of difficulty breathing (some describe it as feeling a conscious need to breathe more deeply)—particularly in the last trimester, when the expanding uterus presses against the diaphragm, crowding the lungs. Relief usually arrives when lightening occurs (when the fetus settles back down into the pelvis, in first pregnancies generally two to three weeks before delivery). In the meantime, you may find it easier to breathe if you sit straight up instead of slumped over, sleep in a semi-propped-up position, and avoid overexertion.

Women who carry "low" throughout their pregnancies may never experience such exaggerated shortness of breath, and that's normal too.

Shortness of breath that is severe, however, and is accompanied by rapid breathing, blueness of lips and fingertips, chest pain, and/or rapid pulse isn't normal and requires an immediate call to the doctor or trip to the emergency room.

NOT SO FUNNY RIB TICKLING

"It feels as though my son has his feet jammed up into my rib cage—and it really hurts."

In the later months, when fetuses can't always get comfortable in their cramped quarters, they often do seem to find a snug niche for their feet between their mother's ribs, and that's one kind of rib tickling that doesn't tickle. Changing your own position may convince him to change his. A few Dromedary Droops (page 192) may dislodge him. Or try taking a deep breath while you raise one arm over your head, then exhale while you drop your arm; repeat a few times with each arm.

If none of these tactics work, hang in there. When your little pain-in-the-ribs engages, or drops into your pelvis, which usually happens two or three weeks before delivery in first pregnancies (though not until labor begins in subsequent ones), he probably won't be able to get his toes up quite so high.

STRESS INCONTINENCE

"I've started leaking urine occasionally. Is something wrong?"

In the last trimester, some women start to leak a little urine—usually only when they laugh (or cough, or sneeze). This is called stress incontinence, and is the result of the mounting pressure of the growing uterus on the bladder. Kegel exercises (see page 190), which are also useful for firming up pelvic muscles for delivery and postpartum recovery, may help control incontinence. But, because there's a slight chance the leak is amniotic fluid, report it to your doctor.

YOUR WEIGHT GAIN AND THE BABY'S SIZE

"I've gained so much weight that I'm afraid the baby will be very big and difficult to deliver."

Just because you've gained a lot of weight doesn't necessarily mean your baby has. A 35- to 40-pound weight gain can yield a 6- or 7-pound baby, or an even smaller one if the weight was gained largely on junk food. On the average, however, a larger weight gain produces a larger baby. Your baby's size may also be influenced by your own birthweight (if you were born large or small, your baby will tend to be too) and by your prepregnancy weight (in general, heavier women have heavier babies). By palpating your abdomen and measuring the height of your fundus (the top of the uterus), your practitioner will be able to give you some idea of your baby's size, though such "guess-timates" can be off by a pound or more. A sonogram may more accurately gauge size, but it may be off too.

Even if your baby is large, that doesn't automatically portend a difficult delivery. Though a 6- or 7-pound baby often makes its way out faster than an 8- or 9-pounder, many women are able to deliver a bigger baby vaginally and without complications. The determining factor, as in any delivery, is whether the baby's head (its largest part) can fit through the mother's pelvis. At one time, x-rays were routinely used to try to determine whether or not a mismatch between the fetal head and the mother's pelvis (cephalopelvic disproportion, or CPD) existed. But experience and research have shown that an x-ray is not an accurate predictor of CPD, partly because it can't foresee to what extent the fetal head will mold in order to squeeze through the birth canal. Though the risk of an x-ray is slight, it is recommended only rarely, when benefits outweigh that risk.

More commonly today, when there is some suspicion of cephalopelvic disproportion (sometimes also called fetopelvic disproportion), the practitioner will allow the mother to go into labor naturally. This trial of labor is carefully monitored, and if the fetal head descends and the cervix dilates at a normal rate, then the labor will be permitted to continue. If labor doesn't progress, it may, when appropriate, get a boost with the administration of oxytocin. If no progress is made, a cesarean will usually be required.

HOW YOU'RE CARRYING

"Everyone says I seem to be carrying small and low for the eighth month. Could it be that my baby isn't growing properly?"

It would be a good idea to make earplugs and blinders a part of every pregnant woman's maternity wardrobe. Wearing them for nine months would enable her to avoid the worry generated by the misguided commentary and advice of relatives and friends—even strangers—and prevent invidious comparisons of her belly to those of other pregnant women who are larger, smaller, lower, or higher.

Just as no two prepregnant figures are proportioned in precisely the same fashion, no two pregnant silhouettes are identical. How you carry, both in size and shape, is dependent on whether you started out tall or short, thin or not-so-thin, petite or voluptuous. And it is seldom an indication of the size of the baby you're carrying. A petite woman carrying low and small may give birth to a larger infant than a bigger-boned woman carrying high and wide.

The only accurate assessments of your baby's progress and well-being are likely to come from your practitioner. When you're not in his or her office, keep your earplugs in and your blinders on—and you'll have a lot less to worry about.

PRESENTATION AND POSITION OF THE BABY

"My doctor says the baby is in a breech position. How will this affect my labor and delivery?"

It's never too early to prepare yourself for the possibility of a breech birth, but it's definitely too early now to resign yourself to one. Most babies settle into a head-down position between the 32nd and 36th weeks, but a few keep their parents and doctors guessing until only a few days before delivery.

Some nurse-midwives recommend doing exercises in the last eight weeks, designed to encourage a breech baby to turn. There's no medical proof that these exercises work, but there's also none to suggest that they do any harm.

When a fetus is still in the breech position near term, a physician may attempt external cephalic version (ECV), applying his or her hands to the mother's abdomen and gently, with ultrasound guidance, trying to shift the fetus to the head-down position. The condition of the fetus is monitored continuously to be sure that the umbilical cord isn't accidentally compressed or the placenta disturbed. The procedure is best performed before labor begins or very early in labor, when the uterus is still relatively relaxed. Once turned, most fetuses stay head down, but a few do revert to breech before delivery.

When successful (as it is more than half the time), ECV can reduce the likelihood that a cesarean delivery will be necessary. For this reason ECV has become popular, with a majority of physicians using it at least occasionally. Some, however, hesitate to use it because of the possibility of complica-

Carrying Baby, Eighth Month

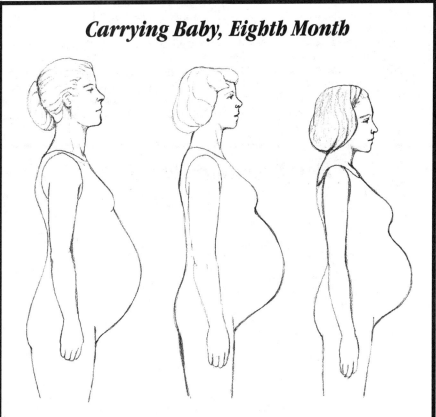

These are just three of the very different ways that a woman may carry near the end of her eighth month. The variations are even greater than before. Depending on the size and position of your baby, as well as your own size and weight gain, you may be carrying higher, lower, bigger, smaller, wider, or more compactly.

tions. Only a physician who has been trained to do ECV—and is prepared to do an emergency c-section if a problem arises—should attempt it.

Breeches are more common when the fetus is smaller than average and not cradled snugly in the uterus, when the uterus is unusually shaped, when there is an excess of amniotic fluid, when there is more than one fetus, and when the uterus is relatively relaxed because of having been stretched during previous pregnancies. If your baby is one of the 3% or 4% in breech position at term, you should discuss the delivery possibilities with your physician (nurse-midwives do not usually handle breech births). You may be able to have a normal vaginal delivery, or, depending on various conditions, you may indeed have to undergo a cesarean. (Which is *not* the end of the world, and for which eventuality every pregnant woman should be prepared anyway. See page 307.)

There appears to be little strong scientific evidence pointing to either vaginal or cesarean as the better way to deliver a breech baby. Vaginal deliveries are believed to be perfectly safe in about one-third to one-half of breech births, but *only* if the doctor is experienced in the proper procedure for such deliveries. Some studies of vaginal breech deliveries show that the potential risk is not always from the delivery itself, but from the reason for the breech: for example, the baby is premature or undersize, there are multiple fetuses, or there is some other congenital problem.

Some physicians routinely perform cesarean sections for breech presentations, believing this is the safest route to follow for the baby (in this malpractice climate, it can also be the best route for the doctors themselves, since they avoid the possibility of being blamed for a baby being harmed because a c-section was not performed). Others, persuaded by their

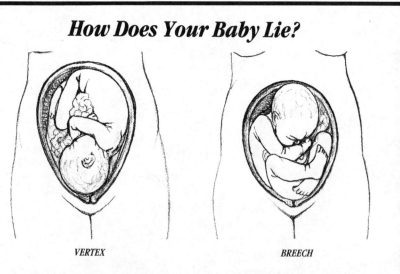

How Does Your Baby Lie?

VERTEX   BREECH

About 96 out of every 100 babies present head first (vertex). The rest are usually in one or another breech position (buttocks first). The complete breech is illustrated here. The frank breech, in which the baby's legs are folded straight up, is the easiest breech to deliver vaginally.

own experience as well as studies that show that mode of delivery doesn't affect outcome in breech deliveries, permit a trial of labor under the following conditions:

❖ The baby is a frank breech (the legs are folded flat up against the face).

❖ The baby is determined to be small enough (usually under 8½ pounds) for easy passage, but not so small (under 5½ pounds) that a vaginal delivery would be risky. Usually, breech babies under 36 weeks are delivered by cesarean.

❖ There is no evidence of placenta previa, prolapsed umbilical cord, or fetal distress that can't be easily remedied.

❖ The mother has no obstetrical or medical problem that could complicate a vaginal delivery, appears to have an adequate-size pelvis, and has no history of previous difficult or traumatic deliveries. Some physicians add the requirement that the mother be under 35.

❖ The presenting part is engaged (has descended into the pelvis) as labor begins.

❖ The fetal head is not hyperextended, but rather the chin is tucked down toward the chest.

❖ Everything (and everyone) is in readiness for an emergency surgical delivery if one should suddenly become necessary.

When a vaginal delivery is to be attempted, labor is carefully monitored in a surgically equipped delivery suite. If all goes well, it is allowed to continue. If the cervix dilates too slowly or if other problems arise, the doctor and surgical team are ready to perform a cesarean section in a matter of minutes. Continuous electronic fetal monitoring is absolutely essential.

Sometimes an epidural (see page 229) is administered to prevent the mother from bearing down too hard before she is fully dilated (which might lead to the cord being compressed between the baby and the pelvis). Occasionally, general anesthesia is administered to the mother when the baby is halfway delivered, to permit rapid completion of the birth by the physician. Forceps may be used to keep the head properly flexed, and to help deliver the head without pulling too much on the body or neck. A wide episiotomy is often routinely made to facilitate the process.

Sometimes when a cesarean is scheduled, labor progresses so quickly that the baby's buttocks slip into the pelvis before surgery is begun. In that case, most doctors will attempt a vaginal delivery rather than a rushed and difficult cesarean.

"How can I tell if my baby is lying the right way for delivery?"

Playing "name that bump" (trying to figure out which are shoulders, elbows, and bottom) may be better evening entertainment than TV, but it's not the most accurate way of determining your baby's position. Your doctor or nurse-midwife can probably get a better idea than you, by palpating your abdomen with the flat of his or her trained hands for recognizable baby parts. The baby's back, for instance, is usually a smooth, convex contour opposite a bunch of little irregularities which are the "small parts"—hands, feet, elbows. In the eighth month, the head has usually settled near your pelvis; it is round, firm, and—when pushed down—bounces back without the rest of the body moving. The baby's bottom is a less regular shape, and softer, than the head. The location of the baby's heartbeat is another clue to its position—if the presentation is head first, the heartbeat will usually be heard in the lower half of your abdomen; it will be loudest if the baby's back is toward your front. If there's any doubt about the position, a sonogram may be used for verification.

YOUR SAFETY DURING CHILDBIRTH

"I know medical science has taken most of the risk out of giving birth, but I'm still afraid of dying during delivery."

There was a time when mothers routinely risked their lives to have children; they still do in some areas of the world. In the United States today, the risk to maternal life in labor and delivery is virtually non-existent. Fewer than 1 in 10,000 women die in childbirth. And this figure includes not only women with chronic heart conditions and other serious illnesses, but those who give birth in backwoods shacks and dingy tenements, without medical assistance.

In short, even if your pregnancy falls into the highest-risk category—and certainly if it doesn't—you stand a lot better chance of surviving labor and delivery than you do a trip to the supermarket in your car, or a stroll across a busy street.

ADEQUACY FOR DELIVERY

"I'm 5 feet tall and very petite. I'm afraid I'll have trouble delivering a baby."

Fortunately, when it comes to giving birth, it's what's inside, not what's outside, that counts. The size and shape of your pelvis in relation to the size of your baby's head is what determines how difficult your labor will be. And you can't always tell a

pelvis by its cover. A short, slight woman can have a roomier pelvis than a tall, stocky woman. Your practitioner can make an educated guess about its size—usually using measurements taken at your first prenatal exam. If there's some concern that your baby's head is too large to fit through your pelvis while you're in labor, a sonogram may be done.

Of course, in general the overall size of the pelvis, as of all bony structures, is smaller in people of smaller stature. For example, Asian women usually have smaller pelvises than Nordic women. Luckily nature, in its wisdom, rarely presents an Asian woman with a Nordic-size baby—even when the father is a 6-foot fullback. Instead, all things being equal, babies are generally fairly well matched to the size of their mothers.

TWIN LABOR AND DELIVERY

"I'm expecting twins. How will my labor and delivery be different from that of other women?"

There may not be any differences—other than the fact that you'll reap twice the reward for your efforts. Many twin deliveries turn out to be normal, vaginal, and uncomplicated.[2]

However, it's not surprising that there is more potential for complications during the delivery of twins. In most cases the problems don't arise in the first phase of labor, which is actually shorter, on the average, in twin deliveries than in singleton ones. (And though active labor and the pushing

---

2. With each increase in the number of fetuses, however, the likelihood of a surgical delivery increases.

phase are usually longer, the total time from the first contraction to the birth of the babies is generally shorter.) Though most twins can be delivered vaginally (sometimes with the use of forceps to avoid putting the babies through excessive trauma), it is usually recommended that an anesthesiologist be on hand in case a cesarean is needed. A pediatrician or a neonatologist usually stands by too, ready to deal with any immediate problems in the newborns. Often both fetuses are monitored, one externally and the other internally, with scalp electrodes.

With twins, as you will soon find out, you can always expect the unexpected. And this can start at delivery. Because there is more than one baby, and possibly more than one set of circumstances, there may be more than one type of delivery. Perhaps, after the first baby arrives easily via the vaginal route, the second, lying crosswise and unturnable, has to be extracted abdominally. Perhaps though the first infant's amniotic sac ruptures spontaneously, the other twin's has to be ruptured artificially.

In most cases, the second twin comes along within 20 minutes of its sibling. If number two is a slowpoke, the physician may administer oxytocin or use forceps to facilitate delivery, or he or she may perform a cesarean. Once both twins are born, the placenta or placentas usually separate quickly. But sometimes their actual delivery is slow and requires some help from the physician.

BANKING YOUR OWN BLOOD

"I'm worried about the possibility of needing a transfusion during delivery and receiving contaminated blood. Can I store my own blood beforehand?"

First of all, there is very little likelihood you will need a blood transfusion. Only 1% of vaginal deliveries and 2% of cesareans require one. A woman typically loses only 1 to 2 cups of blood (½ to 1 pint) during vaginal childbirth and 2 to 4 cups with a cesarean. This loss presents no problem since in pregnancy the blood volume is up 40% to 50% anyway. Second, the risk of contracting AIDS or hepatitis B or C (the diseases most commonly transmitted through the blood) from a transfusion in the U.S. today is very low (estimated to be anywhere from 1 in 40,000 to 1 in 250,000), since all donated blood is screened by some very accurate (though not foolproof) tests. Third, because facilities for autologous (self) blood donations are limited and priority is given to those about to undergo major high-risk surgery, women who are about to deliver may not even be accepted for such a donation.

If, however, you have reason to believe that you may be at high risk for blood loss during delivery because your blood does not clot normally, because you are scheduled for a cesarean delivery, or for some other reason, speak to your doctor about the possibility of making an autologous blood donation. (Donating the blood late in pregnancy could be a problem because it could lower your blood volume excessively or lead to anemia.) Or plan to have a relative or friend with compatible blood make a directed donation (one to a specific person) just prior to delivery or standing by at the time of delivery just in case. Not every hospital is equipped for or willing to oblige with directed donations, and personnel may point out that the risk of contracting AIDS from a blood transfusion isn't any lower when the donation is from a friend or family member than when it's from the general blood supply.

HAVING A CESAREAN SECTION

"My doctor just told me I will have to have a cesarean. But I'm afraid the surgery will be dangerous."

Though popular lore has it that the cesarean section got its name because Julius Caesar came into the world via abdominal delivery, that's virtually impossible. Julius might have survived such an operation, but his mother wouldn't have—and it is known that Mrs. Caesar lived for many years after his birth.

Today, however, cesareans are nearly as safe as vaginal deliveries for the mother, and in difficult deliveries or when there's fetal distress, they are often the safest delivery mode for the baby. Even though it is technically considered major surgery, a cesarean carries relatively minor risks—much closer to those of a tonsillectomy than of a gall bladder operation, for instance.

Learning all you can about cesarean sections before delivery—from your doctor, in your childbirth class (a special class on cesareans is ideal), and through reading—will help to prepare you and to ease your fears.

"The doctor says I may have to have a cesarean section. I'm worried that this may be dangerous for the baby."

Chances are that if you have a cesarean, your baby will be at least as safe, and possibly safer, than if you had had a vaginal delivery. Every year thousands of babies who might not have survived the perilous journey through the birth canal (or might have survived impaired) are lifted from their mothers' abdomens sound and unscathed.

Though there has been some speculation that cesareans are somehow harmful to babies, there's no hard evidence that this is so. Of course a higher proportion of cesarean babies are found to have medical problems, but these problems are most often due to the distress that necessitated the operation, not to the operation itself. Many of these infants would not have made it through a natural delivery.

In most ways, babies delivered via cesarean don't differ from those delivered vaginally—though cesarean babies do have the edge in initial appearance. Because they don't have to accommodate to the narrow confines of the pelvis, they usually have nicely rounded, not pointy, heads.

Apgar scores, which rate an infant's condition one and five minutes after birth, are comparable in babies born vaginally and those born by cesarean. Cesarean-born babies do have the slight disadvantage of not having some of the excess mucus squeezed out of their respiratory tracts in the birthing process, but this mucus can be easily suctioned after delivery. Very, very rarely is any serious damage sustained by a baby during cesarean delivery—much more rarely than during vaginal deliveries. They are, however, at higher risk of respiratory problems if they do not go through labor at all.

The most likely kind of damage a baby delivered abdominally might suffer is psychological—not from the delivery itself, but because of the mother's attitude toward it. Occasionally a mother who has had a cesarean will subconsciously harbor resentment toward the baby who she feels deprived her of her finest hour and brought such insult to her body.[3] She may allow the jealousy she feels toward mothers who've delivered vaginally, and the guilt she feels about "failing," interfere with the establishment of a

---

3. Women who deliver vaginally may also resent their babies, almost always temporarily, because of the pain of delivery.

good relationship with her baby. Or she may incorrectly assume that the cesarean-born infant is unusually fragile (few are) and become overprotective. If she develops such feelings, the mother should try to confront and resolve them, seeking professional help if necessary.

But often, destructive attitudes can be avoided right from the start. First, by recognizing that the method by which a baby is delivered in no way reflects on either the mother or the child; a woman is no less a mother and her baby is no less the fruit of her womb when there is a cesarean birth rather than a vaginal one. Second, by making sure there is an opportunity for you and your baby to have time together as early as possible. Long before you go into labor, let your doctor know that if you have a cesarean you would like to be able to hold or even nurse the baby on the operating table, or if that's not possible, in the recovery room. If you wait until delivery day to state your case, you may not have the strength or opportunity to make it. Planning ahead also gives you the chance to question contrary hospital rules, such as those requiring every cesarean-delivered newborn, even healthy ones, to spend some time in the neonatal intensive care unit. If you present a strong argument in a rational, nonhysterical way, you may be able to effect a change in, or an exception to, the rules.

If, good intentions notwithstanding, you turn out to be too weak to participate in any serious mother-baby bonding (and many women are, whether they've had abdominal or vaginal deliveries), or if your baby needs to be observed or cared for in the neonatal intensive care unit for a while, don't panic. There is no evidence, despite the hoopla the concept has aroused in the past, that bonding *must* begin immediately after birth (see page 382).

"I so much want a natural birth; but it seems like everybody is having a cesarean these days and I'm terrified I'll have to have one too."

Not quite "everybody" is having a cesarean these days—but far more women are than ever before. In the early 1960s your chances of having a cesarean would have been 1 in 20. Today they are nearly 1 in 4 (higher in some hospitals, lower in others), and if your pregnancy is in a high-risk category, as high as 1 in 3.

Why such a substantial increase? Many point an accusing finger at the medical community: at the occasional doctor who schedules a cesarean during office hours rather than be awakened at 3 A.M. or who, at the slightest medical pretext, jumps at the chance to collect the higher fee a cesarean commands. (The fact that insurance carriers usually pick up the tab assuages any guilt.) And at the malpractice-shy physician, who performs a cesarean to cover him- or herself when a vaginal delivery shows even the slightest potential for problems. (More suits against obstetricians are instituted for *not* performing a cesarean—and consequently getting a bad result—than for performing one.) Add the physicians who decide to do a cesarean the instant a negative reading is picked up on the fetal monitor (without double-checking to be sure the baby, and not the fetal monitor, is in trouble), and it would appear that bad medicine is to blame.

But the major reason for the increase in the cesarean rate is not bad medicine, but *good* medicine: Cesareans save the lives of babies who might not or cannot safely be delivered vaginally. Most doctors perform cesareans not for convenience, or for the money, or for fear of malpractice, but because they believe that in certain circumstances this surgery is the best way to protect the baby.

Several changes in obstetrical practice have also contributed to the increase in cesareans. First of all, mid-forceps delivery (see page 286) is used less frequently than in the past because of doubts about the safety of reaching up into the vaginal canal with a metal implement to extract a recalcitrant fetus by the head.[4] Second, cesarean delivery has become an extremely quick and safe option—and in most instances mothers can be awake to see their babies born. Third, the fetal monitor, and a variety of tests, can more accurately (though not infallibly) indicate when a fetus is in trouble and needs to be delivered in a hurry. Fourth, the current trend among expectant mothers toward higher than recommended weight gains (over 35 pounds) has led to a greater number of large babies, who are sometimes more difficult to deliver vaginally. Then there is the trend toward noninterventionist obstetrics—letting nature set its own pace, rather than hurrying it by rupturing membranes, using oxytocin, or employing forceps—with the result that labors have more of a chance of stalling. In addition, there are the increasing ranks of women with chronic medical problems who are able to have successful pregnancies but require cesarean deliveries. Finally, a major, and now recognized as largely unnecessary, factor in the burgeoning c-section rate is the repeat cesarean.

In spite of many legitimate reasons for c-sections, there is general agreement in the medical community that a significant number of unnecessary cesareans are presently being performed. In order to reverse this trend, many insurers, hospitals, medical groups, and other individuals and agencies are requiring or encouraging second opinions, when feasible, before a cesarean is performed; a trial of labor for all women who have previously had cesareans to see if they can deliver vaginally (see page 23); better training of physicians in interpretation of fetal monitor readings, so that surgery won't be performed unnecessarily; vaginal deliveries for many breech babies; greater patience with slow labor and with the pushing phase, assuming mother and baby are doing well, before resorting to surgery; the judicious use of oxytocin to get arrested labor moving again; and the use of a variety of more reliable fetal assessment techniques (such as fetal scalp blood sampling, biophysical profile, or acoustical stimulation) to confirm fetal distress that may be suspected from readings on a fetal monitor. Some hospitals now fax ambiguous fetal monitor strips to consultants to get an immediate expert opinion on the condition of the fetus. Others have found that instituting a peer review system—wherein all first-time cesareans are carefully studied on a case-by-case basis and doctors found to be doing unnecessary cesareans face disciplinary action—greatly reduces the cesarean rate. It is also generally agreed that better training of residents in vaginal birth after cesarean (VBAC), external cephalic version (ECV), and the vaginal delivery of breech babies would help reduce the number of cesareans done in this country. But in the case of VBAC, physicians will need the cooperation of mothers as well. Some women who've had one or more cesareans refuse to go through a trial labor again—either because they're concerned about the risks of a vaginal delivery or because they just don't want to have to face another long and painful labor.

---

4. That the rate of mid-forceps deliveries and cesareans are linked is clear in comparing rates of each in the U.S. (where cesarean rates are high and mid-forceps rates low) and Great Britain (where mid-forceps rates are high and cesareans lower).

Most women won't know whether or not they will have a cesarean until they are well into labor. There are, however, several advance indications that point to the possibility:

❖ Cephalopelvic disproportion (when a fetus's head is too large to pass through its mother's pelvis; see page 240), suggested either by the size of the baby on ultrasound examination or by a previous difficult delivery.

❖ A fetal illness or abnormality that makes labor and vaginal delivery unacceptably risky or traumatic.

❖ A previous cesarean (see page 22), if the reason for it still exists (maternal disease or an abnormal pelvis, for example) or a vertical incision was made in the uterus.

❖ Maternal hypertension (page 330) or kidney disease, because the mother may be unable to tolerate the stress of labor.

Cesarean Questions to Discuss With Your Doctor

❖ Will it be possible, assuming it isn't an emergency situation, to try other alternatives before a cesarean is resorted to? For example, oxytocin to stimulate contractions, or squatting to make pushing more effective?

❖ If the reason for the proposed c-section is a breech presentation, will trying to turn the baby in the uterus (external cephalic version) be tried first?

❖ What kinds of anesthesia might be used? A general anesthesia, which puts you to sleep, is usually necessary when time is of the essence, but spinal or epidural anesthesia will allow you to remain awake during a nonemergency abdominal delivery. (See All About Childbirth Medication, page 226.)

❖ Does he or she routinely use a low transverse incision in the uterus whenever possible, so that a vaginal delivery can be attempted next time around? You may also want to know, for cosmetic reasons, if the abdominal incision (which is unrelated to that in the uterus) is usually low, or "bikini."

❖ Can your coach be present if you are awake? If you are asleep?

❖ Can your nurse-midwife (if you have one) be with you too?

❖ Will you and your husband be able to hold the baby immediately after birth (if you are awake and all is well), and will you be able to nurse in the recovery room? If you're asleep, will your husband be able to hold the baby?

❖ If the baby doesn't need special care, can he or she room-in with you? Can your husband stay overnight to help you out?

❖ After an uncomplicated cesarean birth, how much recovery time will you need both in and out of the hospital? What physical discomforts and limitations can you expect to experience?

❖ If the fetal monitor suggests the baby may be in trouble, will other tests (such as checking a fetal scalp blood sample, or evaluating the fetal response to sound or pressure; see page 263) be used to verify the monitor readings before a cesarean is decided upon? Will it be possible to get a second opinion?

Hospitals and Cesarean Rates

Cesarean rates vary from hospital to hospital. Many major medical centers have very high rates because they do a lot of high-risk deliveries. But some small community hospitals also have high rates because they don't have the staff on hand at all hours to do an emergency cesarean; if there's some question that a vaginal delivery might not succeed, the anesthesiologist and others needed for the surgery are called in and a cesarean is performed before an emergency arises. A larger hospital can take a wait-and-see attitude. Discuss the cesarean rate at your hospital with your practitioner, and ask whether there are any special procedures in place to discourage unnecessary cesarean deliveries.

❖ Unusual fetal presentation, such as breech (buttocks or feet first) or transverse (crosswise, with the shoulder first), which can make a vaginal delivery difficult or impossible (see page 236).

A cesarean may be scheduled before labor begins for a variety of reasons, including:

❖ Maternal diabetes, in cases where preterm delivery is deemed necessary and it is found that the cervix is not ripe enough for the induction of labor.

❖ Active maternal herpes infection (page 35) is present as labor begins, to prevent the infection being passed to the fetus during a vaginal birth.

❖ Placenta previa (when the placenta partially or completely blocks the cervical opening) to head off labor, which can result in hemorrhage if the placenta detaches prematurely (see page 356).

❖ Abruptio placenta (page 358), when there is an extensive separation of the placenta from the uterine wall and the fetus is in danger.

Cesareans may also be scheduled before labor when prompt delivery is necessary and either there is no time to induce labor or it is believed that mother and/or baby will be unable to tolerate its stresses. Any of the following might necessitate such a delivery:

❖ Preeclampsia or eclampsia (page 351) that doesn't respond to treatment.

❖ A postmature fetus (two or more weeks overdue; see page 262), when the uterine environment has begun to deteriorate.

❖ Fetal or maternal distress, due to any cause.

In most cases, however, it isn't until active labor that the possible need for a cesarean becomes apparent. Then the most likely reasons include:

❖ Failure of labor to progress (the cervix hasn't dilated quickly enough) after 16 to 18 hours (some physicians will wait longer).[5]

❖ Fetal distress, signaled by the fetal monitor or other tests of fetal well-being (see page 263).

❖ A prolapsed umbilical cord (page 360), which if compressed could cut off oxygen to the fetus, causing fetal distress.

5. In such cases, some physicians will try to give sluggish contractions a boost with oxytocin before resorting to a cesarean.

❖ Previously undiagnosed cases of placenta previa or abruptio placenta, particularly if there is a risk of hemorrhage.

If cesareans are so safe, and sometimes lifesaving, why do most of us dread the prospect of having one? Partly because major surgery, even when it's routine and almost risk-free, is still a little scary; but mostly because we spend months preparing ourselves for natural childbirth, and we usually enter the labor room utterly unprepared for the very real possibility that we'll have a cesarean instead. For nine months we block that unpleasant possibility out of our minds. We devour childbirth primers, but we bypass the chapters on cesarean section. We ask dozens of questions about natural delivery in childbirth class, but not one about surgical birth. We look forward to holding our husband's hand as we pant and push our baby into the world—not to lying passively, and possibly unconscious, as sterile instruments slice into our abdomen to extract the baby like a hot appendix. When suddenly faced with a cesarean, we feel deprived of control over the birth of our baby. As we see it, medical technology has taken over, ushering in frustration, disap-pointment, anger, and guilt.

But that's not how it has to be. Not if you are as prepared for an abdominal delivery as for a vaginal one, if you recognize that both can be beautiful, and if you focus on the product of childbirth rather than the process.

Several steps taken now can make the prospect of a cesarean less ominous and the reality more fulfilling. Even if you have no reason to believe that you might end up needing a cesarean, be sure that at least one session on the subject is included in your childbirth preparation course. If you do have some reason to believe a cesarean section might be necessary, try to take a full preparatory course. Do some reading on your own, too.

If your obstetrician decides in advance that a cesarean will be necessary, be sure to ask for a detailed explanation of the reasons. Ask if there are any alternatives, such as a trial of labor—in which, once labor begins spontaneously, you would be allowed to continue as long as it progressed normally. (This option may not be available in a small hospital that doesn't have the facilities for an emergency c-section should it be needed; some have suggested such hospitals shouldn't do deliveries at all.) If you come away from your consultation

Making the Cesarean Birth a Family Affair

Family-centered cesarean birth is becoming more commonplace across the country, with the vast majority of practitioners and hospitals relaxing the usual surgical rules for cesarean deliveries. During a nonemergency cesarean, most now make it possible for the mother to be awake, the father to be in attendance, and the new family to get to know each other in the period just after birth, just as they would after an uncomplicated vaginal delivery. Studies show that this "normalizing" of surgical delivery helps couples feel better about the experience, reduces the possibility of postpartum depression and low self-esteem in the mother (both of which are more likely to be a problem after cesarean delivery), and allows the bonding process to begin sooner.

wondering whether the major reason a cesarean has been recommended is physician convenience, you should ask for, and get, another opinion.

Whether you're preparing for a scheduled cesarean or just for the possibility of one, there are a number of issues you might want to talk over with your doctor or the on-call physician your nurse-midwife uses (see page 245). Don't be put off by assurances that you aren't likely to need one; explain that you want to be prepared, just in case. Let the doctor know if you would like to be part of the decision-making team should a cesarean seem necessary.

Of course most pregnant women would not select a cesarean as their delivery of choice, and better than 3 out of 4 will end up delivering vaginally. But for those who don't, there's no reason for disappointment or feelings of guilt or failure. Any delivery (vaginal or abdominal, medicated or unmedicated) that yields a healthy mother and baby is an unqualified success.

TRAVEL SAFETY

"I've got an important business trip scheduled this month. Is it safe for me to travel, or should I cancel?"

If you can possibly avoid traveling in the last trimester, do. Not only is traveling in late pregnancy uncomfortable, it can be hazardous—since you could suddenly go into labor (premature labor can't always be predicted) hundreds or thousands of miles from your doctor. The threat of labor occurring thousands of feet in the air (and hours away from landing) is enough to keep airlines from allowing pregnant women in their ninth month to fly without a doctor's letter of permission. And such a letter may prove difficult to obtain, since most physi-

cians don't recommend travel in the last trimester, particularly in the eighth and ninth months. If you must travel, refer to the tips on page 180. It's particularly important to secure the name of a reputable obstetrician at your destination.

DRIVING

"Should I still drive?"

Long car trips (lasting more than an hour) are probably too exhausting late in pregnancy, no matter who's driving. If you must take a longer trip, however, and have your practitioner's okay, be sure to stop every hour or two to get up and walk around. Driving shorter distances is fine up until delivery day, as long as you're not experiencing any dizzy spells and as long as you can still fit behind the wheel. Don't, however, try to drive yourself to the hospital while in labor. And don't forget—on any car trip, whether you are driver or passenger—fasten your seat belt.

BRAXTON HICKS CONTRACTIONS

"Every once in a while my uterus seems to bunch up and harden. What's going on?"

These are probably Braxton Hicks contractions, which usually begin to rehearse the pregnant uterus for labor sometime after the 20th week of pregnancy. These contractions are felt earlier and are more intense in women who have had a previous pregnancy. In effect, your uterus is flexing its muscles, warming up in preparation for the real contractions, which will normally push your baby out at term.

You'll feel these practice contractions as a painless (but possibly uncomfortable) tightening of your uterus, beginning at the top and gradually spreading downward before relaxing. They usually last about 30 seconds (ample time to practice your breathing exercises), but may last as long as 2 minutes or more.

As pregnancy draws to a close in the ninth month, Braxton Hicks contractions may become more frequent, intense—sometimes even painful— and thus more difficult to distinguish from true labor contractions (see Prelabor, False Labor, Real Labor, page 268). Though they're not efficient enough to deliver your baby, Braxton Hicks contractions may get the prebirth processes of effacement and early dilatation started, thereby giving you a leg up on labor before it even begins.

To relieve any discomfort you may feel during these contractions, try lying down and relaxing, or getting up and walking around. Changing your position may stop the contractions completely.

Though Braxton Hicks contractions are not true labor, they may be difficult for you to differentiate from preterm uterine activity of the kind that precedes premature labor. So be sure to describe the contractions to your practitioner at your next visit. Report them immediately if they are very frequent (more than 4 per hour) and/or are accompanied by pain (back, abdominal, or pelvic) or by any kind of unusual vaginal discharge, or if you are at high risk for premature labor (see page 218).

BATHING

"My mother says I shouldn't take a bath after the 34th week. My doctor says it's okay. Who's right?"

This is one case where mother doesn't know best. Though well intentioned, she is misinformed. It's likely that she is basing her warning on the orders she got from her doctor when she was pregnant with you. Most doctors 20 or 30 years ago believed that dirty bath water could travel up the vagina to the cervix in pregnancy and cause an infection. But while further research remains to be done, doctors today believe that water does not enter the vagina unless it is forced, as in douching; thus, worry about infection from bathwater is not justified. Even if water does enter the vagina, the cervical mucous plug that seals the entrance to the uterus effectively protects the membranes that surround the fetus, the amniotic fluid, and the fetus itself from invading infectious organisms. Therefore, most doctors permit tub baths in normal pregnancies up until the membranes rupture or the mucous plug has been expelled. Showers are usually permitted right up to delivery.

Baths and showers, however, aren't totally risk free, particularly in the last trimester when ungainliness can lead to slips and falls. To avoid such mishaps, bathe with care; be sure your tub or shower has a nonslip surface or use a slip-resistant mat; and have someone nearby, if possible, to help you in and out of the tub.

RELATIONSHIP WITH YOUR SPOUSE

"The baby isn't even born yet, and already my relationship with my husband seems to be changing. We're both so wrapped up in the upcoming birth and the baby—instead of in each other, the way we used to be."

All marriages, to differing degrees, undergo some alterations in dynamics and a reshuffling of priorities after baby makes three, but studies show that the shock of this upheaval is usually less stressful if the couple begins the process during pregnancy. So, though the change you're noticing in your relationship may not seem like a change for the better, it's one you're better off experiencing now, rather than after your baby is born. Couples who romanticize the notion of a cozy threesome, and who don't anticipate at least some disintegration or disruption of their romance, often find the reality of life with a demanding newborn harder to deal with.

But while it's very normal—and healthy—to be wrapped up in the pregnancy and your expected extra-special delivery, you shouldn't let this new facet of your life completely block out the others, especially your relationship. Now is the time to learn to combine the care and feeding of your baby with the care and feeding of your marriage. Regularly reinforce romance. Once a week, do something together—see a movie, have dinner out, visit a museum—that has nothing to do with childbirth or babies. While you're layette shopping, stop in the men's department and buy a little something special (and unexpected) for your husband. When you leave the practitioner's office after your next visit, surprise him with a pair of tickets for his favorite opera or sports event. At dinner now and then, ask about his day, talk about yours, discuss the day's headlines—all without indulging in baby talk even once. None of this will make the wonderful event any less special, but it will remind you both that there's more to life than Lamaze and layettes.

Keeping this in mind now will make it easier to keep the love light burning later, when you're taking turns walking the floor at 2 A.M. (Tips to fan the flame can be found in *What to Expect the First Year.*) And that love light is,

after all, what will make the cozy nest you're busily preparing for your baby a bright, happy, and secure one.

MAKING LOVE NOW

"I'm confused. I hear a lot of conflicting information about sexual intercourse in the last weeks of pregnancy."

The problem is that existing medical evidence on the subject is confusing and conflicting. It is widely believed that neither intercourse nor orgasm alone precipitates labor unless conditions are ripe (though many impatient-to-deliver couples have enjoyed trying to prove otherwise). For that reason, many physicians and midwives allow patients with normal pregnancies to make love—assuming they're still interested—right up until delivery day. And most couples apparently can do so without any problems arising.

There does, however, seem to be some risk of sexual intercourse triggering premature labor, at least in women at high risk for preterm delivery (such as those carrying multiple fetuses, those who start effacing and dilating early, and those with a history of premature labor). Intercourse also seems to be related to premature rupture of the amniotic membranes, particularly when they are already inflamed, and to infection, both prenatal (of the amniotic sac or amniotic fluid) and postpartum. To help prevent possible infection, as well as possible premature contractions produced by exposure of the cervix to the irritant prostaglandins in semen, many physicians recommend the use of condoms during intercourse in the last eight weeks of pregnancy.

Ease your confusion by checking with your practitioner to see what the latest medical consensus is. If you get a green light, then by all means make love—if you want to and feel comfortable about it. If the light is red (and it will be if you are at high risk for premature delivery, have placenta previa or abruptio, are experiencing unexplained bleeding, or if your membranes have ruptured), then foster intimacy in other ways. Try a romantic rendezvous at a candlelit restaurant or walking hand-in-hand under the stars. Or an evening at home snuggling in bed or under an afghan in front of the TV, hugging and kissing on the sofa, or soaping each other in the shower. Or use massage—of the neck, back, feet, and of course belly and genitals—as the medium.

WHAT IT'S IMPORTANT TO KNOW:
FACTS ABOUT BREASTFEEDING

At the turn of the century, nearly every baby was fed at the breast; there was no other choice. But in the early 1900s, women began to demand rights they'd never had—to vote, to work, to smoke cigarettes, to let down or bob their hair, to peel off confining undergarments, and to set their sights outside the kitchen and the nursery. Breastfeeding was old-fashioned, it was restricting, and it represented all that women sought freedom from. To be a modern woman was to bottle-feed. And by the 1950s, the only remaining breastfeeders (besides our senior author and an assortment of bohemian stragglers) were those with whom emancipation hadn't yet caught up.

Ironically, it was the revitalized women's movement of the 1960s and '70s that brought breastfeeding back into vogue. Women wanted not only freedom but control—control of their lives, control of their bodies. They knew that control was gained with knowledge, and knowledge told them that breastfeeding was best—for their babies and, on the whole, for themselves. Today there is clearly a back-to-breast trend.

WHY BREAST IS BEST

There is no question but that given normal circumstances, breast-feeding provides the perfect food and food delivery system for human infants:

❖ Human breast milk contains at least 100 ingredients that are not found in cow's milk and that cannot be exactly duplicated in commercial formulas. Breast milk is individualized for each infant; raw materials are selected from the mother's bloodstream as needed, altering the milk's composition from day to day, feeding to feeding, as the baby grows and changes. The nutrients are matched to infant needs. Variations from breast milk in homemade cow's milk formulas can lead to nutritional deficiencies.

❖ Breast milk is more digestible than cow's milk. The proportion of protein in mother's milk is lower (1.5%) than in cow's milk (3.5%), making it easier for the infant to handle. The protein itself is mostly lactalbumin, which is more nutritious and digestible than the major protein component of cow's milk, caseinogen. The fat content of both milks are similar, but the fat in mother's milk is more easily digested by the baby.

❖ Breast milk is less likely to cause overweight in infants, and obesity later in life.

❖ Virtually no baby is allergic to breast milk (though some can have allergic reactions to a certain food or foods in their mothers' diets, including milk). Beta-lactoglobulin, a substance contained in cow's milk, can trigger an allergic response and, following the formation of antibodies, can even cause anaphylactic shock (a life-threatening allergic reaction) in infants—which some suspect could be a contributing factor in some cases of sudden infant death syndrome (or crib death). Soy milk formulas, which are often substituted when an infant is allergic to cow's milk, stray even farther in composition from what nature intended.

❖ Nursed babies are almost never constipated, because of the easier digestibility of breast milk. They also rarely have diarrhea—since breast milk seems both to destroy some diarrhea-causing organisms and to encourage the growth of beneficial flora in the digestive tract, which further discourage digestive upset. On a purely esthetic note, the bowel movements of a breastfed baby are sweeter-smelling (at least until solids are introduced) and less apt to cause diaper rash.

❖ Breast milk contains one-third the mineral salts of cow's milk. The extra sodium in cow's milk is difficult for baby's kidneys to handle.

❖ Breast milk contains less phosphorus. The higher phosphorus content of cow's milk is linked to a decreased calcium level in the formula-fed infant's blood.

❖ Breastfed babies are less subject to illness in the first year of life. Protection is partially provided by the transfer of immune factors in breast milk and in the premilk substance, colostrum.

❖ Nursing at the breast, because it requires more effort than sucking on a bottle, encourages optimum development of jaws, teeth, and palate.

❖ Breast milk is safe. There is no risk of contamination or spoilage.

❖ Breastfeeding is convenient. It requires no advance planning or packing, no equipment; it is always available (in the car, on an airplane, in the middle of the night) and at just the right temperature. When mother and baby aren't together (if the mother works outside the home, for instance), milk may be expressed in advance and stored in the freezer for bottle feedings as needed.

❖ Breastfeeding is economical. There are no bottles, sterilizers, or formula to buy; there are no half-emptied bottles or opened cans of formula to waste. And the nutritious diet needed for nursing (see page 392) probably costs less than a typical American diet saturated with empty but expensive fast-food calories.

❖ Breastfeeding reduces a woman's risk of developing breast cancer before menopause (though it seems to have no effect on later breast cancer).

❖ Nursing helps speed the shrinking of the uterus back to its prepregnant size and decreases the flow of lochia (the postpartum vaginal discharge).

❖ Lactation suppresses ovulation and menstruation, at least to some degree. Though it shouldn't be relied on for birth control, it may postpone resumption of a woman's periods for months, or at least for as long as she nurses.

❖ Nursing can help burn off the fat accumulated during pregnancy. If a woman is careful to consume only enough calories to keep her milk supply and energy up (see page 392), and makes certain that all those calories come from nutritious foods, she can fill all of her infant's nutritional needs while recovering her own figure.

❖ Breastfeeding enforces rest periods for the new mother—particularly important during the first six postpartum weeks.

❖ Nursing in public is becoming more acceptable. With a little discretion and a big napkin, both mother and baby can dine at the same restaurant table.

❖ Breastfeeding brings mother and baby together, skin to skin, at least six to eight times a day. The emotional gratification, the intimacy, the sharing of love and pleasure, can be very fulfilling.

(A note to mothers of twins: All the advantages of breastfeeding are doubled for you. See page 395 for tips that can make breastfeeding easier.)

WHY SOME PREFER THE BOTTLE

Just as there were holdouts against bottle-feeding 30 years ago, there are women today who choose not to nurse. And though the advantages of bottle-feeding seem to be dwarfed by those of breastfeeding, they can be real and convincing for some women.

❖ Bottle-feeding doesn't tie the mother down to her baby. She's able to work outside the home, shop, go out in the evening, even sleep through the night—because someone else can feed the baby.

❖ Bottle-feeding allows the father to share the feeding responsibilities and its bonding benefits more easily. (Although the father of a breastfed baby can derive the same benefits, assuming his baby will take a bottle at all, by feeding a bottle of expressed mother's milk.)

❖ Bottle-feeding doesn't interfere with a couple's sex life (except when baby wakes up for a feeding at the wrong time). Breastfeeding, on the other hand, can. First, because lactation hormones can keep the vagina relatively dry; and second, because leaky breasts during lovemaking are a turn-off to some couples. For bottle-feeding couples, the breasts can play their sensual role rather than their utilitarian one.

❖ Bottle-feeding doesn't dictate your diet or cramp your eating style. You can eat all the garlic, spicy foods, and cabbage you want, and you don't have to drink even one glass of milk.

❖ Bottle-feeding may be preferable for a woman who is squeamish about having such intimate contact with her infant and uncomfortable about the possibility of nursing in public. Or for a woman who feels she is too high-strung or impatient to breastfeed.

MAKING THE CHOICE

For more and more women today, the choice is clear. Some know they will opt for breast over bottle long before they even decide to become pregnant. Others, who never gave it much thought before pregnancy, choose breastfeeding once they've read up on its many benefits. Some women teeter on the brink of indecision right through pregnancy and even delivery. A few women, convinced that nursing isn't for them, still can't shake the nagging feeling that they ought to do it anyway.

For all undecided women, we have one suggestion: Try it—you may like it. You can always quit if you don't, but at least you will have eased those nagging doubts. Best of all, you and your baby will have reaped some of the most important benefits of breastfeeding, if just for a brief time.

Give breastfeeding a fair trial, though. The first few weeks are always difficult, even for the most ardent breastfeeders. Some experts suggest that a full month, or even 6 weeks, of nursing is needed to establish a successful feeding relationship and to give a mother time to decide whether she likes it or not.

WHEN YOU CAN'T OR SHOULDN'T BREASTFEED

Unfortunately, the option of breastfeeding isn't open to every new mother. Some women can't or shouldn't nurse their newborns. The reasons may be emotional or physical, due to mother's health or the baby's, temporary or long-term.[6] The most

common maternal factors making breastfeeding ill-advised include:

❖ Serious debilitating illness (such as cardiac or kidney impairment, or severe anemia) or extreme underweight.

❖ Serious infection, such as tuberculosis.

❖ Conditions that require medications that pass into the breast milk and might be harmful to the baby, such as antithyroid, anticancer, or antihypertensive drugs; lithium, tranquilizers, or sedatives. If you take any kind of medication, check with your physician before beginning breastfeeding.[7]

❖ AIDS, which can be transmitted via body fluids, including breast milk.

❖ Drug abuse—including the use of tranquilizers, cocaine, heroin, methadone, marijuana, and heavy use of caffeine or alcohol.[8]

❖ A deep-seated aversion to the idea of breastfeeding.

Conditions in the newborn that interfere with breastfeeding include:

❖ Disorders, such as lactose intolerance or phenylketonuria (PKU), in which neither human *nor* cow's milk can be digested.

---

6. There have been some suggestions that, in families with a history of premenopausal breast cancer, the condition might be passed on from mother to daughter through a virus in the breast milk. This theory is unsubstantiated, and it appears that women with such family histories, and even those who have had cancer in one breast, can safely and successfully breastfeed their babies.

7. A temporary need for medication, such as penicillin, even at the time you begin nursing, need not necessarily eliminate the chances of your breastfeeding. It may be possible to start the baby on formula temporarily, express milk to get your milk supply going, and as soon as the medication is discontinued, switch to breastfeeding.

8. Smokers who nurse will pass nicotine along to their babies, and should quit. If they don't quit, they should try to cut back—but they should not use smoking as an excuse not to breastfeed.

❖ Cleft lip and/or cleft palate, and other mouth deformities that make sucking at the breast difficult. Sometimes, there are no contraindications to breastfeeding, but it just doesn't work. The milk supply is just inadequate, sometimes because of insufficient glandular tissue in the breast. When this happens, a mother should not feel guilty, but recognize that bottle feeding can work, too.

BOTTLE-FEEDING WITH LOVE

Though breastfeeding is a good experience for both mother and child, there is no reason why bottle-feeding can't be too. Millions of happy, healthy babies have been raised on the bottle. When you can't, or don't wish to, breastfeed, the danger lies not in the bottle, but in the possibility that you might communicate any frustration or guilt you feel to your baby. Know that, with but a little extra effort, love can be passed from mother to child through the bottle as well as through the breast. Make every feeding a time to cuddle your baby, just as you would if you were nursing (don't prop the bottle). And when it's practical, make skin-to-skin contact by opening your shirt and letting the baby rest against your bare breast while feeding.

Considering Cord Blood Banking

Though it is still experimental and quite expensive, some parents are deciding to have blood from their newborn's umbilical cord harvested and stored in case the stem cells should be needed at a future time for the treatment of serious disease (such as leukemia and other cancers, sickle cell anemia and other blood disorders) in the child or another family member. Cord blood harvesting is completely safe for mother and child and holds a lot of promise. If you think you might be interested having this done, speak to your practitioner about the possibility. If you decide to go ahead, be sure the blood is stored with a reliable blood bank that will be scrupulous about keeping your child's blood for your child or other family usage. Get prices, including yearly storage fees, up front.

13
The Ninth Month

WHAT YOU CAN EXPECT AT
THIS MONTH'S CHECKUPS

After about the 36th week, you will see your practitioner weekly. Both the tenor and the content of these examinations will be reminders that you are getting closer to D-day. In general, you can expect your practitioner to check the following, though there may be variations depending upon your particular needs and upon your practitioner's style of practice:[1]

❖ Weight (gain generally slows down or ceases) and blood pressure (it may be slightly higher than it was at mid-pregnancy)

❖ Urine, for sugar and protein

❖ Fetal heartbeat

❖ Height of fundus

❖ Fetal size (you may get a rough weight estimate), presentation (head or buttocks first?), position (facing to the front or to the back?), and descent (is presenting part engaged?)

❖ Feet and hands for edema (swelling), and legs for varicose veins

❖ Cervix (by internal examination, usually sometime after the 38th week) for effacement and dilatation, or where appropriate, for repeat cultures of the cervix

❖ Symptoms you have been experiencing, especially unusual ones

❖ Frequency and duration of Braxton Hicks contractions, as reported by you

❖ Questions and problems you want to discuss, particularly those related to labor and delivery—have a list ready

❖ You can also expect to receive instructions from your practitioner as to when to call if you think you are in labor; if you don't, ask for them.

---

1. See Appendix for an explanation of the procedures and tests performed.

WHAT YOU MAY BE FEELING

You may experience all of these symptoms at one time or another, or only a few of them. Some may have continued from last month, others may be new. Still others may hardly be noticed because you are used to them and/or because they are eclipsed by new and more exciting signs indicating that labor may not be far off.

PHYSICALLY:

❖ Changes in fetal activity (more squirming and less kicking, as the fetus has progressively less room to move around in)

❖ Vaginal discharge (leukorrhea) becomes heavier and contains more mucus, which may be streaked red with blood or tinged brown or pink after intercourse or a pelvic exam

❖ Constipation

❖ Heartburn, indigestion, flatulence, bloating

❖ Occasional headaches, faintness, dizziness

❖ Nasal congestion and occasional nosebleeds; ear stuffiness

❖ Bleeding gums

❖ Leg cramps during sleep

❖ Increased backache and heaviness

❖ Buttock and pelvic discomfort and achiness

❖ Increased swelling of ankles and feet, and occasionally of hands and face

❖ Itchy abdomen, protruding navel

❖ Varicose veins of the legs

WHAT YOU MAY LOOK LIKE

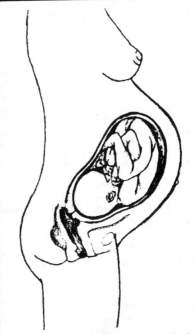

Final preparations are being made for birth, which can safely take place any time now. Lungs are mature. About 2 inches and 2½ pounds are added to baby's length and weight (the average baby will be 20 inches, 7½ pounds at term). More confined, and possibly engaged in the pelvis, the fetus may seem less active.

❖ Hemorrhoids

❖ Easier breathing after the baby drops

❖ More frequent urination after the baby drops

❖ Increased difficulty sleeping

❖ More frequent and more intense Braxton Hicks contractions (some may be painful)

❖ Increasing clumsiness and difficulty getting around

❖ Colostrum, either leaking or expressable from breasts (though this premilk substance may not appear until after delivery)

❖ Fatigue or extra energy, or alternate periods of each

❖ Increase in appetite, or loss of appetite

EMOTIONALLY:

❖ More excitement, more anxiety,

more apprehension, more absent-mindedness

❖ Relief that you're almost there

❖ Irritability and oversensitivity (especially with people who keep saying: "Are *you* still around?")

❖ Impatience and restlessness

❖ Dreaming and fantasizing about the baby

WHAT YOU MAY BE CONCERNED ABOUT

CHANGES IN FETAL MOVEMENTS

"My baby used to kick so vigorously; now he isn't kicking, just squirming."

When you first heard from your baby, way back in the fifth month, there was ample room in the uterus for acrobatics—and lots of kicking and punching. Now that conditions are getting a little cramped, gymnastics are curtailed. In this uterine straightjacket, there is room for little more than turning, twisting, and wiggling. And once the head is firmly engaged in the pelvis, baby will be even less mobile. It's not important what kind of fetal movement you feel at this stage, as long as you note activity every day. If, however, you feel no activity (see below) or a sudden spurt of very panicky activity, check with your doctor.

"I've hardly felt the baby kick at all this afternoon. Should I be alarmed?"

It could be that your baby has settled down for a nap, or that you've been too busy or too active to notice his or

her movements. For reassurance, check for activity in a more formal way, by performing the test on page 202. It's a good idea to repeat this test routinely a couple of times each day throughout the last trimester. Ten or more movements during each test period mean that your baby's activity level is normal. Fewer suggests that medical evaluation might be necessary to determine the cause of the inactivity—so contact your practitioner at once. Though a baby who is relatively inactive in the womb can be perfectly healthy, inactivity sometimes indicates fetal distress. Picking up this distress early through fetal movement testing and intervening medically can often prevent serious consequences.

"I've read that fetal movements are supposed to slow down as delivery approaches. My baby seems more active than ever. Could that mean he's going to be hyperactive?"

Before birth is too soon to start worrying about hyperactivity. Studies show that fetuses who are very active in the womb are no more likely than quieter fetuses to be hyperactive in childhood, though they may well turn out to be very active children.

Recent research also contradicts the notion that the average fetus becomes lazy just before delivery. In late pregnancy, there is generally a gradual decline in the number of movements (from about 25 to 40 an hour at 30 weeks to 20 to 30 at term), probably related to tighter quarters, a decrease in amniotic fluid, and improved fetal coordination. But unless you're counting, you're not likely to notice a significant difference.

FEAR OF ANOTHER LONG LABOR

"I had a 48-hour labor my first time around, and finally delivered after 4½ hours of pushing. Though we both came out of it okay, I dread going through that torture again."

Anyone brave enough to go back into the ring after such a challenging first round deserves a break. And chances are good that you'll get one. Second and subsequent labors and deliveries are usually easier and shorter than first ones—often dramatically so. Less resistance will be met from your now roomier birth canal and your laxer musculature, and though the process won't be effortless (it rarely is), it may well be less of an ordeal. The most marked difference may be in the amount of pushing you have to do; second babies often pop out in a matter of minutes rather than hours.

Of course, though your odds of an easier childbirth are significantly improved the second time around, there are no sure bets in the labor and delivery rooms. Short of a crystal ball,

there's no way to predict precisely what each labor will bring.

BLEEDING OR SPOTTING

"Right after my husband and I made love this morning, I began to bleed. Does this mean that labor is beginning—or is the baby in some kind of danger?"

Any new symptom in the ninth month immediately raises one of two questions—or both: Is it time? Is something wrong? Bleeding and spotting are two such anxiety-provoking events. What they indicate depends on the type of bleeding and the circumstances that surround it:

❖ Pinkish-stained or red-streaked mucus appearing soon after intercourse or a vaginal examination, or brownish-tinged mucus or brownish spotting appearing within 48 hours after the same, is probably just a result of the sensitive cervix being bruised or manipulated. This is normal and not a danger sign—although it should be reported to your practitioner. He or she may advise abstinence from intercourse until delivery.

❖ Bright red bleeding or persistent spotting could be originating at the placenta and requires immediate medical evaluation. Call your practitioner at once. If he or she can't be reached, have someone take you to the hospital.

❖ Pinkish- or brownish-tinged or bloody mucus accompanied by contractions or other signs of oncoming labor (see Prelabor, False Labor, Real Labor, page 268), whether it follows intercourse or not, could be signaling the start of labor. Put in a call to your practitioner.

LIGHTENING AND ENGAGEMENT

"If I'm past my 38th week and haven't dropped, does it mean I'm going to be late?"

"**D**ropping," also called "lightening," occurs when the fetus descends into the pelvic cavity. In first pregnancies, this lightening generally takes place two to four weeks before delivery. In women who have had children previously, it rarely occurs until they go into labor. But as with almost every aspect of pregnancy, exceptions to the rules are the rule. A first-time mother can drop four weeks before her due date and deliver two weeks "late," or she can go into labor without having dropped at all.

Often, lightening is quite apparent. The pregnant woman notes that her belly seems to be lower and tilted farther forward. The happy consequences: as the upward pressure of the uterus on the diaphragm is relieved, taking a deep breath becomes easier, and with the stomach less crowded, eating a full meal becomes more comfortable. These welcome changes are offset by the discomforts caused by pressure on the bladder, the pelvic joints, and the perineal area: increased frequency of urination, difficult mobility, a sensation of increased perineal pressure, and sometimes pain. Sharp little shocks or twinges may be felt when the fetal head presses on the pelvic floor. Some women sense a rolling in the pelvis when the baby's head turns. And often, because her center of gravity has again shifted, a pregnant woman feels more off balance once lightening has occurred.

It is possible, however, for lightening to occur without your realizing it. If, for instance, you were carrying low to begin with, your pregnant silhouette might not alter noticeably. Or if you never experienced difficulty breathing or getting a full meal down, you might not notice any obvious change.

Lightening is a sign that the presenting part, usually the fetal head, is engaged in the upper portion of the bony pelvis. Your practitioner will rely on two basic indicators to determine whether or not your baby's head is engaged: on internal examination, the presenting part is felt in the pelvis; on palpating the head externally, it is found to be fixed in position, no longer "floating."

How far the presenting part has progressed through the pelvis is measured in "stations," each a centimeter long. A fully engaged baby is said to be at "zero (or 0) station"—that is, the fetal head has descended to the level of the ischial spines (prominent bony landmarks on either side of the midpelvis). A baby who has just begun to descend may be at -4 or -5 station. Once delivery begins, the head continues on through the pelvis past 0 to $+1$, $+2$, and so on, until it begins to "crown" at the external vaginal opening at $+5$. Though a woman who goes into labor at 0 station probably has less pushing ahead than the woman at -3, this isn't invariably true, since station isn't the only factor affecting the progression of labor.

Though the engagement of the fetal head strongly suggests that the baby can get through the pelvis without difficulty, it's no guarantee; conversely, a fetus that is still floating going into labor is not necessarily going to have trouble. And in fact, the majority of fetuses that haven't yet engaged when labor begins come through the pelvis smoothly. This is particularly true in women who have already delivered one or more babies previously.

WHEN YOU WILL DELIVER

"Can the doctor tell exactly how close I am to going into labor?"

No. And don't you believe it if he or she tells you otherwise. There are clues that labor may soon begin, which your practitioner begins to look for in the ninth month. Has lightening or engagement taken place? What level, or station, in the pelvis has the baby's presenting part descended to? Have effacement (thinning of the cervix) and dilatation (opening of the cervix) begun?

But "soon" can mean anywhere from an hour to three weeks or more. Ask the woman whose euphoria at being told by her practitioner, "You'll be in labor by this evening," dissolves into depression as weeks more of pregnancy pass with nary a contraction.

A practitioner's prognostication that, since effacement and dilatation haven't yet begun, labor is weeks away can be equally unreliable—as women will testify who, upon hearing such a prediction, have dragged home from the doctor's office resigned to another long month of pregnancy, only to give birth by the following morning.

The fact is that engagement, effacement, and dilatation can occur gradually, over a period of weeks or even a month or more in some women. In others they can occur in a matter of hours. No one, no matter how well trained, can accurately predict the onset of labor—because no one knows exactly what triggers it. (That's why most practitioners are as loath to venture guesses on when you will deliver as on whether it's going to be a girl or a boy.)

So like every pregnant woman before you, you'll just have to play the waiting game, knowing for certain only that your day, or night, will come—sometime.

LABOR AND DELIVERY ROOMS

"I'm very uneasy about going into the hospital and having my baby in unfamiliar surroundings."

The labor and delivery floor is by far the happiest in the hospital. Still, if you don't know what to expect, you can arrive filled with trepidation. Most hospitals allow—in fact, encourage—advance tours of the labor and delivery suite by expectant

Do-It-Yourself Labor Induction?

One study showed that women who, from 39 weeks on, stimulated their nipples for three hours or more daily were much less likely to carry past their due dates. In the study women stimulated the nipple, areola, and breast with the balls of their fingertips, 15 minutes a breast, alternating breasts, for one hour three times a day. Creams or lotions were optional as was a husband's help. The problem is that not only is this technique time- and energy-consuming, but without careful medical supervision, it can be risky. It can produce very strong contractions (much as oxytocin can), which could lead to trouble. So *do not try this technique unless your practitioner recommends it.*

couples. Inquire when you make your reservation. If tours aren't routine, ask your practitioner if he or she can arrange a visit for you. Some hospitals have video tapes of the labor and delivery areas that you can borrow. You can also stop in during visiting hours, and though you won't see the actual labor and delivery area, you can see what patient rooms look like in the postpartum section, and also take a good look at the nursery. Besides making you feel more comfortable, this will give you the opportunity to see what a newborn looks like before you hold your own in your arms.

Labor and delivery rooms vary from hospital to hospital. Some are very sterile and businesslike; others are more homey. Birthing rooms are becoming more and more common and boast the at-home look, with rocking chairs, bright pictures on the walls, curtains on the windows, and birthing beds that look more as if they came out of an Ethan Allen showroom than a hospital supply catalogue.

But although it's nice to be in pleasant surroundings, in the long run it won't be the artistic flair of the hospital's interior decorator but the skill and caring of the medical personnel that will be important to your well-being and that of your baby.

THE OVERDUE BABY

"I'm a week overdue and my doctor's arranged to give me a non-stress test. Is it possible that I might never go into labor on my own?"

The magic date is circled in red on the calendar; every day of the 40 weeks that precede it is crossed off with great anticipation. Then, at long last, the big day arrives—and, as in about half of all pregnancies, the baby doesn't. Anticipation dissolves into discouragement. The baby carriage

and crib sit empty for yet another day. And then a week. And then, in 10% of pregnancies, most often those of first-time mothers, two weeks. Will this pregnancy never end?

Though women who have reached the 42nd week might find it hard to believe, no pregnancy on record ever went on forever—even before the advent of labor induction. (It's true an occasional pregnancy progresses to the 44th week or even slightly beyond, but today a large majority are induced before they go much past the 42nd.)

Studies show that about 70% of apparent post-term pregnancies aren't post-term at all. They are only believed to be late because of a miscalculation of the time of conception, usually thanks to faulty recollection of the exact date of the last menstrual period. And in fact, when ultrasound examination is used to confirm the due date, diagnoses of post-term pregnancy drop dramatically from the long-held estimate of 10% to about 2%.

When a pregnant woman appears to be post-term (technically 42 weeks or more, though some doctors will take action sooner), the practitioner, in evaluating the situation, considers two major factors: One, is the estimated due date accurate? He or she can be reasonably sure that it is if throughout the pregnancy the dating correlated with such physical findings as the size of the uterus and the height of the fundus (the top of the uterus), and with the timing of the first fetal movements felt by the mother and the first fetal heartbeats detected by the examiner. Early pregnancy ultrasound or blood tests for hCG levels (see page 5) may be looked at to further confirm the correct gestational age.

The second factor usually considered is whether the fetus is continuing to thrive. Many babies continue to grow and thrive well into the tenth

How Is Baby Doing?

Doctors are daily discovering new ways of determining how the unborn baby is faring in the uterus. These tests may be performed at any time in pregnancy when there is some concern, or at 41 or 42 weeks when the baby is presumed overdue. The most common are:

At-Home Fetal Movement Assessment. A mother's record of fetal movements (see page 280), though not foolproof, can furnish some indication of her baby's condition and can be used to screen for possible problems. If the mother fails to note adequate activity, other tests are then performed.

The Non-Stress Test (NST). The mother is hooked up to the fetal monitor just as she would be if she were in labor, and the response of the fetal heart to fetal movements can be observed. If, during the non-stress test, the heart rate doesn't react to movement or the baby doesn't move at all, or if other abnormalities are noted, fetal distress may be present. A weakness of the NST (and of electronic fetal monitoring) is that the accuracy of the test depends on the skill of the person interpreting it.

Fetal Acoustical Stimulation (FAS), or Vibroacoustic Stimulation. This non-stress test evaluates the reaction of the fetus to sound or vibrations and has been found to be more accurate than the traditional non-stress tests.

The Stress Test, or Oxytocin Challenge Test (OCT). A test used to evaluate the reactivity of the fetal heart to uterine contractions. In this somewhat more complex and time-consuming test (it may take up to three hours), the mother is hooked up to a fetal monitor. If contractions are not occurring frequently enough on their own, they are given a push via the intravenous administration of oxytocin, or by stimulation of the mother's nipples (with hot towels and, if necessary, manually by the mother). Fetal response to contractions indicates the probable condition of fetus and placenta. This rough simulation of the conditions of labor allows a prediction to be made about whether or not the fetus can safely remain in the uterus or, if necessary, meet the strenous demands of true labor.

A Biophysical Profile (BPP). A BPP is compiled by means of ultrasound and evaluates fetal movement, fetal breathing, and the quantity of amniotic fluid. Normal movements, breathing, and adequate amniotic fluid are a sign that baby is probably okay. When combined with an assessment of the fetal heart rate, the BPP provides a very clear picture of the baby's condition.

The "Modified" Biophysical Profile. This combination of the results of a biophysical profile (above) with a non-stress test (see below) provides an accurate assessment of fetal well-being.

Other Tests of Fetal Well-Being. These include: serial ultrasound to document fetal growth; amniotic fluid volume check by ultrasound (decreased volume may signal placental insufficiency); amniotic fluid sampling (through amniocentesis; page 44); Doppler velocimetry (which measures the velocity of blood flow through the umbilical cord); the "fetal admissions test" (combining FAS with an assessment of the amniotic fluid volume), used early in labor to predict potential fetal problems; fetal electrocardiography (to assess the fetal heart, usually via an electrode attached to the scalp); fetal scalp stimulation (which tests fetal reaction to pressure on or pinching of the scalp); and fetal scalp blood sampling.

month (although this can be a problem if the baby becomes too large during this time to pass easily through the mother's pelvis). Occasionally, however, the once ideal environment in the uterus begins to deteriorate. The aging placenta fails to supply adequate nutrition and oxygen, and production of amniotic fluid drops, dangerously reducing levels of fluid in the uterus. Under these conditions, it becomes difficult for the fetus to continue to do well.

Babies born after spending time in such an environment are called post-mature. They are thin, with skin that is dry, cracked, peeling, loose, and wrinkled and has lost the cheesy vernix coating common in term newborns. Being "older" than other new arrivals, they have longer nails and more abundant hair, and are generally open-eyed and alert. Those with longer stays in a deteriorating uterus may have greenish (meconium) staining of the skin and umbilical cord. Those who have been in the post-term uterus the longest display yellow staining, and are the most at risk during labor or even before.

Both because they are usually larger than 40-week babies, with wider head circumferences, and because they may be somewhat compromised by insufficient oxygen and nutrition or by possibly having inhaled meconium, postmature babies are at increased risk of having a difficult labor and are more likely to be delivered by cesarean. They may also need some special care in the neonatal intensive care nursery for a short time after birth. Still, those born at 42 weeks after uncomplicated pregnancies are at no greater risk of permanent problems than babies born at 40 weeks.

When it has been determined with certainty that a pregnancy is past 41 weeks, and on examination the cervix is found to be ripe (soft), many practitioners will choose to induce labor (see page 273). Delivery by induction or cesarean will also be initiated, whether the cervix is ripe or not, if complications such as hypertension (chronic or pregnancy-induced) or diabetes threaten the mother, or if meconium staining, suspected inadequate fetal growth, or other problems threaten the fetus. If the cervix is not ripe, the practitioner may choose to try to ripen it by administering a drug, such as prostaglandin E_2 (usually via vaginal suppositories or gel), before inducing. Or he or she may choose to wait it out a little longer, performing one or more tests (see page 263) to see if the fetus is still doing okay in the uterus, and repeating these tests once or twice a week until labor begins.

Some practitioners will wait until 42 weeks or even a bit more before deciding to circumvent Mother Nature—assuming the fetus continues to pass its tests and the mother is doing well. If at any point test results indicate placental insufficiency or inadequate levels of amniotic fluid, or if there are any other signs that either mother or baby is in trouble, the practitioner will take action and, depending upon the situation, induce labor or perform a cesarean section. Fortunately for anxious expectant mothers, few pregnancies are allowed to go more than a matter of days beyond 42 confirmed weeks.

A couple of ways of reducing the likelihood of having a post-term baby are sometimes recommended, but both have their drawbacks. One—daily nipple stimulation—can be handled by the mother at home (see page 261), but is risky because it could trigger overly strong contractions. The other—stripping of the fetal membranes—calls for the manual separating of the chorionic membranes surrounding the fetus from the lower section of the uterus and must be performed by the practitioner. Many physicians believe stripping the mem-

What to Take to the Hospital

For the Labor or Birthing Room

❖ This book.

❖ A watch or clock with a second hand for timing contractions.

❖ A radio or a cassette player equipped with your favorite tapes, if music soothes and relaxes you.

❖ A camera, tape recorder, and/or video equipment, if you don't trust your memory to capture the moment (and if the hospital rules allow media coverage of births).

❖ Powder, lotions, oils, or anything else you'd like to be massaged with.

❖ A small paper bag, to breathe into in case you begin to hyperventilate during your breathing exercises.

❖ A tennis ball or plastic rolling pin, for firm counter-massage should lower backache be a problem.

❖ Sugarless lollipops to keep your mouth moist (though sugar-full candies are usually recommended, they will only make you thirstier and more dehydrated).

❖ Heavy socks, in case your feet become cold.

❖ A hairbrush, if having someone brush your hair is comforting.

❖ A washcloth for sponging down with, though the hospital may provide this (don't bring a white one, which might accidentally end up in the hospital laundry).

❖ A sandwich or other snack for Dad (a coach who faints from hunger can't be very useful).

❖ A bottle of champagne or bubbly cider labeled with your name, for celebrating (your coach can ask the nurse to put it in the fridge), though depending on the hour you deliver, you may be more in the mood for an orange juice toast.

For the Hospital Room

❖ A robe and/or nightgowns, if you'd rather wear your own than the hospital's. Be forewarned, however, that though pretty nightgowns can boost your spirits, they may get bled on and permanently stained. Ditto bathrobes. A good compromise might be a favorite bedjacket to wear over the hospital gown.

❖ Perfume, powder, or whatever else makes you feel fresh.

❖ Toiletries, including shampoo, toothbrush, toothpaste, lotion (your skin may be dry from a loss of fluids), a bar of soap in a carrying case, deodorant, hairbrush, hand mirror, makeup, and any other essentials of beauty and hygiene.

❖ Sanitary napkins, preferably the adhesive variety, though pads are usually provided by the hospital.

❖ Playing cards, books (including what-to-name-your-baby books if you're leaving that decision for the last minute), and other distractions.

❖ Packs of raisins, nuts, whole-wheat crackers, and other healthy snacks to keep you healthy and regular in spite of a hospital diet.

❖ A going-home outfit for you, keeping in mind that you'll still be sporting a sizable abdomen.

❖ A going-home outfit for baby—a kimono or stretch suit, T-shirt, booties, a receiving blanket, and a heavy bunting or blanket if it's cold; diapers will probably be provided by the hospital, but take along an extra, just in case. An infant car seat.

❖ A copy of *What to Expect the First Year.*

branes is not advisable because of the risks of rupturing them or causing infection.

MEMBRANES RUPTURING IN PUBLIC

"I live in fear of my membranes rupturing in public."

Y ou're not alone in your fear. The idea of the "bag of waters" breaking on a bus or in a crowded department store is as mortifying to most pregnant women as that of losing bladder control in public. One woman reportedly became so obsessed with her worry that she began carrying a jar of pickles in her handbag, ready to be dropped at the first telltale trickle of amniotic fluid.

But before you start rummaging through your cupboards for the garlic dills, there are two things you should know. First, the rupture of membranes before labor begins is uncommon—occurring in less than 15% of pregnancies. And once they do break, the flow of amniotic fluid is unlikely to be heavy except when you are lying down (something you aren't likely to do in public). When you are walking or sitting, the fetal head tends to block the opening of the uterus like a cork in a wine bottle.

And second, should your membranes rupture and the amniotic fluid gush suddenly, you can be sure that those around you will not point, shake disapproving heads, or—worse—chuckle. Instead they will (as you would if you were a bystander) either offer you assistance or discreetly ignore you. Keep in mind, after all, that no one is likely to overlook the fact that you're pregnant and therefore to mistake amniotic fluid for anything else.

Some women whose membranes rupture prior to labor never experience a gushing of amniotic fluid when their membranes rupture—partly because of the cork effect, partly because there are no contractions to force the fluid out. All they notice is a trickle, either constant or intermittent.

Wearing a panty liner in the last weeks may give you a sense of security, as well as keeping you fresher as your vaginal discharge (leukorrhea) increases.

BREASTFEEDING

"My breasts are very small and my nipples are flat. Will I be able to breastfeed?"

A s far as hungry babies are concerned, satisfaction comes in all kinds of packages. Breasts don't have to be centerfold-shaped or -sized, and they can come equipped with almost any kind of nipple—small and flat, large and pointy, even inverted. All combinations of breasts and nipples have the capacity to produce and dispense milk—the quantity and quality of which are not in the least dependent on outward appearance. Unfortunately, because so many fallacies and old wives' tales exist about what kinds of breasts can and cannot satisfy a baby, many women are unnecessarily discouraged from breastfeeding.

Inverted nipples that don't become erect with sexual stimulation generally need some special priming prior to childbirth. The use of breast shells, available in many maternity and infant supply shops, which provide a gentle suction, is the best way to "pull out" inverted nipples. At first they should be worn for only short intervals morning and evening; gradually the time they are worn can be extended to a full day. A manual breast pump used several times a day can also help to correct inverted nipples, but do not use a pump if it stimulates uterine contractions or if you are at high risk for premature delivery.

Some experts recommend that all women who expect to nurse try to prepare their breasts in advance by expressing a small amount of colostrum from the nipples daily from the eighth month on (though not every woman will be able to do this) and by pulling, twisting, or rolling the nipples between forefinger and thumb—also daily—to toughen them. Others say that nursing comes naturally to nipples, without special preparation.

"My mother says she had milk leaking from her breasts by this time; I don't. Does this mean I won't have any milk?"

The thin, yellowish discharge that some pregnant women can express, or may notice leaking from their breasts, is not milk. It is a pre-milk called colostrum. Richer in protein and lower in fat and milk sugar than the breast milk that comes three or four days after delivery, it contains antibodies that may be important in protecting the baby against disease.

Many women, however, don't have any noticeable colostrum until after delivery. (Even then, they may not be aware of it.) This in no way predicts a lack of milk or difficulty in nursing.

MOTHERING

"Now that the baby's arrival is so close, I'm beginning to worry about taking care of it. I've never even held a newborn before."

Women are not born mothers, instinctively knowing how to rock a crying baby to sleep, change a diaper, or give a bath. Motherhood—parenthood, for that matter—is a learned art, one that requires plenty of practice to make perfect (or even near-perfect). A hundred years ago, that practice commonly took place at an early age, when female children learned to care for younger siblings—much as they learned to bake bread and mend socks.

Today, a high percentage of fully grown women have never kneaded bread dough, taken a needle to a worn sock, or held—let alone taken care of—an infant. Their training for motherhood comes on the job, with a little help from books, magazines, and, if they're lucky enough to find one at their local hospital, a baby-care class. Which means that for the first week or two, the baby may do more crying than sleeping, the diapers may leak, and many a tear may be shed over the "no-more-tears" lather. Slowly but surely, however, the new mother begins to feel like an old pro. Her trepidation turns to assurance. The baby she was afraid to hold (won't it break?) is now cradled casually in her left arm while her right sets the table or pushes the vacuum cleaner. Dispensing vitamin drops, giving baths, slipping squirming arms and legs into sleepers, have ceased to be dreaded ordeals. They, like all the daily tasks of parenting, have become second nature. She's a mother, and—difficult though it may be to imagine—you will be one, too.

Though nothing can make those first days with a first baby easy, starting the learning process before delivery can make them seem a little less overwhelming. Any of the following should help: visit a newborn nursery and view the most recent arrivals; hold, diaper, and soothe a friend's new baby; read up on a baby's first year; and take a class in parenting a newborn.

WHAT IT'S IMPORTANT TO KNOW:
PRELABOR, FALSE LABOR, REAL LABOR

It always seems so simple on TV. Somewhere around 3 A.M., the pregnant woman sits up in bed, puts a knowing hand on her belly, and reaches over to rouse her sleeping husband with a calm, almost serene, "It's time, honey."

But how, we wonder, does this woman know it's time? How does she recognize labor with such cool, clinical confidence when she's never *been* in labor before? What makes her so sure she's not going to get to the hospital, be examined by the resident, and be found to be uneffaced, undilated, and nowhere near her time? That she won't be sent home—amid snickers from the night shift—just as pregnant as when she arrived?

On our side of the screen, we're more likely to awaken at 3 A.M. with complete uncertainty. Are these really labor pains, or just more Braxton Hicks? Should I turn on the light and start timing? Should I bother to wake my husband? Do I call the doctor in the middle of the night to report what might really be false labor? If I do and it isn't time, will I turn out to be the pregnant woman who cried "labor" once too often, and will anybody take me seriously when it's for real? Or will I be the only woman in my childbirth class not to recognize labor? Will I leave for the hospital too late, maybe giving birth in a taxicab? The questions multiply faster than the contractions.

The fact is that most women, worry though they might, *don't* end up misjudging the onset of their labor. The vast majority, thanks to instinct, luck, or no-doubt-about-it killer contractions, show up at the hospital neither too early nor too late, but at just about the right time. Still, there's no reason to leave your deliberations up to chance. Becoming familiar in advance with the signs of prelabor, false labor, and real labor will help to allay the concerns and clear up the confusion when those contractions (or are they?) begin.

No one knows exactly what triggers labor. A group of natural substances produced by the body, called prostaglandins (PGs), are believed to be very important in the process. PGs produced by the uterus during pregnancy are known to increase during spontaneous term labor; they stimulate uterine muscle activity and trigger oxytocin release by the pituitary gland, both important factors in the initiation of labor. And prostaglandin inhibitors, such as aspirin, can delay the onset of labor. Probably a combination of fetal, placental, and maternal factors are responsible for setting labor into motion.

PRELABOR SYMPTOMS

The physical changes of prelabor can precede real labor by a full month or more—or by only an hour or so. Prelabor is characterized by the beginning of cervical effacement and dilatation, which your practitioner can confirm, as well as by a wide variety of related signs that you may notice yourself:

Lightening and Engagement. Usually somewhere between two and four weeks before the onset of labor in first-time mothers, the fetus begins to descend into the pelvis. This milestone is rarely reached in second or later births until labor has actually commenced.

Sensations of Increasing Pressure in the Pelvis and Rectum.
Crampiness and groin pain are particularly common in second and later pregnancies. Persistent low backache may also be present.

Loss of Weight or Cessation of Weight Gain.
In general, weight gain slows in the ninth month; as labor approaches, some women lose up to 2 or 3 pounds.

A Change in Energy Levels.
Some ninth-monthers find that they are increasingly fatigued. Others experience energy spurts. An uncontrollable urge to scrub floors and wash woodwork has been related to the "nesting instinct"—in which the female of the species prepares the nest for the impending arrival.

A Change in Vaginal Discharge.
You may find that your discharge increases and thickens.

Loss of Mucous Plug.
As the cervix begins to thin and open, the "cork" of mucus that seals the opening of the uterus becomes dislodged. This gelatinous chunk of mucus can be passed through the vagina a week or two before the first real contractions, or just as labor begins.

Pink, or Bloody, Show.
As the cervix effaces and dilates, capillaries frequently rupture, tinting the mucus pink or streaking it with blood. This "show" usually means labor will start within 24 hours—but it could be as much as several days away.

Intensification of Braxton Hicks Contractions.
These practice contractions may become more frequent and stronger, even painful.

Diarrhea.
Some women experience loose bowel movements just prior to the onset of labor.

FALSE LABOR SYMPTOMS

Real labor probably has not begun if:

❖ Contractions are not regular and don't increase in frequency or severity.

❖ Pain is in the lower abdomen rather than the lower back.

❖ Contractions subside if you walk around or change your position.

❖ Show, if any, is brownish.[2] (Often the result of an internal exam or intercourse within the past 48 hours.)

❖ Fetal movements intensify briefly with contractions. (Let practitioner know if activity becomes frantic.)

REAL LABOR SYMPTOMS

When contractions of prelabor are replaced by stronger, more painful, and more frequent ones, the question arises: "Is this the real thing or false labor?" It is probably real if:

❖ The contractions intensify, rather than ease up, with activity and aren't relieved by a change in position.

❖ Pain begins in the lower back and spreads to the lower abdomen; it may also radiate to the legs. Contractions may feel like gastrointestinal upset and be accompanied by diarrhea.

---

2. Bright red blood requires immediate consultation with your practitioner.

❖ Contractions become progressively more frequent and painful, and generally (but not always) more regular. (This progression isn't absolute—not every contraction will necessarily be more painful or longer than the previous one, but their general intensity does build up as real labor progresses. Nor does frequency always increase in regular, perfectly even intervals— but it does increase.)

❖ Show is present and pinkish or blood-streaked.

❖ Membranes rupture. In 15% of labors the waters break—in a gush or a trickle—before labor begins.

WHEN TO CALL THE DOCTOR

When in doubt, call. Even if you've checked and rechecked the above lists, you may still be unsure whether you're really in labor. If you *are* unsure, call your practitioner, unless you'd like an unplanned home birth. He or she will probably be able to tell from the sound of your voice, as you talk through a contraction, whether it's the real thing. (But only if you don't try to cover up the pain in the name of stoicism or good manners.) Fear of embarrassment if it turns out not to be labor shouldn't prevent your calling your practitioner. If it does turn out to be a false alarm, nobody's going to snicker. You wouldn't be the first patient to misjudge her labor signs—and you certainly won't be the last.

❖ Call anytime, night or day, if all signs indicate that you're ready to go to the hospital. Don't let an overdeveloped sense of guilt or politeness keep you from waking your practitioner up in the middle of the night, or disturbing his or her weekend at home. People who deliver babies for a living don't expect to work only 9 to 5.

❖ Your practitioner has probably specified that you should call when your contractions have reached a particular frequency—say 5, 8, or 10 minutes apart. Call when at least some are that frequent. Don't wait for perfectly even intervals; they may never come.

❖ Your practitioner has probably also instructed you about when to call if your membranes rupture, or if you think they have ruptured, but labor has not begun. Follow these instructions unless: your due date is still several weeks away; you know your baby is small or is not engaged in the pelvis; or the amniotic fluid is stained greenish brown. In these cases, call immediately.

❖ Don't assume that if you're not sure it's real labor, it isn't. Err on the side of caution; call.

Best Medicine for Labor?

Recent studies show that when a woman in labor is supported, encouraged, touched, soothed, and kept abreast of what is happening by an experienced mother, or "doula," the number of cesarean and forceps deliveries, the need for anesthesia, the rate of complications, and even the length of labor can be reduced.

14
Labor and Delivery

It takes nine months to make a baby, and only a matter of hours to bring one out into the world. Yet it's those hours that seem to occupy the minds of expectant women most—more questions, fears, and concerns revolve around the processes of labor and delivery than around any other aspect of pregnancy. When will it start? More important, when will it end? Will I be able to tolerate the pain? Will I have to have an enema? A fetal monitor? An episiotomy? What if I don't make any pro-

gress? What if I progress so quickly that I don't even have time to get to the hospital?

You'll find answers to your questions and reassurance for your fears and concerns in the following chapter. These, teamed with a lot of support from your partner and your birth attendants, and the knowledge that labor and delivery have never been safer and more manageable than they are today, should help prepare you for most anything that labor and delivery might bring your way.

WHAT YOU MAY BE CONCERNED ABOUT

BLOODY SHOW

'I have a pink mucous discharge. Does it mean labor's about to start?''

Don't send your husband out for the cigars yet. Passage of a "bloody show," a mucous discharge tinged pink or brown with blood, is often a sign that your cervix is effacing and/or dilating and that the process that leads to delivery is beginning. But it's a process with an erratic timetable that will keep you in suspense until the first contractions. Labor could be one, two, or even three

weeks away, with your cervix continuing to dilate gradually over that time. Or it could be less than an hour away.

If your discharge should suddenly become bright red or seems to amount to more than an ounce of blood, contact your practitioner immediately. Bleeding could indicate premature separation of the placenta or placenta previa, which require prompt medical attention.

RUPTURE OF MEMBRANES

"I woke up in the middle of the night with

*a wet bed. Did I lose control of my blad-
der, or did my membranes rupture?"*

A sniff of your sheets will probably
clue you in. If the wet spot smells
sort of sweet and not like ammonia,
it's likely to be amniotic fluid. Another clue: You'll probably still be
leaking the pale, straw-colored amniotic fluid (which won't run dry because it continues to be produced until delivery, replacing itself every three
hours). When you stand up or sit
down, however, the baby's head may
act like a cork and stop up the leak
temporarily.

Whether or not there continues to
be leakage, if you suspect your membranes have ruptured, you should call
your practitioner. Until you've con-
tacted him or her, act as though your
membranes have indeed ruptured (see
below).

*"My water just broke, but I haven't had
any contractions. When is labor going to
start, and what should I do in the meantime?"*

The majority of pregnant women
whose membranes rupture prior
to labor feel their first contractions
within 12 hours; most others feel
them within 24 hours. About 1 in 10,
however, take longer to go into labor.
Because, as time passes, the risk of
infection to baby and/or mother
through the ruptured amniotic sac increases, most physicians will induce
labor with oxytocin within 24 hours
of the rupture if a woman is at or near
her due date, though a few wait as
little as 6 hours to induce. Recent
studies show that, when the pregnancy reaches this point, there is no
advantage in delaying induction beyond 24 hours, and a definite disadvantage: an increased risk of infection
(see page 359).

If you experience a trickle or flow
of fluid from your vagina, call your
doctor or nurse-midwife. In the
meantime, keep the vaginal area as
clean as possible, to avoid infection.
Don't take a bath or have sexual relations; use sanitary napkins (not a tampon) to absorb the flow of amniotic
fluid; don't try to do your own internal exam; and wipe front to back at
the toilet.

Rarely, in premature rupture of the
membranes (most often when the
baby is breech or premature), when
the presenting part is not yet engaged
in the pelvis, the umbilical cord becomes "prolapsed"—it is swept into
the neck of the uterus (the cervix), or
even into the vagina, with the gush of
amniotic fluid. If you can see a loop of
umbilical cord showing at your vaginal opening, or think you feel something inside your vagina, see page 360
and get immediate medical attention.

DARKENED AMNIOTIC FLUID (MECONIUM STAINING)

*"My membranes ruptured, and the fluid is
greenish-brown. What does this mean?"*

Your amniotic fluid is probably
stained with meconium, which
is a greenish-brown substance that
comes from your baby's digestive
tract. Ordinarily, meconium is passed
after birth as the baby's first stool. But
sometimes—particularly when the fetus has been under stress in the womb,
and very often when the baby is
postmature—it is passed prior to birth
into the amniotic fluid.

Meconium staining alone is not a
sure sign of fetal distress, but because
it suggests the possibility, notify your
practitioner immediately.

INDUCTION OF LABOR

"My doctor wants to induce labor. I'm upset because I had wanted a natural delivery."

Though some doctors 20 years ago believed it was safe to routinely induce labor in their patients so that birth would come at a convenient time, doctors today rarely induce without good cause. This has come about partly because the FDA has withdrawn approval of elective (not absolutely necessary) use of the drug oxytocin, with which labor is induced, and partly for fear of malpractice suits should something go wrong. But it has come about mostly because they recognize that, when possible, it's best to let nature take its time taking its course.

In close to 1 in 3 deliveries, however, nature may need a little prodding. There are a variety of situations in which it is necessary to deliver a baby before nature appears ready and willing to do so. In some cases, a cesarean section is the best way to do this. In others, when time is not of the essence, both mother and baby are deemed able to tolerate the stresses of labor, and the practitioner has reason to believe that a normal vaginal delivery is possible, induction is usually the first choice. For example:

❖ When labor is weak or erratic, or has stalled.

❖ When a fetus isn't thriving (because of inadequate nourishment, poor placental function, postmaturity, or any other reason) and is mature enough to do well outside the uterus.

❖ When a stress or non-stress test suggests that the placenta is no longer functioning optimally and the uterine environment is no longer healthy.

❖ When there is premature rupture of the membranes at term (see page 359).

❖ When a pregnancy has gone two or more weeks past a due date that is considered accurate (see page 262).

❖ When the mother has diabetes and the placenta is deteriorating prematurely, or when it's feared her baby will be very large—and thus difficult to deliver—if carried to term.

❖ When the mother has preeclampsia (toxemia) that cannot be controlled with bed rest and medication, and delivery is necessary for her sake and/or her baby's.

❖ When the mother has a chronic or acute illness, such as high blood pressure or kidney disease, that threatens her well-being or that of her baby if the pregnancy continues.

❖ When the fetus is afflicted with severe Rh disease which necessitates early delivery.

Occasionally, all that's required to induce labor is for the physician to artificially rupture the membranes (bag of waters) that surround the fetus. If the cervix is not ripe, pain relief medication may be given during this procedure. Some practitioners will give the mother a dose of mineral oil and/or have her attempt nipple self-stimulation to get contractions going. Prostaglandin E_2 suppositories or gel may be used to help ripen the cervix. But in most cases, the administration of oxytocin turns out to be necessary to consistently activate the uterus.

Oxytocin is a hormone produced naturally by the maternal pituitary gland throughout pregnancy. As pregnancy progresses, the uterus becomes more and more sensitive to the hormone, although it isn't clear whether it plays a significant role in the triggering of natural labor. It is known that the hormone may be released by the pregnant woman when her nipples are stimulated, causing the uterus to contract—which is why nipple stimulation sometimes works to trigger labor. The administration of oxytocin (trade name, Pitocin), however, is a more reliable method of induction. When the cervix is ripe, oxytocin is capable of initiating a labor that closely mimics one that occurs naturally. When the cervix isn't ripe, induction may be carried out (assuming there is time) over a two- or three-day course, to allow gradual ripening. Or efforts may be made to ripen the cervix by using prostaglandin E_2 or to open it manually by using graduated dilators before induction is begun. These procedures can improve the chances for a spontaneous vaginal delivery within 24 hours.

To induce labor, oxytocin is administered through an intravenous IV drip with an infusion pump. This is the safest and easiest route to controlling the rate of administration. The IV is introduced via a needle in the arm or the back of the hand, and connected by tubing to two bottles. One bottle contains unmedicated intravenous fluid, and the other contains the oxytocin. By routing the oxytocin into the primary tubing through an infusion pump, it is possible to precisely control the dosage. Usually the induction begins slowly, with very little oxytocin being infused into the mother, and the reactions of the uterus and the fetus carefully monitored. (A doctor or nurse must be in attendance at all times during induction.) The rate of infusion is increased gradually until effective contractions are established. Should the woman's uterus prove extremely sensitive to the drug and be overstimulated into either too long or too powerful contractions, this method allows the infusion rate to be reduced or discontin-

ued entirely by switching the IV to the primary tubing bottle of unmedicated solution.

Contractions usually begin after 30 minutes in women who are at or close to term, and they're generally more regular and more frequent than those of a naturally occurring labor, right from the start. If, after six to eight hours of oxytocin administration, labor hasn't begun or progressed, the procedure will probably be terminated in favor of an alternative approach, usually a cesarean section. Treatment may also be terminated if contractions become well established and continue on their own.

Induction of labor is inappropriate when immediate delivery is necessary or when there is any doubt that the fetus can fit through the mother's pelvis; the procedure also is avoided when the placenta is near or covering the opening of the uterus (placenta previa), when the woman is judged to be in false labor, and, generally, in women who have had five or more previous births or who have a vertical scar from a past cesarean section, since they are at greater risk for uterine rupture. Some physicians will also not attempt induction when a woman is carrying multiple fetuses or when a baby is in the breech position. The American College of Obstetricians and Gynecologists recommends that when labor is induced with oxytocin the physician be ready and available to perform an emergency cesarean, if one is needed.

Some women find the sudden onset of hard labor that usually occurs with induction unpleasant; some even feel cheated by the artificially shortened duration of their laboring experience. Others enjoy such down-to-business births. With their coach at their side, they go through their induced labor otherwise naturally, using all the breathing exercises and other coping mechanisms learned in childbirth classes. And so can anyone who keeps in mind that labor, no matter how it's triggered, is labor.

HAVING A SHORT LABOR

"Can a short labor actually be harmful to the baby?"

Short labor isn't always as short as it seems. Often the expectant mother has been having painless contractions for hours, days, even weeks, which have been dilating her cervix gradually. By the time she feels the first contraction, she is well into the transition stage of labor (see the stages of childbirth, beginning on page 288). This slow-buildup, quick-resolution labor places no extra strain on the fetus, and may be even less stressful than the average 12-hour labor.

Occasionally the cervix dilates very rapidly, accomplishing in a matter of minutes what most cervixes (particularly those of first-time mothers) take hours to do. But even with this abrupt, or precipitous, kind of labor (one that takes three hours or less from start to finish), there is rarely any threat to the baby. There is no evidence to support the notion that an infant must go through a minimum amount of labor in order to arrive in good condition.

Once in a great while, however, an extremely rapid labor does deprive the fetus of oxygen or other needed gases, or results in tearing or other damage to cervix, vagina, or perineum in the mother. So, if your labor seems to start with a bang—with contractions strong and close together—get to the hospital quickly. Medication may be helpful in slowing contractions a bit and easing the pressure on the fetus and on your own body.

CALLING YOUR PRACTITIONER DURING LABOR

"I just started getting contractions and they're coming every three or four minutes. I feel silly calling the doctor, who said we should spend the first several hours of labor at home."

Most first-time mothers-to-be (whose labors often begin slowly, with a gradual buildup of contractions) *can* safely count on spending the first several hours at home. But if your contractions start off strong—lasting at least 45 seconds and coming more often than every five minutes—and/or you've delivered a baby before, your first several hours of labor may very well be your last. Chances are that much of the first stage of labor has passed painlessly, and that your cervix has dilated significantly during that time. This would mean that not calling your doctor—and chancing a dramatic dash to the hospital at the last minute—would be considerably sillier than picking up the phone now.

Before you do, however, it is best to have timed several consecutive contractions. Be clear and specific about their frequency, duration, and strength when you report them. Don't try to minimize your discomfort when you describe it by trying to maintain a calm voice. (Your practitioner is used to judging the phase of labor in part by the sound of a woman's voice as she talks through a contraction.)

If you feel you're ready but your practitioner doesn't seem to think so, don't take "wait" for an answer. Ask if you can go to the hospital and have your progress checked. (See When to Call the Doctor in Prelabor, False Labor, Real Labor, page 268.) You can take your suitcase along "just in case," but be ready to turn around and go home if you've only just begun to dilate.

BACK LABOR

"The pain in my back since my labor began is so bad that I don't see how I'll be able to make it through delivery."

Technically, "back labor" occurs when the fetus is in a posterior (or occipitoposterior) position, with the back of its head pressing against the mother's sacrum—the rear boundary of the pelvis. It's possible, however, to experience back labor when the baby is not in this position, or to continue to experience it after the baby has turned from a posterior to an anterior position—possibly because the area has become a focus of tension.

When you're having this kind of pain—which often doesn't let up between contractions and becomes excruciating during them—the cause is not a crucial consideration. How to relieve it, even slightly, is. There are several measures that may help; all are at least worth trying:

❖ Taking the pressure off your back. Try changing your position—walk around (though this may not be humanly possible once contractions are coming fast and furiously), crouch or squat, get down on all fours, or do whatever is most comfortable and least painful for you. If you feel you can't move and would prefer to be lying down, lie on your side, with your back well rounded.

❖ Heat or cold, applied by your coach or attendant. Use a hot-water bottle wrapped in a towel, warm compresses, a heating pad, or ice packs or cold compresses—whichever soothes best.

❖ Counterpressure. Have your coach experiment with different ways of applying pressure to the area of greatest pain, or to adjacent areas, to find one or more that seem to help. He can try his knuckles, or the heel of one hand reinforced by pressure from the other hand on top of it, using direct pressure or a firm circular motion. Pressure can be applied while you are sitting or while you are lying on your side. The relief you may get from really intense counterpressure will be well worth any black-and-blue marks you find the morning after.

❖ Acupressure. This is probably the oldest form of pain relief—and you don't have to be Chinese to try it. In the case of back labor, it involves applying strong finger pressure just below the center of the ball of the foot.

❖ Aggressive massage to the area may spell relief either in place of counterpressure or alternated with it. A rolling pin or a tennis ball can be used for especially firm massage (although you will probably be a little sore afterward). Oil or powder can be applied periodically to avoid irritation.

IRREGULAR CONTRACTIONS

"In class we were told not to go to the hospital until the contractions were regular and five minutes apart. Mine are less than five minutes apart, but they aren't at all regular. I don't know what to do."

Just as no two women have exactly the same fingerprints, no two women have exactly the same labors. The labor often described in books, in childbirth education classes, and by practitioners is what is typical—and close to what many women can expect. But far from every labor is true-to-textbook, with contractions regularly spaced and predictably progressive.

If you are having strong, long (40 to 60 seconds), frequent (five minutes apart or less) contractions, even if they vary considerably in length and time elapsed between them, do not wait for them to become "regular" before calling your practitioner or heading for the hospital—no matter what you've heard or read. It's possible that your contractions are about as regular as they are going to get, and that you are well into the active phase of your labor. Waste no time in calling your practitioner and getting to the hospital; she who hesitates in a case like this could end up with an unscheduled home birth.

NOT GETTING TO THE HOSPITAL IN TIME

"I'm afraid that I won't get to the hospital in time."

Fortunately, most surprise deliveries take place in the movies and on television. In real life, deliveries, especially those of first-time mothers,

rarely occur without ample warning. But once in a great while, a woman who has had no labor pains, or just erratic ones, suddenly feels an overwhelming urge to bear down; often she mistakes it for a need to go to the bathroom.

Just in case you might turn out to be one of these women, it's a good idea for both you and your husband to become familiar with the basics of an emergency home delivery (see pages 279 and 281). But don't spend a lot of time worrying about this very remote possibility.

ENEMAS

"I've heard that enemas early in labor aren't really necessary, and that they interfere with natural birth."

Enemas were, until fairly recently, not a matter of patient choice. They were administered routinely in early labor, as part of the hospital admissions procedure. The theory was, and still is in some hospitals, that emptying the bowels before delivery eliminates the possibility of fecal matter in the rectum hindering the baby's descent through the birth canal, and prevents contamination of the sterile birthing setup by involuntary evacuation of feces during the pushing stage

Emergency Delivery En Route to the Hospital

1. If you're in your own car and delivery is imminent, pull over. If you have a CB or car phone, call for help. If not, turn on your hazard warning lights or turning signal. If someone stops to help, ask him or her to get to a phone and call 911 or the local emergency medical squad. If you're in a cab, ask

the driver to radio for help.
2. If possible, you should help the mother into the back of the car. Place a coat, jacket, or blanket under her. Then proceed as on page 281. As soon as delivery is completed, continue to the nearest hospital in a hurry.

of labor. In addition, this precaution may spare the laboring woman "embarrassment" and lessen her inhibitions about pushing.

This way of thinking is less in favor today. It is recognized that compression of the birth canal is not likely to be a problem if a woman has had a bowel movement in the past 24 hours, or if no hard fecal mass is felt in her rectum on internal examination. And the use during delivery of disposable sterile gauze pads to whisk away any fecal matter that is expelled virtually eliminates the threat of fecal contamination. According to some studies, the possibility of neonatal infection from bowel organisms is highly remote to begin with; others suggest that enemas themselves can actually increase the risk of infection. For these reasons, most hospitals have abandoned the routine enema; others are certain to follow.

If your hospital isn't among these and if the prospect of an enema is one you don't relish, discuss the subject with your practitioner in advance of labor. If you feel strongly that you don't want an enema, he or she may agree to skip it. (But be sure that the decision is relayed to hospital staff.) On the other hand, if you're more uncomfortable with the prospect of moving your bowels on the delivery table (though an enema doesn't guarantee you won't), don't let anyone bully you into accepting the idea that enemas are unnatural and unnecessary. Include your preferences in your birthing plan, if you draw one up (see page 225).

You may be more comfortable taking care of the enema yourself at home, while you're in early labor. But whether it's given at home or in the hospital, a warm water enema may provide the added benefit of boosting sluggish contractions and giving labor a little push.

The entire issue may be academic, however, if your labor begins, as many do, with loose or frequent bowel movements, which may effectively empty the colon; or if you arrive at the hospital in active labor, with contractions so close together that it's barely possible for hospital personnel to get you into a gown, much less give you an enema.

SHAVING THE PUBIC AREA

"I don't like the idea of having my pubic hair shaved. Is it obligatory?"

Though shaving of the pubic area is still a routine "prepping" procedure in some hospitals, it is being utilized less and less. It is most often done simply because it's always been done, not because it is necessary. It was once believed that pubic hair harbored bacteria that could infect the baby as it passed through the vaginal outlet. But since the entire area surrounding the vagina is swabbed with an antiseptic solution prior to delivery, infection of this type is not likely. And in fact, some studies have shown a *higher* rate of infection among women who are shaved prior to delivery than among those who aren't, probably because the small—sometimes microscopic—nicks that even very careful shaving can produce may serve as excellent breeding grounds for bacteria. From the woman's point of view, the humiliation of the shaving itself and the postpartum burning and itching as the hair grows back are additional reasons to object to the procedure.

Some doctors feel that shaving facilitates performing and repairing an episiotomy, by providing a clearer area in which to work. But for them, too, shaving is more likely a matter of habit than conviction. An increasing number of physicians are performing and repairing episiotomies without shav-

Emergency Delivery If You're Alone

1. Try to remain calm.

2. Call 911 (or your local emergency number) for the emergency medical squad. Ask them to call your practitioner.

3. Find a neighbor or someone else to help, if possible.

4. Start panting to keep from bearing down.

5. Wash your hands and the vaginal area, if you can.

6. Spread some clean towels, newspapers, or sheets on a bed, sofa, or the floor, and lie down to await help.

7. If despite your panting the baby starts to arrive before help does, gently ease it out by pushing each time you feel the urge, catching it with your hands.

8. Proceed with steps 10 to 14 on page 281 as best you can.

---

ing the surrounding area—either clipping the hair with scissors or pushing it back as they work.

Whether or not you will be shaved may depend on the practices of your practitioner and the hospital you are delivering at. Increasingly, it is one of the decisions of childbirth that you can, at the very least, be instrumental in making. Don't wait until you arrive at the hospital, however, to make your feelings about shaving known. Discuss them in advance of labor with your practitioner. Include your preferences in your birthing plan (see page 225).

If your practitioner or the hospital insists on your being shaved, ask that they not shave any more than is absolutely necessary. A "mini-prep," which shaves only the hair in the area of any possible incision or tear, is usually sufficient. An alternative to being shaved at the hospital, which you may also want to discuss with your practitioner, is having your mate shave or clip you at home.

ROUTINE IVs

"When we had our visit to the hospital, I saw a woman being wheeled from the delivery room with an IV attached. Is that necessary with a normal labor and delivery?"

Thanks to reruns of *M*A*S*H* and edge-of-your-seat soap operas, we readily associate IVs (intravenous setups) with wounded GIs, rapidly fading heroines with fatal illnesses, and heros soundly thrashed by jealous lovers. But it's hard to associate an IV with normal childbirth.

Yet in many American hospitals, it is routine to administer an IV containing a simple solution of nutrients and fluid to a woman in labor. This is done partly to be certain that the woman does not become dehydrated from lack of fluids or weak from lack of food during labor, partly to provide ready access for medication should the need arise (it can be injected right into the IV bottle or line, instead of into the patient). In these instances, the IV is precautionary.

Some doctors and midwives, on the other hand, prefer to wait until there is a clear need for an IV—for instance, because the labor has been lengthy and the laboring woman is weakening. Check your practitioner's policy in advance, and if you strongly object to having an IV, say so. It may be possible to hold off until the need, if any, arises.

If it's your practitioner's policy to give IVs routinely and there's no room for discussion, or if you end up needing one, don't despair. The IV is only slightly uncomfortable as the needle is inserted and thereafter should barely be noticed. When it's hung on a movable stand, you can take it with you to the bathroom or on a brief constitutional. (If at any point the area becomes sore or painful, inform your practitioner or nurse.)

Though you can't always make the decision about whether or not you should have an IV, you do have a right to know what the IV is infusing into your veins. Ask the nurse or doctor who inserts it. Or have your labor partner read the label on the bottle. Occasionally medication may be ordered without your being consulted. If this happens, ask to speak to your practitioner as soon as possible.

FETAL MONITORING

"My doctor believes in fetal monitoring at all births. I've heard that monitoring can lead to unnecessary cesareans and also makes labor more uncomfortable."

For someone who's spent the first nine months of his or her life floating peacefully in a warm and comforting amniotic bath, the trip through the narrow confines of the maternal pelvis will be no joy ride. Your baby will be squeezed, compressed, pushed, and molded with every contraction.

It is because there is an element of risk in this stressful journey—not to promote maternal discomfort or unnecessary cesareans—that fetal monitors have come into such common use. In some hospitals, all labor and delivery patients are electronically monitored. In virtually every hospital, at least half of the patients— particularly those in high-risk categories, who have meconium-stained amniotic fluid, who are receiving oxytocin, or who are having a difficult labor—are monitored electronically.

A fetal monitor gauges the response of the baby's heartbeat to the contractions of the uterus. The reader of the monitor printout may be able to pick up signs of possible fetal stress and distress through variations from the normal reactions to labor. Sometimes an alarm is preset to go off if such variations occur. Fetal monitoring can be external or internal:

External Monitoring. In this type of monitoring, used most frequently, two devices are strapped to the abdomen. One, an ultrasound transducer, picks up the fetal heartbeat. The other, a pressure-sensitive gauge, measures the intensity and duration of uterine contractions. Both are connected to a monitor, which displays or prints out the readings. This doesn't mean the laboring woman must be confined to bed, hooked up to a machine like Frankenstein's monster, for hours on end. In most cases, monitoring is required only intermittently, and the laboring woman can walk around between readings. Some hospitals may be equipped with portable monitors that can be hooked up to the patient's clothing, allowing her complete freedom to go for a stroll down hospital corridors while it sends data on her baby's well-being back to her bedside or a nursing station.

During the second (pushing) stage of labor, when contractions may come so fast and furiously that it's hard to know when to push and when to hold back, the monitor is able to accurately signal the beginning and end of each contraction. Or the use of the monitor

Emergency Home (or Office) Delivery

1. Try to remain calm. Remember, even if you don't know the first thing about delivering a baby, a mother's body and her baby can do most of the job on their own.

2. Call 911 (or your local emergency number) for the emergency medical squad; ask them to call the doctor or nurse-midwife.

3. The mother should start panting to keep from bearing down.

4. During all the preparations and during the delivery, comfort and reassure the mother.

5. If there's time, wash the vaginal area and your hands with detergent or soap and water.

6. If there's no time to get to a bed or table, place newspapers or clean towels or folded clothing under the buttocks, to provide some height for delivering the baby's shoulders.

7. If there is time, place the mother onto the bed (or desk or table) so that her buttocks are slightly hanging off, her hands under her thighs to keep them elevated. If available, a couple of chairs can support her feet. A few pillows or cushions under shoulders and head will help to raise her to a semi-sitting position, which can aid delivery. If you are awaiting emergency help and the head hasn't appeared, however, lying flat will slow delivery.

8. Protect delivery surfaces, if possible, with a plastic tablecloth, shower curtain, newspapers, towels, and so on. A dishpan or basin can be used to catch the amniotic fluid and blood.

9. As the top of the baby's head begins to appear, instruct the mother to pant or blow (not push), and apply very gentle counterpressure to the head to keep it from popping out suddenly. Let the head emerge gradually—*never* pull

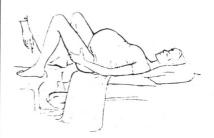

it out. If there is a loop of umbilical cord around the baby's neck, hook a finger under it and gently work it over the baby's head.

10. When the head has been delivered, gently stroke the sides of the nose downward, the neck and under the chin upward, to help expel mucus and amniotic fluid from the nose and mouth.

11. Next take the head gently in two hands and press it very slightly downward (do no pull), asking the mother to push at the same time, to deliver the front shoulder. As the upper arm appears, lift the head carefully, watching for the rear shoulder to deliver. Once the shoulders are free, the rest of the baby should slip out easily.

12. Quickly wrap the baby in blankets, towels, or anything else that is available (preferably something clean; something recently ironed is relatively sterile). Place the baby on the mother's abdomen, or if the cord is long enough (don't tug at it), at her breast.

13. Don't try to pull the placenta out. But if it arrives on its own before the ambulance comes, wrap it in towels or newspaper, and keep it elevated above the level of the baby, if possible. There is no need to try to cut the cord.

14. Keep both mother and baby warm and comfortable until help arrives.

may be all but abandoned during this stage, so as not to interfere with the mother's concentration. In this case, the fetal heart rate is checked periodically with a stethoscope.

Internal Monitoring. When more accurate results are required—such as when fetal distress is suspected—an internal monitor may be used. Since the electrode that transmits a reading of the fetal heartbeat is attached to the fetus's scalp through the cervix, internal monitoring is possible only once the cervix is dilated to at least 1 or 2 centimeters and the membranes have ruptured. Contractions can be measured either with the pressure gauge strapped to the maternal abdomen or with a fluid-filled catheter (tube) inserted into the uterus. Because an internal monitor can't be periodically disconnected and reconnected, it limits mobility somewhat—but changes in position are possible.

Sometimes internal monitoring employs telemetry, which reads and transmits vital signs via radio waves. This technique, pioneered in the space program, allows the patient to be monitored without being confined by equipment. She is totally mobile— able to strike any position she finds comfortable, to go to the bathroom, or even to take a stroll.

Like any invasive medical procedure (one that enters or intrudes upon the body), internal fetal monitoring entails some risk—mostly of infection. In some instances the fetus later develops a rash, or occasionally an abscess, on the site where the electrode was placed, and, very rarely, may even have a permanent bald spot. It may also be possible that the insertion of the electrode causes momentary pain or discomfort to the baby. Because of the risks, though they are slight, internal fetal monitoring is best used when its benefits are significant.

If your fetal monitor—external or internal—signals trouble, don't panic. Most such signals are false alarms. Sometimes the monitor isn't working right; sometimes it is misread. Frequently the abnormal heart rate reading is a result of the mother's position putting pressure on her vena cava or her baby's cord, interfering with blood flow to the fetus. A change in position (to lying on the left side) often rectifies the problem. If administration of oxytocin is causing the problem, reducing the dosage or terminating the infusion completely will generally eliminate it. Oxygen to the mother may also do the trick.

If the abnormal readings continue, several possible steps can be taken. If the danger to the fetus seems great, the physician may opt for an immediate abdominal delivery. Otherwise, some speedy testing will be done to confirm the diagnosis of fetal distress: the amniotic fluid will be checked for meconium; pH levels in a fetal blood sample, taken from the scalp, will be assessed; and/or the response of the fetal heart to sound stimulation, or to pressure on or pinching of the fetal scalp will be evaluated. Since direct access to the fetus is necessary in order for some of these determinations to be made, the membranes must be ruptured artificially at this point, if they haven't already ruptured spontaneously. In addition, the mother's medical and obstetrical history may be reviewed to determine if the fetal heart rate abnormalities are related to maternal infection or chronic disease or to medication the mother is taking, rather than to actual fetal distress. An experienced and knowledgeable obstetrician will take many factors into account before concluding that a baby is actually in trouble. In some cases, the monitor printout may be faxed to an expert for a second opinion. If fetal distress is confirmed, then an immediate cesarean is usually called for. In some cases, the physician may use drugs to try to improve the condition of the fetus in the uterus. When successful, this approach allows additional time for preparing for a cesarean delivery, enhances the chances of delivering an alert baby, and in some cases may even allow a vaginal delivery to continue.

The most recent review of fetal monitoring research suggests that monitoring probably does not save more newborn lives than the old-fashioned nurse-with-a-stethoscope method (checking every 15 minutes during labor and every 5 during delivery)—though it appears to slightly reduce the risk of neonatal seizures, the long-term effects of which seem to be minimal. Still, there are physicians who think it likely that some cases of fetal distress are detected with a monitor that might be missed otherwise. Thus its routine use remains controversial. Because electronic monitoring is expensive, because it is believed to have led to an increase in unnecessary cesareans in some hospitals (largely through misreadings), because some view it as just another technological intrusion into the natural birthing process, and because the impersonal machine replaces the personal ministrations of a nurse, the American College of Obstetricians and Gynecologists seems to be leaning toward a position that monitoring need only be used in high-risk deliveries. Nevertheless, some of the very doctors who are making this recommendation plan to continue monitoring all their patients. So apparently the issues aren't all that clear yet.

How expectant parents respond to electronic fetal monitoring depends a great deal on their attitudes. If they come into the labor or birthing room resentful or fearful of all that isn't "natural," they will probably find the fetal monitor objectionable. If they want the best of both worlds—the natural and the scientific—they will feel reassured and more in control at seeing their baby's heartbeats registering rhythmically on the monitor.

THE SIGHT OF BLOOD

"The sight of blood makes me feel faint. What if I pass out while I'm watching my delivery?"

The sight of blood makes many people feel weak-kneed. But remarkably, though they might faint while watching a film of someone else's delivery, even the most squeamish women manage to get through their own without smelling salts.

First of all, there isn't all that much blood—not much more than you see when you're menstruating (a little more with an episiotomy or a tear). Second, you won't be a spectator at your delivery—you'll be a very active participant, putting every ounce of your concentration and energy into pushing your baby those last few inches. Caught up in the excitement and anticipation (and, let's face it, the pain and fatigue), you are unlikely to notice, much less be unsettled by, any bleeding. Few new mothers would be able to tell you just how much blood, if any, there was at their deliveries.

If you feel strongly that you don't want to see any blood, simply avert your eyes from the mirror (if one has been provided for you) during the episiotomy and at the moment of birth. Instead, just look down past your belly for a good view of your baby as it emerges. From this vantage point, virtually no blood will be visible.

EPISIOTOMY

"My childbirth educator says we shouldn't have episiotomies—they aren't natural. My doctor says that's ridiculous. I don't know whether to have one or not."

To have or not to have an episiotomy? That is the question that has some obstetricians shooting it out with some childbirth educators and nurse-midwives, catching pregnant women in the crossfire.

The minor surgical procedure that is at the center of this heated controversy was originated in Ireland in 1742 to help facilitate difficult births, but it wasn't widely performed until the middle part of this century. Today, the episiotomy (a surgical incision made in the perineum to enlarge the vaginal opening just before the birth of the baby's head) is performed in 80% to 90% of first births, and in about 50% of subsequent deliveries.

There are two basic types of episiotomies: the median and the mediolateral. The median incision is made directly back toward the rectum. In spite of its advantages (it provides more exit space per inch of incision, heals well and is easier to repair, causes less blood loss, and results in less postpartum discomfort or infection), it is less frequently used in the United States because it has a greater risk of tearing completely through to the rectum. To avoid this tearing, most physicians prefer the medio-lateral incision, which slants away from the rectum, especially in first births.

Traditional medical wisdom supports the use of episiotomy for several reasons: Its straight edges are easier to repair than a ragged tear; timed well, it can prevent injury to the muscles of the perineum and vagina; it spares the fetal head from battering against the perineum; and it can shorten the pushing stage of labor by 15 to 30 minutes—particularly advantageous when there is prolonged labor, fetal distress, and/or maternal exhaustion.

Opponents counter that episiotomies are an unnatural, largely unnecessary, technological intrusion into the birth process. They claim that the incision made is often more extensive than tearing would be, and that it results in excessive bleeding, immediate postpartum discomfort, painful in-

tercourse for months afterward, and (sometimes) infection. Instead, they support the use of Kegel exercises (page 190) and local massage for four to six weeks before delivery to prepare and strengthen the perineum for delivery. During labor they recommend warm compresses to lessen perineal discomfort; massage; a standing or squatting position, and exhaling or grunting while pushing to facilitate stretching of the perineum; and avoidance of regional anesthesia, which makes the perineal muscles flaccid. Although all of these measures can improve the odds of a birth occurring without episiotomy, and sometimes without tearing, they don't guarantee such a birth. At birthing centers where they are employed regularly, between 15% and 25% of women have episiotomies, and 25% to 30% of the others tear badly enough to need repair. Another 3% or 4% end up with serious lacerations extending to the rectum.

What hard-liners (those who routinely perform episiotomies, even when they're not needed, and those who routinely refrain from performing them, even when they are needed) fail to recognize is that "to have or not to have an episiotomy" is a question that shouldn't be answered in the classroom or the office—but in the delivery or birthing room, as the baby's head crowns. It is only then that a realistic judgment can be made as to whether or not the perineum can stretch sufficiently to accommodate the baby's head without tearing, and whether not doing an episiotomy will jeopardize fetal or maternal well-being by prolonging labor. The prudent physician or nurse-midwife who has some doubt will generally opt for the episiotomy rather than risk an uncontrolled and difficult-to-repair tear.

If you feel, after reading this, discussing the issue with your practitioner, and weighing the evidence, that you would prefer not to have an episiotomy if at all possible, say so in your birthing plan (page 225) or otherwise make your preference known. But remember that the final decision should be made in the delivery or birthing room, with your well-being and the speedy and safe delivery of your baby the prime considerations.

BEING STRETCHED BY CHILDBIRTH

"The thing that frightens me most is my vagina stretching and tearing. Will I ever be the same again?"

The vagina is a remarkably elastic organ whose accordion-like folds open for childbirth. It is normally so narrow that inserting a tampon may be difficult, yet it can expand to allow the passage of a 7- or 8-pound baby. After birth, over a period of weeks, it returns to almost its original size. For most women the slight increase in roominess is imperceptible and does not interfere with sexual enjoyment. For those who were unusually small before conception, it can be a real plus, as intercourse may become more pleasurable.

The perineum, the area between the vagina and the rectum, is also elastic, but less so than the vagina. In some women, the perineum will stretch enough without tearing to allow the birth of a baby. But in others, it will tear unless an episiotomy is performed by the birth attendant. Stretching may leave the muscles a little slacker than will a carefully timed episiotomy, one in which the perineum wasn't allowed to stretch excessively before the incision was made.

But exercising the muscles of childbirth long before you get to the delivery room may enhance elasticity and certainly will hasten their return to normal tone. Kegel exercises, which strengthen the muscles in the perineal area (see page 190), should be done regularly during pregnancy and for at least six months following childbirth.

Many couples report that sex after delivery is even more satisfying than it was before, thanks to the increased muscular awareness and control the woman has developed as a result of prepared childbirth training. In other words, you may not be the same after childbirth—you may be even better!

Very occasionally, however, in a woman who "just right" before, childbirth does stretch the vagina enough to reduce sexual enjoyment. Often the vaginal muscles tighten up again with the passage of time. Faithfully doing Kegels at frequent intervals during the day—while showering, urinating, washing the dishes, walking the baby, driving the car, sitting at your desk—may help speed the process. If after six months the vagina still seems too slack, medical advice should be sought.

BEING STRAPPED TO THE DELIVERY TABLE

"The idea of being strapped to a table like my mother was terrifies me. Is this really necessary?"

The prospect of being bound, hand and foot, to a delivery table is an appalling one—particularly to women who wish to participate fully in childbirth. Fortunately, though it was once routine procedure, it is virtually unheard of today. Most birthing attendants will simply ask the woman to keep her hands above her waist, away from the area that should remain sterile during the delivery; if she should forget in the middle of a particularly consuming contraction, her coach and the nurse are there to remind her.

Whether or not the woman's feet are up in stirrups during delivery (there's no need for this during labor), and whether her legs are strapped to the stirrups, depends on hospital policy, practitioner preference, and, most of all, the patient's wishes.

The use of stirrups in delivery evolved for several reasons. One, they kept the woman's legs elevated and out of the way so that the doctor had adequate work space. Two, they kept her from involuntarily kicking during a powerful contraction (possibly interfering with the delivery). Finally, they kept her feet out of the area that should remain as sterile as possible.

One reason that stirrups are now used less often in many hospitals—and hardly at all in birthing rooms, where special birthing beds have taken the place of delivery tables—is that a variety of birthing positions have replaced the standard woman-on-her-back-legs-up-and-spread attitude. Another is strong opposition from women who want to retain as much dignity and control as possible during their deliveries. In addition, because woman are now generally better prepared for childbirth, they aren't as likely to thrash around in pain and fear of the unknown. Still many physicians continue to ask their patients to use the stirrups during delivery because they believe this allows room for maneuvering and therefore for a safer delivery.

Discuss this issue with your practitioner in advance, sharing your feelings and listening to his or hers. It is very likely that your wishes will prevail or that, at the very least, a compromise can be reached.

THE USE OF FORCEPS

"I've heard all kinds of horror stories about forceps. What if my doctor wants to use them?"

It was in 1598 that British surgeon Peter Chamberlen the Elder designed the first pair of forceps and used the tong-shaped instrument to ease babies out of the birth canal when a difficult delivery might otherwise cost both mother and infant their lives. Instead of writing himself up in the latest obstetrical journal, however, Dr. Chamberlen kept his discovery a secret—privy only to four generations of Chamberlen medical men and their patients, many of them royalty. Indeed, the use of forceps might have ended forever with the career of the last Chamberlen doctor, had a hidden box of instruments not been uncovered beneath a floorboard in the family's ancestral home in the mid-1800s.

To the minds of some today, the use of forceps should have died with the Chamberlens. But that's not quite a fair assessment. Before cesarean sections became commonplace and safe, forceps delivery was the only way out for a baby stuck in the birth canal. The occasional serious damage caused by the use of forceps was considered a small price to pay for the countless lives saved. The risks were clearly outweighed by the benefits.

But the picture is more complicated. Today, the high-forceps procedure, in which the doctor reaches up into the maternal pelvis to extract a stuck baby, and to which most of the horror stories you've heard are probably attributable, has been totally abandoned in favor of cesarean delivery. But the American College of Obstetricians and Gynecologists and most physicians still see a role for mid-, low-, and outlet forceps deliveries. Such deliveries, the most recent studies show, pose no more risk to mother and baby than cesareans *when carried out properly by someone experienced in forceps use.* Before resorting to a cesarean, many physicians will try the judicious use of forceps when a baby's head is engaged and labor has stalled.

In countries such as Great Britain where this is routine, the rate of cesarean deliveries is, as a consequence, relatively low.

Forceps should be used only when valid indications exist (fetal distress, maternal distress, prolonged labor, prolonged second stage). And all should be in readiness for a cesarean section should a trial of forceps fail.

When forceps are used, a local anesthetic (see page 229) is administered to the mother. Then the curved blunt blades are cradled one at a time around the crowning head, at the temples, and the baby is gently delivered. The vacuum extractor, which suctions the infant out of the birth canal via a metal or plastic cup (less traumatic) applied to the head, is an option that may be used instead of forceps by your practitioner.

If you have any concerns about the possible use of forceps or vacuum extraction during your delivery, discuss them with your practitioner now, before you go into labor. He or she should be able to allay your fears.

THE BABY'S CONDITION

"The doctor said the baby is okay, but her Apgar score was only 7. Is she really all right?"

Your doctor is right. Any Apgar score of 7 or over indicates a baby in good condition. However, most babies with lower scores also turn out to be normal and healthy.

The Apgar test was developed by Dr. Virginia Apgar, a noted anesthesiologist, to enable medical personnel

APGAR TABLE

SIGN	POINTS		
	0	1	2
Appearance (color)*	Pale or blue	Body pink, extremities blue	Pink
Pulse (heartbeat)	Not detectible	Below 100	Over 100
Grimace (reflex irritability)	No response to stimulation	Grimace	Lusty cry
Activity (muscle tone)	Flaccid (no or weak activity)	Some movement of extremities	A lot of activity
Respiration (breathing)	None	Slow, irregular	Good (crying)

*In non-Caucasian children, the color of mucous membranes of the mouth, of the whites of the eyes, and of the lips, palms, hands, and soles of feet will be examined.

to quickly evaluate the condition of a newborn. At 60 seconds after birth, a nurse or doctor checks the infant's *A*ppearance (color), *P*ulse (heartbeat), *G*rimace (reflex), *A*ctivity (muscle tone), and *R*espiration. Hence the acronym APGAR. (See Apgar Table, below.) Those who score between 4 and 6 often need resuscitation—which generally includes suctioning their airways and administering oxygen. Those who score under 4 require more dramatic lifesaving techniques.

The Apgar test is administered once again at five minutes after birth. If the score is 7 or better at this point, the outlook for the infant is very good. If it's low, it means the baby needs some careful watching, but is still very likely to turn out to be fine.

WHAT IT'S IMPORTANT TO KNOW:
THE STAGES OF CHILDBIRTH

Few pregnancies seem as though they could have been lifted right from the pages of an obstetrical text—with morning sickness that vanishes at the end of the first trimester, first fetal movements felt at precisely 20 weeks, and lightening that occurs exactly two weeks before the onset of labor. Likewise, few childbirth experiences mirror the textbook case—commencing with mild regular contractions that progress at a predictable pace to delivery. Yet just as it's helpful to have a general idea of what a typical woman can expect when she's expecting, it's helpful to know what an average childbirth is like—as long as you are prepared for the likelihood of variations that will make your experience yours alone.

Childbirth is divided (more loosely by nature, more formally by obstetrical science) into three stages. The first stage is labor, with its early, active, and transitional phases ending with the full dilation (opening) of the cervix; the second stage is delivery, culminating in the birth of the baby; and the third is delivery of the placenta, or afterbirth. The whole process averages about 14 hours for first-time mothers, about 8 hours for women who have already had children.

Unless labor is cut short by the need for a cesarean, all women who carry to term go through all three phases of the first stage. Some, however, may not recognize that they are in labor until the second, or even the third, phase because their initial contractions are mild or painless. The third phase of labor is complete once the cervix has dilated to a full 10 centimeters. For a very few women, all of dilatation passes unnoticed; they don't realize they're in labor until they feel the urge to push that signals the second, or delivery, stage.

The timing and intensity of contractions can help pinpoint which phase of labor a woman is in at any particular time. Periodic internal exams, to check on the progress of dilatation, will confirm the progress.

If labor doesn't seem to be progressing along the typical course, many doctors will augment Mother Nature's efforts (with oxytocin, for example), and if that fails, will preempt her entirely with a cesarean section. Others may elect to allow more time before taking such action, as long as both mother and baby are doing well.

Labor Positions

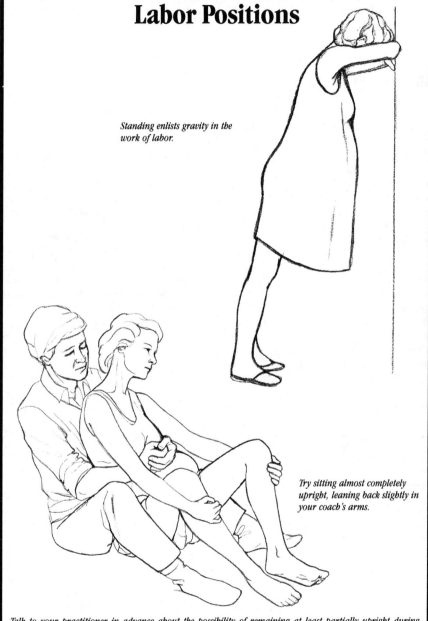

Standing enlists gravity in the work of labor.

Try sitting almost completely upright, leaning back slightly in your coach's arms.

Talk to your practitioner in advance about the possibility of remaining at least partially upright during labor: perhaps standing, walking, or sitting (in a rocking or beanbag chair, or in your husband's arms). Studies show that upright positions can shorten labor by speeding dilatation and descent—though the position that works best and is most comfortable varies from woman to woman. Lying flat on your back can not only slow down labor, but can also compress major blood vessels (especially if you are on a firm surface), possibly interfering with blood flow to the fetus. If you are more comfortable lying down, lie on your side, switching sides and doing pelvic tilts periodically.

THE FIRST STAGE OF CHILDBIRTH: LABOR

THE FIRST PHASE: EARLY OR LATENT LABOR

This is usually the longest and, fortunately, the least intense phase of labor. The dilatation (opening) of the cervix to 3 centimeters and the accompanying effacement (thinning out) that characterize this phase can be reached over a period of days or weeks without noticeable or bothersome contractions, or over a period of two to six hours (and, less commonly, up to 24 hours) of unmistakable labor.

Contractions in this phase usually last 30 to 45 seconds. They are mild to moderately strong, may be regular or irregular (ranging between 5 and 20 minutes apart), and become progressively closer together, but not necessarily in a consistent pattern. Some women don't notice them at all.

You will probably be told to go to the hospital at the end of this phase or the beginning of the next.

What You May Be Feeling or Noticing.
The most common signs and symptoms in this phase include backache (either constant or with each contraction), menstrual-like cramps, indigestion, diarrhea, a sensation of warmth in the abdomen, and bloody show (a blood-tinged mucousy discharge). You may experience all of these, or just one or two. The amniotic membranes may have ruptured before the onset of contractions, but it is more likely that they will rupture sometime during labor itself. (If they don't rupture spontaneously, your practitioner may decide to rupture them artificially sometime after you've gone into active labor.)

Emotionally, you may feel excitement, relief, anticipation, uncertainty, anxiety, fear; some women are relaxed and chatty, others tense and apprehensive.

What You Can Do:
❖ Relax. Your practitioner has probably told you not to call until you are in more active labor. Or he or she may have suggested that you call early on if labor begins during the day or if your membranes rupture. Definitely call, however, if your membranes rupture and the amniotic fluid is murky or greenish, if you have any bright red bleeding, or if you feel no fetal activity (it may be hard to notice because you are distracted by contractions, so you might want to try the test on page 202). Although you may not feel like it, it's best if you, not your coach, make the call and talk to your practitioner. A lot can be lost in third-party translations.

❖ If it's the middle of the night, try to sleep (but not on your back; see page 173 for the recommended sleeping position). It's important to rest now, because you probably won't be able to later on in labor. And you needn't fear that you'll sleep through the next phase—the contractions will be too insistent. If sleep eludes you, don't just lie in bed timing contractions—that'll only make labor seem longer. Instead, get up and do things around the house that will distract you. Clean out a closet; put sheets on the baby's bed; finish packing your bag for the hospital (see page 265); make your coach a sandwich to take along; play solitaire; do a jigsaw puzzle.

❖ If it's daytime, go about your usual routine—as long as it doesn't take you far from home. If you have nothing planned, find something to keep you occupied. Try some of the distractions suggested above, take a walk (gravity aids the work of labor), watch TV, make and freeze a casserole or two for easy postpartum dining. Put your husband on alert, but it's not necessary for him to come running home—yet.

❖ Make yourself comfortable. Take a warm bath (only if your membranes haven't ruptured) or a shower (but be careful not to slip); use a heating pad if your back is aching—but *do not* take aspirin or lie on your back.

❖ Eat a light snack if you're hungry (broth, toast with apple butter, or fruit juice). Don't eat heavily, and avoid hard-to-digest foods, such as meats, dairy products, and fats. Not only will digesting a heavy meal compete with the birthing process for body resources, but a full stomach could cause complications if you should need anesthesia later on.

❖ Time contractions for a half-hour span if they seem to be getting closer than 10 minutes apart, and periodically even if they don't. But don't be a clock watcher.

❖ Remember to urinate frequently to avoid bladder distention, which could inhibit the progress of labor.

❖ Use relaxation techniques if they help, but don't start your breathing exercises yet, or you will become bored and exhausted long before you really need them.

What the Coach Can Do:
❖ Practice timing contractions. The interval between contractions is timed from the beginning of one to the beginning of the next. Time them periodically, and keep a record. When they are coming less than 10 minutes apart, time them more frequently.

❖ Be a calming influence. During this early phase of labor, your most important function is to keep the expectant mother relaxed. And the best way to do this is to keep yourself relaxed, both inside and out. Your own anxiety can be transferred to her unwittingly, communicated not just through words but through touch. Doing some relaxation exercises together or giving her a gentle, unhurried massage may help you both. It's too soon, however, to begin using breathing exercises.

❖ Keep your sense of humor, and help her keep hers; time flies, after all, when you're having fun. It'll be easier to laugh now than when contractions are coming fast and hard.

❖ Help distract the expectant mother. Suggest activities that will help keep both your minds off her labor: reading aloud, playing board games or cards, viewing engrossing (and preferably light) television fare, taking short walks.

❖ Offer comfort, reassurance, and support. She'll need them all from now on.

❖ Keep up your own strength so you'll be able to reinforce hers. Eat periodically (not necessarily in front of her), even if she can't. Prepare a sandwich to bring along to the hospital (but nothing with an overpowering or lingering odor that might make you, or your wife, feel queasy—such as salami or tuna).

If You Aren't Making Progress

Progress in labor is measured by the dilatation, or opening, of the cervix and the descent of the fetus through the pelvis. Good progress is believed to require three main components: strong uterine contractions that effectively dilate the cervix; a baby that can fit through the pelvis and is in position for easy exit; and a pelvis that is sufficiently roomy to permit the passage of the baby.

If one or more of these factors is not present, abnormal (or dysfunctional) labor, in which progress is slow or nonexistent, generally occurs. There are several types of abnormal labor:

Prolonged Latent Phase—when little or no dilatation has occurred after 20 hours of labor in a first-time mother, or after 14 hours in one who has delivered previously. Sometimes progress is slow because labor hasn't really begun and the contractions felt are those of false—not true—labor. Sometimes the reason is overmedication before labor was well established. Sometimes, it is theorized, the cause may be psychological: a woman panics when labor begins, triggering the release of chemicals in the nervous system that interfere with uterine contractions.

In general, the practitioner may suggest stimulating a slow first phase of labor with activity (such as walking) or with just the opposite (sleep and rest, possibly aided by the use of relaxation techniques and, if the laboring woman is too agitated to relax naturally, an alcoholic drink or the administration of a sedative). Such treatment will also help rule out false labor (the contractions of false labor will usually subside with activity or a nap).

Once true latent-phase labor has been established, it may be speeded up with an enema or mineral oil, with walking, or with the administration of oxytocin. (Note: it is important to remember to urinate periodically, as a full bladder can interfere with the baby's descent.) If attempts to stimulate labor are unsuccessful, the practitioner may have to consider the possibility that cephalopelvic disproportion (a mismatch between the fetus's head and the mother's pelvis) exists.

Most physicians will perform a cesarean after 24 or 25 hours (sometimes sooner) if sufficient progress has not been made by that time; some will wait longer, as long as both mother and baby are doing well.

Primary Dysfunction of Active Phase—when the second, or active,

THE SECOND PHASE: ACTIVE LABOR

The second, or active, phase of labor is usually shorter than the first, lasting an average of 2 to 3½ hours (with a wide range of normal). The contractions are more concentrated now, accomplishing more in less time. As they become stronger, longer (40 to 60 seconds, with a dis-

tinct peak of about half that time), and more frequent (generally 3 to 4 minutes apart, though the pattern may not be regular), the cervix dilates to 7 centimeters. There is less time to rest between contractions.

You will probably be in the hospital early in this phase—unless, as occasionally happens, dilatation occurs over a period of a week or two, in which case labor may not be apparent until the next phase (transition).

phase of labor progresses very slowly (less than 1 to 1.2 centimeters of dilatation per hour in women having their first babies, and 1.5 centimeters per hour in those who've had previous deliveries). When any progress, albeit slow, is being made, many practitioners will let the uterus set its own pace—on the theory that the woman will eventually deliver naturally, as two-thirds of those who experience primary dysfunction do. A laboring woman may be able to speed up the work of her uterus by walking, if possible, staying off her back, and keeping her bladder empty. Intravenous fluids will probably be administered during a lengthy labor.

Secondary Arrest of Dilatation— when, during active labor, there is no progress for two hours or more. In about half of these cases, it is estimated, disproportion exists between the fetal head and the pelvis (CPD), necessitating a cesarean delivery. In most other cases, the administration of oxytocin (sometimes along with artificial rupture of the membranes) will reestablish labor, particularly when the cause of the labor slowdown is simply exhaustion. Again, the woman may be able to contribute to the battle against sluggish labor by utilizing gravity when possible (sitting upright, squatting, standing, or walking) and by keeping her bladder empty.

Abnormal Descent of the Fetus— when the baby moves down the birth canal at a rate of less than 1 centimeter per hour in women having their first babies, or 2 centimeters per hour in others. In most such cases delivery will be slow, but otherwise uneventful. Trying to remove with forceps a baby that isn't already at the vaginal outlet, once common practice, is now considered dangerous and unnecessary. Today, stimulation with oxytocin and/or artificial rupture of the membranes is preferred—once CPD and a fetal position that would make vaginal delivery difficult have been ruled out.

Prolonged Second Stage— one that lasts longer than two hours in a first delivery, or slightly less in subsequent deliveries. Many physicians routinely use outlet forceps or perform a cesarean when a second stage goes beyond two hours; others allow the spontaneous vaginal delivery to continue if steady progress is being made and both mother and fetus (whose conditions are being carefully monitored) are doing well. Sometimes the baby's head is gently eased out those last few inches with outlet forceps. Rotation of the head (so that it faces back and will better fit through the pelvis) may also be attempted, either manually or with forceps. Gravity, again, can help; a semi-sitting or semi-squatting position may be most effective for delivery.

What You May Be Feeling or Noticing. The most common signs and symptoms in this phase include increasing discomfort with contractions (you may be unable to talk through them now), increasing backache, leg discomfort, fatigue, increasing bloody show. You may experience all of these, or just one or two. Rupture of the membranes may occur now if it hasn't earlier. (If they don't rupture spontaneously, your practitioner may choose to rupture them artificially sometime during this phase.)

Emotionally, you may feel restless and find it more difficult to relax; or your concentration may become more intense, and you may become completely absorbed in the work at hand. Your confidence may begin to waver, and you may feel as if labor is never going to end; or you may feel excited and encouraged that things are really starting to happen.

What You Can Do:

❖ Start your breathing exercises, if you plan to use them, as soon as contractions become too strong to talk through. (If you have never practiced any of these exercises, some simple breathing suggestions from the nurse may help make you more comfortable.) If the exercises seem to make you uncomfortable or more tense, however, don't feel that you have to use them. Women have given birth without them for centuries.

❖ If your practitioner permits it (some do, particularly if there is no medication being given), drink clear beverages frequently to replace fluids and to keep your mouth moist. If you're uncomfortably hungry, and again if you have your practitioner's okay, have a light snack of a nonfat, non-fibrous food (sorbet, Jell-O, or applesauce, for example). If your practitioner prohibits anything else by mouth, sucking on ice chips can serve to refresh. Some doctors and hospitals, however, discourage even ice chips and use IVs to keep laboring patients hydrated.

❖ Make a concerted effort to relax between contractions. This will become increasingly difficult as they come more frequently, but it will also become increasingly important as your energy reserves are taxed.

❖ Walk around, if possible, or at least change position frequently, seeking those that provide the most comfort. (See page 289 for suggested labor positions.)

❖ Remember to urinate periodically; because of tremendous pelvic pressure, you may not notice the need to empty your bladder.

❖ If you feel you need some pain relief, don't be afraid to discuss it with your attendant. He or she may suggest waiting for 20 minutes or half an hour before actual administration—at which point you may have made so much progress that you won't need it, or you may have found renewed strength and no longer want it.

What the Coach Can Do:

❖ If possible, keep the door of the labor or birthing room closed, the lights low, and the room quiet to promote a restful atmosphere. Soft music, if permitted, may also help. Continue relaxation techniques between contractions. And stay as calm as possible yourself.

❖ Keep track of the contractions. If your wife is on a fetal monitor, ask the practitioner or the nurse to show you how to read it. Later, when contractions are coming one on top of the other, you can alert your wife as each new contraction begins. (The monitor may detect the tensing of the uterus before she can.) You can also encourage her by telling her when each peak is ending. This will give both of you some sense of control over the labor. If there is no monitor, learn to recognize the arrival and departure of contractions with your hand on your wife's abdomen.

❖ Breathe with her through difficult contractions, if that helps her. Don't pressure her to do the breathing exercises if she is uncomfortable with them, they make her tense, or they annoy her.

❖ If she shows any symptoms of hyperventilation (dizziness or lightheadedness, blurred vision, tingling and numbness of fingers and toes), have her exhale into a paper bag (the nurse will be able to supply one if you haven't brought one

On to the Hospital

Getting to the Hospital. Sometime near the end of the early phase or the beginning of the active phase (probably when your contractions are five minutes apart or less, sooner if you live far from the hospital or if this isn't your first baby), your practitioner will tell you to pick up your bag and get going. Getting to the hospital will be easier if you've planned your route in advance, are familiar with parking regulations, and know which entrance will get you to the obstetrical floor most quickly. (If parking is likely to be a problem, taking a cab may be more sensible.) En route, try stretching out on the rear seat with a pillow for your head, your seat belt fastened loosely beneath your belly, and if you have chills, a blanket covering you.

Hospital Admission. Procedures will vary, but you can probably expect something like the following:

❖ If you've preregistered (and it's best if you have), this process will be brief; if you're in active labor, your coach can take care of it.

❖ Once in the labor and delivery suite or birthing unit, you will be taken to a labor or birthing room by your nurse for this shift. Depending on hospital regulations, your husband and other family members may be asked to wait outside while you are being admitted and "prepped." (Note to the coach: This is a good time to make a few priority phone calls, to get a snack, and to arrange for stowing your wife's luggage in her room and for chilling the celebratory champagne. If you aren't called to join your wife within 20 minutes or so, remind someone at the nurses' station that you are waiting. Be prepared for the possibility that you will be asked to put on a sterile gown over your clothes.)

❖ Your nurse will take a brief history, asking, among other things, when the contractions started, how far apart they are, whether your membranes have ruptured, when it was that you last ate.

❖ Your nurse will ask for your signature on routine consent forms.

❖ Your nurse will give you a hospital gown to change into and will request a urine sample. She will check your pulse, blood pressure, respiration, and temperature; look for leaking amniotic fluid, bleeding, or bloody show; listen to the fetal heartbeat with a stethoscope or hook you up to a fetal monitor; and, possibly, evaluate the fetal position and take a fetal blood sample.

❖ Depending on the policies of your doctor and hospital, and possibly, your preferences, your pubic area may be partially shaved, you may be given an enema, and/or an IV may be started.

❖ Your nurse, your practitioner, or a resident doctor will examine you internally to see how dilated and effaced your cervix is. If your membranes haven't ruptured spontaneously and you are at least 3 or 4 centimeters dilated (many practitioners prefer to wait until the cervix has dilated to at least 5 centimeters), your membranes may be artificially ruptured—unless you and your practitioner have decided to leave them intact until later in labor. The procedure is painless; all you will feel is a warm gush of fluid.

If you have any questions that haven't been answered before, now is the time for you or your coach to ask them.

along) or into cupped hands. She should then inhale the exhaled air. After repeating this several times, she should feel better. If she doesn't, inform a nurse or your practitioner at once.

❖ Offer constant verbal reassurance (if it doesn't make your wife more edgy); praise, but don't criticize, her efforts (think what you'd like her to say if your roles were reversed). Particularly if progress is slow, remind her to take her labor one contraction at a time, and that each pain brings her closer to seeing the baby.

❖ Massage her abdomen or back, or use counterpressure or any other techniques you've learned, to make her more comfortable. Take your cues from her; let her tell you what kind of stroking or touching or massage helps. If she prefers not to be touched at all (some women find it annoying), then it might be best to comfort her verbally.

❖ Don't pretend the pain doesn't exist, even if she doesn't complain; she needs your empathy. And don't tell her you know how it feels (you don't).

❖ Remind her to relax between contractions.

❖ Remind her to try to urinate at least once an hour.

❖ Don't take it personally if she doesn't respond to—or even seems irritated by—your attempts to comfort her. A woman's moods during labor are mercurial. Stand by to offer support as she needs and wants it. Remember that your role is important, even if you sometimes feel superfluous.

❖ If it is allowed, be sure she has an ample supply of ice chips to suck on or fluids to sip. From time to time ask her if she would like some.

❖ Use a damp washcloth, wrung out in cold water, to help cool her body and face; refresh it often.

❖ If her feet are cold, offer to get out a pair of socks and help her to put them on.

❖ Continue with distractions she finds helpful (card games, conversation between contractions, reading aloud), encouragement, and support.

❖ Suggest a change of position; walk around with her, if that's possible.

❖ Serve as her go-between with medical personnel as much as possible. Intercept questions that you can answer, ask for explanations of procedures, equipment, any medication, so you'll be able to tell her what's happening. For instance, now might be the time to find out if a mirror will be provided so that she can view the delivery. Be her advocate when necessary, but try to fight her battles quietly, perhaps outside the room, so that she won't be disturbed.

❖ If she requests medication, communicate her request to the nurse or doctor, but suggest a waiting period before the administration. During that time, the practitioner will probably want to discuss the need for medication and do an internal exam to check on the progress of labor anyway. It's possible that an encouraging progress report or some time to think it over may give your wife renewed strength to continue unmedicated. Don't be disappointed, however, if she and the doctor decide that medication is needed. Remember, labor isn't a test of pain endurance that your wife will fail if she asks for or accepts medication.

What Hospital Personnel Will Do:

❖ Provide a relaxed, comfortable, supportive environment and answers to your questions and concerns.

❖ Continue monitoring the baby's condition with a stethoscope or electronic fetal monitor, and through observation of the amniotic fluid (greenish-brown staining is a sign of possible fetal distress). Fetal position may be assessed with external palpation.

❖ Continue checking your blood pressure.

❖ Periodically evaluate the timing and strength of contractions and quantity and quality of bloody discharge. (Pads beneath your buttocks will be replaced as needed.) When there is a change in the pattern or intensity of contractions, or the show becomes more bloody, an internal exam will be done to check the progress of your labor.

❖ Possibly, stimulate labor if it is progressing very slowly, by the use of oxytocin or artificial rupture of the membranes if they are still intact, and if this wasn't done earlier.

❖ Administer sedatives and/or analgesics as needed and desired.

THE THIRD PHASE: ADVANCED ACTIVE OR TRANSITIONAL LABOR

Transition is the most exhausting and demanding phase of labor. Suddenly the intensity of the contractions picks up. They become very strong, two to three minutes apart, and 60 to 90 seconds long—with very intense peaks that last for most of the contraction. Some women, particularly women who have given birth before, experience multiple peaks. You may feel as though the contractions never completely disappear, and that you can't completely relax between them. The final 3 centimeters of dilatation, to a full 10 centimeters, will probably take place in a very short time: on average, 15 minutes to an hour.

What You May Be Feeling or Noticing. In transition, you are likely to feel strong pressure in the lower back and/or perineum. Rectal pressure, with or without an urge to push or move your bowels, may cause you to grunt involuntarily. You may feel either very warm and sweaty or chilled and shaky, or alternate between the two. Your bloody vaginal show will increase as more capillaries in the cervix rupture; your legs may be crampy and cold and may tremble uncontrollably. You may experience nausea and/or vomiting, and drowsiness may overcome you between contractions as oxygen is diverted from your brain to the site of the delivery. Not surprisingly, at this point you may feel exhausted.

Emotionally, you may feel vulnerable and overwhelmed; you're reaching the end of your rope. In addition to frustration over not being able to push yet, you may feel discouraged, irritable, disoriented, restless, and have difficulty concentrating and relaxing (it may seem impossible to do either).

What You Can Do:

❖ Hang in there. By the end of this phase, your cervix will be fully dilated, and it will be time to begin pushing your baby out.

❖ Instead of thinking about the work ahead, try to think about how far you've come.

❖ If you feel the urge to push, pant or blow instead, unless you've been instructed otherwise. Pushing

against a cervix that isn't completely dilated can cause the cervix
to swell, which can delay delivery.

❖ If you don't want anybody to
touch you unnecessarily, if your

coach's once comforting hands
now irritate you, don't hesitate to
let him know.

❖ If you find them useful, use breathing techniques you have learned

Pain Risk Factors

Your perception of pain may be increased by:	It may be decreased by:
Being alone.	Having the company and support of those you love, and/or of experienced medical personnel.
Fatigue.	Being well rested (try not to overdo things during the ninth month); trying to rest and relax between contractions.
Hunger and thirst.	Having light snacks during early labor; sucking ice chips throughout, drinking fluid if permitted.
Thinking about and expecting pain.	Turning your mind to other thoughts and distractions (though not during pushing); thinking of contractions in terms of how much they accomplish, rather than how much they hurt; and remembering that no matter how intense the discomfort, it will be of relatively brief duration.
Anxiety and stress; tensing up during contractions.	Using relaxation or visualization techniques between contractions; concentrating on your breathing or pushing efforts during them.
Fear of the unknown.	Learning as much as you can about childbirth in advance; taking childbirth one contraction at a time; and not worrying about what's to come.
Self-pity.	Thinking about how lucky you are and about the wonderful reward ahead.
Feeling out of control and helpless.	Having good childbirth preparation; knowing enough to feel some measure of control and confidence.

that are appropriate for this stage of labor (or ask the nurse for guidance).

❖ Try to relax between contractions (as much as is humanly possible) with slow, rhythmic chest breathing.

What the Coach Can Do:

❖ Be specific and direct in your instructions, without wasting words. She may find small talk annoying. If she doesn't want your help anymore at some point, don't take it personally. Give her the space she needs for as long as she needs it, but stay nearby in case you can be of help.

❖ Offer lots of encouragement and praise, unless she prefers you to keep quiet. At this moment, eye contact or touch may communicate more expressively than words.

❖ Touch her only if she finds it comforting. Abdominal massage may be offensive now, though counterpressure applied to the small of her back may provide some measure of relief for back discomfort.

❖ Breathe with her through every contraction if it seems to help her through them.

❖ Remind her to take it one contraction at a time. Again, she may need you to warn her when each begins and to tell her as it declines.

❖ Help her relax between contractions, touching her abdomen lightly to show her when a contraction is over. Remind her to use slow, rhythmic breathing.

❖ If her contractions seem to be getting closer and/or she feels the urge to push—and she hasn't been examined recently—inform the nurse or practitioner. She may be fully dilated.

❖ Offer her ice chips frequently, if allowed, and mop her brow with a cool damp cloth often.

What Hospital Personnel May Do:

❖ Continue providing comfort and support.

❖ Continue monitoring your condition and that of the fetus.

❖ Continue noting duration and intensity of contractions, and the progress you are making.

❖ Prepare for delivery, ultimately moving you to a delivery room if you are not delivering in a birthing or labor room.

THE SECOND STAGE OF CHILDBIRTH: PUSHING AND DELIVERY

Up to this point, your active participation in the birth of your child has been negligible. Though you've undeniably taken the brunt of the abuse in the proceedings, your cervix and uterus (and baby) have done most of the work. But now that dilatation is complete, your help is needed to push the baby the remainder of the way through the birth canal and out. This generally takes between half an hour and an hour, but can be accomplished in 10 short minutes or in two, three, or even more very long hours.

The contractions of the second stage are usually more regular than the contractions of transition. They are still about 60 to 90 seconds long, but sometimes farther apart (usually about two to five minutes) and possibly less painful—though sometimes they are more intense. There now should be a well-defined rest period between them, although you may still have trouble recognizing the onset of each contraction.

What You May Be Feeling or Noticing. Common in the second stage is an overwhelming urge to push—although not every woman feels it. You may experience a burst of renewed energy (a second wind) or fatigue; tremendous rectal pressure; very visible contractions, with the uterus rising noticeably with each; an increase in bloody show; a tingling, stretching, burning, or stinging sensation at the vagina as the head crowns; and a slippery wet feeling as the baby emerges.

Emotionally, you may feel relieved that you can now start pushing (though some women feel embarrassed or inhibited); you may also feel exhilarated and excited or, if the pushing stretches on for much more than an hour, frustrated or overwhelmed. In prolonged second stages, the woman's preoccupation is often less with seeing the baby than with getting the ordeal over with; this is a natural, and temporary, reaction, which in no way reflects on her capacity for motherly love.

What You Can Do:

❖ Get into a pushing position (which one will depend upon hospital policy, your practitioner's predilection, the bed or chair you are in, and most important, what is most comfortable and effective for you). A semi-sitting or semi-squatting position is probably the best because it enlists the aid of gravity in the birthing process and may afford you more pushing power.

❖ Give it all you've got. The more efficiently you push, and the more energy you pack into the effort, the more quickly your baby will make the trip through the birth canal. But keep your efforts controlled, coordinating your rhythm closely with the instructions of the practitioner or nurse. Frantic, disorganized pushing wastes energy and accomplishes little.

❖ Don't let inhibition or embarrassment break the pushing rhythm. Since you're bearing down on the whole perineal area, anything that's in your rectum may be pushed out too; trying to avoid this while you're pushing can impede your progress. A little involuntary evacuation (or even a little passage of urine) is experienced by nearly everyone in delivery. No one else in the room will think twice about it, and neither should you. Sterile pads will be used to whisk away any excretion immediately.

❖ Do what comes naturally. Push when you feel the urge, unless otherwise instructed. Take a few deep breaths while the contraction is building; take another and hold it. As the contraction peaks, push with all your might until you can no longer comfortably hold your breath. You may feel as many as five urges to bear down with each contraction. Follow each urge, rather than trying to hold your breath and push through an entire contraction; breath-holding for long periods of time can exhaust you and may deprive the fetus of oxygen. It can also increase the risk of breaking blood vessels in your eyes and face. Taking several deep breaths as the contraction wanes will help restore your respiratory balance. If nothing seems to be coming naturally—and pushing doesn't for every woman—your practitioner

A Baby Is Born

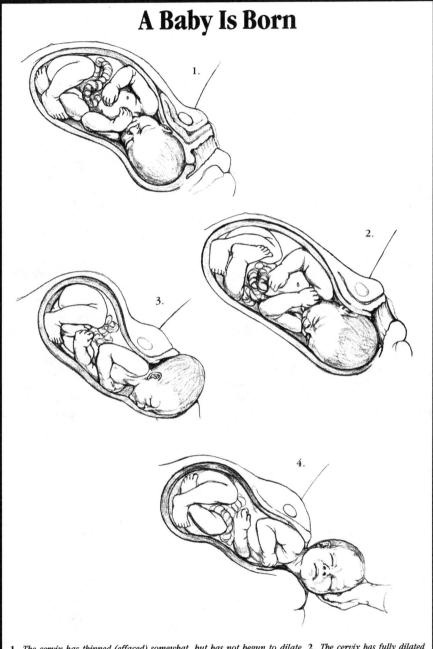

1. *The cervix has thinned (effaced) somewhat, but has not begun to dilate.* **2.** *The cervix has fully dilated and the baby's head has begun to press into the birth canal (vagina).* **3.** *To allow the narrowest diameter of the baby's head to fit through the mother's pelvis, the baby usually turns sometime during labor. Here the slightly molded head has crowned.* **4.** *The head, the baby's broadest part, is out. The rest of the delivery should proceed quickly and smoothly.*

A First Look at Baby

Those who expect their babies to arrive as round and smooth and pink as a Botticelli cherub may be in for a shock. Nine months of soaking in an amniotic bath and a dozen or so hours of compression in a contracting uterus and cramped birth canal take their toll on a newborn's appearance. Those babies who arrived via cesarean section will have a temporary edge as far as appearance goes.

Fortunately, most of the less-lovely newborn characteristics that follow are temporary. One morning, a couple of months after you've brought your wrinkled, slightly scrawny, puffy-eyed bundle home from the hospital, you'll wake to find that the Botticelli cherub has taken its place in the crib.

An Oddly Shaped Head. At birth the infant's head is, proportionately, the largest part of the body, with a circumference as large as the chest. As the baby grows, the rest of the body will catch up. Often the head has molded to fit through the mother's pelvis, giv-ing it an odd, possibly pointed "cone" shape; pressing against an inadequately dilated cervix can further distort the head by raising a lump (called caput succedaneum). The caput will disappear in a day or two, the molding within two weeks—at which point your baby's head will begin to take on that Botticelli roundness.

Newborn Hair. The hair that covers the head at birth may have little resemblance to the hair the baby will have later. Some newborns are virtually bald, some have thick manes, but most have a light cap of soft hair. All will eventually lose their newborn hair (though this may not be apparent), which will gradually be replaced by new growth.

Vernix Caseosa Coating. The cheesy substance that coats the fetus in the uterus is believed to protect the skin from the long exposure to the amniotic fluid. Premature babies have quite a bit of this coating at birth; postmature babies have almost none, except

or nurse will help direct your efforts, and redirect them if you lose your concentration.

❖ Relax your entire body, including your thighs and perineum, as you push. Tenseness works against your pushing efforts.

❖ Stop pushing when you're instructed to (as you may be, to keep the baby's head from being born too rapidly). Pant or blow instead.

❖ Rest between contractions, with the help of your coach and the attendants. If you are really exhausted, especially when the second stage drags on, your practitioner may suggest that you don't push for several contractions so you can rebuild your strength.

❖ Don't become frustrated if you see the baby's head crown, then disappear again. Birthing is a two-steps-forward, one-step-backward proposition.

❖ Remember to keep an eye on the mirror (if one is available). Seeing your baby's head crown (and reaching down and touching it, if your practitioner approves) may give you the inspiration to push when the pushing gets tough. Besides, unless your coach is videotaping, there won't be any replays to watch.

in the folds of their skin and under their fingernails.

Swelling of the Genitals. This is common in both male and female newborns, and is particularly pronounced in boy babies delivered via cesarean. The breasts of newborns, male and female, may also be swollen (occasionally even engorged, secreting a white or pink substance nicknamed "witch's milk") due to stimulation by maternal hormones. The hormones may also stimulate a milky-white, even blood-tinged, vaginal secretion in girls. These effects are not abnormal, and disappear in a week to ten days.

Lanugo. Fine downy hair, called lanugo, may cover the shoulders, back, forehead, and temples of full-term babies. This will usually be shed by the end of the first week. Such hair can be more abundant, and will last longer, in a premature baby.

Puffy Eyes. Swelling around the newborn's eyes is often caused by the eye drops that are used to protect the baby from infection, and disappears within a few days. Caucasian babies' eyes are almost always a slate blue, no matter what color they will be later on. In darker-skinned babies, the eyes are usually brown at birth.

Birthmarks and Skin Lesions. A reddish blotch at the base of the skull, on the eyelid, or on the forehead, called a salmon patch, is very common, especially in Caucasian newborns. Mongolian spots—bluish-gray pigmentation of the deep skin layer that can appear on the back, buttocks, and sometimes the arms and thighs— are more common in Asians, southern Europeans, and blacks. These markings will eventually disappear, usually by the time a child is four years old. Hemangiomas, elevated strawberry-colored birthmarks, vary from tiny to about quarter-size. They will eventually fade to a mottled pearly gray, then disappear entirely. Coffee-with-cream-colored (cafe-au-lait) spots can appear anywhere on the body; they are usually inconspicuous, and don't fade. A variety of rashes, tiny "pimples," and whiteheads may also mar the newborn complexion, but all are temporary.

What the Coach Can Do:

❖ Continue giving comfort and support, but don't feel hurt if your wife doesn't seem to notice you're there. Her energies are necessarily focused elsewhere.

❖ Guide her pushing and breathing, using the cues that you have both become familiar with during childbirth preparation; or relay instructions from the nurse or practitioner.

❖ Don't feel intimidated by the finesse and expertise of the professional medical team around you. Your presence is important, too. And in fact, your whispered "I love you" may be more valuable to her at this stage than anything they can offer.

❖ Help her to relax between the contractions—with soothing words, a cool cloth applied to forehead, neck, and shoulders, and, if feasible, back massage or counterpressure to help ease backache.

❖ If it's allowed, continue to supply ice chips to moisten her parched mouth as needed.

❖ Support her back while she's pushing, if necessary; hold her hand, wipe her brow—or do whatever seems to help her. If she slips out of position, help her back up.

❖ Periodically point out her progress. As the baby begins to crown, remind her to keep an eye on the mirror so she can have visual confirmation of what she is accomplishing; when she's not looking, or if there's no mirror, give her inch-by-inch descriptions. Take her hand and touch the head together for renewed inspiration (with the practitioner's okay).

❖ If you're offered the opportunity to "catch" your baby as it emerges or, later, to cut the cord, don't panic. Both are easy—and you'll get step-by-step directions, support, and backup from the attendants.

What Hospital Personnel May Do:

❖ Move you to the room in which you will deliver, if you aren't already there. If you're in a birthing bed, they'll simply remove the foot of the bed to prepare for delivery.

❖ Give support and direction to you as the delivery progresses.

❖ Continue to check the condition of the fetus periodically, usually by attaching the fetal monitor briefly.

❖ About the time the head crowns, prepare for the delivery—spreading sterile drapes and arranging instruments, donning surgical garments and gloves, sponging the perineal area with antiseptic.

❖ Perform an episiotomy just before the head is delivered, if necessary. First a local anesthetic will probably be injected into the perineum. This will be done at the height of a contraction, when the pressure of the baby's head naturally numbs the area; the incision will also be made at the height of a contraction and, if the perineum is anesthetized, will probably be painless.

❖ Elect to use outlet forceps to ease the baby's head out if the second stage lasts more than two hours (some doctors will wait longer if mother and baby are doing well), if the baby shows signs of difficulty tolerating the stresses of labor, if your medical condition prohibits further pushing, or if progress is being impeded because of a slightly irregular fetal presentation or a slight disproportion between fetus and pelvis. (See Forceps Delivery, page 286.) Usually a regional anesthetic will be administered if an epidural or other block hasn't already been given, because forceps delivery can be painful. If forceps aren't feasible or don't work, a cesarean may be the safest delivery route for baby and you.

❖ Once the head emerges, quickly suction the baby's nose and mouth to remove excess mucus, then assist the shoulders and torso out.

❖ Clamp and cut the umbilical cord, possibly with the newborn lying across your abdomen. Your husband may be asked if he would like to do the snipping. Some practitioners prefer to wait until the placenta is delivered or the cord has stopped pulsating before cutting the cord.

❖ Provide initial protective care for the newborn: evaluate his or her condition, and rate it on the Apgar scale at one minute and five minutes after birth (see page 287); give a brisk, stimulating, and drying rubdown; identify the baby by taking his or her footprints and your fingerprint for hospital records, and by attaching an identifying band to your wrist and/or ankle and that of your baby; administer nonirritating eyedrops, to prevent infection; weigh the baby, and wrap him or her to prevent heat loss. (In some hospitals some of these procedures may be omitted; in others many will be attended to later, in the nursery.)

❖ Show your now cleaned-up baby to you and your husband. Unless there is a problem, you and your husband should be able to hold your baby for some significant period. You may, if you wish to, try

breastfeeding (don't worry if you and/or your baby don't catch on immediately—see Getting Started Breastfeeding, page 388).

❖ When you are finished getting acquainted, they will probably whisk baby off to the nursery (at least temporarily) and transfer you to your room.

THE THIRD STAGE OF CHILDBIRTH: DELIVERY OF THE PLACENTA, OR AFTERBIRTH

The worst is over, the best has already come. All that remains is the tying up of loose ends, so to speak. During this final stage of childbirth (which generally lasts anywhere from five minutes to half an hour or more) the placenta, which has been your baby's life support inside the womb, will be delivered. You will continue to have mild contractions of approximately one minute's duration, though you may not feel them. The squeezing of the uterus separates the placenta from the uterine wall and moves it down into the lower segment of the uterus or into the vagina so you can then push it out. Once the placenta is delivered, any necessary stitching up of episiotomy or tears will be taken care of.

What You May Be Feeling or Noticing.
Now that the work of labor and delivery is done, you may feel fatigue or, conversely, a burst of renewed energy. You are likely to be very thirsty and, especially if labor has been long, hungry. Some women experience chills in this stage; all experience a bloody vaginal discharge (called lochia) comparable to a heavy menstrual period.

For many women, the immediate emotional reaction is a sense of relief.

There may also be exhilaration and talkativeness; elation, tempered by a new sense of responsibility; impatience at having to push out the placenta or submit to the repair of the episiotomy or tear, though you may be too excited or tired to care. Some women feel a strong closeness to their husbands and an immediate bond with their new baby; others feel somewhat detached (who is this stranger sniffing at my breast?), even resentful (how he's made me suffer!), particularly after a difficult delivery. (See pages 267 and 382 for more on bonding and new-mother love.)

What You Can Do:
❖ Help expel the placenta, by pushing when directed.

❖ Be patient during repair of any episiotomy or tears.

❖ Nurse or hold the baby, once the cord is cut. In some hospitals, and under some circumstances, the baby may be kept in a heated bassinette for a while or be held by the father.

❖ Take pride in your accomplishment, relax, and enjoy! And don't forget to thank your coach.

What the Coach Can Do:

❖ Give your wife some well-earned words of praise—and congratulate yourself for a job well done.

❖ Begin bonding with your baby by holding and hugging him or her now.

❖ Don't forget to do some husband-wife bonding, too.

❖ Ask the nurse for some juice for your wife; she may be very thirsty. After she's been rehydrated, and if both of you are in the mood, break out the bubbly.

❖ Take pictures if you've brought your camera, or tape the baby's first cries if you've brought your tape recorder along.

What Hospital Personnel May Do:

❖ Help extract the placenta. The exact procedure will vary depending upon the practitioner and the situation. Some will pull the cord gently with one hand while pressing and kneading the uterus with the other; others will exert downward pressure on the top of the uterus, asking you to push at the appropriate time. Many physicians will use oxytocin, by injection or IV, after delivery of the placenta to encourage uterine contractions, which will speed expulsion of the placenta and minimize bleeding.

❖ Examine the placenta to be sure it is intact. If it isn't, the practitioner will inspect the uterus manually for placental fragments and remove any that remain.

❖ Cut the cord, if it wasn't cut earlier.

❖ Stitch an episiotomy or tear, if any. A local anesthetic (if none was previously given, or if it has worn off) will probably be injected to numb the area. You will feel a pinch.

❖ Check your vagina to remove clots or sponges used during episiotomy repair.

❖ Sponge-bathe the lower part of your body, help you into a clean gown, and help you put on a perineal pad (sanitary napkin) held in place by a belt.

❖ Wheel you into the recovery room, or to your own room. If you're in a birthing bed, they'll put the foot of the bed back on.

❖ Deliver the baby to the nursery for a bath and some additional protective measures. (If you have rooming-in, the baby will be returned as soon as possible.)

BREECH DELIVERY

As far as the mother and coach are concerned, labor and vaginal delivery of a breech baby don't differ much from that of a vertex (head-down) baby; tips for coping and comforting are virtually identical. The activities of the hospital staff will be different, however, and will vary further depending on the type of breech position and the delivery procedure that the practitioner elects to follow.

Up until the second stage, a vaginal breech labor progesses about the same as a vertex labor. But it is always considered a trial labor, allowed to proceed only as long as it progresses normally. Because of the ever-present possibility that a cesarean may become necessary, you will probably be transferred to a delivery/operating room at the end of the first stage. Depending upon your baby's exact breech position, your doctor will determine the safest and most effective way to proceed. (What is most advisable in such a case also depends on the practitioner's experience. Asking a doctor to perform a procedure for breech extraction that you've read or heard about, but with which he or she is not comfortable, is not in your or your baby's best interest.)

A common procedure is to allow the baby to deliver naturally until the legs and lower half of the torso are out. Then a local anesthetic is administered and the shoulders and head are delivered, with or without the aid of forceps.

A vaginal delivery is not likely to be attempted if the baby is in the complete breech (see page 238) or footling breech (with one leg dangling down) position, if the baby's head is extended (facing upward), if the fetus is estimated to be very large or the mother's pelvis inadequate, if the delivery is premature, or if there are signs of fetal distress.

A large episiotomy is often necessary with a breech, but occasionally it can be avoided. The delivery position for a vaginal breech birth will vary, again depending on the situation and on your practitioner's experience. Some find they have more control if the woman is flat on her back, legs up in stirrups.

Once the baby is delivered, the proceedings continue as with a head-first birth.

CESAREAN SECTION: SURGICAL DELIVERY

You won't be able to participate actively at a cesarean delivery the way you would at a vaginal one. In fact, your most important contribution to the comfort and success of your baby's cesarean birth can be made before you arrive at the hospital—possibly before you even know that you're having a cesarean. That contribution is preparation. Being prepared both intellectually and emotionally for a cesarean, in case it should become necessary, will minimize any disappointment you may feel and help make your surgical delivery experience a positive one.

Thanks to regional anesthesia and the liberalization of hospital regulations, most women (and often their husbands) are able to be participants at their cesarean deliveries. Because they aren't preoccupied with pushing or discomfort, they are often able to relax and enjoy the birth—something women delivering vaginally rarely can do. This is what you can expect in a typical cesarean birth:

❖ Your pubic and/or abdominal hair may be shaved, and a catheter (a narrow tube) will be inserted into your bladder to keep it empty and out of the surgeon's way.

❖ In the operating room, sterile drapes will be arranged around your exposed abdomen, which will be washed down with an antiseptic solution. If you are to be awake for the delivery, a screen will be put up at about shoulder level so that you won't have to see the incision being made.

❖ An IV infusion will be started to provide speedy access if additional medication is needed.

❖ Anesthesia will be administered: either an epidural or a spinal block (both of which numb the lower part of your body but don't knock you out) or a general anesthetic (which does put you to sleep—sometimes necessary in an emergency when the baby must be delivered immediately).

❖ If you've had a regional anesthetic and your coach is going to attend the delivery, he will be suited up in sterile garb. He will sit near your head, so that he can give you emotional support and hold your hand; he will have the option of viewing the actual surgery. (Whether or not you know in advance that you are going to have a cesarean, it's a good idea to discuss with your doctor ahead of time the conditions under which your spouse will or won't be allowed to be with you during surgery.) Usually, if general anesthesia is used, the husband will be asked to wait outside the operating room.

❖ If yours is an emergency cesarean, things may move very quickly. Don't be alarmed by the seeming storm of activity around you. Be prepared for the possibility that hospital policy, and concern for the safety of you and your baby, may dictate that your husband leave during the delivery, which will take only about five or ten minutes.

❖ Once the physician is certain that the anesthetic has taken effect, an incision (a cut) is made in the lower abdomen. If you are awake, you may feel a sensation of being "unzipped," but no pain.

❖ A second incision is then made, this time in the lower segment of your uterus. The amniotic sac is opened, and if it hasn't already ruptured, the fluid is suctioned out; you may hear a sort of gurgling or swooshing sound.

❖ The baby is then eased out, either manually or with forceps, usually with an assistant pressing on the upper portion of the uterus. With an epidural (though not likely with a spinal block), you will probably feel some pulling and tugging sensations, as well as some pressure. If you're eager to see your baby's arrival, ask the doctor if the screen can be lowered slightly, which will allow you to see the actual birth, but not the more graphic details.

❖ Your baby's nose and mouth are then suctioned; you'll hear the first cry, and if the cord is long enough, you will be allowed a quick glimpse.

❖ The cord will be quickly clamped and cut, and while the baby is getting the same routine attention that a vaginally delivered infant receives, the doctor removes the placenta.

❖ Now the doctor will quickly do a routine check of your reproductive organs and stitch up the incisions that were made.

❖ An injection of oxytocin may be given intramuscularly or into your IV bottle, to help contract the uterus and thus control bleeding. IV antibiotics may be given to minimize the chances of infection.

❖ Depending upon your condition and the baby's, as well as hospital rules, you may or may not be able to hold the baby right there in the delivery room. If you can't, perhaps your husband can. If the infant has to be whisked away to the ICU nursery, don't fret. This is standard in many hospitals and doesn't necessarily indicate a problem with a baby's condition. And as far as bonding is concerned, later can be just as good as sooner.

Part 3

OF SPECIAL CONCERN

15
If You Get Sick

Every woman expects to succumb to at least a few of the less desirable pregnancy symptoms during her nine-month stint—morning sickness and leg cramps, for instance, or indigestion and exhaustion. But it surprises some to discover that they're also susceptible to symptoms that have nothing at all to do with pregnancy: those associated with such "civilian" sicknesses as colds, flu, gastroenteritis, even measles and mumps. Though most such illnesses do not affect a pregnancy, an occasional one can. Prevention is, of course, the best way to keep that healthy glow of pregnancy going strong. But when it fails, quick and safe treatment, in most cases under the supervision of your doctor, is essential to protect yourself and your baby from complications.

WHAT YOU MAY BE CONCERNED ABOUT

COMING DOWN WITH A COLD OR FLU

"I've got a terrible cold and I'm worried about it affecting my baby."

Most women come down with a cold or the flu at least once during their nine months, and though you may be very uncomfortable, a mild illness like this will not affect your pregnancy. However, the medications that you're probably accustomed to taking for these maladies, such as cold tablets and antihistamines, could. So don't take these or any other medications, including aspirin (see page 320) or megadoses of vitamin C, without your doctor's approval. He or she should be able to tell you which cold treatments are safe in pregnancy and which will work best in your case. None, of course, will cure a cold, but some may relieve its symptoms. (See page 321 for information on taking medication during pregnancy.)

If you've already taken a few doses of one medication or another, don't panic. It's very unlikely any harm was done. But do check with your practitioner if you're concerned.

Fortunately for you and your baby, some of the best cold and flu remedies are the safest ones, too:

❖ Nip the cold in the bud, before it blossoms into a nasty case of bronchitis or another secondary infection. At the very first sneeze, go to bed or at least plan on getting a little extra rest.

❖ When you're lying down or sleeping, keep your head slightly elevated to facilitate breathing.

❖ Don't starve your cold, fever—or baby. Stay on the Best-Odds Diet whether you have an appetite or not, forcing yourself to eat if need be. Be sure to have some citrus fruit or juice every day, but don't take extra vitamin C supplements (beyond that in your pregnancy formula) without medical advice.

❖ Flood yourself with fluids. Fever, sneezes, and a runny nose will cause your body to lose fluids that you and your baby urgently need. Keep a thermos of hot grapefruit juice or orangeade (½ cup unsweetened frozen juice concentrate to 1 quart of hot water) next to your bed, and drink at least one cupful an hour. Also try the Jewish penicillin: chicken soup. Medical researchers have proven that it not only replaces fluids but also helps make cold sufferers more comfortable.

❖ Keep your nasal passages moist with a humidifier (see Appendix), and by spraying the inside of your nose with an atomizer filled with salt water.

❖ If your throat is sore or scratchy, or if you're coughing, gargle with salt water (1 teaspoon of salt to 8 ounces of water) at the temperature of hot, but not scalding, tea.

❖ Bring down a fever naturally. Take cool showers or baths, or sponge with tepid water; drink cool beverages; and wear light bedclothes. If your fever reaches 102 degrees or more, call your doctor immediately (see page 320).

Unfortunately, colds tend to last longer during pregnancy, possibly because the immune system slows down a bit in order to protect the baby (a foreign body) from immunological rejection. If your cold or flu is severe enough to interfere with eating or sleeping, if you're coughing up greenish or yellowish sputum, or if symptoms last more than a week, call your doctor. Also call if you come down with influenza in the last trimester, when flu can lead to severe illness and to premature delivery. Prescribed medication may be needed for your safety and your baby's.

Don't put off calling the doctor or refuse to take a prescribed medication you are assured is safe, because you've heard all drugs are harmful in pregnancy. They aren't.

For that important ounce of prevention (including flu shots), see page 323.

GASTROINTESTINAL ILLS

"I've got a stomach bug, and I can't keep anything down. Will this hurt my baby?"

Fortunately gastroenteritis (an inflammation of the stomach and intestines) usually has a limited life span—often no longer than 24 hours, very rarely longer than 72. And as long as fluid balance is maintained through adequate replacement, even complete lack of solid nourishment for a day or two won't harm your baby.

But the fact that the virus isn't affecting your baby's health doesn't mean that you should ignore it. Take these steps to increase your comfort and speed your recovery while you're waiting for your bug to bug off.

❖ Consult with your doctor. Discuss all of your symptoms, particularly fever, just in case you turn out to have something more than a stomach bug. Call again as instructed, and/or if symptoms last more than 48 hours; treatment may be needed.

❖ Take to your bed, if possible. Bed rest, particularly in a dark, quiet room, seems to reduce symptoms of gastroenteritis.

❖ Replenish lost fluids. Diarrhea and vomiting are extremely dehydrating. And since fluid intake is more important than solid intake for the short term, it's essential to keep the clear liquids coming. Take them in whatever form they're palatable (water, club soda or seltzer, weak decaffeinated tea, orange juice diluted with an equal quantity of water, or if diarrhea isn't also a problem, diluted apple or grape juice), in small sips as often as possible (aim for every 15 minutes). If you can't even keep these down, suck on ice chips or ice cubes. Avoid the traditional cure of sugary soft drinks—this will only prolong your symptoms. Milk may, too.

❖ Modify your diet. Traditional wisdom says that unless you're really hungry, it's probably better to eat nothing for the first 12 hours or so with a stomach virus. More recent research, however, suggests that continuing solids may actually be preferable to semi-starvation. Check with your physician for advice. Whether you continue solids or wait 12 to 24 hours before digging in, keep your diet simple. At first stick to diluted nonacidic fruit juices, clear broths or bouillon, thinned cream of wheat or rice, unbuttered white toast, boiled or steamed converted white rice, boiled or baked potato without the skin, bananas, applesauce, gelatin desserts (make these with unflavored gelatin and fruit juice instead of sugary mixes). Gradually add, as they become appealing to you, cottage cheese, yogurt, chicken, fish, then cooked vegetables and fruit, before returning to your normal diet.

❖ Supplement, when you can. Getting your vitamin insurance is an especially good idea now; so try to take your supplement when it's least likely to come back up. Don't worry, however, if you can't manage to keep it down for a few days or so; no harm will be done.

If others who have eaten with you take ill at the same time or if you have eaten suspicious food in the last few weeks, this may be food poisoning, which needs immediate medical attention. Or if you recently traveled to an exotic destination, parasites or other exotic infectious organisms may be responsible for your distress. Check with your doctor if you suspect anything more than a simple virus.

Of course, even better than trying to cure an illness is preventing it in the first place. So always observe the prevention tips on page 323.

GERMAN MEASLES (RUBELLA)

"I was exposed to German measles on a trip out of the country. Do I have to have an abortion?"

That's a question only 1 out of 7 pregnant women need ever confront. The other six are, happily, immune to rubella, or German measles, having contracted it at some other time in their lives (usually during childhood) or because they were vaccinated against it (usually in early adolescence or when they were married). You may not know whether or not you are immune, but you can find out with a simple test—a rubella antibody titer—which measures the level of antibodies to the virus in your blood and is performed routinely at the first prenatal visit by most practitioners. If this test was not performed, it should be now.

If it turns out you're not immune,

you still needn't consider drastic measures immediately. Exposure alone cannot harm your baby. For the virus to do its damage, you have to contract the illness. The symptoms, which show up two or three weeks after exposure, are usually mild (malaise, slight fever, and swollen glands, followed by a slight rash a day or two later) and may sometimes pass unnoticed. A blood test during that time, however, can show whether or not you have an active infection. By 22 weeks it's possible to test a fetus to see if it has been infected (earlier, the infection may not show up), but this is rarely needed.

Unfortunately there is no way of absolutely preventing an exposed woman from coming down with rubella. Gamma globulin shots were once given routinely, but they have been found to be inconsistent in preventing infection. Should you come down with rubella, you will need to discuss with your doctor all the possible risks to your fetus before making a decision about terminating your pregnancy. It's important to understand that the risks involved decrease as a pregnancy progresses. If a woman is infected in the first month, the chance of her baby developing serious congenital malformation is high, about 35%. By the third month, the risk is down to 10% to 15%. After that the risk is very slight.

Fortunately, the chance of being exposed to rubella in this country is small. Since immunization has become routine in the U.S., the disease is becoming more and more rare here. Still, if you aren't immune and don't contract the disease this time around, avoid the concern entirely in subsequent pregnancies by having your doctor vaccinate you after this delivery. As a precaution, you will be instructed not to become pregnant for two or three months following vaccination. But should you conceive acci-

dentally during this time—or if you were vaccinated early in this pregnancy, before you knew you had conceived—don't worry. Though there is a theoretical risk of fetal damage, there have been no reported cases of birth defects of the type associated with congenital rubella in babies whose mothers were inadvertently vaccinated early in pregnancy or conceived soon after vaccination.

TOXOPLASMOSIS

"Though I've given all the cat-care chores over to my husband, just the very fact that I live with cats makes me worry about toxoplasmosis. How would I know if I came down with the disease?"

You probably wouldn't. Most people who are infected show no symptoms at all, though some do notice mild malaise, slight fever, and swollen glands two or three weeks after exposure, followed by a rash a day or two later.

A blood test for antibodies to *Toxoplasma gondii* is available, but it's not 100% accurate. It doesn't work at all unless you've previously been tested for antibodies. Check with your practitioner to see if you were tested before pregnancy. If you had antibodies then—very likely if you've been living with cats—you're immune and needn't worry about developing an infection now. If you had no antibodies, you are not immune. In that case, it may be recommended that you be tested regularly until you deliver to see if you suddenly test positive, which would indicate a new infection. Because of the lack of accuracy and the infrequency of infection in pregnant women, testing may not be suggested.[1]

---

1. *Do not* try to test yourself; home tests for toxoplasmosis are highly unreliable.

In that unlikely event (in the U.S., only 1 woman in 1,000 is believed to become infected during pregnancy), a thorough discussion of the options with the doctor, a maternal-fetal subspecialist, or possibly with a genetic counselor, should be the next step. The point in a pregnancy at which the infection occurs is a factor to consider. The risk of a fetus becoming infected in the first trimester is relatively small, probably less than 15%, but the risk of serious damage to the fetus is high. In the second trimester, the likelihood of infection is a little higher, but the risk of fetal damage somewhat smaller. In the last trimester the baby is most likely to be infected, but the risk of serious damage is smallest. Only 1 baby in 10,000 is born with severe congenital toxoplasmosis. Early treatment may improve prognosis.

Another factor to consider is whether or not the fetus itself has actually become infected. Recent advances have made it possible to test for fetal infection through amniocentesis, as well as through the examination of a fetal blood and/or amniotic fluid sample, though not usually before 20 to 22 weeks. If there is no fetal infection, the fetus is probably not affected. Finally, it's recommended that if a pregnant woman does show an infection and does not wish to terminate her pregnancy no matter what testing suggests, she should be treated with special antibiotics—possibly for several months. Such treatment appears to greatly reduce the risk of a baby being born with severe problems.

If you weren't tested earlier, then according to the latest research there is no point in testing you now unless you develop symptoms. The tests are not accurate enough to show whether a woman who was never tested before has a new infection or simply shows antibodies from an old infection.

The best "treatment" of toxoplas-mosis is prevention. See page 65 for tips on how to avoid infection.

CYTOMEGALOVIRUS (CMV)

"I teach at a nursery school, and I've been told that I should take a leave of absence during my pregnancy because I could contract cytomegalovirus, which could be harmful to my baby."

Although somewhere between 25% and 60% of all preschoolers carry the cytomegalovirus and can excrete it in saliva, urine, and feces for months or even years, the chances that you will pick up the infection from your young charges and pass it on to your baby with adverse results are small. First of all, the virus is not extremely contagious. Second, most adults were infected in childhood. If you were, you can't "catch" CMV from the children you care for now. (If your CMV becomes reactivated, the risks to your baby are smaller than if you have a new infection during pregnancy.) Third, though roughly 1 in 100 babies is born with the virus, only a small percentage of these actually show any of the ill effects commonly associated with CMV infection in utero, which include jaundice, high-tone deafness, and eye problems.

Still some physicians, like yours, suggest that unless a woman knows for sure that she has already been infected (most people don't have this information unless they are tested prenatally, since CMV usually comes and goes with no obvious symptoms), it's a good idea to take a leave of absence from any job that puts her in daily contact with large numbers of preschoolers, at least for the first 24 weeks of pregnancy, during which the risks to the fetus are the greatest. Others recommend wearing gloves on the job, washing up carefully after changing diapers (which you should do anyway), and resisting kissing the toddlers in your care or eating their leftovers.

Though pregnant women with toddlers of their own may worry about catching CMV in the nursery, the possibility is so remote that the worry is unnecessary. That doesn't mean, of course, that good hygiene in the home should be ignored—it should be practiced whether you're worried about CMV or not.

Should you come down with what seems like flu or mononucleosis (fever, fatigue, swollen lymph glands, sore throat), however, do check with your doctor. Whether these symptoms represent CMV or another illness, they need treatment.

FIFTH DISEASE

"I read that a disease I had never even heard of before—fifth disease—could cause problems in pregnancy."

Fifth disease—technically "erythema infectiosum," caused by the human parvovirus B19—is the fifth of a group of six diseases that cause fever and rash in children. But unlike its sister diseases (such as chicken pox), fifth disease isn't widely known because its symptoms are mild and can go unnoticed—or be totally absent. Fever is present in only 15% to 30% of cases. The rash—which for the first few days gives the cheeks the appearance of having been slapped, then spreads in a lacy pattern to trunk, buttocks, and thighs, recurring on and off (usually in response to heat from the sun or a warm bath) for one to three weeks—is often confused with the rash of rubella and other childhood illnesses. Concentrated exposure from caring for a child sick with fifth disease or from teaching at a school where it is epidemic puts an expectant mother at

greater risk of developing the infection than with casual contact.

Recently fifth disease has been linked to a very slightly increased risk of miscarriage in women who contract it. But since most women of childbearing age are already immune because they were infected as children, infection of pregnant women is not common. If the disease does cause a miscarriage in one pregnancy, however, a repeat miscarriage due to parvovirus is not likely.

Very rarely, fifth disease may lead to an unusual form of fetal anemia, similar to that in Rh disease. For that reason, women who have fifth disease during pregnancy are generally examined periodically with ultrasound to look for the swelling (resulting from fluid retention) in the fetus that is characteristic of this kind of anemia; if it is found, treatment will probably be necessary.

GROUP B STREP

"I read in a magazine that strep B infection in a mother can kill her baby. It's terrifying to think that I might be carrying it around."

Scary headlines sell magazines, but they do a disservice to readers. Though it's true that a baby who contracts a group B streptococcus infection from its mother at birth can become ill and even die, with modern obstetrical practice this doesn't have to happen.

Since there are no symptoms to indicate a woman is carrying the bacteria, there are two recommended approaches for protecting newborns. One is to test (via vaginal swab) all expectant women at 35 to 37 weeks and treat those who are positive with antibiotics during labor. The second is to treat, during labor, high risk women: those in preterm labor, or with a fever, prolonged ruptured membranes (18 hours or more), a prior child with GBS, or GBS in their urine during pregnancy. In most cases this will protect the newborn from becoming infected. If necessary, the baby can also be treated.

So while you shouldn't worry, you should insist that you be tested and that if the test is positive, you are treated during labor.

LYME DISEASE

"I know I live in an area that's high risk for Lyme disease. Is it dangerous to have when you're pregnant."

Lyme disease—which got its name from Lyme, Connecticut, where it was first diagnosed in the U.S.—is most common among those who spend time in woods frequented by deer, mice, or other animals carrying "deer" ticks, but it can also be picked up in forest-free cities via greenery brought from the country or at a farmer's market. Lyme disease can be passed on to the fetus, but whether or not the fetus can suffer permanent harm isn't entirely clear. It is suspected, but not proven, that the disease may be linked to heart defects in the babies of infected mothers.

The best way to protect your baby as well as yourself is by practicing preventive measures. If you are out in woodsy or grassy areas, or if you handle greenery grown in such areas, wear long pants tucked into boots or socks, and long sleeves; use an insect repellent effective for Lyme ticks on your clothing, but *not* on your skin. When you return home, check your skin carefully for ticks (removing them shortly after they attach almost entirely eliminates the possibility of infection) and shower thoroughly.

If you suspect you've been infected, see your doctor immediately. (Early symptoms may include a blotchy bull's-eye rash at the bite site, fatigue, headache, fever and chills, generalized achiness, swollen glands near the site of the bite; other possible symptoms are redness or swelling of the eyes, erratic behavior, sore throat, nonproductive [dry] cough, hives or other allover rash.) Prompt treatment may prevent your passing the infection on to your baby, and your becoming seriously ill.

MEASLES

"I'm a teacher, and a child in our school has the measles. Should I be immunized?"

No. Measles vaccine is not given during pregnancy because of the theoretical risk to the fetus from the vaccine, though there have been no reports of malformations among newborns whose mothers were inadvertently vaccinated. Besides, the odds are good that you are already immune to measles, since most women of childbearing age were vaccinated against the disease as children. If you are not immune (your doctor can run a test to determine whether you are), the risk that you will contract measles is small since most, if not all, of the children in your class have been vaccinated against it and are themselves unlikely to come down with the disease. Also reassuring is the fact that measles, unlike German measles, or rubella, does not appear to cause birth defects, though it may be linked to an increased risk of miscarriage or premature labor and is sometimes quite a severe illness in pregnant women. Still, if you are exposed directly to someone with measles and are not immune, your doctor may administer gammaglobulin during the incubation period—between exposure and the start of symptoms to decrease the severity of the illness.

If a pregnant woman contracts measles near her due date, there is a risk of infection in the newborn, which could be serious. Again, gammaglobulin may be administered to reduce the severity of such an infection.

URINARY TRACT INFECTION

"I'm afraid I have a urinary tract infection."

Urinary tract infections (UTIs) are so common in pregnancy that 10% of pregnant women can expect to develop at least one—and those who have already had one have a 1 in 3 chance of an encore. Most often it will be cystitis, a simple bladder infection. In some women cystitis is without symptoms, or "silent," and is diagnosed only after a routine urine culture. In others, symptoms can range from mild to quite uncomfortable (an urge to urinate frequently, a burning sensation when the urine— sometimes only a drop or two—is passed, sharp lower abdominal pain).

Regardless of whether there are symptoms or not, once an infection is diagnosed it should be treated promptly by a physician, with an antibiotic approved for use during pregnancy.[2] Finishing the prescription is vital to preventing a recurrence; don't be tempted to discontinue treatment once you're feeling better.

In 20% to 40% of cases, untreated bladder infection during pregnancy progresses to kidney infection (pyelonephritis), which is more of a threat to mother and baby. This occurs most often in the last trimester, and can lead to preterm labor. The symptoms are the same as those of cystitis but are frequently accompanied by fe-

---

2. Do not take a medication previously prescribed for you or for anyone else, even if it was prescribed for a urinary tract infection.

ver (often as high as 103 degrees), chills, blood in the urine, and backache (in the midback or on one or both sides). Should you experience these symptoms, notify your doctor *immediately.* Antibiotics can generally cure a kidney infection, but hospitalization for intravenous administration will probably be necessary.

Many physicians today try to head off kidney infection by screening pregnant women, at their first visit, for susceptibility. If a culture of the urine turns up bacteria (and it does in about 7% to 10% of pregnant women), antibiotics are administered to prevent the development of cystitis or pyelonephritis.

There are some home remedies and preventives that may also help ward off UTI; used in conjunction with medical treatment, they may help speed recovery when infection occurs:

❖ Drink plenty of fluids, especially water. Unsweetened citrus and cranberry juices may also be beneficial.Avoid coffee and tea (even decaffeinated varieties) and alcohol.

❖ Wash your vaginal area well before intercourse; empty your bladder just before and after intercourse.

❖ Every time you urinate, take the time to be sure your bladder is thoroughly emptied. Leaning forward when you urinate may help to ensure that you empty your bladder completely. Also, it sometimes helps to "double void"; after you urinate, wait five minutes, then try to urinate again. And don't put off urinating—chronically "holding it in" increasing susceptibility to infection.

❖ Wear cotton-crotch underwear and pantyhose, and avoid wearing tight under or outer pants. Don't wear pantyhose under slacks. And sleep without panties on.

❖ Keep the vaginal and perineal areas meticulously clean. Wash daily (shower rather than bathe) and avoid bubble bath; perfumed powders, soaps, sprays, detergents, toilet tissue; hot tubs and improperly chlorinated pools. Wipe front to back after using the toilet. And ask your practitioner about an antibacterial cleanser.

❖ Eat unsweetened yogurt or frozen yogurt that contains active cultures when taking antibiotics, to help restore the balance of bacteria.

❖ Keep your resistance high by eating a nutritious low-sugar diet (see Best-Odds Diet, page 80), getting plenty of rest, not working to the point of fatigue, and not letting your life get too stressful.

HEPATITIS

"One of the toddlers in the day care center where I work was just diagnosed as having hepatitis A. If I get it, could it affect my pregnancy?"

Hepatitis A is very common (nearly 1 in 3 children comes down with it before the age of five), is almost always a mild disease (often with no notable symptoms), and is not known to be passed on to a fetus or newborn. So it should not affect your pregnancy. Still, you are better off not contracting an infection of any kind. Since hepatitis A is passed by the fecal-oral route, be sure to wash your hands after changing diapers or taking your young charges to the bathroom, as well as before eating. You might also ask your physician about immunization against hepatitis A.

"Is hepatitis B contagious? My husband came down with a case of it, which is strange because he isn't in a high-risk category."

Not really so strange. While about 6 in 10 hepatitis B victims fall into the so-called high-risk categories,[3] 1 in 3 cases occurs in those with no known risk factors. Since this liver infection, which is most common during the childbearing years of 15 to 39, can be passed from mother to fetus, it's of concern to expectant parents. And since it's transmissible from person to person, it's of particular concern to you. To prevent your becoming infected, you and your husband should take special precautions: no sharing of toothbrushes, razors, or other personal items, and abstention from sexual intercourse. Unlike hepatitis A, for which everyone in the home may be given preventive shots to forestall infection, with hepatitis B only the spouse (or sexual partner) is immunized. So ask your doctor about immunization.

If you haven't been tested for hepatitis B and experience any of its symptoms (yellowing of the skin or whites of the eyes, along with vomiting, abdominal pain, and loss of appetite), ask your doctor about being tested. A test may be a good idea even if you have no symptoms, since many cases of hepatitis are so mild that no symptoms, or only stomach-flu-like ones, are noted.[4]

When an expectant mother (or any-

---

3. At highest risk of hepatitis B, which is transmitted through blood and body fluids, are IV drug users, homosexual men, and heterosexuals with more than one partner in a six-month period. Also at risk are health-care workers and immigrants from China, Southeast Asia, and other high-prevalence areas. Vaccination is available and is recommended for these groups.

4. It's now recommended that all pregnant women be tested for hepatitis B. If a woman tests positive, her family will usually be immunized and her newborn treated with vaccine and immune globulin.

one else) has an active hepatitis B infection, bed rest and a nutritious diet are the mainstays of treatment. Alcoholic beverages must be avoided, but that applies to pregnant women in general anyway. The patient's blood is checked periodically to monitor the progress of the disease. In 95% of cases, full recovery can be expected; in the others, the disease may become very severe or chronic.

If the hepatitis B virus is present in the mother at delivery, bathing the newborn as soon as possible to remove all traces of maternal blood and secretions, and administering hepatitis B vaccine and immune globulin within 12 hours of birth, usually prevent the infection taking hold in the baby. Treatment is repeated at 1 and 6 months, and the child is usually tested at 12 to 15 months to be sure that the therapy has been effective.

There are other forms of hepatitis, such as C and E (also known as non-A non-B), as well as the recently discovered G. At present it isn't clear whether or not these can be transmitted from mother to child during pregnancy or childbirth.

MUMPS

"A co-worker just came down with mumps. I don't know if I ever had the disease. Would it be dangerous to get it now that I'm expecting?"

Mumps in pregnancy is rare because most young adults today either had the disease or were immunized against it as children. If you can, check with your parents or the doctor who cared for you as a child to see if you are in this category. If you're not, you still may not come down with mumps because it is not highly contagious. Nevertheless, because the disease appears to trigger uterine contractions and thus can lead to

miscarriage in early pregnancy or to premature labor later, you should be alert for the first symptoms of the disease (possibly vague pain, fever, and loss of appetite before the salivary, or parotid, glands become swollen; then ear pain and pain on chewing or on taking acidic or sour food or drink). Notify your doctor of such symptoms immediately, because prompt treatment can reduce the chance of problems developing.

CHICKEN POX (VARICELLA)

"My toddler was exposed to chicken pox at her day care center. If she comes down with it, could the baby I'm now carrying be hurt?"

Not likely. Well insulated from the rest of the world, the fetus can't contract chicken pox, or varicella, from a third party—only from its mother. And you would have to catch it first, which may very well be impossible. There is only a small chance that you didn't have the infection as a child (85% to 95% of today's adult population has had it) and are not already immune. Ask your mother, or check your health records to find out whether you have had chicken pox. If you can't find out for sure, ask your practitioner to run a test to see if you are immune.

Though the chances of your becoming infected are slim even if you aren't immune (about 1 to 5 in 10,000), an injection of varicella-zoster immune globulin (VZIG) within 96 hours of exposure may be recommended. It isn't clear whether or not this will protect the baby should you come down with chicken pox anyway, but it should minimize complications for you, which is significant, since this mild childhood disease can be quite severe in adults, sometimes causing varicella pneumonia. (Whether or not it is even more severe in pregnant women is a matter of debate.) If you should be hit with a severe case, treatment with an antiviral drug may be begun to reduce the risk of complications.

There is a risk of damage to the fetus when the mother is infected, but it is a small one. Even if a fetus is exposed when most vulnerable—during the first half of pregnancy—recent research shows that there's only a 2% chance of its developing the defects typical of congenital varicella syndrome. When the exposure occurs in the second half of pregnancy, fetal damage is extremely rare.

Chicken pox once again becomes a threat close to term, when a maternal infection can lead to a baby being born with neonatal varicella. The risk is reduced if delivery doesn't occur until the mother develops antibodies and passes them to the fetus through the placenta, which may take 1 to 2 weeks. But if a mother develops chicken pox within 4 or 5 days of delivery, there's a 15% to 30% chance her newborn will arrive infected and will develop the characteristic rash within a week or so. Since neonatal varicella can be extremely serious, VZIG is usually given to the baby. The risk of the newborn being infected is small if maternal infection occurs between 5 and 21 days before delivery, and serious consequences from the disease at that point are rare.

Incidentally, shingles, or herpes zoster, which is a reactivation of the chicken pox virus in someone who had the disease earlier, does not appear to be harmful to a developing fetus, probably because the mother and thus the baby already have antibodies to the virus.

Once the now experimental varicella vaccine is approved for general use, women who are not immune will probably be routinely vaccinated

prior to conception, effectively eliminating the issue of chicken pox in pregnancy.

FEVER

"I'm running a fever. Should I take aspirin to bring it down?"

During most of your life, fever needn't be feared or fought. In fact, it is one of the body's most powerful allies in the war against infection. During pregnancy, however, an increase of body temperature to over 104 degrees for a day or more can cause birth defects—particularly during weeks three to seven of pregnancy. Damage may occasionally occur when a temperature as low as 102 degrees is sustained for two or more days. So bringing a fever down promptly—rather than letting it run its course—becomes the safest way to go.

How best to bring a fever down will depend on how high it has gone up, and on your practitioner's recommendations. Call your doctor the same day if you're running a fever of between 100 and 102 degrees; call immediately if it's 102 or higher. For a temperature under 102, home remedies, such as a cool bath (see Appendix), may do the trick without medication. For a higher temperature related to a bacterial infection, acetaminophen teamed with an antibiotic (there are several that are considered safe for use during pregnancy) will probably be prescribed. Aspirin should not be routinely taken for fever (see below).

TAKING ASPIRIN AND NONASPIRIN

"Last week I took two aspirins for a pounding headache, and now I read that

aspirin can cause birth defects. I'm a nervous wreck."

Of the millions of Americans who opened their medicine cabinets today and reached for a bottle of aspirin, few thought twice—or even once—about its safety. And for most people, occasional aspirin use is not only helpful but perfectly harmless. But during pregnancy, there is concern that aspirin, like many other ordinarily innocuous over-the-counter remedies, may be hazardous.

If you've unwittingly taken one or two aspirins on one, or even a few, occasions in the first two trimesters, don't worry—there is no evidence they will hurt your baby. It's estimated that 1 in every 2 pregnant women takes at least one dose of aspirin during pregnancy, with seemingly no ill effect. For the rest of your pregnancy, however, it's advisable to treat aspirin as you would any other drug, taking it only when absolutely necessary and only when recommended by a practitioner who knows you're pregnant.

Aspirin use is most risky in the third trimester, when even one dose can interfere with fetal growth and cause other problems. Because it is an anti-prostaglandin, and prostaglandins are involved in the mechanism of labor, aspirin can prolong both pregnancy and labor and lead to other complications during delivery. And since it interferes with blood-clotting, aspirin taken during the two weeks before delivery can increase the risk of hemorrhage at delivery and even bleeding problems in the newborn.

Carefully, medically supervised administration of less than half a regular-strength aspirin a day may be useful in treating immunological conditions (such as lupus). Recent studies have raised questions, however, about routinely using low-dose aspirin to prevent preeclampsia or intrauterine growth retardation in high-risk women.

Indiscriminately popping aspirin substitutes in place of aspirin isn't the logical solution in pregnancy. Though the moderate use of acetaminophen (Tylenol, Datril, Anacin III) in pregnancy appears to pose no problem, it too should be taken only when necessary, and *only* with the approval of your practitioner.

Ibuprofen (Advil, Nuprin, Medipren) is a relatively new entry in the pain reliever sweepstakes. Similar to aspirin in some ways, it may trigger a cross reaction in those sensitive to aspirin. Though there have been no reports of problems when ibuprofen is used early in pregnancy, its use in the last trimester can result in problems in the unborn child, a prolonged pregnancy, and/or a prolonged labor. Because of this risk, don't use this medication at all in the last three months of pregnancy, and use it earlier only if recommended by a physician who knows you are pregnant. (But don't worry about the ibuprofen you took before you found out you were pregnant.)

While caution is imperative in considering the use of these medications, avoiding their use entirely is unwarranted. There are times when pain can not be relieved or a fever brought down in any other way. The most sensible course in pregnancy is first to try to use nondrug remedies (see Appendix) for pain or low-grade fever, and then to resort to nonaspirin acetaminophen products—under medical supervision—if those methods fail.

TAKING MEDICATIONS

"How do I know which medicines, if any, are safe to take during pregnancy, and which aren't?"

No drug, prescription or over-the-counter, is 100% safe for 100% of the people 100% of the time. And when you're pregnant, every time you take a drug there are two individuals at risk, one very small and vulnerable. Although a few drugs have been shown to be particularly hazardous to a developing fetus, many drugs have been used safely during pregnancy, and there are situations in which medication is absolutely essential to life and/or health. Whether you will take a particular medication at a particular time during pregnancy is something you and your physician will have to decide by weighing the drug's potential risks against the benefits it offers. In any case, the general rule should be: take medication only on the advice of a physician who knows you are pregnant, and only when it is absolutely necessary.

Which drug you take in a specific situation will depend on the latest information available on drug safety in pregnancy. The many lists of safe, possibly safe, possibly unsafe, and definitely unsafe drugs may provide some assistance, but most are outdated and unreliable by the time they're published. Package inserts and labels are of limited use, since most warn not to use the product during pregnancy without a physician's orders, even when the product is believed safe. Your best sources of information will be:

❖ A well-informed physician (not all are familiar with drug safety in pregnancy); a maternal-fetal medicine subspecialist may be particularly helpful.

❖ The Food and Drug Administration—contact your regional office or write to the Public Health Service, FDA, Parklawn Building, 5600 Fisher's Lane, Rockville, MD 20857.

❖ The March of Dimes—try your local office first, or contact the National Foundation/March of Dimes,

1275 Mamaroneck Avenue, White Plains, NY 10605.

Once you've made certain that a prescribed drug is considered safe for use during pregnancy, don't hesitate to take it because you're still afraid it might somehow harm your baby. It won't—but delaying treatment might.

If you do need some kind of medication during pregnancy, follow these steps for increased benefit and reduced risk:

❖ Discuss with your physician the possibility of taking the medication in the smallest effective doses for the shortest possible time.

❖ Take the medication when it's going to benefit you the most—a cold medication at night, for instance, so it will help you sleep.

❖ Follow package or doctor's directions carefully. Some medications must be taken on an empty stomach; some should be taken with food or milk. If your physician hasn't given you any instructions, ask your pharmacist for particulars.

❖ Explore nondrug remedies, and use them to supplement the drug therapy—eliminating as many offending allergens from your home as you can, for instance, so your physician can reduce the amount of prescribed antihistamine you take.

❖ Make sure the medication gets where it's supposed to by taking a sip of water before you swallow a capsule or tablet, to make it go down more easily, and by drinking a full glass afterward, to ensure that it is washed speedily down to where it will be absorbed. Taking the medication while sitting or standing, rather than lying down or propped up, may also help speed its passage.

HERBAL CURES

"I wouldn't think of taking any drugs during pregnancy. But would it be all right to substitute medicinal herbs?"

Medicinal herbs *are* drugs—often very powerful ones. Some are so powerful that they're used in laboratories to produce prescription medicines. Others have been used for generations in some societies to induce abortions, and some have been linked to miscarriage. Even in a seemingly soothing cup of tea, some herbs are capable of producing such symptoms as diarrhea, vomiting, and heart palpitations. The use of herbal medicines presents an added risk that isn't present when the remedies come from the drugstore. They are not made under quality-controlled conditions, and may be dangerously strong or impotently weak. They may also contain harmful contaminants, including such allergens as insect parts, pollens, and molds, and even such toxic agents as lead or arsenic.

So treat medicinal herbs as you would any drugs during pregnancy. Do not take them except on the advice of your doctor. If you are experiencing any symptoms that need treatment, check with your practitioner instead of trying to self treat.

Also avoid herbal teas. If you've been drinking herbal teas up until now, don't worry. They obviously haven't made you ill or caused problems in your pregnancy. But from now on, avoid them unless prescribed by your doctor. If you're hankering for the taste of a favorite herbal tea, concoct your own potion by adding any of the following to boiling water or decaffeinated tea: orange, apple, pineapple, or other fruit juice; raspberry, strawberry, orange, or other jam or marmalade; slices of lemon, lime, orange, apple, pear, or other fruit; mint leaves, cinnamon, nutmeg, cloves, or other spices. And never make tea from a plant growing in your backyard unless you are absolutely certain what it is and that it is safe to use in pregnancy.

WHAT IT'S IMPORTANT TO KNOW: STAYING WELL

In pregnancy, because of the potentially harmful effects of both illness and medication on the unborn baby, the proverbial ounce of prevention is worth far more than a pound of cure. The following suggestions will increase your odds of staying well, whether you're pregnant or not.

❖ Ideally, you should have gotten your immunizations up to date before you conceived (see page 425). If that wasn't done, ask about the results of your rubella (German measles) test to see if you are immune or susceptible to the disease. If you're not immune, try to avoid contact with anyone infected. Also ask about flu shots if flu season is approaching. They can be given during pregnancy and greatly reduce the chances of your coming down with influenza.

❖ Keep your resistance up. Eat the best diet possible (see the Best-Odds Diet, page 80); get enough sleep and adequate exercise; and don't run yourself down by running yourself ragged.

❖ Avoid sick people like the plague. Try to stay away from anyone who has a cold, flu, stomach virus, or anything else noticeably contagious. Distance yourself from coughers on the bus, avoid lunching with a colleague who's complaining of a sore throat, and evade the handshake of a friend with a runny nose (germs as well as greetings can be exchanged in a handshake). Also avoid crowded or cramped indoor spaces when you can. Wash your hands thoroughly after exposure to crowds or riding on public transportation—especially before touching your mouth, nose, or eyes.

❖ At home, limit contact with sick children or a sick spouse as much as possible (have other family members, a sitter, or a nonpregnant friend play nursemaid). Avoid finishing up their lunches, drinking from their cups, and kissing them on the face. Wash your hands after any contact with the patients, their linens, or soiled tissues, especially before touching your own eyes, nose, or mouth. See that they wash their hands frequently, too, and that they cover their mouths when they cough or sneeze. Use disinfectant, such as Lysol spray, on telephones and other surfaces they handle. Isolate contaminated toothbrushes, and replace them when the illness is over.

❖ If your own child or a child you regularly spend time with develops a rash of any kind, avoid close contact and call your doctor at once unless you already know that you are immune to rubella. (German measles), chicken pox, fifth disease, and CMV (cytomegalovirus).

❖ To avoid food poisoning, practice safe food preparation and storage habits: keeping hot foods hot and cold foods cold, refrigerating leftovers quickly (perishables should be discarded after standing out for two hours or more), and discarding questionable items. Use nonporous surfaces (such as Formica, glass, stainless steel) rather than porous ones (wood or plastic with dirt-collecting gashes) for food preparation, and keep them scrupulously clean. Hands, too, should be washed before food is handled and after touching raw meat, fish, or eggs. Always cook meats, fish, and poultry thoroughly, and if there is a threat of salmonella in your area, do the same with eggs (eggs that are certified "fresh" and kept refrigerated in the market are the safest). Avoid unpasteurized juices and dairy products (including milk and soft cheeses), which can cause very serious illness. Also avoid eating in restaurants that seem to ignore basic sanitation rules (perishable foods are kept at room temperature, kitchen workers and waiters handle food directly with their hands, bathrooms are unclean, and so on).

❖ Keep pets in good health, updating their immunizations as necessary. If you have a cat, take the precautions to avoid toxoplasmosis (page 65).

❖ Avoid outdoor areas where Lyme disease is prevalent, or be sure to protect yourself adequately (see page 316).

❖ Don't share toothbrushes or other personal items.

16
Coping With a Chronic Condition

Anyone who's lived with a chronic condition knows that life can get pretty complicated, what with the special diets, the medications, and the medical monitoring. Anyone who's lived with a chronic condition while being pregnant knows that those complications can double, with the special diet needing to be modified, the medications altered, and the medical monitoring stepped up.

In the past there was another complication for women with chronic conditions who became pregnant: ma-jor risk to themselves and their babies. Today, happily, thanks to many scientific advances, that complication is much less common and most chronic conditions *are* compatible with pregnancy. Still, special precautions are necessary on the part of both the mother and her medical providers. This chapter outlines those precautions for the most common chronic conditions. Where the recommendations in this chapter differ from your doctor's, be sure to follow those of your doctor, since they probably have been tailored to your personal needs.

WHAT YOU MAY BE CONCERNED ABOUT

DIABETES

"I'm a diabetic, and I'm concerned about the effect of my condition on my baby."

Until recently, getting pregnant was a risky business for the diabetic woman, and even riskier for her unborn baby. Today, with expert medical care and guidance and scrupulous self care (ideally beginning before conception), a woman with diabetes has just about as good a chance of having a successful pregnancy and healthy baby as any other woman. In fact, diabetic women in one study took such excellent care of themselves throughout their pregnancies that they and their babies had even *fewer* problems than their nondiabetic counterparts.

Making your diabetic pregnancy a success will take a good deal of effort on your part, but the reward—a healthy baby—will make it well worthwhile.

Research has proved that the key to successfully managing a diabetic pregnancy is maintaining euglycemia (normal blood glucose levels). The availability in the past few years of home monitoring, split-dose administration of insulin, and even insulin pumps has made this increasingly possible.

Whether you came into pregnancy a diabetic or developed gestational diabetes along the way, all of the following considerations will be important in working toward a safe pregnancy and a healthy baby.[1]

Doctor's Orders. You will probably see your obstetrician (as well as your internist or endocrinologist) more often than do other expectant moms. You will be given many more orders, and will have to be far more scrupulous in following them.

Good Diet. A diet geared to your personal requirements should be carefully planned with your physician, a nutritionist, or a nurse-practitioner with expertise in diabetes. The diet will probably be high in complex carbohydrates, particularly beans (about half your daily calories should be from carbohydrates), moderate in protein (20% of caloric intake), low in cholesterol and fat (30% of caloric intake, no more than 10% saturated), and contain no sugary sweets. Plenty of dietary fiber will be important (40

to 70 grams daily are recommended), since some studies show that fiber may reduce insulin requirements in diabetic pregnancies. Calories may be restricted, particularly if you are overweight.

The extent of your carbohydrate restriction will depend on the way your body reacts to particular foods. Some women can handle fruit and fruit juices; others experience sharp blood sugar increases on consuming them, in which case they have to get more of their carbohydrates from vegetable, grain, and legume sources than from fruits (and may not be able to partake of certain Best-Odds treats). To maintain normal blood sugar levels, you will have to be particularly careful to get enough carbohydrates in the morning. Snacks will also be important, and ideally they should include both a complex carbohydrate (such as whole-grain bread) and a protein (such as meat or cheese). Your caloric requirement, like that of other pregnant women, will increase by about 300 calories a day over what you needed before pregnancy, and your protein requirement by about 30 grams (an average serving of meat or fish). Skipping meals or snacks can dangerously lower blood sugar, so be sure to eat regularly.

Pregnancy is not a time to be lax about your diet, although exhaustion may tempt you to be. It is, rather, an ideal time to get your dietary act together—for you and for your baby. Perfecting dietary control in a diabetic pregnancy is so important that many specialists recommend in-hospital training for diabetic women prior to conception or early in pregnancy. In some cases, in-hospital training may also be recommended for women who develop diabetes as pregnancy progresses (gestational diabetes).

If morning sickness is a problem at any time during pregnancy, try not to let it interfere with nourishing your

1. These are components of a typical diabetic pregnancy program. The one laid out for you by your physician or medical team may differ and is the one you should follow. If you are not already pregnant, your physician will start you on a special program to ready you for conception.

Safe Exercise Heart Rate for Diabetic Pregnancies

It is usually recommended that pregnant women with diabetes not exercise beyond 70% of the maximum safe heart rate for their age group, which is determined by subtracting one's age from 220, then multiplying the result by .70. If you are 30, for example, you would figure it this way: 220 − 30 = 190; then .70 × 190 = 133. This means that 133 beats per minute would be your upper safe limit of exercise intensity, the level you should not exceed.

baby and keeping your blood sugar stable.[2] Never fast or skip meals; eating regularly is essential. If you have trouble getting down three large meals, take six to eight small ones, regularly spaced and carefully planned. (See page 105 for some general tips on dealing with morning sickness.)

Sensible Weight Gain. It's best to try to reach your ideal weight before conception (something to remember if you plan another pregnancy). But if you start your pregnancy overweight, don't plan on using the gestational period for slimming down. Getting sufficient calories is vital to your baby's well-being. Weight gain should progress according to the guidelines set by your physician, usually 25 to 30 pounds during the nine months.

Exercise. A moderate exercise program will give you more energy, aid in regulating your blood sugar, and help you get in shape for delivery. But it must be planned in conjunction with your medication schedule and diet plan by or with the help of your medical team. If you experience no other

medical or pregnancy complications and are physically fit, such moderate exercise as brisk walking, swimming, and light stationary biking (but not jogging) will likely be suggested. Only light exercise (such as leisurely walking) will be allowed if you were out of condition prior to pregnancy or if there are any signs of problems with your diabetes, your pregnancy, or your baby's growth.

Precautions you may be asked to observe when exercising include taking a snack, such as milk, before your workout; not allowing your heart rate (pulse) during exercise to exceed 70% of the maximum safe heart rate for your age (see box); and never exercising in a warm environment (with temperatures in the 80s or higher). If you are on insulin, you will probably be advised to avoid injecting insulin into the parts of the body being exercised (your legs, for example, if you're walking) and not to reduce your insulin intake prior to exercise.

Rest. Especially in the third trimester, adequate rest is very important. Avoid overtaxing your energies, and try to take some time off during the middle of the day for putting your feet up or napping. If you have a job, especially a demanding one, your doctor may recommend that you begin your maternity leave early.

---

2. If nausea and vomiting interfere with eating, check with your physician about adjusting your insulin intake.

Medication Regulation. If diet and exercise alone do not control your blood sugar, you will probably be put on insulin. If you had been taking oral medication for diabetes prior to conception, you will be switched to injected insulin, which is less likely to adversely affect your fetus, for the duration of your pregnancy. If you need insulin for the first time, you may be hospitalized briefly so that your blood sugar can be stabilized under close medical supervision. Since levels of the pregnancy hormones that work against insulin increase as pregnancy progresses, your insulin dose may have to be adjusted upward periodically. The dose may also have to be recalculated as your size and your baby's size change, or if you are ill or under emotional strain.

Blood Sugar Regulation. You may have to test your blood sugar (with a simple finger-prick method) at least four or as often as ten times a day (possibly before and after meals) to be sure it is remaining at normal levels (euglycemia). To maintain such levels, you will have to eat regularly (no meal skipping), adjust your diet and exercise as needed, and, if necessary, take medication. If you were insulin dependent before pregnancy, you may be more subject to hypoglycemic (low blood sugar) episodes than when you were not pregnant, especially in the first trimester. You may also be asked to check your urine for ketones.

Reduction of Other Risk Factors. Since risk in pregnancy is cumulative—the more risk factors, the higher the risk—you should endeavor to eliminate or minimize as many as possible. (See Reducing Risk, page 50.)

Careful Monitoring. Don't be alarmed if your physician orders a great many tests for you (in and out of the hospital), especially during the third trimester, or even suggests hospitalization for the final weeks of your pregnancy. This doesn't mean something is wrong, only that he or she wants to be sure that everything stays right. The tests will primarily be directed toward regular evaluation of your condition and that of your baby, in order to determine the optimal time for delivery and whether any other intervention is needed.

You will probably have regular eye exams to check the condition of your retinas and blood tests to evaluate your kidneys (retinal and kidney problems tend to worsen during pregnancy, but usually return to pre-pregnancy states after delivery). The condition of your baby and the placenta will probably be evaluated through stress and/or non-stress tests (see page 263), biophysical profiles, amniocentesis (to determine lung maturity and readiness for delivery), and sonography (to size up your baby to be sure it's growing as it should be and so that delivery can be accomplished before he or she's too big for vaginal delivery).

You may be asked to monitor fetal movements yourself three times a day (see page 202 for one way to do this). If you don't feel any fetal movement on testing, call your doctor immediately.

Don't panic if your baby is placed in a neonatal intensive care unit immediately after delivery. This is routine procedure in most hospitals for infants of diabetic mothers. Your baby will be observed for respiratory problems (which are unlikely if the lungs were tested and found to be mature enough for delivery) and for hypoglycemia (which, though more common in babies of diabetics, responds quickly and completely to treatment).

Elective Early Delivery. Because babies of many diabetics tend to be too large for full-term vaginal delivery (particularly when euglycemia has not been maintained throughout pregnancy); because their placentas often begin to deteriorate early (robbing the fetus of vital nutrients and oxygen during the last weeks); and because they are subject to acidosis (abnormal acid-base balance in the blood) and other problems, they are often delivered before term, generally at about 38 or 39 weeks. The various tests mentioned above help the physician to decide when to induce labor or perform a cesarean—late enough so that the fetal lungs are sufficiently mature to function outside the womb, not so late that fetal safety has been jeopardized. Women who developed gestational diabetes, as well as women with pre-existing mild diabetes and sometimes even those with very well-controlled moderate disease, can often carry to term safely.

ASTHMA

"I've been an asthmatic since childhood. I'm concerned that the attacks and the drugs I take for them might harm my baby."

While it's true that a severe asthmatic condition does put a pregnancy at higher risk, studies have shown that this risk can be almost completely eliminated. Asthmatics who are under close, expert medical supervision (preferably by their internist and/or allergist in collaboration with their obstetrician) throughout their pregnancies have as good a chance of having normal pregnancies and healthy babies as nonasthmatics. But though asthma, if controlled, has only a minimal effect on pregnancy, pregnancy often has a considerable effect on asthma. With about one-third of pregnant asthmatics, the effect is positive—their asthma improves. In another third, their condition stays about the same. In the remaining third (usually those with the most severe disease) the asthma worsens, generally after the fourth month.

Whether your asthma is mild or severe, you and your baby will benefit if you get the condition under control before conception or at least early in pregnancy. The following steps will help:

❖ If you smoke, quit immediately. See page 55 for how-to tips.

❖ Identify environmental triggers. The most common offenders are pollens, animal danders (you may need to board your pet at a friend's), dusts, and molds. Tobacco smoke, household cleaning products, and perfumes can also provoke a reaction, and it's a good idea to steer clear of them. (See Allergies, page 157, for tips on avoiding allergens.) If you were started on allergy shots before pregnancy, this treatment will probably be continued. If necessary, such therapy may be begun during pregnancy. Attacks can also be brought on by exercise; these can usually be prevented by taking the medication prescribed by your doctor for this purpose prior to exertion.

❖ Try to avoid colds, flu, and other respiratory infections. (See page 323.) Your doctor may give you medication to ward off an asthma attack at the beginning of a mild cold, and will probably want to treat any but the most minor respiratory infections with antibiotics. You may also be immunized against influenza and pneumococcal infections.

❖ If you have an asthma attack, treat it immediately with your prescribed medication, to avoid depriving the fetus of oxygen. If the medication doesn't help, head for the nearest emergency room or call your doctor immediately.

❖ Take only drugs that have been prescribed by your physician *during your pregnancy,* and take them only as prescribed *for pregnancy use.* If your symptoms are mild, you may not require medication. If they are moderate to severe, there are several medications, both inhaled and ingested, that are considered to be "probably safe" for the fetus. The risks of taking these medications, if any, are quite small compared to the benefits of preventing fetal hypoxia (oxygen deprivation). And as an added benefit, some of these medications actually appear to reduce the risk of pre-eclampsia (see page 204) as well.

❖ Reduce other pregnancy risk factors. Since pregnancy risks are cumulative, you should endeavor to eliminate or minimize as many as possible. (See Reducing Risk in Any Pregnancy, page 50.)

The normal breathlessness that afflicts a majority of women in late pregnancy (see page 234) may be alarming to the asthmatic mother-to-be, but it is not dangerous. However, in the last trimester, as breathing becomes more labored because of the enlarged uterus crowding the lungs, pregnant asthmatics may notice a worsening of asthmatic flare-ups. Prompt treatment is especially important during such attacks.

The tendency toward allergies and asthma is inherited, and so it is wise for asthmatics to postpone exposing their babies to potential food allergens by breastfeeding exclusively for at least six months, thereby delaying the onset of allergic sensitization in their children and possibly reducing their long-term risk of allergy.

CHRONIC HYPERTENSION

"I've had hypertension for years. How will my high blood pressure affect my pregnancy?"

Since increasing numbers of women are choosing to conceive in their 30s and 40s and hypertension (high blood pressure) is more common as one gets older, the condition is showing up in more and more pregnant women. So you're not alone. Still, yours is considered a high-risk pregnancy (see page 339), which means that you will be seeing your doctor or doctors more often (preferably beginning with pre-pregnancy counseling), and will have to follow their advice more faithfully. But assuming that your blood pressure remains under control, with good medical and self care, it is very likely that both you and your baby will come through pregnancy well. Recent studies show that even those hypertensive women who have some kidney impairment can usually have successful pregnancies.

All of the following can help increase the odds of a successful pregnancy:

Relaxation. Pay more than just passing attention to the kinds of relaxation exercises mentioned on page 114. Try, too, any others that are recommended by your physician, such as biofeedback. Studies have shown that relaxation can help lower high blood pressure.

Blood Pressure Monitoring. You may be advised to take your own blood pressure daily, using a home blood pressure kit. Take it when you are most relaxed.

Good Diet. Following the Best-Odds Diet is particularly important. It may also be advisable to increase fruits and vegetables to eight to ten servings and cut sodium intake; both these dietary tactics have been shown to reduce hypertension. Adequate calcium intake may also help.

Adequate Fluid. Though your first instinct on experiencing a slight swelling of your feet and ankles because of fluid retention may be to cut down on your fluid intake, you should really do just the opposite. Drinking more water (up to a gallon a day), rather than less, will help flush out the excess.

Plenty of Rest. Take rest breaks, preferably with your feet up, both morning and afternoon. If you work at a high-stress job, consider giving it up until after the baby arrives. If you have your hands full at home with other children, get help—paid or volunteer.

Prescribed Medication. If you have been taking medication to control your blood pressure, your physician may okay your continuing it, or he or she may prescribe one that is considered to be safer in pregnancy. There are several blood-pressure-regulating drugs that appear to be safe when taken as directed. Low doses of aspirin, once thought to be helpful, have been shown not to be effective.

Attention to Your Body. Be alert to signs of pregnancy complications (see page 117), and contact your physician immediately if you experience any of them.

Close Medical Monitoring. Your physician will probably schedule more frequent visits for you than for other expectant mothers, and may subject you to many more tests.

If your blood pressure is very high and remains high in spite of medication, and/or you have protein in your urine early on or such serious side effects as retinal hemorrhages, severely impaired kidney function, or an enlarged heart, the risks of an unfavorable outcome to your pregnancy increase. In such a case, you may, in consultation with your physicians, have to weigh risks against benefits before deciding to attempt a pregnancy or continue with one already under way.

MULTIPLE SCLEROSIS

"I was diagnosed several years ago as having multiple sclerosis. I've only had two episodes, and they were relatively mild. Will the MS affect my pregnancy? Will my pregnancy affect my MS?"

Multiple sclerosis appears to have little if any effect on pregnancy. Nevertheless, early and regular prenatal care, coupled with regular visits to your neurologist, is a must. Iron supplements will probably be prescribed to prevent anemia and if necessary, stool softeners to combat constipation. Because urinary tract infections are more common in pregnancy, and because they could cause MS symptoms to flare, you may be given antibiotics as a preventive measure if you have a history of UTIs. Labor and delivery are not usually affected by MS, either. Epidural anesthesia, if needed, appears to be safe for use during both.

Nor does pregnancy seem to have much effect on MS. In fact, during pregnancy most women with MS find that their condition stabilizes, though in the later months, as weight gain increases, those with preexisting gait problems may find these exacerbated. If steroids are needed, prednisone in low to moderate doses is considered safe to use. Some other medications used for MS are less so; be sure to have your doctor check out the safety for use in pregnancy of any medication before you take it.

Though risk of relapse doesn't seem to increase during pregnancy, it does in the first six months postpartum. This risk, however, doesn't appear to be as serious as once supposed or to affect the overall lifetime relapse rate or the extent of ultimate disability. To reduce the risk of postpartum relapse, take your iron supplements as prescribed, and try to minimize stress, get adequate rest, and avoid infection and raising your temperature unduly (as in exercise or a hot tub). Going back to work early in the postpartum period may increase both exhaustion and stress, so discuss the risks with your doctor before deciding to return.

Breastfeeding will be possible, even if you occasionally need to take steroid medication; in small doses, very little of the drug passes into the breast milk. If you have to take large doses temporarily, you can pump your milk and discard it, giving your baby formula or previously pumped milk until the drug is gone from your milk. If breastfeeding is stressful for you, consider switching to bottle feeding, partially or completely—and don't feel guilty about your decision. Babies do very well on a good formula.

Most MS mothers manage to stay active for 25 years or more after their diseases are diagnosed, and are able to carry out childcare chores without difficulty. However, if MS does interfere with your functioning while your child is young, see page 334 for tips on baby care for disabled parents.[3]

AN EATING DISORDER

'I've been fighting bulimia for the last ten years. I thought I'd be able to stop the bingeing/purging cycle now that I'm pregnant, but I can't seem to. Will it hurt my baby?''

Not if you get help right away. The fact that you've been bulimic (or anorectic) for a number of years puts your baby and your body at a disadvantage right off the bat—your nutritional reserves are probably low. Fortunately, early in pregnancy the need for nourishment is less than it will be later on, so you have the chance to make up for the abuse done to your body before it can damage your baby.

There has been very little research in the area of eating disorders and pregnancy, partly because these disorders cause disrupted menstrual cycles, reducing the number of women with such problems who become pregnant in the first place. But the studies that have been done suggest the following:

❖ A pregnant woman with an eating disorder who gets help in getting it under control is as likely as anyone else to have a healthy baby—all other things being equal.

❖ It is important that the practitioner who is caring for her pregnancy be informed of the eating disorder.

❖ Counseling from a professional who is experienced in treating eating disorders is advisable for anyone who suffers from such a problem, but it is essential for the woman who is pregnant. Support groups may also be helpful.

❖ The laxatives, diuretics, and other drugs taken by bulimics are harmful to a developing fetus if the mother continues taking them once she learns she's pregnant. They draw off nutrients and fluids from the mother's body before they

3. Many women with MS are concerned about passing the disease on to their children. Though there is a genetic component to the disease, placing these children at increased risk of being affected as adults, the risk is really quite small. Between 90% and 95% of children of MS mothers remain MS free. If you are concerned nevertheless, see a genetic counselor.

can be utilized to nourish her baby (and later to produce milk); and they may lead to fetal abnormality. These medications, like all others, should not be used by any pregnant woman unless prescribed by a physician who is aware of the pregnancy.

It is also clear that it is necessary for you, and anyone else with an eating disorder, to understand the dynamics of weight gain in pregnancy. Keep in mind the following:

❖ The pregnant shape is beautiful, not fat and repugnant. Whereas excess fat may ordinarily be unhealthy and unattractive, pregnancy weight gain is vital to your baby's growth and well-being as well as to your own health.

❖ Gaining a moderate amount of weight each week in the second and third trimesters of pregnancy is not only normal, it's desirable (see page 147). If you stay within the recommended guidelines (which are higher in those who begin pregnancy underweight), you will be able to lose the weight easily after the baby arrives.

❖ If the weight is gained on high-quality foods as recommended in the Best-Odds Diet, the chances of having a healthy baby increase considerably, as do the chances that you'll recover your figure faster postpartum.

❖ Exercise can help avoid excessive weight gain, and can ensure that what weight is gained ends up in the right places—but it should be exercise appropriate for a pregnant woman (see page 189).

❖ All of the weight gain of pregnancy does not drop off in the first few days after delivery. With sensible eating, the average woman returns to close to her prepregnancy weight about six weeks after delivery, though for some women the weight loss process takes longer. If negative feelings about your body image cause you to slip back into bingeing and purging during the postpartum period (which could interfere with your ability to recover from childbirth, to parent effectively, and to produce milk if you choose to breastfeed), it's important that you continue professional counseling with someone experienced in the treatment of eating disorders or get help if you hadn't previously.

If you cannot seem to refrain from bingeing, vomiting, diuretics or laxatives, or practicing semi-starvation, you should discuss with your physician the possibility of hospitalization until you get your disease under control. If this isn't acceptable, you may want to consider whether this is the right time for you to be pregnant.

PHYSICAL DISABILITY

"I'm a paraplegic because of a spinal-cord injury, and I'm confined to a wheelchair. In spite of a lot of dire warnings and our own fears, my husband and I have wanted a baby for a long while. I've finally become pregnant. Now what?"

Like every pregnant woman, you'll need to deal with first things first: selecting a practitioner. And like every pregnant woman who falls into a high-risk category, your practitioner should ideally be an obstetrician or maternal-fetal subspecialist who has experience dealing with women who face the same challenges and potential risks as you do. If such a person isn't available in your area, you need a doctor who is willing to learn "on the job," and who is able to offer the wholehearted support you and your husband will need. Toward the end of your pregnancy you will also have to start looking for a pediatrician or family doctor who will be supportive of you as a physically challenged parent.

Just which special measures will be necessary to make your pregnancy successful will depend on your physical limitations. In any case, restricting your weight gain to within the recommended range (25 to 35 pounds) will help to minimize the stress on your body. Eating the best possible diet will improve your general physical well-being while decreasing the likelihood of pregnancy complications. And keeping up your physical therapy will help ensure that you have maximum strength and mobility when the baby arrives. It should be reassuring to know that, though pregnancy may be more difficult for you than for other pregnant women, it should not be any more stressful for your baby. There is no evidence of an increase in fetal abnormality among babies of spinal-cord injury patients (or of those with other physical disabilities not related to hereditary or systemic disease).

Women with spinal-cord injuries are more susceptible to such pregnancy problems as kidney infections and bladder difficulties, palpitations and sweating, anemia, and muscle spasms. Childbirth, too, may pose special problems, though in most cases a vaginal delivery will be possible. Because uterine contractions will probably be painless, you will have to be instructed to note other signs of impending labor.

Long before your due date, devise a fail-safe plan for getting to the hospital—one that takes into account the fact that you may be home alone when labor strikes (you may want to plan to leave for the hospital early in labor to avoid any problems caused by delays en route); prepare the hospital staff for your special needs; and be sure you will be able to get around the obstetrical unit in your wheelchair.

Parenting is always a challenge. It will be even more so for you and your husband. Planning ahead will help you meet this challenge more successfully. Make any necessary modifications to your home to make child care easier (you might try to contact other physically disabled mothers to see what tricks they've learned); sign on help (paid or otherwise) to at least get you started; enlist your spouse in the preparations for your baby's arrival, and divide up the household chores and baby care tasks for when baby comes home. Be creative. You don't have to do things "by the book"—do them in the way that works best for you. Breastfeeding, if it's possible, will make life simpler—you won't have to fuss with sterilizing, rush off to the kitchen to prepare a bottle when baby starts to cry, or shop for formula. A diaper service (they can deliver cloth or disposable diapers) will also save effort and time. The changing table should be tailored for you to use from your wheelchair, and the crib should have a drop side so you can take baby in and out easily. If you are going to be the one to bathe baby (though this is a job fathers often like and do well), you will have to arrange a baby tub on an accessible table. Since daily tub baths aren't a must, you can sponge baby on the changing table or on your lap on alternate days. A baby carrier may be a convenient way for you to carry your baby around, leaving your hands free to control your chair. Joining a support group of parents with disabilities can be not only a source of comfort and strength but also a gold mine of ideas and advice.[4]

---

4. For additional practical parenting advice, get a copy of *Aids and Adaptations for Parents with Physical or Sensory Disabilities* by T. Conine et. al (Vancouver, Canada: School of Rehabilitation Medicine, University of British Columbia, 1988).

It won't be easy, for you or for your husband, who may have to be a more-than-equal partner in parenting. But knowing that you're not the first to do it—and that the vast majority of those who have done it before you have reported that the satisfactions are more than worth the struggles—should be reassuring.

EPILEPSY

"I'm epileptic, and I just found out I'm pregnant. Will my baby be okay?"

With expert medical care, preferably beginning before conception, for both your epilepsy and your pregnancy, the odds are very much with you and your baby; epileptics have a 90% chance of having a healthy baby. If you haven't yet begun seeing an obstetrician, do so as soon as possible. And inform the physician who cares for your epilepsy of your pregnancy; close supervision of your condition, and possibly frequent adjustment of medication levels, will be necessary.

Epileptic mothers-to-be don't seem to have an increased incidence of such serious pregnancy and childbirth complications as miscarriage, pre-eclampsia, and premature birth, but they are more likely to experience excessive nausea and vomiting (hyperemesis).

It's believed that the slight increase in the incidence of certain birth defects in the children of epileptic mothers is in great measure attributable to the use of certain anticonvulsant medications during pregnancy, though some appear related to the epilepsy itself. Ideally, a woman with epilepsy should discuss with her doctor ahead of time the possibility of being weaned from her medications prior to conception. If she has to continue medication, it may be possible to switch to a less risky drug (phenobarbital, for example.) Though some women may worry that the medication they take for their epilepsy will harm their baby, not taking it and having frequent seizures may be more dangerous to the unborn child than any medication. Taking just one antiepileptic medication at the lowest effective dose appears to be safest for pregnant women with epilepsy.

Since the greatest risk of abnormalities developing exists during the first three months, there is little reason to worry about the effects of medication after that. Sometimes ultrasound or alpha-fetoprotein tests can determine early in pregnancy whether the fetus has been affected. If you've been taking valproic acid (Depakene), the doctor may want to look specifically for neural-tube defects, such as spina bifida.

Epileptic women often develop folate-deficiency anemia (which research shows may also be related to neural-tube defects in their babies), and so many doctors will prescribe a folic acid supplement for pregnant epileptics even though it may rarely increase the number of seizures. Vitamin D supplementation may also be recommended for women on certain anticonvulsants. During the last two months of pregnancy, a vitamin K supplement may be prescribed to reduce the increased risk of hemorrhage in the newborn. Alternatively, the baby will be given an injection of the vitamin at birth.

Most epileptic women find that pregnancy does not have a negative effect on their epilepsy. Half experience no change in their disease, and a smaller percentage find that seizures become less frequent and milder. A few find, however, that their seizures become more frequent and severe. This may be because of individual differences, or because medication has been vomited or overly diluted in the excess body fluid of pregnancy. The problem of losing medication by vomiting can often be minimized by taking a time-release anticonvulsant before going to bed, which allows the medication to build up before vomiting begins in the morning. Ask your doctor about the appropriateness of such a drug for you. If the problem is overdilution of the medication, it may be necessary for your doctor to readjust the dosage.

Once your baby arrives, if you want to breastfeed, it shouldn't be a problem. Most epilepsy medications pass into the breast milk in such low doses that they are unlikely to affect a nursing baby. But do check with your baby's doctor to be sure the specific medications you are taking are okay. And if your breastfed baby becomes unusually sleepy after you've taken a medication, report this to the doctor. A change may be necessary.

PHENYLKETONURIA (PKU)

"I was born with PKU. My doctors let me get off a low-phenylalanine diet when I was in my teens, and I was fine. But when I discussed getting pregnant with my obstetrician, she said I should go back on the diet and stay on it for my entire pregnancy. Should I take her advice even though I feel perfectly fine on a regular diet?"

Not only should you take her advice, you should thank her for it. It has only recently been recognized that pregnant women with phenylketonuria (PKU) who are *not* on a low-phenylalanine diet put their babies at great risk of being born too small, with small head circumferences, malformations, and possible brain damage. Ideally, as your doctor recommended, the special diet should be resumed before conception and blood levels of phenylalanine kept low

through delivery. The phenylalanine-free milk substitute and measured amounts of other foods permitted on this diet should be supplemented with micronutrients (zinc, copper, etc.) that might otherwise be absent from it. And, of course, all foods sweetened with aspartame (Equal or NutraSweet) are absolutely off-limits.

Though this diet isn't appealing, most mothers feel it's clearly worth the sacrifice to protect their developing babies from harm. If in spite of this incentive, you find yourself slipping off the diet, try to get some professional help from a therapist who is familiar with your type of problem. If counseling doesn't help, you should consider whether it is fair to continue the pregnancy with such heavy odds against your baby.

CORONARY ARTERY DISEASE (CAD)

"My doctor warned me not to get pregnant because I have coronary artery disease. But I did accidentally, and I don't want to abort. I want this baby more than anything."

Your situation isn't as unique as it once might have been. CAD, which is seen more often as women grow older, is becoming more common in pregnancy as more women opt to have their babies at a later age.

Whether or not it's safe for you to continue your pregnancy depends on the nature of your disease. If your disease is mild (you have no limitations on physical activity, and ordinary activity doesn't cause undue fatigue, palpitations, breathlessness, or angina) or moderate (you have slight limitations on physical activity, are completely comfortable at rest, but do experience symptoms with ordinary physical activity), chances are good that you can, under very close medical supervision, safely carry a pregnancy to term. If your disease is severe (you have marked limitations on physical activity, even very light activity causes symptoms, though you are comfortable at rest) or very severe (any physical activity causes discomfort, symptoms are noted even at rest), your doctor will probably tell you that carrying this baby will put your life at risk.

You and your husband will have to decide, with the help of your doctor, just how to proceed. When making that decision, keep in mind that if you don't survive the pregnancy, your baby probably won't either. But even if terminating this pregnancy turns out to be necessary in order to save your life, you aren't necessarily doomed to a life of childlessness. It's possible that your heart condition may be correctable (through open-heart surgery, for example), so that you will be able to go through a future pregnancy safely. If surgery isn't an option, perhaps adoption is, assuming you have the strength for childrearing.

If your cardiologist believes you can weather pregnancy safely, you will probably be given some very strict instructions. They will vary depending on your condition, but they may include:

❖ Avoiding physical and emotional stress; in some cases you may be asked to limit your activities for the duration of your pregnancy, possibly even to stay in bed.

❖ Taking your medication faithfully (be sure it's one that is safe for your baby; many appear to be).

❖ Watching your diet carefully so that you don't gain excess weight, which can put additional strain on your heart.

❖ Eating a low-cholesterol, low-saturated-fat, low-overall-fat diet if

your condition requires it, but not a no-fat diet; some fat is essential for healthy fetal development. Moderate sodium restriction (about 2,000 milligrams a day) is usually recommended, but greater restriction isn't. An iron supplement is generally prescribed.

❖ Wearing pressure-graded support pantyhose, to help reduce the pooling of blood in your legs.

❖ Quitting smoking, if you smoke.

Toward the end of your pregnancy, you are likely to begin undergoing frequent ultrasound scans and non-stress tests, so that the physician can keep abreast of your baby's condition. The tests will also help assure you that everything's okay.

If you pass through pregnancy without heart or lung complications, you're not likely to encounter problems during labor and delivery. Nor are you more likely to need a cesarean than other mothers. Outlet forceps (under local anesthesia; see page 286) may be used, however, to reduce the stress of labor and speed the final stage of delivery.

SICKLE-CELL ANEMIA

"I have sickle-cell disease, and I just found out that I'm pregnant. Will my baby be okay?"

Not too many years ago, the answer would not have been reassuring. Today, however, thanks to major medical advances, women with sickle-cell disease have a very good chance of coming through childbirth safely and of winding up with a healthy baby. Even those women with such sickle-cell complications as heart or kidney disease are often able to have a successful pregnancy.

Pregnancy for the woman with sickle-cell anemia, however, is usually classified as high risk. Because of the added stress on her body, her chances of having a sickle-cell crisis increase; and because of the disease the risks of certain pregnancy complications, such as miscarriage and preterm delivery, also increase. Preeclampsia, or toxemia, is also more common in women with sickle-cell anemia, but whether this is because they have sickle cell or because they're black and more subject to hypertension isn't clear.

The prognosis for both you and your baby will be best if you receive state-of-the-art medical care. You should have prenatal checkups more frequently than other pregnant patients—possibly every two to three weeks up to the 32nd week, and every week thereafter. Ideally your obstetrician should be familiar with sickle-cell disease and should work closely with a knowledgeable maternal-fetal subspecialist, internist, or hematologist. It's likely that prenatal vitamin and iron supplements will be prescribed. And probably at least once (usually in early labor or just prior to delivery), and possibly periodically throughout pregnancy (though this treatment is controversial), you will be given a blood transfusion. You are as likely as other mothers to have a vaginal delivery. Postpartum, you may be given antibiotics to prevent infection.

If both parents carry a gene for sickle-cell anemia, the risk that their baby will inherit a serious form of the disease is increased. Early in your pregnancy (if not prior to conception), your husband should be screened for the sickle-cell trait. If he turns out to be a carrier, you may want to see a genetic counselor, and possibly to undergo prenatal diagnosis (see page 42) to see if the fetus is affected.

SYSTEMIC LUPUS ERYTHEMATOSUS (SLE)

"My lupus has been pretty quiet lately. I just became pregnant. Is this likely to bring a flare-up? Will my baby get lupus?"

There's a lot that's still unknown about systemic lupus erythematosus (SLE), an autoimmune disease that affects primarily women between the ages of 15 and 64, black women more often than white. The studies that have been done seem to indicate that pregnancy doesn't affect the long-term course of lupus. During pregnancy itself, some women find their condition improves, others find it worsens. What happens in one pregnancy doesn't predict what will happen in subsequent ones. In the postpartum period, there does appear to be an increase in flare-ups.

The effect of SLE on the pregnancy, however, isn't absolutely clear. It does seem that the women who do best are those who, like you, conceive during a quiet period in their disease. Though their risk of pregnancy loss is slightly increased, their chances of having a healthy baby are excellent. Those with the poorest prognosis are those women with SLE who have severe kidney impairment (ideally, kidney function should have been stable for at least six months before conception) or who have what is called the lupus anticoagulant in their blood. No matter what the severity of a pregnant woman's lupus, it is extremely unlikely that her baby would be born with lupus.

If needed for arthritic symptoms or by women with the lupus anticoagulant, and if taken at the lowest effective doses, both daily doses of aspirin and the steroid prednisone seem to reduce overall risk. Many steroids are safe to use in pregnancy—some because they don't cross the placenta. Some that do cross the placenta are nevertheless safe, and some may actually benefit the fetus by hastening lung maturity.

Because of your lupus, your pregnancy care will be more complicated than most, with more, and more frequent, tests and possibly more limitations. But with you, your obstetrician or maternal-fetal subspecialist, and the physician who treats your lupus all working together, the odds are very much in favor of a happy outcome that will make it all worthwhile.

WHAT IT'S IMPORTANT TO KNOW:
LIVING WITH THE HIGH-RISK OR PROBLEM PREGNANCY

Pregnancy is a "normal" process to be experienced, not an illness to be treated—so the popular gestational dogma goes these days. But if yours is a high-risk pregnancy, you're all too aware that it's not universally true. For many women pregnancy is a time of fear, anxiety, constant medical care, frequent hospitalization, and a feeling that "no one else knows what it's like." Other expectant couples are living with joy and anticipation, but the couple in a high-risk pregnancy may live with:

Fear. While other parents are excitedly preparing for the birth of their baby at the end of nine months, high-risk parents may just be hoping that the fetus they are nurturing will still be alive tomorrow.

Resentment. A woman who is used to being independent may resent her sudden total dependence, especially if her activities are restricted ("Why me? Why do I have to give up my job? Why do I have to stay in bed?"). The anger may be aimed at the baby, at her spouse, or elsewhere. Her husband, of course, may have his own share of resentments ("Why does she get all the attention? Why do I have to do all the work? Does she really have to stay

in bed—and do I really have to stay home with her every evening?"). There may be unspoken resentments, too, about the high cost of her medical care and the lack of lovemaking, if it is restricted.

Guilt. A woman may agonize over what she may have done to make this a high-risk pregnancy, or to lose previous pregnancies, even though in the vast majority of cases, her actions aren't the cause at all. She may worry that she's just being lazy, staying in bed or leaving her job early. She may fear that she's destroying her relationship with her husband or with her other children. Her husband may be saddled with guilt too; he may feel bad that his wife is doing all the suffering, or he may feel remorse for the resentments he's harboring.

Feelings of Inadequacy. A woman who can't have a "normal" pregnancy may consider herself somehow lacking.

Constant Pressure. The high-risk expectant parent often has to keep her pregnancy and its requirements in mind every moment of every day; she'll need to pause almost constantly to ask herself "Can I do this? Is that allowed?" There may be a special diet, activity restrictions or even total bed rest, frequent examinations and tests.

Marital Stress. Any kind of crisis puts stress on a marriage, but a high-risk pregnancy often adds the stress of limited or prohibited sexual intercourse, which may make it hard for the couple to achieve intimacy. There may be added stress from the high cost of a high-risk pregnancy (much of which may not be reimbursed by insurance) and from the loss of income if the expectant mother can't continue working.

Though the ultimate rewards can make all the efforts more than worthwhile, it can be an undeniably tough nine months for the high-risk couple. The following may help make the going a little easier:

Financial Planning. As other parents save for college, you'll need to save for your baby's safe delivery. Knowing in advance that yours will be a high-risk, and thus an expensive, pregnancy is ideal, but it isn't always possible, at least not the first time. If it is, it makes sense to shop around for the best available insurance plan, and to forgo expensive vacations and other lifestyle frills so you can sock away some of the needed cash before the pregnancy begins. If it isn't, start taking belt-tightening steps as soon as you discover your situation.

Social Planning. If your pregnancy requires bed rest, partial or complete, don't resign yourselves to the hermit's life. Invite your best friends to supper in the bedroom (order pizza in and have your husband whip up some Mock Sangrias). Or ask friends in to play Monopoly, Scrabble, or cards, or to view a film that's just come out on video. If you have to miss an important family event, a friend's wedding, or your company's annual party, have your husband attend and record (in

his head, on tape, on video, or with a camera) the goings-on so he can share them with you later. If your sister is getting married 1,000 miles away and the doctor has vetoed traveling, videotape a message of love to her, or write a special poem to be read at the reception. Ask her to videotape the ceremony so you can share it.

Filling Time. Weeks, or even months, in bed may sound like a life sentence. But it can also be a time to do all the things you haven't had time for in your hectic life. Read those bestsellers everyone's been talking about, or some of the old classics that you never got around to enjoying. Join a video club that offers a good selection and good prices (how many other people ever have the time to take advantage of those "two-films-for-the-price-of-one" offers?). Study a foreign language, listen to a good book if you're tired of reading, or cultivate a new interest via audio tapes. Learn to knit or crochet or embroider—and make something for yourself, your husband, your mom, or your doctor if you're too superstitious to make something for your baby. If you're permitted to sit up, get a laptop computer and organize your financial life. Keep a journal of your thoughts, both the good and the bad, as a way both to pass the time and to work out your resentments. Collect some of the best catalogs, and do your shopping by phone or mail.

Childbirth Preparation. If you can't go to Lamaze classes, ask your husband to go and tape them, or to take notes and report on them verbally. If your bedroom is large and the class is small, ask if the others would mind holding at least one session at your home. Though you may feel that learning about normal childbirth may jinx yours, it will be important for you to be as well informed as possible. Read what you can on the subject in this book and elsewhere; even view a childbirth video or two. And though you may feel that you'd rather not know, learn all you can, too, about what delivery is like for someone with your particular problem—from your doctor as well as from books.

Mutual Support. A high-risk pregnancy, particularly when there are a lot of restrictions, is a real test of a marriage. You'll be going through a period of months where many of the normal pleasures of marriage are missing (sex, going out together, weekend trips, for example) and where even the joy 'of expecting a baby is marred and muddled. To be sure you end up with a healthy baby and a healthy marriage, each of you will have to think about the other's needs. The expectant mother's will be most obvious. She will need support in everything, from sticking to a restricted diet to sticking to restricted activities. But the needs of the father, who must be providing a lot of this support, may be neglected as a result. Even from her bedridden or otherwise depressingly restricted position, she has to recognize his feelings and let him know how truly important he is in all that is going on.

Sexual Sublimating. Making love doesn't always have to mean sexual intercourse. Read about how to achieve intimacy in pregnancy even when the doctor says "no sex" (page 168).

Getting Support. As with so many of life's crises, being able to talk to others in the same position as yours can help immeasurably. See below for tips that can help.

MOMS HELPING MOMS

Often a woman who has a high-risk or difficult pregnancy, or who has experienced a pregnancy loss, feels that she is unlike everyone else; she is acutely aware that her pregnancy experience is very different from those of her "normal" friends. If you feel this way, you may find comfort and support in a group of women who have had experiences similar to yours.

Discussions may cover such topics as feeling guilty about not being able to have a normal pregnancy; coping with being confined at home or in the hospital; concern over subsequent pregnancies; grieving over the loss of a baby; finding sources of emotional support; dealing with feelings of alienation. A lot of practical advice is also exchanged at support groups—managing your household when confined to bed; keeping your family going when you have a baby in intensive care; getting the best care for a particular disorder. And continuing with such a group after you feel better also helps you bring your own experience full circle, and helps with your healing while you support other women in need.

If you think you might benefit from a support group, try to find out if there is one in your area (check with your hospital, doctors, midwives, nurses). If there isn't and you have the energy, consider collecting the names of women in similar situations and starting a group yourself.

If you are bedridden and can't attend a support group, try phone meetings with other expectant mothers in bed, hold a meeting at your home occasionally, and subscribe to "LeftSide Lines," the newsletter for women with complicated pregnancies (Sidelines, 2805 Park Place, Laguna Beach, CA 92651).

17
When Something Goes Wrong

Considering the incredibly intricate processes that are involved in the creation of a baby, from the impeccably precise divisions of a fertilized egg to the dramatic transformation of a shapeless bundle of cells into a tiny human form, it's nothing short of miraculous that all goes right most of the time. And it's not surprising that very occasionally something goes wrong— because of genetics, environmental factors, a combination of the two, or just a quirk of nature. Modern medicine, modern sanitation, and an understanding of the significance of diet and lifestyle have all overwhelmingly improved the odds that a pregnancy (and the labor and delivery that follow) will be completed successfully and safely, but some risk still exists. Fortunately, with today's technology on our side, even when something does go wrong, early diagnosis and intervention can often right it.[1]

An obstetrical complication, whether it happens suddenly or was expected, complicates a woman's life as well as her pregnancy. Tips on coping with pregnancy problems that supplement the following medical explanations are under "Living with the High-Risk or Problem Pregnancy," page 339.

Most women go through pregnancy and childbirth without any complications. This chapter, which describes the most common complications, their symptoms and treatments, is not for them. *It should be read only by those women who have a suspected or diagnosed complication; and even then reading should be confined to the problem at issue. Casual reading could lead to not-so-casual, and unnecessary, worrying.*

1. Most complications that can occur during the postpartum period are covered in *What to Expect the First Year.*

CONDITIONS THAT MAY CAUSE CONCERN DURING PREGNANCY

HYPEREMESIS GRAVIDARUM

What Is It? This exaggerated form of morning sickness probably occurs in fewer than 1 in 200 pregnancies. Hyperemesis gravidarum, or excessive vomiting of pregnancy, is more common in first-time mothers, in women who are carrying multiple fetuses, and in women who suffered from the condition during a past pregnancy. Psychological stress may be a factor, but so is the sensitivity of the vomiting center in the brain, which seems to vary from person to person.

Signs and Symptoms. The nausea and vomiting of early pregnancy is unusually frequent and severe, and may linger longer—sometimes for the full nine months. If untreated, the frequent vomiting can lead to malnutrition, dehydration, and possibly harm to the health of mother or baby. Severe abdominal pain with morning sickness could mean gall bladder or pancreatic involvement and requires prompt medical attention.

Treatment. Milder cases may be controlled with dietary measures, rest, antacids, and antiemetic (antivomiting) medication,[2] but if vomiting continues and adequate weight is not being gained, hospitalization may be necessary. Further tests may be run to rule out nonpregnancy-related causes

---

2. Do not take any antivomiting medication without your doctor's approval. Since some of these drugs interact adversely with other drugs, be sure to let your doctor know about any medication you are presently taking before an antiemetic is prescribed.

of vomiting, such as gastritis, an intestinal blockage, or an ulcer. The patient's room may be darkened and her visitors limited to reduce stimulation; she may receive psychotherapy in an effort to reduce tension. If necessary, intravenous feeding may be given, along with an antiemetic. When fluid balance is restored (usually within 24 to 48 hours), a clear liquid diet is begun. If this is tolerated, the patient graduates to six small meals a day. If she still can't keep food down, intravenous feeding may be continued, though some food by mouth will still be encouraged. Occasionally, when the problem persists for long enough to threaten the proper nutrition of the fetus, special nutrients will be added to the intravenous fluids to allow a complete resting of the gastrointestinal tract for a matter of weeks. This is known as IV hyperalimentation. Only very rarely, when the mother's life is in danger, does termination of the pregnancy need to be considered.

ECTOPIC PREGNANCY

What Is It? A pregnancy that implants outside the uterus, most often in a fallopian tube. Early diagnosis and treatment are very effective. Without them, the pregnancy will continue to grow in the tube and the tube will eventually burst, destroying its ability to carry fertilized eggs on their way to the uterus in future conceptions. An uncared-for ruptured tube could also threaten the mother's life.

Signs and Symptoms. Colicky (spasmodic), crampy pain with tenderness, starting on one side and often spreading throughout the abdomen; pain may worsen on straining of bowels, coughing, or moving. Often, brown vaginal spotting or light bleeding, intermittent or continuous, which may precede pain by several days or weeks. Sometimes, nausea and vomiting, dizziness or weakness, shoulder pain, and/or rectal pressure. If the tube ruptures, heavy bleeding may begin, signs of shock (rapid, weak pulse, clammy skin, and fainting) are common, and pain becomes very sharp and steady for a short time before diffusing throughout the pelvic region.

Treatment. Getting to the hospital immediately is important. New techniques for early diagnosis and treatment of tubal pregnancy have removed most of the risk for the mother while greatly improving the chances of preserving her fertility.

Diagnosis is usually made through a combination of two procedures: (1) a series of highly sensitive pregnancy tests that track the level of the hor-

---

Bleeding in Early Pregnancy

Bleeding in early pregnancy does not necessarily indicate anything serious, but as a precaution, it should always be reported to your practitioner. Be precise in describing the bleeding: Is it intermittent or persistent? When did it start? Is the color bright or dark red, brownish or pink? Is it heavy enough to soak a sanitary pad in an hour, just occasional spotting, or somewhere in between? Is there any unusual odor? Do any tissue fragments (bits of solid material) seem to have been passed with the blood? (If so, try to save them in a jar or plastic bag.) Be sure to report, too, any accompanying symptoms, such as excessive nausea and vomiting, cramps or pain of any kind, fever, weakness, and so on.

Spotting or staining that is not accompanied by such symptoms is not considered an emergency situation; if it begins in the middle of the night, you can wait until morning to call the doctor. Any other kind of bleeding suggests a prompt call or, if the doctor is unavailable, a trip to the ER.

The two most common causes of first-trimester bleeding, neither of which is an indication of trouble, are:

Normal implantation of the pregnancy in the uterine wall. Such bleeding, which sometimes occurs when the fertilized egg attaches itself to the wall of the uterus, is brief and light.

Hormonal changes at the time menstruation would ordinarily have occurred. Bleeding is usually light, though an occasional woman experiences what seems like an actual period.

Less common, and more worrisome, causes of early bleeding include:

Miscarriage. Usually, heavy bleeding is accompanied by abdominal pain and possibly the passage of embryonic material (see page 346). A brownish discharge may indicate a missed miscarriage (see page 113). Sometimes, when the ovum doesn't develop (a blighted ovum), the sac is empty and no embryonic material is passed.

Ectopic pregnancy. Brown vaginal spotting or light bleeding, intermittent or persistent, is accompanied by abdominal and/or shoulder pain, which can often be quite severe (see page 343).

Trophoblastic disease. A continuous or intermittent brownish discharge is the prime symptom (see page 348).

Often, however, the actual cause of bleeding in the first trimester remains unidentified and the pregnancy continues to a happy conclusion.

Bleeding in Mid- or Late Pregnancy

Light or spotty bleeding in the second or third trimester is generally not a cause for concern. It is often the result of trauma to the increasingly sensitive cervix during an internal exam or sexual intercourse, or simply of causes unknown. Occasionally, however, it is a sign that immediate medical attention is needed. Since only your practitioner can determine the cause, he or she should be notified if you experience any bleeding— immediately if bleeding is heavy, the same day even if it is only spotty and there are no accompanying symptoms.

The most common causes of serious bleeding are:

Placenta previa, or low-lying placenta. Bleeding is usually bright red and painless. It most often starts spontaneously, though it can also be triggered by coughing, straining, or sexual intercourse. It can be light or heavy, and it usually stops, only to recur later on in pregnancy. See page 356 for further information.

Abruptio placenta, or premature separation of the placenta. Bleeding may be as light as a light menstrual flow, as heavy as a heavy one, or much heavier, depending on the degree of separation. The discharge may or may not contain clots. The intensity of the accompanying cramping, pain, and abdominal tenderness will also depend on the degree of separation. With a major separation, signs of shock from blood loss may be evident. See page 358.

Late miscarriage. When miscarriage is threatening, the discharge may at first be pink or brown; when bleeding is heavy and accompanied by pain, a miscarriage may be imminent. See page 347.

Premature labor. Labor is considered premature when it begins after the 20th week but before the 37th. A mucousy bloody discharge accompanied by contractions could signal preterm labor. See page 361.

mone hCG in the mother's blood (if the levels of hCG fall or fail to rise as the pregnancy progresses, an abnormal pregnancy, possibly in a fallopian tube, is suspected); and (2) high-resolution ultrasound to visualize the uterus and the fallopian tubes (the absence of a gestational sac in the uterus and, though this isn't always visible, a pregnancy developing in a fallopian tube are indications of ectopic pregnancy). If there is any doubt, confirmation is most often made by viewing the tubes directly, by means of a tiny laparoscope inserted through the navel. High-tech diagnostic tools such as these have made early diagnosis of ectopic pregnancies possible, catching 80% of them before they rupture.

Successful treatment of an ectopic pregnancy is also dependent on high-tech medicine. Laparoscopy, via two tiny incisions, one in the navel for the insertion of the viewing instrument, the laparoscope, and another lower in the abdomen for the surgical instruments, is usually the surgical choice because it allows for a much shorter hospital stay and a more rapid recovery period. Depending on the circumstances, lasers or electrocautery may be used to remove the pregnancy from the fallopian tube. More recently, the drug methotrexate has been used as an alternative to surgery. It destroys the pregnancy by halting cell growth.

Unless the fallopian tube has irreparable damage, it is usually possible to save it, improving the chances of a successful pregnancy in the future. Since residual material from a pregnancy left in the tube could damage it, a followup test of hCG levels is performed to be sure that the entire tubal pregnancy was removed.

EARLY MISCARRIAGE, OR SPONTANEOUS ABORTION

What Is It? A miscarriage, also called a spontaneous abortion, is the spontaneous expulsion from the uterus of an embryo or fetus before it is able to live outside the uterus. A miscarriage in

---

If You've Had a Miscarriage

Though it is hard for parents to accept it at the time, when a miscarriage *does* occur it is usually a blessing. Early miscarriage is generally a natural selection process in which a defective embryo or fetus (defective because of environmental factors, such as radiation or drugs; because of poor implantation in the uterus; because of genetic abnormality, maternal infection, random accident, or other unknown reasons) is discarded, probably because it is incapable of survival or is overwhelmingly defective.

All that said, losing a baby, even this early, is traumatic. But don't let guilt compound your misery—*a miscarriage is not your fault*. Do allow yourself to grieve. Sharing your feelings with your spouse, your practitioner, a friend, will help. In some communities, there are support groups for couples who have experienced pregnancy loss. Ask your practitioner if he or she knows of one in your area, or inquire at your hospital. This may be especially important if you've experienced more than one pregnancy loss. For more suggestions on coping with your loss, see page 366.

Possibly the best therapy is getting pregnant again as soon as it is safe. But before you do, discuss possible causes of the miscarriage with your doctor. Most often, miscarriage is simply a random one-time occurrence caused by chromosomal abnormality, infec-

tion, chemical or other teratogenic exposure, or chance, and is not likely to recur. Repeat miscarriages (more than two) are often related to hormonal insufficiency in the mother or to the mother's immune system rejecting a "foreign" intruder, the embryo. In both these situations, treatment when you conceive again, or even before, can often prevent a recurrence. Rarely, repeated miscarriages are due to genetic factors that are detectable by prepregnancy chromosome tests of both husband and wife. Check with your doctor about whether such tests are indicated in your case.

Whatever the cause of your miscarriage, many doctors suggest waiting three to six months before trying to conceive again, though sexual relations can often be resumed after six weeks. (Use reliable contraception, preferably of the barrier type—condom, diaphragm—when you get your doctor's okay.) Take advantage of this waiting period—spend it improving your diet and your health habits. Happily, the odds are excellent that next time around you'll have a normal pregnancy and a healthy baby. Most women who have had one miscarriage do not become habitual aborters. In fact a miscarriage is an assurance of fertility, and the great majority of women who lose a pregnancy this way go on to complete one.

the first trimester is referred to as an early miscarriage. Early miscarriage is very common (many doctors believe that virtually every woman will have at least one sometime in her reproductive years), occurring in as many as 40% of conceptions. Most occur so early that pregnancy is not even suspected yet; so these miscarriages often go unnoticed, passing for an unusually heavy and crampy period. Early miscarriage is usually related to a chromosomal or other genetic abnormality in the embryo; to the mother's body failing to produce an adequate supply of pregnancy hormones; or to her having an immune reaction to the embryo.

Signs and Symptoms. Most often, bleeding with cramps or pain in the center of the lower abdomen. Sometimes, severe pain or persistent pain that lasts 24 hours or more unaccompanied by bleeding; heavy bleeding (like a menstrual period) without pain; persistent light staining (that continues for 3 days or more). Clots or grayish matter may be passed as the miscarriage actually begins.

Treatment. If, on examination, the doctor finds that the cervix is dilated, it will be assumed that a miscarriage has occurred or is in progress. In such a case nothing can be done to prevent the loss. In many cases the embryo or fetus will already have died prior to the onset of miscarriage, triggering the spontaneous abortion.

On the other hand, if the fetus is shown to be alive through either ultrasound or a Doppler device and there is no dilatation, the chances are very good that the threatened miscarriage will not occur. Some physicians will suggest no particular treatment on the theory that a doomed pregnancy will abort, therapy or no, and a healthy pregnancy will hang in there (also with or without therapy). Others—

particularly when a woman has had a history of miscarriage or when it is believed that implantation is imperfect—will impose bed rest and restrictions on activities, including sexual intercourse. Female hormones, once given routinely for early bleeding, are now rarely used because there is doubt about their efficacy and concern over the potential harm to the fetus if the pregnancy continues. In very unusual cases, however, patients with a history of miscarriages who have shown evidence of producing too little of the hormone may benefit from progesterone administration.

Sometimes, when a miscarriage does occur, it isn't complete—only parts of the placenta, sac, and embryo are expelled. If you've had, or believe you've had, a miscarriage, and bleeding and/or pain continues, phone your doctor immediately. A D and C (dilation and curettage) will probably be required to stop the bleeding. It's a simple but important procedure, in which the cervix is dilated and any remaining fetal or placental tissue is scraped or suctioned out. Your physician will probably want to evaluate the material for clues to the cause of the miscarriage.

LATE MISCARRIAGE

What Is It? Any spontaneous expulsion of a fetus between the end of the first trimester and the 20th week is termed a late miscarriage. (After the 20th week, when the fetus may be able to live outside the uterus—even if only with a lot of help from the neonatal nursery staff and equipment—the event is labeled a preterm birth.[3]

3. When a baby is born dead after the 20th week, it's usually described as a stillbirth rather than a miscarriage. The definitions of late miscarriage and stillbirth may vary from state to state.

The cause of late miscarriage is usually related to the mother's health, the condition of her cervix or uterus, her exposure to certain drugs or other toxic substances, or to problems of the placenta (see page 177).

Signs and Symptoms. A pink discharge for several days, or a scant brown discharge for several weeks, indicates a threatened miscarriage. Heavier bleeding, especially when accompanied by cramping, probably means a miscarriage is inevitable.

Treatment. For a threatened late miscarriage, bed rest is often prescribed. If the spotting stops, this is taken as an indication that it wasn't related to miscarriage, and a resumption of normal activity is usually permitted. If the cervix has started to dilate, a diagnosis of incompetent cervix may be made and cerclage (stitching closed of the cervix) may prevent miscarriage.

Once the heavy bleeding and cramping that signal a miscarriage begin, the treatment is aimed at protecting the mother's health. Hospitalization may be required to prevent hemorrhaging. If cramping and bleeding continue following a miscarriage, a D and C may be necessary to remove anything that remains of the pregnancy.

If the cause of a late miscarriage can be determined, it may be possible to prevent a repeat of the tragedy. If a previously undiagnosed incompetent cervix was responsible, future miscarriages can be prevented by cerclage early in pregnancy, before the cervix begins to dilate. If hormonal insufficiency was to blame, hormone replacement may allow future pregnancies to progress to term. If chronic disease, such as diabetes or hypertension, is responsible, better control can be established. Acute infection or malnutrition can be prevented or treated. And an abnormally shaped uterus or

one that is distorted by the growth of fibroids or other benign tumors can, in some instances, be corrected by surgery.

TROPHOBLASTIC DISEASE (HYDATIDIFORM MOLE)

What Is It? In roughly 1 in 2,000 pregnancies in the United States, more often in women over 45 than in younger mothers, the trophoblast—the layer of cells that line the gestational sac and normally give rise to the chorionic villi—convert into a mass of clear tapioca-like vesicles instead of into a healthy placenta. Without its placental support system, the fertilized ovum deteriorates. Known as trophoblastic disease or hydatidiform mole, the condition is probably caused by a chromosomal abnormality in the fertilized egg.

Signs and Symptoms. The first sign of a molar pregnancy is usually an intermittent, though sometimes continuous, brownish discharge. Frequently the normal morning sickness of pregnancy becomes abnormally severe. As the pregnancy progresses, 1 in 5 women may pass a few of these tiny vesicles through the vagina. By the beginning of the second trimester, the uterus is larger than expected and feels doughy rather than firm; no fetal heartbeat can be detected. Preeclampsia (elevated blood pressure, excessive swelling, and protein in the urine), or in some cases loss of weight and other indications of increased thyroid activity, may also be seen. The definitive diagnosis will depend on an ultrasound exam, which will show the absence of embryonic or fetal tissue and the uterus distended with these small vesicles. The ovaries may also be enlarged because of the accompanying high levels of hCG.

Treatment. The cervix is dilated and the contents of the uterus are carefully evacuated, as in a missed miscarriage or a therapeutic abortion. Follow-up is important, since about 10% to 15% of molar pregnancies don't stop growing immediately. If blood hCG levels fail to return to normal, a repeat D and C is performed. If hCG levels remain elevated after a second procedure, the physician will check for a new pregnancy or for spread of the molar tissue to the vagina or lungs, which may be treated with chemotherapy. Rarely, a molar pregnancy becomes malignant (see choriocarcinoma, page 350), so close medical follow-up is especially important (this condition is potentially curable with early diagnosis and treatment).

It is generally recommended that attempts to conceive again following a molar pregnancy be postponed for one to two years. Careful monitoring of a new pregnancy is vital because of the possibility of another mole developing. Since there is some very tentative evidence that links trophoblastic disease to an inadequate intake of animal protein and vitamin A, strict ad-

When a Serious Fetal Defect Is Detected

It's the nightmare of everyone who undergoes any kind of prenatal diagnosis: something actually does turn out to be wrong, so wrong that termination of the pregnancy may have to be considered. The fact that such a nightmare becomes a reality only rarely is no consolation to the couples who receive that dreaded abnormal report.

Before you do consider terminating your pregnancy, you should be sure that the diagnosis is correct and that all your options are clear. Get a second opinion, preferably from a genetic counselor or a specialist in maternal-fetal medicine.

If the pregnancy is to be terminated, you may find that comfort is hard to come by. Well-meaning friends and relatives may not understand what you're going through and may underplay what you view as a tragedy with comments like "It's for the best" or "You can try again." Professional support—from your doctor, a therapist, a social worker, or a genetic counselor—may be necessary to help you deal with this difficult situation. Accepting it won't be easy. You'll probably go through all or most of the other stages of grieving—denial, anger, bargaining, depression—before you reach acceptance.

Often, couples who get bad news saddle themselves with an added, and unnecessary, burden: guilt. It's important to realize that birth defects are most often a matter of chance. You wouldn't knowingly hurt your baby, and if you did so unknowingly, you aren't to blame. See page 366 for additional counsel on dealing with the loss of a baby.

If you decide to terminate but are upset about doing so, it may help you to keep in mind that if this diagnosis were not made prenatally, you would have carried your baby, getting to know and love it, for nine months, only to lose it shortly after birth. Or you would have delivered a baby who lingered for months or years, but with no semblance of life as we know it. Instead, by the time your due date rolls around you may have had the opportunity to become pregnant once again—this time, hopefully, with a healthy baby. That in no way, of course, takes away your right to mourn for the loss of this one.

herence to the Protein and Green Leafy and Yellow Vegetables and Yellow Fruit requirements of the Best-Odds Diet (see page 80) should begin before conceiving again, and should continue throughout any subsequent pregnancy.

PARTIAL MOLAR PREGNANCY

What Is It? In a partial molar pregnancy, as in a complete molar pregnancy (above), there is abnormal development of the trophoblast. With a partial mole, however, identifiable embryonic or fetal tissue is present. If the fetus survives, it is often growth-retarded and likely to have a variety of congenital abnormalities, such as webbed (or connected) fingers and toes (syndactyly) and water on the brain (hydrocephalus). If a normal baby is born, it usually turns out that it was part of a multiple pregnancy, with the mole belonging to a twin that had deteriorated.

Signs and Symptoms. These are similar to those of an incomplete or missed abortion. There is usually irregular vaginal bleeding, usually no fetal heartbeat, and a uterus that is either small or normal for the length of the pregnancy. Only a small percentage of women with partial molar pregnancies have an enlarged uterus, as is common in a complete molar pregnancy. Ultrasound and hCG levels are used to diagnose a partial mole.

Treatment. Follow-up and treatment are similar to that for a complete molar pregnancy, and a new pregnancy is not recommended until hormone levels have been normal for six months. Most women can have healthy babies after having had a partial molar pregnancy, but since the risk of a repeat exists, early ultrasound examination is important in future pregnancies to rule out that possibility.

CHORIOCARCINOMA

What Is It? Choriocarcinoma is an extremely rare cancer related directly to pregnancy. About half the cases develop when there is a hydatidiform mole (page 348), 30% to 40% following a miscarriage, and 10% to 20% after a normal pregnancy.

Signs and Symptoms. The signs of the disease include intermittent bleeding following a miscarriage, a pregnancy, or the removal of a mole, along with elevated hCG levels and a tumor in the vagina, uterus, or lungs.

Treatment. Chemotherapy. With early diagnosis and treatment, survival is the norm and fertility is unaffected, though it is usually recommended that pregnancy be deferred for two years after treatment is complete.

GESTATIONAL DIABETES

What Is It? A temporary condition, similar to other types of diabetes, in which the body does not produce adequate amounts of insulin to deal with the increased blood sugar of pregnancy. (See page 152.)

Diabetes, both the kind that begins in pregnancy and the kind that started before conception, is generally not dangerous for either the fetus or the mother—*if* it is controlled. But if excessive sugar is allowed to circulate in a mother's blood, and thus to enter the fetal circulation through the placenta, potential problems for both mother and baby are serious.

Signs and Symptoms. The first sign may be sugar in the urine, but there may also be unusual thirst, frequent and very copious urination (as distinguished from the also frequent but usually light voiding of early pregnancy), and fatigue (which may be difficult to differentiate from pregnancy fatigue).

Treatment. Fortunately, virtually all of the potential risks associated with diabetes in pregnancy can be eliminated through the scrupulous control of blood sugar levels achieved by good medical and self care. If doctor's instructions are followed (see page 326 for recommended care), the diabetic mother and her baby will have almost as good a chance to come through pregnancy and childbirth well as any other mother and baby.

CHORIOAMNIONITIS

What Is It? This infection of the amniotic fluid and fetal membranes is diagnosed in only 1 in 100 pregnancies, but it is suspected that the true incidence may be much higher. The infection is believed to be a major cause of premature rupture of the membranes as well as of premature labor.

Signs and Symptoms. In some cases, chorioamnionitis is asymptomatic (has no symptoms), particularly at first. Diagnosis is complicated by the fact that there is no simple test that can confirm the presence of infection. Often, the first sign of chorioamnionitis is rapid heartbeat (tachycardia) in the mother. This may also be caused by dehydration, medication, low blood pressure, or anxiety, but should in any case be reported to the practitioner. Then a fever over 100.4 degrees develops, and in many cases there is uterine tenderness. If the membranes have ruptured, there may also be a foul odor from the amniotic fluid; if they are intact, there may be

an unpleasant-smelling vaginal discharge, originating in the cervix. Lab tests will reveal an increased white blood count (a sign that the body is fighting an infection). The fetus may score low on a biophysical profile (see page 263), indicating some distress.

Treatment. Chorioamnionitis can be caused by a wide range of microorganisms, and the treatment will depend upon the particular organism involved as well as on the condition of the mother and the fetus. Usually other reasons for the symptoms will be ruled out, lab tests to try to determine the type of infectious organism involved will be ordered, and the fetus will be monitored before treatment is begun. If the pregnancy is near term and the membranes have ruptured, and/or if the fetus or mother is in trouble, a prompt delivery is generally the preferred course. If the fetus is extremely immature and unlikely to survive outside the uterus and it is acceptable to delay delivery, large amounts of antibiotics that can cross the placenta are given, while the situation is carefully monitored. Delivery is postponed until the fetus is more mature or the condition of mother or baby begins to deteriorate.

Recent medical advances allowing for more rapid diagnosis and treatment have greatly reduced the risk of chorioamnionitis to both mother and baby; further improvement of diagnostic tools teamed with a better understanding of how to prevent such infections in the first place will reduce these risks even further.

PREECLAMPSIA (PREGNANCY-INDUCED HYPERTENSION)

What Is It? Also called toxemia, preeclampsia is a pregnancy-related form of high blood pressure. No one knows what causes PIH, or why it develops most often in first-time moms-to-be, although some research links it to poor nutrition. Studies suggesting tiny doses of aspirin or large doses of calcium might help have not held up. Toxic substances have been found in the blood of women who become preeclamptic. In a test tube, these substances damage human endothelial cells (the cells that line the blood vessels). It's theorized that they are produced by the body as an immune, or defensive, reaction to a foreign intruder—the baby—when the mechanism that is supposed to work to suppress such a reaction during pregnancy is absent or fails. Further research into this theory may lead to better ways of dealing with toxemia.

Signs and Symptoms. Initially: swelling of hands and face with sudden excessive weight gain (both related to water retention); high blood pressure (140/90 or more in a woman who has never before had high blood pressure)[4]; and protein in the urine. The condition can progress quickly to the severe stage, characterized by a further increase in blood pressure (usually to 160/110 or higher), increased quantities of protein in the urine, blurred vision, headaches, all-over itching, irritability, scanty urine output, confusion, severe gastric pain, and/or abnormal liver or kidney function and blood platelet test results. Untreated, severe preeclampsia can in turn progress very quickly to the very serious eclampsia, characterized by convulsions, and sometimes coma.

Preeclampsia occurs in 5% to 10%

4. In the HELLP syndrome form of toxemia the blood pressure doesn't always go up, but there is usually severe upper mid-abdominal pain, nausea, and possibly unexplained vomiting. Blood tests show Hemolysis, Elevated Liver enzymes, and Low Platelet count.

of pregnancies and, *if it goes untreated,* can lead to permanent damage to the nervous system, the blood vessels, or the kidneys in the mother and growth retardation (because of a reduced blood supply through the placenta) or oxygen deprivation in the baby. Fortunately, in women who are receiving regular medical care, the disease is almost invariably caught early on and treated successfully, avoiding the rare bad outcome.

Occasionally preeclampsia, or pregnancy-induced hypertension, doesn't appear until labor and delivery, or even until the postpartum period. Such a sudden increase in blood pressure may be merely a reaction to stress or may be true preeclampsia. Therefore women who exhibit such elevations of blood pressure are watched very carefully with frequent checks not just of their blood pressure, but of their urine (for protein), their reflexes, and their blood chemistry.

Treatment. Treatment will vary according to the severity of the disease, the condition of both mother and baby, the length of the pregnancy, and the doctor's judgment.

With mild disease, the woman who is near term and whose cervix is ripe (softened and thinned) is usually induced without delay. The woman who isn't is usually hospitalized for complete bed rest (lying on the left side is best) and close observation, usually without diuretics, blood pressure medication, or drastic sodium restriction. In some very mild cases, bed rest at home may be permitted once blood pressure is normalized. If she is allowed to go home, the mother must be monitored by a visiting nurse and must make frequent visits to the doctor's office. She is informed of the danger signs—severe headache, visual disturbances, or upper or mid-abdominal pain—that may warn her that her condition is worsening, and she is expected to seek emergency medical attention immediately should she experience any of them.

Whether the mother is in the hospital or at home, the baby's condition will be assessed regularly: fetal movements will be checked daily, stress and non-stress tests, ultrasound, amniocentesis, and other procedures will be performed as needed. If at any point the mother's condition worsens or the tests of the fetus indicate the baby would be better off outside the uterus, the mother's condition will be evaluated to determine the best mode of delivery. If the cervix is favorable and the baby is not in acute distress, a vaginal induction of labor is ordinarily decided upon. Otherwise a cesarean will be recommended.

Generally a woman with preeclampsia, even mild preeclampsia, will not be allowed to go past her due date (40 weeks), since post-term the environment in the uterus begins to deteriorate more rapidly than normal. Depending on the circumstances, labor will be induced or the baby will be delivered by cesarean.

The prognosis for a pregnant woman with mild preeclampsia is very good when the medical care is appropriate, and pregnancy outcome is virtually the same as for a woman with normal blood pressure.

With severe disease, or if a mild preeclampsia progresses, the treatment is usually more aggressive. Intravenous magnesium sulfate is begun promptly because it almost always prevents convulsions, one of the most serious complications of the disease. (The side effects of this treatment are uncomfortable, but not usually serious.) If the fetus is close to term, and/or if its lungs are determined to be mature, immediate delivery is usually the recommended route. If the fetus is preterm, but at least 28 weeks old, many doctors will still choose to deliver immediately because they believe

it is best for both mother (in order to normalize her blood pressure and improve her general condition) and baby (who they feel will be better off continuing growth in a neonatal intensive care unit than in the less than hospitable environment in its mother's uterus). Women with such severe disease are best delivered in a tertiary hospital (a major medical center), where optimum maternal support as well as neonatal care for the premature infant are available.

Some doctors, however, prefer a more conservative approach (hospital bed rest, medication, and close monitoring of mother and baby) to give the fetus more time to develop before birth, though it isn't clear if this is really a more beneficial approach. Some will administer steroids to the fetus to try to speed lung maturity before delivery, but there is debate over whether or not this is effective. If the mother's blood pressure can't be controlled or there are signs of maternal or fetal deterioration, conservative methods will be abandoned in favor of immediate delivery.

Between 24 and 28 weeks, virtually all physicians try conservative management of preeclampsia, even when it's severe, in order to give the fetus a little more time in the uterus. Before 24 weeks (when the fetus is rarely able to live outside of the uterus and when severe preeclampsia is fortunately uncommon), delivering the pregnancy is sometimes necessary to reverse the preeclamptic process, even though the baby has no chance of survival.

With appropriate and prompt medical care, the chances of a favorable outcome for the preeclamptic mother and, except in rare instances, for her baby are very good.

In 97% of the women with preeclampsia who do not also have chronic hypertension, blood pressure returns to normal following delivery. The drop takes place for the majority of new mothers within the first 24 hours after childbirth, and for most of the others within the first week. If blood pressure doesn't return to normal by the six-week checkup, the doctor will look for underlying disease.

ECLAMPSIA

What Is It? Eclampsia, which can occur before, during, or after childbirth, is the final stage of toxemia syndrome-preeclampsia/eclampsia. It is very unusual for this stage to be reached when good medical care is given.

Signs and Symptoms. Convulsions and/or coma. These are often preceded by spiking blood pressure, seriously increased levels of protein in the urine, and exaggerated reflex reactions, as well as severe headache, nausea or vomiting, irritability, restlessness and twitching, upper abdominal pain, visual disturbances, drowsiness, fever, or rapid heartbeat.

Treatment. The patient is prevented from injuring herself during the convulsions. Oxygen and drugs to arrest the seizures will be administered; the patient's environment will be kept as free of stimuli, such as light and noise, as possible. Labor will generally be

induced or a cesarean-section performed when the patient is stable. With optimum care the survival rate is 98%, and the majority of patients rapidly return to normal after delivery, though careful follow-up is necessary to be certain blood pressure returns to normal.

INTRAUTERINE GROWTH RETARDATION (IUGR)

What Is It? Sometimes when the uterine environment is not ideal—because of maternal illness, maternal lifestyle, placental inadequacy, or other factors—a fetus doesn't grow as rapidly as it should. Without intervention, that baby will be born, whether prematurely or at term, small for gestational age (also called small for date). But if IUGR is diagnosed prenatally, as it often is when a mother is receiving regular medical care, steps are taken that may reverse it.

IUGR is more common in first pregnancies and in fifth and subsequent ones. It's also somewhat more common among women who are under 17 or over 34.

Signs and Symptoms. Carrying small is *not* usually a tip-off to IUGR—as

Lowering the Risks for the Baby at Risk

If there is any reason to believe that a baby may be less than perfectly healthy at birth, it is important to be sure that he or she comes into the world under the best of all possible conditions. In most cases, this means being delivered in a tertiary hospital, one that is equipped to handle the most serious of newborn emergencies. (Studies show that this is preferable to moving a sick baby after birth.) If yours is a high-risk pregnancy that puts your baby at serious risk, talk to your doctor about arranging to deliver in a tertiary medical center, and then make the necessary arrangements to get there when the time comes. Specially equipped ambulances or even helicopters may be available to transport you there in a hurry, if necessary.

Repeat Low-Birthweight Babies

A mother who has already had a low-birthweight baby has only a slightly increased risk of having another one—and to her advantage, statistics show that each subsequent baby is actually likely to be a bit heavier than the preceding one. Whether or not her subsequent babies will be small depends to a great extent on the reason her first baby was small and whether or not the same factor, or factors, exists the next time she conceives (see page 354).

Whether or not the cause of her previous baby's IUGR is known, the woman who is planning to become pregnant or who has already become pregnant again should pay extra attention to all the factors that can reduce the risk this time around; see page 50.

carrying large, or having gained a lot of weight, is not necessarily a sign that the baby is big. In most cases there are no outward symptoms that might alert a mother to the problem. The practitioner may, after measuring the abdomen with a tape measure, suspect that the uterus or fetus is small for date. The diagnosis can be confirmed, or ruled out, with an ultrasound examination.

Treatment. In some instances, the factors that might lead to a baby failing to thrive in the uterus are easily identifiable and, once identified, can be modified or eliminated. These include inadequate prenatal care (finding a practitioner early and seeing him or her regularly can reduce risk considerably); poor diet and/or inadequate weight gain (a well-balanced pregnancy diet, such as the Best-Odds Diet on page 80, can help remedy both these problems); cigarette smoking (the sooner a mother quits, the better her baby's chances of coming into the world at a fighting weight); alcohol or other substance abuse (professional help may be needed for some women to deal with these problems before they affect their babies).

Certain maternal factors that contribute to poor fetal growth can't be eliminated, but they can be controlled to minimize any threat to a baby's growth. These factors include chronic illness (diabetes, high blood pressure, lung or kidney disease); illnesses related to pregnancy (anemia, preeclampsia); and acute illnesses not related to pregnancy (urinary tract infections). To learn how these are treated in pregnancy, see the specific conditions.

For intervention to be effective, some other risk factors must be altered before pregnancy begins. These include significantly low maternal weight (putting on some weight and improving nutritional status before conceiving again can help); susceptibility to rubella (immunization eliminates the risk); inadequate spacing between pregnancies (less than six months between the end of one pregnancy and the beginning of the next may shortchange the next baby, although excellent nutrition, lots of rest, and top-notch medical care will go a long way toward improving uterine conditions if such a pregnancy has already begun); a malformed uterus or other problems with reproductive or urinary organs (surgery or other therapy may remedy these); exposures to toxic substances or environments, including occupational hazards (see page 72).

` Some factors that make a woman somewhat more likely to have a baby who does not grow well are difficult or impossible to alter. These include being poor, uneducated, and/or unmarried (probably because circumstances make it less likely that a woman will receive optimum nourishment and prenatal care); DES exposure before birth (page 40); living at a high altitude (though risk is only very slightly increased); having had a previous low-birthweight baby, a baby who has a birth defect, or multiple miscarriages; carrying twins, triplets, or more; having first- or second-trimester bleeding, placental problems (such as placenta previa or abruptio placenta), or very severe nausea and vomiting that continues after the third month; having too much or too little amniotic fluid, abnormal hemoglobin, or premature rupture of the membranes; or Rh isoimmunization (see page 33). Having been small at birth yourself also puts you at an increased risk of having a small baby. But in almost every instance, optimum nutrition and the elimination of any other existing risk factors can improve the chances for normal fetal growth.

Since most babies who are delivered early are small (though they may be an appropriate size for their gestational age and don't necessarily suffer from IUGR), altering the factors that lead to premature labor and halting premature labor when it begins or is anticipated (see page 218) can have a major impact on the risk of having a low-birthweight baby.

Recent research has turned up a variety of additional factors that may be involved in producing a too-small baby. These include stress (physical, including fatigue, and possibly psychological); inadequate increase in the mother's blood plasma volume; and progesterone deficiency.

When preventive measures fail and

IUGR is diagnosed, a variety of approaches may be tried to deal with the problem, depending on the suspected cause. Among the procedures that may be beneficial are bed rest in the hospital, especially if the home environment is less than ideal; improved nutrition, with an emphasis on protein, calories, and iron, and intravenous feedings if necessary; medications to improve placental blood flow or to correct a diagnosed problem that may be contributing to the IUGR; and finally, prompt delivery of the fetus if the intrauterine environment is very poor and can't be improved.

Even when prevention and treatment are unsuccessful and a baby is born smaller than normal, chances of survival and even excellent health are increasingly good thanks to the miracles of modern medicine. And low-birthweight babies often eventually catch up in both growth and development to their higher-birthweight peers.

PLACENTA PREVIA

What Is It? Placenta previa sounds like a disease of the placenta, but it isn't that at all. It refers to the position of the placenta, not its condition. In placenta previa, the placenta is attached in the lower half of the uterus, covering, partially covering, or touching the edge of the os, or mouth of the uterus. In early pregnancy a low-lying placenta is fairly common; but as pregnancy progresses and the uterus grows, the placenta in most cases moves upward.[5] Even when it doesn't move up, it is unlikely to cause a serious problem unless it actually touches

---

5. Even low-lying placentas diagnosed fairly late in pregnancy may occasionally continue to move upward, allowing for a normal delivery at term.

the cervical os. In the small percentage of cases in which it does touch the os, it can cause problems late in pregnancy and at delivery. The closer to the os the placenta is situated, the greater the possibility of hemorrhage. When the placenta blocks the cervix partially or completely, vaginal delivery is usually impossible.

The risk of having placenta previa is higher in women who have scarring of the uterine wall from previous pregnancies, cesareans, uterine surgery, or D and Cs following miscarriage. The need for greater placental surface area due to an increased need for oxygen or nutrients on behalf of the fetus (because of smoking, living at a high altitude, or carrying more than one fetus) may also increase the risk of placenta previa.

Signs and Symptoms. Painless bleeding as the placenta pulls away from the stretching lower portion of the uterus, occasionally before the 28th week but most often between the 34th and 38th, is the most common sign of placenta previa, though an estimated 7% to 30% of women with low-lying placentas don't bleed at all before delivery. The bleeding is usually bright red, not associated with significant abdominal pain or tenderness, and spontaneous in onset, though it can also be triggered by coughing, straining, or sexual intercourse. It can be light or heavy, and often stops, only to recur later. Because the placenta is blocking their way, fetuses with low-lying placentas do not usually "drop" into the pelvis in preparation for delivery.

In women who have no symptoms, the condition may be discovered during a routine ultrasound exam or may not be found until delivery.

When bleeding is present and placenta previa suspected, diagnosis is usually made by ultrasound.

Treatment. Because most early cases of low-lying placenta correct themselves long before delivery (see page 187) and never cause a problem, the condition doesn't require treatment before the 20th week. After that time, when there are no symptoms, the woman with a diagnosed placenta previa may be put on a modified activity schedule with increased bed rest. When there is bleeding, hospitalization is imperative in order to evaluate the condition of mother and baby, and if necessary to try to stabilize them. If the bleeding stops or is very light, conservative treatment is usually recommended. This consists of hospitalization, including bed rest with bathroom privileges, careful monitoring, supplementation with iron and possibly vitamin C, and transfusions as needed until the fetus is mature enough for delivery. A high-fiber diet with stool softeners may be prescribed to reduce the need to strain at the toilet. Occasionally a mother who has had no bleeding for a week, has easy access to the hospital (within 15 minutes' travel time), can be relied upon to stay in bed, and can find an adult who can be with her 24 hours a day (and if necessary drive her to the hospital in a hurry) may be allowed to go home and follow a similar restricted regimen.

The goal is to try to keep the pregnancy going until at least 36 weeks. At that point, if testing finds the lungs mature, the baby may be delivered by cesarean to reduce the risk of massive hemorrhage. Of course, if before that time the mother and/or her baby is endangered by the bleeding, delivery will be postponed no longer, even if this means the baby will be premature. Thanks to the skill and caring of topnotch neonatal intensive care units, most of these babies will do much better connected to lifesaving equipment in the NICU than connected to a bleeding placenta in the uterus.

Roughly 3 in 4 women with diagnosed placenta previa will be delivered by cesarean section before labor starts. If the condition isn't discovered until labor has begun, bleeding is mild, and the placenta is not blocking the cervix, vaginal delivery may be attempted. In either case, results are usually good; though placenta previa once posed a very serious threat, nearly 99% of mothers today come through it okay, as do almost as many of their babies.

PLACENTA ACCRETA

What Is It? Occasionally the placenta grows into the deeper layers of the uterine wall and becomes firmly attached. Depending on how deeply the placental cells invade, the condition may also be called placenta percreta or placenta increta. This condition is most common in women who have scarring of the uterine wall from previous surgeries or deliveries and especially in those with placenta previa or a prior cesarean.

Signs and Symptoms. During the third stage of childbirth, the placenta will not separate from the uterine wall.

Treatment. In most cases the placenta must be removed surgically to stop the bleeding. When the bleeding cannot be controlled by tying off the exposed blood vessels, removal of the entire uterus may be necessary.

ABRUPTIO PLACENTA

What Is It? This condition, in which the placenta separates, or abrupts, from the uterus prematurely, is responsible for roughly 1 in 4 cases of late-pregnancy bleeding. It is more common in older mothers who have had babies before, and in those who

smoke, have hypertension (chronic or pregnancy-induced), have been taking aspirin late in pregnancy, or have had a previous premature separation of the placenta. A short umbilical cord or trauma due to an accident[6] is occasionally the cause of an abruption.

Signs and Symptoms. When the separation is small, bleeding may be as light as a light menstrual flow or as heavy as a heavy one, and may or may not contain clots. There may also be cramping or a mild ache in the abdomen, and uterine tenderness. Occasionally, particularly when there has been trauma to the abdomen, there may be no bleeding at all.

With a moderate separation, bleeding is heavier, the abdomen is tender and firm, and abdominal pain may be more severe, stemming in part from strong uterine contractions. Both mother and baby may show signs of blood loss.

When more than half the placenta separates from the uterine wall, an emergency situation exists for both mother and baby. The symptoms are similar to those for a moderate separation, but more extreme.

The diagnosis is made using patient history, physical examination, and observation of uterine contractions and the fetal response to them. Ultrasound is helpful, but only about half of abruptions can actually be seen on ultrasound.

Treatment. When the separation is small, bed rest often stops the bleed-

---

6. If you sustain an injury and have any signs of abruption, call your doctor immediately. If you have no such signs, do a test for fetal movement after the accident (page 202). Repeat the test after several hours, and again two or three times during the next two days. Signs of abruption and fetal distress may not show up for 24 to 48 hours.

ing and the mother can usually resume her normal routine, with some restriction on activity, a few days later. Though it's not usual, there is the possibility of a repeat bleeding episode or even of a hemorrhage, so close medical supervision for the rest of the pregnancy is necessary. If signs of trouble recur and the baby is near term, delivery may be carried out.

In most cases, a moderate separation also responds to bed rest. But often transfusions and other emergency treatment may also be needed. Careful monitoring of both mother and baby is necessary, and if either shows signs of distress, delivery without delay may be essential.

When the separation is severe, prompt medical action, including transfusions and immediate delivery, is imperative.

At one time the outlook was bleak for both mothers and their babies when a placenta separated prematurely. Today, with expert and prompt medical care, virtually all the mothers with placental abruption and better than 90% of their babies will survive the crisis.

PREMATURE RUPTURE OF THE MEMBRANES (PROM)

What Is It? PROM refers to the rupture of the chorionic membranes, or "bag of waters," before contractions begin. This can happen just hours before the baby is due, or weeks or even months earlier. Why one woman's membranes spontaneously rupture early and another's don't rupture even during labor, and have to be ruptured artificially, isn't clear. There is speculation, however, that the enzyme collagenase, produced by certain bacteria, plays a role by reducing the strength and elasticity of the membranes surrounding the fetus.

Signs and Symptoms. Leaking or gushing of fluid from the vagina; the flow is heavier when the woman is lying down. The practitioner's check of the vagina reveals fluid that is alkaline (rather than acid, as would be the case with urine) coming from the cervix.

Treatment. Most doctors agree that initially, for anywhere from a few hours to a full day, the expectant mother whose membranes rupture prematurely should be closely observed, and that during that time the baby's condition should be evaluated and the mother monitored for contractions and the possibility of infection. During the initial evaluation, the mother is ordinarily admitted to the hospital for bed rest and careful monitoring of her condition and the baby's. Her temperature and white blood count will be checked periodically so that doctors can take action immediately should infection develop, which can lead to premature delivery. A culture from the cervix may be also taken to check for infection, and in some cases intravenous antibiotics will be given even before the results of the culture are in to prevent any infection from moving into the now open amniotic sac. If contractions begin and the fetus is believed to be immature, medication may be given to try to halt them. As long as both mother and baby are all right, this conservative course may be continued until the baby is deemed mature enough for safe delivery. If at any point mother or baby is thought to be in danger, delivery will be carried out promptly. Rarely the break in the membranes heals and the leakage of amniotic fluid stops on its own. If that happens, the mother may be allowed to go home and resume her normal routine while remaining on the alert for signs of further leakage.

Most doctors will try to delay delivery until 33 or 34 weeks of pregnancy.

At that point some will induce labor; others will continue to try to postpone delivery until 37 weeks. (To help them decide whether or not to induce labor, some will perform amniocentesis or check the amniotic fluid in the vagina to determine the maturity of the baby's lungs.) If PROM occurs at 37 weeks or later most physicians will induce, since at this point the negligible risk to the fetus is far outweighed by the risk of infection that comes with a delay of as little as 24 to 36 hours.

With good care, both mother and baby should be fine, though if the baby is premature a long stay in the NICU and other problems may complicate the picture.

CORD PROLAPSE

What Is It? The umbilical cord is a baby's lifeline in the uterus. Occasionally, when the amniotic membranes rupture, the cord slips, or prolapses, through the cervix or even well into the vaginal canal, carried by the rush of amniotic fluid. It then becomes vulnerable to compression by the baby's presenting part as it presses through the cervix and down the canal during delivery. If the cord does become compressed, the vital supply of oxygen to the fetus can be reduced or even cut off. Prolapse is most common in premature labors (because the presenting part of the fetus is so small it doesn't completely fill the pelvis) or when a part other than the head, especially a foot, presents first (because a foot, for example, takes up less space than a head, allowing the cord to slip down). Prolapse is also more common when the membranes rupture before labor begins, rather than after.

Signs and Symptoms. An umbilical cord can prolapse so far that it may be seen hanging from the vagina, or it may just be felt as "something in there." If it becomes compressed, any distress is likely to be evident on the fetal monitor or other tests of fetal well-being.

Treatment. If you should actually see or feel your baby's umbilical cord in your vagina, or you suspect it might have prolapsed, get on your hands and knees to reduce pressure on the cord. If the cord protrudes, support it gently (don't press or squeeze) with warm wet gauze pads or a clean towel or diaper. Have someone rush you to the hospital, or call 911 or your local emergency number. Prompt treatment is vital.

At the hospital, a saline solution may be injected into your bladder to cushion the cord; a cord that is outside the vagina may be tucked back in and held in place by a special sterile tampon; and drugs may be given to stop labor while you are readied for an emergency cesarean section.

VENOUS THROMBOSIS

What Is It? A blood clot that develops in a vein. Women are more susceptible to clots during pregnancy, delivery, and particularly in the postpartum period. This happens because nature, worried about too much bleeding at childbirth, tends to increase the blood's clotting ability—occasionally too much—and because the enlarged uterus makes it difficult for blood in the lower body to return to the heart. Clots in superficial veins (thrombophlebitis) occur in about 1 or 2 in every 100 pregnancies. Deep vein thrombosis, which if untreated can result in the clot moving to the lungs and threatening the patient's life, is fortunately much less common. Women who are at a somewhat increased risk of developing clots are those who have had previous clots;

are over 30; have had three or more previous deliveries; have been confined to bed for long periods; are overweight, anemic, or have varicose veins; or have undergone mid-forceps or cesarean delivery.

Signs and Symptoms. In superficial thrombophlebitis there is usually a tender, reddened area that runs in a line over a vein that is near the surface in the thigh or calf. In deep vein thrombosis, the leg may feel heavy or painful, there may be tenderness in the calf or thigh, swelling (ranging from slight to severe), distention of the superficial veins, and calf pain on flexing the foot (turning the toes up toward the chin). Ultrasound or other methods may be used to diagnose the blood clot. Any such symptoms, as well as any other unusual leg symptoms, unexplained fever, or speeded up heartbeat should be reported to the practitioner. If the blood clot (embolus) has moved to the lungs, there may be chest pain, coughing with frothy, blood-stained sputum, speeded up heartbeat and breathing rate, blueness of lips and fingertips, and fever. These symptoms require immediate medical attention.

Treatment. The best treatment is prevention: wear support hose if you are prone to blood clots; avoid sitting for more than an hour or so without walking about and stretching your legs; exercise your legs if you are confined to bed; and don't sleep or exercise while lying flat on your back. Once diagnosed, treatment will depend on the degree and type of clot. A superficial thrombus will be treated with rest, leg elevation, local ointments, moist heat, an elastic compression stocking, and possibly, postpartum, with aspirin. With deep vein thrombosis, an anticoagulant drug (almost always heparin) is given, usually

intravenously for a week or 10 days, then under the skin until labor starts, at which point the drug is discontinued. Several hours after delivery it is resumed once more, and continued for the first few weeks postpartum. With a pulmonary embolus, drugs and surgery may be needed, as well as treatment for any accompanying side effects.

PRETERM OR PREMATURE LABOR

What Is It? Labor that begins after the age of viability (20 weeks in most states) and before the 37th week (when the baby is considered full term). There are a wide range of risk factors associated with preterm labor (see page 218), but what causes labor to begin early is not fully understood at present.

Signs and Symptoms. Menstrual-like cramps, with or without diarrhea, nausea, or indigestion; lower back pain or pressure; an achiness or pressure in the pelvis, thighs, or groin; a watery or pinkish or brownish discharge possibly preceded by the passage of a thick, gelatinous mucus plug; and/or a trickle or flow of amniotic fluid from the vagina.

Treatment. Prompt medical attention to the above symptoms is important since treatment (see below) can occasionally halt or postpone premature labor, and each day a baby remains in the uterus the better its chances of survival. Only when the mother and/or child are endangered is no attempt made to postpone early delivery.

Postponement or prevention of the

onset of premature labor can often be achieved through limitations on sexual intercourse and other physical activities, bed rest, and if necessary hospitalization. In about half the cases of women who have early strong contractions but no bleeding and a single live fetus, hospitalized bed rest alone, without medication, will check contractions. If the membranes are also intact and the cervix has not effaced or dilated, 3 out of 4 of these women will carry to term. Tocolytic agents (drugs that relax the uterus and have the potential to halt contractions) may be administered to improve these odds, but new research has raised questions about their safety and effectiveness. If infection is thought to have triggered labor, antibiotics may also be given. When early delivery is imminent, corticosteroids (but not with TRH) can help speed maturation of the fetus and reduce complications. Magnesium sulfate may be given to help prevent cerebral palsy in the newborn.

CONDITIONS THAT MAY CAUSE CONCERN DURING CHILDBIRTH

UTERINE INVERSION

What Is It? Rarely, the placenta doesn't detach completely after delivery of a baby and when it emerges, it pulls the top, or fundus, of the uterus with it—in effect very much like pulling a sock inside out.

Signs and Symptoms. Symptoms of uterine inversion include excessive bleeding and sometimes signs of shock in the mother. The practitioner, pressing down on the abdomen, will not be able to feel the uterus, and in a complete inversion, part of it will be visible in the vagina. Women at slightly higher risk for an inverted uterus (though the risk is still extremely small) are those who have had many prior births or a prolonged labor (over 24 hours); those who have the placenta implanted across the top (fundus) of the uterus or abnormally attached to it; and those who were given magnesium sulfate during labor. The uterus may also invert if it is overly relaxed or if the fundus isn't held in place while the placenta is coaxed out in the third stage of childbirth.

Treatment. In most cases the uterus can be replaced by hand, though sometimes other techniques are used. Intravenous fluid and blood transfusions may be needed if blood loss has been great. Drugs (such as magnesium sulfate) may be given to relax the uterus even further in order to facilitate the replacement. If fragments of placenta remain in the uterus, they may be removed before or after the uterus is replaced. In very rare cases, the uterus can't be replaced manually and abdominal surgery is necessary.

After replacement, pressure will usually be kept on the abdomen to keep the uterus in place, and oxytocin or other drugs given to firm it so it won't reinvert. Antibiotics may be given to prevent infection.

Since a woman who has had one uterine inversion is at an increased risk for another, your practitioner should be informed if you've had an inversion in the past.

UTERINE RUPTURE

What Is It? Rarely, the uterus ruptures or tears during pregnancy or labor (most often during labor). A scar in the uterine wall is the largest single cause of rupture. The scar may be the result of a prior cesarean section with a classic vertical incision; a repaired uterine rupture; uterine surgery (to correct its shape or remove fibroids); or previous uterine perforation. Extremely violent contractions (spontaneous or induced) can also lead to rupture; but this is rare, particularly in a first pregnancy, without a predisposing scar. Rupture is more common in women who have already had five or more children, have a very distended uterus (because of multiple fetuses or excess amniotic fluid), have had difficult labor previously, or are experiencing difficulties in their present delivery (particularly shoulder dystocia, see below, or midforceps delivery). Abnormalities related to the placenta (such as a placenta that separates prematurely or that is attached deeply in the uterine wall) or to fetal position (such as a fetus lying crosswise), as well as severe trauma to the abdomen (as from a knife or a bullet), can increase the risk of uterine rupture.

Signs and Symptoms. Uterine rupture is not a complication that the average pregnant woman need be concerned about. But women who are at increased risk of rupture, because of a scarred uterus or any of the other factors above, should know the possible warning signs, just in case: severe abdominal pain, fainting, hyperventilation (deep, fast breathing), rapid heartbeat, restlessness, and agitation. If you experience such symptoms, which are more severe when the rupture is in the upper half of the uterus, seek immediate emergency medical attention. The first sign of actual rupture is usually a searing pain in the abdomen, accompanied by a feeling that something inside is "ripping." This is generally followed by a brief

period of relief, then diffuse abdominal pain and tenderness. Unless the rupture is in the lower segment of the uterus, contractions will generally cease. There may or may not be vaginal bleeding. The fetus will be more easily felt through the abdomen and may show signs of distress.

Treatment. Immediate surgical delivery is necessary, followed by repair of the uterus, is possible. If damage is extensive, a hysterectomy may be required. Sometimes a rupture isn't recognized until hemorrhaging occurs after delivery. Again, the uterus may be repaired or removed.

After a rupture, the mother is closely monitored to be sure complications don't occur, and antibiotics may be given to prevent infection. Depending on the situation, she may be allowed out of bed in as few as six hours or not for several days.

SHOULDER DYSTOCIA

What Is It? Dystocia is labor that doesn't progress; in shoulder dystocia labor doesn't progress because the baby's shoulders become stuck on their way through the birth canal after the head has been delivered.

Signs and Symptoms. Delivery stalls after the head emerges and before the shoulders are out. This can occur unexpectedly in a labor that to that point seemed absolutely normal.

Treatment. A variety of approaches may be used to rescue the baby whose shoulder is impacted in the pelvis, including performing an extra-large episiotomy; trying to rotate the baby and maneuver the back shoulder out first; hyperflexing the mother's knees up on her abdomen; applying moderate pressure to the top of the uterus

First Aid for the Fetus

In late pregnancy, absence of fetal activity could be a sign that something is wrong (for a home test, see page 202). Since diminishing activity (generally judged to mean fewer than ten movements in a two-hour period) is often noted before the fetus actually succumbs, it should be reported immediately to your practitioner. If he or she is not available, have someone take you to the emergency room or the labor and delivery area of your local hospital immediately. With prompt action it is sometimes possible to resuscitate the fetus.

and the pelvis; attempting various other maneuvers to force the shoulders out, including breaking the baby's collarbone. If possible (and rarely is it so), it may be preferable to tuck the baby's head back into the vagina and perform a cesarean section.

FETAL DISTRESS

What Is It? The term is used to describe a situation in which the fetus is believed to be in jeopardy, most often because of decreased oxygen flow. The distress may be caused by a variety of problems, including the mother's position putting pressure on major blood vessels; maternal illness (anemia, hypertension, heart disease), abnormally low blood pressure, or shock; placental insufficiency, degeneration, or premature separation; cord compression; prolonged or excessive uterine activity; or fetal infection, malformation, hemorrhage, or anemia.

Signs and Symptoms. The precise signals sent by the fetus vary with the cause of the distress. The mother may notice a change in fetal movement patterns or an absence of movement. The practitioner can pick up heartbeat changes typical of fetal distress with a Doppler stethoscope or on the fetal monitor.

Treatment. When fetal distress is confirmed (see page 280), immediate delivery is usually indicated. If vaginal delivery is not imminent, then an emergency cesarean is usually performed. In some cases the physician may elect to resuscitate the baby in the uterus before doing a cesarean delivery, to decrease the risk that it will suffer from oxygen deprivation. This is usually done by giving the mother medication to slow contractions, which will increase oxygen to the fetus; to dilate the mother's blood vessels and raise her heart rate, which will also enhance blood flow.

VAGINAL AND CERVICAL LACERATIONS

What Are They? Tears in the vagina and/or cervix, which can range from minor to extensive. These occur only occasionally during labor and delivery.

Signs and Symptoms. Excessive bleeding may be the most obvious symptom, though the lacerations may also be evident to the practitioner after the delivery.

Treatment. Generally, all lacerations that are longer than 2 centimeters or that continue to bleed heavily are sutured (stitched). A local anesthetic may be given first, if one wasn't administered during delivery.

POSTPARTUM HEMORRHAGE

What Is It? Postpartum hemorrhage, or heavy bleeding that is difficult to stem, is a very serious but uncommon complication. When treated promptly, it is rarely the life-threatening situation it once was. Excessive bleeding may occur if the uterus is too relaxed and doesn't contract because of a long, exhausting labor; a traumatic delivery; a uterus that was overdistended because of multiple births, a large baby, or excess amniotic fluid; an oddly shaped placenta, or one that separated prematurely; fibroids that prevent symmetrical contraction of the uterus; or a generally weakened condition of the mother at the time of delivery (due to, for example, anemia, preeclampsia, or extreme fatigue).

Excessive bleeding, or hemorrhage, can occur immediately postpartum because of unrepaired lacerations to the uterus, cervix, vagina, or somewhere else in the pelvis or because the uterus has ruptured or inverted (been turned inside out). It can occur up to a week or two after delivery when fragments of the placenta are retained in, or adhere to, the uterus. Infection can also cause postpartum hemorrhage, right after delivery or weeks later. Postpartum hemorrhage occurs more frequently in women who had placenta previa or abruptio placenta prior to delivery. Rarely, the cause of the hemorrhage is a previously undiagnosed bleeding disorder in the mother that is genetic or is caused by the use of aspirin or other drugs that can interfere with blood clotting.

Signs and Symptoms. Abnormal bleeding after delivery: bleeding that saturates more than one pad an hour for more than a few hours or is bright red any time after the fourth postpartum day, especially if it doesn't slow down when you do; a foul smell to your lochia; large blood clots (lemon-size or larger); pain and/or swelling in the lower abdominal area beyond the first few days after delivery.

Treatment. Depending on the cause of the hemorrhage, the physician may try one or more of the following to stem the bleeding: uterine massage to encourage the uterus to contract; the administration of drugs (such as oxytocin, ergometrine, or prostaglandins) to promote the contraction of the uterus; search for and repair of any lacerations; removal of any retained placental fragments. If bleeding isn't quickly arrested, further measures will be taken: intravenous fluids and, if necessary, transfusion; the administration of blood-clotting agents if failure of the blood to coagulate is the problem, and of antibiotics to prevent infection. Rarely, packing of the uterus with gauze to stem bleeding for 6 to 24 hours or the ligation, or tying off, of the major artery in the uterus will be needed. When all attempts to stop the bleeding fail, the removal of the uterus is necessary.

The odds are very good that treatment of postpartum hemorrhage will be successful, and that the new mother will recover quickly.

POSTPARTUM INFECTION

What Is It? An infection related to childbirth, rare in women who are receiving good medical care and have had an uncomplicated vaginal delivery. The most common postpartum infection is endometritis, infection of the endometrium (lining) of the uterus, which is vulnerable after the detachment of the placenta. Endometritis is more likely to occur after a cesarean section that followed a prolonged labor or early rupture of the membranes. It is also more likely to occur if a fragment of the placenta has been retained in the uterus. Also possible is an infection of a laceration to the cervix, vagina, or vulva.

Signs and Symptoms. These vary according to the site of origin. A slight fever, vague lower abdominal pain, and sometimes a foul-smelling vaginal discharge characterize an infection of the endometrium. With infection of a laceration, there will usually be pain and tenderness in the area; sometimes a foul-smelling, thick discharge; abdominal or side pain; or difficult urination. In certain types of infection, the fever spikes as high as 105 degrees and there are chills, headache, malaise. On occasion, there are no obvious symptoms but fever. Any fever postpartum should be reported to your doctor.

Treatment. Treatment with antibiotics is very effective, but it should begin quickly. A culture may be taken to determine the causative organism so that the right antibiotic can be prescribed.

COPING WITH PREGNANCY LOSS

Demise in the Uterus. When you don't hear from your baby for several hours or more, it's natural to fear the worst. And the worst is, of course, that your unborn baby has died. Fortunately, that's rarely the case. But when it does happen, it can be devastating.

You are likely to be in a fog of disbelief and grief after being told that your baby's heartbeat can't be located and that it has died in the uterus. It may be difficult or even impossible for you to carry on with your normal life while carrying around a fetus that is no longer living, and studies show that a woman is much more likely to suffer severe depression after the delivery of a stillborn if the delivery is delayed more than three days after the death is diagnosed. For this reason, your mental state will be taken into account while doctors decide what to do next. If labor is imminent, or has already started, your stillborn baby will probably be delivered normally. If labor isn't clearly about to start, the decision whether or not to induce it immediately, or to allow you to return home until it begins spontaneously, will depend on how far you are from your due date, and on your physical as well as your mental state.

The grieving process you will go through if your fetus has died in utero will probably be very similar to that of parents whose baby has died during or after birth (see below), although sometimes holding the fetus or having a funeral may not be possible or practical.

Death During or After Birth. Sometimes the death occurs during labor or delivery, sometimes just after delivery. Either way, your world comes crashing down. You've waited for this baby for nearly nine months. You've dreamed about it, felt it kick and hiccup, heard its heartbeat. You've picked out a crib, ordered a tiny layette, prepared your friends, family, and life for the new arrival—and now you're going home empty-handed.

There's probably no greater pain

than that inflicted by the loss of a child. And though nothing can banish the hurt you're feeling, there are steps you can take now to make the future more bearable, and to lessen the inevitable depression that follows such a tragedy.

❖ See your baby, hold your baby, name your baby. Grieving is a vital step in accepting and recovering from your loss, but you can't grieve for a nameless child you've never seen. Even if your child is malformed, experts advise that it is better to see him or her than not to, because what is imagined is usually worse than the reality. Holding and naming your baby will make the death more real to you, and ultimately easier to deal with. So will arranging for a funeral and burial, which will also give you another opportunity to say goodbye. And the grave will provide a permanent site where you can visit your baby in future years.

❖ Discuss autopsy findings and other details with the doctor to harden the reality of what happened and to aid you in the grieving process. You may have been given a lot of details in the delivery room, but medications, your hormonal status, and the shock you felt probably prevented you from fully understanding them.

❖ If possible, ask not to be sedated in the hours after you hear the news. Though it will ease your pain momentarily, sedation will tend to blur your recollections and the reality of what happened. This makes it harder to get on with your grieving, as well as depriving you and your spouse of the chance to support each other.

❖ Save a photo (many hospitals take them) or other mementos, so that you'll have some tangible reminders to cherish when you think about your lost baby in the future. As morbid as this may sound, experts say it helps. Try to focus on positive attributes—big eyes and long lashes, beautiful hands and delicate fingers, a headful of hair.

❖ Ask friends or relatives not to remove all vestiges of the preparations you made for baby at home. Tell them you will do it yourself. As well-meaning as their gestures might be, coming home to a house that looks as though a baby was never expected will only add to any tendency to deny what has happened.

❖ Cry—for as long and as often as you feel you need to. Crying is part of the mourning process. If you don't cry now, it will remain unfinished business that you may find you have to attend to later.

❖ Expect a difficult time. For a while you may feel depressed, empty; experience intense sadness; have trouble sleeping; fight with your husband and neglect your other children; even imagine you hear your baby crying in the middle of the night. You will probably feel the need to be a child yourself, to be loved, coddled, and cared for. All this is normal.

❖ Recognize that fathers grieve too, but that their grief may in some cases be or appear to be shorter-lived and/or less intense, partly because, unlike mothers, they haven't carried their baby inside them for so many months. And they often have different ways of dealing with their distress. They may, for example, try to bottle it up, to be strong for their wives. But then the pain often comes out in other ways: bad temper, irresponsibility, loss of interest in life—or they may use alcohol in an attempt to feel better.

Unfortunately, a grieving father may not be much help to his wife, nor she to him, and both may need to seek support elsewhere.

❖ **Don't face the world alone.** If you're putting off getting back into circulation because you dread the friendly faces asking, "Oh, what did you have?" take a friend who can field the questions for you on the first several trips to the supermarket, bank, and so on. Be sure that those at work, at church or synagogue, at other organizations in which you're active, are informed before you return so you don't have to do any difficult explaining.

❖ Expect that some friends and family may not know how to respond, and may withdraw for a while. Others, in trying to help, may make thoughtless statements like "I know just how you feel," or "Oh, you can have another baby," or "It's a good thing the baby died before you became attached to it." They don't understand that no one who hasn't lost a baby can know how it feels, that another baby can never take the place of the one you lost, or that parents can become attached to a baby long before birth, sometimes even before conception. If you are hearing such comments frequently, ask a close friend or

When Multiple Fetuses Aren't Thriving

Twins, triplets, and quadruplets, not surprisingly, are more prone to poor fetal growth than singletons, especially in the third trimester. That's why multiple gestations are followed very closely with series of ultrasound checks from the 20th week on. If one or more fetuses are growing poorly, intensive surveillance, usually in the hospital, is needed. The babies will be delivered promptly either when it is determined that the lungs of the larger (or largest) fetus are mature or when it becomes risky for the smaller fetus to continue to remain in the uterus. Fortunately, such circumstances arise very infrequently.*

Nature often attends to such situations on her own. It's believed that

*If you are carrying more than one fetus, be sure to follow the Best-Odds Diet faithfully, with the additions for multiple pregnancies recommended on page 145. This will improve the odds that all your fetuses will thrive.

each year thousands more multiple births are conceived than are born. Early in these pregnancies, because the mother's body is unable to support so many fetuses, generally all but one die, often leaving no visible evidence that they ever existed. Sometimes, however, the multiple fetuses continue to struggle on together, all of them suffering, none of them doing well enough to survive. Then, since Mother Nature hasn't taken the initiative, it may be necessary for medical science to take over and salvage one or two rather then letting them all perish.

Usually there is no way a mother can tell that one or more of the fetuses she is carrying is not doing well. But her physician, using ultrasound and other sophisticated diagnostic techniques, can generally assess the condition of the unborn children.

When it's determined that multiple fetuses aren't doing well, and it is too early to deliver them safely, the medical solution is usually to recommend removing one or more of the fetuses (usually those doing least well) from

relative to explain your feelings and to indicate that you would rather that people just say they are sorry about your loss.

❖ Expect your pain to lessen over time. At first there will be only bad days, then a few good days among them; eventually there will be more good days than bad. But be prepared for the possibility that the pain will never go away entirely. The grieving process, with nightmares and intrusive recollections, is often not fully completed for as long as two years, but the worst is usually over in three to six months after the loss. If after six to nine months your grief remains the center of your universe, if you lose interest in everything else and can't seem to function, seek help. Seek help, too, if from the beginning you haven't been able to grieve at all.

❖ Seek support. Like many other parents, you may derive strength from joining a self-help group for parents who have lost infants. But beware of letting such a group become a way of sustaining your rage or grief. If after a year you're still having problems coming to terms with your loss (sooner, if you're having trouble functioning), you should seek individual therapy.

---

the uterus so that the remaining fetus or fetuses have a better chance of surviving. This procedure may also be recommended if one of the fetuses is seriously malformed (lacking part or all of the brain, for example).

Some physicians reserve such pregnancy reduction for situations where there are four or more fetuses; others will reduce triplets as well, when it seems appropriate. Some researchers suggest that since up until the end of the first trimester nature may still spontaneously reduce the number of fetuses, the best time to consider a reduction is at the end of this time.

If pregnancy reduction is suggested, the expectant parents are faced with the difficult task of deciding whether or not to let the doctors go ahead with this procedure. Before they make their decision, they should get a second opinion to be sure that the evaluation of the tests on their fetuses is accurate. Then they should discuss the risk that all the fetuses may be lost as a result of the procedure with their physician. This risk is lower, of course, when the surgeon has had a great deal of experience and success with the procedure.

Finally, if religion plays an important part in a couple's life, getting some advice from spiritual as well as medical advisors is a good idea. It will probably also be necessary to talk to a specialist in medical ethics (check with your local hospital), a genetic counselor, a maternal-fetal subspecialist, or another counselor familiar with this issue. In these discussions, they will probably find that most ethicists (even some Catholic theologians) believe that trying to save one baby is preferable to letting them all die. (On the other hand, many would question performing a reduction simply for the sake of convenience—because the family doesn't have room for four cribs, for example.) Reading "When a Serious Fetal Defect Is Detected" (page 349) and "Coping with Pregnancy Loss" (page 366) may be helpful.

Once a couple has made their decision, they should accept that it was the best one they could make. If it doesn't go as they'd hoped, they shouldn't blame themselves.

❖ Limit the use of tranquilizers and sedatives. Although they may seem helpful at first, they can interfere with the grieving process—and can also make you dependent on them.

❖ Turn to religion if you find it comforting. Some bereaved parents feel too angry with God to do this, but for many faith is a great solace.

❖ Don't expect that having another baby will resolve any unresolved grief. Do become pregnant again, if that's what you both want—first observing whatever waiting period the doctor recommends. But don't try to conceive in order to feel better, assuage guilt or anger, or gain peace of mind. It won't work, and it could put an unfair burden on

Loss of One Twin

The parent who loses one twin (or more babies, in the case of triplets or quads) has to face celebrating a birth and mourning a death at the same time. If you are in this position, you may feel too depressed to either mourn your lost child or enjoy your living one—both vitally important processes. Typically, the feeling is "I should be thrilled I have one baby, but I'm so upset, I can't take care of him." Understanding why you feel the way you do may help you to feel better:

❖ You've lost the excitement and prestige of being the parent of twins, a fantasy you may have been playing out for months since your multiple pregnancy was diagnosed. Even if you didn't know in advance about the twins, you may feel cheated. Don't feel guilty if you do; your disappointment is normal. Let yourself mourn this loss as well as the loss of your baby.

❖ You feel it will be difficult and embarrassing to explain that you only have one baby to friends and family who have been eagerly awaiting the twins with you. To ease this burden, enlist a friend or relative to spread the word. When you first go out of the house with the baby, take someone with you who can help explain the situation to people you may run into, if you don't feel up to it.

❖ You may feel inadequate as a woman or as a mother because you lost one of your babies, particularly if they were conceived through the use of fertility agents or IVF or GIFT (gamete intrafallopian transfer). Of course, what happened had nothing to do with your value as a woman or mother.

❖ You feel you are somehow being punished—because you really couldn't have taken care of two children, or because you wanted a boy more than a girl (or vice versa), or because you really didn't want twins. Though such guilt is common in parents who experience a pregnancy loss, it is completely unwarranted.

❖ You are concerned that as your surviving infant grows—at birthdays, the first step, the first "ma-ma" and "da-da"—you will be reminded of the lost child and of what could have been. And it's true that you will be. It will help if you and your spouse share your feelings with each other on these occasions, and not try to suppress them.

❖ You worry that your child, as he or she grows older, will be tormented by the loss. Though some surviving twins do seem to feel that someone is missing or appear lonelier than other children, your child should

any new arrival. Any decision about your future fertility—either to have another baby or to undergo sterilization—should be postponed until the period of deepest sorrow has passed.

❖ Recognize that guilt can compound grief and make adjusting to a loss more difficult. If you feel that the loss of your baby was your punishment for having been ambivalent about your pregnancy, or for lacking the nurturing or other qualities necessary for motherhood, seek professional support to help you understand that such feelings are in no way responsible for your loss. Seek help, too, if you feel insecure about your womanhood and now

not suffer because of the loss unless you make an issue of it. Providing lots of love and attention will help ensure a secure, happy youngster.

❖ In trying to help, friends and family may overdo the fanfare when welcoming your living child and maintain a polite silence on the topic of your dead one. Or they may tell you to forget the lost child and appreciate your living one. These insensitive attitudes can anger and upset you. Let people know that you need to grieve for the lost baby as well as rejoice in the live one.

❖ You haven't been allowed, or haven't allowed yourself, to grieve. But grieve you must, or you will never come to terms with your loss. Take the steps for grieving parents described on page 366, so that you can more easily accept your baby's death as a reality.

❖ You believe that to enjoy your surviving baby is somehow disloyal to your dead one. Shake this feeling, though it's a natural one. Loving the sibling that your lost baby spent all those months cuddled up with in your uterus is a way of honoring that child, certainly something he or she would have wanted. On the other hand, idealizing the dead baby and making the living one compete with this idealized image could be quite damaging. If you are uncomfortable about having a christening or a circumcision or other baby-welcoming event for the surviving baby, consider holding a memorial ceremony or farewell for the dead baby first or at the same time.

❖ You're experiencing postpartum depression. It's normal, whether you've lost a child or not, for hormones in chaos to make everything harder to deal with and feelings more conflicted. See page 398 for tips on dealing with postpartum depression.

❖ You're afraid that the loss you've experienced and your consequent depression will damage your relationship with your husband. This is very unlikely if you share feelings, both positive and negative, with each other. One study showed that fully 90% of parents who have gone through this experience have found that their marriage was strengthened by helping each other pull through the mourning period.

❖ You feel guilty that your ambivalence is making it difficult for you to care for your baby. Remind yourself that you have no reason to feel guilty about having feelings that are completely normal.

Give yourself some time. Chances are that you'll soon feel better and, if you let yourself, will be able to begin to truly enjoy your new baby.

Why?

The philosophical question "Why?" may never be answered.* But it is usually helpful to the grieving parents to attach some reality to the tragedy by learning about the physical causes of the death of a fetus or newborn. Often the baby looks perfectly normal, and the only way to uncover the cause of death is to carefully examine the history of the pregnancy and do a complete examination of the fetus or baby. If the fetus died in utero or was stillborn, histological examination of the placenta by a pathologist is also important. At first it may not seem that knowing the cause of death will make acceptance of the loss easier, but in the long run it will. Knowing what happened doesn't really tell you why it happened to you and your baby, but it puts a closure on the event, and it will help you prepare for a future pregnancy.

Of course sometimes it's impossible to determine what went wrong, and in that case the grieving couple have to accept the event in light of their own personal philosophy. They may look upon it as God's will, or as a random occurrence over which humans have no control. In any case, the loss of a baby should never be viewed as punishment.

---

*For help in thinking about this question, see *When Bad Things Happen to Good People* by Harold S. Kushner.

believe your doubts have been confirmed (you couldn't produce a live baby), or if you feel you have failed your family and friends. If you feel guilty even thinking about getting your life back to normal because you sense it would be disloyal to your dead baby, it may help to ask your baby, in spirit, for forgiveness or for permission to enjoy life again.

Part 4

LAST BUT NOT LEAST:

Postpartum, Fathers, and the Next Baby

18
Postpartum: The First Week

WHAT YOU MAY BE FEELING

During the first week postpartum, depending on the type of delivery you had (easy or difficult, vaginal or cesarean) and other individual factors, you may experience all, or only some, of the following:

PHYSICALLY:

❖ Bloody vaginal discharge (lochia), turning pinkish toward week's end

❖ Abdominal cramps (afterpains) as uterus contracts

❖ Exhaustion

❖ Perineal discomfort, pain, numbness, if you had a vaginal delivery, especially if you had stitches (pain is worse with sneezing and coughing)

❖ Incisional pain and, later, numbness in the area, if you had a cesarean (especially a first one)

❖ Discomfort sitting and walking if you had a repair of an episiotomy or tear or a cesarean

❖ Difficulty urinating for a day or two; difficulty and discomfort with bowel movements for the first few days; constipation

❖ General soreness, especially if pushing was difficult

❖ Bloodshot eyes; black-and-blue marks around eyes, cheeks, elsewhere, from vigorous pushing

❖ Sweating, possibly profuse, after the first couple of days

❖ Breast discomfort and engorgement about the third or fourth day postpartum

❖ Sore or cracked nipples, if you are breastfeeding

EMOTIONALLY:

❖ Elation, depression, or swings between the two

❖ Feelings of inadequacy and trepidation about mothering, especially if you're breastfeeding

❖ Frustration, if you're still in the hospital and would like to leave

❖ Little interest in sex or, less commonly, increased desire (intercourse won't be okayed until at least four weeks postpartum)

WHAT YOU MAY BE CONCERNED ABOUT

BLEEDING

"I'd been told to expect a bloody discharge after delivery, but when I got out of bed for the first time and saw the blood running down my legs, I was really frightened."

Don't be alarmed. This discharge of leftover blood, mucus, and tissue from your uterus, known as lochia, is normally as heavy as (sometimes even heavier than) a menstrual period for the first three postpartum days. And though it'll probably seem more copious than it really is, it may total up to two cups before it begins to taper off. A sudden gush on getting out of bed in the first few days is common, and no cause for concern. And since blood and an occasional blood clot are the predominant ingredients of lochia during the immediate postpartum period, your discharge will be quite red for two or three days, gradually turning to a watery pink, then to brown, and finally to a yellowish white over the next week or two. Sanitary napkins, not tampons, should be used to absorb the flow, which may continue on and off for as long as six weeks.

Breastfeeding and the intramuscular or intravenous administration of oxytocin (routinely ordered by some doctors following delivery) may reduce the flow of lochia by encouraging uterine contractions and helping to shrink the uterus back to normal size more quickly. The contraction of the uterus after delivery is important because it pinches off exposed blood vessels at the site where the placenta separated from the uterus, preventing hemorrhage. If the uterus is too relaxed and doesn't contract, excessive bleeding occurs. If while you are in the hospital, you notice any signs of postpartum hemorrhage listed on page 381 (some of which may also indicate infection), notify a nurse immediately. If any of these signs occur once you are home, call your practitioner immediately; if you can't reach him or her, go to the emergency room (at the hospital in which you delivered, if possible) immediately. To learn how postpartum hemorrhage is treated, see page 365.

YOUR POSTPARTUM CONDITION

"I look and feel as though I've been in a boxing ring rather than in a delivery room. How come?"

You probably worked harder birthing your child than most boxers work in the ring. So it isn't surprising that, thanks to powerful contractions and strenuous pushing during delivery, you look and feel as though you've gone several rounds. Many women do, particularly following a labor that was long and/or difficult. Not uncommon postpartum are:

❖ Black or bloodshot eyes (dark glasses will do a cover-up job in public until the eyes return to normal; and cold compresses for 10 minutes several times a day may hasten that return).

❖ Bruises, ranging from tiny dots on the cheek to larger hematomas, or black and blue marks, on the face or upper chest area.

❖ Soreness at the site of incisions (episiotomy or cesarean) or repairs.

❖ Pelvic soreness as a result of stretching (see page 285).

❖ Difficulty taking a deep breath because of overexertion of the chest muscles during strenuous pushing (hot baths, showers, or a heating pad may reduce discomfort).

❖ Pain and tenderness in the area of the coccyx (tailbone) either because of injury to the muscles of the pelvic floor or because the tailbone is actually fractured (heat and massage may help).

❖ General all-over achiness (again, heat may help).

Though looking and feeling as though you've taken a beating is normal postpartum, you should report any of the above or any other unusual symptoms you notice to the nurse or your practitioner without delay.

AFTERPAINS

"I've been having cramp-like pains in my abdomen, especially when I'm nursing."

These are probably "afterpains," which are believed to be caused by the contractions of the uterus as it makes its normal descent back into the pelvis following birth. The contractions are more likely to be felt by, and be more intense in, women whose uterine musculature is flaccid (lacking in tone) because of previous births or excessive stretching (as with twins).

Afterpains can be more pronounced during nursing, when contraction-stimulating oxytocin is released. Mild analgesics may be prescribed if necessary, but the pain should subside naturally within four to seven days. If analgesics don't relieve the symptoms, or if they persist for more than a week, see your practitioner to rule out other postpartum problems, including infection.

PAIN IN THE PERINEAL AREA

"I didn't have an episiotomy, and I didn't tear. Why am I so sore?"

You can't expect some 7 pounds of baby to pass by the perineum unnoticed. Even if the perineum was left intact during the baby's arrival, the area has still been stretched, bruised, and generally traumatized; and discomfort, ranging from mild to not-so-mild, is the very normal result.

"My episiotomy site is so sore, I'm afraid my stitches are infected. But how can I tell?"

The perineal soreness experienced by all vaginal deliverees is likely to be compounded if the perineum was torn or surgically cut. Like any freshly repaired wound, the site of an episiotomy or laceration will take time to heal—usually seven to ten days. Pain alone during this time, unless it is very severe, is not an indication that an infection has developed.

Infection is possible, but very unlikely if good perineal care has been practiced. While you're in the hospital, a nurse will check the perineum at least once daily to be certain that there is no inflammation or other indication of infection. She will also instruct you in postpartum perineal hygiene, which is important in preventing infection not only of the repair site but of the genital tract as well (puerperal fever). For this reason, the same precautions apply for those who were neither torn nor had an episiotomy. Follow this ten-day plan for the care of the perineum:

❖ Use a fresh sanitary pad at least every four to six hours. Secure it snugly so that it doesn't slide back and forth.

❖ Remove the pad front to back to avoid dragging germs from the rectum toward the vagina.

❖ Pour or squirt warm water (or an antiseptic solution, if one was recommended by your practitioner) over the perineum after urinating or defecating. Pat dry with gauze pads, or with the paper wipes that come with some hospital-provided sanitary pads, always from front to back.

❖ Keep your hands off the area until healing is complete.

Though discomfort is likely to be greater if you've had a repair (with itchiness around the stitches possibly accompanying soreness), suggestions for relief are usually welcomed by all recently delivered mothers:

❖ Warm sitz baths, hot compresses, or heat lamp exposure.

❖ Chilled witch hazel on a sterile gauze pad, or a surgical glove filled with crushed ice, applied to the site.

❖ Local anesthetics in the form of sprays, creams, or pads; mild pain relievers may be prescribed by your physician.

❖ Lying on your side; avoiding long periods of standing or sitting, to decrease strain on the area. Sitting on a pillow or inflated tube may help, as may tightening your buttocks before sitting.

1. Use a heat lamp only under supervision in the hospital; to use at home, ask for instructions from your practitioner on how to avoid burns.

❖ Doing Kegel exercises (see page 190) as frequently as possible after delivery, and right through the postpartum period, to stimulate circulation to the area, which will promote healing and improve muscle tone. (Don't be alarmed if you can't feel yourself doing them; the area will be numb right after delivery. Feeling will return to the perineum gradually over the next few weeks.)

DIFFICULTY WITH URINATION

"It's been several hours since I gave birth, and I haven't been able to urinate yet."

Difficulty in passing urine during the first 24 postpartum hours is common. Some women feel no urge at all; others feel the urge but are unable to fulfill it. Still others do urinate, but with accompanying pain and burning. There are a host of reasons why bladder function often becomes such an effort after delivery:

❖ The holding capacity of the bladder increases because it suddenly has more room to expand—thus the need for urination may be less frequent.

❖ The bladder may have been traumatized or bruised during delivery, due to pressure created by the fetus, and become temporarily paralyzed. Even when it's full, it may not send the necessary signals of urgency.

❖ Drugs or anesthesia may decrease the sensitivity of the bladder or the alertness of the mother to its signals.

❖ Pain in the perineal area may cause reflex spasms in the urethra, making urination difficult. Edema

378

(swelling) of the perineum may also interfere with urination.

❖ Any number of psychological factors may inhibit urination—fear of pain on voiding, lack of privacy, embarrassment or discomfort over using a bedpan or needing assistance at the toilet.

❖ The sensitivity of the site of an episiotomy or laceration repair can cause burning and/or pain with urination. (Burning may be alleviated somewhat by standing astride the toilet while urinating so that the flow comes straight down, without touching sore spots.)

As difficult as urination may be after delivery, it's essential that the bladder be emptied within six to eight hours—to avoid urinary tract infection, loss of muscle tone in the bladder from overdistension, and bleeding due to the bladder hindering the proper descent of the uterus. Therefore, the nurse will ask you frequently after delivery if you've urinated. She may request that you void for the first time postpartum into a container, so that she can measure your output, and may palpate your bladder to make sure it's not distended.

If you haven't urinated within eight hours or so, your physician may order a catheter (a tube inserted into your urethra) to empty the bladder of urine. You may be able to avoid this with the following:

❖ Take a walk. Getting up from bed and going for a stroll as soon after delivery as you're allowed will help get your bladder (and your bowels) moving.

❖ If you're uncomfortable with an audience, have the nurse wait outside the bathroom while you urinate. She can come back in when you've finished, to give you a demonstration of perineal hygiene.

❖ If you're too weak to walk to the bathroom and must use a bedpan, ask for privacy; be sure the nurse has warmed the pan (if it's metal) and given you warm water to pour over the perineal area (which may stimulate the urge); and sit on the pan instead of lying on it.

❖ Warm the area in a sitz bath or chill it with ice packs, whichever seems to induce urgency for you.

❖ Turn the water on while you try. Running the water in the sink really does help encourage your own faucet to flow.

After 24 hours, the problem of too little becomes one of too much. Postpartum women begin urinating frequently and copiously as the excess body fluids of pregnancy are excreted. If urinating is still difficult, or if output is scant during the next few days, it's possible you have a urinary tract infection. The symptoms of simple cystitis (bladder infection) include pain and/or burning with urination that continues even after the sensitivity of the episiotomy or laceration repair has lessened; frequency and urgency with little urine passed; and, sometimes, a low-grade fever. Symptoms of a kidney infection are more severe, and may include a fever of 101 to 104 degrees and back pain on one or both sides—usually in addition to the symptoms of cystitis. Your physician will want to begin antibiotic treatment specific to the infection-causing organism, if infection is confirmed. You can help speed recovery by drinking plenty of extra fluids. (Also see page 317.)

HAVING A BOWEL MOVEMENT

"I delivered almost a week ago and I haven't had a bowel movement yet. Al-

though I've felt the urge, I've been too afraid that straining would open my episiotomy."

The passage of the first bowel movement after childbirth is a milestone in the postpartum period. Every day that precedes it may be fraught with increasing emotional and physical discomfort.

Several physiological factors may interfere with the return of normal bowel function after delivery. For one thing, the abdominal muscles that assist in elimination have been stretched during childbirth, making them flaccid and possibly ineffective. For another, the bowel itself may have been traumatized by delivery, leaving it sluggish. And, of course, it may have been emptied before or during delivery, and probably remained empty because no solid food was taken for the duration of labor.

But perhaps the most potent inhibitors of postpartum bowel activity are psychological: the unfounded fear of splitting open the stitches; the natural embarrassment over the lack of privacy in the hospital; and the pressure to perform, which often makes performance all the more elusive.

Although reregulating your system is rarely effortless, it isn't necessary to suffer helplessly. There are steps you can take to resolve the problem:

Don't Worry. Nothing keeps you from moving your bowels more effectively than worrying about moving your bowels. Don't worry about opening the stitches—you won't. And don't worry if it takes a few days to get things moving; that's okay, too.

Request Roughage. Select whole grains and fresh fruits and vegetables from the hospital menu, if possible. Supplement the hospital diet, which many patients find constipating, with bowel-stimulating food brought in

from outside. Apples, raisins and other dried fruit, nuts, bran muffins, and small boxes of bran cereal will help. Chocolate—so often a gift to hospital patients—will only worsen constipation.

Keep the Liquids Coming. Not only must you compensate for fluids lost during labor and delivery, you must take in additional liquids—especially water and fruit juices—to help soften stool if you're constipated.

Get Off Your Bottom. You won't be running marathons the day after delivery, but you should be able to take short strolls through the corridors. An inactive body encourages inactive bowels. Kegel exercises, which can be practiced in your bed almost immediately after delivery, will help tone up not only the perineum but also the rectum.

Don't Strain. Straining won't break your stitches open, but it can lead to hemorrhoids. If you do have hemorrhoids, you may find relief with sitz baths, topical anesthetics, suppositories, or hot or cold compresses.

The first few bowel movements may pass with great discomfort. But as stools soften and you become more regular, the discomfort will ease and eventually end.

EXCESSIVE PERSPIRATION

"I've been waking up at night soaked with perspiration. Is this normal?"

What your doctor may call diaphoresis (but is more commonly referred to as perspiration or sweating) is one of the ways the body rids itself of pregnancy-accumulated fluids during the week following delivery. Often perspiration continues to be a problem for several weeks, because of the postpartum hormonal adjustments. Don't worry about it; but do make sure essential fluids are replaced—particularly if you're breastfeeding—by taking extra liquids. An absorbent towel over your pillow may help make you more comfortable if you do most of your perspiring during the night.

As a precaution, it's a good idea to take your temperature, and to report it to your doctor if it's over 100 degrees.

ADEQUACY OF YOUR MILK SUPPLY

"It's been two days since I delivered, and nothing comes out of my breasts when I squeeze them, not even colostrum. I'm worried that my baby is starving."

Not only is your baby not starving, he or she isn't even hungry yet. Babies aren't born with an appetite, or with immediate nutritional needs. And by the time your baby begins to hunger for a breast full of milk (on the third or fourth postpartum day), you will undoubtedly be able to oblige.

Which isn't to say that your breasts are empty now. Colostrum (which provides your baby with enough nourishment for now and with important antibodies his or her own body can't yet produce, while helping to empty the digestive system of excess mucus and the bowels of meconium) is definitely present in the tiny amounts necessary. (A teaspoon or so per feeding is all your baby needs at this point.) But until the third or fourth postpartum day, when your breasts begin to swell and feel full (indicating the milk has come in), it's not that easy to express manually. Even a day-old baby, with no previous experience, is better equipped to extract this premilk than you are.

ENGORGED BREASTS

"My milk finally came in, leaving my breasts swollen to three times their normal size—and so hard, engorged, and painful that I can't bear to put on a bra. Is this what I have to look forward to until I wean my baby?"

If painfully tender, granite-hard breasts the size of an exotic dancer's were indeed what mothers had to look forward to for the duration of the breastfeeding experience, most babies would be weaned before they entered their second week of life. The engorgement, caused by the milk's arrival, can make nursing agonizing for the mother and, if the nipples are flattened by the swelling, frustrating for the baby. The condition can be aggravated when the initial feeding doesn't begin until 24 to 36 hours after birth, as is common in some hospitals.

Happily, the engorgement and its distressing effects gradually diminish once a well-coordinated milk supply-and-demand system is established—within a matter of days. Nipple soreness, too—which usually peaks at about the 20th feeding—generally diminishes rapidly as the nipples toughen up from frequent nursing. Some women, particularly those with fair skin, may also experience nipple cracking and bleeding. This, with proper care (see page 393), is also only temporary.

Until nursing becomes as gratifying and fulfilling as you had hoped it would be—and, believe it or not, painless—there are some steps you can take to reduce the discomfort and speed the establishment of a good milk supply (see Getting Started Breastfeeding, page 388).

When to Call Your Practitioner

During the first six postpartum weeks, there remains the possibility of a post-childbirth complication. It could be signaled by one or more of the following, all of which require *immediate* consultation with your practitioner:

❖ Bleeding that saturates more than one pad an hour for more than a few hours. Have someone take you to the emergency room, or call 911 or your local emergency medical squad, if you can't reach your doctor immediately. En route or while waiting for emergency help to arrive, lie down and keep an ice pack (or a securely tied plastic bag filled with ice cubes and a couple of paper towels to absorb the melting ice) on your lower abdomen (directly over your uterus, if you can locate it, or at the focus of the pain), if possible.

❖ Bright red bleeding any time after the fourth postpartum day. But don't worry about an occasional bloody tinge to your discharge, a brief episode of painless bleeding at about three weeks postpartum, or an increased flow that slows down when you do.

❖ Lochia that has a foul odor. It should smell like a normal menstrual flow.

❖ Large (lemon-size or larger) blood clots in the lochia. Occasional small clots in the first few days, however, are normal.

❖ An absence of lochia during the first two weeks postpartum.

❖ Pain or discomfort, with or without swelling, in the lower abdominal area beyond the first few days after delivery.

❖ After the first 24 hours, a temperature of over 100 degrees for more than a day. But a brief temperature elevation up to 100.4 degrees right after delivery (due to dehydration) or a low-grade fever at the time your milk comes in is of no concern.

❖ Sharp chest pain, which could indicate a blood clot in the lungs. Call 911 or your local emergency medical squad if you can't reach your doctor immediately.

❖ Localized pain, tenderness, and warmth in your calf or thigh, with or without redness, swelling, and pain when you flex your foot—which could be signs of a blood clot in a leg vein (page 360). Rest, with your leg elevated, while you try to reach your doctor.

❖ A lump or hardened area in a breast once engorgement has subsided, which could indicate a clogged milk duct. Begin home treatment (see page 393) while waiting to reach the doctor.

❖ Localized pain, swelling, redness, heat, and tenderness in a breast once engorgement has subsided, which could be signs of mastitis or breast infection. Begin home treatment (page 394) while waiting to reach the doctor.

❖ Localized swelling and/or redness, heat, and oozing at the site of a cesarean incision.

❖ Difficult urination; pain or burning when urinating; a frequent urge to urinate that yields little result; scanty and/or dark urine. Drink plenty of water while trying to reach the doctor.

❖ Depression that affects your ability to cope, or that doesn't subside after a few days; feelings of anger toward your baby, particularly if those feelings are accompanied by violent urges.

ENGORGEMENT IF YOU'RE NOT BREASTFEEDING

"I'm not nursing. I understand that drying up the milk can be painful."

Whether you nurse or not, your breasts will become engorged (overfilled) with milk on the third or fourth postpartum day. This can be uncomfortable, even painful. However, it is blessedly temporary.

Some physicians used to rely on hormones or other drugs to suppress lactation. But because the drugs have serious side effects and are not reliable (they sometimes fail to relieve engorgement, and if they do, it frequently returns when the medication is discontinued), the FDA's Fertility and Maternal Health Advisory Committee has recommended against their use. Since postpartum breast engorgement is a natural process, it is best to let nature resolve it, which it always does eventually.

The breasts are designed to produce milk only as needed. If the milk isn't used, production ceases. Though sporadic leaking may continue for several days, or even weeks, severe engorgement shouldn't last more than 12 to 24 hours. During this time, ice packs, mild pain relievers, a supportive bra, and squeezing a few drops of milk from the breast when engorgement is severe may help. Avoid hot showers, which stimulate milk production.

BONDING

"My new son was premature and I won't get to hold him for at least two weeks. Will it be too late for good bonding?"

Bonding, the process of attachment between a mother and her newborn child, has in recent years become a *cause célèbre* in childbirth circles. The term originated in the 1970s, when some studies began to show that the separation of an infant from its mother immediately after birth posed a threat both to their lifelong relationship and to the infant's future relationships with others. Some very positive changes in post-childbirth procedure have come about because of this work. Today, many hospitals permit new mothers to hold their babies moments after birth, and to cuddle and nurse them for anywhere from ten minutes to an hour or more, instead of whisking the newborns off to the nursery the moment the cord is cut.

But as sometimes happens with the popularization of a good idea, the concept of bonding soon became misunderstood and abused (one of the doctors who published the first book on the subject later said: "I wish we'd never written the statement"), with some unfortunate results. Mothers who have surgical deliveries and are unable to see their babies at birth worry that their parent-child relationship will be forever tarnished. The same worry haunts parents whose babies must be in neonatal intensive care for several days or weeks, giving them little bonding opportunity. So frantic have some parents become about the necessity for instant bonding that they are demanding it even at risk to their infants.

Of course, initial bonding in the delivery room is nice. This early meeting of mother and baby gives them a chance to make contact, skin to skin, eye to eye. It's the first step in the development of a lasting parent-child bond. But only the *first* step. And it doesn't have to take place at the moment of birth. It can take place later in a hospital bed, or through the portholes of an incubator, or even weeks later at home. When your parents were born, they probably saw little of their mothers and even less of their fathers until they went home—usually ten days after birth—and the vast majority of this "deprived" generation grew up with strong, loving family ties. Mothers who had the chance to bond at birth with one child and not with another usually report no difference in their feelings toward the children. And adoptive parents, who often don't meet their babies until hospital discharge (or even much later) manage to foster strong bonds. Some experts believe, in fact, that bonding doesn't really take place until somewhere in the second half of the baby's first year. Certainly it is a complex process that isn't accomplished in minutes.

It's never too late to tie the bonds that bind. So, instead of wasting energy regretting the time you've lost, prepare to make the most of the lifetime of mothering you have ahead.

"I've been told that bonding brings mother and child closer together, but every time I hold my baby, she seems like a stranger to me."

L ove at first sight is a concept that flourishes in romantic books and movies but rarely materializes in real life. The kind of love that lasts a lifetime usually requires time, nurturing, and plenty of patience to develop and deepen. And that's as true for the love between a newborn and its parents as it is between a man and a woman.

Physical closeness between mother and child immediately after birth does not guarantee instant emotional closeness. Feelings of affection don't flow as quickly and surely as lochia; those first few postpartum seconds aren't automatically bathed in the glow of maternal love. In fact, the first sensation a woman experiences after birth is far more likely to be relief than love—relief that the baby is normal and, especially if her labor was difficult, that the ordeal is over. It's not at all unusual to see that squalling and unsociable infant as a stranger—with very little connection to the cozy, idealized little fetus you carried for nine months—and to feel little more than neutral toward him or her. One study found that it took an average of over two weeks (and often as long as nine weeks) for mothers to begin having positive feelings toward their newborns.

Just how a woman reacts to her newborn at their first meeting may depend on a variety of factors: the length and intensity of her labor; whether she received tranquilizers and/or anesthetics during labor; her previous experience (or lack of it) with infants; her feelings about having a child; her relationship with her husband; extraneous worries that may preoccupy her; her general health; and, probably most important of all, her personality. *Your* reaction is normal for *you*.

And as long as you feel an increasing sense of comfort and attachment as the days go by, you can relax. Some of the best relationships get off to the slowest starts. Give yourself and your baby a chance to get to know and appreciate each other, and let the love grow naturally and unhurriedly.

If you don't feel a growing closeness after a few weeks, or if you feel anger or antipathy toward your baby, discuss these feelings with your pediatrician. It's important to work them out early on, to prevent lasting damage to your relationship.

ROOMING-IN

"In childbirth class, having the baby room-in with me sounded like heaven. Since I gave birth, it's been more like hell. I can't get the baby to stop crying— yet what kind of mother would I be if I asked the nurse to take her?"

Y ou would be a very human mother. You've just completed the more-than-Herculean task (Hercules couldn't have done it) of giving birth and are about to embark on an even greater challenge: child rearing. Needing a few days' rest in between is nothing to feel guilty about.

Of course, some women handle rooming-in with ease. They may have had easy deliveries that left them feeling exhilarated instead of exhausted. Or they may have had experience caring for newborns, their own or other people's. For these women, an inconsolable infant at 3 A.M. may not be a joy, but it's not a nightmare, either. For a woman who's been without sleep for 48 hours, however, whose body has been left limp from an enervating labor, and who's never been closer to a baby than a diaper ad, such predawn bouts can leave her wondering tearfully: "Why did I ever decide to become a mother?"

Playing the martyr can raise motherly resentments against the baby, feelings the baby will be likely to sense. If, instead, the baby is sent back to the nursery between feedings at night, mother and child, both well rested, may have a better chance to get acquainted when morning comes.

Full-time rooming-in is a wonderful new option in family-centered maternity care—but it's not for everyone. You are *not* a failure or a bad mother if you don't enjoy, or feel too tired for, rooming-in. Don't be pushed into it if you don't think you want it; and once you've committed yourself, don't feel you can't change your mind. Partial rooming-in (during the day but not at night) may be a good solution for you. Or you might prefer to get a good night's sleep the first night and start rooming-in on the second.

Be flexible. Be more concerned with the quality of the time you spend with your baby in the hospital than the quantity. Round-the-clock rooming-in will begin soon enough at home. And by then, if you are sensible now, you should be emotionally and physically ready to deal with it.

GOING HOME

"My labor was almost effortless, and I feel great. Why should I have to stay in the hospital if I have nothing to recover from?"

C hances are *you* don't have to stay in the hospital. Though ten-day hospital stays were once considered a necessary precaution after giving birth, it's now recognized that a woman who's had an uncomplicated delivery really doesn't need any hospitalization. Your baby, on the other hand, does need some observation to be certain everything is all right before discharge. So you will probably have to stay in the hospital at least eight hours, possibly 24 or more, depending on your newborn's condition.

Of course, no one can hold you or your baby hostage in the hospital against your will. You have the right to sign yourself and your baby out of the hospital AMA (against medical advice) at any time—if you take full legal, written responsibility for the possible consequences. But unless you have a degree in medicine, it would be extremely unwise to play doctor. If either your pediatrician or obstetrician recommends a prolonged stay, ask for an explanation—but do follow their professional advice. And try to make the best of your extended sojourn, getting as much rest as you can while you still have the chance.

Even if your doctors authorize your early release, you'd be wise to think twice if you don't have full-time help (either hired or volunteer) waiting for you. It's important to rest postpartum—in the hospital or at home.

"I had a rough labor and a major epi-siotomy, and I feel awful. But my doctor told me I have to go home this afternoon, even though I only gave birth early this morning."

Physicians are put in a difficult po-sition these days. Under pressure from hospitals and insurance pro-viders, many are forced to discharge patients from the hospital sooner than their medical judgment dictates, some-times as early as eight hours after de-livery. If you really feel unwell and unready to go home, say so. Insist that you (or your husband or other family member) see the hospital's patient ad-vocate or administrator and explain that you do not feel up to going home. You may be able to persuade them that discharging you would be unwise. Or they may allow you to stay AMA (against medical advice), in which case you, and not your insurance carrier, will probably have to foot the bill.

If you are sent home early in spite of your efforts, ask that the fact that you were discharged against your own wishes be noted on your chart. When you get home, be certain that you have someone with you round the clock (a family member, a friend, or a hired baby nurse), get plenty of bed rest (pretend you're still in the hospi-tal), and pay close attention to your body's signals (keeping in mind the signs and symptoms of postpartum problems; see page 381).

"Is discharge less than 24 hours after birth safe for my baby?"

The practice is new and controver-sial and the answer is not ab-solutely clear. What is clear, however, is that the decision of when to go home is best made on a case by case basis. Early discharge is safest when a an infant is full term, of an appropriate weight, feeding well, going home with a parent (or parents) who knows the basics and is well enough to provide care, and will be seen by the doctor at two or three days after birth. If these requirements aren't met or if for any other reason you have concerns about early discharge, speak to your child's doctor.

RECOVERY FROM A CESAREAN SECTION

"How different will my recuperation be from that of a woman with a vaginal delivery?"

Recovery from a cesarean section is similar to recovery from any ma-jor abdominal surgery—with a de-lightful difference: Instead of losing an old gallbladder or appendix, you gain a brand-new baby.

Of course there's another differ-ence, slightly less delightful. In addi-tion to recovering from surgery, you'll also be recovering from childbirth. Except for a neatly intact perineum, you'll experience all the same post-partum discomforts you would have had if you'd delivered vaginally—afterpains, lochia, breast engorge-ment, fatigue, hormonal changes, hair loss, excessive perspiration, and the baby blues. (See this chapter and the next for tips on how to deal with all of these.)

As for your surgical recovery, you can expect the following in the re-covery room:

Anesthesia Aftereffects. Until your an-esthesia wears off, you will be ob-served carefully in the recovery room. You may be very shaky and sensitive to temperature change. If you've had a general anesthetic, your memory of this time may be fuzzy or totally ab-sent. Since everyone responds differ-ently to drugs—and each drug is different—whether you are clear-headed and alert in a few hours or not for a day or two will depend upon you and upon the medications you were given. If you feel disoriented, or have hallucinations or bad dreams, your coach or an understanding nurse can help you get back to reality when you waken.

It will take longer for spinal or epidural anesthesia to wear off—which they usually do from the toes up. You will be encouraged to wiggle your toes and move your feet as soon as you can. If you've had a spinal block, you will have to stay flat on your back for about 8 to 12 hours. You may be allowed to have both your husband and your baby visit with you in the recovery room.

Pain Around Your Incision. Once the anesthesia wears off, your wound, like any wound, is going to hurt—though just how much depends on many factors, including your personal pain threshold and how many cesareans you've had. (The first is usually the most uncomfortable.) You will probably be given pain relief medication as needed, which may make you feel woozy or drugged. It will also allow you to get some needed sleep. You needn't be concerned if you're nursing; the medication won't pass into your colostrum, and by the time your milk comes in, you probably won't need any medication.

Possibly, Nausea, With or Without Vomiting. This isn't always a problem, but if it is, you may be given an antiemetic preparation to prevent vomiting. (If you vomit easily, you might want to talk to your doctor about giving you such a medication before nausea appears.)

Breathing and Coughing Exercises. These help rid your system of any leftover general anesthetic, and help to expand your lungs and keep them clear to prevent pneumonia. Such necessary lung calisthenics may be very uncomfortable if you do them correctly. You may be able to minimize this discomfort by "splinting" your incision with a pillow.

Regular Evaluations of Your Condition. A nurse will check your vital signs (temperature, blood pressure, pulse, respiration), your urinary output and vaginal flow, the dressing on your incision, and the firmness and level of your uterus (as it shrinks in size and makes its way back into the pelvis). She will also check your IV and urinary catheter.

Once you have been moved to your hospital room, you can expect:

Continuing Evaluation of Your Condition. Your vital signs, your urinary output and vaginal flow, your dressing, and your uterus, as well as your IV and catheter (as long as they remain in place) will be checked regularly.

Removal of the Catheter After 24 Hours. Urination may be difficult, so try the tips on page 377. If they don't work, the catheter may be reinserted until you can urinate by yourself.

Afterpains. These start about 12 to 24 hours after delivery. See page 376 for more about these occasional uncomfortable contractions.

Removal of the IV. About 24 hours after surgery, or when your bowels begin to show signs of activity (by producing gas), your IV will be discontinued and you will be allowed some fluids by mouth. Over the next few days, you will probably be able to progress to soft foods, and then to a normal diet. Even if you feel as though you are starving, don't try to circumvent doctor's orders by having someone sneak in a Big Mac. Take it easy getting back to your normal diet. If you are breastfeeding, be sure to get plenty of fluids.

Referred Shoulder Pain. Irritation of the diaphragm following surgery can cause a few hours of sharp shoulder pain. An analgesic may help.

Possible Constipation. It may be a few days until you have a bowel movement, and that's all right. A stool softener or mild laxative may be prescribed to help move things along. Try some of the tips given on page 378, but exclude the roughage for the first few days. If you haven't had a movement by the fourth or fifth day, you may be given a laxative, an enema, or a suppository.

Encouragement to Exercise. Before you are out of bed, you will be encouraged to wiggle your toes, flex your calves, bend your feet up at the ankles, push against the end of the bed with your feet, and turn from side to side. You can also try these: (1) Lie flat on your back, bend one knee, and then extend the other leg while tightening your abdomen slightly. Slide the bent leg slowly back down; repeat with the other leg. (2) Lie on your back, knees pulled up, feet flat on the bed, and raise your head for about 30 seconds. (3) On your back, knees bent, tighten your abdomen, and reach with one arm across your body to the other side of the bed, at about waist level. Reverse. These exercises are intended to improve circulation, especially in your legs, and prevent the development of blood clots. (But be prepared for some of these to be quite painful, at least for the first 24 hours or so.)

To Get Up Between 8 and 24 Hours after Surgery. With the help of the nurse, you'll sit up first, supported by the raised head of the bed. Then, using your hands for support, you will slide your legs over the side of the bed and dangle them for a few minutes. Then, slowly, you'll be helped to step down on the floor, your hands still on the bed. If you feel dizzy (which is normal), sit right back down. Steady yourself for a few more minutes before taking a couple of steps. Those steps may be extremely painful. Stand as straight as you can, though the temptation to hunch over to ease the discomfort may be great. (This difficulty in getting around is temporary; in fact, you may soon find yourself more mobile than the vaginal deliveree next door—and you will certainly have the edge in sitting.)

To Wear Elastic Stockings. These improve circulation and are also intended to prevent blood clots in the legs.

Abdominal Discomfort. As your digestive tract (temporarily put out of business by surgery) begins to function again, trapped gas can cause considerable pain, especially when it presses against your incision line. The discomfort may be worse when you laugh, cough, or sneeze. Tell the nurse or doctor about your problem and they will suggest some possible remedies. Narcotics are not usually recommended because they can prolong the problem, which ordinarily lasts just a day or two. You may get a small enema or a suppository to help release the gas. Or you may be advised to walk up and down the corridor. Lying on your left side or on your back, your knees drawn up, taking deep breaths while holding your incision, may help. If the pain remains severe, a tube may be inserted in your rectum to allow the gas to escape.

Time with Your Baby. You can't lift the baby yet, but you can cuddle and feed him or her. (If you're nursing, place the baby on a pillow over your incision.) Depending on how you feel, and on hospital regulations, you may be able to have modified rooming-in. Some hospitals even allow full rooming-in.

Sponge Baths. Until the stitches are removed (or absorbed), you probably won't be allowed a real bath or shower.

Removal of Stitches. If your stitches or clips aren't self-absorbing, they will be removed about four or five days after delivery. And although the procedure isn't very painful, you may find it uncomfortable. When the dressing is off, look at the incision with the nurse or doctor; ask how soon you can expect the area to heal, which changes will be normal, and which might require medical attention.

In most cases, you can expect to go home three to five days postpartum.

WHAT IT'S IMPORTANT TO KNOW:
GETTING STARTED BREASTFEEDING

Ever since Eve put Cain to suckle for the first time, breastfeeding has been coming naturally to mothers and newborns. Right?

Well, not always—at least not immediately. Though nursing does come naturally, it comes naturally a little later for some mothers and babies than for others. Sometimes there are physical factors that foil those first few attempts; at other times it's just a simple lack of experience on the part of both participants. But whatever might be keeping your baby and your breasts apart, it won't be long before they're in perfect synch—as long as you don't give up first. Some of the most mutually satisfying breast-baby relationships begin with several days of fumbling, of bungled efforts, and of tears on both sides.

Knowing just what to expect and how to deal with setbacks can help ease the mutual adjustment:

❖ Start as soon as possible after birth. Right in the delivery room is best, when that's feasible. (See Breastfeeding Basics, page 389.) But sometimes mother's not in any condition to nurse, sometimes baby isn't—neither of which means they won't be able to start successfully later. (Even if you and the baby feel well, this first nursing experience won't necessarily go smoothly. You both have a lot to learn.)

❖ Don't let hospital bureaucracy break your tentative connection because of insensitivity, ignorance, and unnecessary rules. Enlist the support of your doctor in advance to be sure that you will be allowed to nurse in the delivery room if all goes normally. Also, arrange for full or partial rooming-in, or for a demand-feeding schedule (having the nursery bring the baby when he or she is hungry) if the staff will oblige. If the baby is with you all day, this may mean limiting visiting privileges to just your husband, which is probably for the best anyway since it allows the three of you to get to know each other while maintaining the relaxed atmosphere needed for nursing. Or you could have the nursery take the baby during visiting hours.

Breastfeeding Basics

1. Get into a comfortable position.

2. Position your baby facing your nipple.

3. Support your breast with your free hand, your thumb on top, fingers beneath. But keep your fingers off the areola, which your baby has to grasp.

4. Gently tickle the baby's lips with your nipple until the mouth is opened wide. Then move your breast closer.

5. Don't stuff the nipple in an unwilling mouth; let your baby take the initiative.

6. Be sure the baby latches on to both the nipple and the areola. Sucking on just the nipple won't compress the milk glands and can cause soreness and cracking. Also be sure that it is the nipple that the baby is busily milking. Some infants are so eager to suck that they will latch on to any part of the breast (even if no milk is forthcoming), and this gumming of sensitive tissue can cause a painful bruise.

7. If your breast is blocking your baby's nose, lightly depress the breast with your finger. But be sure not to pull loose your baby's grip on the areola.

8. You can assure yourself that your baby is suckling if there is a strong steady rhythmic motion visible in his or her cheek.

9. If your baby has finished suckling but is still holding on to the breast, pulling it out abruptly can cause injury to the nipple. Instead, break the suction first by depressing the breast or by putting your finger into the corner of the baby's mouth to admit some air.

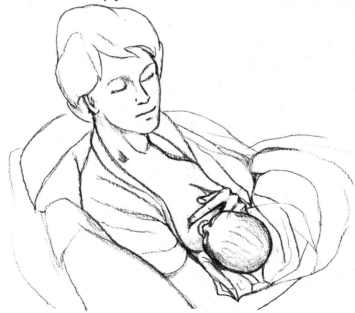

Whatever is comfortable for you and the baby is a good position as long as baby is directly facing your nipple. Prop with pillows as needed to avoid stress.

❖ Don't let sleeping babies lie if it means that they'll sleep through a feeding. If you have rooming-in, you're not likely to have a problem with this. You'll be able to demand-feed the baby when he or she is hungry and let the baby sleep when he or she's sleepy. If you're dependent on the nursery staff to bring the baby—on their schedule, not junior's—you may find that feeding time is over before the baby wakes. Don't let this happen. If the baby isn't awake on arrival at your room, wake him or her. This sounds crueler than it actually is. Gently set the baby on the bed in a sitting position, one hand holding up the chin, the other supporting the back. Next, bend the baby forward at the waist. The moment he or she stirs, quickly adopt the nursing position. If your baby is swaddled, loosen the blanket so he or she can be close to you.

❖ Be patient if your baby is still recovering from delivery. If you received anesthesia or had a prolonged, difficult labor, you can expect your baby to be drowsy and sluggish at the breast for a few days. This is no reflection on you, your nursing ability, or your baby. There's no danger the baby will starve in the meantime, since newborns have little need for nourishment during the first days of life. What they do need, though, is nurturing. Cuddling at the breast is just as important as suckling.

Baby and Breast—A Perfect Feeding Team

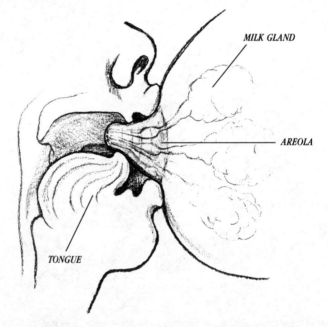

MILK GLAND

AREOLA

TONGUE

Be sure that the nursing baby has the areola and not just the nipple in his or her mouth. This way the milk can be efficiently and, eventually, painlessly extracted.

❖ Make sure your baby's appetite and sucking instinct aren't sabotaged between feedings. It's routine in some hospital nurseries to quiet a crying baby between mother's feedings with a bottle of sugar water. This can have a twofold detrimental effect. First, it satisfies the baby's still-delicate appetite for hours. Later, when brought to you for feeding, if your baby doesn't want to nurse, and your breasts aren't stimulated to produce milk, a vicious cycle will have begun. Second, because the rubber nipple requires less effort, the baby's sucking reflex becomes lazy. Faced with the greater challenge of tackling the breast, he or she may just give up. *Don't let anyone talk you into the sugar water.* Give strict orders—through your pediatrician —that supplementary feedings are not to be given to your baby in the nursery unless medically necessary.[2]

❖ Don't try to feed a screaming baby. It's hard enough for an inexperienced suckler to find the nipple when calm. When your baby is overexcited, it may be impossible. Rock and soothe him or her before you start nursing.

❖ If you're having trouble establishing breastfeeding, ask for assistance from hospital personnel or from your practitioner. If you are lucky, a lactation specialist will join you at your first baby feeding to provide hands-on instruction, helpful hints, and perhaps literature. If this is not a policy in your hospital (or you are somehow bypassed), you can find empathy and advice by calling your local La Leche League chapter.

❖ No matter how frustrating nursing becomes, try to stay calm. Start out as relaxed as you can. Clear out the visitors 15 minutes before feeding time, and don't think about your hospital bill or anything else that might upset you. Then try to remain cool throughout the nursing period, no matter how badly it's going. Tension not only hampers your ability to give milk, it can cause anxiety in your baby. An infant is extremely sensitive to and reacts to its mother's moods.

WHEN THE MILK COMES IN

Just when you and your baby seem to be getting the hang of it, your milk comes in. Up until now, your baby has been getting tiny amounts of colostrum (premilk), and your breasts have been quite comfortable. Then, within a few hours, your breasts become swollen, hard, and painful. Nursing is difficult for the baby and agonizing for you.[3] Fortunately, this period of engorgement is brief. While it lasts, there are a variety of ways of relieving it and the accompanying discomfort:

❖ Nurse more often (at least eight to ten times a day), for shorter periods—a four-hour schedule can lead to engorgement, and 20-minute nursing periods to sore nipples; both make nursing difficult in the long run for mother and baby. Start

---

2. You may also want to discuss with your pediatrician the pros and cons of a pacifier being given to your baby in the nursery. On the one hand, it could get him or her hooked on a rubber nipple; on the other, it may be comforting when there's no one to cuddle with in the middle of the night.

3. A few lucky new mothers don't experience engorgement when their milk comes in, possibly because their babies were vigorous nursers from birth; there is also less engorgement with subsequent babies.

off with 5 minutes on each breast, gradually building up to 15 minutes on each by the third or fourth day.

❖ Don't be tempted to skip or skimp on a feeding because of pain. The less your baby sucks, the more en-

gorged you will become. Don't favor one breast because it is less sore or because the nipple isn't cracked; the only way to toughen up nipples is to use them. Use both breasts at every feeding, even if only for a few minutes—but nurse from the

Best-Odds Nursing Diet

The levels of protein, fat, and carbohydrates in your breast milk aren't usually affected by the levels of these nutrients in your diet; however, levels of some vitamins are (A and B_{12}, for example). But though the quality of your milk isn't always directly related to the quality of your diet, the quantity of milk usually is. Women whose diets are deficient in protein and/or calories, for example, may produce milk of good composition but in smaller amounts. To make good breast milk, and plenty of it, continue taking your pregnancy (or pregnancy/lactation) vitamin-mineral supplement, and adhere closely to the Best-Odds Diet on page 80, with modifications:

❖ Increase your caloric intake to about 500 calories per day over your prepregnancy requirements. This is flexible, and as during pregnancy, you can let your scale be your guide. If you have a lot of fat stores from pregnancy (or before), you can take fewer calories, as the fat will be burned to produce milk (and you will lose weight). If you are underweight, you will probably need more than 500 additional calories daily (the recommended daily allowance assumes some use of fat stores, which you don't have). No matter what your weight, you may find that you need still more calories as the baby grows and demands more milk. Again, you will be able to determine this by checking your

scale. If your weight starts dipping below the ideal, increase your daily intake.

❖ Increase your calcium requirement to five servings per day.

❖ Reduce your protein intake to three servings per day.

❖ Drink at least eight glasses of fluids (milk, water, broths or soups, and juices); take more during hot weather and if you've been perspiring a lot. (Though it's all right to drink moderate amounts of tea or coffee, and an occasional alcoholic beverage, don't count them in your fluid allowance since they have a dehydrating effect.) Excess is not best, however; flooding yourself with fluid (more than 12 glasses per day) can paradoxically *slow* milk production. Thirst and urinary output can help you gauge your needs.

❖ Splurge occasionally. You've served your nine-month sentence of abstinence; you're entitled to your just desserts, at least once in a while. The key is moderation. Small amounts of sugar won't interfere with milk production, but a steady diet of sweets can, by dulling your appetite for necessary nutrients. Ditto for other nutritionally superfluous foods, such as potato chips, french fries, white bread; eat them only *after* you've fulfilled your nutritional obligations.

less sore one first, since the baby will suck more vigorously when hungry. If both nipples are equally sore (or not sore at all), start off the feeding with the breast you used last. Be sure to position your baby correctly to reduce nipple soreness.

❖ Use a breast pump on each breast before nursing to lessen the engorgement so that your baby can get a better hold on the nipple, and to get milk flow started.

❖ Use ice packs to reduce engorgement. Or a hot shower or hot soaks, if you find them more soothing.

❖ Support is important in a nursing bra, but pressure against your sore and engorged breasts can be painful. Whenever leaking isn't a problem—and especially after nursing—leave the flaps of your nursing bra open.

SORE NIPPLES

Tender nipples sometimes compound the difficulties of early nursing. Most toughen up quickly. But in some women, particularly those who are fair-skinned, the nipples become sore and cracked. To relieve the discomfort:

❖ Expose sore or cracked nipples to the air as much as possible. Protect them from clothing and other irritations and surround them with a cushion of air by wearing breast shells (not shields).

❖ Let nature—and not the cosmetic companies—take care of your nipples. Nipples are naturally protected and lubricated by sweat glands and skin oils. A commercial preparation should be used only when nipple cracking is severe, and

then should be as pure as possible. Ultra-purified, medical grade lanolin, A & D ointment, or Vitamin E (squeezed from capsules) may be useful, but avoid petroleum-based products and petroleum jelly itself (Vaseline). Wash nipples only with water—never with soap, alcohol, tincture of benzoin, or pre-moistened towelettes—whether your nipples are sore or not: Your baby is already protected from your germs, and the milk itself is clean.

❖ Vary your nursing position so a different part of the nipple will be compressed at each feeding; but always keep baby facing your breasts.

❖ Relax for 15 minutes or so before feeding. Relaxation will enhance the let-down of milk, whereas tension will only hinder it.

OCCASIONAL COMPLICATIONS

Once nursing is established, it generally continues uneventfully until weaning. But once in a while, complications occur, among them:

Clogged Milk Ducts. Sometimes a milk duct clogs, causing milk to back up. Since this condition (characterized by a small, red, and tender lump on the breast) can lead to infection, it's important to try to remedy it quickly. The best way to do this is to offer the affected breast first at each feeding, and to let your baby empty it as completely as possible. If he or she doesn't do the job, any remaining milk should be expressed by hand or with a breast pump. Keep pressure off the duct by making sure your bra is not too tight, and by varying your nursing positions to put pressure on different ducts. Also, check to see if dried milk is blocking the nipple after nursing. If so, clean it off with sterile cotton dipped in boiled and cooled water. Do not use this time to wean the baby; discontinuing nursing now will only compound your problem.

Breast Infection. A more serious complication of breastfeeding is mastitis, or breast infection, which can occur in one or both breasts, most often between the 10th and 28th postpartum day, in an estimated 7% to 10% of mothers—usually first-timers. The factors that can combine to cause mastitis are failure to empty breasts completely of milk at each nursing, germs gaining entrance into the milk ducts through a crack or fissure in the nipple (usually from the baby's mouth), and lowered resistance in the mother due to stress, fatigue, and inadequate nutrition.

The most common symptoms of mastitis are severe soreness, hardness, redness, heat, and swelling of the breast, with generalized chills and a fever of about 101 to 102 degrees. If you develop some of these symptoms, contact your doctor. Prompt medical treatment is necessary, and may include bed rest, antibiotics, pain relievers, increased fluid intake, and ice or moist heat applications. During treatment you should continue to nurse. Since the baby's germs probably caused the infection in the first place, they won't harm him or her. And emptying the breast will help to prevent clogged milk ducts. Nurse first on the infected breast, and empty it with a pump if the baby doesn't. If the pain is so excruciating that you can't nurse,

try pumping your breasts while lying in a tub of warm water with your breasts floating comfortably. Don't use an electric pump.

Delay in treating mastitis could lead to the development of a breast abscess, the symptoms of which include excruciating, throbbing pain; localized swelling, tenderness, and heat in the area of the abscess; and temperature swings between 100 and 103 degrees. Treatment includes antibiotics and, generally, surgical drainage under anesthesia. Breastfeeding with the affected breast must be halted, and a breast pump should be used regularly to empty it until healing is complete and breastfeeding can be resumed. In the meantime, nursing can continue on the unaffected breast.

Don't let breast and nursing problems with your first baby discourage you from nursing future babies. Engorgement and nipple soreness are far less common with subsequent births.

BREASTFEEDING AFTER A CESAREAN

How soon you can breastfeed your newborn after a surgical delivery will depend on how you feel and how your baby is doing. If you are both in good shape, you can probably introduce baby to breast in the delivery room after the surgery is completed, or in the recovery room shortly afterward. If you're groggy from general anesthesia or your baby needs imme-

---

Medication and Breastfeeding

Be sure to tell any physician who prescribes medication for you that you are nursing your baby. Many medications are safe to use when nursing; some others are not. It is usually best to take medication just after you finish a feeding, so that levels in your milk will be lowest when you nurse again.

diate care in the nursery, you may have to wait. If after 12 hours you still haven't been able to get together with your baby, you should probably inquire about using a pump to express milk (at this point it is actually premilk, or colostrum) to get lactation started.

You may find breastfeeding after a cesarean uncomfortable at first—most mothers do. It will be less so if you try to avoid putting pressure on the incision: place a pillow on your lap under the baby; lie on your side; or use the football hold, again supported by a pillow, to nurse. Both the afterpains you experience as you nurse (see page 376) and the soreness at the site of the incision are normal and will lessen in the days ahead.

BREASTFEEDING TWINS

Breastfeeding, like just about every aspect of caring for newborn twins, seems as though it will be impossible until you get into the rhythm of it. Once you have a routine, it is not only possible but very rewarding. To successfully nurse twins, you should:

❖ Fulfill all the dietary recommendations for lactating mothers (see the Best-Odds Nursing Diet), with these additions: 400 to 500 calories above your prepregnancy needs for *each* baby you are nursing (you may need to increase your caloric intake as the babies grow bigger and hun-

grier, or decrease it if you supplement nursing with formula and/or solids, or if you have considerable fat reserves you would like to burn); an additional serving of protein (for a total of four) and an additional serving of calcium (six total) or a calcium supplement.

❖ Drink 8 to 12 cups of fluid a day—but not more, because too much may suppress milk production.

❖ Get as much help as you can with housework, meal preparation, and infant care, in order to conserve your energy.

❖ Explore the various feeding options: nurse one baby, bottle-feed the other; alternate feedings of bottle and breast with each baby; or nurse each separately (which can take ten hours or more a day), or both together. Combining individual and group feedings, and giving each infant at least one private feeding a day, is a good compromise that encourages mother-baby closeness. Father might give a bottle to the other baby at these feedings. Such relief bottles, given by the father or another helper, can be either formula or expressed milk.

❖ Recognize that the twins have different personalities, needs, and nursing patterns, and don't try to treat them identically. Keep records to be sure both are fed at each feeding.

19
Postpartum: The First Six Weeks

WHAT YOU MAY BE FEELING

During the first six weeks post-partum, depending on the type of delivery you had (easy or difficult, vaginal or cesarean), how much help you have at home, and other individual factors, you may experience all, or only some, of the following:

PHYSICALLY:

❖ Continued vaginal discharge (lochia), turning brownish, then yellowish-white

❖ Fatigue

❖ Some pain, discomfort, and numbness in the perineum, if you had a vaginal delivery (especially if you had stitches)

❖ Diminishing incisional pain, continuing numbness, if you had a cesarean delivery (especially if it was your first)

❖ Continued constipation (although this should be easing up)

❖ Gradual flattening of your abdomen as your uterus recedes into the pelvis (but only exercise will bring you fully back to prepregnancy shape)

❖ Gradual loss of weight

❖ Breast discomfort and nipple soreness until breastfeeding is well established

❖ Achiness in arms and neck (from carrying the baby)

❖ Hair loss

EMOTIONALLY:

❖ Elation, depression, or swings between the two

❖ A sense of being overwhelmed, a growing feeling of confidence, or swings between the two

❖ Decreased or increased sexual desire

WHAT YOU CAN EXPECT AT YOUR POSTPARTUM CHECKUP

Your practitioner will probably schedule you for a checkup four to six weeks postpartum.[1] During that visit, you can expect the following to be checked, though the exact content of the visit will vary depending upon what your particular needs are and your practitioner's style of practice.

❖ Blood pressure

❖ Weight, which will probably be down by 17 to 20 pounds or more

❖ Your uterus, to see if it has returned to prepregnant shape, size, and location

❖ Your cervix, which will be on its way back to its prepregnant state, but will still be somewhat engorged and its surface possibly eroded

❖ Your vagina, which will have contracted and regained much of its muscle tone

❖ The episiotomy or laceration repair site, if any; or, if you had a cesarean delivery, the site of your incision

❖ Your breasts, for any abnormalities

❖ Hemorrhoids or varicose veins, if you have either

❖ Questions or problems you want to discuss—have a list ready

At this visit, the practitioner will also discuss with you the method of birth control that you will be using. If you plan on using a diaphragm and your cervix has recovered sufficiently, you will be fitted for one; if not, you may have to use condoms until you can be fitted. If you're not breastfeeding and plan to take birth control pills, they may be prescribed now.

WHAT YOU MAY BE CONCERNED ABOUT

FEVER

"I've just returned home from the hospital and I'm running a fever of about 101 degrees. Could it be related to childbirth?"

Thanks to Dr. Ignaz Semmelweiss, the chances of a new mother developing childbed (or puerperal) fever today are extremely slight. It was in 1847 that this young Viennese physician discovered that if birth attendants washed their hands before delivering babies, the risk of childbirth-related infection could be greatly reduced (though at the time, his theory was considered so outlandish that he was driven from his post, ostracized, and later died a broken man). And thanks to Sir Alexander Fleming, the British scientist who developed the first infection-fighting antibiotics, the occasional case that does occur is easily cured.

The most severe cases of infection usually begin within 24 hours of delivery. A fever on the third or fourth

---

1. If you had a cesarean, your physician may also check your incision at about three weeks postpartum.

day, when you are already at home, could possibly be a sign of postpartum infection—but it could also be caused by a virus or other minor problem. A low-grade fever (of about 100 degrees) occasionally accompanies engorgement when your milk first comes in. Report any fever that lasts more than four hours during the first three postpartum weeks to the doctor—even if it's accompanied by obvious cold or flu symptoms or vomiting—so that its cause can be diagnosed and any necessary treatment started. See page 365 if postpartum infection is suspected or diagnosed.

DEPRESSION

"I have everything I have always wanted: a wonderful husband, a beautiful new baby—why do I feel so blue?"

Why should roughly one half of all new mothers be so miserable during one of the happiest times of their lives? That's the paradox of postpartum depression, for which experts have yet to provide any definitive explanations or solutions.

Hormones, so often the culprit fingered in the case of a woman's mood swings, may offer some rationale. Levels of estrogen and progesterone drop precipitously after childbirth and may trigger depression, just as hormonal fluctuations prior to menstruation may do. The fact that sensitivity to hormonal fluctuations varies from woman to woman is believed to explain at least partially why, though all women experience the same shift in hormone levels after delivery, only about 50% suffer from postpartum depression.

But there are a host of other factors that probably contribute to the postpartum blues—which are most common around the third day after delivery, but which can strike at any time

during the first year, and which afflict second-time mothers more often than first-timers:

The Shift from Center Stage to Backstage. Your baby is now the star of the show. Visitors would rather run to the nursery than sit at your bedside inquiring after your health. This change in status will accompany you home; the pregnant princess is now the postpartum Cinderella.

Hospitalization. When you're eager to get home and begin mothering, you may be frustrated by the lack of control you have over your life and your baby's in the hospital.

Going Home. It's not unusual to feel overwhelmed and overworked by the responsibilities that greet you (particularly if you have other children and no help).

Exhaustion. Fatigue from a strenuous labor and from too little sleep in the hospital is compounded by the rigors of caring for a newborn, and often contributes to the feeling that you aren't equal to the demands of motherhood.

A Sense of Disappointment in the Baby. He or she's so small, so red, so puffy, so unresponsive—not quite the all-smiles Ivory Snow baby you'd pictured. Resultant guilt adds to depression.

A Sense of Disappointment in the Birth and/or in Yourself. If unrealistic expectations of an idealized childbirth experience weren't realized, you may feel (unnecessarily) that you've somehow failed.

A Feeling of Anticlimax. Childbirth—the big event you'd schooled for and looked forward to—is over.

Feelings of Inadequacy. A novice mother may wonder, "Why did I have a baby if I can't take care of it?"

A Sense of Mourning for the Old You. Your carefree, possibly career-oriented, self has died (at least temporarily) with your baby's birth.

Unhappiness over Your Looks. Before you were fat and pregnant; now you're just fat. You can't stand wearing maternity clothes, but nothing else fits.

Probably the only good thing that can be said about postpartum depression is that it doesn't last very long—about 48 hours for most women. And though there's no cure other than the passage of time, there are ways of fading those baby blues:

❖ If the blues arrive at the hospital, try to have your husband bring in a special dinner for the two of you; limit visitors if their chattering grates on your nerves, have more of them if they cheer you up. If it's the hospital that's getting you down, inquire about early discharge. (See Going Home, page 384.)

❖ Fight fatigue by accepting help from others, by being less compulsive about doing things that can wait, by trying to squeeze in a nap or rest period when your baby is sleeping. Use feeding times as rest periods, nursing or bottle-feeding in bed or in a comfortable chair with your feet up.

❖ Follow the Best-Odds Nursing Diet (see page 392) to keep your strength up (minus 500 calories and three calcium servings if you're not breastfeeding). Avoid sugar (especially combined with chocolate), which can act as a depressant.

❖ Occasionally unwind with your husband over a cocktail after the baby's evening feeding, but be careful not to overdo—too much can lead to morning-after depression.

❖ Treat yourself to dinner out, if possible. If not, make believe. Order dinner in (or let your husband cook), dress up, create a restaurant ambiance with candlelight and soft music. And keep your sense of humor handy, in case the baby decides to interrupt your romantic interlude.

❖ Look good so you'll feel good. Walking around in a robe all day with unkempt hair would depress anyone. Shower before your husband leaves in the morning (or you may not have a chance again); comb your hair; put on makeup if you ordinarily wear it. Buy an attractive new outfit (washable, of course) that fits loosely now but can be belted so that it continues to fit as you lose weight.

❖ Get out of the house. Go for a walk with the baby or, if someone volunteers to sit, without the baby. Exercise helps chase away the baby blues and will help you get rid of any postpartum flab that might be adding to your depression. But don't do too much too soon.

❖ If you think your misery might like some company, get together with any new mothers you know, and share your feelings with them. If you don't have any newly delivered friends, make some. Ask your pediatrician for names of new mothers in your neighborhood, or contact women who were in your childbirth class, possibly organizing a weekly after-birth reunion. Or join a postpartum exercise class.

❖ If yours is the kind of misery that would rather be by itself, indulge in some solitude. Though depression usually feeds on itself, some experts believe that this is not true of the postpartum variety. If going out with cheerful people, or having cheerful people visit, makes you feel worse—don't do it. Don't, however, leave your husband out in the cold. Communication in the immediate postpartum period is vital for you both. (Husbands, too, are susceptible to postpartum depression, and yours may need you as much as you need him.)

Severe postpartum depression, which requires professional therapy, is extremely rare—affecting fewer than 1 in 1,000 women. If your depression persists for more than two weeks and is accompanied by sleeplessness, lack of appetite, a feeling of hopelessness and helplessness—even suicidal urges or violent or aggressive feelings toward the baby—seek counseling promptly.

"I feel terrific, and have since the moment I delivered three weeks ago. Is all this good feeling building up to one terrific case of letdown?"

It's an unfortunate fact that feeling good doesn't get the kind of attention that feeling bad does. There's no shortage of articles in magazines and newspapers, or chapters in books, about the 50% of newly delivered women who suffer from postpartum depression; but there's little or nothing written about the other 50% who feel terrific after giving birth.

Baby blues are common, but they're by no means an absolute requirement of the postpartum period. And there's no reason to believe that you're in for an emotional crash just because you've been feeling buoyant. Since the majority of baby blues cases occur within the first postpartum week, it's pretty safe to assume you've escaped them. If you'd like to play it even safer

(or if you'd like to prevent depression occurring when you wean), see the tips for fading those baby blues, above.

The fact that you're not suffering from postpartum depression, however, doesn't mean your family has escaped this problem completely. Studies show that while new fathers are unlikely to be depressed when their wives are, their risk of falling into a postpartum slump increases dramatically when the new mother is feeling great. So be sure that your husband isn't experiencing the baby blues. And if he is, use some of the tips on page 398 to help him over them. If his depression persists, or if it is so severe that it interferes with his work and other activities, then be sure that he seeks professional help.

RETURNING TO PREPREGNANCY WEIGHT AND SHAPE

"I knew I wouldn't be ready for a bikini right after delivery, but I still look six months pregnant a week later."

Though childbearing produces more rapid weight loss than the Scarsdale, Stillman, and Mayo Clinic diets combined (an average of 12 pounds at delivery), most women don't find it quite rapid enough. Particularly after they catch a glimpse of their postpartum silhouettes in the mirror—which can still look distressingly pregnant. But happily, most will be able to pack away their maternity jeans within a month or two.

Of course, how quickly you return to your prepregnant shape and weight will depend on how many pounds and inches you put on during pregnancy. Women who gained 25 pounds or so should be able to shed the weight, without dieting, by the end of the second month. Others will find that delivery won't make thighs and hips thickened by overindulgence during pregnancy magically disappear. But sticking to the Best-Odds Nursing Diet (see page 392) if they are breastfeeding (or to the Diet minus the 500 extra nursing calories and the extra calcium serving[2] if they are not) should start them on the way to slow, steady weight loss. After the first six weeks, non-nursers can go on a good, well-balanced reducing diet, such as Weight Watchers. Nursing mothers with considerable amounts of excess body fat can cut their caloric intake somewhat without cutting into milk production and also lose weight. They will usually take off any remaining excess poundage when they wean their babies.

Getting back into shape is a problem even for those women who didn't gain excess weight. No one comes out of the delivery room looking much slimmer than when they went in. Part of the reason for that protruding postpartum abdomen is the still-enlarged uterus, which will be reduced to prepregnancy size by the end of six weeks, reducing your abdominal girth in the process. (You can follow the progress of your uterus by asking the nurse or your practitioner to show you how to palpate it in your abdomen. When you can no longer feel it, it has slipped back into the pelvis.) Another reason for your bloated belly is leftover fluids, 5 pounds or so of which will flush out within a few days after delivery. But the rest of the problem is stretched-out abdominal muscles and skin, which may sag for a

lifetime unless a concerted exercise effort is made. (See Getting Back into Shape, page 408.)

BREAST MILK

"Does everything I eat, drink, or take get into my breast milk? Could any of it harm my baby?"

Feeding your baby outside the womb doesn't demand quite as Spartan an existence as feeding him or her inside did. But as long as you're breastfeeding, a certain amount of restraint in what goes into you will ensure that everything that goes into your baby is safe.

The basic fat-protein-carbohydrate composition of human milk isn't dependent on what a mother eats. If a mother doesn't eat enough calories and protein to produce milk, her body's stores will be tapped and the baby will be fed—until the stores run out. Some vitamin deficiencies in the mother's diet will, however, affect the vitamin content of her breast milk. So will excesses of some vitamins. A wide variety of substances, from medications to seasonings, can also show up in milk, with varying results.

To keep breast milk safe and healthful:

❖ Follow the Best-Odds Nursing Diet (page 392).

❖ Avoid foods to which your baby seems sensitive. Garlic, onion, cabbage, dairy products, and chocolate are common offenders, causing bothersome gas in some, though by no means all, babies. Infants with discriminating palates may also be displeased by the taste a strong seasoning may impart.

❖ Take a vitamin supplement especially formulated for pregnant and/ or lactating mothers. Do not take

---

2. It may be a good idea for women who are not nursing to continue to get adequate calcium to prevent the development of osteoporosis later in life. If necessary, take a calcium supplement to get your intake up to 1,200 mg daily.

any other vitamins without the advice of your physician.

❖ Do not smoke. Many of the toxic substances in tobacco enter the bloodstream, and eventually your milk. (Besides, smoking near the baby can cause respiratory problems for him or her and may even be associated with sudden infant death syndrome, or crib death.)

❖ Do not take any medications or recreational drugs without consulting your physician. Most drugs pass into the breast milk, and even in small doses can be harmful to a tiny infant. (Particularly dangerous are antithyroid, antihypertensive, and anticancer drugs; penicillin[3]; narcotic drugs, including heroin, methadone, and prescription painkillers; marijuana and cocaine; tranquilizers, barbiturates and sedatives; lithium; hormones, such as most birth control pills; radioactive iodine; bromides.) Often, safe substitutes can be found for a medication you must take; or perhaps a particular medication can be discontinued for the duration of nursing. (Do make sure that any doctor who prescribes a medication for you is aware that you are breastfeeding.)

❖ Avoid alcohol entirely, or have a single drink only rarely. Daily imbibing or binge drinking can make baby drowsy, depress the nervous system, and may slow motor development and reduce your milk supply.

❖ Restrict your intake of caffeine. One cup of caffeinated coffee or tea a day probably won't affect your baby. Six cups could make him or her jittery.

❖ Don't take laxatives to promote regularity (some of them will have a laxative effect on your baby); increase your fiber intake instead.

❖ Take aspirin or aspirin substitutes only with your practitioner's approval, but don't take more than the recommended dose, and don't take the drugs frequently.

❖ Avoid excessive amounts of chemicals in the foods you eat, and opt for the foods that are close to their natural state. Read labels to steer clear of foods composed largely of synthetic chemicals.[4] Avoid saccharin, since it passes into the breast milk and has been shown in animal studies to cause cancer. Aspartame, on the other hand, seems to pass into the breast milk in only small quantities and appears safe to use. But be sure the foods you consume that contain aspartame aren't full of a lot of other chemicals.

❖ Minimize your ingestion of incidental pesticides. A certain amount of pesticide residue in your diet (from produce, for example), and thus in your breast milk, is inevitable—and not proven to be harmful to a nursing infant. But though hysteria about possible breast milk contamination is unwarranted, it's prudent to keep your baby's exposure to pesticides as low as you can without giving up eating. Peel vegetables and fruits or scrub with detergent and water; eat low-fat milk products, lean meats, white-meat poultry with the skin removed, and limited amounts of organ meats. (The pesticides ingested by animals are stored in fat, skin, and possibly organs.)

❖ Avoid eating any fish that might be

---

3. Exposure to penicillin at this early age could lead to a baby developing a sensitivity, or allergy, to the drug.

4. See *What to Eat When You're Expecting* for a list of safe, unsafe, and questionable chemicals used in foods.

contaminated. (The same rules for safe fish and seafood consumption that apply to pregnant women apply to lactating women; see page 130.)

LONG-TERM CESAREAN RECOVERY

"I am just now going home, four days after a cesarean. What can I expect?"

To Need Plenty of Help. Paid help is best for the first week, but if that's not possible, ask your husband, mother, or another relative to lend a hand. It's best not to do any lifting (including the baby) or any housework, at least for the first week. If you must lift the baby, lift from waist level, so you use your arms, not your abdomen. Bend at the knees, not at the waist.

Little or No Pain. But if you do hurt, a mild pain reliever should help. Don't take medication, however, if you are breastfeeding, unless it has been approved by your doctor.

Progressive Improvement. Your scar will be sore and sensitive for a few weeks, but will improve steadily. A light dressing may protect it from irritation and you will probably be more comfortable wearing loose clothing. Occasional sensations of pulling or twitching and other brief pains in the region of the scar are a normal part of healing and will eventually subside. Itchiness may follow. The numbness of the abdomen around the scar will last longer, possibly several months. Lumpiness in the scar tissue will probably diminish (unless you tend to get that kind of scar), and the scar may turn pink or purple before it finally fades.

If pain becomes persistent, if the area around the incision turns an an-gry red, or if a brown, gray, green, or yellow discharge oozes from the wound, call your doctor. The incision may have become infected. (A small amount of clear fluid discharge may be normal, but report it to your physician anyway.)

To Wait at Least Four Weeks Before Resuming Sexual Intercourse. Depending on how your incision is healing and when your cervix returns to normal, your doctor may recommend that you wait anywhere from four to six weeks for actual intercourse (though other kinds of lovemaking are certainly permissible). See page 404 for tips on making postpartum intercourse more successful. You are, incidentally, much more likely to find resumption of intercourse comfortable than are women who delivered vaginally.

To Be Able to Start Exercising Once You Are Free of Pain. Since the muscle tone of your perineum probably hasn't been compromised, you may not need to do Kegel exercises, though they can benefit anyone. Concentrate instead on those that tighten the abdominal muscles. (See Getting Back into Shape, page 408.) Make "slow and steady" your motto; get into a program gradually and continue it daily. Expect it to take several months before you're back to your old self.

RESUMING SEXUAL RELATIONS

"My doctor says I have to wait six weeks before having sex. Friends say that isn't necessary."

It's fairly safe to assume that your doctor is more familiar with your medical condition than your friends are. And his or her restriction is probably based on what's best for you, taking into consideration the kind of labor and delivery you had, whether or not you had an episiotomy or laceration, and the speed of healing and recovery. Some practitioners, of course, apply the six-week rule routinely to all their postpartum patients, regardless of condition. If you think that's the case with your doctor and you're feeling up to making love, ask if he or she will consider bending the rule for you. This will be possible only if your cervix has healed and the lochia has stopped. And, for your own comfort, you probably will also want to wait until intercourse no longer causes discomfort in your perineal area.

Should your plea be denied, however, it's wise to follow your doctor's orders. Waiting the full six weeks can't hurt (at least not physically), while not waiting might.

LACK OF INTEREST IN MAKING LOVE

"Ever since the baby was born I just don't feel very interested in sex."

Sex takes energy, concentration, and time—all of which are in particularly short supply in the lives of new parents. Your libido—and your husband's—must regularly compete with sleepless nights, exhausting days, dirty diapers, and an endlessly demanding baby. Your body is still recuperating from the trauma of childbearing; your hormones are readjusting. Fears (of pain, of doing some damage internally, of not being the same, of becoming pregnant again too soon) may plague you. If you are breastfeeding, this may unconsciously be satisfying your sexual needs. Or making love may stimulate uncomfortable leakage of milk. All in all, it's not surprising—

and perfectly normal—if your sexual appetite, no matter how voracious it once was, is temporarily suppressed. (On the other hand, some women have strong sexual drives now, particularly in the immediate postpartum period, when there is engorgement of the genital region.)

If your problem is lack of interest, there are many ways to make making love good again. Which ones will work for you will depend on you, your husband, and your problems:

Make Time Your Ally. It takes at least six weeks for your body to heal, and sometimes much longer—especially if you had a difficult delivery or a cesarean. Your hormonal balance won't be back to normal until you start menstruating, which, if you are breastfeeding, may not be for many months. Even if the doctor's given you the go-ahead, don't feel obligated to make love if it doesn't feel good, emotionally or physically. And when you do, start slowly, possibly with cuddling and petting but no penetration.

Don't Be Discouraged by Pain. Many women are surprised and disheartened to find that postpartum intercourse can really hurt. If you've had an episiotomy or a laceration, there may be discomfort (ranging from slight to severe) for weeks, even months, after the stitches have healed. You may also have pain with intercourse, although it may be less severe, if you delivered with the perineum intact—and even if you've had a cesarean. Until the pain eases, you can try to minimize it in the ways described in Easing Back into Sex, facing page.

Find Alternative Means of Gratification. If intercourse isn't pleasurable yet, seek sexual satisfaction through mutual masturbation or oral sex. Or if you're both too pooped to pop, find pleasure in just being together. There's

Easing Back into Sex

Lubricate. Lowered hormone levels during the postpartum period (which may not rise in the nursing mother until her baby is either partially or totally weaned) can make the vagina uncomfortably dry. Use a lubricating cream, like K-Y Jelly, until your own natural secretions return.

Medicate, If Necessary. Your practitioner may prescribe an estrogen cream to lessen pain and tenderness.

Inebriate. Don't get drunk, of course (since too much alcohol can interfere with sexual enjoyment and perfor-

mance, and if you're breastfeeding can be harmful to your baby), but do feel free to enjoy a glass of wine with your husband before making love, to help both of you relax physically and emotionally. It will also dull some of your pain, plus lessen your fear of feeling it and his fear of causing it. Or use other relaxation techniques to banish fear.

Vary Positions. Side-to-side or woman-on-top positions allow more control of penetration and put less pressure on the episiotomy site. Experiment to find what works best for you.

---

absolutely nothing wrong (and everything right) about lying in bed together, cuddling, kissing, and swapping baby stories.

Keep Your Expectations Realistic. Don't expect simultaneous orgasms the first time you make love after delivery. Some usually orgasmic women don't have orgasms at all for several weeks, or even longer. With love and patience, sex will eventually be as satisfying as ever—or more so.

Readjust Your Sex Life to Dovetail with Your Life with the Baby. When your companionable two becomes a crowded three, you can no longer make love when and where you want to. Instead you'll have to either grab it when you can (if the baby is napping at 3 o'clock on Saturday afternoon, drop everything) or make a point of planning ahead. Don't feel that unspontaneous sex can't be fun. Instead, think of the advance planning as giving you the opportunity to look forward to making love (the baby will be asleep at 8—can't wait!). Accept interruptions—there will be many—with a

sense of humor, and try to start again where you left off as soon as possible. And should sex turn out to be less frequent than before, strive for quality, not quantity.

Don't Be a Perfectionist. A lot of postpartum exhaustion is natural; learning to become parents is certainly taxing. But some of it is unnecessary, often caused by trying to do too much too soon. Pack away your white gloves and forgo the dusting sometimes. Use frozen vegetables instead of fresh. Cut some dispensable corners, so that you occasionally have sufficient energy left for loving.

Communicate. A really good sexual relationship must be built on trust, understanding, and communication. If, for instance, you're too wrapped up in motherhood one night to feel sexy, don't beg off with a headache. Be honest. A husband who's been included in parenting since conception is most likely to understand. If intercourse is painful, don't be a martyr. Explain to your spouse what hurts, what feels good, what you'd rather put off until another time.

Don't Worry. Despite how you may be feeling now, you will live to love again, with as much passion and pleasure as ever. (And because shared parenthood can often bring couples closer together, you may find the flame not only rekindled, but burning brighter than before.) Worry now can only put an unnecessary damper on your sexual relationship.

BECOMING PREGNANT AGAIN

"I thought that breastfeeding was a form of birth control. Now I hear you can get pregnant while nursing, even before you start menstruating again."

How completely you can rely on nursing as a means of birth control depends on how completely devastated you would be if you became pregnant again now. If you're like most brand-new parents, tummy-to-tummy pregnancies just months apart are not your idea of perfect family planning. And if that is indeed the case, breastfeeding by itself shouldn't be relied on for contraception.

It's true that on the average, women who nurse resume normal menstrual cycles later than those who don't. In nonlactating mothers menstruation usually begins somewhere between four and eight weeks after delivery, whereas in lactating women the average is somewhere between three and four months. As usual, however, averages are deceptive. Nursing women have been known to begin menstruating as early as 6 weeks and as late as 18 months postpartum. The problem is, there's no sure way to predict when you will again begin menstruating, though several variables can influence the timing. For example, frequency of

feeding (more than three times a day seems to suppress ovulation better), duration of nursing (the longer you nurse, the greater the delay in ovulation), and whether or not feedings are being supplemented (your baby's taking bottles, solids, even water, can interfere with the ovulation-suppressing effect of nursing).

Why worry about birth control before that first menstrual period? Because the point at which you ovulate for the first time after delivery is as unpredictable as when you menstruate. Some women have a sterile first period; that is, they don't ovulate during that cycle. Others ovulate before the period, and therefore can go from pregnancy to pregnancy without ever having had a menstrual period. Since you don't know which will come first, the period or the egg, caution in the form of contraception is highly advisable. For information on choosing birth control methods, see *What to Expect the First Year.*

Of course accidents can happen. Medical science has yet to develop a method of contraception (with the possible exception of sterilization) that is 100% effective. So even if you've been using contraception— and especially if you haven't been— pregnancy is still a possibility. Unfortunately, the first symptom of pregnancy you would ordinarily look for (absence of menstruation) will not be apparent if you've been nursing and not menstruating. But because of hormonal changes (there are different sets of hormones in operation during pregnancy and lactation), your milk supply will probably diminish noticeably soon after a new pregnancy is established. You might, in addition, experience any or all of the other symptoms of pregnancy (see page 2). Of course, if you do have any suspicion that you might be pregnant, the best thing to do is to visit your practitioner as soon as possible. If you are pregnant, you can continue breastfeeding as long as you feel up to it. But you will need plenty of rest and good nutrition. And after delivery, the new baby should have nursing priority.

HAIR LOSS

"My hair seems to be falling out suddenly."

D on't order a hairpiece. This hair fall is normal, and will stop well in advance of baldness. Ordinarily the average head sheds 100 hairs a day, which are being continually replaced. During pregnancy (as when you're taking oral contraceptives), the hormonal changes keep those hairs from falling out. But the reprieve is only temporary. Those hairs are slated to go, and they will—within three to six months of delivery (or after you stop taking the Pill). Some women who are breastfeeding exclusively find that hair fall doesn't begin until they wean their baby or supplement the nursing with formula or solids.

To keep what hair you do have healthy, be sure to stay on the Best-Odds Postpartum diet, to continue your pregnancy vitamin supplement, and to treat your hair with kindness. That means shampooing only when necessary, using a conditioner to reduce the need to untangle, using a wide-toothed comb if you do have to untangle, and avoiding the application of heat (with blow dryers, curling irons, or hot rollers). It may also be a good idea to avoid further damage by postponing permanents, hair colorings, and hair relaxing treatments until your tresses seem back to normal.

Just because you lost a lot of hair following this pregnancy doesn't mean you will if there's a next time. Your body's reaction to each pregnancy, as you are sure to find out, can be very different.

TAKING TUB BATHS

"I seem to be getting a lot of contradictory advice about whether or not tub baths are all right in the postpartum period. Are they?"

A t one time, new mothers weren't permitted to set foot in a tub until at least one month after delivery, because of fear of infection from the bathwater. Today, because it's known that still bathwater does not enter the vagina, infection from bathing is no longer considered a threat. Some physicians, in fact, recommend tub baths in the hospital (when a tub is available) because they believe bathing removes lochia from the perineum—and from between the folds of the labia—more efficiently than showering. In addition, the warm water is comforting to the episiotomy site, relieves soreness and edema in the area, and soothes hemorrhoids.

Still, your doctor may prefer that you hold off on bathing until you are home, or even later. If you're eager to bathe (especially if you have no shower at home), discuss the issue with him or her. You may be able to get a dispensation.

If you do bathe during the first week or two following delivery, be sure the tub is scrubbed meticulously before it's filled. (But be sure you're not the one who does the scrubbing.) And get help getting into and out of the tub during the first few postpartum days, when you're still likely to be shaky.

EXHAUSTION

"It's nearly two months since I had the baby, but I feel more tired than ever. Could I be sick?"

M any a new mother has dragged herself into her doctor's office and complained of overwhelming chronic fatigue—convinced that she's fallen victim to some fatal malady. The nearly invariable diagnosis? A classic case of motherhood.

Rare is the mother who escapes this maternal fatigue syndrome, characterized by tiredness that never seems to ease up and an almost total lack of energy. And it's not surprising. There's no other job as emotionally and physically taxing as that of being a mother. The strain and pressures are not, as in most other jobs, limited to eight hours a day or five days a week. (And mothers don't get lunch hours or coffee breaks, either.) Motherhood for first-timers also adds the stress inherent in any new job: there's always something new to learn, mistakes to be made, problems to solve. If all this isn't enough to produce symptoms, add the energy that goes into breastfeeding, the strength sapped by toting around a rapidly growing infant and accompanying paraphernalia, and night after night of broken sleep.

Check with your doctor to be sure there is no physical cause for your exhaustion. If you get a clean bill of health, be assured that time, experience, and your baby sleeping through the night will gradually help relieve much of your fatigue. And once your body adjusts to the new demands, your energy level should pick up a bit, too. In the meantime, try the tips for relieving postpartum depression (page 398), which is closely tied to fatigue.

WHAT IT'S IMPORTANT TO KNOW: GETTING BACK INTO SHAPE

I t's one thing to look six months pregnant when you *are* six months pregnant, and quite another to look it when you've already delivered. Yet most women can expect to be wheeled out of the delivery room not much trimmer than when they were wheeled in—with a little bundle in their arms and several still around their middles. As for the pencil-thin skirts optimistically packed for the going-home trip, they're likely to stay packed, with maternity jeans the depressing substitute.

How soon after you become a new mother will you stop looking like a mother-to-be? With active exercise, that old prepregnancy figure (or a newly slender one) is only a couple of months away.

"Who needs exercise?" you may wonder. "I've been in perpetual motion since I got home from the hospital. Doesn't that count?"

Unfortunately, not much. Exhausting as it is, that kind of activity won't tighten up the perineal and abdominal muscles that have been left saggy by pregnancy. Only an exercise program will.

You can start a postpartum exercise program as early as 24 hours after delivery. But be careful not to overdo it. The following is geared for healthy women who've had uncomplicated vaginal deliveries. If you've had a surgical or a traumatic one, check with your doctor before beginning.

GROUND RULES

❖ Start each session with the least strenuous exercise, as a warm-up.

❖ Keep your exercise sessions brief and frequent, rather than doing one long session a day (this tones muscles better).

❖ If you have the time and really enjoy exercise, take a class for new mothers or buy a postpartum exercise book and develop an extensive program. If those prospects are unappealing, doing just a few simple routines regularly can also get you back into shape, especially if you gear them directly to problem areas, such as abdomen, thighs, buttocks, and so on.

❖ Do exercises slowly, and don't do a rapid series of repetitions with inadequate recovery time after each.

❖ Rest briefly between exercises (the muscle buildup occurs then, not while you are in motion).

❖ Don't do more than recommended, even if you feel you can.

❖ Quit before you feel tired: If you overdo it, you usually won't feel it until the next day—by which time you may be unable to exercise at all.

❖ Don't let mothering stop you from mothering yourself—your baby will love lying on your chest as you exercise.

❖ Do not do knee-chest exercises, full sit-ups, or double-leg lifts during the six-week postpartum period.

Kegel exercises can be done in any comfortable position. All the others are done in the basic position: lying on your back, knees bent, feet about 12 inches apart, soles flat on the floor; your head and shoulders should be supported by cushions, and your arms resting flat at your sides (see page 190). The early exercises can be done in bed; the others are best done on a harder surface, such as the floor. (An exercise mat is a good investment because the baby can try his or her first tentative crawls on it later.)

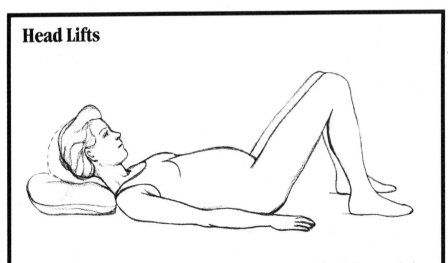

Head Lifts

Assume the basic position. Take a deep breath; then raise your head very slightly, exhaling as you do. Lower your head slowly, and inhale. Raise your head a little more each day, gradually working up to lifting your shoulders slightly off the floor. Don't try full sit-ups for at least three or four weeks—and then only if you have always had very good abdominal muscle tone.

PHASE ONE: 24 HOURS AFTER DELIVERY

Kegel Exercises. You can resume these exercises immediately after delivery (see page 190 for directions, if you haven't done them before), though you won't be able to feel yourself doing them at first. You can do them on your back in bed, while sitting up or walking, while feeding the baby or talking to friends, or in a warm bath. Work up to 25 repetitions four to six times a day and continue for the rest of your life for good pelvic health.

Deep Diaphragmatic Breathing. In the basic position, place your hands on your abdomen so you can feel it rise as you inhale slowly through your nose; tighten the abdominal muscles as you exhale slowly through your mouth. Start with just two or three deep breaths at a time, to prevent hyperventilating. (Signs that you've overdone it are dizziness or faintness, tingling, or blurred vision. See page 294 for tips on dealing with hyperventilation.)

PHASE TWO: THREE DAYS AFTER DELIVERY

Three days after you deliver, you can begin doing more serious exercises—but only if you are sure that the pair of vertical muscles of your abdominal wall (called the recti abdominis) have not separated during pregnancy. Fairly common, especially in women who have had several children, this separation (or diastasis) will get worse if you do anything even mildly strenuous before it heals. Ask your nurse or doctor about the condition of these muscles, or examine them yourself this way: As you lie in the basic position, raise your head slightly with your arms extended forward; then feel for a soft lump below your navel. Such a lump indicates a separation.

You may be able to help correct a diastasis, if you have one, with this exercise: Assume the basic position; inhale. Now cross your hands over your abdomen, using your fingers to draw the sides of your abdominal

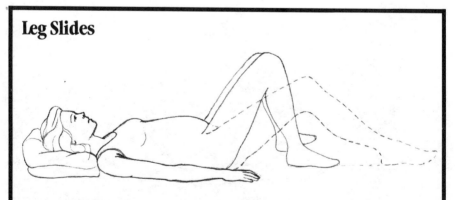

Leg Slides

Assume the basic position. Slowly extend both legs until they are flat on the floor. Slide your right foot, flat on the floor, back toward your buttocks. Keep the small of your back against the floor. Slide your leg back down. Repeat with your left foot. Start with three or four slides per side, and increase gradually until you can do a dozen or more comfortably. After three weeks, move to a modified leg lift (lifting one leg at a time slightly off the floor and lowering it again very slowly), if it is comfortable.

muscles together as you breathe out while raising your head slowly. Inhale as you lower your head slowly. Repeat three or four times, twice a day. When the separation has closed, or if you've never had one, move on to the exercises described here: Head Lifts, Leg Slides, and Pelvic Tilts.

The Pelvic Tilt (see illustration, page 191). Lie on your back in the basic position. Inhale as you press the small of your back against the floor. Then exhale, and relax. Repeat 3 or 4 times to start, increasing gradually to 12, and then 24.

PHASE THREE: AFTER YOUR POSTPARTUM CHECKUP

Now, with your practitioner's permission, you can resume a more active exercise schedule. You can gradually return to, or begin, a program that includes walking, jogging, swimming, aerobics, bicycling, or similar activities. But don't try to do too much too soon. A postpartum exercise class run by a qualified instructor may be the best way to begin.

Exercise postpartum will do more than flatten your tummy and tighten your perineum. The perineal exercises will help you avoid stress incontinence (leaking of urine), a dropping (prolapse) of pelvic organs, and sexual difficulties. Abdominal exercises will reduce the risk of backache, varicose veins, leg cramps, edema, and the formation of blood clots in the veins (thrombi), as well as improve circulation. Regular exercise will also promote healing of your traumatized uterine, abdominal, and pelvic muscles, and hasten their return to normal tone. Planned activity will also help the pregnancy- and delivery-loosened joints return to normal, and will prevent further weakening and strain. Finally, exercise can have a psychological benefit (ask any runner), improving your ability to handle stress and to relax—and minimizing the chance of postpartum blues.

20
Fathers Are Expectant, Too

Mothers- and fathers-to-be to-day share not only the joys of pregnancy, childbirth, and childrearing, but the worries as well; and the chances are good that there is considerable overlap in what concerns each member of your expectant (or newly delivered) team. Yet fathers are entitled to a few worries of their own—and to some very special reassurance, not only during the pregnancy and the birth, but in the postpartum period as well.

And so this chapter—dedicated to the equal, but often neglected, partner-in-reproduction. But it isn't intended for fathers' eyes only—any more than the rest of the book is intended only for mothers'. An expectant mother can gain some valuable insights into what her spouse is feeling, fearing, and hoping by reading this chapter; an expectant father can better understand the physical and emotional changes his wife will undergo during pregnancy, childbirth, and postpartum while at the same time better preparing himself for his own role in the unfolding drama by reading the rest of the book.

WHAT YOU MAY BE CONCERNED ABOUT

FEELING LEFT OUT

"So much attention has been focused on my wife since she became pregnant that I hardly feel I have anything to do with it."

In generations past, the male involvement in the reproductive process ended once his sperm had fertilized his wife's ovum. Fathers-to-be watched pregnancy from afar, and childbirth not at all.

Great strides have undeniably been made in the past decade for fathers' rights. But social re-education hasn't changed the fact that pregnancy takes place within a woman's body. Or the fact that some fathers are lost in what is still largely a woman's shuffle and end up feeling forgotten, left out— even jealous of their wives.

Sometimes the woman is unwittingly responsible, sometimes the man is. Either way, it's vital that the father's feelings are resolved before resentment grows and is allowed to spoil what should be one of the most wonderful experiences of *both* parents' lives. The best way to accomplish this is for you to get involved in as many aspects of your wife's pregnancy as you can:

See an Obstetrician (or Midwife). Your wife's—as often as she does, if possible. Most practitioners will encourage the husband to attend the monthly appointment. If your schedule won't permit a monthly visit, perhaps you can arrange to attend the landmark appointments (when the heartbeat will first be heard, for instance) and prenatal tests (especially the sonogram, when you can see the baby).

Act Pregnant. You don't have to show up for work in maternity clothes or start drinking a quart of milk a day. But you can do your wife's pregnancy exercise routine with her; give up junk food for nine months; quit smoking, if you're a smoker. And when someone offers you a drink, tell them, "No thanks, we're pregnant."

Get an Education. Even Harvard Ph.D.s have a lot to learn when it comes to pregnancy and childbirth. Read as many books and articles as you can. Attend childbirth classes with your wife; attend classes for fathers, if they are available in your community. Talk to friends and colleagues who've become new fathers recently.

Make Contact with Your Baby. Your wife may have the edge in getting to know the baby prenatally because it's comfortably ensconced in her uterus, but that doesn't mean that you can't start to get to know the new family member, too. Talk, read, sing to your baby frequently; he or she can hear your voice now, and will recognize it after delivery. Enjoy baby's kicks and squirms by resting your hand or your cheek on your wife's naked abdomen each night—it's a nice way to share intimacy with her, too.

Shop for a Layette. And a crib, and a stroller. Help your wife decorate the nursery. In general, become active in picking out, planning, and preparing for the baby's arrival.

Talk It Out. Your wife may be leaving you out unintentionally—she may not even be aware that you'd like to be more involved. It's very likely that she'd be as happy to make you a part of her pregnancy as you would to be a part of it.

FEAR OF SEX

"Even though the doctor has assured us that sex is safe throughout pregnancy, I often have trouble following through for fear of hurting my wife or the baby."

Never is sex more a mind-over-matter situation—for both partners—than during pregnancy. This is true particularly as gestation advances and the mind (and libido) must confront a very sizable matter: the expanding pregnant belly and its precious contents.

Fortunately, you can put your mind to rest over the matter. As vulnerable as mother and baby may seem to an anxious father contemplating intercourse, in a normally progressing low-risk pregnancy, neither one is. (There are a few caveats, particularly in the last two months, detailed in Making Love During Pregnancy, page 164.)

Not only can making love to your wife not do her any harm (assuming the caveats are observed), but because pregnancy is a time for emotional and physical closeness, it can do her a world of good. And as for your baby, though basically oblivious to the whole event, he or she may be pacified by the gentle rocking motion of intercourse and of the contracting uterus during orgasm.

MOODINESS

"Ever since we got the positive pregnancy test, my wife and I seem to be going through opposite mood swings. When she's feeling good, I'm feeling down, and vice versa."

More studies recently have been focusing on the "pregnant" father because it's becoming more and more apparent that even though he doesn't carry the fetus, he can experience many of the prenatal symptoms that are common in pregnant women. Depression, during pregnancy and postpartum, is one of those symptoms. Although in about 1 in 10 cases both parents succumb to depression at the same time, most of the time the depression occurs in just one partner at a time. This may be because signs of depression in a loved one give us the inner strength to rise above our own feelings and to become supportive.

You needn't worry about your pregnancy depression—it's common and likely to be self-limiting—but you should take steps to relieve it. Keep active and try not giving in to your down feelings; talk your feelings over with your wife (if she seems up to listening), with a friend who recently became a father, or even with your own father; avoid alcohol and other drugs, which can aggravate depression and mood swings; and prepare for the baby both mentally and practically (by participating in shopping, painting the nursery, arranging your finances, etc.). You can also try some of the other tips recommended for mothers experiencing prenatal depression (see page 104). If nothing works, and your depression deepens and begins to interfere with your work and other aspects of your life, then seek professional help—from a member of the clergy, from your physician, from a therapist, or from a psychiatrist.

IMPATIENCE WITH YOUR WIFE'S MOOD SWINGS

"I know it's my wife's hormonal changes that are making her so weepy and volatile. But I don't know how much longer I can be patient."

If patience is a virtue, you're going to have to be very virtuous for the rest of your wife's pregnancy. Although the stabilization of hormone levels by the fourth month eases the pronounced premenstrual-like weepiness and moodiness of early pregnancy, the stresses of being pregnant continue. And many women continue to be subject to sudden bursts of emotion and feelings of vulnerability right up to delivery. It doubtless won't be easy, and at times you may find it close to impossible. But there's also little doubt that your efforts will pay off. Touchiness met with understanding will dissipate faster than touchiness met with anger and frustration; shoulders offered to your wife for a 15-minute cry won't have to carry around the weight of her unvented anxiety for days at a time.

Try to keep in mind that pregnancy is *not* a permanent condition, and that the changes in your wife's emotional status are as transient as the changes in her figure.

Be aware, too, that postpartum depression can also afflict dads, and these same tips can help lift you out of the baby blues later.

SYMPATHY SYMPTOMS

"If it's my wife who's pregnant, why am I having morning sickness?"

You may well be among the estimated 11% to 65% (depending on the study) of expectant fathers who suffer from the couvade syndrome during their wives' pregnancies. The symptoms of couvade (which comes from the French for "to hatch") most often appear in the third month and again at delivery, and can mimic virtually all the normal symptoms of pregnancy—including nausea and vomiting, abdominal pain, appetite changes, weight gain, food cravings, constipation, leg cramps, dizziness, fatigue, and mood swings.

Many theories have been suggested to explain couvade—all, some, or none of which may be appropriate to you: sympathy for and identification with the pregnant wife; jealousy over being left out, and a resultant desire for attention; guilt over being responsible for putting the wife in such an uncomfortable situation; stress from living with a woman who's become irritable, moody, and possibly off-limits sexually; and anxiety over the impending addition to the family.

Of course your symptoms could also indicate illness, so it's a good idea to see a doctor. But should an examination show no physical problem, couvade is a likely diagnosis. The underlying cause, if you can identify it, may offer a clue to the cure. For instance, if the cause is jealousy, becoming more involved in your wife's pregnancy may relieve your morning sickness. Or if it's anxiety over handling a newborn for the first time, taking a course in infant care, reading a copy of *What to Expect the First Year*, or spending some time with a friend's baby might prove helpful.

Even if you can't put your finger on any one cause for your symptoms, talking out your feelings about pregnancy, childbirth, and parenthood with your wife may alleviate your sympathy pains. So might discussing them with other expectant parents in your childbirth class. Should none of this help, be assured that your reactions are normal, and that all symptoms that don't go away during pregnancy will disappear soon after delivery.

Equally normal, of course, is the father who doesn't have a sick day during his wife's pregnancy. Not suffering from morning sickness or not putting on weight doesn't mean an expectant father doesn't empathize and identify with his wife.

ANXIETY OVER YOUR WIFE'S HEALTH

"I know pregnancy and childbirth are safe today, yet I still can't stop worrying that something will happen to my wife."

There's something undeniably vulnerable about a pregnant woman —and something very natural about your desire, as a loving husband, to want to protect your wife from any possible harm. But you can relax. Your wife is in virtually no danger. Women very, very rarely die as a result of pregnancy or childbirth anymore— and the vast majority of those who do haven't had the benefits of prenatal care or adequate nourishment.

But even though pregnancy doesn't pose a serious physical threat to your wife, you can help make it a safer and more comfortable experience for her: by making sure she gets the best medical care possible and that she eats the best possible diet (see Chapter 4); by letting her get extra rest while you do the laundry, make dinner, or clean the house; and by giving her the kind of emotional support she can't get from anyone else (no matter how far obstetrical science advances, pregnant women will always be *emotionally* vulnerable).

ANXIETY OVER THE BABY'S HEALTH

"I'm so afraid that something will be wrong with the baby, I can't even sleep at night."

Mothers-to-be by no means hold a corner on the worry market. And like almost every expectant mother, virtually every expectant father worries about his unborn baby's health and well-being. Happily, nearly all such worry is needless. The odds that your baby will be born both alive and completely normal are overwhelming—far better than was the case in previous generations.

Happily, too, you don't have to just sit back and hope for the best. You can actually take some steps to help ensure your baby's good health:

❖ Be sure your wife gets good medical care from the very beginning of her pregnancy; be sure she keeps all her prenatal appointments and follows her practitioner's orders.

❖ Encourage her to follow the Best-Odds Diet, which will significantly better the odds of having a healthy baby. If you follow it with her, not only will she be more likely to stay faithful to it, but you'll earn the added benefit of better health yourself.

❖ Make certain that she abstains from alcohol, drugs, and tobacco. Research shows you can best help her do this by abstaining yourself, at least when you are with her. If you think this is a big sacrifice, consider all the sacrifices she's making to have your baby.

❖ Reduce both physical and emotional stress in her life as much as possible. Help around the house, take over some of the chores that have traditionally been hers, encourage her to reduce her work load if her life is too frantic. If your social calendar is usually filled to overflowing, see that it's cut back and that more evenings are spent at home relaxing. If they work for both of you, try doing some relaxation exercises (see page 114) together.

❖ Become familiar with the signs of possible trouble in pregnancy (see page 117), and later in the postpartum period (page 381). If your wife seems to be experiencing any of these, make sure that the appropriate action is taken promptly. If necessary, make the call to her doctor or take her to the emergency room. She may be too embarrassed or too sick to take the needed steps herself.

❖ Share your fears with your wife, and let her share hers with you. This will serve to unburden you both, or at least make your burden of worries easier to carry.

Of course, even the most reassuring statistics and the best preventive measures probably won't be able to banish all your worries; only the birth of a healthy baby will do that. But knowing you're doing all you can toward that important end will make the waiting—and the sleeping—a little easier.

ANXIETY OVER LIFE CHANGES

"Ever since I saw him on a sonogram, I've

been looking forward to our son's birth. But I've also been worrying about whether I'll like being a father."

You and probably every first-time father-to-be in history. At least as much, and possibly even more, than the expectant mother, the expectant father worries about impending parenthood and about the effect it will have on his life. The most common areas of concern include:

Can I Afford a Larger Family? Especially today, when childrearing costs are going through the roof (as are the costs of maintaining or enlarging that roof), many fathers-to-be lose sleep over this very legitimate question. But once the baby comes, they often find that the alteration of priorities makes available the money that's needed for the newborn. Opting for breastfeeding over bottle-feeding if that's possible, accepting all hand-me-downs that are offered (new clothes start to look like hand-me-downs after a few spitting-up episodes, anyway), letting friends and family know which gifts you really need rather than allowing them to fill baby's shelves with silver spoons and other dust-gatherers, can all help reduce the cost of caring for the new arrival. If the new mother is planning not to go back to her job right away and this concerns you from a financial standpoint, recognize that weighed against the costs of quality child care, a business wardrobe, and commuting, the amount of income lost may really be minimal.

Will I Be a Good Father? Few people are born good fathers (or mothers, for that matter). They learn to meet the challenge in time through on-the-job training, persistence, and love. But if you feel you'll be more comfortable with the tasks at hand if you're formally prepared, by all means take a parenting class—if one is available in

your area—to learn how to diaper, bathe, feed, hold, dress, and play with your baby. If a class isn't available, or if you have an unquenchable thirst for such preparation, dive into a pile of childcare books.

How Will We Divide the Child Care? This wasn't an issue for fathers a generation or two ago, when child care was widely considered woman's work. But most of today's fathers are aware, to some degree, that parenting is a two-person job (at least when there are two parents), although they're not exactly sure what the division of labor should be. Don't wait until baby needs his first midnight diaper change or his first bath to decide this question. Start negotiating now. Some details may change once you really start operating as parents (she committed to the diaper changes but you turn out to be more proficient at it), but exploring the options in theory now will make you feel more confident about how baby care is going to work in practice later.

Will We Have to Give Up Our Social Lives? You won't have to give up your social life entirely after baby is born, but you should expect it to change somewhat—at least if both of you plan to be active participants in parenting. A new baby does, and should, take center stage, pushing some old lifestyle habits at least temporarily aside. Parties, movies, and shows may have to be squeezed in between feedings; dinners for two in your favorite restaurant may come less frequently, with more meals being taken in "family" restaurants that tolerate squirming infants. Your taste in friends may change, too; couples without children may suddenly have little in common with you and you may start gravitating toward other stroller-pushers for empathetic companionship.

Will Our Husband-Wife Relationship Change? Every set of new parents finds that their relationship undergoes some change after childbirth. And anticipating this change during pregnancy is an important first step in dealing with it postpartum. No longer will being alone together be as simple as closing the blinds and taking the phone off the hook; from the moment baby comes home from the hospital, spontaneous intimacy and complete privacy will be precious, often unattainable, commodities. Romance may have to be planned (for the two hours grandma's taken him to the park, for instance) rather than spur of the moment, and interruptions may be the rule (you can't take a baby off the hook). But as long as you both take the trouble to make time for each other—whether that means skipping your favorite television show so that you can share a late dinner after baby's in bed, or giving up Saturday golf with the guys so you can make love during baby's morning nap—your relationship will weather the changes well. Many couples, in fact, find that becoming a threesome ultimately deepens; strengthens; and improves their twosome. (For more tips on nurturing your relationship as you nurture your baby, see *What to Expect the First Year.*)

YOUR WIFE'S LOOKS

"As petty as this might seem, I'm afraid my wife's going to get fat and flabby during pregnancy, and stay that way afterward."

If it were in your wife's obstetrical interest to gain 50 pounds with pregnancy, you (and the countless other expectant husbands who share your "petty" concern) would have no option, of course, but to accept fat and flab as the price of a healthy baby.

But such calories-are-no-object weight gains just aren't medically justifiable —and can, in fact, lead to unnecessary complications during both pregnancy and delivery. A moderate, steady, carefully monitored weight increase of between 25 and 35 pounds, gained on a diet of highly nutritious food, gives your baby the best odds for healthy development and safe delivery—and your wife the speediest return to slenderness after childbirth. (See the Best-Odds Diet, page 80; Weight Gain, page 147).

Sticking to a rigid diet even for two weeks isn't easy. Sticking to one for nine months can be close to impossible, unless the dieter has the support, understanding, and assistance of those close to her. In the case of your wife, that's you. Not only do many husbands fail to provide their wives with that help, they may unwittingly sabotage their efforts. Husbands have probably done more to undermine their wives' diets than Hershey's and Sara Lee put together—either by bringing temptation into the house, ordering it in restaurants, or even offering it directly to their wives ("Come on—one bite won't hurt!").

With the following tips, you'll be able to become your wife's best ally in her campaign to gain weight moderately and eat sensibly during pregnancy—while protecting your own selfish interests (a slim wife):

Lead Your Wife Not into Temptation. If you must indulge in dietary indiscretion, do so out of your home and away from your wife. You can't expect her to live happily on broiled meats, steamed vegetables, and fresh fruit while you gorge on burgers, fries, and Heavenly Hash ice cream beside her.

Practice What You Preach to Her. What's good for the goose and the gosling is good for the gander, too. Your staying close to the Best-Odds

Diet (recognizing that you don't need all that protein or calcium) will not only support your wife, but probably will benefit your health as well.

Don't Be Too Preachy. If she slips, nagging will only help her to fall faster and farther. Remind, don't remonstrate. Prod her conscience, don't try to become it. Signal her quietly when in public, rather than making a pointed announcement to all within earshot about her ordering her chicken breaded and fried. Most important, do it with a sense of humor and a lot of love.

Accentuate the Positive. Nothing will undermine her willpower like a faltering ego. So make a point of building her up, admiring her new pregnant shape, commenting often on how pregnancy becomes her.

Exercise with Her. It's much more fun for two to tango—or to follow a pregnancy exercise program. Proper exercise during pregnancy is important not only for keeping your wife (and you) trim, but also for getting her in good shape for labor and delivery.

FALLING APART DURING LABOR

"I'm afraid I'll faint or become ill during the delivery."

Few fathers enter the delivery room without fear. Even obstetricians who've assisted at births of thousands of other people's babies can experience a sudden loss of self-confidence when confronted with their own baby's delivery.

Yet very few of these fears—of freezing, falling apart, fainting, or becoming sick to the stomach while watching the delivery—are ever realized. And though being prepared for the birth (by taking childbirth education classes, for instance) generally makes the experience more satisfying, even most unprepared fathers come through labor and delivery better than they'd thought they would. One study of fathers who attended their babies' births with no previous preparation found that though 70% expected that the delivery would be a frightening, unpleasant, and negative experience, all described it afterward in highly positive terms.

But like anything new and unfamiliar, childbirth becomes less frightening and intimidating if you know what to expect. So become an expert on the subject. Read the entire chapter on labor and delivery, beginning on page 288. Attend childbirth education classes, watching the labor and delivery films with your eyes open. Visit the hospital ahead of time so that you'll be acquainted with the technology that's used in labor and delivery rooms. Talk to friends who have recently become first-time parents. You will probably find they had the same anxieties beforehand but came through feeling terrific.

Though it's important to get an education, it's also important to remember that childbirth isn't the final exam in your childbirth education course. Don't feel that you must perform perfectly (as some women feel obligated to) at the delivery. Nurses and doctors won't be evaluating your every move or comparing you to the husband next door. More important, neither will your wife. She won't care if you forget every coaching technique you learned in class. Your being beside her, holding her hand, urging her on, providing the comfort of a familiar face and touch, will do her more good than having Drs. Lamaze, Bradley, and Dick-Reade themselves at her bedside.

"I would really rather not be at the birth, but I feel pressured to be there."

Just because it's currently in vogue in the birthing business for fathers to attend births doesn't mean it's mandatory. Studies have shown that fathers who don't attend births don't have less meaningful relationships with their offspring than fathers who do; just as fathers who don't bond with their babies immediately after birth don't seem automatically to become less loving parents. What's important is that you do what's right for you and your wife. If it doesn't feel right for you to attend the delivery, for whatever reason, you would probably do more harm than good to all concerned by being there. Ignore those who try to pressure you into a decision that would be wrong for you. Remember, more generations of fathers *haven't* seen their babies born than *have*—with no ill effects.

However, that's not to say that attending the birth of your child is not a worthwhile experience, or one you should forgo without careful consideration. Though it's important that you not let anyone else make up your mind for you, it's equally important that you not make up—and close—your mind until the last minute. Go through all the preparations: accompany your wife on her prenatal visits, take childbirth classes, do extensive reading. Many once-hesitant fathers find that familiarity with labor and delivery breeds a new perspective, which allows them to feel comfortable enough with childbirth to attend and participate fully.

Others, however, still end up deciding that being at the birth would be counterproductive for themselves and their spouses. Still others decide to give labor a try but find, sometime before or during delivery, that they'd rather step outside. All should feel free to follow their instincts, with the reassurance that doing so won't reflect in any way on their capacity for fathering.

"My wife is having a planned cesarean. Hospital regulations won't allow me to be there, and I'm afraid that our new family won't get off to the best start."

If you made the decision to be at the birth only to discover that the decision wasn't yours to make (as in the case of a cesarean in a hospital that doesn't permit husbands to attend), don't give up without a civilized fight. With the support of your wife's obstetrician (if such support is forthcoming), try first to persuade hospital officials to bend—or even change—the regulations. (It may help to remind them that a majority of hospitals now allow fathers to be present at non-emergency surgical deliveries.) If your campaign is unsuccessful (or if a hasty delivery precludes your presence), you have every right to be disappointed. But you have no right to let that disappointment taint the joy that should surround the birth of your child. Your not being at the birth can threaten your relationship with your baby only if you let it, by harboring feelings of guilt, resentment, or frustration.

BONDING

"My wife had a last-minute cesarean and I wasn't allowed to be with her. I didn't hold the baby for 24 hours and I'm afraid I didn't bond with him."

Until the 1960s, few fathers ever witnessed the birth of their children, and since the word "bonding" originated only in the 1970s, none were ever even aware that the possibility of bonding with their offspring existed. But such a lack of enlightenment didn't stop generations of loving father-son and father-daughter relationships from developing. Conversely, every father who attends his child's birth and is allowed to hold him or her immediately isn't automatically guaranteed a lifetime of closeness with his offspring.

Being with your wife during delivery is ideal, and being deprived of that opportunity is reason for disappointment—particularly if you spent months training together for childbirth. But it's no reason to expect a less than fulfilling relationship with your baby. What really bonds you with your baby is daily loving contact—changing diapers, giving baths, feeding, cuddling, lullabying. Your child will never know that you didn't share in the moment of birth, but will know if you aren't there when he or she needs you from then on.

EXCLUSION DURING BREASTFEEDING

"My wife is breastfeeding our son. There's a closeness between them that I can't seem to share, and I feel left out."

There are certain immutable biological aspects of parenting that exclude the father: he can't be pregnant, he can't labor and deliver, and he can't breastfeed. But, as millions of new fathers discover each year, a man's natural physical limitations don't have to relegate him to spectator status. You can share in nearly all the joys, expectations, trials, and tribulations of your wife's pregnancy, labor, and delivery—from the first kick to the last push—as an active, supportive participant. And though you'll never be able to put your baby to the breast (at least not with the kind of results the baby's looking for), you *can* share in the feeding process:

Be Your Baby's Supplementary Feeder. There's more than one way to feed a baby. And though you can't nurse, you can be the one to give any supplementary bottles. Not only will it give your wife a break (whether in the middle of the night or in the middle of dinner), it will give you extra opportunities for closeness with your baby. Don't waste the opportunity by propping the bottle up to the baby's mouth. Strike a nursing position, with the bottle where your wife's breast would be and your baby snuggled close to you.

Don't Sleep Through the Night Until Your Baby Does. Sharing in the joys of feeding also means sharing in the sleepless nights. Even if you're not giving supplementary bottles, you can become a part of nighttime feeding rituals. You can be the one to take the baby out of the crib, do any necessary diaper changing, deliver him for his feeding, and return him to bed once he has fallen asleep again.

Watch in Wonder, and Appreciate. There can be enormous satisfaction in simply watching the miracle of breastfeeding—as there is in watching the miracle of birth. Instead of feeling left out, feel privileged to be a witness to the love that passes between your wife and your baby as they nurse.

Participate in All Other Daily Rituals. Nursing is the *only* daily chore limited to mothers. And chances are that if you make at least one other chore your responsibility (or as many as possible) you'll be too busy to be jealous.

FEELING UNSEXY AFTER DELIVERY

"The delivery was absolutely miraculous to watch. But seeing our baby come out

of my wife's vagina seems to have turned me off sexually."

Human sexual response, compared to that of other animals, is extremely delicate. It's at the mercy not only of the body but of the mind as well. And the mind can, at times, play merciless havoc with it. One of those times, as you probably already know, is during pregnancy. Another, as you seem to be discovering, is during the postpartum period.

It's very possible that the cause of your sudden sexual ambivalence has nothing to do with having seen your baby delivered. Most brand-new fathers find both the spirit and the flesh somewhat less willing after delivery (although there's nothing abnormal about those who don't), for many very understandable reasons: fatigue, especially if the baby still isn't sleeping through the night; uneasiness about having a third person in your home; fear that he or she will awake crying at the first caress (particularly if the baby is sharing your room); concern that you may hurt your wife by having intercourse before her body is thoroughly healed; and finally, a general physical and mental preoccupation with your newborn, which sensibly concentrates your energies where they are most needed at this stage of your lives.

In other words, it's probably just as well that you aren't feeling sexually motivated, particularly if your wife (like many women in the immediate postpartum period) isn't feeling emotionally or physically up to it either. Just how long it will take for your interest, and hers, to return is impossible to predict. As with all matters sexual, there is a wide range of what is "normal." For some couples, desire will precede even the doctor's go-ahead at six weeks. For others, six months can pass before l'amour and le bébé begin to coexist harmoniously in

the same home. (Some women find desire lacking until they stop breastfeeding, but that doesn't mean they can't enjoy the intimacy of intercourse with the man they love.)

Some fathers, even if they've been prepared for the childbirth experience, do come out of it feeling that their "territory" has been "violated," that the special place that had been meant for loving has suddenly taken on a practical purpose. But as the days pass, that feeling usually does too. The father begins to realize that the vagina has two functions, equally important and miraculous. Neither excludes the other, and in fact they are very much interconnected. He also comes to recognize that the vagina is a vehicle for childbirth only briefly, while it is a source of pleasure for himself and his wife for a lifetime.

If the sexual urge doesn't return and its absence begins to cause tension, professional counseling is probably needed.

"Before the baby, my wife's breasts were a focus of sexual pleasure—for both of us. Now that she's breastfeeding, they seem too functional to be sexy."

Like the vagina, breasts were designed to serve both a practical and a sexual purpose (which, from a strictly procreative standpoint, is also practical). And though these purposes aren't mutually exclusive in the long run, they can conflict temporarily during lactation.

Some couples find breastfeeding a sexual turn-on. Others, for esthetic reasons (leaking milk, for instance) or because they feel uncomfortable about using the baby's source of nourishment for their sexual pleasure, find it a very definite turn-off.

Whatever turns you on—or off—is what is normal for you. If you feel that your wife's breasts are too functional to be sexy now, don't try to force yourself to feel otherwise. Leave them out of sexual foreplay for now, with the reassurance that you will feel differently once the baby has been weaned. Be sure, however, to be open and honest with your wife; taking a sudden, unexplained hands-off approach to her breasts could leave her feeling unappealing. Be careful, also, not to harbor any resentment against the baby for using "your" breasts; try to think of nursing as a temporary "loan" instead.

21
Preparing for the Next Baby

In the best of all possible worlds, we would be able to plan life to our precise specifications. In the real world, where most of us live, the best-laid plans often give way to the unexpected twists and turns of fate, over which we have precious little control—leaving us to accept, and to make the best of, what comes our way.

In the best of all possible pregnancies, we would know in advance when we would conceive and could make all the changes and adjustments in our lifestyle to help ensure that our baby has the best of all possible odds of being born alive and well. Such advance planning is a luxury that many women (because of menstrual irregularity and/or the frailties of contraception) may never be able to indulge in. And as has been stressed throughout this book, what a woman does before she realizes she's pregnant (a few drinks, a few dietary indiscretions, a dental x-ray) ordinarily does little to affect her baby's odds. Few women act pregnant from the moment of conception, and yet the vast majority give birth to normal, healthy babies.

But it would be remiss not to outline a plan for the best of all possible pregnancies—because the possibility does exist for an increasing number of women, as family planning techniques become more reliable. The plan is appropriate whether you're already in the process of trying to conceive or you're just thinking ahead. Although it's never too late to start taking care of your body, it's also never too early. And in fact, your good prepregnancy care will benefit not only your own children but your children's children. Act now, and:

Get a Thorough Physical. Both you and your husband should see your internist or family doctor. An exam will pick up any problems that need to be corrected beforehand, or that will need to be monitored during pregnancy. Also take care of allergy shots, minor elective surgery, and anything else medical—major or minor—that you've been putting off. (If you start allergy desensitization now, you will probably be able to continue once you conceive.)

See Your Dentist. Make an appointment for a thorough examination and cleaning. Have any necessary work, including x-rays, fillings, and dental or periodontal surgery, completed now.

Select a Practitioner—and Have a Pre-pregnancy Exam. It's easier to choose a practitioner now, in an unhurried manner, than when that first prenatal checkup is hanging over your head. (See Chapter 1 for your options.) Even if you think you might like to use a certified nurse-midwife, you should still have a gynecologist or family physician whose medical opinion you respect perform this examination to screen your planned pregnancy for high-risk potential. If your history and/or the physical findings suggest such potential, you will need the care of an obstetrician or even a maternal-fetal medicine subspecialist during your pregnancy. See page 8 for tips on choosing a practitioner.

Correct any Gynecological or Other Health Problems. Now is the time to be checked and/or treated for conditions that might interfere with pregnancy, such as polyps, cysts, benign tumors, an over- or underactive thyroid, endometriosis, or recurrent urinary tract infections. If you know, or suspect, that your mother took diethylstilbestrol (DES) when she was pregnant with you, tell the doctor, so your reproductive organs can be carefully examined—with colposcopy (which allows close visual examination of vagina and cervix) if necessary. If you've had a previous pregnancy problem, such as a miscarriage or premature delivery, discuss the measures that can be taken to head off a repeat. Even if you're sure you couldn't have a sexually transmitted disease, ask for tests for syphilis, gonorrhea, chlamydia, and herpes. Get treatment, if needed. If it is appropriate, have a test for HIV (the AIDS virus), but be sure to arrange for counseling in the unlikely event the results are positive.

Other tests that may be recommended before you conceive include hemoglobin or hematocrit (to test for anemia); Rh (to see if you are positive or negative); urine (to check for protein or sugar); TB skin test (if you live in a high-incidence area); hepatitis B (if you are in a high-risk category, such as a health care worker); possibly, cytomegalovirus and varicella antibody titer (to determine whether or not you are immune to CMV and chicken pox). If a test shows a medical problem, make certain that you get appropriate treatment before you try to conceive.

If you have a cat or regularly eat raw or rare meat or drink unpasteurized milk, a toxoplasmosis antibody titer may also be recommended. If you are found to be immune, you needn't worry about this problem now or during your pregnancy. If you're not, start taking the precautions on page 65 now.

Start Keeping Track. Your chances of conceiving when you want to will be much greater if you have intercourse during the fertile part of your cycle. Knowing exactly when you conceived will also make establishing an estimated date of delivery easier. To keep track, note the first day of each menstrual period on a handy calendar or diary; also try to note when you ovulate. Ovulation generally occurs at the midpoint of the cycle (on the 14th day of a 28 day cycle, for instance), but is less easy to predict in women with irregular cycles. The physical signs of ovulation are readily apparent to some women, more elusive to others (your basal body temperature, taken first thing in the morning, reaches its low point of the month then abruptly rises; your vaginal mucus is clear, jelly-like, and can be pulled into strings; your normally pink cervix turns bluish; and you may experience mittelshmerz—a brief period of pain on one side of your back or the other). If you're among the latter, appear to be ovulating irregularly, or are having trouble conceiving, home ovulation predictor kits are available to help you pinpoint ovulation; check with your practitioner for a recommendation.

Update Immunizations. If you haven't had a tetanus shot in the past ten years, have one now. You should also be sure you are immune to rubella (German measles), either through having had the disease or through vaccination. Ask your doctor for the appropriate blood test before you conceive. If you turn out not to be immune, you should get immunized and then wait three months before attempting to conceive (but don't panic if you accidentally conceive earlier—any risk is purely theoretical; see page 313). If you have never been immunized for measles and haven't had the disease or if you are at high risk for hepatitis B, immunization may be recommended now.

Have a Genetic Screening. If either of you has any genetic disorder (for example cystic fibrosis, Down synrome, muscular dystrophy, PKU, spina bifida, or other birth defects) in your personal history or among blood relatives, see a genetic counselor or a maternal-fetal medicine subspecialist. You should also be tested for any genetic disease common to your ethnic background: Tay-Sachs disease if either of you is of Jewish-European (Ashkenazi) or French Canadian descent; sickle-cell trait if you are of African descent; one of the thalassemias if you are of Greek, Italian, Southeast Asian, or Philippino origin. Previous obstetrical difficulties (such as two or more miscarriages, a stillbirth, a long period of infertility, or a child with a birth defect) or being married to a cousin or other blood relative are also reasons to seek genetic counseling.

Evaluate Your Birth Control Method. If you are using a method of birth control that might present some risk (however slight) to a future pregnancy, change it before you start trying to conceive. Birth control pills should be discontinued several months before conception, if possible, to allow your reproductive

system to go through at least two normal cycles before you start making a baby. The IUD should be removed before you begin trying. Since the risks of spermicides are as yet unclear, playing it extra safe means discontinuing their use (alone or with a diaphragm or condom) one month to six weeks before you want to become pregnant. The birth control method to switch to for the interim: the condom (used with care and without spermicide).

Get Any Other Medical Condition Under Control. If you have diabetes, asthma, a heart condition, or any other chronic illness, be sure that you have your doctor's okay to become pregnant, that your condition is under control before you conceive, and that you start taking optimum care of yourself now (see Chapter 16). If you were a PKU baby (ask your mother if you aren't sure, or check your medical records), then begin a phenylalanine-free diet (distasteful as it may be) before conceiving (see page 336) and continue it through pregnancy.

Improve Your Diet. First of all, be sure you are getting enough folic acid. Studies show that inadequate quantities of the vitamin in a woman's diet, even before she conceives, can lead to defects of the neural tube in developing infants. Folic acid is found in whole grains and green leafy vegetables. It is now, by law, also added to most refined grains. Also start eliminating junk food and refined sugars from your diet, and increase whole grains, fruits, and vegetables (especially green leafies and yellows). Use the Best-Odds Diet, page 80, for a good basic food plan, but you will need only three calcium and two protein servings daily until you conceive.

If you have any unusual dietary habits (such as a taste for laundry starch or clay), suffer or have suffered from an eating disorder (such as anorexia nervosa or bulimia), or are on a special diet (macrobiotic, diabetic, or any other), inform your practitioner.

Get as Close to Your Ideal Weight as Possible. Add or cut calories as needed. Any weight changes, however, should be achieved sensibly, using the Best-Odds Diet, even if it means putting off conception for another couple of months. Strenuous dieting can result in a nutritional deficit—not good for your pregnancy. If you've been on a crash diet recently, give your body a few months to get your body back into balance before you try to conceive.

Improve Your Husband's Diet. The better your husband's nutrition, the healthier his sperm. His diet should mirror your prepregnancy diet, with caloric intake adjusted to accommodate his weight and activity. If he's a diabetic, he should get his blood sugar under control.

Take a Vitamin-Mineral Supplement Formulated for Pregnancy. Although many grains are now fortified with folic acid, it's still a good idea to take a pregnancy supplement containing the vitamin while you are trying to conceive. If you are taking other nutritional supplements, however, stop before conceiving, since excesses of certain nutrients can be hazardous.

Shape Up, But Keep Cool. An exercise program will tone and strengthen your muscles in preparation for the challenging tasks of carrying and delivering your baby-to-be. It will also help you take off excess weight. Avoid becoming overheated during workouts, however, when you begin trying to conceive, since this can lead to a potentially harmful increase in body temperature. Avoid hot tubs and direct exposure to heating pads and electric blankets for the same reason. Keep in mind, too, that while exercise is good

for you, you *can* get too much of a good thing. Excessive exercise can interfere with ovulation—and if you don't ovulate, you can't conceive.

Avoid Unnecessary Exposure to Radiation. If x-rays are necessary for medical reasons, be sure that your reproductive organs are protected (unless they are being targeted) and that the lowest doses possible are used. Once you start trying to conceive, keep in mind that you might have succeeded. Inform any physician treating you with radiation, or technicians taking x-rays, that you could be pregnant, and ask them to take all necessary precautions. Only radiation exposure that is absolutely required for your health or the baby's should be permitted (see page 66).

Avoid Excessive Exposure to Hazardous Chemicals. Some (though far from all) chemicals, usually only in very large doses, are potentially harmful to your husband's sperm and your ova before conception, and later to a developing embryo or fetus. Though the risk is in most cases slight, both of you should play it safe by avoiding potentially hazardous exposure on the job. Special care should be taken in certain fields (medicine and dentistry, art, photography, transportation, farming and landscaping, construction, hairdressing and cosmetology, dry cleaning, and some factory work). Contact the Occupational Safety and Health Administration for the latest information on job safety and pregnancy; also see page 72. In some cases it may be wise to change jobs or to take special precautions before trying to conceive.

Because elevated lead levels when you conceive could pose problems for your baby, you should be tested if you have been exposed to lead in the workplace or elsewhere, such as in your water supply. If your blood levels are high, experts recommend chelation therapy to remove the lead from

LAST BUT NOT LEAST

the blood, and then reduced exposure before conception is attempted. Avoid, too, excessive exposure to household toxins (see page 67).

Cut Back on Caffeine. Moderating (and gradually cutting out, if possible) your intake of coffee, tea, and colas now will spare you the symptoms of withdrawal once you're pregnant. In addition, there's some recent evidence that women who consume more than one cup of brewed coffee or the equivalent in other caffeinated beverages (tea or soft drinks containing caffeine) daily are less likely to become pregnant. Whether this is because caffeine has a biological effect on fertility or because caffeine use is often part of the type of high-stress lifestyle that can compromise a couple's chances of conceiving is unclear. Regardless, it's a good idea to cut down.

Limit Your Intake of Over-the-Counter Drugs. Since most nonprescription medications carry warnings about use in pregnancy, consult your physician before taking them once you start trying to conceive. Don't douche without a doctor's Rx, since douching can interfere with getting pregnant.

Check the Safety of Any Prescripton Drugs You Take. Certain medications used in the treatment of chronic illnesses or disorders are linked with the development of birth defects; if you're taking any medication now, consult with your physician. Potentially harmful drugs should be discontinued at least a month (for some, three to six months) before you begin trying to have a baby, with a safe alternative therapy standing in until pregnancy is over (or the baby is weaned if the drug also poses a threat to the nursing infant).

Avoid Illicit Drugs. All so-called recreational drugs, including cocaine, crack, marijuana, and heroin, can be dangerous to your pregnancy. To vary-

ing degrees they can prevent your conceiving, and then if you do succeed, they are potentially harmful to the fetus and also increase the risks of miscarriage, prematurity, and stillbirths. If you use drugs, casually or regularly, stop all use immediately. If you can't stop, seek help (see Appendix) before trying to conceive.

Get Your Husband to Give Up Illicit Drugs and Reduce Alcohol Consumption. All the answers are not yet in, but research is beginning to show that the use of drugs (including excessive amounts of alcohol) by the father prior to conception could prevent pregnancy or lead to a poor pregnancy outcome. The mechanisms aren't clear, but drugs can apparently damage sperm as well as reduce their number, can alter testicular function and reduce testosterone levels, and are excreted in the semen. If your husband is unable to quit, he should seek help through Alcoholics Anonymous or in- or outpatient treatment.

Cut Down on Alcohol Consumption. Although a daily drink will not be harmful in your pregnancy-preparation phase, avoid heavy drinking, which can interfere with fertility by disrupting your menstrual cycle. Once you start trying to conceive, stop drinking altogether (see page 52).

Quit Smoking. Both of you. Tobacco not only is hazardous to your pregnancy (see page 54) and increases the risk of SIDS and possibly cancer in the baby, but it can also reduce fertility in both men and women, foiling attempts to conceive. A smoke-free environment is one of the best pre-birthday gifts you can give your baby.

Relax. This is perhaps the most important of all. Getting tense and uptight about conception could prevent you from conceiving at all.

Appendix

COMMON TESTS DURING PREGNANCY*

TEST AND WHEN PERFORMED	PROCEDURE	REASON
Blood type; first visit, unless already known from previous pregnancy or test	Examination of blood drawn from your arm.	To determine blood and Rh type in case blood transfusion is needed at some point, and to be prepared for the possibility of Rh incompatibility (see page 37). Testing will also be done for the Kell factor; Kell factor incompatibility is much rarer.
Sugar (glucose) in the urine; at each visit	A specially treated stick, dipped in a specimen of your urine, shows presence of sugar.	While an occasional increase in sugar is normal in pregnancy (see page 152), persistent high levels could indicate hyperglycemia; further tests will determine if gestational diabetes is present, requiring special diet and care.
Albumin (protein) in the urine; at each visit	A special strip, dipped in a urine specimen, shows presence of albumin (protein).	High albumin levels could be related to toxemia; if routine test shows increase, a 24-hour test may be ordered.
Bacteria in urine; first visit	Urine specimen is examined in lab.	Bacteria in urine could indicate susceptibility to infection; treatment may be initiated.

*Your practitioner may omit some of these tests or add others, depending upon your condition and his or her professional opinion. Do not use self-tests without your doctor's okay; do not use a test that is not approved by the FDA.

TEST AND WHEN PERFORMED	PROCEDURE	REASON
Blood pressure; at each visit	Blood pressure is measured with cuff and stethoscope, or with an electronic device.	A sudden rise in your normal blood pressure of more than 30 points in the upper (systolic) range, or 15 in the lower (diastolic) range, could be warning of complication such as pre-eclampsia (pages 204,351).
Hematocrit or hemoglobin; first visit and often fourth month (repeated if values are low or anemia diagnosed)	Blood drawn from arm or from pricked finger is examined.	Values are slightly reduced in pregnancy, but abnormally low levels require further examination and treatment.
Rubella titer; first visit	Blood drawn from your arm is tested for levels of antibodies to rubella.	High levels of rubella (German measles) antibodies in your blood indicate you are immune to the disease; if you aren't immune, it is important to avoid exposure to the disease— particularly in your first trimester—and to be immunized before another pregnancy.
Pap smear; first visit	Cervical secretions are collected on a swab and examined under a microscope for abnormal cells.	Abnormal cells could, on further study, turn out to be malignant, requiring treatment.
Glucose tolerance test; fifth month; usually earlier and more often in diabetics	Examination of a series of blood samples, taken before and after a special glucose drink.	Abnormal levels of glucose in blood may indicate inadequate insulin and the presence of diabetes.
VDRL; first visit, sometimes again in seventh or eighth month	Blood drawn from your arm is tested.	To test for syphilis infection; if present, prompt treatment will prevent harm to fetus.
Gonorrhea culture; first visit†	Vaginal secretions are collected on a swab and cultured in the lab.	If gonococcus is present, treatment will prevent eye infection in baby at birth.

†Tests for genital herpes may also be done at the first visit.

TEST AND WHEN PERFORMED	PROCEDURE	REASON
Test for chlamydia; preconception or first visit	Area around cervix, urethra, or rectum is swabbed to pick up possible infectious organisms.	Chlamydia in the mother must be treated to prevent infection in newborn.
Test for HIV (human immunodeficiency virus); preconception or first visit.	Blood drawn from your arm is examined for anti-bodies to HIV.	Diagnosis and treatment can help mother and reduce the risk of HIV being passed to fetus.
Drug screen; preconception or first visit	Urine specimen is examined for signs of illicit drug use. Sometimes a blood sample is used.	Any abuse of drugs during pregnancy is hazardous to the fetus and should be promptly treated.
Group B streptococcus swab; 35 to 37 weeks	A sample of material from cervix is examined for strep B.	If strep B is present, mother is treated as labor begins or when membranes rupture, to prevent infection of newborn.
Hepatitis B screen; usually late in second trimester	Blood sample drawn from your arm is evaluated.	To uncover hepatitis B infection, so mother can be treated prenatally and infant immediately after birth.

See individual conditions (diabetes, hepatitis B, etc.) for more information.

NON-DRUG TREATMENTS DURING PREGNANCY

SYMPTOMS	TREATMENT	PROCEDURE
Aching back	Warmth	Take a long warm (not hot-as-you-can-stand-it) bath, morning and evening. Apply a heating pad wrapped in a towel for up to 20 minutes, 3 or 4 times a day.
	Preventive measures	Exercise, proper body mechanics, good posture; see page 174.

SYMPTOMS	TREATMENT	PROCEDURE
Bruises due to injury	Ice pack	Use a commercial ice pack you store in the freezer; a plastic bag filled with ice cubes and a few paper towels to absorb the melting ice, closed with a twist tie or rubber band; or an unopened can of frozen juice or package of vegetables. Apply for 30 minutes; repeat 30 minutes later if swelling or pain persists, and as needed.
	Cold compresses	Dip a soft cloth in a basin of ice cubes and cold water, wring it out, and place over affected site. Re-chill when cold dissipates.
Bruises on hands, wrists, feet	Cold soaks	Place a tray or two of ice cubes in a basin (a Styrofoam bucket or cooler is best) of cold water and immerse the injured part for 30 minutes; repeat 30 minutes later if necessary.
Burns	Cold compresses	See Bruises. Do not apply ice directly to a burn.
Burns on hands, wrists, feet	Cold soaks	See Bruises.
Colds	Saline nose drops	Use a commercial preparation or a solution of ¼ teaspoon salt in 8 ounces water (measure carefully). Put a few drops in each nostril, wait 5 to 10 minutes and blow your nose.
	Vicks VapoRub	Follow package directions.
	Additional fluids	Drink 8 ounces liquid every hour, including water, juices, soups. Hot

SYMPTOMS	TREATMENT	PROCEDURE
		fluids, particularly chicken soup, are best. Limit milk intake only if recommended by your doctor.
	Inhalation	Use a steam vaporizer, humidifier, or steaming kettle; prepare a tent by draping a sheet over an open umbrella which is resting on a chair back; place humidifier on chair.

Keeping Moist

Hot dry air can contribute to dry skin, coughing, and possibly to an increase in colds and other respiratory ailments. Adding moisture to your home can help reduce this problem, but how you do this can make a difference. Sometimes the suggested cure can do more harm than good.

Vaporizers and humidifiers, for example, have to be chosen and used with caution. Steam vaporizers manufactured since the 1970s are safe and effective, although if young children are around, the vaporizer must be carefully positioned out of reach. Cold-mist humidifiers, which became popular because they didn't present a burn hazard, encourage bacterial growth and spread germs, and should not be used at all. Ultrasonic humidifiers spew tiny particles of bacteria and other impurities from the water into the air and can cause allergic reactions or illness if they are not cleaned daily, and if plain tap water (rather than unfiltered or undistilled water) is used in them. Pans of water on radiators can add small amounts of moisture to the air but, again, could be a burn risk for small children. A steaming kettle under a tent also presents a burn problem and should be used with care for brief periods only.

Manufacturers have been attempting to produce safer humidifiers. Warm-mist humidifiers (which boil the water before mixing it with cool water to produce a mist) and wicking humidifiers (which use wicks to remove impurities) appear to release fewer germs than older cool-mist units. All humidifiers should be drained and cleaned before storing, and should be thoroughly cleaned before being used again.

No matter which method you use to add humidity to your home, limit the time of operation. Don't humidify around the clock—among other things, this can encourage the growth of molds on plants and furniture. Instead, try not to let the air in your home become dry and overheated in the first place. To do this, keep the indoor temperature under 68 degrees in cold weather. And don't make your home totally airtight—allow some leakage through windows or doors, for example, by eliminating weatherstripping. (This will also minimize hazards from indoor pollutants, such as radon.)

SYMPTOMS	TREATMENT	PROCEDURE
Colds (con't.)		Spend 15 minutes 3 or 4 times a day under tent; extend the time to 30 minutes if you aren't too uncomfortable. (Don't stay under tent if you become uncomfortably warm.) Keep the humidifier near your bedside when you are sleeping or resting.
Coughing, due to colds or flu	Inhalation	See Colds.*
	Additional fluids	See Colds.
Diarrhea	Additional fluids	Drink 8 ounces liquid every hour, including water, diluted fruit juice (but not prune juice), soups. Take milk as recommended by your practitioner. (See page 311.)
Fever	Cooling bath	Use a tub of tepid water and gradually cool it by adding ice cubes— stopping immediately if shivering begins.
	Sponge bath	Soak towels in bowl containing 2 quarts water, 1 pint rubbing alcohol, and 1 quart ice cubes; apply cold towels to the skin. Use a plastic sheet to catch drips. Stop if shivering begins. Call your doctor immediately for fevers of 102°F or higher.
Hemorrhoids	Sitz bath	Sit in enough hot water (hotter than your usual

*See "Keeping Moist," page 433. Though steam inhalation has long been a standard in treating coughs and colds, there is now some question as to whether it is really effective.

SYMPTOMS	TREATMENT	PROCEDURE
		bath) to cover the affected area for 20 to 30 minutes, 2 or 3 times daily.
Itchy abdomen or skin elsewhere	Baking soda and ammonia paste	Mix ½ cup baking soda with enough household ammonia to make a paste (avoid breathing the fumes); apply to itchy skin. Check any persistent skin problems with your practitioner.
	Preventive measures	Avoid long hot showers and baths, and soaps that are drying. Use a good moisturizer, spread on while you are still damp from the shower. For moisturizing indoor air, see page 433.
Itchy eye discharge	Warm soaks	Use a cloth dipped in warm, not hot, water (test it for comfort on your inner forearm), and apply to your eye for 5 or 10 minutes every 3 hours.
Muscle soreness, injury	Ice pack, cold compresses, or cold soaks for first 24 to 48 hours	See Bruises.
	After 48 hours, hot soaks, warm baths, or heating pad	Wet a towel thoroughly in warm water, then wring it out and place it over the affected site, covering all completely with a plastic bag. Place a heating pad over the plastic at a medium setting, being careful that it does not touch the wet towel. Apply for 1 hour twice daily.
Nasal congestion due to colds	Saline nose drops	See Colds.

SYMPTOMS	TREATMENT	PROCEDURE
	Additional fluids	See Colds.
Sinusitis	Alternating hot and cold compresses	Dip a cloth in hot water, wring it out, and apply to the painful area until the heat dissipates, about 30 seconds; then apply a cold compress until the cold dissipates. Continue alternating heat and cold for 10 minutes, 4 times daily.
Sore or scratchy throat	Gargle	Dissolve 1 teaspoon salt in 8 ounces hot water (the temperature of tea) and gargle for 5 minutes; repeat as needed, or every 2 hours.

BEST-ODDS CALORIE AND FAT REQUIREMENTS

Calorie and fat requirements vary according to an individual's weight and level of activity; factors such as metabolism also come into play. Though the following are merely rough guidelines, they can help you plan your daily fat intake during pregnancy. These servings take into account the fact that you will get at least one fat serving a day in dribs and drabs from "low-fat" foods.

Your Ideal Weight (pounds)	Your Activity Level*	Daily Calorie Needs†	Maximum Fat Intake (grams)	Maximum Full Fat Servings
100	1	1,500	50	2 ½
100	2	1,800	60	3 ½
100	3	2,500	83	5
125	1	1,800	60	3 ½
125	2	2,175	72	4
125	3	3,050	101	6
150	1	2,100	70	4
150	2	2,550	85	5
150	3	3,600	120	7 ½

*Score your activity level this way: 1 sedentary, 2 moderately active, 3 extremely active; very few pregnant women will fall into the extremely active category.
†See page 83.

SOURCES AND RESOURCES

American College of Nurse-Midwives. For information on nurse-midwifery: 818 Connecticut Ave., NW, Suite 900, Washington, DC 20006; (202) 728-9860; Fax (202) 728-9897; E-mail: infoacnm.org; Web site: www.midwife.org.

March of Dimes Resource Center. For information on pre-pregnancy and pregnancy; birth defects; genetics; drug use and environmental hazards during pregnancy: (888) MODIMES (toll free); (914) 997-4764; Fax (914) 997-4763; on line URL:http://www.modimes.org; e-mail resourcecenter@modimes.org.

The American College of Obstetricians and Gynecologists (ACOG) Resource Center. For information on pregnancy and women's health: 409 12th Street, S.W. Washington DC 20024. Enclose a stamped, self-addressed, business-size envelope along with the subject of your request.

Maternal and Child Health Center. Disseminates information to both the public and professionals: (202) 625-8410.

March of Dimes Birth Defects Foundation, Community Services Division. Provides information on prenatal hazards: 1275 Mamaroneck Avenue, White Plains, NY 10705: (914) 428-7100 or your local chapter.

Healthy Mother, Healthy Babies Coalition. Provides information on pregnancy safety: 121 North Washington Street, Suite 300, Alexandria, VA 22314: (703) 836-6110.

City- or state-sponsored pregnancy, women's health, health, or environmental hotlines. Provides information and referrals: check your local telephone directory (avoid hotlines that are sponsored by private clinics unless referred by your practitioner).

Pesticide Hotline. Provides information on pesticides and their safe use, for the public and professionals: (800) 858-7378.

National Council on Alcoholism. Provides information and materials: 733 Third Avenue, New York, NY 10017; (800) NCA-CALL or your local or state affiliate.

Alcoholics Anonymous. Provides information and materials: 468 Park Avenue South, New York, NY 10016; for referral to nearby AA meetings, check Alcoholics Anonymous listing in your local directory.

National Cocaine Hotline. Information and referrals for cocaine users and their families: (800) COCAINE.

National Institute on Drug Abuse. Information and referrals for drug abusers and their families: (800) 662-HELP.

National Library of Medicine. Provides a list of 300 health hotlines: 8600 Rockville Pike, Bethesda, MD 20894; ATTN: Health Hotlines: (301) 496-6308.

Department of Health and Human Services. Provides information on prenatal care: (800) 311-2229 or (800) 311-BABY.

The National Coalition of Hispanic Health and Human Services Organizations. For information on pregnancy and prenatal care in Spanish: (800) 504-7081.

Pregnancy Notes

Prenatal Test Results

Weekly Weight Gain

Week 1:	Week 22:
Week 2:	Week 23:
Week 3:	Week 24:
Week 4:	Week 25:
Week 5:	Week 26:
Week 6:	Week 27:
Week 7:	Week 28:
Week 8:	Week 29:
Week 9:	Week 30:
Week 10:	Week 31:
Week 11:	Week 32:
Week 12:	Week 33:
Week 13:	Week 34:
Week 14:	Week 35:
Week 15:	Week 36:
Week 16:	Week 37:
Week 17:	Week 38:
Week 18:	Week 39:
Week 19:	Week 40:
Week 20:	Week 41:
Week 21:	Week 42:

First Month

First Month

Second Month

Second Month

Third Month

Third Month

Fourth Month

Fourth Month

Fifth Month

Fifth Month

Sixth Month

Sixth Month

Seventh Month

Seventh Month

_____
_____
_____
_____
_____
_____
_____
_____
_____
_____
_____
_____
_____
_____
_____
_____
_____
_____
_____
_____
_____
_____
_____
_____
_____
_____
_____
_____
_____
_____
_____

Eighth Month

Eighth Month

Ninth Month

Ninth Month

Labor and Delivery

Postpartum

INDEX

A

AA (Alcoholics Anonymous), 437
Abdomen
  itchy, 204
  itchy, treatment of, 434
  pain in, 109, 112, 117, 177
  see also, What You May Look Like
  sleeping on, 173
Abdominal muscles, postpartum, 411
Abortion, induced
  following rubella exposure, 312
  opposition to, and prenatal diagnosis, 42
  and prenatal diagnosis, 43
  previous, and pregnancy, 18
Abortion, spontaneous, 111, 177, 346, 347
  see also, Miscarriage
Abruptio placenta, 358
  and cesarean delivery, 246
  signs of, 358
  treatment of, 359
Abscess, breast, 394
Absent-mindedness, 155
Accidents
  concern about, 222
  and injury, 222
  and miscarriage, 111
  prevention of, 133
  when to seek help following, 222
Acetaminophen use in pregnancy, 321
Acne flare-ups, 122
Acquired immune deficiency syndrome (AIDS), 37
  testing for, 38, 431
Active (second) phase of labor, 292
Acupressure, in labor, 276

Acupuncture, for pain relief in childbirth, 231
Acute mountain sickness (AMS), 181
Advice, unwanted, 163
Aerobics, 190
AFP, see MSAFP screening
Afterpains, 376
Age, maternal
  and amniocentesis, 44
  and baby's health, 30
  and pregnancy, 28
  and prenatal testing, 30
Age, paternal
  and baby's health, 30
  and Down Syndrome, 30
  and prenatal testing, 30
Aids, 37
  test for, 431
Airbags, 133
Air pollution, 71
Air, moisturizing of, 433
Airplane travel, 182
Albumin, test for, in urine, 429
Alcohol, 52
  abstaining from, 53
  and breastfeeding, 402
  effects of, on fetus, 53
  effects of, on pregnancy, 53
  and premature labor, 218
  substitutes for, 52
  use, preconception, 428
Alcoholics Anonymous, 437
Allergies, 157
  aggravation of, 157
  dealing with, 157
Allergy shots, 329
Alpha-fetoprotein screening, 47
Altitude, high
  living at, and pregnancy, 32
  travel to, 181
Amenorrhea, as a sign of pregnancy, 3
American College of Nurse-Midwives, 12

American College of Obstetricians and Gynecologists, 88, 283
American Society for Psychoprophylaxis in Obstetrics, 212
Ammonia-baking soda paste, 434
Amniocentesis, 44
  complications from, 45
  reasons for, 44
  safety of, 44
Amniotic fluid
  assessment of volume, 263
  identification of, 271
  infection of, 351
  meconium staining of, 272
  sampling of, 263
Amniotic sac, rupture of, see Membranes, amniotic
Analgesics for childbirth pain, 228
Anemia, 154
Anesthesia
  for dental work, 179
  general, 230
  regional, 229
Anorectics, and pregnancy, 332
Apgar score, 287
Appearance, 160
  see also, What You May Look Like
Areola
  in breastfeeding, 390
  darkening of, 108
Aspartame, 62
Aspirin
  and breast milk, 402
  use in pregnancy, 320
Aspirin substitutes, 321
ASPO, 212
Asthma, 329
Attachment, infant-parent, 382
Autosafety, 133
Aversions, food, 124

B

Baby
  ambivalence about, 162,
    383
  anxiety about, 110, 115,
    216
  birth of, 301
  bonding with, 382
  condition of, at birth, 287
  first look at, 302
  life with, 189
  loss of, 366
  and maternal love, 383
  responsibility for, 221
  size, and diabetes, 329
  size, and maternal weight
    gain, 235
Baby roulette, 76
Back
  exercises to strengthen,
    175
  exercising on, 190
  sleeping on, 173
Back pain, 173
  in labor, 269, 276
  lower, 222
  non-drug treatments for,
    431
  prevention of, 174
  relief of, 174
Bacteria in urine, testing for,
  317, 429
Baking soda-ammonia paste,
  434
Basic exercise position, 190
Baths
  for fever, 434
  in last six weeks, 249
  postpartum, 407
Bed rest, living with, 339
Belly, sleeping on, 173
Bending and lifting, 174
Best-Odds Diet, 80
  basic principles of, 81
  for breastfeeding, 392
  calorie and fat
    requirements in, 436
  cheating on, 129
  daily requirements in, 83
  Food Selection Groups for,
    89
Best-Odds Fries, 93

Beta-carotene
  foods rich in, 91
  need for, in pregnancy, 85
Bicycling, 197
Biophysical profile (BPP), 263
Biotin, 88
Birth control
  altering, preconception,
    426
  need for, postpartum, 406
Birth control
  altering, preconception,
    426
  need for, postpartum, 406
Birth control pills, and
    pregnancy, 39
Birth defects, 24
  correction of, 43, 216
  prenatal diagnosis of, 42
  see also, Genetic defects,
    24
Birth of baby (stages in), 301
Birthing
  alternatives, 12
  bed, 12
  centers, 12
  chair, 12
  plan, 225
  rooms, 12
Birthmarks, in newborn, 303
Bladder
  after lightening, 260
  in first trimester, 107
  postpartum, 377
Bleeding
  in early pregnancy, 344
  in mid or late pregnancy,
    345
  in ninth month, 259
  postpartum, 365, 375
  rectal, 203
  related to sexual
    intercourse, 166
  vaginal, 117, 344, 345,
    375
Blood
  banking your own, 241
  concern about transfusions
    of, 241
  at delivery, 283
Blood clot, in vein, 360
Blood pressure
  changes in, during
    pregnancy, 152

chronic high, 330
high, in preeclampsia, 352
low, 172
measuring of, 430
Blood sugar
  and fainting or dizziness,
    172
  and fatigue, 103
  and morning sickness,
    105
  in gestational diabetes,
    153, 350
  low, 103, 105, 172
  regulation of, in diabetes,
    328
Blood type, Rh, 33
Blood type, tests for, 429
Bloody show, 269, 270, 271
Bonding
  father-baby, 420
  mother-baby, 382
Boron, 86
Bottle feeding
  benefits of, 253
  succeeding at, 255
Bowel movement, postpartum,
  378
Bradley method of childbirth,
  213
Bran Muffins, 94
Braxton Hicks contractions,
  248
Breast milk
  adequacy of, 380
  benefits of, 251
  contamination of, 401
Breastfeeding, 251
  after cesarean, 394
  as birth control, 406
  basics, 389
  benefits of, 251
  Best-Odds Diet for, 392
  contraindications for, 254
  deciding about, 253
  getting started, 388
  and medication, 254
  positions for, 389
  twins, 395
Breast changes
  in first trimester, 108
  postpartum, 108
  as a sign of pregnancy, 3
  in subsequent pregnancies,
    108

Breasts
    abscess in, 394
    clogged milk ducts in, 393
    drying up of, postpartum,
        382
    engorgement of, 380, 382
    infection in, 394
    leakage from, 267
    painful, 380
    preparation of, for nursing,
        267
    in sexual relations, 422
    size of, and breastfeeding,
        266
Breath, shortness of, 234
    in asthma, 329
Breathlessness, 155
    in asthma, 330
    in third trimester, 234
Breech presentation, 236, 238
    delivery options with, 238
    turning of fetus in, 237
    vaginal delivery with, 306
Bruises, treatment of, 431,
        432
Bulimia, 332
Burns, treatment of, 432

C

Caffeine
    breaking the habit of, 60
    and breastfeeding, 402
    minimizing withdrawal
        from, 61
    preconception, 427
    safety of, in pregnancy, 60
Calcium
    Food Selection Group, 90
    and leg cramps, 202
    requirements in pregnancy,
        85
    snacks high in, 91
    in supplements, 88
    in vegetarian diet, 127
Calisthenics, 191, 197
Calories
    burning of, with exercise,
        194
    individual requirements,
        436
    need for, in pregnancy, 83

    quality of, 81
Caput succedaneum, 302
Car travel, 183
Carbohydrates, 82
    in Best-Odds Diet, 86
    Food Selection Group, 91
    importance of complex, 82
Carbon monoxide
    in air pollution, 71
    in tobacco smoke, 56
Carpal tunnel syndrome, 200
Carrying, different ways of,
        236
    in eighth month, 237
    in fifth month, 188
Catheter, urinary
    with anesthesia, 229
    in cesarean recovery, 386
    postpartum, 378
Cats, and toxoplasmosis, 64
Caudal block, 230
Cephalopelvic disproportion,
        240, 292
Cerclage, 20
Cereals and grains, 86, 91
Certified Nurse-Midwife, 10
    in birthing center, 12
    independent, 11
    see also, Practitioner
Cervical lacerations, 364
Cervix
    changes in, as a sign of
        pregnancy, 3, 4
    dilatation of, 261
    dilatation of, in labor,
        290, 292, 297
    dilatation of, in prolonged
        labor, 292
    effacement of, 261
    incompetent, 20
Cesarean section, 242, 307
    being prepared for, 247
    breastfeeding after, 394
    coach at, 308
    effects of, on baby, 242
    emergency, 308
    exercise following, 387, 403
    family-centered, 247
    fear of having, 243
    and hospitals, 246
    indications for, 245
    long-term recovery from,
        403

    pain following, 386, 387,
        403
    questions to ask your
        doctor about, 245
    reasons for increase in,
        244
    recovery from, 385
    removal of stitches in,
        388
    repeat, safety of, 22
    safety of, 242
    scar of, 403
    sexual relations following,
        403
    typical procedure during,
        307
    vaginal birth after (VBAC),
        23
Chamberlen, Peter, 286
Checkups, 118
    importance of, 116
    initial, 100
    preconception, 424
    schedule of, 116
    see also, What You Can
        Expect at This Month's
        Checkup
Checkups, dental, 118, 180,
        424
Chemicals
    in breast milk, 402
    exposure to, in pregnancy,
        74
    exposure, preconception,
        427
    in fish, 130
    in food, 129
    in meat and poultry, 131
Chicken pox, 319
Childbed fever, *see,* Postpartum
    Infection
Childbirth,
    alternatives in, 12
    concerns about, 208
    difficulty in previous, 22
    family-centered care
        during, 12
    by Leboyer method, 12
    pain of, 206
    and pelvic size, 240
    underwater, 12
    vaginal stretching during,
        285

Childbirth education, 209
  benefits of, 210
  choosing a class for, 211
  different approaches to,
    212
  sources of information on,
    212
Childbirth medication, 226
  deciding about, 232
  need for, 227
  reducing risk of, 227
  types of, 228
Childbirth stages, 288
  first stage (labor), 290
  second stage (delivery),
    299
  third stage (delivery of
    placenta), 305
Childcare responsibilities, 417
Children, carrying
  in first trimester, 116
  in second trimester, 176
Chlamydia, 36
  test for, 431
Chloasma, 178
Cholesterol in pregnancy, 126
Chorioamnionitis, 351
Choriocarcinoma, 350
Chorionic villus sampling, 48
  safety of, 49
Chromium, 88
Chromosomal abnormalities,
    28, 44
Chronic illness in pregnancy,
    325
  living with, 339
  preparing for, 426
Cigarettes, 54
  see also, Smoking
Cleaning products, safety of,
    67
Clumsiness, 206
Coach
  at cesarean delivery, 308
  at emergency delivery,
    308
  responsibilities of, 291,
    294, 299, 303, 306
Cocaine, 59
  hotline, 437
Cold compresses, for injury,
    432
Cold soaks, for injury, 432

Colds, 310
  non-drug treatments for,
    432
Colostrum (premilk), 380
  absence of, prenatally, 267
  leakage, in ninth month,
    267
  leakage, during
    lovemaking, 165
Complexion problems, 122
Complications
  of childbirth, 362
  in past pregnancies, 22
  of pregnancy, 342
  postpartum, 365
Conception, concern about,
    406
Constipation, 135
  dealing with, 135
  during travel, 182
  and hemorrhoids, 203
  lack of, 136
Contraceptives, conceiving
    while using, 38, 39
Contractions
  Braxton Hicks, 248
  in false labor, 269
  in first phase of labor,
    290
  halting premature, 362
  irregular, 276
  postpartum, 376
  prelabor, 269
  premature, 221
  in second phase of labor,
    292
  in third phase of labor,
    297
  in true labor, 269
Copper, in supplements, 88
Cord blood storage, 255
Cord prolapse, 360
Cord, *see,* Umbilical cord
Cordocentesis, 51
Coronary artery disease, 336
Corpus luteum cyst, 146
Coughing
  of blood, 117
  night time, 156
  non-drug treatment of,
    434
Counterpressure, in labor,
    276

Couvade, 415
Crack use in pregnancy, 60
Cramps, abdominal
  after orgasm, 143
  in early miscarriage, 112
  in ectopic pregnancy, 110
  in late miscarriage, 177
  in prelabor, 269
  postpartum, 376
  from stretching ligaments,
    178
Cravings, food, 124
  as a sign of pregnancy, 3
Cyst, ovarian, 146
Cyst, choroid plexus, 169
Cystic fibrosis, 41
Cystitis, 317
  postpartum, 378
Cytomegalovirus (CMV), 314

D

Daily Dozen, Best-Odds, 83
Daiquiri, Mock Strawberry,
    98
Daydreams, 223
DES daughters, 40
Death
  fear of, 240
  of fetus, 366
  of newborn, 366

Delivery
  after due date, 262
  description of, 304
  embarrassment during,
    208, 300
  emergency, 277, 279
  positions for, 300
  predicting time of, 261
  strapping down during,
    285
  see also, Childbirth
Delivery rooms, 261
Demerol, 229
Dental checkup
  preconception, 424
  in pregnancy, 180
Dental problems
  frequency of, in pregnancy,
    179
  prevention of, 180

Dental work
  anesthesia for, 179
  diet following, 179
  preconception, 424
  x-rays for, 180
Depression
  absence of, postpartum, 400
  dealing with, 398
  during pregnancy, 104
  in father, 414
  postpartum, 398
Diabetes, 325
  diet for, 326
  exercise heart rate in, 327
  gestational, 153, 350
  proper care of, 326
  symptoms of, 350
Diagnosis of pregnancy, 2
Diaphoresis, 379
Diaphragmatic breathing, 410
Diarrhea
  with gastroenteritis, 311
  in prelabor, 269
  treatment of, 311, 434
Diastasis, of abdominal muscle, 411
Diet
  Best-Odds, 80
  Best-Odds Nursing, 392
  with a cold, 310
  effects of, in pregnancy, 80
  as a family affair, 83
  with gastroenteritis, 312
  improving, preconception, 426
  meatless, 126
  vegetarian, 127
Diet pills, use of, 60
Diethylstilbestrol (DES)
  and ectopic pregnancy, 109, 110
  effect of prenatal exposure to, 40
Dilatation, 261
  see also, Cervix
Diving, 197
Dizziness, 172
  when to call the doctor, 117
  with hyperventilation, 294
Doctor, see, Practitioner

Doppler velocimetry test, 263
Double-the-Milk Shake, 95
Doula, 270
Down syndrome
  and father's age, 30
  and mother's age, 28
  testing for, 30
Dreams, 223
Driving, 248
Dromedary Droop, 192
Dropping (lightening), 260
Drug use in pregnancy
  alcohol, 52
  and breastfeeding, 402
  cocaine, 59
  heroin, 60
  marijuana, 58
  narcotics, 60
  nicotine, 54
  other drugs, 60
  preconception, 428
  and premature labor, 218
  testing for, 431
  see also, Medication
Dry skin, prevention of, 435
Due date, 6
  calculating your, 7
  delivery past, 262
  determining accuracy of, 7
Dysfunctional labor, 292
Dystocia, 363

E

Eating disorders, 332
Eating in pregnancy, see, Best-Odds Diet
Eating out, 183, 184
Echocardiography, 51
Eclampsia, 354
Ectopic pregnancy, 109, 343
  factors in, 110
  signs of, 343
  symptoms of, 110
  treatment of, 343
EDD (Estimated date of delivery), 6
Edema (swelling)
  of feet and ankles, 217
  of hands and face, 217
  when to call practitioner for, 117

Effacement, 261
Efficient eating, 81
Electric blankets, safety of, 65
Electrocardiography, 263
Electromagnetic fields, 66
Emergency delivery
  alone, 279
  at home or office, 281
  en route, 277
Emotions, in pregnancy, 104
  1st month, 102
  2nd month, 119
  3rd month, 135
  4th month, 151
  5th month, 171
  6th month, 200
  7th month, 215
  8th month, 234
  9th month, 258
  father's, 414
  father's reaction to, 414
Enemas in labor, 277
Engagement of fetus in pelvis, 260, 268
Environmental hazards
  air pollution, 71
  household cleaning products, 67
  insecticides, 69
  microwaves, 64
  paint, 70
  tap water, 68
Epidural block, 229
Epilepsy, 335
Episiotomy, 283
  infection following, 376
  pain following, 376
Equal, 62
Erythema infectiosum, 315
Estimated date of delivery, 6
  see also, Due date
Exercise, in pregnancy, 189
  benefits of, 190
  choosing the right, 197
  classes for, 194
  developing a program for, 192
  moderation in, 195
  overheating during, 196
  to prevent constipation, 136
  relaxation, 114, 193
  restrictions on, 198

safety during, 195
while sedentary, 194
Exercise, postpartum, 408
Exercise, preconception, 427
Exhaustion, postpartum, 407
External cephalic version, 237
External fetal monitoring, 280
Eyes
  problems with, in
    pregnancy, 186
  problems with,
    postpartum, 375
  treatment of itchy, 435

F

FAS (fetal alcohol syndrome),
  53
Face
  bruises on, postpartum,
    375
  swelling of, 217
Fainting, 172
  when to call practitioner
    for, 117
Falls, 222
False labor, signs of, 269
Family, and Best-Odds Diet,
  83
Family history, and pregnancy,
  24, 25
Family physician, 9
  see also, Practitioner
Family size, and pregnancy,
  27
Family-centered care, 12
Fantasies, 223
Fast food, 128
Fasting in pregnancy, 81
Fat
  Food Selection Group, 92
  individual requirements,
    436
  requirement in pregnancy,
    87
Father, 412
  age of, and baby's health,
    30
  alcohol use by,
    preconception, 428
  anxieties of, 412–421
  and breastfeeding, 421

and childcare, 221, 417,
  421
drug use by,
  preconception, 428
impatience of, 414
moods of, 414
nausea in, 415
presence at birth of, 420
presence of, at cesarean,
  308
smoking by, 57, 428
sympathy symptoms of,
  415
Fatigue
  dealing with, 102
  extreme, in anemia, 216
  in first trimester, 102
  increasing, in seventh
    month, 215
  postpartum, 407
  in second trimester, 171
FDA (Food and Drug
  Administration), 322
Feelings, *see,* What You May
  Be Feeling; *see also,*
  Emotions
Feet
  changes in, 176
  problems with, 176
  swelling of, 217
Fetal Acoustical Stimulation,
  263
Fetal activity, *see,* Fetal
  movement
Fetal alcohol effect, 53
Fetal alcohol syndrome (FAS),
  53
Fetal blood sampling, 51
Fetal defect
  coping with discovery of,
    349
  see also, Genetic defects
Fetal development
  1st month, 101
  2nd month, 121
  3rd month, 135
  4th month, 151
  5th month, 171
  6th month, 200
  7th month, 215
  8th month, 234
  9th month, 257
Fetal distress, 364

on fetal monitor, 282
meconium staining in, 272
signs of, 364
tests for, 263
treatment of, 364
Fetal heartbeat
  as a measure of well being,
    263
  in diagnosing pregnancy, 5
  hearing, for first time, 142
  in labor, 280
Fetal lung maturity, 44, 361
Fetal monitoring, 280
  abnormal readings on, 282
  external, 280
  internal, 282
Fetal movement
  absence of, before twenty-
    eighth week, 159
  absence of, in ninth
    month, 258
  assessment of, 263
  changes in, in ninth
    month, 258
  with false labor, 269
  first recognition of, 159
  in labor, 290
  in late pregnancy, 364
  pain caused by, 202, 235
  in second trimester, 201
  test for, 202
  as a sign of pregnancy, 4,
    5
  and twins, 202
  variations in, 202
  very active, 202
  when to call practitioner
    about, 117
Fetal scalp blood sample, 263,
  283
Fetal skin sampling, 51
Fetoscopy, 47
Fetus
  death of, 111, 366
  hiccups in, 223
  impaired growth in, 354
  and intercourse, 143, 218
  outside influences on, 187
  position of, 236
  prenatal treatment of, 43
  size of, and mother's
    weight gain, 235
  stimulation of, 187

worry about condition of,
115
see also, Baby
Fever
non-drug treatment of,
321, 434
postpartum, 397
in pregnancy, 320
when to call practitioner
for, 117, 381
Fiber, 86
in Best-Odds Diet, 82
importance of, in diabetes,
326
postpartum, 379
to prevent constipation,
135
Fibroids and pregnancy, 19
Fifth Disease, 315
Fig Bars, 96
Figure
changes in, in early
pregnancy, 122
concerns about losing, 122
regaining, postpartum,
400, 408
in second trimester, 160
Financial worries, 417
Fingernails, 176, 178
Fish, safety of, 130
Flatulence, 137
Flu, 310, 323
Fluids
and breastfeeding, 392
and exercise, 194
for diarrhea, 434
need for, in pregnancy, 87
to prevent constipation,
136, 379
for treatment of colds, 432
Flying
occupational risks of, 74
during travel, 182
Folic acid, 88, 426, 427
Food
contamination, 132
processing of, 82
safe preparation of, 132
safety of, 129, 324
Food and Drug Administration,
322
Food aversions, 124
Food cravings, 124

as a sign of pregnancy, 3
Food Selection Groups, 91
Foot problems, 176
See also, Feet
Forceps, 286
Forgetfulness, 155
Fries, Best-Odds, 93
Fruited Yogurt, 98
Fruits and vegetables
chemical residues on, 131
Food Selection Groups for, 91
requirements for, 85, 86
Fruity Oatmeal Cookies, 96

G

Gall bladder, 343
Gamete intrafallopian transfer, 31
Gamper method of childbirth,
212
Gas, intestinal, 137
Gassy foods, 137
Gastrointestinal illness, 311
General anesthesia, 230
Genetic counseling, 40
preconception, 426
Genetic defects
counseling about possible,
40
family history of, 24, 25
options on diagnosis of, 43
risk of baby with, 41
transmission of, 41
Genital warts, 37
Genitals
engorgement of, in
pregnancy, 165
swelling of, in newborn,
303
German measles, 312
immunization for, 313
Gestational diabetes, 153, 350
symptoms of, 153
GIFT, 31
Glucose
levels of, in blood, 153
test for, in urine, 429
tolerance test, 153
in the urine, 152
see also, Blood sugar
Glucose tolerance test, 430
Gonorrhea, 36

test for, 430
Grains
Food Selection Groups, 91
in protein combinations,
97
requirements for, in
pregnancy, 86
Grantly-Dick Read method of
childbirth, 212
Green leafy vegetables
Food Selection Group for,
91
requirements for, in
pregnancy, 85
Group B strep, 315
testing for, 431
Gums
bleeding of, 179
nodule on, 180
preventive care of, 180
Gynecological history, effect
of on pregnancy, 18

H

Habits, changing, 63
Hair
excess growth of, 176
loss of, postpartum, 407
in newborn, 302
Hair dyes and permanents,
155
Hands
burning and tingling, 201
carpal tunnel syndrome
of, 200
pain and numbness in,
200
pins and needles in, 201
red palms on, 178
swelling of, 217
tingling in, 201
HCG
in post-date deliveries,
262
screening, for prenatal
diagnosis, 51
testing for, 4, 5
Head
fetal and maternal pelvis,
240
molding of newborn, 302

Head lifts, 409
Head, fetal, molding of, 302
Headache, 138
  hunger, 139
  migraine, 139
  non-drug treatment of,
    138
  in preeclampsia, 204
  sinus related, 139
  when to call the doctor
    for, 117, 139
Health care work and
  pregnancy, 73
Healthy Mothers, Healthy
  Babies, 437
Hearing, fetal, 187
Heart disease
  congenital, 41
  and pregnancy, 336
Heartbeat, fetal
  hearing, 142
  as a measure of well being,
    263
Heartburn, 123
Heat
  application of, for
    backache, 431
  danger of exercising in,
    196
Heat rash, 179
Heating pad
  safety of, 65
  for treating injury, 435
HELLP syndrome, 352
Hematocrit, 430
Hemoglobin, 430
Hemophilia, 41, 44
Hemorrhage, postpartum, 365
Hemorrhoids
  in pregnancy, 203
  treatment of, 434
Hepatitis A, 318
Hepatitis B
  carrier for, 38
  infection of spouse with,
    318
  routing testing for, 172
  testing for, 431
Hepatitis C and E, 319
Herbal medicines, 323
Heroin use in pregnancy, 60
Herpes, genital, 35
  and need for cesarean, 246

test for, 430
Hiccups, fetal, 223
High altitude, 32, 181
High blood pressure, 152
  chronic, 330
  in preeclampsia, 352
High-risk pregnancy
  choosing obstetrician for, ,
    9
  living with, 339
  lowering the risk of, for
    baby, 354
  and marital stress, 340
  self-help groups in, 341
  see also, Chapers 16, 17
HIV, 37, 431
Home birth
  by choice, 12
  emergency, 281
Home pregnancy test, 4
Home, going, postpartum, 384
Honey, 82
Hormonal imbalance, and
  premature labor, 219
Horseback riding, 197
Hospital
  admission to, 295
  concerns about, 261
  getting to, 295
  going home from, 384
  length of stay at, 384
  not getting to in time, 277
  rooming-in at, 383
  touring of, in advance,
    261
  what to take to, 265
Hot soaks, for treating injury,
  435
Hot tubs, safety of, 65
Hotlines, health, 437
Household products, safety of,
  67
Human chorionic gonadotropin
  (hCG)
  in post-date deliveries,
    262
  screening, for prenatal
    diagnosis, 51
  testing for, 4, 5
Human parvovirus B_{19}, 314
Humidification, of indoor air,
  433
Humidifier, 433

Hunger headache, 139
Hunter's syndrome, 44
Huntington's chorea, 41, 44
Hydatidiform mole, 348
Hyperemesis gravidarum, 343
Hypertension, 152
  chronic, 330
  in preeclampsia, 204, 352
Hyperventilation, in labor,
  294
Hypnosis, for relief in
  childbirth, 231
Hypotension, and dizziness,
  172
Hypotension, postural, 159

I

Ibuprofen, use in pregnancy,
  321
Ice, for injury, 431
Illness in pregnancy, 310
  chronic, 325
  prevention of, 323
Immunization, 323
  for rubella, 313
  for travel, in pregnancy,
    181
  updating, prepregnancy,
    425
Implantation and multiple
  abortions, 111
Incompetent cervix, 20
  and late miscarriage, 177
  and premature labor, 219
Indigestion, 123
Induction of labor, 273
  do-it-yourself, 261
  procedures for, 273
  reasons for, 273
  reasons to avoid, 274
Infant mortality rate, 216
Infant, *see,* Baby
Infection
  of amniotic membranes,
    351
  breast, 394
  postpartum, 365
  and sexual intercourse,
    250
Influenza, 310, 323
Inhalants, as childbirth

medication, 229
Inhalation, as non-drug
    treatment, 433
Inherited disorders, *see,*
    Genetic disorders
Injury
    accidental, 222
    muscle, treatment of, 435
Insecticides, safety of, 69
Insulin
    production of, in
        pregnancy, 153
    use of, in pregnancy, 328
Intercourse, sexual
    bleeding related to, 166
    changing interest in, 142
    cramping following, 143
    fears relating to, 166
    and the fetus, 166, 219
    in last weeks of pregnancy,
        250
    and miscarriage, 166
    positions for, 168
    and premature delivery,
        166, 167
    restrictions on, 168
Internal fetal monitoring, 282
International Association for
    Medical Assistance to
    Travelers, 182
International Childbirth
    Education Association,
    12, 212
Intrauterine device (IUD)
    and ectopic pregnancy, 110
    and miscarriage, 111
    and pregnancy, 38
Intrauterine growth
    retardation, 354
    see also, Low-birthweight
        baby
Intravenous fluids (IV)
    in cesarean section, 307
    in labor, 279
    removal of, after cesarean,
        386
Invitro fertilization, and
    pregnancy, 31
Iodine, in supplements, 88
Iron
    deficiency (anemia), 154
    foods rich in, 92
    requirement for, in

pregnancy, 86
    supplementation, 86, 154
    in supplements, 88
Itching
    of abdomen, 204
    of skin, 178, 352
    treatment for, 434
    see also, Skin
IUD, and pregnancy, 38
IUGR, 354
IVF, 31
IVs, *see,* Intravenous fluids

J

Jaundice, in newborn, 384
Job risks in pregnancy, 72
    see also, Work
Jogging, 197
Junk food, 127

K

Kegel exercise
    benefits of, 192
    how to perform, 190
    postpartum, 410
Kell factor, test for, 429
Kennedy, Ethel, 22
Kicking, baby, 159, 201, 258
    see also, Fetal movement
Kidney disease, 246
Kidney infection
    postpartum, 378
    in pregnancy, 317

L

Labels, nutrition, 132
Labor
    back, 276
    comfortable positions for,
        289
    describing, to practitioner,
        275
    duration of, 290
    false, 269
    first phase of (early or
        latent), 290
    induction of, 273

pain of, 269
    premature, 218, 361
    recognizing, 268
    second phase of (active),
        292
    signs of impending, 268
    symptoms of, 269
    third phase of,
        (transitional), 297
    very short (precipitous),
        275
    when to call practitioner
        in, 270, 275
Labor and delivery, 271
    concerns about, 208
    fear of lengthy, 259
Labor and delivery rooms, 261
Labor pain, relief for
    acupressure, 276
    acupuncture, 231
    counterpressure, 276
    deciding about, 232
    distraction, 231
    hypnosis, 231
    medication, 226, 228
    physical therapy, 231
    TENS, 231
Labor, abnormal, 292
    dysfunctional or arrested,
        292
    and cesarean section, 276
    and induction, 273
    prolonged, 292
    shoulder dystocia in, 363
Lacerations, postpartum, 364
Lactation, *see,* Breastfeeding
Lactation, suppression of, 382
Lactose intolerance, 125
Lamaze, 212
Lanugo, 303
Latent (first) phase of labor,
    290
Lead exposure, 68
Leboyer, Frederick, and
    nonviolent childbirth,
    12
Leg
    cramps, 202
    pain, 222
Leg lifts, 196
Leg slides, 410
Legumes
    Food Selection Group, 91

in protein combinations,
97
requirements for, 86
Leukorrhea, 158
Life, first feeling of, 159
Lifting
best positions for, 174
on the job, 206
of other children, 116,
176
Ligament pain, abdominal,
178
Lightening, 260
Linea nigra, 178
Listeria, 324
Lochia, 375
Love, mother-baby, 383
Lovemaking, *see,* Making love,
164
Low-birthweight baby, 224,
354
chances of repeat, 355
reducing risk of, 224
Low-blood pressure, 172
Low-blood sugar, 103, 105,
172
LSD use in pregnancy, 60
Lupus, 338
Lyme disease, 316

M

Magnesium, 86
in supplements, 88
Magnetic resonance imaging,
51
Making love, 164
cramps after orgasm and,
143
enjoyment of, 168
lack of interest in,
postpartum, 404
in the last weeks of
pregnancy, 250
oral sex in, 143
restrictions on, in
pregnancy, 168
resumption of, postpartum,
403
symptoms affecting, 165
variations in desire for,
142

Malpractice,
and cesareans, 243
protecting yourself against,
16
Manganese, 88
Mannitol, 130
March of Dimes, 322, 437
Marijuana use in pregnancy,
58
Marriage, changing
relationships in, 249,
418
Mask of pregnancy, 178
Massage, in labor, 276
Mastitis, 394
Maternal age, 28, 30, 44, 220
Maternal and Child Health
Center, 437
Maternal distress, and
cesarean, 246
Maternal safety, in childbirth,
240
Maternal serum alpha-
fetoprotein test, 47
Maternity Centers, 11
Maternity clothes, 161
Measles, 316
Measles, German, 312
Meat
chemicals in, 131
raw, 64
Meatless diet, 126
Meconium staining of amniotic
fluid, 272
Medication
and breastfeeding, 254,
402
for childbirth, 226
for epilepsy, 335
need for, during labor,
296
preconception, 428
safe use of, 321
weighing risk vs. benefit,
in use of, 322
Membranes, amniotic,
infection, of, 351
Membranes, rupture of, 271,
272
before labor begins, 272
to induce labor, 273
premature,359
and prolapsed cord, 272

in public, 266
recognizing, 271
restriction following, 272
when to call practitioner
about, 270
Menstrual periods
absence of, as a sign of
pregnancy, 3
irregular, and due date, 7
Meperidine hydrochloride, 229
Metabolism, change in, 217
Methadone use in pregnancy, 60
Microwave exposure, 64
Midwife, *see* Certified Nurse-
Midwife
Milk
aversion, 125
intolerance, 125
raw, and toxoplasmosis, 64
Milk ducts, clogged, 393
Milk Shake, Double-the, 95
Mineral oil, to induce labor,
273
Minerals, trace, 86, 88
Mini-prep, for delivery, 279
Miscarriage, 111, 346, 177,
347
coping with, 346
Miscarriage, early, 111, 346,
347
coping with, 346
factors related to, 111
fear of, 113
and previous abortions, 111
signs of, 112, 347
treatment of, 347
water beds and, 66
what to do if you suspect,
113
when to call the doctor
for, 112
Miscarriage, late, 177, 347
prevention of, 177, 348
signs of, 348
symptoms of, 177
treatment of, 348
Mock Strawberry Daiquiri, 98
Molar pregnancy, 348
Molybdenum, 88
Mood swings, 104
Morning sickness, 104
absence of, 104

dealing with, 105
  in father, 415
  severe, 343
  as a sign of pregnancy, 3
Mother, single, 28
Mothering
  alone, 28
  concerns about, 189, 221,
    267
  and physical disability,
    334
  and sexuality, 167
Movements, fetal, *see,* Fetal
    movements
MSAFP screening, 47
MSG, 131
Mucous discharge, 158
Mucous plug, loss of, 269
Mucus, blood-tinged, 259,
    269, 270
Muffins, Bran, 94
Multiple gestations, 143, 368
  and sexual intercourse,
    168
  see also, Twins, 143
Multiple sclerosis (MS), 331
Mumps, 319
Muscle injury, treatment of,
    435
Music, influence of, on fetus,
    188
Myomas (tumors) of uterus,
    177

N

Nails
  changes in, 178
  fast growth of, 176
Narcotics, use in pregnancy,
    60
Nasal congestion, treatment
    of, 435
Nasal stuffiness, 156
National Academy of Sciences,
    88
National Cocaine Hotline, 437
National Council on
    Alcoholism, 437
National Institute of
    Occupational Safety
    and Health, 74

National Institute on Drug
    Abuse, 437
National Library of Medicine,
    437
Nausea
  in ectopic pregnancy, 110
  following general
    anesthesia, 386
  in morning sickness, 105
Navel, protruding, 257
Neck relaxing exercise, 193
Neural tube defect
  reducing risk of, 427
  testing for, 44, 47
Newborn, 287, 302
  see also, Baby
Niacin, in supplements, 88
Night sweats, 217
Nipple stimulation to induce
    labor, 261
Nipples
  inverted, 266
  sore, 380, 393
Nitrates and nitrites, 131
Nitrous oxide, 229
Noise
  and headaches, 139
  pollution, 75
Non-aspirin, use in pregnancy,
    321
Non-drug treatments, 431
Non-stress test, 263
Nonspecific vaginitis (NSV), 37
Nosebleeds, 156
Nurse-Midwife, *see* Certified
    Nurse-Midwife
Nursing, *see* Breastfeeding
Nutrasweet, 62
Nutrition in pregnancy, 80
  inadequate, and preterm
    labor, 219
  see also, Best-Odds Diet;
    Diet
Nutrition labels, reading, 132
Nutritional supplements, *see,*
    Vitamin and mineral
    supplements

O

Oatmeal Cookies, Fruity, 96
Oatmeal, Power-Packed, 94

Obesity and pregnancy, 34
Obstetrical history
  and present pregnancy, 18
  repeating itself, 21
  taken at first visit, 100
Obstetrician, 9
  for high-risk pregnancy, 9
  see also, Practitioner
Occupational risks in
    pregnancy, 72
Occupational Safety and
    Health Administration,
    74
Oral contraceptives, and
    pregnancy, 39
Oral sex, 143
Organ donation, 43
Organic produce, 131
Orgasm
  changes in, 142, 165
  cramp after, 143
  effects on fetus of, 218
  and miscarriage, 166
  and premature labor, 166,
    167
  safety of, 143
  and uterine contractions,
    167
  uterine contractions
    following, 218
Overdue baby, 262
Overheating
  and exercise, 196
  and fainting or dizziness,
    172
  in pregnancy, 217
Overweight, *see,* Obesity
Ovulation
  and due date, 7
  pinpointing for conception,
    425
Oxytocin
  challenge test (OCT), 263
  for induction of labor, 273
  postpartum, 375

P

Pain
  abdominal, 109, 112, 117,
    177
  back, 173

factors that increase/
decrease, 298
fear of, in childbirth, 206
from fetal kicking, 202,
235
following cesarean, 386,
387
hand, 200
leg, 222
lower back, 222
perineal, postpartum, 376
postpartum, 376
relief, in labor, 226
when to call practitioner
about, 117, 381
Pain relief
aspirin and nonaspirin for,
320
in childbirth, 226
postpartum, 377, 386
Paint fumes, safety of, 70
Palms, reddened, 178
Pancakes, Whole-Wheat
Buttermilk, 95
Pap smear, 430
Parenthood
concerns about, 189, 221,
267, 417
dreams about, 223
and sexuality, 167
single, 28
Partial molar pregnancy, 350
Patient-practitioner
partnership, 15
PCP use in pregnancy, 60
Pelvic inflammatory disease
(PID) and ectopic
pregnancy, 109
Pelvic tilt, 191, 411
Pelvic toning (Kegels), 190,
192, 410
Pelvis
adequacy of, for delivery,
240
engagement of fetus in,
260
Perineum
care of, postpartum, 377
and episiotomy, 284
pain in, postpartum, 376
stretching of, in childbirth,
285
Periods, *see,* Menstrual periods

Permanent waves, safety of,
155
Perspiration, excessive
postpartum, 379
in pregnancy, 179, 218
Pesticide hotline, 437
Pets, allergy to, 157
Ph, of fetal scalp sample, 283
Phenergan, 229
Phenylketonuria (PKU), 336
Physical activity
and miscarriage, 111
strenuous, and preterm
labor, 219
strenuous, at work, 205
strenuous, during exercise,
195
Physical disability and
pregnancy, 333
Physical examination
first month, 100
see also, Checkups
Physical stress, at work, 75
Physical therapy for pain relief
in childbirth, 231
Physician, *see,* Practitioner
Pill, the, 39
Pitocin, *see,* Oxytocin
PKU and pregnancy, 336
Placenta
abruptio, 358
accreta, 358
delivery of, 305
development of, 102
low-lying, 187, 357
premature separation of,
358
Placenta previa, 356
and sexual intercourse,
168
signs of, 357
treatment of, 357
Plants, as air cleaners, 71
Position of fetus, 236, 239
Positions
for delivery, 300
for intercourse in
pregnancy, 168
for labor, 289
Post-term delivery, 262
dealing with, 265
Postpartum, 374, 396
bleeding, 375

bowel movements, 378
condition, 375
depression, 398
difficulty urinating, 377
exercise, 408
exhaustion, 407
fever, 397
figure, 400, 408
the first six weeks, 396
the first week, 374
hemorrhage, 365
infection, 365
pain, 376, 386, 387
perspiration, 379
vaginal discharge, 375
weight loss, 400
Postural hypotension, 172
Potassium, 86
Poultry, chemicals in, 131
Power-Packed Oatmeal, 94
Practitioner
changing your, 17
disagree with your, 17
finding a, 11
first prenatal visit to, 100
reporting symptoms to, 15
selecting a, 8
type of practice of, 10
working with your, 15
Practitioner, when to call
during pregnancy, 117
in labor, 270, 275
postpartum, 381
for suspected ectopic
pregnancy, 110
for suspected miscarriage,
112, 177
Preconception preparation,
424
Preeclampsia, 204, 351
signs of, 352
and swelling of hands and
face, 217
treatment of, 352
Pregnancy
and age, 28
ambivalence toward, 162
changing lifestyle in, 63
chronic illness and, 325
close spacing of, 25
complications, 342
complications in past, 22
diagnosis of, 2

duration of, 262
environmental risks in, 76
and family history, 24, 25
and family size, 27
illness during, 310
new, postpartum, 406
perspective on perils in, 59
preparing for, 424
reducing risk in, 50
second or subsequent, 22
signs of, 2
uncomfortable past, 21
Pregnancy loss, 366
Pregnancy reduction, 368
Pregnancy tests, 2
blood, 5
false negative, 6
home, 4
increasing accuracy of, 6
urine, 5
Pregnancy-induced
hypertension (PIH), 204, 351
see also, Preeclampsia
Prelabor, signs of, 268
Premature labor, 218, 361
contributing factors to, 218
postponement of, 361
reducing risk of, 218
signs of, 221, 361
treatment of, 361
Premature rupture of
membranes (PROM), 359
Premilk (colostrum), 380
Prenatal diagnosis
amniocentesis, 44
chorionic villus sampling, 48
fetoscopy, 47
MSAFP screening, 47
miscellaneous types of, 51
and opposition to abortion, 42
reasons for, 43
ultrasound, 45
Prenatal treatment of fetus, 43
Prenatal visits, see, Checkups
Presentation of fetus, 236
Preterm labor, 218, 361
see also, Premature labor

Produce
chemical residues on, 131
organic, 131
Prolapsed cord, 360
Prostaglandin E, to ripen
cervix, 273
Protein
dairy combinations, 97
Food Selection Group, 89
requirements in pregnancy, 84
snacks, 90
vegetarian, 97
Protein (albumin) in the
urine, 351, 429
Protein supplements
(powdered, liquid), 85
Provera, 39, 76
Pruritic urticarial papules and
plaques (PUPP), 223
Ptyalism, 107
PUPP, 223
Pudendal block, 229
Puerperal fever, see,
Postpartum infection, 365
Pushing stage of childbirth, 299
Pyelonephritis, 317

Q

Quickening, 159

R

Raw meat, and toxoplasmosis, 64
Raw milk, and toxoplasmosis, 64
Recipes, 93
Rectal bleeding, 203
Recti abdominis, 411
Regional nerve blocks, for
childbirth pain, 229
Relationship with spouse,
changes in, 249
Relaxation exercises, 114, 191
for the neck, 193
Religious belief
and abortion, 42

and medical care, 32
and pregnancy reduction, 369
Resources, for health
information, 437
Responsibilities of parenthood, 221
Restaurants, eating in, 184
Rh factor, test for, 429
Rh incompatibility, 33
and induction of labor, 273
Rib, pain in, 235
Riboflavin, 86
in supplements, 88
Risk vs. benefit, 77
Rooming-in, 383
Roughage, see, Fiber
Rubella, 312
immunization for, 313
titer test, 430
Rupture of membranes, 266, 271
see also, Membranes,
amniotic; Membranes,
rupture of

S

Saccharin, 62
Safety, in pregnancy, 133
Saline nose drops, 432
Saliva, excessive, 107
Salt, need for, in pregnancy, 87
Sangria, Virgin, 98
Saunas, safety of, 65
Sciatica, 222
Seat belt use in pregnancy, 186
Sedative use in pregnancy, 60
Selenium, 86
Self-help groups, 341
Sexual desire, changes in, 142, 164, 404, 421
Sexual relations
easing into, postpartum, 405
father's lack of interest in
postpartum, 421
lack of interest in,
postpartum, 404

resuming postpartum, 403
see also, Making love
Sexually transmitted diseases
AIDS, 37
chlamydia, 36
genital herpes, 35
gonorrhea, 36
NSV, 37
Syphilis, 36
venereal warts, 37
Shape (while carrying), 236
Shaving pubic area in labor,
278
Shoes
for pregnancy, 176
to prevent backache, 174
for safety, 133
for travel, 182
Shortness of breath
in asthma, 329
in third trimester, 234
Shoulder dystocia, 363
Sickle-cell anemia, 337
inheritance of, 338
and pregnancy, 337
testing for, 41, 44
Simpson, Dr. James Young, 226
Single mothering, 28
Sinus headache, 139
treatment of, 435
Sitz bath, 434
Skating, 197
Skiing, 197
Skin
blotchiness, blueness of,
178
changes in pigmentation of,
178
dry, prevention of, 435
eruptions in third trimester,
222
heat rash on, 179
in newborn, 303
itchy, on abdomen, 204
problems in early
pregnancy, 122
rashes, 223
redness and itching of, 178
sun block for, 178
tags, 179
treatment of itchy, 434
Sleep
best positions for, 173

problems, 140
Smoking, 54
allergy to, passive, 158
and breastfeeding, 402
breaking the habit of, 55
effects of other people's,
57
effects of, on pregnancy,
54
father's, 57
long-term effects of, 56,
58
postpartum, 402
preconception, 428
and premature labor, 218
Snacks, 90, 91, 106
Social life, changes in, 417
Sonogram, *see,* Ultrasound
Sorbitol, 130
Sore throat, 310
treatment of, 436
Soup, Cream of Tomato, 93
Spacing of pregnancies, 25
Spermicides, and pregnancy,
39
Spider nevi, 120
Spina bifida, 44, 47
Spinal block, 230
Spinal-cord injuries, 334
Sponge bath, for fever, 434
Spontaneous abortion, *see,*
Miscarriage
Sports, competitive or contact,
197
Sports, participating in, 186
see also, Exercise
Spouse, changing relationship
with, 249
Sprinting, 197
Squatting
in delivery, 300
in labor, 289
STDs, 35, 36, 37
see also, Sexually
transmitted diseases
Standing
in labor, 289
on the job, 204, 205
to prevent backache, 175
Station, of presenting part,
260
Steam room, 65
Stillbirth, 347

Stirrups, use of during delivery,
285
Stomach "flu," 311
Strep, Group B, 315, 431
Stress, 113
dealing with, 114
and premature labor, 220
Stress incontinence, 235
Stress test for fetus, 263
Stretch marks, 141
Stretching, and backache, 175
Sugar, 82
in the blood, 153
regulation of, in the blood,
329
test for, in the blood, 153
test for, in urine, 429
types of, 82
in the urine, 152
Sugar substitutes, 62
aspartame, 130
saccharin, 130
sorbitol and mannitol, 130
Sun block, 178
Surgical delivery, *see,* Forceps;
Cesarean section
Sweating, *see,* Perspiration
Sweeteners, 62, 130
Swelling
of feet and ankles, 217
of hands and face, 217
of hands, face, eyes, 117
Swimming, 197
Symptoms
of complications, in
pregnancy, 117
of complications,
postpartum, 381
of pregnancy, *see,* What
You May Be Feeling
Syphilis, 36
test for, 430
Systemic Lupus Erythematosus,
338

T

Tailbone pain, 376
Tailor exercises, 195
Tay-Sach's disease, 41, 44
TENS, 231
Teeth, in pregnancy, 179

Telangiectases, 120
Telemetry, fetal monitoring
    with, 282
Tennis, 197
Teratogen susceptibility, 76
Tests
    at first prenatal visit, 101
    of fetal well-being, 263
    pregnancy, 2
    prenatal diagnostic, 42
    routine, in pregnancy, 429
Thalassemias, 41
Thalidomide, 76
Thiamine, in supplements, 88
Thirst, when to call
    practitioner for, 117
Throat, sore, 310
    treatment of, 436
Thrombophlebitis, 360
Tiredness, *see,* Fatigue
Tobacco, 54
    see also, Smoking
Tobacco smoke, allergy to, 158
Tocolytic agents, 362
Tomato Soup, Cream of, 93
Toxemia, 204, 351
    see also, Preeclampsia
Toxoplasmosis, 313
    effects of, on fetus, 313
    prevention of, 64
Train travel, 183
Tranquilizers
    as childbirth medication,
        229
    use of, in pregnancy, 60
Transcutaneous electrical
    nerve stimulation
    (TENS), 231
Transitional (third) phase of
    labor, 297
Travel
    to high altitudes, 181
    immunization for, 181
    medical information on,
        182
    safety in third trimester,
        248
    safety of water, during,
        182
    in second trimester, 180
    tips for, 181
Treatments, non-drug, 431
    see also, individual illnesses

Trophoblastic disease, 348
Tubal pregnancy, 109
    see also, Ectopic pregnancy
Tumors, uterine, 177
Twins
    breastfeeding of, 395
    concern about safety of,
        144
    diagnosing, 143, 202
    disappointment over, 146
    labor and delivery with,
        240
    loss of one, 370
    special needs of, 144
    weight gain with, 145
    when one isn't thriving,
        368
Tylenol, *see* Acetaminophen

U

Ultrasound, 45
    for determining
        cephalopelvic
        disproportion, 240
    for determining fetal
        position/presentation,
        240
    for diagnosing pregnancy, 5
    reasons for, 45
    safety of, 45
Umbilical cord
    blood banking, 255
    blood sampling, 51
    cutting of, 304, 306, 308
    prolapse of, 360
Underwater births, 12
Urinary incontinence, 235
Urinary tract infection, 317
    postpartum, 378
Urination
    burning, painful, 117
    delayed, and triggering of
        contractions, 221
    difficulty with postpartum,
        377
    frequent, as a sign of
        pregnancy, 3
    frequent, in first trimester,
        107
    inability to control, 235
    more frequent, after

    lightening, 260
    no increase in, 108
Urine
    blood in, 235
    sugar in, 152
    test for sugar in, 429
Uterine incision, in cesarean,
    23
Uterine inversion, 362
Uterine irritability, 219
Uterine rupture, 362
Uterus
    abnormalities of, 177, 220
    changing shape/position
        of, *see* What You May
        Look Like
    enlargement of, as a sign
        of pregnancy, 4
    inversion of, 362
    postpartum, 376, 401
    rupture of, 362
    "tilted," 133

V

Vacuum extraction, 287
Vagina
    bleeding from, *see,* Bleeding
    changes in, after childbirth,
        285
    leaking of fluid from, 117
    postpartum care of, 376
Vaginal discharge
    bloody, *see,* Bleeding
    in early miscarriage, 111
    in false labor, 269
    in late miscarriage, 177
    in pregnancy, 158
    in prelabor, 269
    and intercourse, 165
    as a sign of infection, 158
    in true labor, 270, 271
Vaginal infection, 158
Vaginal lacerations, 364
Vaginitis, 158
Vaporizer, 433
Varicella, 319
Varicose veins
    of legs, 120
    of rectum, 203
    of vulva, 120
VBAC, 23

VDRL, 430
VDTs, 72
Vegetables and fruits
    chemical residues on, 131
    Food Selection Groups for,
        91
    requirements for, 85, 86
Vegetarian diet, 127
    complete protein
        combinations for, 97
Veins
    spider, 120
    varicose, 120, 203
    visible, 120
    visible, in breasts, 108
Venereal warts, 37
Venous changes in pregnancy,
    108, 120
Venous thrombosis, 360
Vernix caseosa, on newborn,
    302
Version, in breech
    presentation, 237
Vertex presentation, 238
Vicks Vaporub, 432
Video display terminals, 72
Virgin Sangria, 98
Vision problems
    in preeclampsia, 204, 352
    in pregnancy, 186
    when to call the doctor
        for, 117
Vistaril, 229
Vitamin A
    in supplements, 88
    need for, in pregnancy, 85
    overdose of, 89
Vitamin B$_6$, 86
Vitamin B$_{12}$
    in supplements, 88
    in vegetarian diet, 127
Vitamin C
    Food Selection Group, 90
    in supplements, 88
    in vegetarian diet, 127
    requirements in pregnancy,
        85
Vitamin D
    overdose of, 89
    in supplements, 88
    in vegetarian diet, 127
Vitamin E, 86
    in supplements, 88

Vitamin and mineral
    supplements
    difficulty with, 109
    need for, in lactation, 392,
        401
    need for, in pregnancy,
        88, 109
    need for, preconception,
        427
    pregnancy formula for, 88
Vomiting
    in ectopic pregnancy, 110
    with gastroenteritis, 311
    in morning sickness, 105
    severe, 343
    treatment of, 311
    when to call the doctor
        for, 117
Vulva, varicose veins of, 120

W

Waistline expansion, 122
Walking
    in labor, 289, 291, 294
    as pregnancy exercise, 197
Warm soaks, for itchy eyes,
    435
Warm, feeling, 217
Warts, genital, 37
Water beds, 66
Water, drinking
    safety of, 68
    during travel, 182
    see also, Fluids
Weight gain, 147
    and baby's size, 235
    and backache, 174
    breakdown of, 148
    for diabetics, 327
    effects of, on pregnancy,
        147
    in first trimester, 137
    inadequate, and preterm
        labor, 219
    in multiple gestations,
        145
    in ninth month, 269
    in obese women, 34
    in second trimester, 148
    in third trimester, 148
    recommended, 148

recommended rate of, 148
shedding of, postpartum,
    400
sudden, 117
with twins, 145
for underweight women,
    148
Weight loss, postpartum, 400
Weight, excess, and pregnancy,
    34
What You Can Expect at This
    Month's Checkup
    1st month, 100
    2nd month, 119
    3rd month, 134
    4th month, 150
    5th month, 170
    6th month, 199
    7th month, 214
    8th month, 233
    9th month, 256
    postpartum, 397
What You May Be Feeling
    1st month, 102
    2nd month, 119
    3rd month, 134
    4th month, 150
    5th month, 170
    6th month, 199
    7th month, 214
    8th month, 233
    9th month, 257
    after delivery, 305
    during pushing stage of
        childbirth, 300
    in labor, 290, 293, 297
    postpartum, first week,
        374
    postpartum, six weeks,
        396
What You May Look Like
    1st month, 101
    2nd month, 121
    3rd month, 135
    4th month, 151
    5th month, 171
    6th month, 200
    7th month, 215
    8th month, 234
    9th month, 257
Whole grains
    requirements for, in
        pregnancy, 86

Whole-Wheat Buttermilk
     Pancakes, 95
Work
     continuing at after baby
          arrives, 221
     continuing at, during
          pregnancy, 204
     reducing physical stress at,
          205
     risks of certain types of, 72
     standing at, 204
     strenuous, 204
Worry
     about second pregnancy,
          26

about AIDS, 37
about baby, 110, 115, 216
about miscarriage, 113
about pain of childbirth,
     206
about dying, 240

X

X-rays
     dental, 67
     to diagnose cephalopelvic
          disproportion, 235
     effects on fetus of, 66

exposure to,
     preconception, 427
risk of working with, 74
safety guidelines for, 67

Y

Yogurt, Fruited, 98

Z

Zinc, 86
     in supplements, 88

Afterword

Now that you have read *What to Expect When You're Expecting,* you can see that every pregnancy (like every expectant parent) is different, that there are few hard and fast rules about what you can (or should) expect. You have learned that today we can control much of what happens in our pregnancies and childbirths—through the way we utilize medical care, the way we eat, through our lifestyles—making our chances of having a healthy baby better than those of any generation of parents in history. And we hope you have benefited from the fact that, though all of us worry, accurate information can go a long way toward easing our anxieties.

We hope that this book will answer all of your questions, quiet your fears, help you sleep better at night. We hope that by knowing what you can *really* expect, both the expectation and the reality will become more manageable, more exciting, and more truly fulfilling.

In our preparation and research for this book, we strove to leave no question unanswered. We relied not only on our personal experiences but also on those of the hundreds of pregnant parents we surveyed and interviewed. But since the variations of what expectant couples worry about are great, we're likely to have missed a few questions. If we overlooked any of yours, we'd like to know. That way we'll be able to include your concerns (and reassurances for them) in our next edition—in plenty of time, we hope, for *your* next edition.

Wishing you the happiest of pregnancies and the most joyous of outcomes,

Arlene Eisenberg
Heidi E. Murkoff
Sandee E. Hathaway

Also from Arlene Eisenberg, Heidi E. Murkoff, and Sandee E. Hathaway, B.S.N.

❖ ❖ ❖

WHAT TO EXPECT THE FIRST YEAR

The reassuring and comprehensive month-by-month guide to child care in the first year.

"Unquestionably the best book for parents of infants in their first year of life that I have had the pleasure to read."
—Morris Green, M.D., Perry W. Lesh Professor of Pediatrics, Indiana University Medical Center

❖ ❖

WHAT TO EXPECT THE TODDLER YEARS

An all-inclusive guide for the parent of toddlers.

"A first-rate accomplishment . . . I can hardly imagine a parent's question that goes unanswered in these pages."
—Mark D. Widome, M.D., M.P.H.
Professor of Pediatrics, Pennsylvania State University

❖ ❖

WHAT TO EAT WHEN YOU'RE EXPECTING

Best-odds diet, 100 recipes, and everything you need to know to nourish a healthy pregnancy.

"They've done it again! The authors of What to Expect When You're Expecting *have written another book that obstetricians can respect and expectant mothers can love . . . Not only is this book medically accurate, it's easy to follow."*
—Richard Aubry, M.D.

Available at your local retailer. For more information, write to Workman Publishing Company, Inc., 708 Broadway, New York, NY 10003

Additional praise for
WHAT TO EXPECT THE FIRST YEAR

"It is amazingly complete, detailed, and up-to-the-minute not only in its medical information but in addressing the questions posed by today's parents. Although the authors answer every question I have ever heard a parent ask (and some I have not yet heard), they have consistently avoided the 'one size fits all' cookbook answers that so often are simply not helpful. Rather, in a manner that respects the intelligence of parents and has my stunned admiration, they manage to convey information in a highly readable manner that permits the parent to fit the information to his or her own style and baby...With this book in hand parents will feel reassured, competent, well-informed, and confident that they can cope expertly with the first year of life...The authors are to be warmly congratulated on their major contribution to enhancing parentcraft. It is a book to enjoy!"

—Dr. Morris Green,
continued from the backcover

"WHAT TO EXPECT THE FIRST YEAR is a splendid book. The information it contains is accurate and up-to-date, and is presented in a format that is easy to read and understand. The book meets a real need for a reliable resource for parents interested in being more knowledgeable and confident during that important first year of their child's life."

A. Earl Mgebroff, M.D.,
Clinical Associate Professor
of Family Practice,
University of Texas Health
Science Center

"Straight forward, accurate, and empathetic descriptions of both the delights and problems in the first year. Filled with wonderfully sensible advice."

Michael A. Levi, M.D.
Assistant Professor of
Pediatrics, New York State
School of Medicine

Also available from Arlene Eisenberg, Heidi E. Murkoff, and Sandee E. Hathaway, B.S.N.

WHAT TO EXPECT WHEN YOU'RE EXPECTING
WHAT TO EAT WHEN YOU'RE EXPECTING
THE **WHAT TO EXPECT WHEN YOU'RE EXPECTING**
PREGNANCY ORGANIZER
WHAT TO EXPECT THE TODDLER YEARS

What To Expect The First Year

What To Expect The First Year

❖ ❖ ❖

Arlene Eisenberg
Heidi E. Murkoff
Sandee E. Hathaway, B.S.N.

❖ ❖ ❖

Workman Publishing, New York

Library of Congress Cataloging-in-Publication Data
Eisenberg, Arlene. What to expect the first year.
Includes index. 1. Infants. 2. Child rearing. 3. Infants–Care.
I. Murkoff, Heidi Eisenberg. II. Hathaway, Sandee
Eisenberg. III. Title.
HQ774.E47   1988   649'.122   87-40647
ISBN 0-89480-577-0 (pbk.)

"What Your Baby May Be Doing This Month," adapted from DDST © 1978.
W.K. Frankenburg, M.D., by permission of the author.

Cover illustration: Judith Cheng
Book illustration: Marika Hahn

Workman books are available at special discounts when purchased in bulk for
premiums and sales promotions as well as for fund-raising or educational use.
Special editions or book excerpts can also be created to specification. For details,
contact the Special Sales Director at the address below.

Workman Publishing Company, Inc.
708 Broadway
New York, NY 10003

Manufactured in the United States of America
First printing February 1989

88 87 86 85 84 83 82 81 80 79

Note: All children are unique and this book is not intended to substitute for
the advice of your pediatrician or other physician who should be consulted
on infant matters, especially when a baby shows any sign of illness or
unusual behavior.

DEDICATION

To Emma and Wyatt, Rachel and Ethan
for the magical, memorable first years each of you gave us

To our partners in parenting, Howard, Erik, and Tim
without whom we couldn't have made it through those first years

A MILLION THANKS

If there's anyone who needs more help than parents during the first year of a baby's life, it's authors writing a book about the first year of a baby's life. We've been fortunate to be able to get all the help we've needed—from dozens of academics, doctors in practice, other professionals, and parents. We thank them all for the valuable contributions they've made to this work.

Thanks particularly to pediatrician Henry Harris, M.D., and obstetrician Richard Aubry, M.D., our trusted medical advisers, for taking the time to read the manuscript and for giving us the benefit of their knowledge, wisdom, and insight.

Very special thanks to very special doctors Max Kahn, Michael Levi, Michael Traister, and Herb Lazarus, who among them waded heroically through the manuscript in their very spare, spare time. And to Kathy Lawrence and Eve Coulson, who took time out of their busy mothering schedules to read the manuscript and give us their comments.

Thanks, too, to the many other professionals and friends who read pertinent portions of the manuscript and/or offered their expertise, including Ronald L. Poland, M.D.; Michael Lewis, Ph.D.; Alfred T. Lane, M.D.; Irving J. Selikoff, M.D. and Jerrold Abraham, M.D.; Deborah Campbell, M.D.; Barbara Hogan; Judy Lee; Ken Gorfinkle and Doris Ullendorf; Dina Rosenfeld and Howard Berkowitz, M.D.; Richard Weisman, M.D.; Steven M. Silverman, American Red Cross (Greater Boston Region); John J. Caravollas, D.D.S.; Paul Leonard, EMTA; the other Sandy Hathaway, R.N.; Lisa Shulz; Phil Sherman, mohel; Bonnie Cowan; Mary Lewis, Consumer Product Safety Commission; Michelle Weber and Jeff Moulter; Mort Lebow; Bill Delay; Marvin Eiger, M.D., and Sally Wendkos Olds. And thanks to the American Heart Association, the March of Dimes, the American College of Obstetrics and Gynecology, the American Academy of Pediatrics, and *Contemporary Pediatrics,* for their invaluable help and mountains of information.

To David and Shana Roskies, Sarah Jacobs and David Kronfeld, Susan and David Kramer, Ann Wimpfheimer and Baruch Bokser, Herb and Judy Seaman, Bilick Shelly Bazes and Rueven Weiss, Nessa Rapoport and Toby Kahn, Linda and David Shriner-Kahn, Pearl Beck and David Fisher, Alan Nadler and Diane Sharon, Sharon and Michael Strassfeld, Betsy and David Teutsch, and countless other parents for sharing their concerns with us, so that we could share them with our readers.

To Marika Hahn for her lovely illustrations.

To the entire Workman Publishing crew, for their tireless support and good humor, but especially to Suzanne Rafer for caring as much as we do. And to Kathy Herlihy-Paoli, Mary Wilkinson, Lisa Hollander, Shannon Ryan, Barbara Scott-Goodman, Bert Snyder, Janet Harris, Ina Stern, Saundra Pearson, Steve Garvan, Linda Randel, Jim Joseph, Andrea Glickson, Chip Duckett, and all those who helped this book to come to fruition and get a good healthy start. And to Peter Workman, without whom none of this could ever happen.

To Elise and Arnold Goodman, our agents and friends, who had the good sense to bring us to Workman in the first place.

To Mimi and Gramps, who taught us the importance of love in parenting.

To the caring parents and good friends who participated in our classes and seminars and taught us so much. And, finally, to the many readers of *What to Expect When You're Expecting* who asked that we write this book.

Contents

FOREWORD: A Word From the Doctor xxi

INTRODUCTION: Why This Book Was Conceived xxiii
What Your Baby May Be Doing This Month

PART ONE: The First Year 1

CHAPTER ONE: Get Ready, Get Set 2

FEEDING YOUR BABY: Breast or Bottle? 2
Facts Favoring Breastfeeding • Facts Favoring Bottle Feeding • Factoring in Feelings • *Breastfeeding Myths* • *Adoption and Breastfeeding* • When You Can't or Shouldn't Breastfeed

WHAT YOU MAY BE CONCERNED ABOUT 10
Coping With Motherhood • A Changing Lifestyle • Whether or not to Go Back to Work • Dad Taking Time Off • Grandparents • A Lack of Grandparents • Considering a Baby Nurse • Other Sources of Help • Circumcision • Which Diapers to Use • Quitting Smoking • A Name for Baby • Preparing the Family Pet • Preparing Your Breasts for Breastfeeding

WHAT IT'S IMPORTANT TO KNOW: Selecting the Right Physician 25
Pediatrician or Family Physician • What Kind of Practice Is Perfect? • Finding Dr. Right • Making Sure Dr. Right Is Right for You • The Prenatal Interview • Your Partnership With Dr. Right • *Prepaid Medicine*

CHAPTER TWO: Buying for Baby 35
First Wardrobe • Linen Wardrobe • Toiletries • Medicine Chest • Feeding Supplies • Furnishings • Outing Equipment • Nice to Have • You Will Need, or May Want, Later • What to Take to the Hospital • *Going Home*

CHAPTER THREE: Your Newborn Baby 45

WHAT YOUR BABY MAY BE DOING 45
WHAT YOU CAN EXPECT AT THE HOSPITAL CHECKUPS 45
Portrait of a Newborn • Apgar Test • Your Newborn's Reflexes • *Apgar Table* • *The Brazelton Neonatal Behavioral Assessment Scale*

FEEDING YOUR BABY: Getting Started 49
    Getting Started Breastfeeding • *Breastfeeding Basics* • Getting Started
    Bottle Feeding • Selecting a Formula • Safe Bottle Feeding • Bottle
    Feeding With Love • *Sterilizing Techniques* • Bottle Feeding With Ease •
    Tips for Successful Feeding Sessions

WHAT YOU MAY BE CONCERNED ABOUT 60
    Sleeping Through Meals • Not Sleeping After Meals • Birthweight •
    Bonding • Rooming-In • Baby's Not Getting Enough to Eat • Baby's
    Sleepiness • Pain Medication • Baby's Looks • Eye Color • Gagging and
    Choking • Startling • Quivering Chin • Birthmarks • Complexion
    Problems • Mouth Cysts or Spots • Early Teeth • Thrush • Weight Loss •
    Jaundice • Pacifier Use • Stool Color • Eye Discharge

WHAT IT'S IMPORTANT TO KNOW: The Baby Care Primer 73
    Bathing Baby • Burping Baby • Diapering Baby • *Safe Seating* • Dressing
    Baby • Ear Care • Lifting and Carrying Baby • Nail Trimming • Nose
    Care • Outings With Baby • Penis Care • Shampooing Baby • Swaddling
    Baby • Umbilical Stump Care • *Baby Business*

CHAPTER FOUR: The First Month 89

WHAT YOUR BABY MAY BE DOING 89

WHAT YOU CAN EXPECT AT THIS MONTH'S CHECKUP 90

FEEDING YOUR BABY THIS MONTH: Expressing Breast Milk 91
    Why Mothers Express Milk • Techniques for Expressing Breast Milk •
    How to Express Breast Milk • Collecting and Storing Breast Milk

WHAT YOU MAY BE CONCERNED ABOUT 95
    "Breaking" Baby • Infant Acne • Hearing • Vision • Spitting Up • Swad-
    dling • Having Enough Breast Milk • Your Breastfed Baby Not Thriving •
    Double the Trouble, Double the Fun • The Fontanels • Nursing Blisters •
    Healing of the Umbilical Cord • Umbilical Hernia • Sneezing • Crossed
    Eyes • Teary Eyes • First Smiles • Keeping Baby the Right Temperature •
    Taking Baby Out • Exposure to Outsiders • Skin Color Changes • Feeding
    Schedule • Hiccups • Bowel Movements • Constipation • Explosive Bowel
    Movements • Passing Gas • Milk Allergy • Using Detergent on Baby's
    Clothes • Restless Sleep • Sleeping Patterns • Noise When Baby Is Sleep-
    ing • Pacifier • Checking Baby's Breathing • Mixing Up of Night and Day •
    Better Sleep for Baby • Sleeping Positions • Moving a Sleeping Baby to
    Bed • Crying • Colic • *Prescription for Colic* • Helping Siblings Live With
    Colic • Surviving Colic • *Coping With Crying* • *Comforting the Crier* •
    When to Check Crying With the Doctor • Spoiling Baby • Blood in Spitup •
    Changing Your Mind About Breastfeeding • Photo Flashes • Loud
    Music • Vitamin Supplements • Circumcision Care • Swollen Scrotum •
    Hypospadias • *Keeping Baby Safe*

WHAT IT'S IMPORTANT TO KNOW: Babies Develop Differently 137

CHAPTER FIVE: The Second Month 140

WHAT YOUR BABY MAY BE DOING 140

WHAT YOU CAN EXPECT AT THIS MONTH'S CHECKUP 141
FEEDING YOUR BABY THIS MONTH: Supplementary Bottles 142
Why Supplement? • How to Supplement • *Emergency Cache* • Supplementing When Baby Isn't Thriving
WHAT YOU MAY BE CONCERNED ABOUT 144
Cradle Cap • Smiling • Cooing • Crooked Feet • Comparing Babies • Using a Baby Carrier • Immunization • *What You Should Know About DTP* • *Immunization Time Frame Recommended by the AAP* • Flu Immunization • Undescended Testicles • Hernia • Inverted Nipples • Rejection of the Breast • Favoring One Breast • Difficult Baby • *Do You Have a Difficult Baby?* • *How Do You Talk to a Baby?* • A Second Language • Baby Talk
WHAT IT'S IMPORTANT TO KNOW: Stimulating Your Baby in the Early Months 163
Creating a Good Environment • Practical Tips for Learning and Playing

CHAPTER SIX: The Third Month 169

WHAT YOUR BABY MAY BE DOING 169
WHAT YOU CAN EXPECT AT THIS MONTH'S CHECKUPS 170
FEEDING YOUR BABY THIS MONTH: Nursing While Working Outside the Home 170
Making Nursing and Employment Work
WHAT YOU MAY BE CONCERNED ABOUT 173
Establishing a Regular Schedule • Putting Baby to Bed • Not Sleeping Through the Night • Still Using a Pacifier • Spastic Movements • Giving Baby Cow's Milk • Diaper Rash • Penis Sore • Sudden Infant Death Syndrome • *What is SIDS?* • *Reporting Breathing Emergencies to Your Doctor* • Early Weaning • Sharing a Room With Baby • Sharing a Bed • Roughhousing • Fewer Bowel Movements • Leaving Baby With a Sitter • Being Tied Down by a Nursing Baby • *Baby-Sitter Check List*
WHAT IT'S IMPORTANT TO KNOW: The Right Caretakers for Baby 190
In-Home Care • Group Day Care • Home Day Care • *Your Child as a Barometer of Child Care* • Corporate Day Care • Babies on the Job • When Your Child Is Sick

CHAPTER SEVEN: The Fourth Month 200

WHAT YOUR BABY MAY BE DOING 200
WHAT YOU CAN EXPECT AT THIS MONTH'S CHECKUP 201
FEEDING YOUR BABY THIS MONTH: Thinking About Solids 202
WHAT YOU MAY BE CONCERNED ABOUT 203
Wriggling at Changing Time • Propping Baby • Baby's Standing • Thumb Sucking • Chubby Baby • Thin Baby • *How Does Your Baby Grow?* • Heart Murmur • Black Stool • Baby Massage • Exercise
WHAT IT'S IMPORTANT TO KNOW: Playthings for Baby 212

CHAPTER EIGHT: The Fifth Month 215

WHAT YOUR BABY MAY BE DOING 215
WHAT YOU CAN EXPECT AT THIS MONTH'S CHECKUP 216
FEEDING YOUR BABY THIS MONTH: Starting Solids 216
  Opening Night—and Beyond • Foods to Premiere With • *Good Early Foods to Offer Baby* • Expanding Baby's Repertoire • Best-Odds Diet for Beginners • *No Honey for Your Little Honey* • The Infant Daily Dozen • *Double-Duty Jars*
WHAT YOU MAY BE CONCERNED ABOUT 223
  Teething • *Teething Chart* • Chronic Cough • Ear Pulling • Naps • Eczema • Using a Back Carrier • Gratuitous Advice • Starting the Cup • *Feeding Baby Safely* • Food Allergies • Walkers • Jumpers • Feeding Chairs • *Safety Tips for Feeding Chairs*
WHAT IT'S IMPORTANT TO KNOW: Environmental Hazards and Your Baby 236
  Household Pesticides • Lead • *EPA Hotline* • Otherwise Contaminated Water • Polluted Indoor Air • *Unsafe Play Sand* • Contaminants in Food • *What to Keep Out of the Mouths of Babes* • *Food Hazards in Perspective* • *Organic Foods—Boon or Bane? An Apple a Day? Not Any More* • Your Role as a Consumer

CHAPTER NINE: The Sixth Month 245

WHAT YOUR BABY MAY BE DOING 245
WHAT YOU CAN EXPECT AT THIS MONTH'S CHECKUP 246
FEEDING YOUR BABY THIS MONTH: Commercial or Home-Prepared Baby Foods 247
  Commercial Baby Food • Home-Prepared Baby Foods
WHAT YOU MAY BE CONCERNED ABOUT 249
  Changes in Bowel Movements • Bottle Rejection • Shoes for Baby • Bathing in the Big Tub • Bath Fears • Brushing Baby's Teeth • *Baby's First Toothbrush* • Giving Baby Cow's Milk • Baby-Bottle Mouth • Anemia • Vegetarian Diet • Salt Intake • *Sodium Content of Foods Fed to Babies* • The Whole-Grain Habit • Early Rising • Still Not Sleeping Through the Night • Crying It Out • *Another Route to Sleeping Through the Night?*
WHAT IT'S IMPORTANT TO KNOW: Stimulating Your Older Baby 263
  How Do You Speak to Your Baby Now?

CHAPTER TEN: The Seventh Month 266

WHAT YOUR BABY MAY BE DOING 266
WHAT YOU CAN EXPECT AT THIS MONTH'S CHECKUPS 267
FEEDING YOUR BABY THIS MONTH: Moving Up From Strained Foods 267
WHAT YOU MAY BE CONCERNED ABOUT 268
  Biting Nipples • Spoiling Babies • Baby's Still Not Sleeping Through the Night • Grandparents Spoiling Baby • Is My Baby Gifted? • Snacking • Grazing • Not Sitting Yet • Tooth Stains • Baby's Misbehaving With You

WHAT IT'S IMPORTANT TO KNOW: Raising a Superbaby 275

CHAPTER ELEVEN: The Eight Month 278

WHAT YOUR BABY MAY BE DOING 278
WHAT YOU CAN EXPECT AT THIS MONTH'S CHECKUP 279
FEEDING YOUR BABY THIS MONTH: Finally—Finger Foods 279
WHAT YOU MAY BE CONCERNED ABOUT 281
    Baby's First Words • Baby's Not Crawling Yet • Scooting • Messy House •
    Eating off the Floor • Eating Dirt—and Worse • Erections • Discovering
    Genitals • Getting Dirty • Rough Play • Playpen Use • Reading to Baby •
    Left- or Right-handedness • Childproofing Your Home
WHAT IT'S IMPORTANT TO KNOW: Making Home Safe for Baby 292
    Poison Control • Safety Equipment • Red Light on Greenery

CHAPTER TWELVE: The Ninth Month 303

WHAT YOUR BABY MAY BE DOING 303
WHAT YOU CAN EXPECT AT THIS MONTH'S CHECKUP 304
FEEDING YOUR BABY THIS MONTH: Establishing Good Habits Now 305
WHAT YOU MAY BE CONCERNED ABOUT 307
    Feeding Baby at the Table • Walking too Early • Pulling Up • Fear of
    Strangers • Security Objects • Flat Feet • No Teeth • Still Hairless • Loss
    of Interest in Nursing • Fussy Eating Habits • Self-Feeding • Changes in
    Sleep Patterns • Slow Development • Strange Stools • Baby and Bikes
WHAT IT'S IMPORTANT TO KNOW: Games Babies Play 318

CHAPTER THIRTEEN: The Tenth Month 321

WHAT YOUR BABY MAY BE DOING 321
WHAT YOU CAN EXPECT AT THIS MONTH'S CHECKUP 322
FEEDING YOUR BABY THIS MONTH: Thinking About Weaning 322
WHAT YOU MAY BE CONCERNED ABOUT 325
    Messy Eating Habits • Head Banging, Rocking, and Rolling • Blinking •
    Hair Rolling and Pulling • Teeth Grinding • Breath Holding • Toilet
    Training • Starting Classes • Shoes for Walking • Biting • Hair Care •
    Fears
WHAT IT'S IMPORTANT TO KNOW: The Beginnings of Discipline 335
    To Spank or not to Spank

CHAPTER FOURTEEN: The Eleventh Month 341

WHAT YOUR BABY MAY BE DOING 341
WHAT YOU CAN EXPECT AT THIS MONTH'S CHECKUP 342
FEEDING YOUR BABY THIS MONTH: Weaning Your Baby From
the Breast 342
    Keeping Yourself Comfortable

WHAT YOU MAY BE CONCERNED ABOUT 344
        Bowed Legs • Unclear Speech • Parental Nudity • Falls • Not Pulling Up
        Yet • Cholesterol in Baby's Diet • *Raising a Healthy Heart* • Growth
        Swings • *Fats: The Good, the Best, and the Bad*
WHAT IT'S IMPORTANT TO KNOW: Helping Baby to Talk 351

CHAPTER FIFTEEN: The Twelfth Month 355

WHAT YOUR BABY MAY BE DOING 355
WHAT YOU CAN EXPECT AT THIS MONTH'S CHECKUP 356
FEEDING YOUR BABY THIS MONTH: The Best-Odds Toddler Diet 357
        The Best-Odds Nine Basic Principles • The Best-Odds Daily Dozen—for
        Toddlers • *Milk Sense* • *Vegetarian Protein Combinations for Toddlers* •
        Dairy Protein Combinations for Toddlers
WHAT YOU MAY BE CONCERNED ABOUT 363
        The First Birthday Party • Not Yet Walking • Attachment to the Bottle •
        Putting the Weaned Baby to Bed • Waking Up at Night • Shyness • Social
        Backwardness • Sharing • Hitting • "Forgetting" a Skill • A Drop in
        Appetite • Baby's Getting Adequate Nutrition • Increase in Appetite •
        Refusing to Self-Feed • Unpredictability • Increased Separation Anxiety •
        Nonverbal Language • Gender Differences • Switching to a Bed • Watch-
        ing TV • Hyperactivity • Negativisim
WHAT IT'S IMPORTANT TO KNOW: Stimulating the Toddler 380
        Safety Reminder

PART TWO: Of Special Concern 383

CHAPTER SIXTEEN: A Baby for All Seasons 384

FEEDING YOUR BABY: 'Round the Calendar 384
WHAT YOU MAY BE CONCERNED ABOUT IN SUMMER OR
SUMMERY WEATHER 385
        Keeping Baby Cool • Heatstroke • Too Much Sun • *What to Look for in*
        Selecting a Sunscreen • Insect Bites • Summer Safety • Water Babies •
        Weaning in Summer • *Drownproofing Your Family* • Food Spoilage •
        Swollen Cheeks
WHAT YOU MAY BE CONCERNED ABOUT IN WINTER OR
WINTRY WEATHER 393
        Keeping Baby Warm • *Changeable Weather* • Frostbite • Snow Burn •
        Keeping Baby Warm Indoors • Dry Skin • Fireplace Fires • Holiday
        Hazards • Safe Gift Giving
WHAT IT'S IMPORTANT TO KNOW: The Season for Travel 397
        Planning Ahead • Packing Wisely • Getting There Is Half the Fun •
        High Altitudes • At Hotels and Motels—or Other Homes Away From
        Home • Restaurant Survival • Having Fun

CHAPTER SEVENTEEN: **When Baby Is Sick** 406

Before Calling the Doctor • *Mother's Intuition* • How Much Rest for a
Sick Baby? • Feeding a Sick Baby • When Medication Is Needed • *The
Chicken Soup Cure*

THE MOST COMMON INFANT HEALTH PROBLEMS 413

Allergies • *Treating Baby's Symptoms* • *Respiratory Sounds You Don't
Have to Worry About* • The Common Cold or Upper Respiratory
Infection (URI) • *The Sudden Cough* • Constipation • Diarrhea • Middle-
Ear Inflammation (Otitis Media) • *Your Baby's Health History*

WHAT IT'S IMPORTANT TO KNOW: **All About Fever** 426

Taking Baby's Temperature • Evaluating a Fever • Treating a Fever •
Handling Febrile Convulsions • *Aspirin or Non-Aspirin?* • *Know Your
Baby*

CHAPTER EIGHTEEN: **First Aid Do's and Don'ts** 434

(A gray color bar has been placed at the top of this chapter so that it
may be identified and turned to quickly.)

Abdominal Injuries • Bites • Bleeding • Bleeding, Internal • Broken
Bones or Fractures • Bruises, Skin • Burns and Scalds • *Be Prepared* •
Chemical Burns • Convulsions • Cuts • Dislocations • Dog Bites •
Drowning • Ear Injuries • Electric Shock • Eye Injury • Fainting •
Finger and Toe Injuries • *Treating a Young Patient* • Frostbite • Head
Injuries • Heat Injuries • Hypothermia • Insect Bites • Lip, Split or Cut •
Mouth Injuries • Nose Injuries • Poisoning • Puncture Wounds • Scrapes •
Severed Limb or Digit • Shock • Skin Wounds • Splinters or Slivers •
Sunburn • Teeth, Injury to • Toe Injuries • Tongue, Injury to • *Label
Your Ipecac*

RESUSCITATION TECHNIQUES FOR BABIES 448

Resuscitation: Rescue Breathing • Cardiopulmonary Resuscitation (CPR):
Babies Under One Year • Cardiopulmonary Resuscitation (CPR):
Babies Over One Year • When Baby Is Choking • *The Unsuspected
Inhaled Object*

CHAPTER NINETEEN: **The Low-Birthweight Baby** 457

FEEDING BABY: **Nutrition for the Preterm or Low-Birthweight Infant** 458

Portrait of a Premie • *Expressing Milk for a Premature Baby*

WHAT YOU MAY BE CONCERNED ABOUT 461

Getting Optimum Care • *The Neonatal Intensive Care Unit or Intensive
Care Nursery* • Lack of Bonding • Intrauterine Growth Retardation •
Long Hospitalization • Siblings • Breastfeeding • Catching Up •
Handling Baby • Guilt • Permanent Problems • Car Seats • A Repeat
With the Next Baby • *Special Care Tips for Preterm Babies*

WHAT IT'S IMPORTANT TO KNOW: **Health Problems Common in
Low-Birthweight Babies**. 472

CHAPTER TWENTY: The Baby With Problems 475

FEEDING BABY: Can Diet Make a Difference? 476
WHAT YOU MAY BE CONCERNED ABOUT 476
Feeling Responsible • Feeling Angry • Not Loving the Baby • What to
Tell Others • Handling It All • *Be a Friend in Deed* • Getting the Right
Diagnosis • Whether or not to Accept Treatment • Getting the Best
Care and Treatment • Effect of Baby on Siblings • Effects on Your
Marriage • A Repeat With the Next Baby • A Different Birth Defect
Next Time
**WHAT IT'S IMPORTANT TO KNOW: The Most Common Birth
Disorders** 485
Aids—Perinatal • Anencephaly • Autism • Cancer • Celiac Disease •
Cerebral Palsy • Cleft Lip and/or Palate • Clubfoot • Congenital Heart
Defect • Cystic Fibrosis (CF) • Deformation • Down Syndrome • Fetal
Alcohol Syndrome (FAS) • Hydrocephalus (Water on the Brain) •
Malformation • PKU (Phenylketonuria) • Pyloric Stenosis • Sickle-Cell
Anemia • *How Defects Are Inherited* • *When a Baby Dies* • Rh Disease •
Spina Bifida (Open Spine) • Tay-Sachs Disease • Thalassemia •
Tracheal-Esophageal Fistula

CHAPTER TWENTY-ONE: The Adopted Baby 499

WHAT YOU MAY BE CONCERNED ABOUT 499
Getting Ready • Not Feeling Like a Parent • Feeling Inadequate • Loving
the Baby • Baby's Crying a Lot • Postadoption Blues • Not Being Able to
Breastfeed • Grandparents' Attitudes • Unknown Health Problems • Dealing With Friends and Family • Telling Baby

CHAPTER TWENTY-TWO: The First Postpartum Days 507

WHAT YOU MAY BE FEELING 507
WHAT TO EXPECT AT YOUR IN-HOSPITAL CHECKUPS 508
WHAT YOU SHOULD BE EATING: Surviving Hospital Food 509
WHAT YOU MAY BE CONCERNED ABOUT 511
Feelings of Failure • Broken Tailbone • Black and Bloodshot eyes •
Abdominal Cramping • *When to Call Your Practitioner* • Chest Pain •
Bleeding • Thrombophlebitis • Pain in the Perineal Area • *Perineal Care* •
Getting Out of Bed • Difficulty With Urination • Having a Bowel Move-
ment • Hemorrhoids • Excessive Perspiration • Engorged Breasts • Drying
Up Your Milk • Hospital Confusion • Going Home • Recovery From a
Cesarean Secton
WHAT IT'S IMPORTANT TO KNOW: Getting Back Into Shape 525
Guidelines for Safe and Sane Postpartum Exercise • *Heart Rate Guide-
lines for Postpartum Exercise* • A Postpartum Exercise Program • *Kegel
Exercises* • *Note to Adoptive Mothers* • *Phase Two: The Exercises*

CHAPTER TWENTY-THREE: Surviving the First Six Weeks....... 533

WHAT YOU MAY BE FEELING 533
WHAT YOU CAN EXPECT AT YOUR SIX-WEEK CHECKUP 534
WHAT YOU SHOULD BE EATING: The Best-Odds Postpartum Diet 534
Nine Basic Diet Principles for New Mothers • The Best-Odds Daily
Dozen for Postpartum and Breastfeeding • If You're Not Breastfeeding
WHAT YOU MAY BE CONCERNED ABOUT............................. 540
Getting Everything Done • Not Being in Control • Regaining Your Figure •
Sharing Baby Care • Depression • Feeling Inadequate • Visitors • Doing
Things Right • Postpartum Tub Baths • Time Spent Breastfeeding • Con-
tamination of Breast Milk • Sore Nipples • Leaking and Spraying •
Mastitis • Lump in Breast • Hair Loss • Renewed Bleeding • Postpartum
Infection/Fever • Long-Term Cesarean Recovery • Resuming Sexual
Relations
WHAT IT'S IMPORTANT TO KNOW: Making Love Again 560
Why the Lack of Interest? • *Easing Back Into Sex* • What Can You Do
About It?

CHAPTER TWENTY-FOUR: Enjoying the First Year 564

WHAT YOU MAY BE FEELING 564
WHAT YOU MAY BE EATING: The Best-Odds for a Healthy Future 564
WHAT YOU MAY BE CONCERNED ABOUT............................. 565
Finding Outside Interests • Leaving Baby With a Sitter • Stretched Vagina •
Return of Menstruation • Getting Pregnant Again • *Oral Contraceptive
Warning Signs* • *IUD Warning Signs* • *Calculating the Calendar Rhythm
Method* • *The Basal Body Temperature* • Diagnosing a New Pregnancy •
Exhaustion • Aches and Pains • Urinary Incontinence • Friendships •
Different Mothering Styles • Breastfeeding During Illness • Persistent
Depression • Finding Time for Yourself • Baby Forgetting You • Quality
Time • Finding Time for Romance • Jealousy of Daddy's Attention to
Baby • Jealousy of Daddy's Parenting Skills • Feeling Unappreciated as a
Woman • Thinking About the Next Baby
WHAT IT'S IMPORTANT TO KNOW: To Work or Not to Work............... 587
When to Return to Your Job

CHAPTER TWENTY-FIVE: Becoming a Father.................... 591

WHAT YOU MAY BE CONCERNED ABOUT 591
Your Diet and Your Baby • A Disappointing Delivery • Bonding • Wife's
Postpartum Depression • Your Depression • Feeling Unsexy • Exclusion
From Breastfeeding • Jealousy of Mother's Attention to Baby • Feeling
Inadequate as a Father • Handling Baby • Baby's Crying • Unfair Burden •
Not Enough Time to Spend With Baby

CHAPTER TWENTY-SIX: From Only Child to Older Child 601

WHAT YOU MAY BE CONCERNED ABOUT............................. 602
   Preparing an Older Child • Siblings at the Birth • Separation and Hospital
   Visits • Easing the Homecoming • Open Resentment • Your Own Resent-
   ment • Explaining Genital Differences • Nursing in Front of an Older
   Child • The Older Child Who Wants to Nurse • Regressive Behavior •
   The Older Sibling Hurting the New Baby • Avoiding Jealousy • Lack of
   Jealousy • Sibling Attachment • Escalating Warfare

PART THREE: Ready Reference 617

BEST-ODDS RECIPES 618

FOR THE FIRST YEAR AND BEYOND 618
   Super Cereal • Fruited Cheese Bread • *Low-Sodium Baking Powder* •
   Pumpkin Muffins • Pancake Faces • Golden-Nugget Oatmeal Flapjacks
   • Croque Bébé • Banana French Toast • Cottage Cheese Sundae • Funny
   Fingers • Baby's First Cake • Golden Cake • Dried Apricot Purée • First
   Birthday Cake • Cream Cheese Frosting • Oatmeal Raisin Cookies •
   Apple-Cranberry Cubes • Banana-Orange Gel • Peachy Yogurt

COMMON HOME REMEDIES 627
   Cold Compresses • Cold Soaks • Cool Compresses • Eye Soaks •
   Dosage Chart for Common Infant-Fever Medication • Heating Pad • Hot
   Compresses • Hot Soaks • Hot-Water Bottle • Humidifier • Ice Pack •
   Ice Water • Increased Fluids • Nasal Aspiration • Salt-Water Irrigation •
   Steam • Warm Compresses

COMMON CHILDHOOD ILLNESSES 630

HEIGHT AND WEIGHT CHARTS 650

INDEX 653

A WORD FROM THE DOCTOR

A new baby is fun and exciting, but anxiety provoking, too. At the outset, the responsibilities of new parenthood loom awesomely large. But that natural insecurity and concern are manageable with reassuring advice, down-to-earth information, and an occasional good night's sleep. *What to Expect the First Year* guarantees two out of three, and as such is a welcome extension of my role as counselor to parents with a new baby.

I'm impressed with the authors' medical accuracy, and with the sensible way it's translated into useful mother-to-mother advice. Anticipatory guidance—on feeding, colic, crawling, safety, and day-to-day crisis control—is the heart of pediatrics. During pregnancy, you probably found the reassurance and easily accessed answers you needed in *What to Expect When You're Expecting*. This book picks up where that one left off, telling you what you need to know when you need to know it: as baby grows, one month at a time.

Pediatrics has changed dramatically since I began practicing and teaching it at Albert Einstein Medical Center 25 years ago. Not just in hi-tech diagnosis, treatment, and management of disease. The new mothers and fathers I see today are more advanced, too—more challenging, better informed, more searching and sophisticated in their questions. For them, this lively, comprehensive, and well-organized book is just what the pediatrician ordered.

I was pleased when the American Academy of Pediatrics asked me as an AAP national media spokesman to review the manuscript. One of its three authors is a grandmother, and today's pediatrician, too, assumes that role. Solving a rare diagnostic dilemma may be the pediatric challenge we enjoy most. But in practice, the day to day essence of our work is surrogate grandparenting. With the old extended family virtually dismantled, grandmothers are jogging, sculpting, golfing, traveling, and starting new careers. For the anticipatory guidance grandma once dispensed, parents now turn to their pediatricians.

That kind of guidance is so indispensable that last year, on a trip to China to evaluate pediatric practices, I was astonished at its absence. When I commented to my host pediatricians, "I notice you don't give any advice on child development or mothers' everyday problems," they looked at me oddly. "That's true," said the senior physician, "We're too busy." It wasn't until I was invited to his home for lunch and two sets of grandparents descended from their rooms to join us for tea that I understood. "There's our answer," I exclaimed to my wife. "Chinese parents don't need pediatricians for advice on feeding and toilet training. They've got live-in grandmothers."

The advice in *What to Expect the First Year,"* I'm happy to say, is a lot more up-to-date, informative, and authoritative than grandma's. I've never seen a popular pediatrics book as strong on diet and nutrition. The recommendations of AAP committees on nutrition and early childhood—with the new concerns about cholesterol, obesity, and fitness—receive excellent support on these pages. The information on "What Your Baby Should Be Doing This Month" should be wonderfully helpful. And the guidance on the three major parent-child combat zones (sleeping, feeding, and stool-gazing) deserves the thorough, well-balanced treatment it receives—more attention than many busy pediatricians can manage to give.

In short, I'm delighted that so thorough and useful a book—one which I suspect will be to parents of the 80s and 90s what Spock was to those of the 50s and 60s—

has been published at last. How glad? I plan to hand a copy to every new mother who comes through my office door.

Read it. Enjoy it. You can rely on it. *What to Expect the First Year*—a book by mothers—is first-rate. It won't replace your pediatrician, but it will make his or her life easier, and its well-researched counsel will save you a lot of anxiety.

Henry Harris, M.D.,
Fellow of the American Academy of Pediatrics,
Albert Einstein Medical Center, New York

WHY THIS BOOK WAS CONCEIVED

It seemed so simple and so certain. I would walk into the hospital pregnant and walk out a mother. The role that had come naturally to thousands of generations of women would surely come naturally to me—courtesy of my endocrine glands, which would magically endow me with all the expertise I needed to care for my baby and all the milk I needed to feed her.

Emma's cord had barely been cut when I tested the efficacy of that theory for the first time; it seemed faulty, to say the least. Not only weren't my feelings on cradling my brand-new daughter, still damp from amniotic fluid and ruddy with my blood, less glowing than I'd expected, they were more ambivalent than I'd ever imagined. Why didn't I feel close to her? Why didn't she seem to feel close to me? And why— oh, why—didn't she stop crying? More faults surfaced as I lifted my gown and aimed Emma's swollen face at my breast. Instinct seemed sorely lacking on both sides. My attempts at maneuvering my breast into her mouth were completely ineffectual; her attempts to take hold of the nipple and suckle (she invariably took hold and then let it go) were equally futile.

Nor did matters improve on our arrival home; my ineptitude was evident everywhere and all the time. When I changed her diaper, when I burped her, when I tried to get her to eat or sleep, when I bathed her and dressed her. In the next few weeks, I cried almost as much as Emma did. No mean feat, considering her colic.

Surely I was the most imcompetent mother ever. Or so I thought—until I started talking to other mothers. Feelings of incompetence rivaling mine were, I discovered, rampant among those spending their first weeks as parents. As were the worries (I'd thought I had the market cornered on these, too). Worries that baby wasn't eating enough and was sleeping too much. Worries about the blotchiness of baby's skin and the looseness of baby's bowel movements. Worries about the risks of exposing baby to strangers and their germs, and the risks of immunizing against disease.

Like other new mothers, I turned to every conceivable source for reassurance and guidance—baby books, magazines, more experienced family members, friends who'd been through it before. Each had something to offer, but the sum total of the information they could provide (most of which was contradictory anyway) couldn't answer a fraction of my questions. My baby's pediatricians probably could have answered most of them, but none of them was willing to move in with Emma, my husband Erik, and me.

And so, just as *What to Expect When You're Expecting* was born out of a need for practical, easily accessible, month-by-month information and day-to-day reassurance during the nine months of pregnancy, *What to Expect the First Year* was born out of the same needs during the first twelve months of parenting.

What to Expect the First Year is designed to make the first year easier (it will never be *easy*), to guide you—and your spouse and older children—through the hundreds of problems, crises, and transitions that are an inevitable part of the first year, with the understanding and empathy of those who've gone through it themselves and the benefit of the latest medical information.[1] It strives to take into account the

---

1. For the reader's convenience, we've repeated some material in chapters 1, 22, 23, 24, and 25 that previously appeared in *What to Expect When You're Expecting.*

WHAT YOUR BABY MAY BE DOING THIS MONTH

All parents want to know if their babies are developing well. The problem is that when they compare their babies to the "average" baby of the same age, they find that their own children are usually ahead or behind—few are exactly average. To help you determine whether your baby's development fits within the wide range of normal rather than just into the limited range of "average," we've developed a monthly span of achievements into which virtually all babies fall, based on the Denver Developmental Screening Tests and on the Clinical Linguistic Auditory Milestones (CLAMS). In any one month, a full 90% of all babies will have mastered the achievements in the first category, "What your baby should be able to do." About 75% will have gained command of those in the second category, "What your baby will probably be able to do." Roughly half will have accomplished the feats in the third category, "What your baby may possibly be able to do." And about 25% will have pulled off the exploits in the last category, "What your baby may

even be able to do."

Most parents will find their babies achieving in several different categories at any one time. A few may find their offspring staying constantly in the same category. Some may find their baby's development uneven—slow one month, making a big leap the next. All can relax in the knowledge that their babies are perfectly normal.

Only when a baby is not achieving what a child of the same age "should be able to do" on a consistent basis, need a parent be concerned and consult the doctor. Even then, no problem may exist.

Use the What Your Baby May Be Doing sections of the book to check progress monthly, if you like. But don't use them to make judgments about your baby's abilities now or in the future. They are not predictive. If checking your baby against such lists becomes anxiety provoking rather than reassuring, by all means ignore them. Your baby will develop just as well if you never look at them—and you may be happier.

individual differences among mothers and among babies—as with pregnancies, wide ranges of "normal" exist. It allows for variations in parenting styles, too, since far more often than not when it comes to babycare decisions, there is no one "right" way to proceed.[2] It trusts a mother's instincts, but recognizes that she often doesn't trust them herself. And most of all it reassures that almost everything a mother feels and almost everything a baby does is normal—even if it's not what the mother next door is feeling or what the baby next door is doing.

I survived the first year. In fact, as my weeks on the job turned to months, and Emma and I settled into our roles more comfortably, I began to enjoy mothering. So much so that not long after, I decided to become a mother again. Five years later I (and my co-author and sister, Sandee, who has also made the trip through the first twelve months twice during this time) realize how true it is that the good things in life—chief among them children—don't come easily, but that they are most emphatically worth the effort.

It is to that effort—and to you who are about to make it—that we dedicate *What to Expect the First Year.*

Heidi E. Murkoff
New York City

2. Of course, when it comes to medical decisions, mother doesn't always know best, and even with a book such as this, you should not attempt to be your baby's doctor. Consult the physician who cares for your baby before making any decision concerning his or her health.

What To Expect The First Year

PART ONE

The First Year

CHAPTER ONE

Get Ready, Get Set

After nearly nine months of waiting, there's finally a light at the end of the tunnel (perhaps, even, effacement and dilatation at the end of the cervix). But with just weeks to go before B-Day arrives, have you yet come to terms with your baby coming to term? Will you be ready for your baby's arrival when he or she's ready to arrive?

Even for a former Girl Scout, there's no way to be prepared completely, both physically and psychologically, for the time when baby makes three (or more). But there are a myriad of steps that can be taken—from selecting the right crib to selecting the right doctor, from deciding between breast and bottle to deciding between cloth diapers and disposables, from preparing yourself for the new arrival to preparing the family dog—to make the transition a smoother one. The flurry of activity as you prepare for the birth will occasionally seem frenzied, but you'll find it good preparation for the even more hectic pace that awaits you afterward.

FEEDING YOUR BABY: Breast or Bottle?

For many women, there is no question. When they close their eyes and summon up a daydreamed snapshot of life with baby, they clearly see themselves suckling their infant-to-be at the breast or, just as clearly, cuddling their newborn as it feeds from the latest nursing bottle. Whatever their reasons—emotional, medical, practical—they made up their minds about baby feeding decisively and early in pregnancy, perhaps even before it began.

For other women, however, the picture is not well focused. Maybe they can't see themselves breastfeeding, but they've heard so much about how breast milk is better for baby that they can't see themselves bottle feeding either. Maybe their mother is encouraging them to use the bottle as she did, while friends are pushing for the breast. Maybe they'd really like to try breastfeeding but are afraid it's not practical because they'll be going back to work soon after baby arrives. Or maybe it's the expectant father's mixed feelings that are giving the mother-to-be second thoughts.

No matter what's causing the ambivalence or confusion, the best way to bring the picture into focus is to look at the facts while exploring the feelings of everyone involved. First of all, what are the facts?

FACTS FAVORING BREASTFEEDING

Pediatricians, obstetricians, nurse-midwives, even manufacturers of infant formulas, agree that breastfeeding is best. No matter how far technology advances, there will always be some things that Nature does better. Among them: formulate the best food and best food delivery system for babies—one that is at the same time good for mothers. As Oliver Wendell Holmes the Elder said well over a century ago, "A pair of substantial mammary glands has the advantage over the two hemispheres of the most learned professor's brain in the art of compounding a nutritious fluid for infants." Breastfeeding advantages include:

Milk that is individualized for your baby. Human breast milk contains at least a hundred ingredients that are not found in cow's milk and that can't be synthesized in the laboratory. Moreover, unlike formula, the composition of breast milk changes

constantly to meet a baby's ever-changing needs: it's different in the morning than it is in the late afternoon; different at one month than it is at seven; different for a premature baby than for a term baby.

Better digestibility. Breast milk is designed for a human baby's sensitive and still-developing digestive system, rather than for a young calf's. Its protein (mostly lactalbumin) and its fat are more easily handled by the baby than are the protein (mostly caseinogen) and fat in cow's milk. The practical result: breastfed babies may be less likely to suffer from colic, gas, and excessive spitting up.

Less sodium and protein. Since breast milk is lower than cow's milk in both of these nutrients, it puts less stress on the fledgling kidneys of the newborn.

Better absorption of calcium. This increased absorption is probably due, in part, to breast milk's lower levels of phosphorus, a mineral that, in excess, interferes with the utilization of calcium.

Less risk of allergy. Babies are almost never allergic to breast milk. Though an infant may be sensitive to something a mother has eaten that has passed into her milk (including cow's milk), he or she virtually always tolerates mother's milk, itself, well. On the other hand, better than 1 out of 10 infants, after an initial exposure, turn out to be allergic to cow's milk formula. (A switch to a soy or hydrolysate formula usually solves the problem—though such formulas stray even further from the composition of human milk than cow's milk.[1])

No problems with constipation or diarrhea. Because of breast milk's naturally laxative effect, infants who nurse are often notoriously prolific when it comes to filling the diaper pail, and constipation is virtually unheard of among them. Also, though their

---

1. Soy *milks*, however, are not nutritionally adequate and should not be used for infant feeding.

movements are generally very loose, diarrhea is rarely a problem. Breast milk appears to reduce the risk of digestive upset in two ways: first, by directly destroying a number of the causative harmful microorganisms; and second, by inhibiting their growth via encouraging the growth of the beneficial microorganisms that keep them in check.

Less risk of diaper rash. The breastfed baby's sweet-smelling movements are less likely to cause diaper rash, but this advantage (as well as the less objectionable odor) disappears once solids are introduced.

Better health for baby. Every time breastfed infants suckle at their mother's breasts, from the first time to the last, they are getting a healthy dose of antibodies to bolster their immunity to disease. In general, they will come down with fewer colds, ear infections, and other illnesses than do bottle-fed infants, and will usually recover more quickly and with fewer complications. They are also hospitalized less often. And one recent study suggests that there may also be a decreased risk of childhood cancer in breastfed babies.

Less obesity. Oftentimes, breastfed infants are less chubby than their bottle-fed peers. That is, in part, because breastfeeding puts baby's appetite in charge of consumption. With bottle feeding, on the other hand, baby may be urged to continue until the bottle is empty. In addition, breast milk is actually calorie controlled. The hind milk, the milk that a baby gets at the end of a nursing session, is higher in calories than that at the beginning, and tends to make a baby feel full—a signal to stop sucking. Be aware, however, that the breastfed baby who is offered the breast too often—every time he or she is cranky, for instance—can gain too quickly.

More sucking satisfaction. A baby can continue sucking at an empty breast, but not at an empty bottle, for optimum sucking enjoyment.

Possibly improved cholesterol metabolism. Studies are unclear, but there has been some evidence that breastfed babies have lower cholesterol levels as adults, perhaps because of improved metabolism.

Better mouth development. Mother's nipples and baby's mouth are a perfect match (though it often doesn't seem so the first time mother and baby try to work together). Even the most scientifically designed substitute nipple fails to give a baby's jaws, gums, and teeth the workout he or she would get at mother's breast—a workout that ensures optimum oral development. And since there is no forward thrust of the tongue, as with sucking on a bottle, breastfed babies are less prone to orthodontic problems than those raised on the bottle.

Convenience. Breast milk is always in stock, ready to use, clean, and consistently at the perfect temperature. It's the ultimate convenience food. No formula to run out of, shop for, or lug around, no bottles to sterilize or refill, no cans to open, no feedings to warm. Wherever you are—in bed, on the road, at a restaurant, on the beach—all the nourishment your baby needs is always ready and waiting. Should baby and mother be apart, for the night, the day, or even the weekend, breast milk can be expressed in advance and stored in the refrigerator or freezer for bottle feedings.

Lower cost. Breast milk is free, whereas bottle feeding can be an expensive proposition (and a wasteful one, since half-used bottles or opened cans often end up being dumped down the kitchen sink). Though it's true that a nursing mother needs slightly more food than a non-nursing one, the cost of this more ample diet needn't be high. If it's chosen with an eye toward nutrition, as it should be, it can in fact be a bargain. A carton of low-fat milk is less expensive than a bottle of cherry cola; a bowl of shredded wheat and fresh fruit is less expensive than a Danish pastry; a homemade juice popsicle is less expensive than a store-bought, sugar-sweetened one.

Quicker recovery for mother. Breastfeeding is better for mother's body. All your motivations for breastfeeding needn't be selfless ones. Because breastfeeding is part of the natural cycle of pregnancy-childbirth-mothering, it is designed to be good not just for baby, but for you as well. It will help your uterus shrink back to prepregnancy size more quickly (that's the increased cramping a mother feels during the first postpartum days as her baby suckles), which in turn will reduce your flow of lochia (the postpartum discharge) more rapidly. And it will help you shed leftover pregnancy pounds by burning upwards of 500 extra calories a day. Some of those pounds, you may remember, were laid down in the form of fat reserves especially to help you produce milk; now's your chance to use them. (But beware of burning your fat too quickly; see page 536.)

Some protection against pregnancy. A nursing mother is generally granted a reprieve from "that time of the month" problems for many months postpartum. Ovulation and menstruation are suppressed in most lactating women at least until their babies begin to take significant supplementation (whether in the form of formula or solids), often until weaning, and sometimes for several months afterward. (Which is not, unfortunately, to say that you can't become pregnant. Since ovulation can quietly precede your first postpartum period, you can never be certain as to when the protection you've been receiving from breastfeeding will cease. See page 569 for birth control information.)

Possibly a reduction in the risk of breast cancer. Though breastfeeding does not seem to confer protection from breast cancer that occurs after menopause, there does seem to be some evidence to suggest that it may reduce the risk of breast cancer occurring earlier.

Enforced rest periods. Breastfeeding ensures frequent breaks in your day, especially at first (sometimes, more frequent than you'd like). Whether or not you feel you have the time to relax, your postpartum body needs the time off your feet that breastfeeding forces you to take.

Less complicated nighttime feedings. Even parents who can't get enough of their adorable infants during the day don't look forward to seeing them at 2 A.M. (or at any other time between midnight and dawn). But baby's nighttime waking can be a lot more tolerable (you may even enjoy it as a time of special closeness) when comfort is as close as your breasts, instead of far off in the kitchen refrigerator, needing to be warmed and poured into a bottle. (It's even easier on mom if dad completes the transfer of baby from crib to breast and back again.)

Strong mother-baby relationships. As almost any mother who's ever breastfed will tell you, the breastfeeding benefit you're likely to treasure most is the bond it builds between mother and child. There's skin-to-skin and eye-to-eye contact, and the opportunity to cuddle, baby-babble, and coo at your wonderful new arrival. True, you can reap the same pleasures when bottle feeding, but you've got to make more of a conscious effort (see page 55), since you may frequently be faced with the temptation to relegate the task to others when you're tired, for example, or to prop the bottle when you're busy.

FACTS FAVORING BOTTLE FEEDING

If there were no advantages to bottle feeding, no one capable of breastfeeding would ever turn to formula. But there are some very real advantages, and for some mothers (and some fathers) they outweigh the many benefits of breastfeeding:

Longer satisfaction for baby. Infant formula made from cow's milk is more difficult to digest than breast milk, and the large rubbery curds it forms stay in a baby's stomach longer, giving a feeling of satiety that can last several hours, extending the period between feedings to three or four hours even early on. Because, on the other hand, breast milk is so easily and quickly digested, many nursing newborns feed so often that it sometimes seems as though they're permanently attached to their mothers' breasts. Though this frequent nursing isn't for naught—it stimulates the production of milk and improves the supply—it can be draining.

Easy monitoring of intake. You know just how much a bottle-fed baby is taking. Because breasts aren't calibrated to measure baby's intake, the inexperienced nursing mother often worries that her newborn isn't getting enough to eat. The bottle-feeding mother has no such problem—a glance at the bottle tells her exactly what she wants to know. (This can be a disadvantage, however, if anxious mothers push babies to take more than they want.)

More freedom. Bottle feeding doesn't tie a mother down. Want to take in dinner and a show with your husband? Or even get away for a romantic weekend? Grandma will likely be more than happy to baby-sit and take charge of the feeding honors. Intend to go back to work part-time when baby is three months old? No weaning or expressing breast milk will be necessary. Just tell the sitter where the bottles and formula are, and you're off.

More participation for father. Dads can share in the pleasures of baby feeding when baby is bottle fed in a way that's impossible with the breastfed infant. (Some dads of breastfed babies actually feel cheated.)

More participation for older siblings. There's little that gives an older child as much a feeling of taking care of "his or her new baby" as giving a bottle.

Fewer demands. The woman exhausted by a difficult labor may be delighted to have the option of not getting up for middle-of-the-night feedings, or even those at 6 A.M. Father, grandma, baby nurse—or anyone else on hand—can take those over until she's stronger. There is also less of a physical drain on mother's resources if she doesn't have to produce breast milk.

No interference with fashion. A bottle-feeding mother can dress as she pleases. The nursing mother's wardrobe is not quite as limited as it was when she was pregnant, but most of the time she won't be able to put fashion before practicality. Whenever she will be nursing, she'll have to forgo one-piece dresses that don't button up the front. (Try accommodating a hungry baby by lifting your dress over your head and you'll see why.)

Less restriction on birth control methods. While a breastfeeding mother has to limit her choice of contraception to those methods that won't hurt her baby (see page 569), the bottle-feeding mom has no such restrictions.

Fewer dietary demands and restrictions. A bottle-feeding mother can stop eating for two. Unlike the nursing mom, she can stop taking in extra protein and calcium, and she can forget about her prenatal vitamin supplements. (Though unless she's one of the rare women who has trouble eating enough to keep weight on, she may be less happy about having to relinquish the extra calories a nursing mother can keep enjoying until weaning.) She can have a few drinks at a party, take aspirin for headaches or medication prescribed by her doctor for allergies, eat all the spicy foods she wants—without worrying about the possible effect on her baby. After the first six weeks postpartum (though not before, when her body is still in the recovery phase), she can diet strenuously, but intelligently, to take off any pregnancy weight that lingers. This is something that the breastfeeding mother can't do until baby is weaned—though, because of the calories milk production requires, she may not have to diet at all to reach her goal.

Less stressful feeding in public. Bottle feeding can be done in public without embarrassment or dishabille. While the nursing mother may receive curious or disapproving glances when she chooses to breastfeed in public, no one will look twice or askance at a woman bottle feeding her baby. Neither will the bottle-feeding mother need to worry about the sometimes awkward procedure of redressing (refastening bra flaps, retucking in shirts, rebuttoning buttons) after the feeding is done.

No interference with lovemaking. After nine months of making love under somewhat less than ideal conditions, many couples look forward to picking up where they left off before conception. For the breastfeeding woman, a vagina left dry by the hormonal changes of lactation, teamed with sore nipples and leaky breasts, can sometimes make this an impossible dream for months to come. For the bottle-feeding mother, nothing (except for an unexpectedly awake and crying baby) need stand between her and her mate.

FACTORING IN FEELINGS

The facts are before you; you've read them and reread them, considered them and reconsidered them. And yet, perhaps, you're still left undecided. That's because, as with many other decisions you're making these days, the decision between breast and bottle doesn't just depend on facts. It depends a great deal on how you—and your husband—feel.

Do you feel that you really want to breastfeed, but believe it's impractical because you're planning to go back to work soon after your baby is born? Don't let circumstances deprive you and your baby of the experience. A few weeks of nursing are better than none at all; both of you stand to benefit from even the briefest encounter with it. And with a little extra dedication and planning, you may be able to work out a system for continuing to breastfeed even after you've returned to your job (see page 170).

Do you feel fundamentally negative about breastfeeding, yet find the facts in favor of it too convincing to ignore? Here again, you might give nursing a try. If your feelings don't take a shift toward the positive, you can quit. At least your baby will have reaped the benefits of breastfeeding for a short time (which is better than no time at all), and you'll know that you tried, erasing those nagging doubts. (Don't quit before you've given nursing your best shot, however. A really fair trial would last at least a month, or better six weeks, since it usually takes that long to establish a good nursing relationship even under the best of circumstances.)

Do you have a deep-seated aversion to breastfeeding, feeling totally uncomfortable about every aspect of it, from having to bare your breast (not quite literally, of course) in public to the very idea of putting your child at your bosom to suckle? Or have you previously breastfed and not enjoyed it? If your feelings about breastfeeding are purely negative, and if, for you, these feelings far outweigh the facts favoring it, then bottle feeding will very likely be best for you and your baby. That may also be true if your feelings are *fairly* negative and the facts of your life (such as a planned early return to work) mitigate against breastfeeding. In either case, you should make the decision to turn to a bottle without feeling guilty.

Do you fear that you won't be able to nurse because of a high-strung (can't-sit-still) temperament, but agree that breast milk is best for baby? Again, you have nothing to lose by trying, and you have everything to gain should your personality turn out to be more compatible with breastfeeding than you'd speculated. Don't judge the situation too early in the game, however. Even women ordinarily graced with Madonna-like calm can find the first few weeks of breastfeeding a time of high anxiety. Many women, however, are surprised, once a smoothly working breastfeeding relationship is established, to find that nursing is relaxing—the hormones released as baby suckles actually enhance relaxation, and the experience itself is one of the healthiest routes to tension relief. (At the beginning, give yourself the best chance of success by using relaxation techniques before putting your newborn to breast.) Keep in mind that you can always switch to the bottle later, should your initial instincts prove correct.

Does your husband feel jealous or repelled at the thought of your breastfeeding—though you yourself would like to nurse? If he does, have him read the facts, too. They may persuade him that his loss, which, after all, is only a temporary one, or his distaste, which will also be temporary, will be baby's gain. Also have him read the section on breastfeeding in Chapter 25 (Becoming a Father). If his mind remains made up against breastfeeding, however, and yours resolved for it, you'll need to do some further negotiating to break the impasse and come up with a solution that suits you both.

BREASTFEEDING MYTHS

■ **MYTH: You can't breastfeed if you have small breasts or flat nipples.**

Reality: In no way does outward appearance affect the production of milk or a mother's ability to dispense it. Breasts and nipples of all shapes and sizes can satisfy a hungry baby. Inverted nipples that don't become erect when stimulated may need some advance preparation to make them fully functional; see page 24.

■ **MYTH: Breastfeeding is a lot of trouble.**

Reality: Never again will it be so easy to feed your child. Breasts, unlike bottles, are ready when baby is. You don't have to remember to take them with you when you're planning a day at the beach, lug them in a tote bag, or worry about the milk inside them spoiling in the hot sun.

■ **MYTH: Breastfeeding ties you down.**

Reality: It's true that breastfeeding is naturally better suited to mothers who plan to be with their babies most of the time. But those who are willing to make the effort to express and store milk, or who prefer to supplement with formula, can satisfy their need to work—or see a movie, or go to an all-day seminar—and their desire to breastfeed. And when it comes to stepping out with baby, it's the breastfeeding mother who is more mobile, always having an ample supply of food along no matter where she goes or how long she plans to stay.

■ **MYTH: Breastfeeding will ruin your breasts.**

Reality: Much to the surprise of many people, breastfeeding doesn't seem to permanently affect the shape or size of your breasts at all. Because of hereditary factors, age, poor support (going braless), or excessive weight gain during pregnancy, your breasts may be less firm after having a child. But breastfeeding won't be to blame.

■ **MYTH: Breastfeeding excludes father.**

Reality: A father who wants to be involved in the care of his nursing infant can find ample opportunity—for bathing, diapering, holding, rocking, playing with, and, once solids are introduced, sending "trains through the tunnel."

As in the making of any important marital decision, there are two good approaches: one is compromise; the other is giving the decision to the partner who cares the most about or has the most at stake in a particular issue. A compromise might be for you to breastfeed, but only for three months. Or if it's your nursing in public that bothers your husband, you might agree to breastfeed in private only, and to supplement with a bottle when privacy isn't available. If compromise won't work, then try the other approach. If the chance to nurse means everything to you, ask your husband to concede this point. If he is the more adamant one (a less likely scenario), give in to him.

Some women find breastfeeding an overwhelmingly positive experience, joyful and exhilarating; when it comes time to wean baby (especially if it's the last baby), tears and a bout with depression are common. Others nurse their babies because they know it's best, but feel little more than ambivalence while they do it. Still others never learn to tolerate, never mind enjoy, breastfeeding. But you aren't likely to know where you fall along the spectrum until you've actually held your baby to your breast. Many women who begin to breastfeed out of duty continue to do it out of love. Many who, before baby arrives, are thoroughly appalled at the thought of engaging in such an intimate act in the company of strangers live to eat their words and to lift their shirts with aplomb at the sound of baby's first cry—on an airplane, in a crowded park, at a ritzy restaurant.

In the end, however, if you opt not to breastfeed (with or without a trial run),

don't feel guilty. Almost nothing you do for your baby is right if it doesn't feel right for you—and that includes breastfeeding. Even babies who were born yesterday are wise enough to sense feelings of uneasiness in their mothers; a bottle given lovingly can be better for your infant than a breast offered grudgingly.

WHEN YOU CAN'T OR SHOULDN'T BREASTFEED

For some women, the pros and cons of breastfeeding and bottle feeding are academic. They don't have the option of nursing their new babies, because of either their own health or their baby's. If your medical history includes any of the following, you will almost certainly be advised not to breastfeed:

- Serious debilitating illness (such as heart or kidney disease, or severe anemia), or extreme underweight (your body needs fat stores to produce milk).

- Serious infection, such as HIV/AIDS, TB, and possibly hepatitis B. (You may be able to nurse in spite of the hepatitis if your baby is treated postpartum with gamma globulin and hepatitis B vaccine.)

- A condition requiring regular medication that passes into the breast milk and might be harmful to the baby, such as antithyroid, anticancer, or antihypertensive drugs; lithium, tranquilizers, or sedatives. (The need for temporary medication should not, however, interfere with breastfeeding; see page 553.)

ADOPTION AND BREASTFEEDING

Though few adopting mothers would consider it an option, it is indeed occasionally possible to breastfeed an adopted child. This can work only if plenty of advance planning and preparation is undertaken, and if the baby will be picked up within a few days after birth. See page 503 for tips on breastfeeding an adopted baby.

■ Present drug abuse—including the use of tranquilizers, amphetamines, barbiturates, or other pills, heroin, methadone, cocaine, marijuana, tobacco, and the moderate or heavy use of caffeine or alcohol.

■ Inadequate glandular tissue in the breasts (this has nothing to do with the size of your breasts) or damage to the nerve supply to the nipple (as from injury or surgery). In some cases you may be able to attempt breastfeeding, under careful medical supervision to be certain your baby is thriving. If you've had surgery for breast cancer in one breast, ask your doctor about the possibility of nursing from the other. From present information it isn't clear whether it is safe or not, though it does appear that a mother does not transmit cancer-causing substances to her baby through breast milk. Future research may be able to tell us more about the safety of breastfeeding following cancer surgery.[2]

There are also conditions of the newborn that can interfere with breastfeeding:

■ A metabolic disorder, such as PKU or lactose intolerance, that makes the baby unable to digest human milk.

■ A deformity, such as cleft lip and/or cleft palate, that makes suckling at the breast difficult or impossible. (However, in some cases, especially when only cleft lip is present, it is possible to breastfeed. Ask to see a lactation consultant before you make a feeding decision. It may also be feasible to express breast milk until after surgery, and to begin breastfeeding then.)

If you can't breastfeed, or if you just don't wish to, be assured that a commercial baby formula will almost certainly nourish your baby adequately (rare exceptions would include infants with multiple allergies who require special formulas). Millions of healthy, happy babies (possibly, you among them) have been raised on the bottle, and your baby can be, too, especially if you remember to make bottle feeding as loving an affair as breastfeeding.

WHAT YOU MAY BE CONCERNED ABOUT

COPING WITH MOTHERHOOD

"Everything's ready for the baby—except me. I just can't picture myself as a mother."

Even those women who pictured themselves as mothers from the first time they changed a Betsy-Wetsy or dried Tiny Tears' eyes often start to doubt the validity of their calling when it threatens to become

a round-the-clock reality. Those who spurned dolls for relationships with trucks and soccer balls, mowed lawns instead of baby-sitting, and rarely gave passing strollers more than a passing glance until the day their pregnancy test came back positive may face delivery day with even greater trepidation.

But not only is this ninth-month crumbling of confidence normal, it's healthy. Strolling into motherhood blithely self-assured may only set you up for a swift and unsettling comedown when the task turns out to be more overwhelming than you'd imagined. A little anxiety (a recognition that life with baby will include some difficult, even some seemingly impossible, days and nights) and uncertainty will help you

---

2. Many experts recommend a woman wait three to five years after breast cancer surgery before becoming pregnant and breastfeeding because of the fear that the hormones stimulated might activate cancer cells during this period when the risk of the recurrence of the cancer is greatest.

head off postpartum reality shock.

So if you don't feel ready for motherhood, don't worry. But do prepare. Read at least the first few chapters in this book and everything else you can about newborns and infants (always keeping in mind that babies don't always go "by the book"). Spend some time, if possible, with newborns or young babies; try holding them, even diapering them; talk to their parents about the pleasures and frustrations of caring for an infant. Take a parenting course, if one's available in your area. Thousands have been developed in recent years—by hospitals and medical groups, universities and schools, religious institutions and private entrepreneurs—in response to the demand of parents wanting to learn more about the toughest job they may ever have to handle.

Most of all, realize that mothers are not born—they're created on the job. A woman who's gained some experience with other people's infants may be somewhat more comfortable at first than the totally inexperienced new mother, but by the six-week checkup it will be difficult to tell them apart. And the still-pregnant women in the waiting room will envy them both their skill and poise as mothers.

Remember, too, that we all have gained some experience in child rearing, if only from observation. We have all watched parents—our own as well as friends' and strangers'—at work and silently programmed our own mental computers. A mother slaps her toddler in the supermarket and you say to yourself, "I'll never do that," or another jogs with her baby in a stroller through the park and you say, "That's what I'll do."

A CHANGING LIFESTYLE

"I really look forward to having my baby. But I worry that the lifestyle my husband and I have grown accustomed to will be totally disrupted."

For your mother's generation, a change in lifestyle wasn't an issue. Most young couples married and had children right out of high school or college; they had no chance to develop a child-free adult lifestyle before children appeared on the scene. Having gone directly from their parents' home to their own, the only lifestyle they knew was a family-centered one. Today's mother-to-be is likely to be many years out of school and into an independent, *self*-centered lifestyle—one that may include frequent lunches and dinners out, spontaneous weekends of skiing or boating, late nights of dancing followed by long and leisurely mornings in bed, and a closet full of dry-clean-only clothes. She may also be accustomed to making love when and where the spirit moves (within the realm of good taste, of course).

This lifestyle needn't come to a crashing end. But, realistically, it will need to undergo some radical alterations. Some lunches and dinners may still be taken out, but less often at candlelit French bistros and more often at family-style eateries with high chairs and a high tolerance for peas and carrots ground into the carpeting. Weekends away will no longer be as spontaneous (planning becomes more vital and packing more complicated), but if you've got the will, you'll find the way to get away—usually with baby, occasionally without (if you're bottle feeding or once your breastfed baby is weaned). An early movie or concert may have to replace late night dancing for a while, unless you think you can waltz in for the 2 A.M. feeding and be up again for the 6. And those silk dresses and wool slacks will probably have to be tucked away in the back of the closet for baby-free occasions, so room can be made for washables that can weather baby's spitup and worse. Lovemaking needn't be entirely abandoned, but opportunity will become as critical a factor as mood in determining when you and your husband are intimate.

Nevertheless, if you're like most parents today you won't want to abandon your former style of living entirely and will try to fit baby into it, at least to some extent. Of course, you won't always succeed, especially as baby grows older. While a tiny infant may not object to being dragged hither and yon with mom and dad, a baby even a few months old begins to have social needs and personal preferences of his or her own, and these needs inevitably have to be taken into account as you plan your schedule.

Just how much your lifestyle will have to change will depend a lot on the individual needs of you, your husband, and your baby. And how well you adjust to the changes will depend to a great extent on your own attitudes. If you look at the changes as positive and exciting, then your life will be better and richer than ever. If, however, you're resentful of and resistant to every change mothering brings, then both you and baby (and probably your spouse as well) are in for a very hard time.

WHETHER OR NOT TO GO BACK TO WORK

"Every time I talk to a friend or read an article on the subject, I change my mind about whether or not to go back to work soon after my baby is born."

Today's expectant working woman has it all to look forward to: all the satisfaction of a fulfilling career, all the joy of raising a family—and all the guilt, anxiety, and confusion inherent in deciding which of the two will hold priority in her life after delivery.

But while it seems as though this is a choice you should make now, it really isn't. Deciding while you're still pregnant whether you'll stay home or go back to work (and when) after baby is born is like deciding between a job you're familiar with and one you know nothing about. Instead, assuming you have the options, keep them open until you've spent some time at home with your baby. You may find that nothing

you've ever done—including your job—has ever given you as much satisfaction as does caring for your newborn, and may postpone going back to work indefinitely. Or you may find that, as sweet and adorable as baby is, you're climbing the walls after a month, and may hasten your return to the 9-to-5 life. Or you may find that neither full-time mothering nor full-time working alone fills all your needs, and that you'd like to combine the best of both worlds—by taking a part-time position, if you're lucky enough to find one or savvy enough to create one. (See page 587 for some advice on making the decision once baby appears on the scene.)

DAD TAKING TIME OFF

"My husband wants to take his vacation time when the baby is born. That means there'll be no vacation later in the year. Does this make sense?"

Someday—hopefully sooner than later—this question won't be one that expectant parents will need to ask. Fathers and mothers alike will automatically be granted paternity or maternity leave upon the birth of their babies—just as they already are in many other industrialized nations.

But since that bright day has not yet dawned in the U.S., fathers-to-be who elect to spend the immediate postpartum period at home usually have to give up all or part of their vacation time to do so. This is, of course, a matter of choice and circumstance. While changing diapers and doing laundry may not seem like much of a vacation, to some fathers enjoying those first days as a family can offer more fun than a Mardi Gras, more awe and inspiration than a view of the Grand Canyon, and more memories to cherish than a round-the-world cruise. If your husband feels this way, by all means make the time following baby's arrival vacation time. Be sure, however, that he is fully acquainted in advance with basic household mechanics: laundry, simple cooking, vacuuming, and so on. (Many husbands, of course, are already at least as proficient as, and some are more proficient than, their wives at these chores.)

On the other hand, if you've already enlisted more help than you will need (grandma is coming up from Florida, a younger sister is moving in for two weeks, and/or a baby nurse has been engaged), and the father-to-be would feel like a fifth wheel being around the house during the day and would just as soon get to know his new offspring in the quiet of the night, it may make sense to save those vacation days for a real holiday en famille.

Don't, however, extend invitations to all and sundry to come and help if you and your husband would really rather do it yourselves; it's a wonderful way for mommy, daddy, and baby to become a family.

GRANDPARENTS

"My mother has her bags packed and is ready to fly in the moment the baby arrives 'to give me a hand.' The idea makes me nervous because my mother tends to take over, but I don't want to hurt her feelings and tell her not to come."

Whether it's loving and warm, distant and frosty, or tottering on the brink somewhere in between, a woman's relationship with her mother (or mother-in-law) is one of the most complicated in her life. It becomes even more so when daughter becomes mother, and mother becomes grandmother. Though there may be hundreds of situations in the next couple of decades of parenting and grandparenting when your wishes will come into conflict with your parents', this is the one that will probably set the precedent for those to come.

You and your husband are the ones who should decide who will be around to help out when baby arrives. If you both would rather spend the first week or so alone with your baby, then explain to your mother (and your mother-in-law, too, if necessary) that you and your husband want to get to know the baby and to get more comfortable with him or her before having houseguests. Assure her that you are very eager for her to visit when the baby is a couple of weeks old, reminding her, too, that the baby will be more responsive, interesting, and awake then, anyway. She may feel rejected temporarily, but once she holds her grandchild in her arms, the hurt feelings are sure to melt away, the episode forgotten. What won't be forgotten is that you and your husband are the ones who set the rules for your baby, an important concept to relay to parents and in-laws early. As an old proverb goes: If God had wanted the elderly to raise infants, He would not have invented menopause.

Some new parents, of course, welcome the experience and the set of extra hands that come with a postpartum visit from grandma, particularly when they aren't accompanied by an overbearing, take-charge attitude. Just as those who feel the need to say, "Mother, I'd rather do it myself," shouldn't be plagued by guilt, those who feel they need the help shouldn't have qualms about saying, "I'd rather *not* do it myself."

The expertise that grandparents bring with them is irreplaceable. Whether you feel your parents (or your husband's) did a great job raising you or just a fair one, there is always something to be learned from their experience, even if it's only what not to do. There's no point in reinventing the wheel—or child-care practices—in every generation.

Being open to suggestion, of course, puts you in the position of sometimes (maybe even most of the time) having to disagree. Don't let this stop you from talking over baby preparations, and later baby care, with your mother (or your husband's). She probably disagreed with her own mother (or mother-in-law) when you were born, too—something you can remind her of when she's upset by your rejections. What's *right* in baby care, as in almost any other area, changes from generation to generation, and you should both keep your sense of humor about that. (You'll need it again when your little newborn, twenty or thirty years from now, becomes a mommy or daddy and accuses you of being old-fashioned.)

If you disagree with grandma on an issue—bottle feeding versus breastfeeding, for example—explain your point of view. She may come around when you talk about it, or at least understand why you feel the way you do. Even if she doesn't, your relationship will be better if you are open and share your thoughts and feelings than if you bottle them up.

And remember, if parenthood is a responsibility, grandparenthood is the reward—one you will someday want to enjoy yourself. Be sure you don't deprive your parents of theirs.

A LACK OF GRANDPARENTS

"My husband's parents are deceased. Mine are elderly and live in another state. Sometimes I feel the lack of having family to talk to about my pregnancy and about the baby. I think it will be worse when the baby arrives."

You're not alone in feeling alone. Whereas in generations past the extended family rarely extended beyond the county line, millions of couples in today's mobile society live far from parents and family. Never is this separation more keenly felt than when a new generation is being added.

What helps—besides the telephone—is finding surrogates for family members who are far away or deceased. Churches or synagogues, especially those with a strong sense of community, are a good source of this kind of support. So are parent groups, which sometimes evolve out of childbirth education or exercise classes, or simply develop spontaneously among casual acquaintances. Then there are senior citizens who have as great a need for grandchildren as you do for grandparents. You can find one through seniors groups in your neighborhood and "adopt" each other. Weekly visits and joint outings can give you and your baby a sense of family and give an elderly person or couple a sense of being needed.

If you're worried about not having an experienced grandma around when you come home from the hospital, consider a baby nurse.

CONSIDERING A BABY NURSE

"Some of my friends hired baby nurses when their babies were born. Do I need one, too?"

For many years, baby nurses were a fixture of the upper class; a new mother who could afford to have one wouldn't have thought of being without one. Today, even royalty are changing their share of diapers and taking charge of their share of feedings (though nannies are still employed to tend to the other share), and many new mothers who have the financial resources to hire a baby nurse don't have the desire to do so.

Once you've determined there's enough money in your budget for a baby nurse, you'll need to consider several other factors before deciding whether or not to hire one. Here are some reasons why you might opt for one:

■ To get some hands-on training in baby care. If you haven't had experience or taken a parenting class, and feel you'd rather not learn from the mistakes you make on the job and on your baby, a good baby nurse will be able to instruct in such basics as bathing, burping, diapering, and even breastfeeding. If this is your reason for hiring a nurse, however, be sure that the person you hire is as interested in teaching as you are in learning. Some won't tolerate novice mothers peeping over their shoulders; one with such a dictatorial take-charge attitude can leave you as inexperienced and unsure on her departure as you were on her arrival.

- To avoid getting up in the middle of the night for feedings. If you're bottle feeding and would rather sleep through the night, at least in the early weeks of postpartum fatigue, a baby nurse, on duty 24 hours a day or hired just for nights, can take over this feeding responsibility. (This chore can also be tended to by an obliging father or grandparent.)

- To spend more time with an older child. Some women hire a baby nurse so that they can be more available to their older children, and hopefully spare them the pangs of jealousy that are often provoked by new arrivals. Such a nurse might be hired to work just a few hours a day during the time you want to spend with your older child. If this is your major reason for hiring a nurse, however, bear in mind that her presence will probably only serve to postpone feelings of sibling jealousy; the older child will be in for a dose of reality shock when the nurse leaves and mommy starts her double duty. See page 601 for other ways of coping with the sibling problem.

- To give yourself a chance to recuperate after a cesarean or difficult vaginal birth. Since you probably won't know if you're going to have a difficult time beforehand, it's not a bad idea to do some scouting around for nurses in advance, just in case. If you have the name of a potential nurse or two, or at least have spoken to an agency, you can call shortly after you deliver and have a helper hired before you get home.

A baby nurse may not be the best solution to your postpartum needs if:

- You're breastfeeding. Since a nurse (unless she's a wet nurse) can't feed a nursing baby, and feeding is one of the most time-consuming tasks in the care of a newborn, she may not be much of a help. For the nursing mother, household help—someone to cook, clean, shop, and do laundry—is probably a wiser investment, unless you can find a nurse who will do these chores and also offer breastfeeding instruction.

- You're not comfortable with a stranger living in your home. If the idea of having a non-family member sharing your bathrooms, your kitchen, and your table 24 hours a day makes you uneasy, hire a part-time nurse rather than a live-in, or opt for one of the other sources of help described below.

- You'd rather do it yourself. If you want to be the one to give the first bath, catch sight of the first smile (even if they say it's only gas), soothe your baby through the first bout of crying (even if it's at 2 A.M.), don't hire a nurse, hire household help to free you up for fun with baby.

- You'd like the father to do it, too. If you and your husband want to share baby care, a nurse may get in the way. Even if she is willing to grant mothers some rights, she may not be used to fathers doing anything more than handing out cigars. And may want to keep it that way. If she is willing to share the baby-care workload with both of you, there won't be much left for her to do—except to collect her paycheck, which you could probably spend more sensibly on cleaning help.

If you decide that a baby nurse is right for you, the best way to go about finding one is to ask for recommendations from friends who've used one. Be sure to find out if the nurse in question has the qualifications and qualities you're looking for. Some cook, some don't. Some will do light housework and laundry, others won't. Some are gentle, motherly women who will nurture your innate mothering ability and leave you feeling more confident; others are bossy, cold, and patronizing, and will leave you feeling totally inadequate. Many are licensed practical nurses; some have also been trained specifically in caring for mother as well as baby, in mother-child relations, and in teaching breastfeeding and child-care basics. A personal interview is extremely important, since it's the only way to know whether you are going to feel comfortable with a particular individual. But excellent references (do check them out) are a must.

A nurse hired through an agency should be bonded. It's also important that a nurse—or anyone else you hire who may come in contact with the baby—has been screened for TB.

OTHER SOURCES OF HELP

"With the loss of my income, we just can't afford the expense of a baby nurse. Since I may need a c-section—my baby's in a breech position—I wonder if I will be able to manage without help."

Just because you can't afford—or don't want to hire—a baby nurse doesn't mean you have to go it alone. Most women, in fact, rely on other sources of help, at least one of which is probably available to you:

The new father. If your husband can arrange his schedule so that he can be with you both for the first week or so, he is probably your best baby helper. Together and without outside assistance or inter-ference, you'll both learn more about your baby and baby care than you would any other way. No experience is necessary for the job; you'll both catch on quickly. Do take a baby-care class at your hospital if one is offered and read a child-care book or two before baby arrives to pick up some of the basics beforehand—and feel free to turn to family, friends, the baby's doctor, the hospital nursery staff, La Leche, and other sources of information and advice to fill in the blanks.

A grandma. If you have a mother or mother-in-law whom you'd be comfortable having around on a live-in or come-in basis for the first weeks, this may provide an-other satisfactory solution. Grandmothers have at least a hundred and one uses: they can rock a crying baby, cook a splendid supper, wash and fold the laundry, do the marketing, and much, much more. This kind of arrangement can work particularly

well if you can handle a little well-meant interference good-naturedly. Of course, if the grandma in question has an already busy life and isn't interested in changing diapers, this won't be an option.

Your freezer. You won't be able to put baby on ice when you're tired, but you will be able to pull meals off the ice if you prepared some during the last weeks of pregnancy when, if you weren't working, you may have had too much time on your hands anyway. A few nutritious casseroles, some chicken roasted and ready to reheat, or a prepared pasta sauce will ease the pressure of having to feed the rest of your family nightly—so you can concentrate more on feeding baby (which you may find a full-time job for a while). Don't hesitate to stock up on frozen vegetables, too; they take little preparation time and are at least as nutritious as fresh.

Your favorite take-out. If you don't have the time or the opportunity to prepare meals in advance, you still won't have to cook in those busy postpartum days. Nearly every neighborhood has one or more take-out shops where you can get meats, chicken, sometimes fish, and side dishes ready to heat and eat—and increasingly, fresh salads that require only a fork and an appetite to enjoy. But don't take out fast foods very often. They offer little in the way of nutrition and much in the way of excess fat and sodium.[3]

Then, of course, there's the pizzeria (try to get whole-wheat crust for best nutrition), the Chinese restaurant (order brown rice if it's available), and the local salad bar (favor fresh items over prepared, which are usu-ally slathered in high-fat dressings, and avoid establishments that add sulfites). Cold cereals, canned tuna and salmon, low-fat

---

3. Many fast-food chains now provide nutrition information on request; use these as your guide. Generally, stick to salads, grilled meats, poultry, fish, or pizza, and avoid white buns, fried entrees and sides, other foods very high in sodium and fat, and sugary sweets.

cottage cheese, hard cheese, yogurt, whole-grain breads, and fresh fruits will help to fill the gaps in your meals without any cooking or heavy preparation.[4]

Paper goods. When dinner is over, whether it was prepared in your kitchen or at your local eatery, there are always dishes to do—unless you rely on paper plates, plastic flatware, and disposable cups. Disposables will also come in handy for serving snacks to visitors who have come to admire the baby. (Keep such entertaining to a minimum, however, if you want to survive the postpartum period.)

Cleaning help. If there's one job that most new mothers would gladly relinquish, it's cleaning. Give it up—to a cleaning service, a cleaning person, someone you've used before, or someone new—anyone who can vacuum and dust, mop floors and scour bathrooms, so that you can have more time and energy to devote to baby, your husband, any older children, and yourself. This is a good route for a woman who wants to do most of the newborn care herself (or with her husband), but doesn't want a "She tried to be Superwoman" label pinned to her chart when she's returned to the hospital suffering from complete and total exhaustion.

Remember, even if you hire help, and most especially if you don't, there will inevitably be things that don't get done during those early weeks. As long as getting everybody fed and getting rest for yourself aren't among them, don't worry—and do get used to it. Though a certain amount of order will eventually be restored to your home, life with children will almost always include living with at least a few untied ends.

---

4. A lot of ready-to-eat foods, such as tuna and cottage cheese, are exceptionally high in sodium, so, when possible, look for the low-sodium varieties.

CIRCUMCISION

"I thought that circumcision was routine nowadays, but the pediatrician I'll be using said that it's not really necessary."

Circumcision is probably the oldest medical procedure still performed. Though the most widely known historical record of the practice is in the Old Testament, when Abraham circumcized Isaac, its origins are lost in antiquity, probably going back to before the use of metal tools. Practiced by Moslems and Jews throughout most of history as a sign of their covenant with God, circumcision became widespread in the United States in the late nineteenth century when it was theorized that the removal of the foreskin would make the penis less sensitive (it doesn't), thus making masturbation a less tempting pursuit (it didn't). In the years that followed, many other medical justifications for routine circumcision have been proposed—among others that it might prevent or cure epilepsy, syphilis, asthma, lunacy, and tuberculosis—none of which it apparently does.

Circumcision does reduce the risk of infection of the penis, but careful attention to cleaning under the foreskin once it is retractable will do as well. It also eliminates the risk of phimosis, a condition in which the foreskin remains tight as the child grows and can't be retracted as it normally can in older boys. Phimosis can be extremely painful and sometimes interferes with erection. It is estimated that between 5 and 10% of uncircumcised males have to undergo the discomfort of circumcision some time after infancy because of infection, phimosis, or other problems.

Still, until recently, most of the medical community took the position that there were no "absolute medical indications" that warranted exposing an infant to the surgery, minor though it is. But in 1989, the American Academy of Pediatrics (AAP) task force, after evaluating all the data available, determined that there are medical benefits and advantages to the procedure. The decision was based primarily on new studies that show that compared to circumcised infants, baby boys who are uncircumcised appear to have a 10 times greater risk of urinary tract infection, which can be severe enough to require hospitalization. They found the studies showing a link to penile cancer (possibly because of a higher rate of infection with human papillomavirus) and sexually transmitted diseases, including AIDS, to be less conclusive.

The AAP now recommends that parents make their decisions about circumcision in conjunction with their baby's doctor and based upon a full consideration of medical benefits and risks as well as on esthetic, social, cultural, and religious factors.

Presently more than half of all boys in the U.S. are circumcised, down from more than 80% in the early 1980s. The most common reasons parents give for opting for circumcision, in addition to just "feeling it should be done," include:

■ Religious observance. The religious laws of both Moslems and Jews, rooted in the Bible, require circumcision of the newborn.

■ Cleanliness. Since it's easier to keep a circumcised penis clean, cleanliness is next to godliness as a reason for circumcision in the U.S.

■ The locker-room syndrome. Parents who don't want their sons to feel different from their friends or from their father or brothers often choose circumcision.

■ Appearance. Some feel removal of the foreskin will make their son look better.

■ Health. The hope of reducing the risk of infection, cancer, or other future problems (including possible later circumcision) prompts many to elect to do the surgery immediately.

The reasons why more parents are deciding against circumcision include:

■ The lack of medical necessity. Many question the sense in removing a part of an infant's body without good cause.

■ Fear of bleeding and infection. Though complications, particularly when the procedure is carried out by an experienced physician or a ritual circumciser with medical training, are very rare, many parents are nevertheless apprehensive about the possibility.

■ Concern about pain. There is believed to be some pain connected with circumcision, though it is probably of short duration. (Pain can be minimized by use of a padded restraint chair and a local anesthetic and/or a sugar-coated pacifier.)

■ The wish for the child to be like his uncircumcised father. Another version of the like-father/like-son complex.

■ A belief in children's rights. Some parents wish to leave the decision to the child at a later date.

■ To allow optimal sexual enjoyment. There are those who still believe an uncircumcised penis is more sensitive, though there's no scientific support for this position.

■ Less risk of diaper irritation. It's been suggested that the intact foreskin may protect against diaper rash on the penis.

The risks of circumcision are minimal, but complications can occur. To reduce the risk, be sure the person who is performing the procedure is experienced and, if he's a ritual circumciser, that he is well trained and comes highly recommended. Also be sure that the surgery is not done in the delivery room, but rather when your baby is stabilized, usually after at least 12 to 24 hours. And do not permit cauterization with a metal clamp, which could cause serious burns.

If you remain undecided about circumcision as delivery day approaches, read about circumcision care in Chapter Four, and discuss the issue with the doctor you have chosen for your baby—and possibly with friends who have gone either route.

WHICH DIAPERS TO USE

"Most of my friends are using paper diapers, and they do seem a lot less of a mess than cloth ones. But are they as good for baby?"

Ever since Eve, mothers have had to confront the problem of how to cover baby's bottom. Native American mothers, we are told, kept their babies (and their own backs) dry and comfortable by packing their papoose boards with the shredded, soft insides of cattails.

Luckily, as a mother in the last decades of the twentieth century, you won't have to wade daily into the marshes to choose the softest and most absorbent cattails to pad your Snugli. But you will have to choose among the plethora of ready-to-wraparound-baby possibilities available, ranging from several types of cloth diapers (to launder yourself or order from a diaper service) to a bewildering and ever-changing array of disposables.

The choice that's right for you and your baby may be different from the one that's right for your neighbor and her infant. Personal factors will be of major significance since, scientifically and economically, there's no conclusive winner in the diaper derby. Consider the following in making your choice:

Disposable diapers. Convenience is a major advantage—no dirty diapers to collect, tote around, and pile up for weekly pickup. Disposable diapers also save a certain amount of time and effort; they're faster and easier to put on and take off and require no pins (especially important if your baby is a wriggler). Newer styles are increasingly more absorbent and theoretically less likely to cause diaper rash, they're trimmer, and less apt to leak. These desirable features also add up to a distinct disadvantage: since disposables soak up so much urine and often "feel" dry when they're far from it, parents are less likely to

change diapers frequently enough—and too infrequent changes can lead to diaper rash. Additionally, the new superbreed of diaper keeps babies so comfortable when wet that toilet training may be made more difficult. Also on the minus side is the effect that paper diapers have on the environment (they aren't biodegradable and just add to the collection of clutter on our planet) and the inconvenience of having to shop and lug. This last drawback can be avoided if you order by mail, which is possible with at least one popular brand, or if your local diaper service delivers disposables, which, not insignificantly, are often cheaper than store-bought.

Home-delivered cloth diapers. To those who are reluctant to encase their infants' bottoms in paper and plastic, soft, comfortable, sterilized, and possibly ecologically preferable cotton diapers are appealing, especially when they are delivered to the door weekly. Some studies (those diaper services are fond of quoting) show a lower incidence of diaper rash with such diapers; others (cited by paper-diaper manufacturers) show super absorbent disposables yielding a lower incidence of rash. If cloth diapers are continued into toddlerhood (few parents manage this), toilet training may be easier to accomplish, because direct contact between a wet cloth diaper and skin makes a child very uncomfortable and more aware of having wet.

There are disadvantages, however. Separate waterproof pants are needed to avoid having to change baby, crib, and often mother's clothes, every time baby wets. These pants increase the risk of rash by keeping air out and moisture in, though breathable diaper pants or wraps made of cotton or wool (sometimes with airy mesh linings and/or absorbent foam fillings) can reduce or even eliminate this program. Diaper changes, because of fussing with pins (unless fitted cloth diapers or diaper wraps with Velcro closings are used) and separate pants, are more trouble with cloth diapers, particularly as baby becomes more proficient at squirming. Because absorbency is more limited, double diapers are usually needed at night, and for some heavy wetters, during the day; boys, who concentrate their urine in front, may need paper diaper liners. And then there are the plastic bags of soiled diapers to be carried home from outings and the ever-present pail of dirty diapers, which is never truly odor free.

Home-laundered cloth diapers. These may be the clear loser compared to the other two choices. Because they can't be adequately sanitized, home-laundered diapers are, according to studies, more likely to cause diaper rash. This is compounded by the fact that, as with other cloth diapers, they are almost always used with waterproof pants that further encourage the development of diaper-area irritation. While, like other cloth diapers, they are ecologically sounder than paper, they also present many of the same disadvantages. And though they seem to be far less expensive than either of the other types of diaper, they are, when one considers the cost of soap, water, and power used, only slightly so. In addition, they demand a greater expenditure of time and effort—to soak, wash, dry, and fold them between use.

Some parents decide to use cloth diapers for the first few months, a time when baby usually spends more time at home than on the go, and then move on to disposables. They will often, however, use disposables on outings and, sometimes, at night (because their greater absorbency keeps baby more comfortable longer and may ensure a better night's sleep) from the start.

Whichever diaper you decide on now, you may find that your baby develops diaper rash frequently later. This could point to a sensitivity to your choice. If this occurs, don't fight it—switch. Try a different type of diaper (go from cloth to paper or vice versa) or a different brand of disposable. Also see the tips for treating diaper rash on page 178.

QUITTING SMOKING

"Except for the first few months of pregnancy, when I couldn't smoke because it made me queasy, I never managed to give up smoking—and neither has my husband. How much does smoking around a baby affect him or her?"

Nothing you can buy in a layette department, splurge on in a toy store, or put away into a trust fund can match the gift to your newborn of growing up in a smoke-free environment. Smoking by parents has been linked to an increase in respiratory illnesses (colds, flu, bronchitis, asthma) and ear infections during the first year of life, and impaired lung function and reduced lung capacity. Not only are the children of smokers sick more often than children of nonsmokers, but their illnesses last longer. They are also more likely to be hospitalized in the first three years of life. The more smokers in the household, the more severe the negative effects, since the level of cotinine (a by-product of the metabolism of nicotine) in the blood is directly related to the number of smokers a child is exposed to on a regular basis.

Smoking parents are also more likely to have colicky babies (for the uninitiated, that means a baby who cries, usually inconsolably, for at least two or three hours every day), though the reasons for this aren't clear.

Perhaps worst of all, children of smokers are more likely to become smokers than youngsters whose parents don't smoke. So quitting before you deliver may not only keep your child healthier in childhood, it may, by lessening the chance of smoking later in life, also keep him or her alive and well longer.

If you haven't been able to quit up until now, it obviously won't be easy. As they would with any drug addiction, your body and your mind will align against you. But if you're determined to fight back—for your sake and your baby's—you can triumph over both. And the best time to do it is now, before baby is born. Giving up smoking before delivery will increase the oxygen available to your baby during childbirth; and your newborn will come home from the hospital to clean, breathable air and, if you're breastfeeding, to nicotine-free milk. If you are still in the early months of pregnancy, quitting now will also reduce the risk of premature delivery and of having a low-birthweight baby.

There are many approaches to giving up the cigarette habit. Some are totally inappropriate for the pregnant mother (nicotine chewing gum, for example). Ideal are those that are designed for expectant moms. Help is available from the American Lung Association in the form of their manuals "Freedom from Smoking for You and Your Baby," "Freedom from Smoking in Twenty Days," and "A Lifetime of Freedom from Smoking," a maintenance program.

A NAME FOR BABY

"I've always been unhappy with my name. How can we be sure our son won't be unhappy with the name we choose?"

What's in a name? To a newborn baby, not much. Feed him, clothe him, comfort and entertain him, and you can call him "Rover" for all he'll care. Once friends and the outside world begin to supersede you and the rest of the family as the center of your child's existence, however (usually early in elementary school), antipathy to the name you selected may develop. Though there's no way to guarantee baby will love the name you choose for a lifetime, careful and sensitive selection will lessen the chance of a name turning out to be Trouble.

■ Make sure both you and your spouse like the name—the way it sounds and looks, and the connotations it carries. Ask yourselves, "Would I like it if it were my name?"

■ Select a meaningful name—name your baby after a loved family member, a respected historical or biblical character, a favorite character in literature, or after an important event. Such a name gives the child a sense of belonging, of being part of an extended family or of the greater world.

■ Select a fitting name—one that seems right for your baby. Melanie, for example, which means "black" or "dark," would be fitting for a dark beauty; Dustin, "a fighter," might be appropriate for a boy who made it through a difficult delivery. Or one that symbolizes a quality you wish for him or her, such as Faith or Constance, or Isaac, which means "he will laugh." Or that reflects your feelings about the birth—Joy, for example, or Ian, "gracious gift of God." Such a name can make a child feel extra special—but the choice will often have to wait until your baby is born.

■ How will the name sound to others? Are there any possible hidden meanings or sound-alike words that might someday make the name embarrassing to your child? Check the initials; do they spell something that could make your child the butt of jokes or teasing? The name Anne Sue Smith, for example, could be the source of frequent anguish for a child. What about possible nicknames? Could they trigger childish insults? If you choose a very ethnic name, will the child be living in, and going to school in, an environment in which such a name would be appreciated or made fun of? (If you do pick an unusual ethnic name, be sure it has a pleasing English equivalent in case your child wants to switch later.)

■ Include a middle name so that if your child turns out to be unhappy with his or her first name, the middle name can be substituted.

■ Choose a name that's easy to say and spell. A very unusual name that teachers are always mispronouncing or a very unusual spelling that's always being misspelled will bring your child grief, not compliments.

■ Avoid the trendy or the political. Don't saddle your child with this year's hot name (after a TV or film star or politician who's making every magazine cover); when the famous namesake turns out to be a flash in the pan or worse, the name may become outdated or place your child in a light that is uncomfortable.

■ Use a real name instead of a diminutive (Richard not Rick, Elizabeth instead of Liz). You can use the diminutive form throughout childhood, but your child then has the option of switching to the more dignified version when he or she ventures out into adulthood.

■ If you don't want your child to be one of six Jasons or Jennifers in the class, avoid picking a name from the year's Top Ten. Many newspapers run an annual piece on the subject of popular names, so check the index or call the paper's library. Check out the most popular names by reading the birth announcements, or take a stroll in the playground and listen to the names mothers call their little ones.

■ Consider family feelings, but don't let them dominate. If there's a family name that you don't love but they'd like to see perpetuated, out of either tradition or senti-ment, try it as a middle name, alter it so that it's more appealing to you, choose another form of the same name (most names actu-ally have several forms), or select a name with the same meaning. A good baby name book will be helpful here. And remember, no matter what names you choose, your parents and grandparents will come to love the kids—even if they detest their names at first.

■ Be sure the name or names are euphonic with the last name and with each other. A good general rule: a short last name goes well with a long first name (Susannah Jones) and vice versa (James Janofsky), while two-syllable firsts usually comple-ment two-syllable lasts.

PREPARING THE FAMILY PET

"Our dog is intensely jealous of my af-fections—she always tries to come be-tween me and my husband when we hug. I'm worried about how she'll react to the new baby."

It's hard for a dog who's always been treated like a baby to roll over and play dog when a real baby appears on the scene. But that's exactly what she'll have to do when her place in your heart—and, possibly, your bed—is taken over by that tiny but menac-ing new human you'll soon be bringing home from the hospital. Though a little initial moping around may be unavoidable, you'll want to do whatever you can to pre-vent excessive jealousy and, of course, any aggressive reactions. Start now.

■ Invest in an obedience training program for your dog if she isn't trained already—and even if you've never felt there was the need for it before. Friskiness and over-enthusiasm aren't usually a problem in a childless home, but they could be in one with a new baby. Particularly because the baby's behavior won't be controllable or predictable, your dog's must be. Obedience training won't take the spirit out of your pet, but it will make her more stable, and thus less likely to harm your baby.

■ Get your dog used to babies now, if you can. Invite friends with babies over to the house, or let her (under careful supervision, and if the parent is willing) sniff a baby in the park or be petted by a toddler, so that she can become familiar with their moves.

■ Get your dog used to life with a baby in the house. Use a baby-size doll as a prop in her training (it'll also be helpful in yours). Diaper the doll; carry, sing to, and rock it; "nurse" it; put it to bed in the crib; take it for a walk in the stroller (if you don't mind the neighbors staring). Now and then, play a tape of a baby crying.

■ Get your dog used to sleeping alone, if that's what the postpartum arrangement will be, so that the change doesn't come as a shock. Fix up a comfortable doggie bed in a corner—with a favorite pillow or blanket for company. Everything in your pet's new bed should be washable because once your baby-to-be starts crawling, there's a good chance you will often find baby curled up in doggie's space.

- Take your dog for a complete medical checkup. Be sure that your dog's rabies shots are up-to-date, that she is flea- and tick-free (but don't plan on using a flea collar, unless you are sure it doesn't carry chemicals poisonous to babies and don't use a flea bomb either during pregnancy or after your baby is born). Also be sure to check your dog for worms of any kind.

- If you have new puppies in your home, have them wormed as soon as possible since the worms, which are excreted in the stool (and can remain in the soil for years), can cause serious disease in babies and children.

- If your baby will have a separate room, train your dog to stay out of it while you're not there. A gate to block the doorway will help discourage unsolicited visits. If your baby's crib will be in your room or in a corner of the living room, train your dog not to go under the crib since she could accidentally unlock the side, letting it fall.

- If your dog's feeding station is one your baby will later be able to get to easily, move it to the cellar, garage, or some other area that a curious crawler can be kept out of, since even a pleasant dog can become vicious when her food is threatened. If you live in a small apartment, get your dog on a late-evening feeding schedule and remove her food dish during the day. Don't even leave her food around when the dog is safely outside, because those tasty nuggets taste good not only to canines—many babies love them, too. And use a non-tip water bowl unless you enjoy mopping the floor frequently.

- After delivery, but while you're still in the hospital, have your husband bring home an unwashed piece of clothing your newborn has worn so that your pet can become familiar with the baby's scent. When you arrive home, let your husband hold the baby while you greet your pet. Then to satisfy her curiosity, let the dog sniff the baby—who should be well swaddled, with head and face protected by your arms. Once the baby's snug in the crib, break out a special treat for the dog, and spend a little time alone with her.

- Be attentive to your new baby, of course, but don't act overprotective around your dog. This will only make the animal more jealous and insecure. Instead, as you would with a human sibling (though on a different level, naturally), try to get your pet involved with the new addition and let her know she's still a loved member of the family. Pet her while you nurse, walk her while you take the baby out in the stroller, allow her into the baby's room while you're there. Try to make a point of spending at least five minutes a day with her alone. But should she show even the slightest aggressiveness toward your baby, reprimand her immediately.

- If, despite your efforts to prepare and reassure her, your dog seems hostile toward the new arrival, keep her tied up and away from the baby until you're sure she's worked out her feelings. Just because a dog has never bitten before doesn't mean she's not capable of it under such duress. If tying the dog up only adds to her hostility, you may have to consider finding another home for her. (With male dogs, neutering may reduce aggressiveness.)

"I worry that our tomcat, who has always slept with us, may be jealous of the new baby."

Even friendly cats can undergo personality changes when a baby arrives. And since cats are just as capable of harming an infant as dogs are, with their claws as well as with their jaws, it's as important to make sure that they are well prepared for the family expansion. Most of the above tips for preparing a dog can work for a cat, as well. Be particularly careful to reassure your cat—through plenty of attention— that he is still a family favorite. And because cats usually love to cuddle next to a warm body and can quickly scale the sides of a crib, be sure to attach a net securely over it to keep yours from bedding down with baby—a friendly gesture that could end in tragedy. Also keep a kitten from licking your infant's face or any broken skin.

PREPARING YOUR BREASTS FOR BREASTFEEDING

"I have a friend who insists that I should massage my nipples to toughen them in preparation for nursing. Is that a good idea?"

Female nipples are designed for nursing. And with very few exceptions, they come to the job fully qualified, without the need for prior preparation. In fact, in some cases the procedures recommended for readying the nipples for breastfeeding can do more harm than good. For instance, applying alcohol, witch hazel, or tincture of benzoin can dry the nipples and make them more, rather than less, likely to crack and fissure; even soap can be drying, and its use on the nipples should be avoided during the last trimester of pregnancy and during lactation itself. Using a brush on nipples will also be counterproductive, irritating the tissues and making them more likely to crack under the pressures of nursing.

But while most nipples don't need any preparation for breastfeeding, many women feel more comfortable doing something to improve their chances of succeeding at it than doing nothing. If you feel you

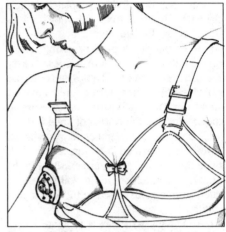

Breast shells are ventilated plastic devices that are available in maternity shops and pharmacies.

would like to do something constructive, have your breasts examined by your obstetrician to see if there are any anatomical features that might interfere with breastfeeding, such as inverted nipples or underdeveloped glandular tissue. Ask if it would be a good idea for you to wear breast shells (see illustration) to help draw out inverted nipples or to massage tender ones to toughen them. But don't undertake nipple massage during pregnancy without your doctor's approval, since nipple stim-

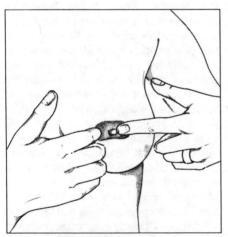 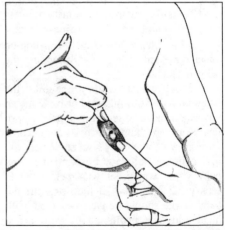

To draw out inverted nipples: Several times daily, place your forefingers at opposite locations on the margins of the areola, then pull outward.

ulation may trigger labor under certain conditions.

With your doctor's okay, you can try any of the following to ready your nipples for your baby's tough gums (though, again, preparation is usually not necessary): rubbing a towel *gently* across them after showering; exposing them to air by walking topless around the house for some time each day; allowing them to rub against your clothing as you go about braless (unless your breasts are heavy and/or prone to sagging) or in a nursing bra with open flaps; rolling them between your thumb and forefinger a couple of times a day, then lubricating them with breast cream, A and D ointment, salad oil or baby oil; expressing a few drops of colostrum, if you can, daily during the last three months; or hav-

ing your husband stimulate your nipples during lovemaking (even if this doesn't work, you'll have fun trying). There's no solid evidence these practices make breastfeeding more comfortable, but they don't seem to do any harm either, and some women find them helpful. Massage and nipple rolling have the added advantage of reducing a woman's inhibitions about handling her breasts—necessary if she's going to be comfortable nursing.

More important than preparing your breasts for breastfeeding is preparing your head. Learn all you can about breastfeeding (take a prenatal course, if possible; read books on the subject), select a pediatrician who strongly advocates it, and find other women who will be able to support you and answer your questions when they arise.

WHAT IT'S IMPORTANT TO KNOW:
Selecting the Right Physician

When you first started shopping around for a practitioner to deliver your baby, it was hard to imagine there was actually going to be a baby to deliver. Now, with tiny but powerful fists, feet, and knees using you regularly as a punching bag, you no longer have any doubts. Not only is there a baby in there—but it's eager to get out. And before it does, you'd better start shopping around for the practitioner who'll care for it: delaying your decision might mean having a stranger care for your baby should you deliver early; no one to ask important questions of during those confusing first days; and no familiar face in case of an emergency.

Assuming you stay in the community and are relatively satisfied with the care, the doctor you choose will be seeing baby—and you—through 16 to 18 years of runny noses, earaches, sore throats, high fevers, upset stomachs, bumps and bruises,

maybe even broken bones, through dramatic physical and psychological developmental milestones that will both thrill and bewilder, through moments you can't now even imagine. You won't be living with your baby's doctor during those years (though there will be times, particularly nights and weekends, when you'll wish you were), but you'll still want someone you feel comfortable and compatible with. Someone you wouldn't hesitate to waken at 2 A.M. when your nine-month-old's fever hits a new high, someone you wouldn't be embarrassed to ask about your six-month-old's sudden fascination with his genitals, someone you would feel free to question when you aren't sure an antibiotic that's been prescribed is necessary.

Before you start securing names, you need to make some basic decisions about the type of doctor you want to care for your baby.

PEDIATRICIAN OR FAMILY PHYSICIAN?

When your mother had a runny nose or a bothersome case of diaper rash, her mother didn't bundle her up and take her to a pediatrician. Chances are she took her to the same doctor who brought her into the world, who treated her father's bursitis and her grandmother's arthritis, who removed her uncle's kidney stones and her cousin's tonsils: the family doctor, a general practitioner (GP), who hung out his shingle after medical school and a single year of internship. Today his breed is virtually extinct, and most runny noses and rashy bottoms are tended to by the pediatrician, a childcare specialist, or by the high-tech successor to the general practitioner—the family physician (FP). Deciding which type of practitioner is for you is your first step toward finding your Dr. Right.[5]

The pediatrician. Babies, children, and, sometimes, adolescents are their business—their only business. Pediatricians have had, in addition to four years of medical school, three years of specialty training. If they are board certified, they have also passed a stringent qualifying exam; those certified after 1988 will be recertified every seven years. The major advantage of selecting a pediatrician for your baby is obvious—since they see only children, and lots of them, they are more familiar than other doctors with what's normal, atypical, and pathological in young patients. They are also more likely to have the answers to the questions that nag new parents, from "Why does he want to nurse all the time?" to "Why isn't she sleeping more?" to "Why does he cry so much?"

A disadvantage is that since pediatricians see only younger members of a fam-

ily, they may not be attuned to the whole family picture (though many are), and may not recognize when a child's problem is rooted in what's going on, either physically or emotionally, with a parent or other family member. Another negative: if the entire family comes down with something that requires medical treatment, it may be necessary to call upon the services of two physicians.

The family physician. Like the pediatrician, the family physician usually has had three years of specialty training following medical school. But an FP residency program is much broader than a pediatric one, covering internal medicine, psychiatry, and obstetrics and gynecology, in addition to pediatrics. Members of the American Academy of Family Practice must take 150 hours of continuing medical education every three years. FPs who are board certified by the American Board of Family Practice (ABFP) have passed a qualifying exam, and must take a recertification exam every six or seven years in addition to continuing to take medical education courses and being subject to periodic review of their office records. The advantage of choosing a family physician is that your entire family can be cared for by the same doctor, one who knows each of you clinically and personally and who can use this information in diagnosis and treatment. If you already have a family physician, adding your baby to the patient roll will have the added advantage of bringing the new family member to an old friend, not a stranger.

The disadvantage: because he or she has had less training and experience in pediatrics than a pediatrician has, a family doctor may be less helpful in dealing with the multitude of well-baby questions you may raise as well as less astute at picking up the obscure diagnosis. To minimize this disadvantage, look for a family physician who sees a lot of babies, not just older children—many do.

---

5. If prenatal diagnosis or family history suggests you may have a baby with a specific health problem (Down syndrome, allergies, asthma), you might consider choosing a pediatrician or family physician with a subspecialty in or at least extensive experience with the problem.

WHAT KIND OF PRACTICE IS PERFECT?

To some patients, the type of practice may be almost as important as the type of physician. There are several options; the one most appealing to you will depend on your personal preferences and priorities.

The solo practitioner. Like the GPs of yesteryear, today's solo practitioners have the opportunity to build close one-to-one relationships with each of their patients. But unlike their predecessors, they aren't likely to be on call round the clock and round the calendar. They'll be around for scheduled appointments (unless called to an emergency), and on call most of the time; but they will take vacations and occasional nights and weekends off, leaving patients who require emergency care or consultation to a covering physician who may be unfamiliar to them. If you do select a solo practitioner, ask about who will be covering at such times, and be sure that in an emergency your child's records will be available even when the doctor is not.

The partnership. Sometimes two doctors are better than one. If one isn't on call, the other almost always is. If you see them in rotation, you and your child often can, thanks to the frequent well-child visits during the first year, build good relationships with both. Though partners will probably concur on most major issues and will likely share similar philosophies of practice, they may occasionally offer different opinions. Having more than one opinion may in some instances be confusing, but hearing two approaches to a particularly confounding problem can be useful. (If one doesn't seem to be able to solve your baby's sleeping problems, maybe the other will.) An important question to ask before deciding on a partnership: can you schedule appointments with the physician of your choice? If not, and if you discover you like one but not the other, you may spend half your visits with a doctor you're not comfortable with. Even if you can choose the preferred doctor for checkups, sick children must usually be seen by whoever is available at the time.

The group practice. If two are good, will three or more be better? In some ways yes, in others no. A group is more likely to be able to provide 24-hour coverage by doctors in the practice, but less likely to ensure close doctor-patient relationships—again, unless you can select the same doctor (or two) for regular checkups. The more physicians a child will be exposed to on well-child and sick-call visits, the longer it may take to feel comfortable with each one, though this will be much less of a problem if all the doctors are warm and caring practitioners. Also a factor here: if you rotate physicians, contradictory advice can either enlighten or confound. In the long run, more important than the number of physicians in a group practice will be the confidence you have in them individually and as a group.

A practice that has a pediatric nurse-practitioner. Any of the above types of practices may include in their ranks a pediatric nurse-practitioner, the equivalent of the nurse-midwife in the obstetrician's office. The pediatric nurse-practitioner, usually a woman, is an RN with additional training (generally at the masters degree level) in her specialty area. She usually handles well-baby checkups, and sometimes the treatment of minor illnesses as well, consulting with her physician colleagues as needed. Problems beyond her scope are referred to one of them. You're likely to favor or object to your baby being cared for by a PNP for many of the same reasons you favored or objected to a nurse-midwife's caring for you during your pregnancy. Like the midwife, the PNP will frequently spend more time with patients at each visit, often devoting as much attention to lifestyle questions as to medical ones.

Fees may in some instances also be lower. But because the level of training is not equal to that of the physician, you may have less confidence in the care your baby is getting. This, however, isn't always a valid concern since many studies have shown that nurse-practitioners and physician's assistants are, on the average, at least as successful as, and sometimes more successful than, physicians at diagnosing and treating minor illnesses.

FINDING DR. RIGHT

For every patient, there is a Dr. Right. Once you know what kind of physician in what type of practice you're looking for, you're ready to start tracking yours down. If your community doesn't have a computer service for matching physicians and patients (a few do), you'll have to rely on more traditional, but usually reliable, sources.

Your obstetrician or midwife. Doctors generally recommend other doctors whose style and philosophy are similar to their own, whose work they are familiar with and respect. So if you've been happy with your pregnancy practitioner, ask for a suggestion. On the other hand, if you've been disappointed, look elsewhere for a recommendation.

An obstetric or pediatric nurse. If you know a nurse who works with pediatricians, in either an office or hospital setting, she's sure to be a good source of information on which doctors are competent, conscientious, caring, and relate well both to parents and children, and which are sloppy, brusque, humorless, and unfriendly. If you don't know a nurse, consider phoning the nursing station on the pediatric floor or the nursery at the hospital where you're going to deliver to seek recommendations.

Parents. No one can tell you more about a doctor's bedside manner than his or her satisfied (or dissatisfied) patients, or, in this case, parents of patients. Recommendations are best when they come from friends or acquaintances who mirror you in temperament and child-rearing philosophy. Otherwise, the very qualities that make them swear by their pediatrican may make you want to swear at him or her.

The local medical society. While these organizations won't recommend one physician over another, they will be able to provide a selection of reputable pediatricians in your area for you to choose from.

Hospital or other referral services. Some hospitals, medical groups, and entrepreneurs have set up referral services to supply the names of doctors in specific specialities. Hospitals recommend doctors who have privileges at their own institution; a referral service may be able to provide, in addition to information about a physician's specialty, training, and board certification, figures on how frequently he or she has been sued for malpractice.

Medical directories. The *American Medical Directory* and the *Directory of Medical Specialties,* often available at your public library or doctor's office, are other bare-bones sources of prospects, providing a way to check credentials (education, training, and affiliations are all listed).

La Leche League. If breastfeeding is a priority and you would particularly like support in this from your pediatrician, your local chapter (see the phone book) can supply you with names.

The Yellow Pages. As a last resort, check under "Pediatrics" or "Family Practice" in the "Grouped by Practice Guide" under "Physicians" in your telephone directory. But keep in mind that these listings are incomplete; many doctors, particularly those who already have thriving practices, opt not to advertise in the Yellow Pages.

MAKING SURE DR. RIGHT IS RIGHT FOR YOU

Procuring a list of names from any of the above sources is a good beginning in your search for Dr. Right. But to narrow down that list to a smaller one of potential candidates made of the "Right" stuff, and finally, to that one practitioner of your health-care dreams, will take a little more investigative phoning and legwork, and personal interviews with a few finalists.

Hospital affiliation. It's advantageous if the doctor you choose is affiliated with a nearby hospital, so that emergency treatment will be easily accessible. And it's nice if that doctor has privileges at the hospital where you are planning to deliver so that he or she can examine your baby before discharge. But don't eliminate from the running a good candidate who doesn't have such an affiliation. Sometimes special permission will be granted for a non-affiliated doctor to see (but not treat) a baby. If not, a staff doctor can perform the hospital exam and arrange for discharge, and you can take baby to see the chosen doctor after you've left the hospital.

Credentials. A Harvard sheepskin looks great on the office wall, but even more important is a residency in pediatrics or family medicine and board certification by either the American Academy of Pediatrics (AAP) or the American Board of Family Practice (ABFP). Pediatricians or family physicians who maintain their status in their professional organizations by sitting periodically for recertification exams are telling you that they are interested both in keeping current medically and in giving their patients the best possible care.

Some doctors charge a fee for a consultation, others don't. During your seventh or eighth month, make appointments with those on your list of finalists and arrive ready to evaluate your prospective baby doctor, taking into account the following:

Office location. Lugging a size-42 belly with you everywhere you go may seem like a struggle now—but it's traveling light compared to what you'll be traveling with after delivery. Going unwalkable distances will no longer be as easy as hopping on a bus, subway, or into a car, and the farther you have to go, particularly in foul weather, the more complicated outings will become. But though a nearby office is certainly a convenience, it can be more—when you're dealing with a sick or injured child, it can mean prompter care and treatment. But keep in mind, when you make your decision, that a truly one-of-a-kind practitioner may be worth a lengthier trip.

Office hours. What constitutes convenient office hours will depend on your own schedules. If one or both of you have 9-to-5 jobs, some early morning, evening, or weekend hours may be a major requirement.

Atmosphere. You can tell a lot about the atmosphere of an office before you even see it. If you're treated curtly on the phone, chances are in-office experiences won't be any more pleasant. If, on the other hand, you're greeted by a cheerful welcoming voice, you're likely to be met with concern and kindness when you come in, panic-stricken, with a sick or injured baby. You can gain further insight when you make your first visit to the office for an interview with the doctor. Is the receptionist friendly, or is her manner as crisp and sterile as her hospital whites? Is the staff responsive to and patient with its young clients, or is communication with them limited to "Get down," "Don't touch," and "Keep quiet"? Is the reception area separate from the waiting area, so you can enjoy some measure of privacy when revealing concerns to and asking questions of office staff?

Decor. A baby doctor needs more than a couple of magazines on the table and a few Expressionist prints on the wall to make the "Right" design statement in his waiting room. On your reconnaissance visit, look for features that will make waiting less painful for both you and your expected: a comfortable play area for toddlers as well as a waiting area for older children; a selection of well-maintained toys and books appropriate for a range of ages; low chairs or other sitting space designed for little bodies. Wallpaper in bold colors and intriguing patterns (orange kangaroos and yellow tigers rather than tastefully understated earth-tone pinstripes) and child-bright pictures (in both the waiting room and the examing rooms) will also give uneasy minds something comforting to focus on while anticipating or experiencing the poking and prodding of a checkup. (But keep in mind, not every good doctor is a Disney buff.) A welcome addition in the family physician's office: separate waiting areas for adults and children.

Waiting time. A forty-five-minute wait when you're pacing with a fussy infant or trying to distract a restless toddler with yet another picture book can be a trying experience for all involved. Yet such waits are not uncommon. For some parents a long wait may merely be an inconvenience; for others it is something their schedules simply can't accommodate.

In trying to gauge the average waiting time in a particular office, don't go by how long *you're* kept waiting for your consultation. Such visits are a courtesy, rather than a medical necessity; screaming infants will (or should) take priority. Instead, ask the receptionist, and if her answer is vague or noncommittal, pose the question to a few waiting parents.

A long average wait can be a sign of disorganization in the office, of overbooking, or of a doctor having more patients than he or she can handle. But it doesn't tell you much about the quality of medical care. Some very good doctors are not very good managers. They may end up spending more time with each patient than allotted (something you will appreciate in the examining room, but not in the waiting room) or may not like to turn down requests to fit sick children into an already full schedule (something you will appreciate when it's your child who's sick).

All waiting doesn't take place in the waiting room. The most uncomfortable wait is often in the examining room, holding an unhappy, undiapered baby, with no space to pace, or trying to distract a frightened toddler without benefit of the toy collection just outside. While long waits in the examining room may not alone be sufficient reason for rejecting a doctor, if they do prove to be a problem, be sure to make a point of letting the nurse know that you would rather do all your waiting in the waiting room.

House calls. Yes, some pediatricians and family physicians still make them. Most of the time, however, as your doctor will probably explain, house calls are not only unnecessary, they aren't best for baby. At the office, a doctor can use equipment and perform tests that can't be stashed in a little black bag. Still, occasions may arise when you will appreciate very much the doctor who is willing to put his or her bedside manner to work literally—as when junior is home from nursery school with a cold, baby's down with a fever and a cough, and you're on duty at home alone in a snowstorm.

Protocol for taking phone queries. If new mothers rushed to the doctor's office every time they had questions about their babies' health or development, their medical bills would skyrocket and physicians' offices would be jammed day and night. That's why most queries are answered and worries assuaged via the telephone. And why you'll want to know in advance how your prospective baby doctor handles such calls. Some parents prefer the call-hour approach: a particular time is set aside each day, during which no patients are seen and distractions are few, for the doctor to field phone calls. This ensures almost immediate access to the doctor—though there may be several bouts with a busy signal or a brief wait for a call back. Other parents find it difficult to confine their worries to between 7 and 8 in the morning or 11 A.M. and noon, or worse, to wait until tomorrow's call-hour for relief of today's worries. They prefer the doctor call-back system: they call when a problem or question arises, and the doctor calls back when there's a free moment between patients. Even if the call back doesn't come for hours (in a non-emergency, of course), callers can at least unburden themselves on—and sometimes be reassured or counseled by—the person who takes the call. And there is the comfort of knowing they will talk to the doctor by the end of the day.

How emergencies are handled. When accidents happen—and they will—how your doctor handles emergencies will be of some consequence. Some doctors instruct parents to take emergencies straight to the emergency room at the local hospital, where the ER staff can provide treatment. Others ask you to call their office first and, depending on the nature of the illness or injury, will see your baby in the office or meet you at the ER. Some physicians are available (unless they're out of town) days, nights, and weekends for emergencies. Others use colleagues or partners to cover for them during off hours.

Matters financial. For all except the very wealthy and the very heavily insured, how financial matters are handled is a prime consideration. Some offices request payment at the time of a visit (unless other arrangements are made in advance); others issue bills. Some offices offer a package deal for first-year care that covers any number of visits. Though the package costs more than the sum of fees for the year's scheduled number of checkups, it is usually a good gamble: you will break even with two or three sick visits, and come out ahead with more. Insurance reimbursement for sick visits, package deal or no, will be handled according to the terms of your coverage.

Payment schedules are also available in some offices, either routinely or under special circumstances, as when financial hardship exists. If you anticipate needing such an arrangement, discuss this with whoever is in charge of billing.

Particularly if finances are tight, you might also want to ask whether routine lab work is done in the office; if so it will probably cost you less than tests sent to an outside laboratory.

Style. When you're in the market for a doctor, as when you're shopping for baby furniture, the style that's right will depend on your style. Do you prefer a doctor who is easygoing and informal, rigid and businesslike, or somewhere in between? Are you most comfortable with a father (or mother) figure who expects to have the last word on everything, or with a doctor who accepts you as a partner and is interested in your opinions? Do you want a doctor who gives the impression of having all the answers, or one who is willing to admit, "I don't know."

Just as there are certain features all parents look for in a crib or a stroller (quality, workmanship, value), there are certain traits they all want in a prospective baby doctor: the ability to listen (without eyeing the next name in the appointment book); an openness to questions and a willingness to respond to them fully and clearly (without becoming defensive or feeling threatened); and, most of all, a genuine fondness for children.

Philosophy. Even in the best of marriages spouses don't always agree, and even in the best of doctor-patient relationships there may be points of difference. But, as with marriages, doctor-patient relationships are most likely to succeed if both partners agree on most major issues. And the ideal time to find out whether you and your prospective baby doctor mesh philosophies is before you make a commitment, at your consultation interview.

Ask about the doctor's positions on

any of the following that you consider important:

▪ Breastfeeding. If you're eager to nurse, a doctor who is only lukewarm toward or confesses to little knowledge of the subject may not provide the support and assistance novice nursers need.
▪ Nutrition. If good nutrition matters to you, beware of the doctor who dismisses the topic with a "don't worry, most kids eat a balanced diet."
▪ Circumcision. Whether you've decided for or against, you'll want a doctor who won't belittle your choice.
▪ Antibiotics. It's a good idea to select a doctor who doesn't prescribe them for every sniffle.
▪ Vegetarianism. If you and your family are non-flesh eaters, it's useful to have a doctor who not only respects that, but knows something about meeting a growing child's nutritional needs on a vegetarian diet.
▪ Early release from the hospital. If that's your desire, you'll want a pediatrician who won't refuse, assuming all is well, to sign baby out with you.
▪ Preventive medicine. If you believe in more than an ounce of prevention, beware the doctor who is grossly overweight, has an ashtray full of cigarette butts on the desk, and nibbles chocolate chip cookies as you speak.

The doctor who has been in practice for any length of time has probably developed some pretty set ideas about child rearing. If you, on the other hand, are new at the game, you may have only the vaguest notion about how you will want to play it (and you will probably make drastic changes in your strategy once the game is underway). With you unsure about your own philosophy and having to judge the doctor's from a short interview, making a perfect match may prove difficult. Still, it's sensible to weed out any candidate whose philosophy seems blatantly contrary to the ideas that have been gestating in your mind during your baby's gestation in your womb.

THE PRENATAL INTERVIEW

Once you've settled on a doctor for your baby, there are probably a number of issues—many of which are examined in this chapter and the next—that you'll want to discuss in a consultation, among them:

Your obstetrical history and family health history. How will these impact on the upcoming delivery and on your new baby's health?

Hospital procedures. What medication will be used in baby's eyes to prevent infection? Which tests are routine after birth? How will jaundice be handled? What are the criteria for early discharge?

Circumcision. What are the pros and cons? Who should perform the procedure and when, if you do opt for it?

Bottle feeding. What type of bottles, nipples, and formula does the doctor recommend?

Breastfeeding. How can your baby's doctor help you get a good start? Can he or she give orders to allow nursing in the delivery room, when feasible; to prohibit the use of pacifiers and supplementary bottles in the nursery; and to facilitate demand feeding if you don't have rooming-in? Can an office visit at one or two weeks postpartum be arranged if you're having difficulty nursing or to assess your progress?

Baby supplies and equipment. Get recommendations on such health supplies as acetaminophen, thermometer, and diaper rash ointment, and on equipment such as cribs, car seats, and strollers.

Suggested reading. Are there any books the doctor would like to specifically recommend, or to steer you away from?

Office etiquette. What should you know about the way the doctor's office operates—for instance, the times that calls are taken or how emergencies are handled?

YOUR PARTNERSHIP WITH DR. RIGHT

Once you've chosen Dr. Right, you can't just drop your baby's health care into his or her lap, sit back with a waiting room magazine, and relax, assured of the right results. As parents, you, and not your doctor, have the most significant impact on your baby's health. If you don't hold up your part of the partnership, even the best of doctors won't be able to provide the best of care for your baby. To be the right patient-parent for Dr. Right, you have a long list of responsibilities of your own.

Follow office etiquette. Be the Amy Vanderbilt of patients: arrive for appointments on time, or if the office perpetually runs late, call half an hour in advance of a scheduled appointment and ask how much later you can safely arrive; try to give at least 24 hours notice when canceling; and keep to arranged payment agreements. Remember, patients (or in this case, parents of patients) are partly responsible for the smooth operation of a doctor's office.

Practice prevention. Though it's wise to select a baby doctor who believes in preventive medicine and concentrates on well-baby care, the burden for keeping baby healthy will fall more heavily on you than on the physician. It's you who must see that baby gets proper nutrition, enjoys a wholesome balance of rest and active play, is not exposed unnecessarily to infection or cigarette smoke, and is kept as safe as possible from accidental injury. It's you who must help your baby establish good health and safety habits (ideally, through your shining example) that can last and give benefit for a lifetime.

Put your worries on paper. Many of the questions you'll come up with between checkups are worthy of your concern without being worthy of a special phone call ("Why doesn't junior have any teeth yet?" or "How can I get him to enjoy his bath?"). Jot these down as they occur to you, before they have a chance to escape in the course of a typically hectic day with baby.

Take notes. The doctor gives you instructions about what to do if your baby has a reaction to her first shots. You get home, she has a fever, and you panic. What was it he said? It's not surprising you've forgotten—the baby was crying after the shot and you could barely hear the instructions as you struggled to redress her, never mind remember them. The remedy for parental memory loss: always bring a pencil and paper to your doctor visits and jot down diagnoses, instructions, and any other information you may want to refer to later. This may not be easy while balancing baby on your lap (that's why two-parent visits are ideal), but it's worth the contortions that may be involved. Or use a tape recorder—with the doctor's okay, of course.

PREPAID MEDICINE

As health maintenance organizations (HMOs) and other prepaid group medical insurance plans proliferate, more and more families are losing the right to choose their physicians. There may be only one pediatrician, or one obstetrician, or one family physician in their neighborhood on the "list." If you find yourself in that position, and are unhappy with the care given by the doctor assigned, let both your employer (or your husband's) and the health plan director know. Be specific in your complaints, but not nasty. Your aim should be to improve the quality of health care offered by the plan; if that doesn't work, perhaps you can persuade the employer to switch to a different plan.

Take notes at telephone "visits," too. Though you're positive you'll remember the name of the over-the-counter ointment the doctor recommended for baby's rash or the dosage of acetaminophen prescribed for teething pain, these details can easily drift from your head when you hang up the phone to the sight of baby smearing potatoes all over the kitchen wall.

Pick up the phone. Thanks to Alexander Graham Bell, the relief for your worries is only a phone call away. But don't use your baby's doctor as a ready reference; before making a call, try to find the answers to your questions in this or in another baby book on your shelf. If you're unsuccessful, however, don't hesitate to call for fear of abusing your telephone privileges. In the early months, baby doctors expect a lot of telephone calls, especially from first-time mothers. Don't call cold, however. Go over the Before Calling the Doctor check list on page 406 and call prepared.

Follow doctor's orders. In any good partnership, both sides contribute what they know or do best. In this partnership, your baby's doctor will be contributing years of training and experience. To get the most benefit from those contributions, it makes sense to take the doctor's advice when feasible, and to inform him or her when you don't intend to or, for some reason, can't. This is particularly vital in medical situations. Say an antibiotic has been prescribed for baby's cough. The baby spits up the medication and won't touch another drop. Since the cough seems a little better anyway, you give up trying to force it down his little throat and don't bother to let the doctor know. Then, two days later, baby's temperature is up, the cough is worse, and playing your baby's doctor has turned out to be a dangerous game. What the doctor would have told you, had you called, is that once the medication is begun the baby may start to improve, but that unless the full course of treatment is completed, the illness can return with greater force. He or she would also have been able to advise you on better ways of getting the medication down or of alternative ways of medicating.

Speak up. To say that it's important to follow doctor's orders is not to say that mother (or father) doesn't sometimes know best—even better than doctor. If you sense the doctor's diagnosis is off or you're afraid the cure prescribed may be worse than the illness, say so, but not in a challenging way. Give the reasons for your concern and ask the doctor to explain the rationale behind his or her position. You may learn something from each other.

Speak up, too, if you've heard about a new form of immunization, a new treatment for colic, or anything else that might benefit your baby. If it's something you've read, bring in the source when possible. Perhaps the doctor has already heard about this advance and can give you additional information for or against it. If the doctor is unfamiliar with it, he or she will probably want to learn more about it before offering an opinion. Be aware however, that medical reporting is notoriously uneven. With your doctor's help, you should be able to sort out the useful from the useless.

Sever an intolerable relationship. Divorcing your baby's doctor (like any divorce) can be very unpleasant. But it's less unpleasant than living with an unsatisfactory relationship—and better for the children. When possible, try to talk out your disagreements and problems with the doctor before severing ties entirely; you may find a misunderstanding rather than serious philosophical differences behind the rift, in which case you may be able to make a fresh start with the same doctor. If the physician you've chosen turns out to truly be Dr. Wrong, you will begin the search for a new doctor a lot wiser and, hopefully, end up with better results. To make sure you don't leave your baby uncovered by a doctor while you shop around again, avoid terminating your relationship with Dr. Wrong until you've found a replacement. When you have, be sure all of your child's medical records are transferred promptly.

CHAPTER TWO

Buying for Baby

You've resisted the temptation for months. Passed wistfully by the Layette Department on your way to Maternity, not daring to run as much as a finger over the lacy rompers and handknit blankets, casting no more than a longing glance at the musical mobiles and cuddly teddies. But now, at long last, with delivery only weeks away, it's not only okay to stop resisting and start buying, it's absolutely necessary.

Do, however, resist the urge to belly up to the counter and put yourself in the hands of the grandmotherly saleswoman who's waiting to sell you everything she has in stock and several other things she's ready to order at the drop of a credit card. Her voice-of-experience sales pitch may make you forget that you'll be getting some hand-me-downs from your sister-in-law, that dozens of gifts will soon come pouring in, and that you will be doing laundry frequently. And you may end up with shopping bags loaded with more tiny outfits, toys, and paraphernalia than your baby will ever be able to use before outgrowing them.

Instead, do your homework before starting your shopping. Calculate your minimum needs (you'll always be able to fill in later) using the shopping list on page 37, and face that saleswoman armed with these basic guidelines:

■ Don't buy a complete layette as espoused by the store or any list; use lists merely as a guide.

■ Keep in mind how many times a week you (or someone else) will be doing the laundry. If you will be washing almost every day, buy the smallest suggested number of items on the list; if you will have to lug loads down to the launderette and can only do it weekly, then buy the largest number.

■ Check off items borrowed or handed down before finalizing your shopping list.

■ If friends and family ask what you'll need, don't be embarrassed to tell them. They really would rather buy you something you'll use than something you'll have to cart back to the store postpartum. Suggest a few items in various price ranges to give them freedom of choice, but don't suggest the same items to different people.

■ Hold off on buying items you won't need right away (a high chair, a baby seat for the bathtub, toys too advanced for infants) and items you may end up not needing (the full quota of pajamas, towels, t-shirt sets) until you've received all your gifts. When they stop coming in, recalculate your needs, and head out for the store once more.

■ Buy mostly 6- to 9-month sizes. You may want a couple of 3-month-size shirts and maybe an outfit or two for dress-up that fit just right, but for the most part it's more practical to roll up sleeves and endure a slightly blousy look for a few weeks until baby starts to fill out the larger sizes. And as irresistible as it may be to unpack your purchases into baby's new dresser, don't do so. Keep all baby clothes (even the set you're planning to take baby home in) tagged or in their original packages. That way, if baby checks in at 10 pounds 6 ounces, your husband, mother, or a friend can exchange at least some of them for 6-month sizes while you're still in the hospital, and the others soon after. Likewise, if your baby arrives early, weighing just 5 pounds, some of the larger sizes can be exchanged.

In general, buy at least one size ahead (most six-month-old babies wear 9- or 12-month sizes, some even wear 18-month sizes), but eyeball before purchasing because some styles (particularly imported ones) can run much larger or smaller than average.

■ Keep the season in mind as you shop. If baby is expected on the cusp of a season, buy just a few tiny items for the immediate weather and larger ones for the weather expected in the months ahead. Continue to consider the seasons as baby grows. That adorable appliquéd sunsuit at half price may be difficult to pass up, but if it's a 12-month size and your baby will be a year old next June, it's a purchase you'll regret.

■ When selecting baby clothes, consider convenience and comfort first, fashion second. Tiny buttons at baby's neckline may be darling, but the struggle to fasten them with baby squirming on the changing table won't be. An organdy party frock may look fetching on the hanger—but may have to stay there if it irritates baby's delicate skin. An imported sailor suit may look smart—until you have to change baby and find no access to the diaper area. Always look for outfits made of soft, easy-care fabrics, with snaps instead of buttons (inconvenient, and should baby manage to chew one off, unsafe), head openings that are roomy (or have snaps at the neck), and bottoms that open conveniently for diaper changing. Shun long strings or ribbons, which are potentially hazardous, and rough seams, which are potentially uncomfortable. Room for growth is another important feature: adjustable shoulder straps, stretch fabrics, undefined waistlines on one-piece garments, elasticized waistlines, double rows of snaps on sleepwear, pants that can be rolled up, wide hems that can be taken down, tucks, pleats, or yokes. Pajamas with "feet" should be the right length, or should have elasticized ankles to keep them in place.

■ If you haven't learned the gender of your baby through ultrasound or amniocentesis, don't buy everything in yellow or green (unless you're mad about those colors), particularly since many infants don't have the complexion to carry off these shades. Both boys and girls can wear reds, blues, and navys. If you wait on some purchases until baby arrives, you'll be able to indulge in some dainty pinks for a daughter or some more distinctly masculine styles for a son. At some stores, you can order a layette and not pick it up until after the baby is born— at which time you can specify the color. This will work only if dad, grandma, or a friend can pick up your order while you're in the hospital, or if it can be delivered before you arrive home.

■ When buying baby furniture, practicality and safety should supersede style. An antique cradle, either purchased or passed down, may lend that heirloom look to the nursery—but you could be setting your baby up for a fall should the bottom not prove strong enough to support his or her weight, or for a lead overdose if the paint job, too, is antique. If you have a dog, a cradle may be too close to the ground for comfort. A plush Rolls-Royce of strollers may evoke a lot of smiles when you walk down the street, but a lot of frowns when you hold up the bus line while struggling to fold it and lug it, baby, and diaper bag, up the steps. For other features to favor in baby furniture, see page 40.

■ When buying toiletries for baby, buy only what you need (see list on page 38), rather than one of everything you see. When comparing products, look for those that are alcohol-free (alcohol is drying to a baby's skin) and contain the fewest artificial colors, preservatives, and other chemical additives. Do not buy baby powders. They serve no medical purpose, can cause irritation if they collect in baby's cracks and crevices, can be dangerous if inhaled, and if they contain talc, may even cause lung cancer down the road.

■ When stocking the medicine chest, however, err on the side of excess, filling it, just in case, with everything you might need in an emergency and hope you'll never have to use. Otherwise, you may find yourself helpless when your baby wakes in the middle of the night burning up with fever and you have no medication on hand to bring it down. Or when he or she is found nibbling on the lovely but poisonous Christmas holly plant a guest has brought and you have nothing in the medicine chest to induce vomiting.

FIRST WARDROBE

3 to 7 undershirts. Open-front, side-snap styles are easiest to use with newborns, but pullovers are smoother and more comfortable; snap-bottom body shirts don't ride up, keeping tummies covered in cold weather.

3 to 8 nightgowns with drawstring bottoms. Drawstrings should be removed as baby becomes more active.[1]

2 to 3 blanket sleepers, for late fall or winter babies. Do not use the bag types once your baby can pull up.

3 to 4 waterproof pants, diaper covers, or diaper wraps, if you're planning to use cloth diapers. If you're using disposables, just one dress-up pair for special occasions.

2 to 3 pairs of booties or socks. Select those that won't kick off easily.

3 to 6 stretchies with feet, for a fall or winter baby, but just 2 or 3 for a late spring or summer arrival.

3 to 6 rompers (one-piece, short-sleeved, snap-at-the-crotch outfits), for a late spring or summer baby.

2 washable bibs. Even before solids are introduced, you'll need these to protect clothes from spitup.

---

1. Clothing for babies and children to sleep in must meet federal standards for flame resistance; they are usually made of synthetic fibers that do not flame up.

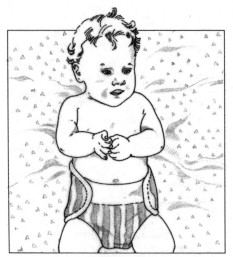

Diaper wraps eliminate the need for pins or rubber pants; they are made of cotton or wool and "breathe," reducing the risk of diaper rash.

1 to 3 sweaters. 1 lightweight sweater will do in summer; heavier ones will be needed in cold weather.

1 to 3 hats. Lightweight with brim (for sun protection) for a summer baby; heavier-weight, and shaped to cover the ears snugly but not too tightly, for a winter baby.

1 bunting or snowsuit bag with attached mitts, for a late fall or winter baby.

LINEN WARDROBE

3 to 6 receiving blankets, depending on season.

3 to 4 fitted sheets each, for crib, cradle, bassinet, and/or carriage.

2 quilted mattress pads, if desired.

2 to 6 waterproof pads, for protecting crib, carriage, laps, and furniture.

2 washable crib or bassinet blankets or comforters. Lightweight for summer; heavier for winter. Avoid long fringes and loose threads.

1 to 2 blankets for carriage or stroller. Just 1 lightweight one for a summer baby.

2 to 3 terry cloth towels, with hoods.

2 to 3 soft washcloths.

1 dozen square cloth diapers, for protecting your shoulders when burping baby, to protect sheets when baby spits up, for emergency bibs, and much more.

Diaper liners for cloth diapers if you like, for heavy wetters or extra nighttime protection.

Diapers. Purchase 2 to 5 dozen prefolded cloth ones, if you are washing your own, or several dozen disposables, if you are using them exclusively (a couple dozen if you will use them only for outings and emergencies). If you are planning on using a diaper service, sign up in the eighth month and they will be ready to deliver as soon as you do.

TOILETRIES

Items needed for diaper changes should be kept on a shelf high enough above the changing table to prevent baby's grabbing for them, but low enough for you to reach easily.

Baby soap or bath liquid, to be used sparingly.

No-tears baby shampoo. For young infants, no-tears baby bath can be used for shampoo.

Baby oil, if desired. This is not a necessary item, unless the doctor prescribes it for cradle cap, and salad oil will often serve as well.

Baby cornstarch, if desired. Not necessary, but nice for warm weather use.

Ointment for diaper rash. Ask the doctor for a recommendation.

Petroleum jelly, such as Vaseline, for lubricating rectal thermometers. Do not use to self-treat diaper rash.

Diaper wipes, for diaper changes, hand washing, and a dozen other uses. But use cotton balls and plain water for cleansing baby's bottom during the first few weeks and whenever diaper rash is a problem.

Sterile cotton balls, for cleaning baby's eyes, for daubing alcohol on the umbilical stump, and for diaper changes in the first few weeks and when baby has a rash.

8 diaper pins, if you're using cloth diapers. Metal heads are better than plastic, which can crack.

Baby nail scissors or clippers.

Baby brush and comb. Use only a wide-toothed comb on wet hair.

MEDICINE CHEST

Have these supplies on hand rather than waiting to buy them as needed. Ask baby's doctor for recommendations. Store them out of reach of infants and children.

Liquid aspirin substitute, such as Baby Tylenol, Tempra, Panadol (all are brands of acetaminophen).

Liquified charcoal, if recommended by your local poison center.

Syrup of Ipecac, in case of accidental poisoning (but do not use without medical advice; see page 448).

Liquid decongestant, infant formula, to be used only if prescribed by the doctor (it is not usually recommended for babies).

Antiseptic cream, such as bacitracin or neomycin, for minor cuts and scrapes.

Hydrogen peroxide, for cleaning cuts.

Calamine lotion or hydrocortisone cream ($1/2\%$), for mosquito bites and itchy rashes.

Rehydration fluid, if the baby's doctor recommends it for treatment of diarrhea; it's not usually needed for breastfed infants.

Sunscreen cream or lotion. Do not use until baby is six months old, unless the doctor suggests otherwise.

Rubbing alcohol, for cleaning thermometers, but not for rubdowns.

Calibrated spoon, dropper, and/ or oral syringe, for administering medications.

Sterile band-aids and gauze pads, in a variety of sizes and shapes.

Adhesive tape, for securing gauze pads.

Tweezers, for pulling out tiny splinters.

Nasal aspirator, a bulb syringe for clearing a stuffy nose (see page 419).

Ear syringe, for removing wax buildup, if baby's doctor recommends it.

Cold mist vaporizer/humidifier. The old-fashioned, hot steam humidifier is not recommended because it can lead to burns.

A thermometer. Best: A standard rectal thermometer or a newer tympanic one. Digital models and temperature strips are less accurate.

Small penlight, to check throat for inflammation or pupils for signs of concussion.

Tongue depressors, for examining the throat.

Heating pad and/or hot-water bottle, for soothing a colicky tummy or relieving sore muscles.

FEEDING SUPPLIES

1 bottle with nipple, for water or an emergency supplementary feeding, if you're breastfeeding exclusively.

4 bottles, 4-ounce size, and **10 to 12 bottles, 8-ounce size, with nipple units,** if you're bottle feeding; 4 to 6, if you're supplementing. Glass bottles are easiest to clean, but are breakable, and are not recommended for use with breast milk. Plastic bottles come in two types: traditional-style reusable and the newer reusable holders with disposable liners, which collapse as baby feeds, minimizing air swallowing.

Nipples come in several shapes (including the more natural orthodontic) and with different hole sizes (smaller for formula and younger babies, larger for juice and older babies). Silicone nipples are odor and taste free, don't get gummy, are dishwasher safe and see-through (so you can see if they're clean). You may want to try several types to see which work best for your baby.

Utensils for formula preparation, if you're bottle feeding. Exactly which items you'll need will depend on the type of formula you plan to use, but the shopping list will usually include bottle and nipple brushes, large Pyrex measuring pitcher, Pyrex measuring cup, can opener, long-handled mixing spoon, and tongs. All should be boilable.

A sterilizer, if you will be bottle feeding, or supplementing early on.

A pacifier, if you decide to use one. Look for sturdy one-piece construction, a shield with ventilation holes (required by the Consumer Product Safety Commission), and orthodontic shape. Like nipples, they also come in easy-to-clean silicone. *Warning:* Never attach a cord or ribbon to a pacifier.

FURNISHINGS

On all items. *Look for:* lead-free paint, if painted; sturdy non-tip construction; smooth edges and rounded corners; safety restraint straps at crotch and waist, where appropriate. *Avoid:* rough edges, sharp points, or small parts that might break loose; exposed hinges or springs; attached strings, cords, or ribbons. Be sure to follow the manufacturer's directions for use and maintenance of all items and to regularly check baby's crib, carriage, and other equipment for loose screws, frayed straps, supports that have snapped, and other signs of wear.

Crib. *Look for:* A label stating Consumer Product Safety Commission (CPSC) standards have been met; bars no more than 2⅜ inches apart, with no splinters or cracks in the wood; mattress level adjustability; minimum rail height of 22 inches when the mattress is at its highest position and the rail is at its lowest setting; steel stabilizing bars; plastic covering on teething rails, if any, tightly secured and unbroken; casters for mobility. *Avoid:* posts or knobs that protrude; crossbars.

Crib mattress. *Look for:* firmness; pocketed-coil innerspring or, if there's a family history of allergy, dense foam (or put an airtight cover over an innerspring); snug fit in crib (with no more than two adult-finger widths between crib and mattress).

Bumpers. *Look for:* snug not floppy fit around entire perimeter of crib; at least 6 ties or sets of snaps for fastening to crib rails.

Bassinet or cradle. Optional, but useful in the early weeks when baby may enjoy the cozy quarters and you may appreciate its mobility (though a carriage can serve the same purpose). *Look for:* firm mattress; sturdy stable base; adequate size to hold your baby (a fragile antique may collapse under the weight of a heavy baby).

Changing space. This can be a table or dresser top designed especially for baby changing, or a makeshift unit put together from things you already have. *Look for:* a comfortable height; washable padding; restraining straps; diaper storage within your reach, toiletry storage out of baby's reach.

Diaper pail, if you will be doing your own diapers (diaper service will provide one, if you use their diapers). *Look for:* easy washability; a tight fitting top that a baby or toddler can't pry open (babies have drowned in water-filled pails and been poisoned by tasting the cake of deodorant).

Chest of drawers, or other storage unit for baby's clothes.

Baby tub. *Look for:* non-skid bottom (or use a towel or stick-ons to keep baby from slipping); easy washability; roomy size (large enough for your baby at four or five months, as well as now); support for baby's head and shoulders; easy portability; easy drainage. *Avoid:* non-removable sponge pads.

Tub seat, for when baby graduates to the big tub. *Look for:* restraining straps; a suction bottom.

Infant seat. *Look for:* wide, sturdy, stable base; non-skid or suction bottom; crotch and waist restraint straps; adequate size (some are too small for any but the tiniest infants); convenient carry handle. *Also nice:* a rocking mechanism; adjustability. Never leave an infant, even a very young one, in such a seat at the edge of a table or counter or near something (such as a wall) he or she could push off from, and never use an infant seat as a car seat.

Toy chest. *Look for:* lightweight lid, removable or with a support mechanism that will keep it from slamming down on a child; smooth edges and corners on metal chests, and no splinters on wooden ones; ventilation holes in lid and sides; no lock or latch. An open bin or toy shelves are preferable for toy storage.

OUTING EQUIPMENT

Stroller. *Look for:* Juvenile Products Manufacturers Association (JPMA) certification seal; a reclining seat, so the stroller can be used when baby is very young as well as for naps when baby is older; a broad non-tip base; large wheels for better maneuverability; good brakes; secure and easy-to-fasten restraining straps; easy foldability (try it); lightweight, if you plan to carry it onto buses or other vehicles often; sun and rain shields; hinges that won't catch curious fingers; comfortable handle height; package rack. When using the stroller, be sure the folding mechanism

is properly locked in the open position and don't overload handles with bags or other items, since they could tip it over.

Combination stroller-carriage. This has some of the advantages of both, but is not as lightweight as a stroller. See stroller and carriage entries for tips on selecting.

Carriage. Many families, especially those living in cramped quarters, or who take most of their outings in a car, don't need or want a carriage. If you do, *look for:* smooth rocking motion; foldability (if that is important to you); maneuverability (be sure it will fit through the doors in your home); a package rack; secure locking devices if top is removable for use as a bassinet. Always be sure a foldable unit is properly locked open when in use; once your baby can sit, propped, always use a baby harness.

Car seat. Even if you don't own a car, you will need a seat if you plan on taking

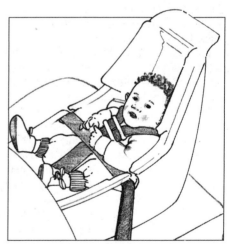

Infant car seat. *This rear facing seat is suitable for infants up to one year old and 20 pounds (some models work for those weighing more; check labels). Some seats can be removed and installed with baby in them and can be used as infant seats indoors.* **Never** *place any rear-facing infant seat in the front seat of an auto equipped with passenger-side airbags.*

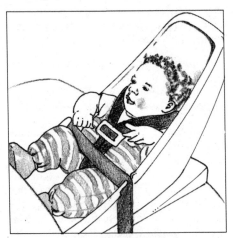

Convertible car seat. *Designed for children from birth to 40 pounds, this unit faces the rear in a semi-reclining position for infant use, then can be switched to an upright, front-facing position when baby is older. Do not use the rear-facing position in a front seat with airbags.*

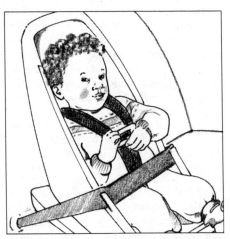

Older babies are ready for forward-facing toddler seats, designed for children over a specific height and weight (see product label). Secured by the auto seat belt, these provide more mobility and visibility. Children should not ride in a booster seat until at least 40 pounds.

baby for drives in anyone else's car. If you rent a car, you can rent a seat along with it, but keep in mind it may not be the best seat available. There are three types—the infant seat, the convertible seat, and the toddler seat—and you should *look for* the following when selecting one: a seat manufactured after January 1, 1981, when strict federal standards went into effect (don't borrow an older one or one that's already been in an accident); ease of installation (preferably without a tether); a one-latch harness, which makes fastening and releasing baby easier (test it yourself to be sure you can handle these maneuvers quickly); comfort and roominess for baby, with adequate visibility and ease of movement for an older infant; adjustability, if you plan to use it as your child grows. For current information, call the Auto Safety Hotline, (800) 424-9393.

Baby carrier. Convenient for carrying a young baby at home or away, leaving your hands free for chores or carrying bundles. *Look for:* a front carrier model (a baby is too young for a back carrier until he or she can sit independently) that is easy to hook up and detach without help; adjustable,

padded straps that don't bind; easy washability; head and shoulder support for baby, and a wide bottom that supports bottom and thighs. A carrier that allows baby to be held face outward when awake is ideal. A sling carrier that puts most of the weight on your hips is better for your back when baby is heavier. Never use a carrier instead of a car seat.

Diaper bag. *Look for:* multiple compartments, at least one waterproof; shoulder strap or back pack style; a zipper closing for main compartment. A detachable changing pad is a plus. See page 84 for how to pack a diaper bag.

NICE TO HAVE

Rocking chair. Great for feeding and calming a baby. *Look for:* sturdy rockers; a comfortable fit (try it).

Intercom. Ideal if baby's room is out of earshot of your bedroom or other parts of the house. *Look for:* portability and safety (no exposed parts that can cause electrocution).

Baby swing. Can often soothe an unhappy baby. *Look for:* secure restraining straps; smooth edges and surfaces; sturdiness; a seat that reclines for a young infant; an activity tray for diversion. *Avoid:* a swing with hinges that can catch little fingers, or small parts that can break off. If the swing is to be attached to a doorway, be sure it will fit yours. Do not use for a baby younger than six weeks.

Portable crib, if you plan on traveling often to places where such equipment will not be available. *Look for:* safety features listed for playpens below.

YOU WILL NEED, OR MAY WANT, LATER

Feeding chair. Available in both high and low models, but high are presently more popular. *Look for:* wide, sturdy, non-tip base; a tray that can be easily removed or locked in place with one hand; a wide lip to catch spills; washability; a seat back high enough to support baby's head; an adjustable foot rest; restraining straps; a secure locking device if the chair folds; JPMA certification.

Portable feeding seat. These are useful when visiting and at restaurants, as well as at home. *Look for:* a locking mechanism to prevent falls; a comfortable seat; a crotch guard to prevent baby's slipping out. Never use such a seat on a glass or pedestal table, or with a chair under it. (For other safety tips, see page 235.)

Playpen. Wooden playpens are better for learning to pull up, but mesh pens are softer if baby falls against the sides. *Look for:* JPMA certification seal; slats no more than 2⅜ inches apart on a wooden pen; fine netting on a mesh pen (it won't catch fingers or buttons); tough vinyl pads that won't tear easily (babies can choke on the torn plastic or on exposed filling); padded metal hinges; a baby-proof collapse mechanism. *Do not* use an accordion-type playpen or leave a mesh pen with the sides down.

Safety gate, for doorways or stairs. *Look for:* rigid mesh or swinging metal construction (not accordion-type, unless it is of a post-1985 design and has safety certification) and a latch that is easy to open and close (or you may neglect to close it).

Walker. Not recommended (see page 233). If used, *look for:* wide, sturdy, non-tip base; secure locking mechanism to safeguard fingers; protective covers for any accessible coil springs; wide three-sided tray for play and protection. *Safest option:* the new stationary or go-around-in-circles walkers.

WHAT TO TAKE TO THE HOSPITAL

Use this as a checklist.

En Route

□ Cash for the cab fare or parking garage
□ Watch or clock with a second hand for timing contractions
□ Notebook and a pen for recording contractions and emotional and physical symptoms

For the Labor or Birthing Room

□ Plenty of change for telephone calls and snack machines
□ Insurance forms
□ Hospital preadmittance forms and information
□ Lotion for massages
□ Small paper bag to remedy hyperventilation
□ Tennis ball or rolling pin for counter-massage during back labor
□ Sugarless lollipops to keep your mouth moist
□ Heavy socks for cold feet
□ Colored washcloth
□ Champagne labeled with your name, for celebrating
□ Sandwiches or other snacks for dad
□ Your address book or a list of family and friends to be called

□ *What to Expect When You're Expecting*[2]

For Your Hospital Room

□ This book
□ Robe and two to three nightgowns (not your best, since they may end up stained by lochia; alternatively, you can use the hospital's)
□ Bed jacket, slippers
□ Perfume, powder, cosmetics, toothbrush, toothpaste
□ Soap, deodorant, skin lotion, shampoo, conditioner
□ Hair brush, hair dryer, curling iron
□ Glasses or contact lenses (with necessary paraphernalia)
□ Sanitary napkins (these will probably be supplied by the hospital)
□ Playing cards, books, magazines, other distractions
□ A baby name book, if you haven't made that decision yet
□ Packs of raisins, nuts, whole-wheat crackers

For Going Home: Mom

□ A roomy outfit to go home in
□ Bra (nursing bra if you plan to breast-feed)
□ Panties and slip
□ Shoes and hosiery
□ Coat or sweater, if necessary
□ Shopping bags to bring home gifts

For Going Home: Baby

□ 2 disposable diapers (though the hospital will probably supply these), or 4 cloth diapers with pins and waterproof pants or wrappers
□ 1 undershirt
□ 1 stretchie or nightgown
□ Socks or booties
□ 1 receiving blanket
□ Sweater and cap in cool weather
□ Bunting or heavy blanket in cold weather (if bunting won't fit in the car seat, strap the baby in, then cover with a blanket)
□ Infant car seat

GOING HOME

In the 1930s, new babies came home from the hospital after ten days, in the '50s after four days, in the '80s after two days. Today you may bring your new infant home within hours of delivery. It's scary, controversial, and not always appropriate. The decision is best made on a case-by-case basis with a physician's input. Early discharge is safest when an infant is full-term; is an appropriate weight; has started feeding well; is going home with a parent (or parents) who knows the basics and is well enough to provide care; and will be seen by the doctor at two or three days after birth. If for any reason you have concerns about early discharge, speak to your child's doctor.

If you and your baby are discharged early, a doctor's visit should be scheduled within the next 48 hours. Also be on the lookout for problems typical of newborns, such as yellowing of the skin* and the whites of the eyes (a sign of jaundice); refusal to eat; dehydration (fewer than six wet diapers in 24 hours, or dark yellow urine); constant crying, or moaning instead of crying; fever; red or purple dots anywhere on the skin.

*To check for jaundice, press your newborn's arm or thigh with your thumb. If the area beneath the pressure turns yellowish rather than white, jaundice may be present.

CHAPTER THREE

Your Newborn Baby

WHAT YOUR BABY MAY BE DOING

Your baby within a few days of birth will probably be able to:

■ lift head briefly when on the tummy

■ move arms and legs on both sides of the body equally well

■ focus on objects within 8 to 15 inches

WHAT YOU CAN EXPECT AT THE HOSPITAL CHECKUPS

Your baby's very first checkup will be in the delivery or birthing room. Here, or later on in the nursery, you can expect that a doctor or nurse will do some or all of the following:

■ Clear baby's airways by suctioning his or her nose (which may be done as soon as the head appears or after the rest of the baby is delivered)

■ Clamp and cut the umbilical cord (antibiotic ointment may be applied to the cord stump, and the clamp is usually left on for at least 24 hours)

■ Check the placenta to be sure it's complete and evaluate its condition

■ Assign baby an Apgar score (rating of baby's condition at one and five minutes after birth; see page 47)

PORTRAIT OF A NEWBORN

Most first-time parents are unprepared for the appearance of the bundle of joy that is handed them at delivery. Despite the oohs and aahs from excited friends and families, most newborns are not cute. The typical new arrival has a head that looks too large for its body (it's about one quarter of the total length), skinny "chicken" legs, and often, unless delivered by cesarean, a battered countenance.

Newborn hair may be sparse or full, it may lay flat or stand up straight in what looks like the latest punk style. When hair is thin, blood vessels in the scalp may appear very prominent and the pulse may be visible at the soft spot, or fontanel on the top of the head.

A newborn's eyes may appear squinty because of the folds at the inner corners and because of swelling from delivery and infection-protecting eye drops. They may also be blood-shot from the pressures of labor. The nose may be flattened and the chin unsymmetrical or pushed in from being squeezed through the pelvis. If it was a particularly tight squeeze, the head may have molded to a point, looking as though baby were wearing a dunce cap.

And/or a bruise, or cephalohematoma, may have been raised on the scalp. (Most of these effects of labor will diminish in a few days, or at most a few weeks.)

Because a newborn's skin is thin, it usually has a pale pinkish caste (even in black babies) from the blood vessels just beneath it. The skin is most often covered with the remains of the vernix caseosa (a cheesy coating) that protects the fetal skin during the time spent soaking in the amniotic fluid, though the later a baby arrives, the less of this coating there is. Many babies, particularly those born early, are also covered with lanugo, a downy prenatal fuzz, usually on the shoulders, back, forehead, and cheeks, that will disappear within the first weeks of life. Because of an infusion of female hormones from the placenta just before birth, many babies, both boys and girls, have swollen breasts and/or genitals. There may even be a milky discharge from the breasts and, in girls, a vaginal discharge (sometimes bloody).

These newborn features will begin to disappear in the weeks to come. And pretty soon, your baby will be picture pretty.

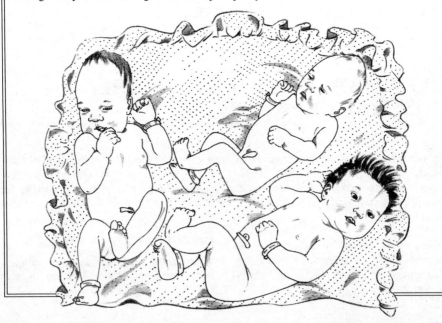

- Administer eyedrops or ointment (silver nitrate or antibiotics; see page 65) to prevent gonococcal or chlamydial infection.
- Count fingers and toes, and note if baby's observable body parts and features appear normal.
- Record passage or lack of passage of urine and/or stools (to help rule out an elimination problem).
- Administer vitamin K injection, to enhance the clotting ability of baby's blood.
- Weigh baby (average weight is 7½ pounds; 95% of new babies weigh between 5½ and 10 pounds).
- Measure baby's length (average length is 20 inches; 95% of newborns are between 18 and 22 inches).
- Measure head circumference (average is 13.8 inches; normal range is from 12.9 to 14.7 inches).
- Obtain blood from infant's heel, to be screened for phenylketonuria (PKU) and hypothyroidism; from the umbilical cord for the Coombs test, to screen for antibodies that would indicate Rh sensitization has occurred; for any other necessary metabolic screening tests (for low blood sugar, for example); for sickle-cell screening.[1]
- Assess gestational age (time spent in the uterus) in babies born before term.

Before your baby leaves the delivery or birthing room, ID bands will be placed on both you and your baby. Baby's footprints and your fingerprint will be obtained for future identification purposes (the ink is washed off your baby's feet, and any residual smudges you may note are only temporary). The baby's doctor, usually of your choosing, will give baby a more complete examination sometime during the next 24 hours; if you (with or without your spouse) can arrange to be present, this is a good time to ask questions. The doctor will check the following:

---

1. Some tests for newborns are mandated in all or most states, and some in a few states; most are more accurate when performed after the first day of life. Federal experts recommend universal sickle-cell screening; most hospitals test black babies only.

- Weight (it will probably have dropped since birth, often by as much as 10% of body weight), head circumference (may be larger, as any molding of the head rounds out), and length (which won't actually have changed, but might seem to have because measuring a baby, who can't stand or cooperate, is a highly inexact procedure)
- Heart sounds and respirations
- Internal organs, such as kidneys, liver, and spleen, by palpation (examining by touch, externally)
- Newborn reflexes
- Hips, for possible dislocation
- Hands, feet, arms, legs, genitals
- Hearing (screening)
- The umbilical stump

APGAR TEST

The first test most babies are given—and which most pass with good scores—is the Apgar, developed by anesthesiologist Virginia Apgar. The scores, recorded at one minute and again at five minutes after birth, reflect the newborn's general condition and are based on observations made in five assessment categories. Babies who score between 7 and 10 are in good to excellent condition, and usually require only routine postdelivery care; those scoring between 4 and 6, in fair condition, may require some resuscitative measures; and those who score under 4, in poor condition, will require immediate and maximal lifesaving efforts. It was once believed that babies whose scores remained low at five minutes were destined to have future neurological problems, but recent research shows that most of these babies turn out to be normal and healthy.

YOUR NEWBORN'S REFLEXES

Startle, or Moro, reflex. Sudden or loud noise or the sensation of falling causes a young baby to extend legs, arms, and

fingers, arch back, and draw head back, then draw arms back, fists clenched, into chest.
Duration: Four to six months.

Babinski reflex. When the sole of the foot is gently stroked from heel to toe, the toes flare upward and foot turns in.
Duration: Between six months and two years, after which toes curl downward.

Rooting reflex. A newborn whose cheek is gently stroked will turn in the direction of the stimulus, mouth open and ready to suckle.
Duration: About three to four months, though it may persist when baby is sleeping.

Walking, or stepping, reflex. Held upright on a table or other flat surface, supported under the arms, a newborn (this works best after the fourth day of life) may lift one leg and then the other taking what seem to be "steps."
Duration: Variable, but typically about

two months. (Existence of this reflex does not forecast early walking.)

Palmar grasping reflex. With baby facing forward, arms flexed, an index finger pressed against his or her palm will cause a flexing of the hand in an attempt to grasp the finger. A newborn's grasp may be powerful enough to support full body weight.
Duration: Three or four months.

Tonic neck reflex. Placed on the back, a young baby will assume a "fencing position," head to one side, with arms and legs on that side extended and opposite limbs flexed.
Duration: It may be present at birth or may appear at about two months, and disappears at about six months.

You can try to elicit these reflexes from your baby, but keep in mind that your results may be less reliable than those of a doctor or other trained examiner and that

APGAR TABLE

SIGN	POINTS		
	0	**1**	**2**
Appearance (color)*	Pale or blue	Body pink, extremities blue	Pink
Pulse (heartbeat)	Not detectible	Below 100	Over 100
Grimace (reflex irritability)	No response to stimulation	Grimace	Lusty cry
Activity (muscle tone)	Flaccid (no or weak activity)	Some movement of extremities	A lot of activity
Respiration (breathing)	None	Slow, irregular	Good (crying)

APGAR acronym devised by L. Joseph Butterfield, MD.

THE BRAZELTON NEONATAL BEHAVIORAL ASSESSMENT SCALE

More complex and more time-consuming to administer than the Apgar test, the Brazelton, developed by baby doctor T. Berry Brazelton, is believed by some to be a better predictor of future development. The thirty-minute assessment—often carried out over several days—uses a variety of stimuli (bells, colors, shapes, rattles, lights) to test the way newborns respond to and cope with their environment. It looks at four types of behavior: interactive (how the baby relates to people, including alertness and cuddliness); motor (including reflexes, muscle tone, hand-mouth activity); control of physiological state (including how well the baby can self-console or be consoled after being upset); and reaction to stress (including the startle reflex). Rather than a baby's average performance during the test, the Brazelton uses the baby's best performance in scoring, and testers make every effort (often enlisting the mother's help) to bring out the best in the newborn subject. Most doctors reserve this test for occasions when they suspect a problem, such as with low birthweight babies or those who show signs of neurological problems.

the response may be affected by factors such as fatigue and hunger. If you fail to induce an appropriate response to one or more of these tests when done at home, chances are the fault lies more with your technique or timing than with your subject. Try again another day, and if you still can't elicit a response, mention the fact to baby's doctor, who probably has already tested your baby successfully and will be happy to repeat them for you at the next office visit. The verified absence of a reflex or its lingering beyond the usual age of disappearance requires further assessment.

FEEDING YOUR BABY: Getting Started

Whether you decide to nourish your infant at bottle or breast, you'll soon realize that feeding time isn't just a time for giving your baby sustenance. It is a time for getting to know and love each other.

GETTING STARTED BREASTFEEDING

They make it look so easy, those nursing mothers you've seen. Without skipping a beat of conversation or a mouthful of salad, they lift their shirts and put their babies to breast. Deftly, nonchalantly, as though it were the most natural process in the world.

Yet the first time you put your baby to your breast, nothing seems to come naturally. Even with all your concentration and most concerted efforts, you can't seem to get the baby to hold on to your nipple, never mind to suck on it. The baby's fussy; you're frustrated; soon you're both in tears. If you're failing at the most basic of mothering functions, you wonder, can failure at the rest of motherhood be far behind?

Don't throw in the nursing bra yet. You're not failing—you're just getting started. Nursing, like most other fundamentals of mothering, is learned, not instinctive. Give yourself and your baby a little time, and it won't be long before you're making it look easy, too. Keeping these pointers in mind will help.

Get an early start. If both you and baby are up to it, and baby isn't whisked off to the nursery, try to nurse in the birthing or delivery room. But don't fret if you and baby aren't successful right off. Trying to force the feeding to happen when you're both exhausted from a difficult delivery only sets the stage for a disappointing experience. Cuddling at the breast can be just as satisfying as nursing in the first few moments of your baby's life. If you don't get around to feeding on the delivery bed, ask to have the baby brought to your room for nursing as soon as possible after all necessary nursery procedures have been completed. Remember, however, that although an early start is ideal, it doesn't guarantee instant success. Plenty of practice will be needed before you and your baby make perfect.

Beat the system. Hospitals are usually run for the greater good—which doesn't always coincide with the needs of the breastfeeding mother and baby. To be sure you aren't thwarted in your efforts by insensitivity, ignorance, or arbitrary regulations, ask your doctor *in advance* to make your preferences (demand feeding, no bottles, no pacifiers) known to the staff or explain them to the nurses in a friendly way. Winning a nursery nurse to your side may be your best route to success. You will, however, need the doctor's support if you have a fever and still want to nurse.

Get together. Breastfeeding can't happen if you and your baby are apart. Thus sharing a room, or rooming-in, can be ideal for a nursing mother, since it doesn't leave her dependent on the nursery staff to bring her baby to her for nursing and ensures that no one will sneak a bottle of plain or glucose water into the infant instead. If you're tired out from a difficult

delivery, or don't feel confident enough yet to deal with the baby on a 24-hour basis, partial rooming-in (having baby with you during the day and in the nursery at night) may be preferable. With this system you can feed your baby on demand during the day, and on the nursery's schedule at night.

If rooming-in isn't available, isn't possible (some hospitals only allow rooming-in in private rooms or when both patients in a shared room want to keep their babies with them), or doesn't appeal to you, you can ask to have the baby brought to you when he or she is awake and hungry rather than at the nursery's convenience. Since this is considered a tall order in most hospitals, your doctor will have to make arrangements in advance. Even then, baby may be brought to you only sporadically, particularly if the nursery is crowded and, as is often the case, understaffed.

If all else fails, you can opt for early discharge so you and baby can room-in at home. If that's not possible, and requests for demand feeding are denied altogether, nurse on the hospital schedule until you do receive your walking papers. But don't let your baby sleep through visits with you. If you're handed a sleepyhead, awaken him or her and get in a few minutes of nursing.

Practice, practice, practice. Consider the feedings before your milk comes in as "dry runs," and don't be concerned that baby is getting very little in the way of nourishment. Your milk supply is tailored to your baby's needs. Right now those needs are minimal—in fact, the newborn stomach can't tolerate a lot of food—and the tiny quantity of colostrum you're producing is just right. Use those initial feeding sessions to work on your nursing technique rather than to fill baby's belly, and be assured that he or she isn't starving while you're both learning.

Take requests. Feeding on demand— when baby is hungry—is always best for a nursing infant. It may only be possible, however, if you're rooming-in, or if the baby nursery is well staffed enough to allow nurses to deliver babies whenever they are hungry. If neither is the case, you'll have to feed whenever you get the chance, which may mean not letting a sleeping babe lie.

Ban the bottle. Consider supplementary feedings of glucose water—routinely offered in some nurseries to breastfed newborns—as sabotage to your nursing efforts. Even a few sips of sugar water will satisfy tender appetites and early sucking needs, leaving baby more sleepy than hungry when brought to you later. You may also find your baby reluctant to struggle with the breast nipple after a few encounters with an artificial nipple, which yields results with a lot less effort. If your baby doesn't nurse, or nurses only briefly or halfheartedly, your breasts won't be stimulated to produce milk, and a cycle almost certainly destined to undermine breastfeeding will have begun.

Though you may be told that breastfeeding newborns need the extra fluids bottled water supplies (since all they're receiving from their mothers is a few teaspoons of colostrum), this is so only if dehydration or hypoglycemia—both very rare—are problems. The practice of giving water in the nursery is most likely to benefit the harried nursery staff; it's less time-consuming for a nurse to put a bottle in a crying baby's mouth than to cart the bassinet down the hall to mommy.

Give it time. No successful breastfeeding relationship was built in a day. Baby is certainly inexperienced, and you are, too, if this is your first time. You both have a lot to learn, and you'll both have to be patient while you learn it. There will be plenty of trial and even more error before supplier and demander are working in concert.

Keep in mind that things may go even more slowly if one or both of you had a difficult time during labor and delivery, or if you had anesthesia; drowsy mothers and sluggish infants may not be up to tackling the art of breastfeeding just yet. Sleep it off (and let baby do the same) before getting serious about the task ahead of you.

Don't go it alone. A hundred years ago, mothers and babies facing first attempts at breastfeeding had a lot of help. Mothers, aunts, and grandmas were usually on hand to pass on their experience; midwives were around to augment the family support. But just because your baby's been delivered in a hospital instead of in a four-poster and because it's likely your mother and aunts not only aren't living nearby but have no breastfeeding experience, you don't have to confront those first breastfeeding encounters alone and unaided. Some hospitals offer breastfeeding classes or individualized instruction, and/or provide written materials. If no one offers help postpartum, ask for it—from a nurse, from your doctor, or from a lactation consultant affiliated with the hospital. If you don't get any help, or you don't get enough, call your local La Leche League (listed in the phone book) for advice or referrals. An early visit (at one or two weeks postpartum) to the baby's doctor to go over your breastfeeding progress is often helpful and reassuring. Talking to mothers who are nursing successfully is too.

Keep your cool. This isn't easy to do when you're a brand-new mother, but it's vital if you want to succeed at breastfeeding. Tension can inhibit the let-down of milk, which means that even if you are producing milk, it may not be dispensed until you relax. If you're feeling edgy, banish visitors from the room fifteen minutes before you're scheduled to feed your baby, or if you're feeding on demand, ask guests to leave as soon as baby begins to appear hungry. Do relaxation exercises if you feel they might help, pick up a book or magazine, switch on the TV, or just close your eyes and listen to soft music for a few minutes. At the cocktail-hour feeding, you might try a glass of bubbly cider to help you unwind. Because a recent study suggests that as little as one glass of wine a day consumed by a nursing mother could slow motor development in their babies, daily alcohol isn't advisable.

BREASTFEEDING BASICS

■ Have a drink. A glass of milk, juice, or water just before or during each feeding will give you the extra fluids you need to produce breast milk. Something stronger (alcoholic, that is) is okay only rarely, and doesn't count toward your fluid intake.

■ Get comfortable. For the first few feedings, lying on your side may work best (see illustration). Later, sitting up in bed or in a chair may be better. But don't lean forward to get the nipple in baby's mouth; instead place

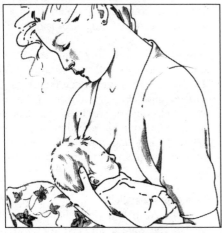

The football hold, good for small babies.

a pillow across your lap to support the arm cradling baby, and to bring him or her up to, and directly facing, your breast. Experiment to find the position most comfortable for you, one you can hold for a long period of time without feeling strained or stiff.

■ Take hold of your breast with your free thumb and forefinger (thumb on top) just above the areola. Holding it this way, bring the nipple toward your baby's lips and tickle them, going from top lip to bottom and back. This should tease the mouth open. But don't tickle or squeeze the cheeks to force the mouth open because baby won't know which way to turn. Once the mouth is open, gently place the nipple in its center so baby can latch on. If necessary, repeat the sequence until baby takes the nipple in his or her mouth. Don't force. Given the chance, your baby will eventually take the initiative.

■ Be sure your baby has a hold on the areola as well as the nipple. Sucking on just the nipple will not only leave your child hungry (because the milk glands that secrete the milk won't be compressed), but it will also make your nipples sore. Be sure, too, that your baby hasn't missed the mark and started sucking on another part of the breast entirely. Newborns are eager to suck even if no milk is forthcoming and can cause a painful bruise

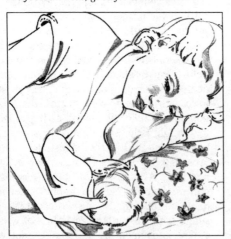

A position that lets you nurse and rest.

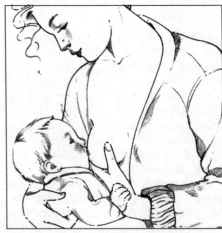

Use your free hand to guide your nipple.

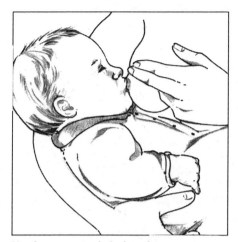

Use fingers to give baby breathing room.

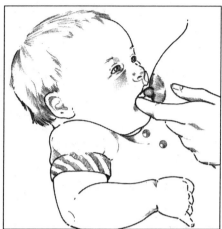

Break suction safely with your forefinger.

by gumming sensitive breast tissue.

■ Be sure your baby isn't sucking his or her own lower lip or tongue. You can check by pulling the lower lip down while nursing. If it does seem to be the tongue that's being suckled, break the suction with your finger, remove your nipple, and make certain the tongue is lowered before you start again. If it's the lip, gently ease it out while baby suckles.

■ Once your baby has a good grip, be sure that his or her nose isn't blocked by your breast. If it is, use your finger to press the breast out of the way and give baby plenty of space to breathe.

■ Watch for a strong, steady, rhythmic motion in baby's cheek, a sign that suckling is in progress. Later, when your milk comes in, you'll want to listen for the sound of swallowing (sometimes even gulping) that assures baby is not suckling in vain. If the milk seems to be coming out so quickly that it is flooding baby's mouth, causing gagging or choking, stop nursing and express a little milk by hand or with a pump to reduce the surplus. If either swollen (engorged) breasts or sore nipples are interfering with nursing, see pages 520 and 555.

■ Nurse for no more than 5 minutes per side at each feeding the first day, 10 the next day, and 15 or more the third. (Some experts okay nursing for as long as baby likes from start.)

Once the milk is in, nurse for 10 minutes on the first breast, and as long as baby wants to on the second, switching back to the first if baby still seems hungry after emptying the second. If baby falls asleep before you switch, a good burp may have him or her sniffing for more.

Start each feeding with alternate breasts. As a reminder, you can fasten a safety pin to your nursing bra on the side you started with at the previous feeding, or you can tuck a nursing pad or tissue in the bra cup on that side. The pad also will absorb any leakage from the breast you're not nursing on.

■ When baby is finished, pat your nipples dry; then, when possible, expose them to the air for ten or fifteen minutes. This will help toughen them, and won't be necessary once nursing is well established.

■ When your milk comes in, nurse often—at least eight or ten times in 24 hours, giving baby both breasts and emptying at least one at each feeding. If baby doesn't nurse vigorously or long enough at any one feeding, and a breast isn't emptied, it may be a good idea to express the remainder (see page 91), especially if your milk supply is scant. The expressed milk can be saved in the refrigerator or freezer for supplementary feedings.

GETTING STARTED BOTTLE FEEDING

Bottle feeding, oddly enough, comes more naturally—or at least more easily—than breastfeeding. Babies have little difficulty learning to suckle from an artificial nipple, and mothers (and fathers, too) have little difficulty at the delivery end. Preparing formula and sterilizing bottles are a little more complicated, but even these skills are mastered without much effort. (See page 39 for information on the types of bottles and nipples available, and for bottle-feeding supplies you will need.)

SELECTING A FORMULA

With the help of your baby's doctor, select a formula that is closest to human milk in composition—types and proportions of proteins, fats, sugars, sodium, and other nutrients should be as similar as possible to those in breast milk. Iron fortified formula (or a nutritional supplement containing iron) is not necessary until four months; fluoride fortification is not needed until six months, and then only if you live in an area without fluoridated water, will not be mixing the formula with fluoridated water, or will not be giving a fluoride supplement. Special formulas are available for babies with milk allergies (see page 114) or metabolic disorders, such as PKU. Commercial formulas come in the following forms:

Ready to use. This comes in 4- and 8-ounce, single-serving bottles and is ready for baby with the addition of a sterilized nipple.

Ready to pour. Available in cans of various sizes, this liquid formula need only be poured into sterilized bottles to be ready for use.

Ready to mix. Less expensive, but a little more time-consuming to prepare, this concentrated liquid or powder is diluted in

bottles of plain or sterilized water. It's available in cans or single-serving packets.

Do not use homemade formula. Formula made from evaporated or fresh milk plus sugar and water will not approximate either human milk or commercial formula, will not adequately nourish your baby, and may impose a severe strain on immature kidneys. *Do not* use any formula or formula-substitute without the approval of your baby's physicians. At least one company has put out a soy beverage that they claimed was a suitable replacement for mother's milk but was later found by the FDA to be nutritionally inadequate.

SAFE BOTTLE FEEDING

At one time, giving a baby a bottle was a risky proposition. Because of poor sanitation and inadequate formulas, bottle-fed babies often didn't thrive and frequently fell ill or even died from infection. Today's commercial baby formulas are designed to imitate mother's milk as much as is scientifically possible and are a safe and appropriate choice in baby feeding. But proper sanitation and correct mixing in the home must be followed in order to be sure the milk you feed your baby is safe.

■ Always check the expiration date on formula; do not buy or use any formula that has expired. Do not buy or use dented, leaky, or otherwise damaged cans or other containers.
■ Wash your hands thoroughly before preparing formula.
■ Before opening, wash the tops of formula cans with detergent and hot water; rinse well and dry. Shake, if required.
■ Use only a sharp, clean can opener, preferably reserved only for opening formula, to open cans of dry formula (a rotary blade is most efficient); wash the opener after each use and check for food or rust deposits before using again. Use a clean punch-type opener to open cans of liquid formula,

making two openings—one large, one small—on opposite sides of the can to make pouring easier. Wash after each use.

■ When preparing bottles of formula, also prepare a bottle or two of sterilized water for use as needed between feedings. When your baby is between one and two months old, your doctor may okay giving water that hasn't been boiled.[2]

■ Wash everything used for baby feeding in a clean dishpan reserved for this purpose, scrubbing with bottle brushes, detergent, and hot water. (New items should be boiled before first use.) Squeeze soapy water through nipple holes, then squeeze hot rinse water through several times. If the holes seem blocked, pierce with a diaper pin. (Clear silicone nipples are easiest to clean.) Rinse all utensils under hot running water.

■ Follow the manufacturer's directions precisely when mixing formula. If they differ from those given by the nursery or your doctor, be sure to ask why before preparing the formula; it may be that the instructions you were given were for a different formula. *Always check cans to see if formula needs to be diluted—diluting a formula that shouldn't be diluted, or not diluting one that should be, could be dangerous.* Continue sterilizing for as long as the doctor recommends—most suggest two or three months, though a few feel washing with hot soapy water is sufficient from the very first. See page 56 for the most common sterilizing techniques.

■ Heat a bottle of formula before using, if necessary, by running hot water over it. (Most babies, however, are just as happy with their formula unheated.) Check the temperature frequently by shaking a few drops on your inner wrist; it's ready for baby when it no longer feels cold—it needn't be warm, just body temperature.

Once warmed, you should use formula immediately, since bacteria multiply rapidly at lukewarm temperatures. Do not heat formula in a microwave oven—the liquid may warm unevenly or the container may remain cool when the formula has gotten hot enough to burn baby's mouth or throat.

■ Do not reuse leftover formula. Any formula remaining after a feeding should be discarded—it's a potential breeding ground for bacteria.

■ Rinse bottles and nipples right after use for easier cleaning.

■ Opened cans or bottles of liquid formula should always be covered tightly and stored in the refrigerator for *no longer* than the times specified on the labels. Cans of dry formula should be covered and stored in a cool, dry place for use within the month.

■ Don't store liquid formula, opened or unopened, at temperatures below 32° or above 95°F. Ideally store it between 45° and 90°F. Don't use formula that has been frozen (soy products freeze more quickly) or that shows white specks or streaks even after shaking.

■ Keep prepared bottles of formula refrigerated until ready to use. If you are traveling away from home, take along ready-to-use bottled formula or bottles of sterile water and single-serving formula packets to mix with them; or store previously prepared bottles in an insulated container or in a plastic bag with a small ice pack or a dozen ice cubes (the formula will stay fresh as long as most of the ice is frozen); or pack the bottles with a small box or can of juice that you've prefrozen (when you or an older child is ready for a snack, the juice will have defrosted and the formula will still be fresh). Do not use formula that is no longer cold to the touch.

BOTTLE FEEDING WITH LOVE

No matter how inept a first-time breastfeeder may be in her attempts to hook her baby up to her nipples, she's not likely to

---

2. If the safety of the tap water in your home is questionable (see page 237), use bottled water that's not distilled (valuable minerals are removed in the distillation process) for preparing formula and for drinking.

have trouble giving her newborn enough skin-to-skin contact—a built-in feature of the breastfeeding system. Unfortunately, it is possible to bottle feed a tiny infant with a minimum of such contact, and many well-meaning but harried bottle-feeding mothers have given in to feeding shortcuts that compromise closeness for convenience. So if there's one area in which beginning bottle feeders have to try harder than novice nursers, it's in making sure they don't lose touch with their babies at feeding time. The

STERILIZING TECHNIQUES

The terminal-heating method for use with concentrated liquid or powder formula. Prepare the formula according to directions in a clean measuring cup or mixing bowl, then pour it into clean bottles. Loosely top bottles with nipples, caps, and collars. Place them on a rack or folded towel in a sterilizer or large pot, and add 3 inches of water. Heat to boiling, then cover and boil for 25 minutes. Remove from the heat. Tighten caps when they are cool enough to handle, and refrigerate until needed. (Refrigerating before cooling may cause film to form on the formula, clogging the nipples at feeding time.) Use within 48 hours.

The aseptic method for use with concentrated liquid or powder formula. Place clean bottles, nipples, collars, caps, mixing spoon, can opener, measuring pitcher, measuring cup and tongs (be sure all these items are boilable) in a rack or on a folded towel in a sterilizer or large pot. Add water to cover and put the lid on the sterilizer or pot. Heat to boiling and boil for five minutes. In another saucepan, measure the amount of water needed for formula. Cover, bring to a boil, and boil for five minutes. Remove from the heat and allow both to cool to room temperature while still covered. Measure formula in a sterilized measuring pitcher and add it to the sterilized water in the saucepan. Pour the blended formula into sterilized bottles; add nipples, collars, and caps using sterilized tongs to avoid contaminating with your hands. Store in a refrigerator for up to 48 hours. Shake before using.

The single-bottle method for use with concentrated liquid or powder formula.

Add specified amounts of water to each clean nursing bottle, then loosely top with nipples and caps. Place on a wire rack or folded towel in a sterilizer or large pot. Add water to level of the water in the bottles. Bring to a boil, cover, and boil for 25 minutes. Remove from the heat. When cool to the touch, remove bottles, tighten caps, and store at room temperature. Use within 48 hours. At feeding time, remove the cap and nipple from one bottle, add the specified quantity of concentrated liquid or powder, replace the cap, and shake well to mix. (Powdered formula will dissolve better in warm water, so you might want to reheat slightly before mixing.)

Ready-to-use-formula methods. Ready-to-use formula requires no mixing. When it comes in ready-to-use bottles, all you need to do is boil the nipples, caps, and collars, tongs, and nipple jar and lid on a wire rack or folded towel in a sterilizer or large covered pot for five minutes. Remove from the heat. When cool, use the tongs to place the nipple units in the sterilized jar or in clean plastic bags. Keep them covered until ready to place on bottles of formula. If formula is stored at room temperature, warming is unnecessary. Shake well and use immediately after opening.

Ready-to-use formula that comes in 8-ounce or quart cans requires sterilization of bottles with nipple units lightly attached. Follow the aseptic method above. When bottles are cooled, tighten collars, and store in a clean place. Add formula when ready to feed, or prepare a full day's supply of bottles, filling them all, and refrigerate. Shake well before using.

following tips will help you to make bottle-feeding sessions as rewarding to both participants as breastfeeding ones:

Don't prop the bottle. For a young baby, who is as hungry for emotional gratification in the form of cuddling as for oral gratification in the form of food, propping is very unsatisfying. And propping has physical as well as emotional drawbacks. Babies are more susceptible to choking when feeding on their backs—a very serious problem when mom isn't around to help. They may also be more susceptible to ear infections in this feeding position, and because they may fall asleep with bottle in mouth, to tooth decay once the first teeth come in.

Limit baby feeders at first. Your baby is just getting used to the idea of sucking on a rubber nipple for nourishment. Because every adult has a different way of holding, handling, and talking to a baby, having many different people (mother, father, grandparents, nurses, other children) give bottles can hamper good feeding adjustment and mother-baby bonding. Initially, try to do most of the feeding yourself with, if necessary, assistance from one other person. Later, when baby becomes proficient, you can let others share in the fun of feeding baby.

Go skin to skin, when possible. There's something special about a baby's cheek touching his mother's breast—for both participants. Even as a bottle feeder you can achieve this by opening your shirt and placing baby next to your chest as you give the bottle. Of course this isn't practical in public, but it works well in private. Or you might want to try a supplemental nutrition system, which allows women who can't nurse but crave the breastfeeding experience to put their infants to the breast (see page 101).

Switch arms. Give your baby a chance to see the world from different perspectives by switching arms at midfeeding. This gives you a chance to relieve the ache that can develop from staying in one position for so long.

Let baby call it quits. If you see only 3 ounces have been emptied when the usual meal is 6 ounces, you may be tempted to push more. Don't. A healthy baby knows when to stop. And it's this kind of pushing that leads to bottle-fed babies being much more likely than breastfeds to become too plump.

Take your time. A nursing baby can keep suckling on a breast long after it's been emptied, just for comfort and sucking satisfaction. Your bottle-fed baby can't do the same with an empty bottle, but there are ways you can supply some of the same satisfactions. Extend the pleasure of the feeding session by socializing once the bottle is drained—assuming the little tyke hasn't dropped off into a milk-induced sleep. If your baby seems to want to continue sucking after each feeding, try using nipples with smaller holes, which will make it necessary to work harder and longer for the same meal, or offer a bottle of water or a pacifier for brief periods. If your baby seems to be fussing for more at meal's end, consider whether you're offering enough formula. Increase it an ounce or two, with the doctor's permission, to see if it's really hunger that's making your baby fretful.

Feel good about bottle feeding. If you were eager to breastfeed and couldn't for some reason, don't feel guilty or frustrated. You can give your baby good nutrition and just as much loving and cuddling with bottle feeding. And your guilt and frustration are feelings you don't want to pass on to your baby.

BOTTLE FEEDING WITH EASE

If you've had some experience bottle feeding a young infant—either a sibling, a baby-sitting charge, or friend's baby—the correct technique will come back to you virtually the moment you hold your baby in your arms. If not, you need to know a few bottle-feeding basics:

■ Let baby know that "formula's on" by stroking his or her cheek with your finger or the tip of the nipple. That will encourage your baby to turn in the direction of the stroke. Then place the nipple gently between baby's lips and, hopefully, sucking will begin.

■ Tilt the bottle up so that formula always fills the nipple completely. If you don't, and air fills part of it, baby will swallow the air and may become gassy—which may make both of you miserable. This precaution isn't, however, necessary if you are using disposable bottle liners, which automatically deflate, eliminating air pockets.

■ Don't be concerned if your baby doesn't seem to take much formula the first few days. The newborn's need for nutrition is minimal at first—a breastfed baby, on orders from Mother Nature, is now getting only a few teaspoonsful of colostrum at each feeding. The nursery will probably give you full 4-ounce bottles, but don't expect them to be drained. A baby who falls asleep after taking just half an ounce or so is probably saying, "I've had enough." But

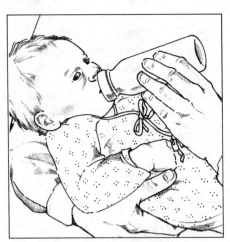

Bottle feeding gives dad and other family members the chance to get close to baby, to use the time for cuddling and interaction; nourishment needn't come from the breast to come with love.

a baby who fusses after taking only a small amount, turns his or her head away, or lets go of the nipple and refuses to take it back again may be in need of a burping. If after a good bubble the nipple is still rejected, the meal is probably over.

How much your baby takes at a feeding will increase as his or her weight does, from just a few ounces up to as many as 8 full ounces, or a total of approximately 32 ounces a day by the time the twelfth week is reached. Don't be concerned if your baby takes a little more or less at each feeding, or each day, as long as weight gain is good.

■ Be certain that formula is coming through the nipple at the right speed. You can check by giving the bottle, turned upside down, a few quick shakes. If milk pours or spurts out, it's flowing too quickly; if just a drop or two escapes, too slowly. If you get a little spray, and then some drops, the flow is just about right. You can also get a clue from observing your baby suck. If your baby seems to work very hard at suckling for a few moments, then seems very frustrated, possibly letting go of the nipple to complain, the flow's too slow. If, on the other hand, there's a lot of gulping and sputtering and milk is always leaking out of the corners of the mouth, it's too fast.

The problem could simply be in the way the cap is fastened. A very tight cap inhibits flow by creating a partial vacuum, and loosening it makes milk flow more easily. If adjusting the cap doesn't seem to correct the flow, the problem is probably in the size of the nipple opening. If the milk is flowing too quickly, the opening is too big. Boiling the nipple for a few minutes may reduce the size of the opening, but if it doesn't, you will have to discard the nipple or put it aside until your baby is much older, and substitute a nipple with a smaller hole. If the flow is too slow, the opening is too small. You can enlarge it by poking the tip with a diaper pin or wide-diameter needle heated to red hot, or by forcing a round wooden toothpick into the opening and boiling the nipple for five minutes. Or make a new hole.

■ Make night feedings less of an ordeal by investing in a bedside bottle holder, which keeps baby's bottle chilled until ready to use and then warms it to room temperature in minutes. Or keep a bottle on ice in baby's room, ready to serve cold or to warm under the bathroom tap when baby starts fussing for a feeding.

TIPS FOR
SUCCESSFUL FEEDING SESSIONS

Feeding a baby in the early weeks isn't an effortless process, no matter what the source of milk. But whether it's a breast or a bottle that will be your newborn's ticket to a full tummy, the guidelines that follow should help make the trip a smoother one:

Minimize the mayhem. You and your baby will both have to concentrate in these early feeding sessions and will fare better with as few distractions as possible. If visitors are banished at feeding times in the hospital, regard the rule a blessing since it will give you the quiet time you need with your baby. If they aren't, consider banishing them yourself. When you get home, try to continue minimizing distractions at baby's mealtimes, at least until you feel comfortable and competent nursing or giving a bottle. Retire to the bedroom to feed baby when you have guests or when the general atmosphere in the living room rivals that of a three-ring circus. Turn off the phone or put on the answering machine at baby's mealtimes; if you have other children, divert their attentions to some quiet activity, or take this opportunity to read them a story.

Make a change. If your baby is relatively calm, you've time for a change. A clean diaper will make for a more comfortable meal and reduce the need for a change right after—a definite plus if your charge has nodded off to dreamland and you'd rather he or she stay there for a while. But don't change during the night if it's not necessary; such a disruption makes falling back to sleep more difficult.

Wash up. Even though you won't be doing the eating, it's your hands that should be washed with soap and water before your baby's meals. If you're breastfeeding, your nipples needn't be washed before each feeding; a once-a-day soapless wash in the shower or tub is sufficient.

Get comfy. Muscular aches and pains are an occupational hazard for new parents who use unaccustomed muscles to carry growing babies around. Feeding baby in an awkward position will only compound the problem. So before putting baby to breast or bottle, be sure you're comfortable, with adequate support for your back and for the arm under baby.

Loosen up. If your baby is tightly swaddled, unwrap him or her so you can cuddle while you feed.

Cool down a screaming baby. A baby who's upset will have trouble getting down to the business of feeding, and even more trouble with the business of digesting. Try a soothing song or a little rocking.

Sound reveille. Some babies are sleepy at mealtimes, and a concerted effort is required to rouse them to the task of nursing at breast or bottle. If your little one is a dinner dozer, try the wake-up techniques on page 60.

Make contact. Cuddle and caress your baby with your hands, your eyes, and your voice. Remember, meals shouldn't fill your baby's daily requirements just for nutrients, but for mother love as well.

Break for a burp. Between breasts or halfway through the bottle, routinely burp your baby. Also try burping if baby seems to want to stop eating prematurely—it may be gas, not food, that's filling the little tummy.

WHAT YOU MAY BE CONCERNED ABOUT

SLEEPING THROUGH MEALS

"The doctor says I should feed my baby every three or four hours, but sometimes I don't hear from him for five or six. Should I wake him up to eat?"

Some babies are perfectly happy to sleep through meals, particularly during the first few days of life. If yours is one of these, try this arousal technique at mealtime: set him in a sitting position on your lap, one hand holding up his chin, the other supporting his back. Now, bend baby forward at the waist. The moment he stirs, assume a nursing position. If he drifts back to sleep before you have the chance to get things started, repeat the sequence. Also try removing swaddling, or even all clothing except for the diaper (very young babies usually don't like being naked); a diaper change; rubbing the area under baby's chin with your finger; tickling his feet; a burp.

If your baby wakens, takes the nipple, then promptly falls asleep, try jiggling the breast or bottle, stroking his cheek, jostling him, or adjusting his position or yours to get the sucking action going again. You may find that in the course of a feeding period you have to jiggle several times to get a full feeding in—some young babies suckle and doze alternately from the start of the meal to the finish. If you're unsuccessful at restarting sucking, try some of the wake-up techniques above. If nothing works, give up and let sleepyhead dream a bit longer. But don't let him go more than five hours between meals right now.

It's okay to let your baby sleep if he drops off to dreamland after only a brief appetizer and attempts at encouraging him to resume sucking fail; a five-minute meal may be all he wanted this time around. It's not, however, a good idea to let your baby nip and nap at fifteen- to thirty-minute intervals all day long. If that seems to be the trend, go all out in your attempts to waken him as soon as he dozes off mid-meal, and try to get in a full-course meal before you let him succumb to sleep once again.

If chronic sleepiness interferes with eating and threatens your baby's well-being (see page 99 for signs of failure to thrive), consult his doctor immediately.

NOT SLEEPING AFTER MEALS

"I'm afraid my baby is going to turn into a little blimp. Almost immediately after I put her down, she's up again crying for food."

Your baby may indeed be destined for the Goodyear fleet if you feed her again immediately after she's had an adequate meal. Babies cry for reasons other than hunger, and it may be that your are misreading her. Consider that she may just be having a little difficulty getting into a deep sleep. Allowed to fend for herself for a couple of minutes, she may accomplish this all by herself. Or maybe your baby isn't ready for sleep after all, is crying out for companionship, and would like to be frolicked with, not fed. Try a little socializing. Or maybe she's just having trouble calming down. Help her by rocking her or try some other soothing technique. Consider, also, that your baby's problem may be gas. In that case, more feeding would only compound it. Try eliciting a burp by putting her over your lap or shoulder and gently rubbing her back. (Be sure to burp her at frequent intervals during feedings.) The problem could also be the way you put her into her crib (see page 120 for tips on how to put a sleeping baby down so she'll stay asleep). Or the problem may just be temporary; she may be going through a growth spurt and need more food.

If you offer your daughter food every

time she cries right after eating, even when not particularly hungry, not only will she be likely to blimp out, but she may develop a snack and snooze habit that will be difficult to break later.

Do be sure, however, that your baby is gaining weight at an adequate rate. If she isn't, she may indeed be crying out of hunger—a sign that you may not be producing enough milk. See page 99 to find out what to do if baby doesn't seem to be thriving.

BIRTHWEIGHT

"My friends all seem to be having babies that weigh 8 and 9 pounds at birth. Mine weighed in at a little over 6½ pounds at full term. She seems so small."

Healthy babies come in all kinds of packages—long and lanky, big and bulky, slight and slender. Though a birthweight of under 5½ pounds full term can mean that baby was not well nourished during gestation, or that growth was otherwise interfered with (for unknown and uncontrollable reasons or because the mother drank, smoked, or took drugs), a petite 6½-pounder can be as vigorous and sound as a chubby 9-pounder.

Many factors affect a baby's size, among them:

The mother's diet during pregnancy. Too little food or too little of the right kinds of food can produce a small baby; too much food, an overly large one.

The mother's pregnancy weight gain. A bigger weight gain may yield a bigger baby, but if the weight was gained on junk food, the baby may be tiny and the mother fat.

The mother's prenatal lifestyle. Smoking, drinking, and drug abuse can all stunt fetal growth.

The mother's health. Poorly controlled diabetes (even the gestational type) can be responsible for an extra-large baby. Toxemia (preeclampsia or eclampsia) or a placenta that is inadequate can interfere with fetal growth, with a tiny newborn the result.

The mother's weight before pregnancy. Heavier women tend to have heavier babies; slight women, lighter ones.

The mother's own birthweight. If the mother weighed in at around 7 pounds, her first baby is likely to, also. If she was very small or very large, her baby will often follow the same pattern.

Genetics. Large parents usually have large babies. If the mother is small and the father is large, the baby is more likely to be on the small side—nature's way of trying to decrease the odds of a difficult delivery. If baby is genetically destined to take after the father, rapid growth spurts during the first year and later on will make up for small birth size.

Baby's sex. Boys, on the average, tend to be a little heavier and longer than girls.

Birth order. First babies are often smaller than subsequent ones.

The number of fetuses. Babies of a multiple pregnancy generally weigh less than singletons.

Race. Oriental, black, and Indian babies are generally smaller than Caucasian babies (although the size differences between black and white babies may be due more to socioeconomic factors than race; middle-class black babies and middle-class white babies are more evenly matched in weight).

BONDING

"I had an emergency cesarean and they whisked my baby away to the ICU before I had a chance to bond with her. I worry that this will affect our relationship."

Bonding at birth is an idea whose time has come—and, by now, should be gone. The theory that a mother-baby relationship will be better when the two spend 16 hours of the first 24 in close loving contact was first suggested in the 1970s. Though recent research has not substantiated it, and even the original propounders of the theory have expressed concern that the concept has been misused, it continues to be popular.

The consequences have been mixed. On the one hand, many hospitals now permit new mothers (and often fathers) to hold their babies moments after birth, to cuddle and nurse them for anywhere from ten minutes to an hour or more, instead of dispatching the newborn off to the nursery the instant the cord is cut. This encounter gives mother and baby a chance to make early contact, skin to skin, eye to eye—certainly a positive change. On the other hand, many moms who've had surgical deliveries or traumatic vaginal births or whose babies arrived in need of special care, and who consequently didn't get to hold their babies immediately after birth, are led to believe that they've missed the chance of a lifetime to foster a close relationship with their offspring. Some become so frantic about the necessity for instant bonding that they demand it even at risk to the health of their infants.

Many experts dispute the idea that parent-child bonding can take place at birth. They believe that the newborn infant is too primitive a creature to bond instantly with anyone; a week or more usually passes before the baby is able to recognize its mother, never mind form a lifelong bond with her. And though the mother isn't too primitive to be capable of initiating an attachment with her baby, there are many reasons why she may not be ready for bonding: exhaustion from a long labor and delivery, grogginess from medication, pain from cramping or an incision, or simply lack of preparation for the experience of holding and caring for a newborn. In addition, there's no solid evidence that a mother-infant attachment has to be firmly established (or even begun) on the first day of life. And there are some who suggest

that it doesn't actually take place until somewhere in the second half of the baby's first year.

Bonding at birth may indeed be part of a long process of mother-baby attachment, but it is only the beginning. And this beginning can just as well take place hours after birth in a hospital bed, or through the portholes of an incubator, or even weeks later at home. When your parents were born, they probably saw little of their mothers and even less of their fathers until they went home (usually ten days after birth), and the vast majority of that "deprived" generation grew up with strong, loving family ties. Mothers who have the chance to bond at birth with one child and not with another usually report no difference in their feelings toward the children. And adoptive parents, who often don't meet their babies until hospital discharge (or even much later), manage to foster strong bonds.

The kind of love that lasts a lifetime can't magically evolve in a few hours, or even a few days. The first moments after birth may become a cherished memory for some, but for others they may turn out to be a disappointment they'd rather forget. Either way, these moments don't indelibly color the character and quality of your future relationship.

The complicated process of parent-child bonding actually begins for parents during pregnancy, when attitudes and feelings toward the baby start developing. The relationship continues to evolve and change all through infancy, childhood, and adolescence, and even into adulthood. So relax. There's lots of time to tie those bonds that bind.

"I've been told that bonding at birth brings mother and baby closer together. I held my new daughter for nearly an hour right after delivery, but she seemed like a stranger to me then, and still does now three days later."

Love at first sight is a concept that flourishes in romantic novels and movies, but rarely materializes in real life. The kind of love that lasts a lifetime usually requires time, nurturing, and plenty of patience to develop and deepen. And that's as true for love between a newborn and parents as it is between a man and woman.

Physical closeness between mother and child immediately after birth does not (in spite of what supporters of "bonding at birth" may tell you) guarantee instant emotional closeness. Those much-touted first postpartum moments aren't automatically bathed in a glow of maternal love. In fact, the first sensation a woman experiences after birth is far more likely to be relief than love—relief that the baby is normal and, especially if her labor was difficult, that the ordeal is over. It's not at all unusual to see that squalling and unsociable infant as a stranger with very little connection to the cozy, idealized Gerber baby you carried for nine months—and to feel little more than neutral toward her. One study found that it took an average of over two weeks (and often as long as nine weeks) for mothers to begin having positive feelings toward their newborns.

Just how a woman reacts to her newborn at their first meeting may depend on a variety of factors: the length and intensity of her labor; whether she received medication during labor; her previous experience (or lack of it) with infants; her feelings about having a child; her relationship with her husband; extraneous worries that may preoccupy her; her general health; and probably most important of all, her personality. *Your* reaction is normal for *you*. And as long as you feel an increasing sense of comfort and attachment as the days go by, you can relax. Some of the best relationships get off to the slowest starts. Give yourself and your baby a chance to get to know and appreciate each other, and let the love grow unhurriedly.

If you don't feel a growing closeness after a few weeks, however, or if you feel anger or antipathy toward your baby, discuss these feelings with your pediatrician.

It's important to work them out early on, to prevent lasting damage to your relationship.

ROOMING-IN

"Having the baby room-in with me sounded like heaven before I gave birth. Now it seems more like hell. I can't get the baby to stop crying—yet what kind of mother would I be if I asked the nurse to take her back to the nursery?"

You would be a very human mother. You've just completed the Herculean task of giving birth, and are about to undertake an even greater challenge: child rearing. Needing a few days of rest in between is nothing to feel guilty about.

Of course, some women handle rooming-in with ease. They may have had deliveries that left them feeling exhilarated instead of exhausted. Or they may have had prior experience caring for newborns, their own or other people's. For these women, an inconsolable infant at 3 A.M. may not be a joy, but it's not a nightmare, either. For a woman who's been without sleep for 48 hours, however, whose body has been left limp from an enervating labor, and who's never been closer to a baby than a diaper ad, such predawn bouts can leave her wondering tearfully: Why did I ever decide to become a mother?

Playing the martyr can raise motherly resentments against the baby, feelings the baby will be likely to sense. If, instead, the baby is sent back to the nursery between feedings at night, mother and child, both well rested, may find getting acquainted easier when morning comes. And morning is a good time to take advantage of one of the major advantages of daytime rooming-in: the chance to learn how to take care of your new baby in a safe environment with experienced help there to advise and assist you if necessary. Even though you've opted to have the baby with you all day, you shouldn't feel you can't call upon the nursery staff for help. That's what they're there for.

When night falls again, try keeping the baby and see how things go; she may surprise you. Or if you're ready for a baby-break, use the good offices of the nursery again. Full-time rooming-in is a wonderful new option in family-centered maternity care—but it's not for everyone. You are *not* a failure or a bad mother if you don't enjoy, or if you feel too tired for, rooming-in. Don't be pushed into it if you don't think you want it; and once you've committed yourself, don't feel you can't change your mind and go part-time.

Be flexible. Focus on the quality of the time you spend with your baby in the hospital rather than the quantity. Round-the-clock rooming-in will begin soon enough at home—with hospitals discharging postpartum patients earlier and earlier, nowadays it could be within 24 to 48 hours. By then, if you don't overdo now, you should be emotionally and physically ready to deal with it.

BABY'S NOT GETTING ENOUGH TO EAT

"It's been two days since I gave birth to my little girl, and nothing comes out of my breasts when I squeeze them, not even colostrum. I'm worried that she's starving."

Not only is your baby not starving, she isn't even hungry yet. Babies aren't born with an appetite, or even with immediate nutritional needs. And by the time your baby begins to get hungry for a breast full of milk, usually around the third or fourth postpartum day, you will very likely be able to oblige. (Occasionally, especially in second-time mothers, breast milk comes in earlier. Rarely, it comes in as late as the seventh day. In such a case, the pediatrician may recommend giving the baby formula after each nursing as a precaution.)

Which isn't to say that your breasts are empty now. Colostrum (which provides your baby with nourishment and with important antibodies her own body can't yet produce, while helping to empty her digestive system of meconium and excess mucus) is almost certainly present, though in very tiny amounts (first feedings average less than a half-teaspoon; by the third day, less than three tablespoons per feeding over ten feedings). But until your breasts begin to swell and feel full, indicating your milk has come in, it's not that easy to express manually—and for some mothers, it isn't easy even then. Even a day-old baby, with no previous experience, is better equipped to extract this premilk than you are.

BABY'S SLEEPINESS

"My new son seemed very alert right after he was born, but ever since he's been sleeping so soundly I can hardly wake him to eat, much less to socialize."

You've waited nine long months to meet your baby; and now that he's here, all he does is sleep. But he's just doing what comes naturally. Wakefulness for the first hour or so after birth followed by a long stretch, often 24 hours, of very sound sleep is the normal newborn pattern (which probably gives him a chance to recover from the fatiguing work of being born).

Don't expect your newborn to become much more stimulating company immediately upon awakening from this beneficial sleep. In the first weeks, his two- to four-hour-long sleeping periods will end abruptly with crying. He will rouse to a semi-awake state to eat, drifting back to sleep when satiated. He will probably even doze while feeding, and it will take a shake of the nipple in his mouth to get him sucking again. He will finally fall more soundly asleep, managing a few last-ditch nibbles at the nipple as you remove it.

He will be truly alert for only about three minutes of every hour during the day, and less (you hope) at night. That allows a total of about an hour a day for active socializing. He's not mature enough to benefit from longer periods of alertness, and his periods of sleep, particularly of REM (or dream state) sleep, apparently help him to mature. Gradually, his periods of wakefulness will grow longer. By the end of the first month, most babies are alert for about two to three hours every day, most of it in one relatively long stretch, usually in the late afternoon. And some of their naps, instead of being two or three hours long, may last as long as six or six and a half hours.

In the meantime, you may continue to be thwarted in your attempts to get to know your baby. But instead of standing over his crib waiting for him to wake up so you can play with him, use his sleeping time to store up some sleep of your own. You'll need it for the days (and nights) ahead, when he'll probably be awake more than you'd like.

PAIN MEDICATION

"I've been having some pretty bad pain from my cesarean incision. My obstetrician has prescribed some pain medication, but I'm afraid to take it because I don't want to drug my little girl with my breast milk."

You're doing your baby more harm if you don't take needed medication than if you do. The tension and exhaustion that can result from unrelieved post-cesarean pain will only hamper your ability to establish a good nursing relationship with your baby (you need to be relaxed) and a good milk supply (you need to be rested). Besides which, the medication will appear only in very minuscule amounts in your colostrum; by the time your milk supply comes in, you probably won't need narcotic pain relief. And if your baby does receive a small dose of medication, she'll sleep it off easily, with no ill effects.

BABY'S LOOKS

"People ask me whether the baby looks like me or my husband. Neither one of us has a pointy head, puffy eyes, an ear that bends forward, and a pushed-in nose. When will he start looking better?"

There's a good reason why two- and three-month-old babies are used to portray newborns in movies and television commercials: most newborns are not exactly photogenic. And though parental love is blinder than most, even parents who are head over heels can't help but notice the many imperfections of their newborn's appearance. Fortunately, most of the newborn characteristics that will keep your baby from co-starring in films and selling diapers on TV are temporary.

The features you're describing weren't inherited from some distant pointy-headed, puffy-eyed, flap-eared relative. They were acquired during your baby's stay in the cramped quarters of your uterus, during the stormy passage through your bony pelvis in preparation for birth, and during his final traumatic trip through the narrow confines of your birth canal during delivery.

If it weren't for the miraculous design of a fetus's head—with the skull bones not fully fused, allowing them to be pushed and molded as the baby makes its descent—there would be many more surgical deliveries. So be thankful for the pointy little head that came with your vaginal delivery, and rest assured that the skull will just as miraculously return to cherubic roundness within a few days or so.

The swelling around your baby's eyes is also due, at least in part, to the beating he took on his fantastic voyage into the world. (Another contributing factor, in babies who have had silver nitrate drops instilled into their eyes, is the irritating effect of this infection-preventing drug.) Some have postulated that this swelling serves as natural protection for newborns, whose eyes are being exposed to light for the first time. The worry that puffy eyes may interfere with a baby's ability to see mommy and daddy, making bonding impossible, is unfounded. Though he can't distinguish one from another, a newborn can make out blurry faces at birth—even through swollen lids.

The bent ear is probably another outcome of the crowding your baby experienced in the uterus. As a fetus grows and becomes more snugly lodged in his mother's cozy amniotic sac, an ear that happens to get pushed forward may stay that way even after birth. But this is only temporary. Taping it back won't help, say the experts, and the tape might cause irritation, but you can speed the return to normal ear positioning by being sure the ear is back against the head when putting baby to sleep on his side. Some ears, of course, are genetically destined to stand out somewhat. Hair will eventually help camouflage this cosmetic problem, and plastic surgery is available for those who wish to eliminate it. (Though it certainly needn't be considered a handicap—remember Clark Gable?)

The pushed-in nose is very likely a result of a tight squeeze during labor and delivery, and should return to normal naturally. But because baby noses are so different from the adult variety (the bridge is broad, almost nonexistent, the shape often nondescript), it may still be a while before you can tell whose nose your baby has.

EYE COLOR

"I was hoping my baby would have green eyes like my husband, but her eyes seem to be a dark grayish color. Is there any chance that they'll turn?"

The favorite guessing game of pregnancy —will it be a boy or a girl?—is replaced by another in the first few months of a baby's life—what color will her eyes turn out to be?

It's definitely too early to call now. Most Caucasian babies are born with dark blue or slate-colored eyes; most black and Oriental infants with dark, usually brown, eyes. While the dark eyes of the darker-skinned babies will stay dark, the eye color of white babies may go through a number of changes (making the betting more lively) before becoming set somewhere between three and six months, or even later.

And since pigmentation of the iris may continue increasing during the entire first year, the depth of color may not be clear until around baby's first birthday.

GAGGING AND CHOKING

"When they brought my baby to me this morning, he seemed to gag and choke and then spit up some liquidy stuff. I hadn't nursed him yet, so it couldn't have been spitup. What's wrong?"

Your baby spent the last nine months, more or less, living in a liquid environment. He didn't breathe air, but he sucked in a lot of fluid. Though a nurse or doctor probably suctioned his airways clear at birth, there may have been additional mucus and fluid in his lungs, and this gagging and choking is your baby's way of clearing out what remains. This is a perfectly normal occurrence.

STARTLING

"I'm worried that there's something wrong with my baby's nervous system. Even when she's sleeping, she'll suddenly seem to jump out of her skin."

Assuming your baby hasn't been overdoing the black coffee, the jumpiness you notice is due to the very normal startle reflex. Also known as the Moro reflex, it may occur for no obvious reason, more frequently in some babies than in others, but most often in response to a loud noise, jolting, or a feeling of falling—as when a young infant is picked up without adequate support. Typically, the baby stiffens her body, flings her arms up and out symmetrically, spreads her usually tightly clenched fists wide open, draws her knees up, then finally brings her arms, fists clenched once again, back to her body in an embracing gesture—all in a matter of seconds. She also may cry out. The Moro is just another of the many protective reflexes with which babies are born, likely a primitive attempt to regain perceived loss of equilibrium.

While the sight of a startled baby often worries parents, a doctor is more likely to be concerned if a baby doesn't startle. Newborns are routinely tested for this reflex, the presence of which is one reassuring sign that the neurological system is functioning well. You'll find that your baby will gradually startle less frequently, and that the reflex will disappear fully somewhere between four and six months. (Your baby may occasionally startle, of course, at any age, but not with the same pattern of reactions.)

QUIVERING CHIN

"Sometimes, especially when he's been crying, my baby's chin quivers."

Though your baby's quivering chin may look like another one of his ingenious inborn ploys for playing at your heartstrings, it's actually a sign that his nervous system, like those of his peers, is not fully mature. Give him the sympathy he's craving, and enjoy the quivering chin while it lasts—which won't be for long.

BIRTHMARKS

"The first thing I noticed about my baby after I saw that she was a girl was the raised bright red blotch on her thigh. Will it ever go away?"

Long before your daughter starts petitioning parental powers for her first bikini, that strawberry birthmark—like most birthmarks—will be a part of her childish past, leaving her thigh ready (even if her father isn't) for beach baring. Of course, looking at a newborn's birthmark, this often seems hard to believe. Sometimes the mark grows a bit before fading, or sometimes it doesn't even appear until some time after birth. And when it does begin to shrink or fade,

the changes from day to day are often difficult to see. For that reason, many doctors document birthmark changes by photographing and measuring the lesion periodically. If your baby's doctor doesn't, you can do so just for your own reassurance.

Birthmarks come in a variety of shapes, colors, and textures and are usually categorized in the following ways:

Strawberry hemangioma. This soft, raised, strawberry red birthmark, as small as a freckle or as large as a coaster, is composed of immature vascular materials that broke away from the circulatory system during fetal development. It may be visible at birth or may seem to appear suddenly during the first few weeks of life, and is so common that 1 out of 10 babies will probably have one. Strawberry birthmarks may grow for a while, but eventually will start to fade to a pearly gray and almost always finally disappear completely, sometime between ages five and ten. Although parents may be tempted to demand treatment for a very obvious strawberry mark, particularly on the face, such birthmarks are best left untreated unless they continue to grow or interfere with a function, such as vision. Treatment apparently can lead to more complications than a more conservative let-it-disappear-on-its-own approach.

If your child's doctor determines treatment is advisable, there are several options. The simplest are compression and massage, both of which seem to hasten involution. More aggressive forms of therapy for strawberry hemangiomas include the administration of steroids, surgery, X-ray or laser therapy, cryotherapy (freezing with dry ice), and injection of hardening agents (such as those used in treating varicose veins). Many experts believe no more than 0.1% of these birthmarks require such radical therapies. When a strawberry, reduced by either treatment or time, leaves a scar or some residual tissue, plastic surgery can usually eliminate it.

Occasionally a strawberry mark may bleed, either spontaneously or because it was scratched or bumped. Applying pressure will stem the flow of blood.

Cavernous hemangioma. This birthmark is less common than the strawberry hemangioma—only 1 or 2 out of every 100 babies has one. Often combined with the strawberry type, it is composed of larger, more mature vascular elements and involves deeper layers of skin. The usually bluish or bluish red lumpy mass, with less distinct borders than strawberry marks, may appear almost flat initially. It grows rapidly in the first six months, then more slowly in the next six. By twelve to eighteen months, it begins to shrink. Fully 50% are gone by age five, 70% by seven, 90% by nine, and 95% by the time the child is ten or twelve. Most often no blemish remains, but occasionally there is a residual scar. The range of possible treatment modes is similar to that for strawberry birthmarks.

Salmon patch or nevus simplex. ("stork bites") These salmon-colored patches can appear on the forehead, the upper eyelids, and around the nose and mouth, but are most often seen at the nape of the neck (this is where the stork carried the baby, thus the nickname "stork bites.") They invariably become lighter during the first two years of life, becoming noticeable only when the child cries or exerts himself. Since more than 95% of the lesions on the face fade completely, these birthmarks cause less concern cosmetically than other birthmarks.

Portwine stain or nevus flammeus. These purplish red birthmarks, which may appear anywhere on the body, are composed of dilated mature capillaries. They are normally present at birth as flat or barely elevated pink or reddish purple lesions. Though they may change color slightly, they don't fade appreciably over time and can be considered permanent. Water-resistant cosmetic creams can be used to cover them, and at about age twelve, laser treatment may be effective in removing them. Rarely, these lesions are associated with an overgrowth of the underlying soft tissue or bone, or when on the face, with abnormalities of brain development. Ask your baby's doctor if you have any concerns.

Café au lait spots. These flat patches on the skin, which can range in color from tan (coffee with a lot of milk) to light brown (coffee with a touch of milk), can turn up anywhere on the body. They are quite common, apparent either at birth or during the first few years of life, and don't disappear. If your child has a large number of café au lait spots (six or more), point this out to his or her doctor.

Mongolian spots. Blue to slate gray, resembling bruises, Mongolian spots may turn up on the buttocks or back, and sometimes the legs and shoulders, of 9 out of 10 children of black, Oriental, or Indian descent. These ill-defined patches are also fairly common in infants of Mediterranean ancestry, but are rare in blond-haired, blue-eyed infants. Though most often present at birth and gone within the first year, occasionally they don't appear until later and/or persist into adulthood.

Congenital pigmented nevi. These moles vary in color from light brown to blackish and may be hairy. Small ones are very common; larger ones, "giant pigmented nevi," are rare, but carry a greater potential for becoming malignant. It is usually recommended that large moles, and suspicious smaller ones, be removed if removal can be accomplished easily, and that those not removed be followed carefully by a doctor familiar with their treatment.

COMPLEXION PROBLEMS

"My baby seems to have little white pimples all over his face. Will scrubbing help to clear them?"

The mother expecting peaches-and-cream smoothness may be dismayed to find a sprinkling of tiny whiteheads across her newborn's face, particularly around the nose and chin, an occasional one or two on the trunk or extremities, or even on the penis. The best treatment for these milia, which are caused by clogging of the newborn's immature oil glands, is no treatment at all. As tempting as it may be to squeeze or scrub them, don't. They'll disappear spontaneously, usually within a few weeks.

"I'm worried about the red blotches with light centers on my baby's face."

Rare is the baby who escapes the neonatal period with skin unscathed. The newborn complexion woe that caught your baby is also one of the most common: toxic erythema. Despite its ominous-sounding name and alarming appearance—blotchy, irregularly shaped, reddened areas with pale centers—toxic erythema is completely benign and short lived. It looks like a collection of insect bites and will disappear without treatment.

MOUTH CYSTS OR SPOTS

"When my baby had her mouth wide open screaming, I noticed a few little white bumps on her gums. Could she be getting teeth?"

Don't alert the media (or the grandparents) yet. While a very occasional baby will sprout a couple of bottom center incisors six months or so before schedule, little white bumps on the gum are much more likely to be tiny fluid-filled papules, or cysts. These cysts are common in newborns and will soon disappear, leaving gums clear in plenty of time for that first toothless grin.

Some babies may also have yellowish white spots on the roof of their mouths at birth. Like the cysts, they are neither uncommon nor of any medical significance in newborns. Dubbed "Epstein's pearls," these spots will disappear without treatment.

EARLY TEETH

"I was shocked to find my baby was born with two front teeth. The doctor says she'll have to have them pulled, which is very upsetting to my husband and me."

Every once in a while, a newborn arrives on the scene with a tooth or two. If these teeth are not well anchored in the gums, they may have to be removed to avoid baby choking on or swallowing them. Early teeth may be preteeth, or extra teeth, which, after they've been removed, will be replaced by primary teeth at the usual time. But more often they are primary teeth, and if they must be extracted, temporary dentures may be needed to stand in for them until their secondary successors come in.

THRUSH

"My baby seems to have a white curd in her mouth. I thought it was spitup milk, but when I tried to brush it away, her mouth started to bleed."

There's a fungus among you—or, more accurately, between you. Though the fungus infection known as thrush is causing problems in your baby's mouth, it probably started its dirty work in your birth canal as a monilial infection—and that's where your baby picked it up. The causative organism is *Candida albicans,* which is a normal inhabitant of the mouth and vagina. Kept in check by other microorganisms, it usually causes no problem. But should this arrangement be upset—by illness, the use of antibiotics, or hormonal changes (such as in pregnancy)—conditions become favorable for the fungus to grow and cause symptoms of infection.

Thrush appears in elevated white patches that look like cottage cheese or milk curds on the insides of a baby's cheeks, and sometimes on the tongue, roof of the mouth, and gums. If the patches are wiped away, a raw red area is exposed, and there may be bleeding. Thrush is most common in newborns, but occasionally an older baby, particularly one taking antibiotics, will become infected. Call the doctor if you suspect thrush.

Though the yeast infection itself is not dangerous, it is painful and can interfere with baby's feeding. Rarely there may be complications if the condition goes untreated by anti-fungal agents.

WEIGHT LOSS

"I expected my baby to lose some weight in the hospital, but she dropped from 7½ pounds to 6 pounds 14 ounces. Isn't that excessive?"

New mothers, eager to start issuing reports on their baby's progress in the weight-gain department, are often disappointed when their babies check out of the hospital weighing considerably less than when they checked in. But nearly all newborns are destined to lose some of their birth weight (usually between 5% and 10%) in the first five days of life—not as a result of fad dieting in the nursery, but because of normal post-delivery fluid loss, which is not immediately recouped since babies need and take in little food during this time. Breastfed babies, who take in only teaspoons at a time of the premilk colostrum, generally lose more than bottle-fed babies. Most newborns have stopped losing by the fifth day and have regained or surpassed their birth weight by ten to fourteen days of age—when you can start issuing those bulletins.

JAUNDICE

"The doctor says my baby is jaundiced and has to spend more time under the bili-lights before she can go home. She says it isn't serious, but anything that keeps a baby in the hospital sounds serious to me."

Walk into any newborn nursery, and you'll

see that more than half the babies have begun to yellow by their second or third days—not with age, but with newborn jaundice. The yellowing, which starts at the head and works its way down to the toes,[3] tinting even the whites of the eyes, comes from an excess of bilirubin in the blood. Bilirubin, the yellow end product of the normal breakdown of oxygen-carrying red blood cells, is usually removed from the bloodstream and processed by the liver, then passed along to the kidneys for elimination. But newborns often produce more bilirubin than their immature livers can handle. As a result, the bilirubin builds up in the blood, causing the yellowish tinge and what is known as normal, or physiologic, newborn jaundice (or icterus).

In physiologic jaundice, yellowing usually begins on the second or third day of life and starts diminishing when the baby is a week or ten days old. It appears a bit later (about the third or fourth day) and lasts longer (often fourteen days or more) in premature babies because of their extremely immature livers. Jaundice is more likely to occur in boys, or in babies who lose a lot of weight right after delivery, in babies who have diabetic mothers, and in babies who arrived via induced labor.

Sometimes a doctor will keep a baby with physiologic jaundice in the hospital a few extra days for observation and treatment. In most cases, the bilirubin levels (determined through blood tests) will gradually diminish, and the baby will go home with a clean bill of health. Rarely, there will be a rapid increase in bilirubin, suggesting that the jaundice may be abnormal, or pathologic.

Pathologic jaundice is extremely uncommon. It usually begins either earlier or later than physiologic jaundice, and levels of bilirubin are higher. When it is present at birth or develops rapidly during the first

3. The process is the same in black- and brown-skinned babies, but the yellowing is visible only in the palms of the hands, the soles of the feet, and the whites of the eyes.

day of life, it may indicate hemolytic disease, caused by blood group incompatibility (as when the baby has a different Rh factor from the mother). Jaundice that doesn't develop until later (usually between one and two weeks after birth) could indicate obstructive jaundice, in which an obstruction in the liver interferes with the processing of bilirubin. Pathologic jaundice can also be caused by other, often hereditary, blood or liver diseases and by a variety of intrauterine and neonatal infections. Treatment to bring down abnormally high levels of bilirubin is important to prevent a buildup of the substance in the brain, a condition known as kernicterus. Signs of kernicterus are weak crying, sluggish reflexes, and poor sucking in a jaundiced infant; untreated, it can lead to permanent brain damage or even death.

Mild physiologic jaundice usually requires no treatment. More severe cases can be treated effectively with phototherapy under an ultraviolet lamp, often called a bili-light. During the treatment, babies are naked and their eyes are covered to protect them from the light's rays. They are also given extra fluids to compensate for the increased water loss through the skin, and may be restricted to the nursery except for feedings. New units, using a fiber-optic pad wrapped around baby's middle, allow more flexibility, sometimes permitting baby to go home with mom.

The treatment of pathologic jaundice will depend on the cause, but may include phototherapy, exchange blood transfusions, or surgery to remove obstructions. New drug therapy with a substance that inhibits bilirubin production, may also be used.

In an older baby or child, jaundice, or yellowing, can indicate anemia, hepatitis, or some other infection or liver malfunction, and should be reported to the doctor as soon as possible.

"I've heard that breastfeeding causes jaundice. My baby is a little jaundiced—should I stop nursing?"

Blood bilirubin levels are, on the average, higher in breastfed babies than in bottle-fed infants and they may stay elevated longer (as long as six weeks). This is believed to be just an exaggerated form of physiologic jaundice and not medically significant. Continuation of breastfeeding is usually recommended, since interrupting it and/or giving glucose water feedings seems to increase rather than decrease bilirubin levels and can also interfere with the establishment of lactation. It's been suggested that breastfeeding in the first hour after birth can reduce bilirubin levels in nursing infants.

True breast-milk jaundice is suspected when levels of bilirubin rise rapidly *late* in the first week of life and other causes of pathologic jaundice have been ruled out. It's believed to be caused by a substance in the breast milk of some women that interferes with the breakdown of bilirubin and is estimated to occur in about 2 out of every 100 breastfed babies. The diagnosis is confirmed by a dramatic drop in bilirubin levels when formula is substituted for breast milk for approximately 36 hours (during which time mom continues to empty her breasts by expressing the milk at feeding times to keep up her milk supply). When breastfeeding is resumed, bilirubin levels usually rise again, but not to previous highs. The condition usually clears up within a few weeks.

PACIFIER USE

"In the nursery they stick a pacifier in the babies' mouths every time they cry. I've always hated seeing older kids with pacifiers, and I'm afraid that will happen to my daughter if she gets started on one now."

Being quieted with a pacifier during the two or three days your baby spends in the hospital nursery will not get her hooked on them. There are, however, some sound reasons why you might prefer that she not be given a pacifier right now:

- If you're nursing, it might cause nipple confusion (sucking on the artificial nipple requires a different motion than suckling at the breast) and interfere with the establishment of breastfeeding.
- Whether you're breast or bottle feeding, your baby may get sufficient sucking satisfaction from the pacifier and refuse to suckle at feeding times.
- Your newborn is better off having her needs attended to when she cries than having a pacifier plugged in.

If you decide you'd rather that the nursery staff not give your baby a pacifier, tell them so. If she's crying and there's no one available to comfort her in the nursery, ask them to bring her to you for a little tender loving care, and perhaps a feeding, which should satisfy sucking needs. Or see if you can switch to rooming-in. If your baby seems to need more sucking once you're at home, and you're considering pacifier use, see page 117.

STOOL COLOR

"When I changed my baby's diaper for the first time, I was shocked to see that his stools were greenish black."

This is only the first of many shocking discoveries you will make in your baby's diapers during the next year or so. And for the most part, what you will be discovering, though occasionally unsettling to the sensibilities, will be completely normal. What you've turned up this time is meconium, the tarry greenish-black substance that gradually filled your baby's intestines during his stay in your uterus. That the meconium is now in his diaper instead of his intestines is a good sign—now you know that his bowels are unobstructed.

Sometime after the first 24 hours, when all the meconium has been passed, you will see transitional stools,[4] which are dark greenish yellow and loose, sometimes "seedy" in texture (particularly among breastfed infants), and may occasionally

contain mucus. There may even be traces of blood in them, probably the result of a baby's swallowing some of his mother's blood during delivery (save any diaper containing blood to show to a nurse or doctor, just to be sure no problem is indicated).

After three or four days of transitional stools, what your baby starts putting out will depend on what you've been putting into him. If it's breast milk, the movements will be golden yellow (like mustard), sometimes loose, even watery, sometimes seedy, mushy, curdly, or the consistency of mustard. If it's formula, the stool will be soft but better formed than a breastfed baby's, and anywhere from pale yellow to yellowish brown, light brown, or brown-green. If the formula is iron-fortified, especially if it is whey rather than casein based, or if baby is taking vitamin drops with iron, the stool may be green, greenish, dark brown, or black.

Whatever you do, don't compare your baby's diapers to those of the baby in the next bassinet. Like fingerprints, no two stools are exactly alike. And unlike fingerprints, they are different not only from baby to baby, but from day to day (even movement to movement) in any one baby. The changes, as you will see when baby moves on to solids, will become more pronounced as his diet becomes more varied.

EYE DISCHARGE

"There's a crusty yellowish discharge on my baby's eyes. Is this an infection?"

This discharge isn't likely to be an infection, but rather the result of the hospital's efforts to prevent a gonococcal infection in your baby's eyes. Once the major cause of blindness, it has been virtually eliminated by this prophylactic treatment. When silver nitrate drops are instilled into a newborn's

---

4. If all meconium in the bowels is passed before a baby is born, as may happen when the fetus is in distress during labor and delivery, the first stools after birth may be transitional.

eyes at birth, however (as they routinely are in many delivery rooms), a chemical conjunctivitis, characterized by swelling and a yellowish discharge that disappears by the fourth or fifth day, develops in about 1 in 5 newborns. Many hospitals now prefer to use antibiotic ointment or drops, which are less likely to trigger an adverse reaction (or to cause a temporary gray stain on the cheek from the drops dripping, another disadvantage of silver nitrate) and can prevent not only gonococcal infection but neonatal chlamydial conjunctivitis as well.

If the swelling and discharge don't clear up, or if they begin any time after the first 24 hours following the administration of the silver nitrate, they may be caused by an infection. So report the symptoms immediately to a nursery nurse or to your baby's doctor. Tearing, swelling, or infection that begins once you are home from the hospital may also be caused by a blocked tear duct (see page 108).

WHAT IT'S IMPORTANT TO KNOW: The Baby Care Primer

Put the diaper on backwards? Take five minutes to get baby in a productive position for a burp? Forget to wash under the arms at bathtime? Don't worry. Babies are not only forgiving—they usually don't even notice. Nevertheless, every new parent wants to do everything, or at least as much as possible, right. This Baby Care Primer will help guide you to that goal. But remember, these are only suggested ways to care for baby. You may come up with some of your own that are even better.

BATHING BABY

Until a baby starts getting down and dirty on all fours, a daily bath isn't a necessity. As long as adequate spot cleaning is done during diaper changes and after feedings, a bath two or three times a week in the precrawling months will keep baby sweet smelling and presentable. Such a light bathing schedule can be particularly welcome in the early weeks when the ritual is often dreaded by both bather and bathee. Babies who don't soon become fond of the bath can continue to be bathed two or three times a week, even when dirt begins to accumulate. Daily spongings, in such critical places as face, neck, hands, and bottom, can stand in between dunks (see page 252 for tips on reducing fear of the bath). For those babies, however, who find it a treat, a daily bath becomes an indispensable ritual.

Just about any time of the day can be the right time for a bath, though bathing just before bedtime will help induce a more relaxed state conducive to sleep. Avoid baths just after or just before a meal, since so much handling on a full tummy could result in spitting up, and baby may not be cooperative on an empty one. Allot plenty of undivided time for the bath, so it needn't be hurried and you won't be tempted to leave baby unattended even for a second to take care of something else. Turn on the telephone answering machine, if you have one, or simply plan on not answering the phone during the bath.

While you are using a portable tub, any room in the house can accommodate the procedure, though with all the splashing and dripping, the kitchen or bath provides the most suitable setting. Your work surface should be at a level that's easy for you to maneuver at, and roomy enough for all the paraphernalia it must hold. For baby's comfort, especially in the early months, turn off fans and air conditioners until the bath is over, and be sure the room you choose is warm (75° to 80° F, if possible) and draft free. If you have a hard time achieving such a temperature range, try warming the bathroom first with shower steam or invest in a safe space heater.

The sponge bath. Until the umbilical cord and circumcision, if any, are healed (a couple of weeks, more or less) tub baths will be taboo, and a washcloth will be your baby's only route to clean. For a thorough sponge bath, follow these steps:

1. Select a bath site. The changing table, a kitchen counter, your bed, or the baby's crib (if the mattress is high enough) are all suitable locations for a sponge bath; simply cover your bed or the crib with a waterproof pad or the counter with a thick towel or pad.

2. Have all of the following ready *before* undressing baby:

- baby soap and shampoo, if you use it
- two washcloths (one will do if you use your hand for soaping)
- sterile cotton balls for cleaning the eyes
- towel, preferably with a hood

- clean diaper and clothing
- ointment for diaper rash, if needed
- rubbing alcohol and cotton balls or alcohol pads for the umbilical cord
- warm water, if you won't be within reach of the sink

3. Get baby ready. If the room is warm, you can remove all of baby's clothing before beginning, covering him or her loosely with a towel while you work (most babies dislike being totally bare); if it's cool, undress each part of the body as you're ready to wash it. No matter what the room temperature, don't take off baby's diaper until it's time to wash the bottom; a naked baby should always be considered armed and dangerous.

4. Begin washing, starting with the cleanest areas of the body and working toward the dirtiest, so that the washcloth and the water you're using will stay clean. Soap with your hands or a washcloth, but use a clean cloth for rinsing. This order of business usually works well:

- Head. Once or twice a week, use soap or baby shampoo, rinsing very thoroughly. On interim days, use just water. A football hold (see illustration, page 52) at the sink's edge

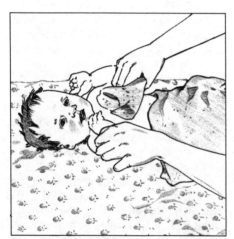

Covering baby's bottom while you wash baby's top keeps baby warm and comfortable while you work; and it protects you, particularly if baby is a boy, from a sudden spurt.

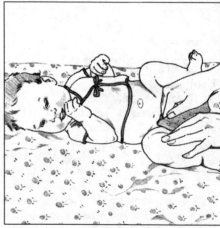

The diaper area will require the most concentrated cleaning effort, and should be saved for last so any germs harbored in the region won't be spread to other parts of the body.

can be the easiest and most comfortable way to rinse baby's head. Towel-dry baby's hair (for most babies this takes just a few seconds) before proceeding.

■ Face. First, using a sterile cotton ball moistened in warm water, clean baby's eyes, wiping gently from the nose outward. Use a fresh ball for each eye. No soap is needed for the face. Wipe around the outer ears, but not inside. Dry all parts of the face.

■ Neck and chest. Soap is not necessary, unless baby is very sweaty or dirty. Be sure to get into those abundant creases. Dry.

■ Arms. Extend the arms to get into the elbow creases, and press the palms to open the fist. The hands will need a bit of soap, but be sure to rinse them well before they are back in baby's mouth. Dry.

■ Back. Turn baby over on the tummy with head to one side, and wash back, being sure not to miss those neck folds. Since this isn't a dirty area, soap probably won't be necessary. Dry, and dress the upper body before continuing if the room is chilly.

■ Legs. Extend the legs to get the back of the knees, though baby will probably resist being unfurled. Dry.

■ Diaper area. Follow special directions for care of the circumcised penis and the umbilical stump (pages 106 and 135) until healing is complete, and instructions for care of the uncircumcised penis on page 85. Wash girls front to back, spreading the labia and cleaning with soap and water. A white vaginal discharge is normal; don't try to scrub it away. Use a fresh section of the cloth and clean water or fresh water poured from a cup to rinse the vagina. Wash boys carefully, getting into all the creases and crevices with soap and water, but don't try to retract the foreskin. Dry the diaper area well, and apply ointment if needed.

5. Diaper and dress baby.

The baby-tub bath. A baby is ready for a tub bath as soon as both umbilical cord stump and circumcision, if any, are healed.

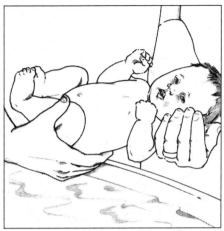

Most babies are very tentative, even tearful, the first few times they're in a tub. So go out of your way to offer support—with reassuring words and a strong, steady grip.

If baby doesn't seem to like being in the water, go back to sponge baths for a few days and try again. Be sure the water temperature is comfortable and that baby is held firmly to combat any innate fear of falling.

1. Select a site for the portable baby tub. The kitchen or bathroom sink or counter or the big tub (though the maneuvering involved when bathing a tiny baby while bending and stretching over a tub can be tricky) are all good candidates. Be sure you will be comfortable and have plenty of room for the tub and bath paraphernalia. The first couple of times you give a tub bath, you might want to omit the soap—soapy babies are slippery babies.

2. Have all of the following ready *before* undressing baby and filling the tub:

■ tub, basin, or sink scrubbed and ready to fill[5].

■ baby soap and shampoo, if you use it

---

5. If you use a sponge pad at the bottom of the tub, be sure to dry it between uses in the sun or in your dryer. Check with the manufacturer for the proper temperature. Towels spread on the bottom of the tub should be washed and dried between baths.

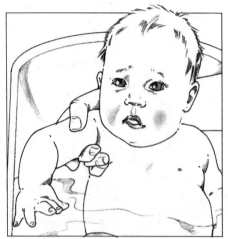

If the tub doesn't offer adequate support for your baby's slippery body and floppy head, you'll need to do so. Gently but firmly does it.

■ two washcloths (one will do if you use your hand for soaping)
■ sterile cotton balls for cleaning the eyes
■ towel, preferably with a hood
■ clean diaper and clothing
■ ointment for diaper rash, if needed
■ as a nice addition, a bath apron of terry cloth with a plastic lining to keep you dry.

3. Run 2 inches of water into the baby

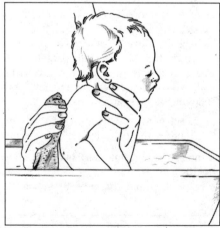

Until baby's neck gains more control over the head, you'll have to hold it steady with one hand while you use your other hand to wash the back.

tub; test with your elbow to be sure it's comfortably warm. Never run the water with baby in the tub because a sudden temperature change might occur. Don't add baby soap or bubble bath to the water, as these can be drying to baby's skin.

4. Undress baby completely.

5. Slip baby gradually into the bath, talking in soothing and reassuring tones to minimize fear, and holding on securely to prevent a startle reflex. Support the neck and head with one hand unless the tub has built-in support, or if your baby seems to prefer your arms to the tub's support, until good head control develops. Hold baby securely in a semireclining position—slipping under suddenly could provide a bad scare.

6. With your free hand, wash baby, working from the cleanest to the dirtiest areas. First, using a sterile cotton ball moistened in warm water, clean baby's eyes, wiping gently from the nose outward. Use a fresh ball for each eye. Then wash face, outer ears, and neck. Though soap won't usually be necessary elsewhere every day (unless your baby tends to have all-over "accidents"), do use it on hands and the diaper area daily. Use it every couple of days on arms, neck, legs, and abdomen as long as baby's skin doesn't seem dry—less often if it does. Apply soap with your hand or with a washcloth. When you've taken care of baby's front parts, turn him or her over your arm to wash back and buttocks.

7. Rinse baby thoroughly with a fresh washcloth.

8. Once or twice a week, wash baby's scalp using mild baby soap or baby shampoo. Rinse very thoroughly and towel dry.

9. Wrap baby in a towel, pat dry, and dress.

BURPING BABY

Milk isn't all baby swallows when sucking on a nipple. Along with that nutritive fluid comes nonnutritive air, which can make a baby feel uncomfortably full before he or

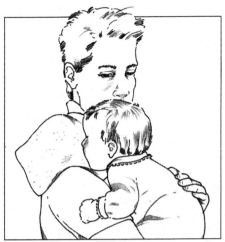

An over-the-shoulder burp yields best results for many babies, but don't forget to protect your clothes.

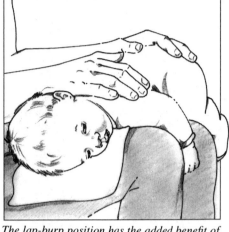

The lap-burp position has the added benefit of being soothing to some colicky infants.

she's finished a meal. That's why burping baby to bring up any excess air that's accumulated—every couple of ounces when bottle feeding, and every five minutes or so (or at least between breasts) when breast-feeding—is such an important part of the feeding process. There are three ways this is commonly done—on your shoulder, face-down on your lap, or sitting up—and it's a good idea to try them all to see which works most efficiently for both you and baby. Though a gentle pat or rub may get the burp up for most babies, some need a slightly firmer hand.

On your shoulder. Hold baby firmly against your shoulder, firmly supporting the buttocks with one hand and patting or rubbing the back with the other.

Face-down on your lap. Turn baby face-down on your lap, stomach over one leg, head resting on the other. Holding him or her securely with one hand, pat or rub with the other.

Sitting up. Sit baby on your lap, head leaning forward, chest supported by your arm as you hold him or her under the armpit. Pat or rub, being sure not to let baby's head flop backward.

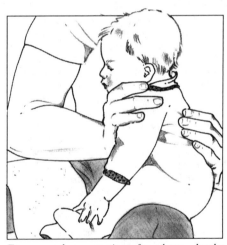

Even a newborn can sit up for a burp—but be sure the head gets adequate support.

DIAPERING BABY

Especially in the early months, the time for a change can come all too often—sometimes hourly during baby's waking hours. But as tedious a chore as it can be for both baby and you, frequent changing (taking place, at the very least, before or after every feeding and whenever there's a bowel movement) is the best way to avoid irritation and diaper rash on baby's sensitive bottom. If you're using disposable diapers, you

SAFE SEATING

New parents taking their babies out for the first time are always careful to bundle them up (often over-bundling them) against the elements, fearful of the consequences of a sudden gust of wind or sprinkle of rain. Yet millions of these same parents fail to protect their offspring where it counts—in the car. Though brief exposure to adverse weather conditions will usually have no ill effect on a newborn, riding unprotected by a safety seat or riding in a safety seat that is improperly anchored can. It is not disease that parents should fear most, but auto accidents—which kill and maim more children yearly than all of the major childhood illnesses combined.

So for that first ride home from the hospital, be sure an infant safety seat is *properly* installed in your car, and baby properly secured in it whenever the car is in motion. Even if your home is literally a few blocks from the hospital, use the seat (most accidents occur within 25 miles of home and not, as is often believed, on superhighways). Don't rely on the fact that you will be driving slowly (a crash at 30 miles per hour creates as much force as a fall from a third-story window). Nor should you rely on your arms to secure your baby, even if you're using a seatbelt (in a crash, your baby would be whipped from your arms and could also be crushed by your body). And remember, too, that you needn't actually crash for severe injury to result—many injuries occur when a car stops short or swerves to avoid an accident.

Getting your baby used to a safety seat from the very first ride will make later acceptance of it almost automatic. And children who ride in safety restraints regularly are not only safer but better behaved during drives—something you'll appreciate when you're riding with a toddler.

In addition to buying a seat that meets federal safety standards (those manufactured since January 1, 1981, do), be sure that you install and use it correctly:

■ Follow manufacturer's directions for installation of the seat and securing of your baby. Check before each ride that the seat is properly secured and the belts or tethers holding it are snugly fastened. Use locking clips, available with most seats, to secure lap/shoulder belts that don't stay tight.

■ Infants should ride in a rear-facing car seat (at a 45-degree angle) until they weigh at least 20 pounds or are a year old. Over 20 pounds, they can ride face forward; over 30 pounds, they can ride in a booster designed for auto use.

■ Place the infant safety seat, if at all possible, in the middle of the back seat—the safest spot in the car (front and side seats are much more vulnerable to impact) and the one with the best belt for installing a child seat. All children under twelve are at risk in the front seat and should ride there only when absolutely necessary and when safely restrained and back as far as possible, but a rear-facing infant seat should *never* be put in the front seat if there is a passenger-side airbag.

■ Be sure that large or heavy objects, such as suitcases, are firmly secured so that they can't become hazardous flying objects during a short stop or crash.

■ Adjust the shoulder harness on the car seat, if it's adjustable, to fit your baby. Be sure all straps fit snugly, and do not use a shield, if any, without the harness straps. For very young babies, pad the sides of the car seat and the area around the head and neck with a rolled blanket or towel to provide support (special cushioned inserts are available for this purpose). If the seat is very deep, placing a rolled towel between baby and the crotch strap will also make baby more comfortable.

■ For older babies, attach soft toys to the seat with plastic links or very short cords—loose toys tend to be flung around the car or dropped, upsetting baby and distracting the driver. Or use toys designed specifically for baby car seat use.

won't be able to use wetness as a gauge; since they absorb so well, disposables don't feel wet until they're seriously saturated. You needn't wake a sleeping baby to change a diaper, however, and unless baby's very wet and uncomfortable or has had a bowel movement, you don't need to change diapers at nighttime feedings; the activity and light involved can interfere with baby's getting back to sleep.

To ensure a change for the better whenever you change your baby's diaper:

1. Before you begin to change a diaper, be sure everything you need is at hand, either on the changing table or, if you're away from home, in your diaper bag. Otherwise, you could end up removing a messy diaper only to find out you have nothing to clean the mess with. You will need all or some of the following:

■ a clean diaper

■ cotton balls and warm water for babies under one month (or those with diaper rash) and a small towel or dry washcloth for drying; diaper wipes for other babies

■ a change of clothes if the diaper has leaked (it happens with the best of them); clean diaper wraps or waterproof pants if you're using cloth diapers

■ ointment, if needed, for diaper rash; lotions and powders are unnecessary, and the latter can be dangerous and can also interfere with the sticking power of the tabs on disposable diapers

■ cornstarch, if needed, to keep baby drier, particularly in hot weather

2. Wash and dry your hands before you begin, if possible, or give them a once-over with a diaper wipe.

3. Have baby entertainment available—live or otherwise. Live shows can be provided by the diaper changer or by siblings, parents, or friends on hand. Other entertainment can come from a mobile hanging over the changing table, a stuffed toy or two in baby's range of vision (and later, within reach), a music box, a mechanical toy—whatever will hold your baby's interest long

enough for you to take off one diaper and put on another. But don't use such items as powder or lotion containers, since an older baby may grab and mouth them.

4. Spread a protective cloth diaper or a changing cloth if you are changing baby anywhere but on a changing table. Wherever you make the change, be careful not to leave baby unattended, not even for a moment. Even strapped to a changing table, your baby shouldn't be out of arm's reach.

5. Unfasten the diaper (pins on cloth diapers, tabs on paper ones), but don't remove it yet. First survey the scene. If there's a bowel movement, use the diaper to wipe most of it away, keeping the diaper over the penis as you work if your baby is a boy. Now fold the diaper under baby with the unsoiled side up to act as a protective surface, and clean baby's front thoroughly with warm water or a wipe, being sure to get into all the creases; then lift both legs, clean the buttocks, and slip the soiled diaper out and a fresh diaper under before releasing the legs. (Keep a fresh diaper over a penis for as much of this process as possible, in self defense.) Pat baby dry if you used water. If you note any irritation or rash, see page 178 for treatment tips.[6]

6. If you're using cloth diapers, they're probably prefolded and ready to use. But you may have to fold them further until your baby is a bit bigger. The extra fabric should be in the front for boys and the back for girls. To avoid sticking baby when using pins, hold your fingers under the layers of diaper as you insert the pin. Sticking the pins in a bar of soap while you're making the change will make them slip more smoothly through the fabric. Once a pin becomes dull, discard it.

If you're using paper diapers, follow the manufacturer's directions (they vary a bit from one brand to another) in order to get the best coverage and protection. Be care-

---

6. Baby boys often get erections during diaper changes; this is perfectly normal, and not a sign that they're being overstimulated.

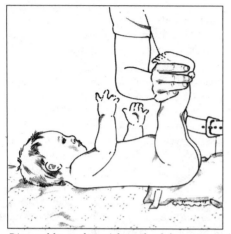
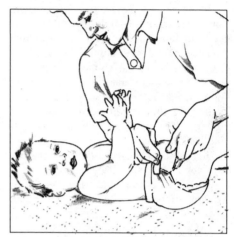

Disposables make quick work of diapering as long as you avoid placing baby's bottom on the adhesive tabs. Once baby is in place, simply bring the front of the diaper through baby's legs and fasten, making sure the tabs are pressed down securely.

ful not to let the tape stick on baby's skin.

Diapers and protective pants should fit snugly to minimize leaks, but not so snugly that they rub or irritate baby's delicate skin. Tell-tale marks will warn you that the diaper is too tight.

Wetness will be less likely to creep up to drench undershirt and clothing on boys if the penis is aimed downward as the diaper is put on. If the umbilical cord is still on, fold the diaper down to expose the raw area to air and keep it from getting wet.

7. Dispose of diapers in a sanitary fashion. When possible, drop any formed stool (there probably won't be any in the diapers of breastfed babies until solids are introduced) into the toilet. Used paper diapers can be folded over, tightly retaped, and tied in a plastic bag for disposal in a trash can. (Using one plastic bag for disposing of an entire day's diapers is sounder ecologically.) Used cloth diapers should be kept in a tightly covered diaper pail (your own, or one supplied by the diaper service) until pickup or wash day. If you are out, they can be held in a plastic bag until you get home.

8. Change baby's clothing and/or bed linen as needed.

9. Wash your hands with soap and water, when possible, or clean them thoroughly with a diaper wipe.

DRESSING BABY

With floppy arms, stubbornly curled-up legs, a head that invariably seems larger than the openings provided by most baby clothes, and an active dislike for being naked, an infant can be a struggle to dress and undress. But there are ways of making these chores less onerous for both of you:

1. Select clothes with easy-on, easy-off features in mind. Wide neck openings or necks with snap closings are best. Sleeves should be fairly loose and a minimum of fastening (particularly up the back) should be necessary. Clothes made of stretch or knit fabrics are often easier to put on than garments with less give.

2. Make changes only when necessary. If you find the odor from frequent spitups offensive, sponge the spots lightly with a diaper wipe rather than changing outfits every time baby has a productive burp. Or try guarding against such incidents by putting a large bib on baby during and after feedings.

3. Dress baby on a flat surface, such as a changing table, bed, or crib mattress. And have some entertainment available.

4. Consider dressing time a social time, too. Light, cheerful conversation can help distract baby from the discomforts and indignities of being dressed and make cooperation more likely. Making a learning game out of pulling on clothes will team distraction with stimulation.

5. Stretch neck openings with your hands before attempting to get baby into a garment. Ease, rather than tug, them on and off, keeping the opening as wide as possible in the process, and trying to avoid snagging the ears or nose. Turn the split second during which baby's head is covered, which might otherwise be scary or uncomfortable, into a game of peekaboo ("Where is mommy? Here she is!" and then, as baby gets old enough to realize that he or she is equally invisible to you, "Where is Janey? Here she is!").

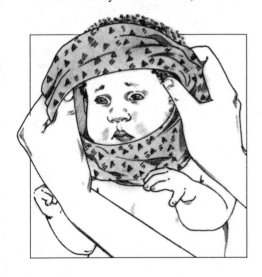

6. With sleeves, try to reach into them and pull baby's hands through, rather than trying to shove rubbery little arms into limp cylinders of cloth. A game here, too ("Where is baby's hand? Here it is!"), will help distract and educate when baby's hands temporarily disappear.

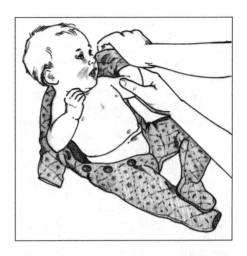

7. When pulling a zipper up or down, draw the garment away from baby's body to avoid pinching the skin.

EAR CARE

The old adage "Never put anything smaller than your elbow in your ears" is advocated not only by grandmothers, but by modern medical authorities as well. They agree that putting anything in the ear that fits— whether it's a dime inserted by a mischievous toddler or a cotton swab inserted by a well-meaning adult—is dangerous. Do wipe your baby's outer ears with a washcloth or cotton ball, but don't try to venture into the ear canal itself with swabs, fingers, or anything else. The ear is naturally self-cleaning, and trying to remove wax by probing may only force it farther into the ear. If wax seems to be accumulating, ask the doctor about it at the next visit.

LIFTING AND CARRYING BABY

For those who have never carried a tiny baby, the experience can, at first, prove very unnerving. But it can be equally unnerving for the baby. After months of being moved gently and securely in the snug uterine cocoon, being plucked up, wafted through the open air, and plunked down can come as quite a shock. Particularly when adequate support isn't provided for the head and neck, this can result in a frightening sensation of falling for baby, and, consequently, a startle reaction. So a good infant carrying technique aims not only at carrying baby in a way that *is* safe, but also in a way that *feels* safe.

You'll eventually develop techniques of carrying your baby that are comfortable for both of you, and carrying will become a completely natural experience. Baby will be casually slung over your shoulder or under your arm as you sort laundry, push the vacuum cleaner, or read labels in the supermarket, yet feel as secure as he or she did in utero. In the awkward interim, however, these tips will help:

Picking baby up. Before you even touch your baby, make your presence known through voice or eye contact. Being lifted unawares by unseen hands to an unknown destination can be unsettling.

Let baby adjust to the switch in support from mattress to arms by slipping your hands under him or her (one under head and neck, the other under bottom) and keeping them there for a few moments be-

fore actually lifting.

Slide the hand under baby's head down the back so that your arm acts as a back and neck support, and your hand cradles the buttocks. Use the other hand to support the legs, and lift baby gently toward your body, caressing as you go. By bending over to bring your body closer, you will limit the distance your baby will have to travel in midair—and the discomfort that comes with it.

Carrying baby comfortably. A small baby can be cradled very nicely in just one arm (with your hand on baby's bottom, and your forearm supporting back, neck and head; see illustration) if you feel secure that way.

With a larger baby, you may both be more comfortable if you keep one hand under legs and buttocks and the other supporting back, neck, and head (your hand encircling baby's arm, your wrist under the head).

Some babies prefer the shoulder carry, all the time or some of the time. It's easy to get baby up there smoothly with one hand on the buttocks, the other under head and neck. Until baby's head becomes self-supporting, you will have to provide

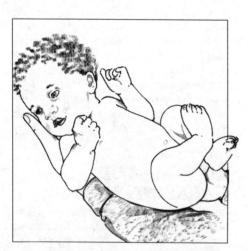

Be sure to carefully support the neck and back with your arm when lifting a baby who is lying face up.

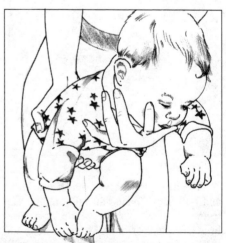

Slip one hand under the chin and neck and the other under the bottom to pick up a baby lying face down.

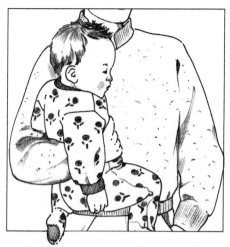

The hip carry leaves the carrier with a free hand.

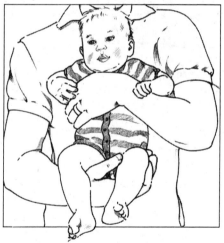

The front carry is a favorite with babies since it allows them a view of the world.

the support. But this can be done even with one hand if you tuck baby's bottom into the crook of your elbow and run your arm up the back with your hand supporting the head and neck.

Even fairly young babies enjoy the front-face carry, in which they can watch the world go by, and many older babies prefer it. Face your baby out, keeping one

hand across his or her chest, pressed back against your own, and the other supporting baby's bottom.

The hip carry gives you freedom to use one hand for chores while carrying an older baby resting on your hip. (Avoid this hold if you have lower-back problems.) Hold baby snugly against your body with one arm, resting his bottom on your hips.

Putting baby back down. Hold baby close to your body as you bend over the crib or carriage (again to limit the midair travel distance), one hand on baby's bottom, one supporting back, neck, and head. Keep hands in place for a few moments until baby feels the comfort and security of the mattress, then slip them out and adjust his or her position for sleeping (see page 120). A few light pats or a bit of gentle hand pressure (depending on what seems to please your baby most), a few parting words if baby's awake, and you're ready to make the break.

NAIL TRIMMING

Although trimming a newborn's tiny fingernails may make most new mothers nervous, it's necessary, nevertheless, because little hands with little control can do a lot of scratching, usually of baby's own face.

An infant's nails are often overgrown at birth, and so soft that cutting through them is nearly as easy as cutting through a piece of paper. Getting your baby to hold still for the procedure won't be so easy, however. Cutting a baby's nails while he's sleeping may work if you've got a sound sleeper or if you don't mind waking him or her. When baby's awake, it's best to trim the nails with the help of an assistant who can hold each hand as you cut. Always use a special baby nail scissor, which has rounded tips—if baby starts to bolt at the wrong moment, no one will be jabbed with a sharp point. To avoid nipping the skin as you clip the nail, press the finger pad down and out of the way as you cut. Even with this precaution you may, however, occasionally draw blood

—most mothers do at one time or another. If you do, apply pressure with a sterile gauze pad until bleeding stops; a band-aid probably won't be needed.

NOSE CARE

As with the inside of the ears, the inside of the nose is self-cleaning and needs no special care. If there is a discharge, wipe the outside, but do not use cotton swabs, twisted tissues, or your fingernail to try to remove material from inside the nose—you may only push the matter back farther into the nose, or even scratch delicate membranes. If baby has a lot of mucus due to a cold, suction it out with an infant nasal aspirator (see page 629).

OUTINGS WITH BABY

Never again will you be able to leave the house empty-handed—at least not when baby's along. In general, you will need some or all of the following whenever you venture forth:

A diaper bag. Don't leave home without it. It can be a bag designed specifically for this purpose or any tote bag you find convenient. Some helpful features include: a built-in changing pad, multiple pockets (including room for your money, license, credit cards), an insulated pocket for bottles, and at least one waterproof compartment. Keep the bag packed and ready, restocking it regularly, so you can just pick up and go.

A changing pad. If your diaper bag doesn't have one, pack a waterproof pad. You can use a towel or a cloth diaper in a pinch, but they won't protect carpeting, beds, or furniture when you're changing baby during a visit.

Diapers. How many depends on how long your outing will be. Always take at least one more than you think you'll need—you'll probably need it. Most people use disposables for outings, but you can use cloth diapers if you prefer.

Diaper wipes. A small convenience pack is easier to carry than a full-size container, but it must be refilled frequently. Or you can use a small plastic sandwich bag to tote a mini-supply. Wipes are handy, incidentally, for washing your own hands before feeding baby and before and after changes, as well as for removing spitup and baby-food stains from clothing or furniture.

Small plastic bags. You'll need these for disposing of dirty disposable diapers, particularly when no trash can is available, as well as for carrying wet and soiled baby clothes home.

A formula feeding. If you are going to be out past the next feeding with a bottle-fed baby, or might be, you'll have to bring a meal along. No refrigeration will be necessary if you take along an unopened bottle of ready-to-use formula (carry a sterilized nipple in a clean plastic bag) or a bottle of sterilized water to which you will add powdered formula. If, however, you bring along formula you've prepared at home, you will have to store it in an insulated container along with a small ice pack or ice cubes.

A shoulder diaper. Your friends may enjoy holding your baby, but not being spit up on. A handy cloth diaper will prevent embarrassing moments and smelly shoulders.

A change of baby clothes. Baby's outfit is picture perfect and you're off to a special family gathering. You arrive, lift your heir from the car seat, and find a pool of loose, mustardy stools has added the "finishing touch." Just one reason why you need to carry along an extra—and for extended outings, two extra—sets of clothing.

An extra blanket or sweater. Particularly in transitional seasons, when temperatures can fluctuate unpredictably, the additional covering will come in handy.

A pacifier, if baby uses one. Carry it in a clean plastic bag.

Entertainment. Something to provide visual stimulation is appropriate for very young babies—particularly for the car seat or stroller. For older babies, light-weight toys they can swat at, poke at, and mouth will fit the bill. Toddlers like books, trucks, dolls, stuffed animals, and small pull-toys.

A sunscreen. Once baby is six months old, a sunscreen is a must year-round (in winter, snow and sun can combine to cause serious burns).

A snack for mom. If you're breastfeed-ing or will be out for a long stretch and may not be able to find a nutritious snack easily, take one along: a piece of fruit; some rounds, sticks, triangles, or cubes of cheese; some whole-grain crackers or bread; a bag of dried fruit. A container or can of fruit juice or a thermos containing a hot or cold drink is a nice addition if your outing will be to a park where no liquid re-freshment is available.

A snack (or two, or three) for baby. Once solids are introduced, bring along jars of baby food (no refrigeration is needed before they're open, no heating up is needed before serving) if you'll be out during mealtime; a spoon stashed in a plastic bag (save the bag to bring the dirty spoon home in); a bib; and plenty of paper towels. Later, a selection of fin-ger foods (nonperishable if you'll be out in hot weather) such as fresh fruit, crack-ers, bread, and breadsticks will ward off hunger between meals, while providing baby with a wholesome activity during your outing. Beware, however, of using snacks to ward off boredom or to keep baby from crying—the pattern of eating for the wrong reasons in childhood can continue as an undesirable habit later on.

Miscellaneous toiletries and first aid items. Depending on any particular health needs your child may have as well as on where you're going, you may also want to carry: diaper rash ointment; baby or regular cornstarch (in hot weather); adhesive strips and antibiotic ointment (especially if your child has begun to get around); medication your baby is taking (if you will be out when the next dose is due; if refrigeration is re-quired, pack with an ice pack in an insu-lated container).

PENIS CARE

The penis is comprised of the cylindrical shaft (most of its length) with a rounded end called the glans. The shaft and the glans are separated by a groove called the sulcus. At the tip of the glans is an opening, the meatus, through which semen and urine flow, though not at the same time. The entire penis—shaft and glans—is covered by a continuous layer of skin, called the foreskin, or prepuce. The foreskin itself is made up of two layers: the outer skin, and a lining similar to a mucous membrane.

At birth, the foreskin is firmly attached to the glans. Over time, foreskin and glans begin to separate, as cells are shed from the surface of each layer. The discarded cells, which are replaced throughout life, ac-cumulate as whitish, cheesy "pearls" that gradually work their way out via the tip of the foreskin.

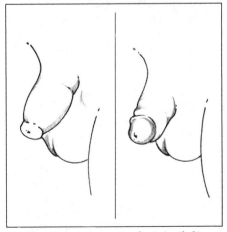

Neither the uncircumcised penis (left) nor the circumcised penis, from which the fore-skin has been removed, requires special care in infancy.

Usually by the end of the second year for 9 out of 10 uncircumcised boys, but sometimes not until five, ten, or more years after birth, foreskin and glans become fully separated. At this point the foreskin can be pushed back, or retracted, away from the glans.

Care of the uncircumcised penis. Contrary to what was once believed, no special care is needed for the uncircumcised penis in infancy—soap and water, applied externally, just as the rest of the body is washed, will keep it clean. It is not only unnecessary to try to forcibly retract the foreskin, or clean under it with cotton swabs, irrigation, or antiseptics—it can actually be harmful. Once the foreskin has clearly separated, you can retract it occasionally and clean under it. By the age of puberty most foreskins will be retractable, and at that time a boy can learn to retract his and clean under it himself.

Care of the circumcised penis. The only care the circumcised penis will ever need, once the incision is healed, is ordinary washing with soap and water. For care during the recovery period, see page 135.

SHAMPOOING BABY

This is a fairly painless process with a young baby. But to help forestall future shampoo problems, avoid getting soap or shampoo in your baby's eyes from the first. Shampoo only once or twice a week, unless cradle cap or a particularly oily scalp requires more frequent head cleanings.

1. Wet baby's hair with a gentle spray from the sink or by pouring a little water from a cup. Add just a drop of baby shampoo or baby soap (more will make rinsing difficult), and rub in lightly to produce a lather.

2. Rinse thoroughly with a gentle spray or two or three cupfuls of clean water.

Older babies, who can stand on their own and have moved up to the big tub, can be shampooed in the tub, but only after the

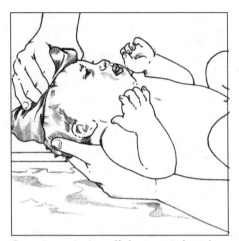

Sometimes rinsing off shampoo is best done with a few gentle wipes with a wash cloth.

bath is over if your child is a girl, since bathing in dirty shampoo water can lead to vaginal infection. The problem, however, is that most children do not like to put their heads back for the shampoo—it makes them feel too vulnerable—and trying to shampoo them this way often ends in tears and tantrums. A spray nozzle, if your tub has one, will give you more control and can be fun for some babies, though others will find it too frightening. A specially designed shampoo visor (available in juvenile-furnishing and toy stores and from mail-order houses) that guards the eyes from flowing water and soap, but leaves the hair exposed for washing, is ideal if your child will wear it—some won't. If your baby resists both sprays and visors, you can continue shampooing (or at least rinsing, after doing the lathering in the tub) at the sink until he or she is more cooperative in the tub. Though the process isn't perfect (and it can grow awkward as the child grows larger), it's quick and consequently minimizes the period of suffering for both of you.

SWADDLING BABY

For some babies, swaddling is soothing and may even reduce crying; others dislike the lack of freedom. If your baby seems to like it, here's how the wrapping's done:

1. Spread a receiving blanket on a crib, a bed, or a changing table, with one corner folded down about 6 inches. Place baby on the blanket diagonally, head above the folded corner.

2. Take the corner near baby's left arm and pull it over the arm and across the baby's body. Lift the right arm, and tuck the blanket corner under baby's back on the right side.

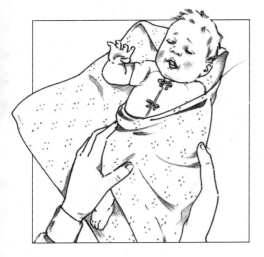

3. Lift the bottom corner and bring it up over baby's body, tucking it into the first swathe.

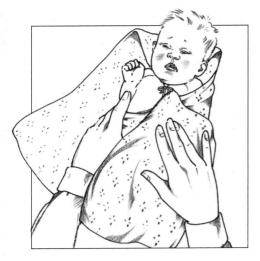

4. Lift the last corner, bring it over baby's right arm, and tuck it in under the back on the left side.

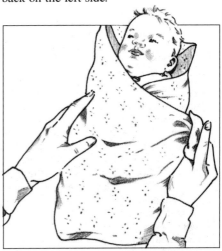

If your baby seems to prefer more hand mobility, do the wrapping below the arms, leaving them free. Because swaddling is confining and can interfere with development in older babies, do not use it once your baby is a month old.

UMBILICAL STUMP CARE

The last remnant of a baby's close attachment to its mother in the uterus is the stump of the umbilical cord. It turns black a few days after birth and can be expected to drop off anywhere between one and four weeks later. You can hasten healing and prevent infection by keeping the area dry and exposed to air. The following will help accomplish this:

1. When putting on baby's diaper, fold the front of it down below the navel to keep urine off and let air in. Fold the shirt up.

2. Skip tub baths and avoid wetting the navel when sponging until the cord falls off.

3. Dab the stump with alcohol (on sterile absorbent cotton balls, sterile gauze squares, or alcohol pads) to help keep the site clean and to hasten drying.

4. If the area around the navel turns red, or the site oozes, call the doctor.

BABY BUSINESS

There are two very important documents that your baby will need periodically throughout life. One is a birth certificate—which will be needed as proof of birth and citizenship when registering for school and applying for a driver's license, passport, marriage license, or social security benefits. Usually, the registering of your baby's birth is handled by the hospital and you receive official notification when the record of the birth is filed. If you don't receive such notification and a copy of the birth certificate within a couple of months, check with the hospital, the local health department, or the state health department to see what's holding it up. When you do receive the birth certificate, examine it carefully to be sure it's accurate—mistakes are sometimes made. If there are errors, or if you hadn't selected a name for your baby before leaving the hospital and want to add it now (you should), call the health department for instructions on how to make the necessary corrections or additions. Once you have a correct birth certificate, make a few copies and file them in a safe place.

The second document that your baby will need is a social security card. Though it isn't likely you're going to put your newborn to work immediately, you'll need the number for other reasons, such as setting up a bank account, investing cash gifts, even purchasing U.S. savings bonds. If you bank baby's savings in your own name and social security number, you will have to pay taxes on the interest at your rate rather than the baby's lower one. To get a social security number for your baby, apply at your local social security office in person or by mail (you will have to send for an application first), submitting a copy of the birth certificate (see, you need it already), plus proof of your own identity, such as a driver's license or passport. It's a good idea to call ahead to see if any other documents are needed. (If you decide your baby doesn't need a social security number now, keep in mind the law requires one by age five.)

CHAPTER FOUR

The First Month

Wʜᴀᴛ ʏᴏᴜʀ ʙᴀʙʏ ᴍᴀʏ ʙᴇ ᴅᴏɪɴɢ:

**By the end of this month, your baby
...should be able to (see Note):**

- lift head briefly when on stomach on a flat surface
- focus on a face

Note: If your baby seems not to have reached one or more of these milestones, check with the doctor. In rare instances the delay could indicate a problem, though in most cases it will turn out to be normal for your baby. Premature infants generally reach milestones later than others of the same birth age, often achieving them closer to their adjusted age (the age they would be if they had been born at term), and sometimes later.

...will probably be able to:

- respond to a bell in some way, such as startling, crying, quieting
- follow an object moved in an arch about 6 inches above face to the midline (straight ahead)

...may possibly be able to:

- on stomach, lift head 45 degrees
- vocalize in ways other than crying (e.g.: cooing)
- follow an object moved in an arch about

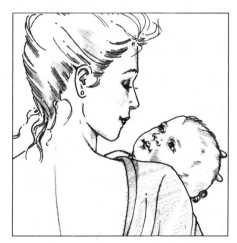

By the end of this month, a baby should be able to focus on a face.

6 inches above face *past* the midline (straight ahead)
- smile in response to your smile

...may even be able to:

- on stomach, lift head 90 degrees

- hold head steady when upright
- bring both hands together
- smile spontaneously
- laugh out loud
- squeal in delight
- follow an object in an arc about 6 inches above the face for 180° (from one side to the other)

WHAT YOU CAN EXPECT AT THIS MONTH'S CHECKUP

Each doctor or nurse-practitioner will have a personal approach to well-baby checkups. The overall organization of the physical exam, as well as the number and type of assessment techniques used and procedures performed will also vary with the individual needs of the child. But in general, you can expect the following at a checkup when your baby is between two and four weeks old. (The first visit may take place earlier under special circumstances, such as when a newborn has had jaundice, was premature, or when there are any problems with the establishment of breastfeeding.)

- Questions about how you and baby and the rest of the family are doing at home, and about baby's eating, sleeping, and general progress.
- Measurement of baby's weight, length, and head circumference, and plotting of progress since birth.
- Vision and hearing assessments.
- A report on results of neonatal screening tests (for PKU, hypothyroidism, and other inborn errors of metabolism), if not given previously. If the doctor doesn't mention the tests, the results were very likely normal, but do ask for them for your own records. If your baby was released from the hospital before these tests were performed, or if they were done before he or she was

72 hours old, they will probably be performed or repeated now.

- A physical exam. The doctor or nurse-practitioner will examine and assess all or most of the following, although some evaluations will be carried out by the experienced eye or hand, without comment:

  □ heart sounds with a stethoscope, and visual check of the heartbeat through the chest wall (ideally, baby shouldn't be crying for this part of the exam)
  □ abdomen, by palpation and/or stethoscope, for any abnormal masses
  □ hips, checking for dislocation by rotating the legs
  □ hands and arms, feet and legs, for normal development and motion
  □ back and spine, for any abnormalities
  □ eyes, with an opthalmoscope and/or a penlight, for normal reflexes and focusing, and for tear duct functioning
  □ ears, with an otoscope, for color, fluid, movement
  □ nose, with otoscope, for color and condition of mucous membranes and abnormalities
  □ mouth and throat, using a wooden tongue depressor, for sores, bumps, color
  □ neck, for normal motion, thyroid and lymph gland size (lymph glands are

more easily felt in infants, and this is normal)

□ underarms, for swollen lymph glands

□ the fontanels (the soft spots), by palpating with the hands

□ respiration and respiratory function, by observation, and sometimes with stethoscope and/or light tapping of chest and back

□ the genitalia, for any abnormalities, such as hernias or undescended testicles; the anus for cracks or fissures; the femoral pulse in the groin, for a strong steady beat

□ the skin, for color, tone, rashes, and lesions, such as birthmarks

□ reflexes specific to baby's age

□ overall movement and behavior, ability to cuddle and relate to adults

■ Guidance about what to expect in the next month in relation to feeding, sleeping, development, and infant safety.

■ Recommendations on vitamin D supplementation, if you are breastfeeding.

Before the visit is over, be sure to:

■ Ask for guidelines for calling when baby is sick. (What would necessitate a call in the middle of the night? How can the doctor be reached outside of regular calling times?)

■ Express any concerns that may have arisen over the past month—about baby's health, behavior, sleep, feeding, and so on.

■ Jot down (or even tape record) information and instructions from the doctor (you're sure to forget them, otherwise).

When you get home, record all pertinent information (baby's weight, length, head circumference, blood type, test results, birthmarks) in a permanent health record.[1]

FEEDING YOUR BABY THIS MONTH: Expressing Breast Milk

You see them in rest rooms all over the country. During intermission at the opera and half time at sports events; in airports, bus depots, and railroad stations; in offices, factories, and shops; in restaurants and department stores; in schools and hospitals. Wherever women work, play, travel, or study, you'll find mothers expressing milk.

WHY MOTHERS EXPRESS MILK

Unlike mothers in primitive societies, who carry their babies in slings at their breasts for convenient round-the-clock nipping, busy mothers in our fast-paced indus-trialized society can't always count on their babies and their breasts being in the same place at the same time. For this, and a host of other reasons, virtually every woman who breastfeeds expresses milk or pumps her breasts at one time or another. Most commonly, breasts are pumped to:

■ Draw out inverted nipples late in pregnancy.

■ Induce lactation in an adopting mother, or in a biological mother whose milk is slow in coming in.

---

1. An appropriate form for recording such information is available from the American Academy of Pediatrics, Division of Publications, 141 Northwest Point Boulevard, Elk Grove Village, IL 60009-0927 (enclose $1.50), or from your baby's doctor.

- Relieve engorgement when the milk comes in.
- Increase or maintain the milk supply.
- Collect milk for interim feedings when working or away from home.
- Prevent clogging from over-full breasts.
- Provide milk for bottle or tube feeding when a baby (premature or otherwise) is too weak to nurse, or has an oral defect that hinders nursing.
- Provide breast milk for a hospitalized sick or premature baby.
- Prevent engorgement and maintain milk supply when nursing is temporarily halted because of illness (mother's or baby's).
- Stimulate relactation, if a mother changes her mind about nursing or if a baby turns out to be allergic to cow's milk after early weaning.

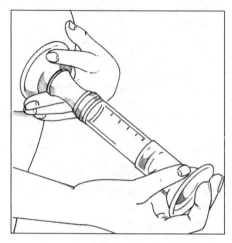

Though tough on the arm that's doing the pumping, the syringe pump is one of the least expensive yet convenient instruments for expressing milk.

TECHNIQUES FOR EXPRESSING BREAST MILK

At one time, the only way to express milk was by hand, a long and tedious process that often failed to produce significant quantities of milk. Today, spurred by the resurgence of breastfeeding, manufacturers are marketing a variety of breast pumps—ranging from simple hand-operated models that cost a few dollars to sophisticated electric ones costing in the thousands of dollars—to make pumping easier and more convenient. Though an occasional mother will still express by hand, at least to relieve engorgement, most will invest in one of the following:

- A bulb or "bicycle-horn" pump, which suctions milk from breasts with each squeeze of the bulb. These are inexpensive—but inefficient, difficult to clean (which could lead to unsanitary milk collection), and uncomfortable to use, often causing sore nipples. Impractical for regularly expressing milk for infant feedings, they can be used to relieve occasional engorgement.

- A trigger-operated pump, which creates suction with each squeeze of the trigger. More expensive than the bulb type, but still very affordable, it has the advantage of requiring only one hand to operate. But, because it requires a great deal of dexterity and strength, women who don't have large strong hands may have trouble using such a pump, and many women may find it difficult to empty the breast opposite their non-dominant hand. Another drawback: the glass construction. Not only are these pumps breakable, but certain immunity-conferring factors from the breast milk may adhere to the glass (they don't adhere to plastic), depriving baby of their benefits.
- A syringe pump, which is composed of two cylinders that fit inside one another. The inner cylinder is placed over the nipple and the outer, when pushed in and pulled out, creates suction that draws milk into it. This type is the most popular because it's fairly simple to use, is moderate in price, easy to clean, portable, and can also double as a feeding bottle. Some allow pressure to be adjusted to more closely mimic an infant's suckling, making expressing milk more comfortable.
- A convertible manual pump, which can

be connected, when desired, to an electrical system. This versatile model offers faster, more efficient operation when electricity is available as well as portability for use away from a power source.

■ A battery-operated pump, which promises portability and efficient operation, but not all models deliver. Moderately priced, they are less powerful than electric models; and the speed at which some eat batteries makes them expensive to use and of questionable practicality. Check with your local La Leche League for the latest scoop on these.

■ An electric pump, which is powerful, fast, and easy to use, leaves a mother's hands free for nursing (on the other breast) or other activities during pumping. They are usually very expensive, often costing from a few hundred to $1,000 or more, but if time is an important consideration, one may be well worth the investment. If portability of a unit will affect your choice, keep in mind that an electric pump is unwieldy at best, but that you can buy a second more portable pump for the road and still get a lot of mileage out of your electric model at home.

Many women rent electric pumps, from either hospitals, pharmacies, or La Leche groups; some buy or rent jointly with other women, or buy them, use them, and then sell them. Insurance plans may cover the cost of purchase or rental if breast milk is prescribed and nursing is not possible, usually when a baby is premature or sick. Personal pump kits (with shield, cup, lid, and tubing) are available, disposable or sterilizable, to make sharing a pump or using a hospital pump more practical.

Before selecting a pump, talk to friends, to someone at La Leche League, a childbirth educator, a lactation consultant, or your baby's doctor (if he or she is conversant with the subject) to learn the pros and cons of various models. If possible, try the one you are considering—by borrowing or renting—before making a purchase. You will want a pump that is easy and convenient to operate, clean, relatively comfortable to use, and, if you will be using it away from home, portable.

HOW TO EXPRESS BREAST MILK

Basic preparations. No matter what method of expressing you choose, you may find it difficult to express milk for the first few days. Making these preparations before getting started will help:

■ Choose a time of the day when your breasts are ordinarily fullest—for most women, that's the morning. Plan on expressing milk for collection about once every three or four hours. Each collection can take from 20 to 40 minutes, and sometimes even longer.

■ Make sure that all your equipment is clean and sterilized according to the manufacturer's directions; washing your pump immediately after each use will make the difficult job of keeping it clean easier. If you use your pump away from home, carry along a bottle brush, detergent, and paper towels for washup.

■ Especially while you are still a novice, select a quiet, comfortably warm environment for pumping, where you won't be interrupted by phones or doorbells, and where you will have some privacy. At work, a private office, an unoccupied meeting room, or the women's lounge can serve as your pumping headquarters. If you're at home, it's ideal if someone else can care for the baby, leaving you free to concentrate on the job at hand.

■ Wash your hands with soap and water, your breasts with water only—don't use soaps, creams, ointments, or anything else on your nipples.

■ Drink a full glass of water, juice, milk, decaffeinated tea or coffee, or soup just before beginning. A warm drink may be more helpful than a cold one for stimulating let-down. Alcoholic beverages don't count toward your fluid quota, but a glass of wine or beer, or a cocktail, no more than twice a day, taken ten to twenty minutes prior to pumping, can be used to help you relax.

▪ Make yourself comfortable, with your feet up, if possible.

▪ Relax for several minutes before beginning. Use meditation or other relaxation techniques, music, TV, or whatever you personally find helps you unwind.

▪ Think about your baby and about nursing or look at baby's photo to help to stimulate let-down. Otherwise, having baby in the room just before you start pumping could do the trick, though ideally someone else should be around to care for baby once you begin. If you're using an electric pump, which leaves your hands free, you can even hold the baby—though many babies balk at being so near and yet so far from being fed. Applying hot soaks to your nipples and breasts for five or ten minutes, taking a hot shower, doing breast massage, or leaning over and shaking your breasts are other ways of enhancing let-down.

▪ If you find you have a lot of difficulty getting results, ask your doctor about an oxytocin nasal spray, which encourages let-down. Use it only as directed.

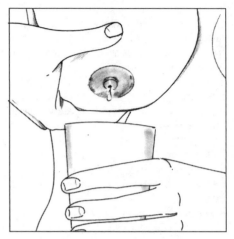

Expressing breast milk by hand is a slow, sometimes painful process. This method is best for expressing only small amounts, as when the breast is too engorged for baby to get a comfortable mouthful.

Expressing milk by hand. To begin, place your hand on one breast, at the edge of the areola, with your thumb opposite the other fingers. Press your hand in toward your chest, gently pressing thumb and forefinger together. (Keep your fingers on the areola only; don't let them slip onto the nipple.) Repeat rhythmically to start milk flowing, rotating your fingers to get to all milk ducts. Repeat with the other breast, massaging in between expressions, as needed. Repeat with the first breast, then do the second again.

If you want to collect the milk expressed, use a wide-topped, sterilized cup under the breast you are working on. You can collect whatever drips from the other by placing a sterilized milk cup over it inside your bra. Collected milk should be poured immediately into sterilized bottles and refrigerated as soon as possible.

Expressing milk with a hand-held or electric pump. Simply follow the directions for the pump you are using. Be patient; it often takes a while to become proficient at pumping. If you want to use a hand pump on one breast while nursing

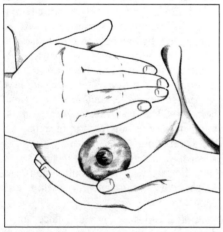

To massage your breast, place one hand underneath your breast, the other on top. Slide the palm of one or both hands from the chest gently toward the nipple and apply mild pressure. Rotate your hands around the breast and repeat in order to reach all the milk ducts.

your baby on the other, either prop the baby at your breast on a pillow (being sure he or she can't tumble off your lap), or have someone else do the pumping as you hold baby. Since you don't have to use your hands to operate an electric pump, you can nurse your baby on one side and pump on the other with ease.

COLLECTING AND STORING BREAST MILK

Plastic containers are better than glass for collecting and storing breast milk, not only because glass is breakable, but also because disease-fighting white blood cells in mother's milk have been shown to cling more to glass than to plastic, making them less available to baby. Many pumps come with containers that can be used as storage and feeding bottles; others allow you to use a standard feeding bottle to collect the milk. Four-ounce bottles are practical for young babies, whose appetites are still small, 8-ounce ones for older babies. A thermos, packed with ice until it is ready to be filled, can be used to keep breast milk fresh when you're away from home—but it may have the drawback of being glass-lined.

Sterilize containers and bottles, or wash them in a dishwasher with temperatures that reach at least 180°F, if milk is going to be kept at room temperature for longer than 30 minutes or stored for more than 48 hours in the refrigerator or freezer. Otherwise, washing thoroughly with hot soapy water and a bottle brush should be sufficient.

Refrigerate expressed milk as soon as you can; if that's not possible, use a sterile container, in which it will stay fresh at room temperature (but away from radiators, sun, or other sources of heat) for as long as six hours. You can store breast milk for up to 48 hours in the refrigerator, or chill for 30 minutes, then freeze. Fill containers for the freezer only three-fourths full to allow for expansion, and label with the date (always use the oldest milk first). Breast milk will stay fresh in the freezer for anywhere from a week or two in a single-door refrigerator, to about three months in a two-door frost-free model that keeps foods frozen solid, to six months in a freezer that maintains a 0° temperature.

To thaw breast milk, shake the bottle under lukewarm tap water; then use within 30 minutes. Or thaw in the refrigerator and use within three hours. Do not thaw in a microwave oven, on the top of the stove, or at room temperature; and do not refreeze. When your baby has finished feeding on a bottle, discard the remaining milk. Also discard any milk that has been stored for periods longer than those recommended above.

If you are going to transport breast milk regularly, invest in an insulated bottle bag, a thermos, or an insulated bag that can hold the bottle and a frozen ice pack.

WHAT YOU MAY BE CONCERNED ABOUT

"BREAKING" BABY

"I'm so afraid of handling the baby— he's so tiny and vulnerable looking."

Newborn babies may look as fragile as china dolls, but they're not. In fact, they're really pretty sturdy. As long as their heads are well supported, they can't be harmed by normal handling—even when it's a little clumsy and tentative, as is often the case when the handling's being done by a first-time parent. You'll gradually learn what's comfortable for your baby and for you, since handling styles vary greatly from parent to parent. Soon you'll be toting your baby as casually as a bag of groceries—and often *with* a bag of groceries.

INFANT ACNE

"I thought babies were supposed to have great complexions. But my two-week-old seems to be breaking out in a terrible case of acne."

As unfair as it might seem, some babies go through bouts with "adolescent" skin before they're days old, let alone teenagers. And actually, many of their complexion problems have the same cause as many of the complexion problems of teenagers: hormones. Except in the case of newborns, it's not their hormones that are causing the problems, but those of their mothers that are still circulating in their systems. Another reason pimples are likely to crop up is that the pores of newborns aren't completely developed, making them easy targets for infiltration by dirt and the resultant blossoming of blemishes.

Don't squeeze, scrub, slather with lotions, or otherwise treat your newborn's acne. Just wash it with water two or three times daily, pat it dry, and it will clear within a few months, leaving no lasting marks.

HEARING

"My baby doesn't seem to react much to noises. In fact, he sleeps right through the dog's barking and my older daughter's tantrums. Could his hearing be impaired?"

It's probably not that your baby doesn't hear the dog barking or his sister screaming, but that he's used to these sounds. Although he saw the world for the first time when he exited your uterus, it wasn't the first time he heard it. Many sounds—from the music you played on the stereo to the honking horns and screeching sirens on the street—penetrated the walls of his peaceful uterine home, and he became accustomed to them.

Most babies will react to loud noise—in early infancy by startling, at about three months by blinking, at about four months by turning toward the source of the sound. But those sounds that have already become a part of the background Muzak of a baby's existence may elicit no response—or one so subtle the untrained eye misses it, such as a change in position or activity.

If you're concerned about your baby's hearing, try this little test: clap your hands behind his head and see if he startles. If he does, you know he can hear. If he doesn't, try again later; children (even newborns) have a wonderful way of ignoring or blocking out their environment at will, and he may have been doing just that. A repeat test may elicit the response you want. If it doesn't, try to observe other ways in which your baby may react to sound: Is he calmed or does he otherwise respond to the soothing sounds of your voice, even when he isn't looking directly at you? Does he respond to singing or music in any way? Does he startle when exposed to an unfamiliar loud noise? If your baby seems never to respond to sound, discuss this with his doctor as soon as it's practical. The earlier a child's hearing deficit is diagnosed and treated, the better the long-range outcome.

Experts disagree on the cost effectiveness of audiological screening of all newborns, but all agree high-risk infants should be evaluated. This includes children who weighed in under 2,500 grams (or 5½ pounds), or who experienced serious complications during or shortly after birth (such as asphyxia, seizures, or intracranial hemorrhage); those exposed prenatally to drugs or infections known to affect hearing (such as rubella); those with a family history of unexplained or inherited deafness; those with visible abnormalities of the ears; and those who are mentally retarded, blind, autistic, or have cerebral palsy.

VISION

"I put a mobile over my baby's crib, hoping the colors would be stimulating. But he doesn't seem to notice it. Could something be wrong with his vision?"

It's more likely there's something wrong with your mobile—at least with where it's hung. A newborn baby focuses best on objects that are between 8 and 14 inches away from his eyes, a range that seems to have been selected by nature not randomly, but by design—it being the distance at which a nursing infant sees his mother's face. Objects closer or farther away from a baby lying in his crib will be nothing but a blur to him, although he will fixate on something distant that is bright or in motion if there is nothing worth looking at within his range of vision.

In addition, he will spend most of his time looking to his right or to his left, rarely focusing straight ahead in the early months. A mobile directly above his crib is not likely to catch his fancy, whereas one hung to one side or the other may. Few babies, however, show any interest at all in mobiles until they are three to four weeks old, and many not until even later.

So your newborn can see, but not the way he will in three or four months. If you want to evaluate your baby's vision, hold a penlight to one side of his line of vision, about 10 to 12 inches from his face. During the first month, a baby will generally focus on the light for a brief period, long enough for you to know he's seeing it. By the end of the first month, some babies will follow as you move the light slowly toward the center of their field of vision. Generally, not until three months will a baby begin to follow an object in a full 180° arc, from one side to the other.

Your baby's eyes will continue maturing during the first year. He probably will be farsighted for several months and not be able to perceive depth well (which may be why he's a perfect candidate for falling off changing tables and beds) until nine months. But though his vision isn't perfect now, he does enjoy looking at things—and this pastime is one of his most important avenues to learning. So provide him with plenty of visual stimuli. But don't overload his circuits—one or two eye-catchers at a time are about all he can handle. And because his attention span is short, change the scenery frequently.

Most young babies like to study faces—even crudely drawn ones. They prefer black-and-white patterns to bright colors; complex objects to simple ones. They love looking at light: a chandelier, a lamp, a window (especially one through which light is filtered via the slats of vertical or horizontal blinds), will all attract their rapt scrutiny; and they are usually happier in a well-lighted room than in a dim one.

Vision screening will be part of your baby's regular checkups. But if you feel that your baby doesn't seem to be focusing on objects or faces or doesn't turn toward the light, mention this to his doctor at the next visit.

SPITTING UP

"My baby spits up so much that I'm worried she's not getting enough nourishment."

Although it may seem all that's going into your daughter is coming back up, that's not likely to be the case. What looks like a mealful of milk to you is probably no more than a tablespoon or two, mixed with saliva and mucus—certainly not enough to interfere with your baby's nourishment. (To see how much a little bit of liquid can look like, spill a couple of tablespoons of milk on your kitchen counter.) The material your baby spits up will be relatively unchanged from the form in which it entered baby's mouth if it only went as far as the esophagus before coming back up. But if it traveled down to the stomach before its return trip, it will look curdled and smell like sour milk.

Most babies spit up at least occasionally; some spit up with every feeding. The process in newborns may be related to an immature sphincter between the esophagus and the stomach and to excess mucus that needs to be cleared. In older babies, spitting up occurs when milk mixed with air is regurgitated with a burp. Sometimes a baby wisely spits up because she's eaten too much.

There are no sure cures for spitting up. But you can try to minimize the air gulping around mealtimes that can contribute to it: don't feed her when she's crying (take a break in the action to calm her down); keep her as upright as possible while feeding and for a while afterward; be sure bottle nipples are neither too large nor too small and that bottles are tilted so that formula (not air) fills the nipple. It may also be helpful to keep your baby from making a pig of herself, and to avoid bouncing her around while she's eating or just afterward (when possible, strap her in a baby seat or stroller for a while). And don't forget to burp her during a meal, instead of waiting until the end of the meal when one big bubble may bring up the works.

Accept, however, that no matter what you do, if your baby's a spitter, she's going to spit—and you're going to have to live with it for at least six months. (The living will be a little neater, however, if you keep a precautionary diaper on your shoulder or lap whenever you're on baby duty.) Most babies ease up on their spitting when they start sitting upright, although a few will continue causing malodorous mayhem well up until their first birthdays.

Ordinary spitting up usually presents no hazards (other than to clothes and furniture).[2] The doctor may recommend a child with *severe* spitting up (gastroesophageal reflux or GER) to sleep on a slant board, possibly on her tummy.

Some kinds of spitting up do, however, signal possible problems. Call the doctor if your baby's spitting up is associated with poor weight gain or prolonged gagging and coughing, or if her vomit is brown or green in color or shoots out two or three feet (projectile vomiting). These could indicate a medical problem, such as an intestinal obstruction (treatable by surgery).

SWADDLING

"I've been trying to keep my baby swaddled, like they showed me in the hospital. But she keeps kicking at the blanket, and it gets undone. Should I stop trying?"

The first few days of life on the outside can be a little disorienting—and even a little scary. After spending nine months snugly enveloped in the uterine cocoon, a newborn must adjust to the suddenly wide-open spaces of her new environment. Many child-care experts feel the transition can be made more comfortable if the security and warmth of the newborn's former home is simulated by swaddling, or bundling, her in a receiving blanket. Swaddling also keeps the infant from being disturbed by her own jerky movements while she sleeps, and keeps her warm in the early days when her thermostat is not at peak efficiency. But don't swaddle in a warm room because overheating is a SIDS risk factor.

Just because all babies are swaddled in the hospital, however, doesn't mean all babies need to be swaddled at home. Many babies will continue to derive comfort from swaddling (and hence will sleep better) for a few weeks, some even longer. It may also help calm some colicky infants. But all eventually outgrow the need for swaddling, usually once they become more active, and make this clear by trying to kick off the wrapping. Some seem not to need it from the start, perfectly content without it or obviously disturbed with it. A good rule: if swaddling seems to feel good to your baby, do it; if it doesn't, don't.

2. Keep a small plastic bottle of water mixed with a little baking soda handy for spitup spot cleaning. Rubbing a cloth moistened with the mixture on spots will keep them from setting and will eliminate most of the odor. Or use a diaper wipe.

HAVING ENOUGH BREAST MILK

"When my milk came in, my breasts were overflowing. Now that the engorgement is gone, I'm not leaking anymore, and I'm worried I don't have enough milk for my son."

Since the human breast doesn't come equipped with ounce calibrations, it's virtually impossible to discern with the eye how adequate your milk supply is. Instead, you'll have to use your baby as a guide. If he seems to be happy, healthy, and gaining weight well, you're producing enough milk. You don't have to spray like a fountain or leak like a faucet to nurse successfully; the only milk that counts is the milk that goes into your baby. If at any time your baby doesn't seem to be thriving, more frequent nursing plus the other tips on page 101 should help you produce more milk.

"My baby was nursing about every three hours and seemed to be doing very well. Now, suddenly, she seems to want to nurse every hour. Could something have happened to my milk supply?"

Unlike a well, a milk supply is unlikely to dry up if it's used regularly. In fact, quite the contrary is true: the more your baby nurses, the more milk your breasts will produce. A much more plausible explanation for your baby's frequent trips to the breast is a growth or appetite spurt. These occur most commonly at three weeks, six weeks, and three months, but can occur at any time during an infant's development. Sometimes, much to parental dismay, even a baby who has been sleeping through the night begins to wake for a middle of the night feeding during a growth spurt. In this case, a baby's active appetite is merely nature's way of ensuring that her mother's body increases milk production to meet her growth needs.

Just relax and keep your breasts handy until the growth spurt passes. Don't be tempted to give your baby formula (or even worse, solids) to appease her appetite, because a decrease in frequency of nursing would have the side effect of cutting down your supply of milk, which is just the opposite of what the baby ordered. Such a pattern—started by baby wanting to nurse more, leading to mother becoming anxious about the adequacy of her milk supply and offering a supplement, followed by a decrease in milk production—is one of the major causes of breastfeeding being abandoned prematurely.

Sometimes a baby begins to demand more daytime feedings temporarily when she begins to sleep through the night, but this too shall pass with time. If, however, your baby continues to want to nurse hourly (or nearly so) for more than a week, check her weight gain and see below. It could mean she's not getting enough to eat.

YOUR BREASTFED BABY NOT THRIVING

"At three weeks, my baby seems skinnier than when he was born. He seems to nurse a lot, so I can't imagine he isn't getting enough milk. What could be wrong?"

If there's anything capable of producing more anxiety than the course of pregnancy weight gain, it's the course of baby's weight gain during the first few months of life. Except, in most cases, pregnant women worry about gaining too much weight, while new mothers worry about their babies gaining too little.

Occasionally, an infant who had a lot of facial swelling at birth begins to look thinner as the swelling goes down. Most, however, have started to fill out by three weeks, looking less like scrawny chickens and more like rounded babies, though those who see a baby every day may be less aware of the change than those who see him less often. In most cases, you can expect a breastfed baby to regain his birthweight by two weeks and then gain roughly 6 to 8 ounces a week for the next couple of months. If you have some doubt about your baby's progress, you might borrow a baby scale and weigh him. Most likely, you will be reassured by your findings. If you still have concerns about your baby's progress, or you can't locate a scale, ask the doctor if you could bring your baby in for an impromptu weighing—to make you feel better and to catch and correct any problems if they turn out to exist.

The fact that your baby is nursing frequently isn't in itself assurance that he's getting all the food he needs; it may, in fact, indicate the opposite. A baby who isn't being satisfied may nurse almost continuously, trying to get enough nourishment. This may be temporary, as when an infant going through a growth spurt is trying to increase his milk supply (see page 99). Or it may indicate a truly inadequate supply. But there are signs you can look for to reassure you that this isn't so for your baby:

He's having at least five large, seedy, mustardy bowel movements a day. Breast-fed newborns may have a movement after every feeding, sometimes as many as a dozen a day. Fewer than five movements a day in the early weeks could indicate inadequate food intake.

His diaper is wet when he's changed before each feeding and the urine is colorless. If a baby urinates fewer than eight to ten times a day or passes urine that is yellow, possibly fishy-smelling, and/or contains urate crystals (these look like powdered brick, give the wet diaper a pinkish red tinge, and are normal before the mother's breast milk comes in but not later), he is not getting enough fluids. Such signs of dehydration may not, however, show up until the problem has become severe.

You hear a lot of gulping and swallowing as your baby nurses. If you don't, he may not be getting much to swallow. Don't worry, however, about relatively silent eating if baby is gaining well.

He seems happy and content after most feedings. A lot of crying and fussing or frantic finger sucking after a full nursing could mean a baby is still hungry. Not all fussing, of course, is related to hunger—after eating, it could also be related to gas or an attempt to push out a bowel movement.

You experienced breast engorgement when your milk came in. Engorgement is a good sign you can produce milk. And breasts that are fuller when you get up in the morning and after four or five hours without nursing than they are after nursing indicate they are filling with milk regularly—and also that your baby is emptying them. If baby is gaining well, however, lack of engorgement need not concern you.

You notice the sensation of let-down and/or experience milk leakage. Different women experience let-down differently (fullness, tingling, tightening, stinging, cramping, lumpiness, with or without actual dripping or spraying), but feeling it, when you start nursing, hear your baby cry, or even just think about him, indicates that milk is coming down from the storage ducts to the nipples ready to be enjoyed by your baby. Not every woman notices let-down when it occurs, but its absence (in combination with signs of baby's failure to thrive) should raise a warning flag in your mind.

You don't start menstruating during the first three months postpartum. The menses usually doesn't return in a woman who is exclusively breastfeeding, particularly in the first three months. Its premature return may be due to lowered hormone levels, reflecting inadequate milk production.

In addition to routine weighing, the doctor may want you to weigh your baby before and after nursing, without changing his diaper in between. That would tell you how many ounces he's taking at a feeding—at least at that feeding—something a bottle-feeding mother knows automatically.

If the doctor's exam shows your baby isn't thriving on breastfeeding, there are a wide range of possible reasons. Some can be remedied:

You are not feeding baby often enough. In this case, increase feedings to at least eight, even ten, in 24 hours. Don't go more than three hours during the day or five at night between feedings (four-hour schedules were devised for bottle-fed babies, not those on the breast). That means waking up a sleeping baby so that he won't miss dinner or feeding a hungry one even if he just finished a meal an hour earlier. If your baby is "happy to starve" (some newborns are) and never demands feeding, it means taking the initiative yourself and setting a busy feeding schedule for him. Frequent nursings will not only help to fill baby's tummy (and fill out his frame), they will also stimulate your milk production.

You're not emptying at least one breast at each feeding. Nursing for at least ten minutes at the first breast should empty it; if your baby accomplishes this task, let him nurse for as long (or as little) as he likes on the second. Remember to alternate the starting breast at each feeding. Switching breasts every five minutes works better for some women (and their babies), because the baby gets the lion cub's share of milk from each before satiety sets in—but be sure to provide a total of at least ten minutes on the first breast. If baby doesn't do the job, empty the breast with a pump to improve milk production.

Your baby is a lazy or ineffective suckler. This may be because he was preterm, is ill, or has abnormal mouth development (such as a cleft palate or tied tongue). The less effective the suckling, the less milk is produced, setting baby up for failure to thrive. Until he's a strong suckler, he will need help stimulating your breasts to provide adequate milk. This can be done with a breast pump, which you can use to empty the breasts after each feeding (save any

milk you collect for future use in bottles). Until milk production is adequate, your doctor will very likely recommend supplemental feedings of formula via bottles or the supplemental nutrition system shown on this page (which has the advantage of not causing nipple confusion by introducing the artificial nipple) following breast feedings.

If your baby tires easily, you may be advised to nurse for only five minutes on each breast, then follow with a supplement of expressed milk or formula given by bottle or the supplemental nutrition system, both of which require less effort by the baby.

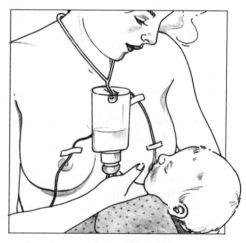

Supplemental Nutrition System: *This vastly useful bit of apparatus can supply baby with supplementary feedings while stimulating mother's milk production. A feeding bottle hangs around the mother's neck; slim tubes leading from the bottle are taped down her breasts, extending slightly past the nipples. The bottle is filled with mother's own milk, collected with a breast pump; with breast milk from a milk bank; or with the formula recommended by the baby's doctor. As baby nurses at the breast, he takes the supplement through the tube. This system avoids the nipple confusion that arises when supplementary feedings are given in a bottle (a baby must learn to suck differently at bottle than at breast) and stimulates the mother to produce more milk even as she is supplementing artificially.*

Your baby hasn't yet learned how to coordinate his jaw muscles for suckling. This ineffective suckler will also need help from a breast pump to stimulate his mother's breasts to begin producing larger quantities of milk. In addition, he will need lessons in improving his suckling technique; the doctor may even recommend physical therapy for him. While your baby is learning, he may need supplemental feedings. For further suggestions on improving suckling technique, call your local La Leche League.

Your nipples are sore or you have a breast infection. Not only can the pain interfere with your desire to nurse, reducing nursing frequency and milk production, it can actually inhibit milk let-down. So take steps to heal sore nipples or cure mastitis (see pages 555 and 556). But do not use a nipple shield, as this can interfere with your baby's ability to latch on to your nipples, compounding your problems.

Your nipples are flat or inverted. It's often difficult for a baby to get a firm hold on such nipples. This situation sets up the negative cycle of not enough suckling, leading to not enough milk, to even less suckling, and less milk. Help baby get a better grip during nursing by taking the areola between your thumb and forefinger and compressing the entire area for his sucking. Use breast shells between feedings to make your nipples easier to draw out, but avoid breast shields during nursing, which, though they can draw nipples out, can prevent baby from properly grasping your nipple and set up a longer-term problem.

Some other factor is interfering with milk let-down. Let-down is a physical function that can be inhibited as well as stimulated by your state of mind. If you're embarrassed or anxious about breastfeeding in general, or in a particular situation, not only can let-down be stifled, but the volume and calorie count of your milk can be affected. So try to feed baby where you are most at ease—in private, if nursing around other people puts you on edge. To help you relax, sit in a comfortable chair, play soft music, have something non-alcoholic to drink (see page 539), try some of the relaxation techniques you learned in childbirth education classes. Massaging the breasts or applying warm soaks just before nursing also encourages let-down. If these aren't effective, ask your baby's doctor about prescribing an oxytocin spray. Though this spray won't increase your milk supply, it will help get the milk you do produce down and out to your baby.

Your baby is getting sucking satisfaction elsewhere. If your baby is getting most of his sucking satisfaction from a pacifier or other non-nutritive source, he may have little interest in the breast. Toss out the pacifier and nurse baby when he seems to want to suck. And don't give him supplementary bottles of water, which not only supply non-nutritive sucking, but can dampen appetites, and, in excess, alter blood sodium levels (see page 137).

You're not burping baby between breasts. A baby who's swallowed air can stop eating before he's had enough because he feels uncomfortably full. Bringing up the air will give him room for more milk. Be sure to burp baby between breasts whether he seems to need it or not, more often if he fusses a lot while nursing.

Your baby is sleeping through the night. An uninterrupted night's sleep is great for mom's looks, but not necessarily for her milk supply. After she undergoes several days of uncomfortable engorgement as baby begins to go seven or eight (or even ten) hours a night without nursing, her milk may begin to diminish, and supplementation may eventually be needed. To avoid this, you may have to wake your baby once in the middle of the night. He shouldn't be going longer than five hours without a feeding at this time.

You've returned to work. Returning to work—and going 8 to 10 hours without nursing during the day—can also decrease the milk supply. One way to prevent this is to express milk at work at least once every four hours you're away from baby.

You're doing too much too soon. Producing breast milk requires a lot of energy. If you're expending yours in other ways and not getting adequate rest, your breast milk supply may diminish. Try a day of almost complete bed rest, followed by three or four days of taking it easy, and see if your baby isn't more satisfied.

You're sleeping on your stomach. When you sleep on your stomach, something a lot of women are eager to do after the later months of pregnancy when they couldn't, you also sleep on your breasts. And the pressure on your breasts could cut down on your milk production—almost as a binder used to prevent lactation would. So turn over, at least partway, to take the pressure off your mammary glands.

You're harboring placental fragments in your uterus. Your body won't accept the fact that you've actually delivered until all the products of pregnancy have been expelled, including all of the placenta. Until it's thoroughly convinced, it may not produce adequate levels of prolactin, the hormone that stimulates milk production. If you have any abnormal bleeding (see page 514) or other signs of retained placental fragments, contact your obstetrician at once. A dilatation and curettage (D and C) could put you and your baby on the right track to successful breastfeeding, while avoiding the danger a retained placenta can pose to your own health.

Even with your best efforts, under the best conditions, with ample support from your doctors, your husband, and your friends, it may turn out that you're still unable to breastfeed successfully. In spite of assurances they may have heard to the contrary, a small percentage of women are simply unable to breastfeed their babies without supplementation, and a very few can't breastfeed at all. The reason may be physical, such as a prolactin deficiency, insufficient mammary glandular tissue, markedly asymmetrical breasts, or damage to the nerves to the nipple caused by breast surgery. Or it could be psychological, due to negative feelings about breastfeeding that can inhibit let-down. Or, occasionally, it may not be pinpointed at all. An early clue that your breasts may not be able to produce adequate milk is their failure to enlarge during pregnancy—though it's not an infallible clue, and may be less reliable in second and subsequent pregnancies than in first ones.

If your baby isn't thriving, and unless the problem appears to be one that can be cleared up in just a few days, his doctor is almost certain to prescribe supplemental formula feedings. Don't despair. What's most important is adequately nourishing your baby, not whether you give breast or bottle. In most cases, when supplementing, you can have the benefits of the direct mother-baby contact that nursing affords by letting baby suckle for pleasure (his and yours) after he's finished his bottle, or by using a supplemental nutrition system.

Ardent breastfeeding advocates may frown at your use of formula; they may recommend that you, instead, radically change your diet, add brewer's yeast, drink beer, or try some other panacea. Though getting the Breastfeeding Daily Dozen (see page 536) is important for keeping up your strength and the quality of your milk, there is no scientific evidence that any dietary manipulations will cure your breastfeeding woes. Try them if you like, but don't let your baby starve while you do.

Once a baby who is not doing well on the breast is put on formula, he almost invariably thrives. In the rare instance that he doesn't, a return trip to the doctor is necessary to see what it is that is interfering with adequate weight gain.

DOUBLE THE TROUBLE, DOUBLE THE FUN

In previous generations, when the stethoscope was an obstetrician's most sophisticated method of prenatal diagnosis, twins often took parents by surprise in the delivery room, leaving no time for the necessary extra preparations. Today, when most expectant parents of twins see double on the ultrasound screen early in pregnancy, mad postpartum dashes to the store for a second set of everything are rare. Though, even with seven or eight month's notice, it may be impossible to prepare completely for the day when babies make four (or if siblings are already on the scene, more). Knowing more about how to plan and what to expect can provide a greater sense of control over what may seem a fundamentally uncontrollable situation.

Be doubly prepared. Since double blessings often come before they're expected, it's a good idea to start organizing for the babies' arrival well in advance of due day. Try to have every childcare item in the house and ready for use before you go to the hospital. (All the preparations suggested in Chapter One for expectant mothers, are doubly important for you.) But while it makes sense to devote a lot of time to preparations, it doesn't make sense to exhaust yourself (particularly if your practitioner has given you specific orders to the contrary). Get plenty of rest before the babies arrive—you can expect it to be a rare luxury once they do.

Double up. Do as much as possible for your babies in tandem. That means waking them at the same time so they can be fed together, putting them in the bath (once they're able to sit in a tub seat) together, walking them in the stroller together. Double bubble the babies together across your lap, or with one on your lap and the other on your shoulder. When you can't manage to double up, alternate. Bathe one one night, the other the next. Or cut down. Bathe them every second or third nights (at an early age daily bathes aren't necessary) and sponge in between.

Split up. The work, that is. When daddy is around, divide the household chores (cooking, cleaning, laundry, marketing) and the babies (you take over one baby, he the other). Be sure that you alternate babies so that both children get to know both parents well, and visa versa.

Try the double-breasted approach. Nursing twins is a physical strain, but eliminates fussing with dozens of bottles and endless ounces of formula. Nursing simultaneously will save time and avoid a daily breastfeeding marathon. You can hold the babies, propped on pillows, in the football position with their feet behind you, or, with one at each breast, their bodies crossed in front of you. Alternate the breast each baby gets at every feeding to avoid creating favorites (and to avoid mismatched breasts, should one baby turn out to be a more proficient sucker than the other). If your milk supply doesn't seem adequate for two, you can nurse one while you bottle feed the other—again alternating from feeding to feeding. To keep up both your energy and your milk supply, be sure to get super nutrition (including 400 to 500 extra calories per baby) and adequate rest.

Plan to have some extra hands on hand, if you're bottle feeding. Bottle feeding twins requires either an extra set of hands or great ingenuity. If you find yourself with two babies and just two hands at feeding time, you can sit on a sofa between the babies with their feet toward the back and hold a bottle for each. Or hold them both in your arms with the bottles in bottle-proppers raised to a comfortable height by pillows. You can also occasionally prop the bottle for one in a baby seat (but never lying down), while you feed the other the traditional way. Feeding them one after the other is another possibility, but one which will significantly cut into the already tiny amount of time you'll have for other activities. Such a procedure will also put the babies on somewhat different napping schedules if they sleep after eating, which can be good if you'd like some time alone with each, or bad if you depend on that tandem sleeping time to get things done for yourself and around the house.

Do half the work. Cut corners on non-essentials. Use paper dishes and take-out food, ignore dust and disorder, rely on paper diapers or diaper service, and easy-care clothes for everyone in the family. Use bibs and rubber pants (if you're determined to use cloth diapers) to protect clothing and cut down on laundry.

Keep twice as many records. Who took what at which feeding, who was bathed yesterday, who's scheduled for today? Unless you keep a log (in a notebook, posted on the nursery wall, or on a blackboard), you're sure to forget. Also make note in a permanent record book of immunizations, illnesses, and so on. Though most of the time, the babies will both get everything that's going around, occasionally only one will—and you may not remember which one.

Sneak sleep. Sleep will necessarily be scarce for the first few months, but it will be scarcer if you allow your babies to waken at random during the night. Instead, when the first cries, wake the second and feed them both. Any time that both your little darlings are napping during the day, catch a few winks yourself—or at least put your feet up.

Double the help. All new mothers need help—you need it twice as much. Accept all the help you can get, from whatever source: spouse, parents, other relatives, friends, local teenagers, paid baby sitters. If you can afford it, hire two baby sitters when you leave your babies during the day. Or sign up two friends or relatives or neighborhood teens. That way, when you take a few hours off, you will know that each of your babies is getting individual attention.

Learn to tune out some of the fussing and crying. You can't be in two places at once, and both you and your twins will have to learn to accept that fact. Pretty soon they will be entertaining each other, giving you more time for other chores.

Double up on equipment. When you don't have another pair of hands around to help, utilize such conveniences as baby carriers (one in the carrier, one in your arms), baby swings (but not until your babies are six weeks old), and infant seats. A playpen is a safe playground for your twins as they get older, and because they'll have each other for company, they will be willing to be relegated to it more often and for longer periods than a singleton. Select a twin stroller to meet your needs (if you will be traversing narrow grocery aisles, for example, a back to front model will be more practical than a side by side one); you will probably find a baby carriage a waste of money. And don't forget that you will need two car seats. (Put one in center front, one in center back, if possible.)

Join a twins network. Parents of twins who've already survived the first few months and more will be your best source of advice and support; be sure to tap them. Find a parents of twins support group in your neighborhood, or if one is lacking, start one—locating members via a notice on your pediatrician's bulletin board. But avoid becoming too clannish, socializing with only the parents of twins and having your babies participate in twins-only playgroups. Though there's something indisputably different about being a twin, excluding your children from relationships with singletons, will discourage normal social development with peers—the majority of whom, of course, will not be twins.

Be doubly alert, once your twins are mobile. Any trouble one baby can get into, two babies can get into—and more often. You'll find, as your babies begin crawling and cruising, that what one of them doesn't think of in the way of mischief, the other will. Consequently, they will need to be watched twice as carefully.

Expect things to get doubly better. The first four months with twins are the hardest; though it never gets easy, handling your twins will become more manageable as you become more adept. Keep in mind, too, that twins are often each other's best company— many have a way of keeping each other busy that mothers of demanding singletons find enviable, and which will free you up more and more in the months and years to come.

THE FONTANELS

*"I'm so nervous when I handle my baby's
head—that soft spot seems so vulnerable.
Sometimes it seems to pulsate, which is
very scary."*

That "soft spot"—actually there are two
and they are called fontanels—is tougher
than it looks. The sturdy membrane covering the fontanels is capable of protecting
the newborn from the probing of even the
most curious sibling fingers, and certainly
from everyday handling.

These openings in the skull, where the
bones haven't yet grown together, aren't
there to make new parents nervous about
handling baby, but for two important reasons. During childbirth, they allow the fetal
head to mold to fit through the birth canal,
something a solidly fused skull couldn't do.
Later, they allow for the tremendous brain
growth of the first year.

The larger of the two openings, the anterior fontanel, is on the top of the newborn's head; it is diamond shaped and may
be as wide as 2 inches. It starts to close
when an infant is six months old and is
usually totally closed by eighteen months.
The fontanel normally appears flat, though
it may bulge a bit when baby cries, and if
baby's hair is sparse and fair, the cerebral
pulse may be visible through it. A depressed anterior fontanel is usually a sign
of dehydration, a warning that the baby
needs to be given fluids promptly. (Call the
baby's doctor immediately to report this
symptom.) A fontanel that bulges persistently may indicate increased pressure
inside the head and also requires immediate medical attention.

The posterior fontanel, a smaller tri-
angular opening toward the back of the
head less than half an inch in diameter,
is much less noticeable, and may be
difficult for you to locate. It is generally
completely closed by the third month.
Fontanels that close prematurely require
medical attention.

NURSING BLISTERS

*"Why does my baby have a blister on her
upper lip? Is she sucking too hard?"*

For a baby with a hearty appetite, there's no
such thing as sucking too hard—although
a new mother with tender nipples may disagree. And though "nursing blisters,"
which develop on the center of the upper
lips of many newborns, both breast and
bottle fed, are caused by vigorous sucking,
they have no medical significance, cause
the infant no discomfort, and will disappear without treatment within a few
months. Sometimes, they even seem to disappear between feedings.

HEALING OF THE UMBILICAL CORD

*"The cord still hasn't fallen off my baby's
belly button, and it looks really awful.
Could it be infected?"*

Healing belly buttons almost always look
and smell worse than they actually are.
What constitutes "perfectly normal" in
medical terms can actually send the weak-
of-knee to the floor as fast as the climactic
scene in a chain-saw horror film.

If you've been taking fastidious care of
the cord stump (see page 88), infection is
unlikely. If, however, you note redness in
the surrounding skin (which could be due
to irritation from alcohol applications as
well as infection) or a discharge from the
navel or from the base of the umbilical
cord, particularly a foul-smelling one,
check with your baby's doctor. If infection
is present, antibiotics will probably be prescribed to clear it up.

The cord, which is shiny and moist at
birth, usually dries up and falls off within a
week or two, but the big event can occur
earlier, or even much later—some babies
don't seem to want to give them up. Until it

does, keep the site dry (no tub baths), exposed to air (turn diaper down and shirt up), and cleaned with alcohol (but try to protect the surrounding skin, perhaps coating with a baby lotion prior to swabbing).

UMBILICAL HERNIA

"Every time she cries, my baby's navel seems to stick out. Our baby's nurse says it's a hernia and wants to wrap a belly band around the baby's middle."

The diagnosis is probably correct, but the treatment is definitely wrong. Prenatally, all babies have an opening in the abdominal wall through which blood vessels extend into the umbilical cord. In some cases (for black babies more often than white) the opening doesn't close completely at birth. When these babies cry or strain, a small coil of intestine bulges through the opening, raising the umbilicus, and often the area around it, in a lump that ranges from fingertip to lemon size. While the appearance of such a lump (especially when it's tagged with the ominous-sounding term "hernia") might be alarming, it's rarely cause for concern. The intestine almost never strangulates in the opening, and in most cases the hernia eventually resolves without intervention. Small openings usually close spontaneously or become inconsipicuous within a few months, large ones by a year and a half or two.

Belly bands (or binders), band-aids, and adhesive-taped coins are outdated and ineffective remedies, and the tape can irritate skin. The best treatment is usually no treatment at all. Though surgery to correct umbilical hernias is simple, safe, and sure, it isn't recommended unless the opening in the abdomen is very large, is growing larger, bothers baby, or upsets mother. Often the pediatrician will suggest waiting until the child is six or seven before considering surgery, because most hernias will have closed by then. If, however, you see

signs of strangulation—the lump does not receed after crying, can't be pushed in, suddenly becomes larger, is tender, baby is vomiting—go to the ER. Immediate surgery may be needed.

Don't confuse a navel that protrudes temporarily (before the cord drops off) or permanently (an "outie") with a hernia. A hernia expands with crying, a protruding navel doesn't.

SNEEZING

"My baby sneezes all the time. He doesn't seem sick, but I'm afraid he's caught a cold."

Hold off on the chicken soup. What your baby's caught isn't likely to be a cold, but some amniotic fluid and excess mucus in his respiratory passages, very common in young babies. And to clear it out, nature has provided him with a protective reflex: sneezing. Frequent sneezing (and coughing, another protective reflex), also helps the newborn to get rid of foreign particles from the environment that make their way to his nose—much as sniffing pepper makes many adults sneeze.

CROSSED EYES

"The swelling is down around my baby's eyes. Now she seems cross-eyed."

Babies are very obliging: they always give their mothers something new to worry about. And most mothers worry plenty when they notice their babies' eyes appear to be crossed. Actually, in most cases, it's simply extra folds of skin at the inner corners of the eyes that make the babies look cross-eyed. When the folds retract as baby grows, the eyes begin to seem more evenly matched.

During the early months, you may also notice that your baby's eyes may not work in perfect unison all the time. These random eye movements mean she's still learning to use her eyes and strengthening her eye muscles; by three months, coordination should be much improved. If it isn't, or if your baby's eyes always seem to be out of synch, then talk to her doctor about the problem. If there is a possibility of strabismus, or true crossed eyes (in which the baby uses just one eye to focus on what she's looking at, and the other just seems aimed anywhere) consultation with a pediatric ophthalmologist is in order. Early treatment is important, because so much that a child learns she learns through her eyes; and because ignoring crossed eyes could lead to amblyopia or "lazy" eye (in which the eye that isn't being used becomes lazy and consequently weaker, from disuse).

TEARY EYES

"At first, there were no tears when my baby cried. Now her eyes seem filled with tears even when she's not crying. And sometimes they overflow."

Tearless crying is common in newborns. It is not until near the end of the first month of life that the fluid that bathes the eye (called tears) begins to be produced in the lacrimal glands over the eyeballs. The fluid normally drains through tiny lacrimal ducts, located at the inner corner of each eye, and into the nose, which is why a lot of crying can make your nose run. The ducts are particularly tiny in infants and in 1 in 100 babies, one or both are blocked at birth.

Since a blocked tear duct doesn't drain properly, tears fill the eyes and often spill over, producing the perpetually "teary-eyed" look even in happy babies. Most clogged ducts will clear up by themselves by the end of the first year without treatment, though your baby's doctor may recommend massaging the ducts to hasten the clearing. (If you do use massage and the baby's eyes become puffy or red, stop massaging and inform the doctor.)

Sometimes there is a small accumulation of yellowish white mucus in the inner corner of the eye with a tear duct blockage, and the lids may be stuck together when baby wakes up in the morning. Mucus and crust can be washed away with cooled boiled water and sterile absorbent cotton balls. A heavy, darker yellow discharge and/or reddening of the whites of the eye, however, may indicate infection and the need for medical attention. The doctor may prescribe antibiotic ointments or drops, and if the duct becomes chronically infected, may refer your baby to an ophthalmologist. The eye doctor may recommend probing the duct with a very thin wire to establish normal tear flow, or may suggest continuing to wait it out, possibly until your child is a year old or so. Very, very rarely, probing doesn't work and surgery is needed.

FIRST SMILES

"Everybody says that my baby's smiles are 'just gas,' but he looks so happy when he does it. Couldn't they be real?"

They read it in books and magazines. They hear it from mothers-in-law, friends with children, their pediatricians, perfect strangers in the park. And yet, no new mother wants to believe that her baby's first smiles are the work of a passing bubble of gas, rather than of a wave of love meant especially for her.

But alas, it appears from scientific evidence so far to be true: most babies don't smile in the true social sense before four to six weeks of age. That doesn't mean that a smile is always "just gas." It also may be a sign of comfort and contentment—many babies smile as they are falling asleep, as they urinate, or when their cheeks are stroked.

When baby does display his first real smile, you'll know it, and you'll melt accordingly. In the meantime, enjoy those glimpses of smiles to come—undeniably adorable no matter what their cause.

KEEPING BABY THE RIGHT TEMPERATURE

"It seems too hot out for a sweater and hat, but when I bring my baby out in just his T-shirt and diaper, everyone on the street complains that he's underdressed."

As far as well-meaning strangers on buses, in stores, and on the street are concerned, new mothers (even if they are on their second or third child) can do no right. So get used to the criticism. But for the most part, don't let it affect how you take care of your baby. Grandmothers and grandmotherly types will go to their graves claiming otherwise, but once a baby's natural thermostat is properly set (within the first few days of life), you needn't dress him any more warmly than you dress yourself. (And in fact, prior to that, too much clothing can be as taxing to the newborn's heat-regulating mechanism as too little.)

So in general, use your own comfort (unless you're the kind of person who's always warm when everybody else is cold, or always cold when everybody else is warm) as a gauge in determining whether baby is comfortable. If you're unsure, don't check his hands for confirmation (as those "well-meaners" will, with disapproving clucks of "See! His hands are cold!"). A baby's hands and feet are usually cooler than the rest of his body, again due to an immature circulatory system. Don't take the fact that your baby sneezes a few times to mean he's cold either; he may sneeze in reaction to sunlight or because he needs to clear his nose. If it's warm out, your baby is not underdressed.

While you needn't listen to strangers, do listen to your baby. Babies will tell you that they are cold (as they tell you most everything else) by fussing or crying. When you get such a message, check the nape of the neck, arms, or trunk (whichever is easiest to reach under baby's clothing) with the back of your hand for a temperature reading. If baby feels comfortably warm, maybe it's a hungry or tired cry you're

hearing. (And if he's sweaty, he's probably overdressed.) If he's cool, add clothing or covering, or turn up the thermostat. If a young baby seems extremely cold, get him to a warm place right away because his body probably can't produce enough heat to rewarm himself even if he has a lot of covering. In the meantime, put him close to the warmth of your body, under your shirt if necessary.

The one part of a baby that needs extra protection in all kinds of weather is his head; partly because a lot of heat is lost from the uncovered head, and partly because most babies have very little protection in the way of hair. On even marginally cool days, a hat is a good idea for a baby under a year old. In hot, sunny weather a hat with a brim will protect baby's head, face, and eyes—but even with this protection exposure to full sun should be no more than fleeting.

A young baby also needs extra protection from heat loss when he's sleeping. In deep sleep his heat-producing mechanism slows down, so in cooler weather bring along an extra blanket or covering for his nap. If he sleeps in a cool room at night, a blanket sleeper or warm quilt will help him stay warm.

When it comes to dressing baby in cold weather, the layered look is not only fashionable, it's sensible. Several light layers of clothing retain body heat more efficiently than one heavy layer, and the outer layers can be peeled off as needed when you walk into an overheated store or board a stuffy bus, or if the weather takes a sudden turn for the warmer.

An occasional baby falls outside the norm for body temperature control—just as the occasional adult does. If your baby seems cooler than you do, or warmer, all the time, then accept that fact. You may find in talking to your in-laws that your spouse was the same way as a baby. That means, for the cooler baby, more coverings and warmer clothes than you would usually need. For the warmer baby (you'll probably discover this because of heat rash even in the winter), it means fewer coverings and lighter clothes.

TAKING BABY OUT

"It's been ten days since I brought my baby home from the hospital, and I'm starting to go stir-crazy cooped up in the house. When can I take her out?"

Unless your hospital and your home are connected by subterranean tunnel, you've taken your baby outside already. And barring a blizzard, a rainstorm, or significantly subfreezing temperatures, you could have conceivably continued to take her outside every day since. Old wives' tales (which continue to be perpetuated by even not-so-old mothers and mothers-in-law) that have kept newborns and new mothers captives in their own homes for two weeks postpartum and more are completely invalid. Any baby hardy enough to leave the hospital is hardy enough to weather a stroll through the park, a trip to the supermarket, even a lengthy excursion to visit grandmother (though in flu season, you might want to limit baby's exposure to indoor crowds, especially for the first month). Assuming you're up to the exercise (you're more likely to need rest than your baby, and should spend a lot of time off your feet for at least the first postpartum week), feel free to plan that first escape from the confines of your home.

When you take baby out, dress her appropriately and always take along an extra covering if there's a possibility of a change for the cooler in the weather. If it's windy or rainy, use a weather shield on the stroller or carriage; if it's very chilly or extremely hot and humid, limit the amount of time your baby spends out of doors—if you're freezing or sweltering, she is too. Avoid more than brief exposure to direct sunlight, even in mild weather. If your outing is in a car, be sure your baby is properly harnessed in her infant safety seat.

EXPOSURE TO OUTSIDERS

"Everybody wants to touch our son. The doorman, the clerk in the supermarket, old women in stores, visitors we have in our home. I'm always worried about germs."

There's nothing that cries out to be squeezed more than a new baby. Baby cheeks, fingers, chin, toes—they're all irresistible. And yet resist is just what most mothers would like outsiders to do when it comes to their newborns.

Your fear of your baby picking up germs this way is a legitimate one. A very young infant is more susceptible to infection because his immune system is still relatively immature and he hasn't had a chance to build up immunities. So, for now at least, politely ask strangers to look but don't touch—particularly the hands, which usually end up in baby's mouth. You can always blame it on the doctor: "The pediatrician said not to let anyone outside the family handle him yet." As for friends and family, ask them to wash their hands before picking up baby, at least for the first month. This should continue indefinitely when those who have a communicable illness handle your baby. And skin-to-skin contact should be avoided with anyone who has a rash or open sores.

No matter what you do or say, expect that every once in a while your baby will have some contact with strangers. All is not lost. If a friendly checker in the supermarket tests your child's grasp on his finger, just pull out a diaper wipe and wash off baby's hands—discreetly, of course.

As your baby gets older, however, he needn't—and shouldn't—be raised in a plastic bubble environment. He needs to be exposed to a wide variety of "bugs" in order to start building up immunities to those common in your community. So loosen up a little and let the germs fall where they may after the first month.

SKIN COLOR CHANGES

"My baby suddenly turned two colors— reddish blue on the bottom and pale on top. What's wrong with her?"

There's probably little more frightening than watching your baby turn color before your eyes. And yet there's virtually nothing to fear when a newborn suddenly takes on a split-color appearance, either side to side or top to bottom. As a result of her immature circulatory system, blood has simply pooled on half of your baby's body. Turn her upside down (or, if the color difference is side by side, over) momentarily, and normal color will be restored.

You may also notice that your baby's hands and feet appear bluish, even though the rest of her body is pink. This, too, is due to immature circulation and usually disappears by the end of the first week.

"Sometimes when I'm changing my new baby I notice his skin seems to be mottled all over. Why?"

Purplish (sometimes more red, sometimes more blue) mottling of a tiny baby's skin is sure to raise questions in his parents' minds. But mottling when a baby is chilled or crying is not at all unusual. These transient changes are yet another sign of an immature circulatory system, visible through baby's still very thin skin. He should outgrow this phenomenon in a few months. In the meantime, when it occurs, check the nape of his neck or his midsection to see if he is too cool. If so, increase his clothing or covering. If not, just relax and wait for the mottling to disappear, as it probably will in a few minutes.

FEEDING SCHEDULE

"I seem to be nursing my new daughter all the time. Whatever happened to the four-hour schedules I've heard about?"

Unfortunately, your baby (and all the other nursing babies you'll notice nipping at their mother's breasts almost continuously in the first few months of life) hasn't heard about the four-hour schedule. Hunger calls and she wants to eat—a lot more often than most "schedules" would permit her to.[3]

Let her—at least for now. Three- and four-hour schedules are based on the needs of bottle-fed newborns, who usually do very well on such regimens. But most breastfed babies need to eat more often than that. First of all, because breast milk is digested more quickly than formula, making them feel hungry again sooner. Second, because frequent nursing helps establish a good milk supply—the foundation of a successful breastfeeding relationship.

Nurse as frequently as baby seems to want to during the early weeks. But if your baby is still demanding food every hour at three weeks of age or so, check with the doctor to see if her weight gain is normal. If it isn't, seek advice from the doctor, and see "Your Breastfed Baby not Thriving," page 99. If she seems to be thriving, however, it's time to start making demands of your own. Hourly nursing is not only too much of an emotional strain for you, it's a physical strain as well, and will probably result in sore nipples and fatigue. Neither is it best for your baby, since she needs longer periods of sleep and longer periods of wakefulness when she isn't eating and when she should be looking at something other than a breast.

Assuming your milk supply is well established, you can start thinking about fitting your baby into a schedule of sorts. Try stretching the periods between feedings (which may also help your baby sleep better at night). When baby wakes crying an

3. Do remember, however, that like labor contractions, intervals between feedings are timed from the beginning of one to the beginning of the next. So a baby who nurses for forty minutes starting at 10 A.M., then sleeps for an hour and twenty minutes before eating again, is on a two-hour schedule, not a one-hour-and-twenty-minute one.

hour after feeding, don't rush to feed her. If she still seems sleepy, try to get her back to sleep without nursing her. Before picking her up, pat or rub her back, turn on a musical toy, and see if she'll drift back off. If not, pick her up, sing softly to her, walk with her, rock her, again with the goal of getting her back to sleep. If she seems alert, don't rush to feed her. Change her, talk to her, distract her in some other way, even take her for a stroll out of doors. She may become so interested in you and the rest of the world that she actually forgets about your breasts—at least for a few minutes.

When you finally do nurse, don't accept the snack-bar approach some babies try to take; encourage her to nurse at least ten minutes on each side—twenty would be even better. If she refuses to nurse this long, start with five minutes on each side so that she fills up with most of the milk from both breasts in ten minutes, then return her to the first breast to continue for as long as she likes. If she falls off to sleep, try to waken her to continue the meal. If you can manage to stretch the periods between nursings a little more each day, eventually you and baby will be on a more reasonable schedule: two to three hours, and eventually four or so. But it should be a schedule based on her hunger, not the clock.

HICCUPS

"My baby gets the hiccups all the time— and for no apparent reason. Do they bother him as much as they do me?"

Some babies aren't just born hiccupers, they're hiccupers before they're born. And chances are, if your baby hiccuped a lot inside of you, he'll hiccup plenty in the first few months on the outside, too. But a newborn's hiccups, unlike the adult variety, don't have a known cause. They are believed to be another of baby's reflexes, though they're frequently triggered by giggling later on. And also unlike adult hiccups, they're not bothersome, at least not to

baby. If they are to you, try letting your baby nurse or suck on a bottle of water, which may quell the attack.

BOWEL MOVEMENTS

"I expected one, maybe two bowel movements a day from my breastfed baby. But she seems to have one in every diaper— sometimes as many as ten a day. And they're very loose. Could she have diarrhea?"

Your baby isn't the first breastfed infant ever who seemed to be aiming to beat the Guinness World Record for dirtying diapers. Not only is such an active elimination pattern not a bad sign in a breastfed newborn, it's a good one. Since the amount that's coming out is related to the amount going in, any breastfeeding mother whose newborn has five or more movements daily can be assured that her baby is getting sufficient nourishment. (Mothers of nursing newborns who have fewer movements should see page 100.) The number of movements progressively decreases and may dwindle down to no more than one a day, or every other day, next month, though some babies continue to have several movements a day for the entire first year. It's not necessary to keep count—the number may vary from day to day, and that's perfectly normal, too.

Normal, too, for breastfed infants is a very soft, sometimes even watery, stool. But diarrhea—frequent stools that are liquidy, smelly, and may contain mucus, often accompanied by fever and/or weight loss— is rare among children who dine on breast milk. If they do get it, they have fewer, smaller movements than bottle babies with diarrhea and recover more quickly, probably because of the antibacterial properties of breast milk.

CONSTIPATION

"I'm worried that my baby is constipated. He's been averaging only one movement every two or three days. Could it be his formula?"

Constipation has been flippantly defined as having movements less often than your mother. But that's an unreliable gauge, since each individual has a personal pattern of elimination, and it's not necessarily a case of "like mother, like child." Some bottle-fed babies go three or four days between movements. But they're not considered to be constipated unless those infrequent movements are firmly formed or come out in hard pellets, or if they cause pain or bleeding (from a fissure or crack in the anus as a result of pushing). If your baby's movements are soft and cause no problems, don't worry. But if you suspect constipation, consult his doctor. It's possible a change in formula or the addition of a couple of tablespoons of diluted prune or other fruit juice to the baby's diet might help. (Citrus juices should not be introduced at this early age, since they are highly allergenic and very acidic.) But don't take any steps such as giving laxatives (especially mineral oil), enemas, or herbal teas without medical advice.

"I thought breastfed babies were never constipated—but my daughter grunts and groans and strains whenever she has a bowel movement."

It's true that breastfed babies are rarely constipated because breast milk is just the right match for the human baby's digestive tract. But it's also true that some have to push and strain to get their movements out, even though the movement comes out soft and seems as though it should have been easy to pass.[4] Why this is so isn't certain. Some have theorized it's because the soft stool of the breastfed baby doesn't put adequate pressure on the anus. Others speculate that the muscles of the anus are neither strong enough nor coordinated enough to eliminate any stool easily. Still others point to the fact that young babies, who usually have bowel movements lying down, get no help from gravity.

Whatever the reason, the difficulty should ease up when solids are added to your baby's diet. But in the meantime, don't worry. And don't use laxatives (especially not mineral oil), enemas, or any other home remedies for the problem—because it really isn't one. When an adult is constipated, walking often helps alleviate the problem; you might try flexing and extending your baby's legs in a bicycling motion while she's on her back to assist her when she seems uncomfortable. And once she starts eating table foods, be sure she gets plenty of whole grains and legumes, fruits, and vegetables—and eventually, exercise.

EXPLOSIVE BOWEL MOVEMENTS

"My son's bowel movements come with such force and such explosive sound, I'm worried that he has some digestive problem. Or maybe something's wrong with my breast milk."

Breastfed newborns are rarely discreet when it comes to making bowel movements. The noisy barrage that fills the room as they fill their diapers can often be heard in the next room, and can alarm first-time parents. Yet these movements and the surprising variety of sounds that punctuate their passing are normal, the result of gas being forcefully expelled from an immature digestive system. Things should quiet down in a month or two.

4. If your breastfed baby has very infrequent bowel movements and is not gaining well, then see page 99 and check with your doctor. It's possible she isn't getting enough to eat and thus has not much to eliminate.

PASSING GAS

"My baby passes gas all day long—very loudly. Could she be having stomach troubles?"

The digestive exclamations that frequently explode from a newborn's tiny bottom, at least as emphatically as the grownup variety, can be unsettling—and sometimes embarrassing—to parents. But, like explosive bowel movements, they are perfectly normal. Once your newborn's digestive system works out the kinks, the gas will pass more quietly and less frequently.

MILK ALLERGY

"My baby is crying a lot, and a friend suggested that he might be allergic to the milk in his formula. How can I tell?"

Though friends are likely to blame excessive crying on a milk allergy, and mothers are so anxious to blame the crying on something other than themselves that they're likely to accept that explanation, doctors are less quick to do so. Milk allergy is the most common food allergy in infants, but it is less common than most people believe. Most doctors believe it an unlikely possibility in a child whose parents don't have allergies, and in one whose only symptom is crying. A baby who is having a severe allergic response to milk will usually vomit frequently and have loose, watery stools, possibly tinged with blood. (It's important to uncover the cause of such symptoms promptly since they can lead to dehydration and a serious chemical imbalance.) Less severe reactions may include occasional vomiting and loose mucous stools. Some babies who are allergic to milk may also have eczema, hives, wheezing, and/or a nasal discharge or stuffiness when exposed to milk protein.

Unfortunately, there's no simple test to determine hypersensitivity (allergy) to milk with any degree of accuracy, except

through trial and error. If you suspect milk allergy, discuss the possibility with your baby's doctor before taking any action. If there is no history of allergy in your family, and if there are no symptoms other than the crying, then it is likely the doctor will suggest you treat the crying spells as ordinary colic (see page 122).

If there are family allergies or symptoms other than crying, a trial change of formula—to hydrolysate (in which the protein is partly broken down or predigested) or soy—may be recommended. A rapid improvement in the colicky behavior and the disappearance of other symptoms, if any, would suggest the possibility of an allergy to milk—or it could just be a coincidence. Reinstating the milk formula is one way of verifying the diagnosis; if the symptoms return with the milk, allergy is likely.

In many cases there's no change when a baby is switched to a soy formula. This may mean he's also allergic to soy, has a medical condition that has nothing to do with milk and that needs to be diagnosed, or simply has an immature digestive system. A switch from soy to hydrolysate formula should help if the baby seems to be sensitive to both soy and milk. In some cases, goat's milk may be recommended, but because it lacks folic acid, look for the type that is fortified with that vitamin.

Very rarely, the problem is an enzyme deficiency—the infant is born unable to produce lactase, the enzyme needed to digest the milk sugar lactose. Such a child has persistent diarrhea from the start, and fails to gain weight. A formula containing little or no lactose will usually resolve the problem. Unlike a temporary lactose intolerance that sometimes develops during a bout with an intestinal bug, a congenital lactase deficiency is usually permanent. The afflicted baby will probably never be able to tolerate ordinary milk products—though he will probably be fine on those that are lactose-reduced.

If the problem is not traced to milk allergy or intolerance, you should probably switch back to a cow's milk formula, since it is the better breast milk substitute.

Infant allergy to cow's milk is usually outgrown by the end of the first year, and almost always by the end of the second. If your baby is taken off cow's milk formula, his doctor may suggest trying it again after six months on a substitute formula, or may suggest waiting until the first birthday.

USING DETERGENT ON BABY'S CLOTHES

"I've been using baby soap flakes to wash my daughter's clothes. But nothing seems to come clean, and I'm also getting tired of doing her loads separately. When can I start using detergent?"

Although manufacturers of special baby laundry soaps wouldn't want it to get around, many babies probably don't need their clothes washed separately from the rest of the family's. Even the kind of high-potency detergents that really get clothes clean, eliminating most stains and odors, aren't irritating to most babies when they're well rinsed. (Rinsing is most thorough, and stain-fighting powers are most effective, with liquid detergents.) An added advantage of using detergents: since they aren't taboo on fire-retardant garments, as soap products are, all of baby's clothes can be tossed in together.

To test your baby's sensitivity to your favorite laundry detergent, add one garment that will be worn close to baby's skin (such as a T-shirt) to your next family load, being careful not to overdo the detergent or underdo the rinse. If baby's skin shows no rash or irritation, feel free to wash her clothes with yours. If a rash does appear, try another detergent, preferably one without colors and fragrances, before deciding you have to stick with soap flakes.

RESTLESS SLEEP

"Our baby, who shares our room, tosses and turns all night. Could our being near be keeping him from sleeping soundly?"

Although the phrase "sleeping like a baby" is often equated with enviably peaceful and restful sleep, particularly by the manufacturers of mattresses and sleep aids, babies' sleep isn't restful at all. Newborns do sleep a lot, but they also wake up a lot in the process. That's because most of their sleep is REM (rapid eye movement) sleep, an active sleep with dreaming and a lot of movement. At the end of each REM sleep period, the sleeper usually awakens briefly. When you hear your baby fuss or whimper at night, it's probably because he's finishing a REM period, not because you share a room with him.

As he gets older, his sleeping patterns will mature. He will have less REM sleep and longer periods of the much sounder "quiet sleep," from which it's harder to rouse him. He will continue to stir and whimper periodically, but less frequently.

Though your being in the same room with baby probably isn't disturbing his sleep at this stage (though it may soon), it certainly is disturbing yours. Not only do you waken at every moan, but you also are tempted to pick him up more often than necessary during the night. Try to ignore your baby's midnight murmurings; pick him up only when he begins to cry steadily and seriously. You'll both sleep better. If you find that difficult, then perhaps you should consider separate sleeping quarters—if you have the space.

Do be alert, however, for sudden waking and crying, unusual restlessness, or other changes in sleeping patterns that don't seem to be related to events in baby's life (such as teething or an overstimulating day). If you note them, check for such signs of illness as fever, appetite loss, or diarrhea (see Chapter 17). Call your doctor if the symptoms persist.

SLEEPING PATTERNS

"I thought newborns were supposed to sleep all the time. Our three-week-old daughter hardly seems to sleep at all."

Newborns often seem not to know what they're "supposed to do." They nurse erratically when they're "supposed to" be on a three- or four-hour schedule, or they sleep 12 hours a day (or 22) when they're "supposed to" sleep 16½ hours. That's because they know what we often forget—that there's almost nothing a baby is supposed to do at any specific time. "Average" babies, who do everything by the book, do exist. But they are in the minority. The 16½ hours that is the average sleeping time for babies in their first month of life takes into account babies who sleep 10 hours a day and others who sleep 23, as well as all those in between. The baby who falls at either end of the spectrum is no less normal than one who falls near the average. Some infants, like some adults, appear to need more sleep than others, some less.

So assuming your baby seems healthy in every way, don't worry about her wakefulness, but do get used to it. Infants who sleep very little tend to grow into children who sleep very little—with parents who, not coincidentally, also sleep very little.

"My baby gets up several times a night. My mother says if I don't get her into a regular sleeping pattern now, she may never develop good sleep habits. She says I should let her cry it out instead of feeding her all night."

Any experienced mother, particularly one who's had difficulty with a baby who wouldn't sleep through the night or who had trouble falling asleep, knows the importance of fostering good sleep habits in children at an early age. But the first month of life is too early. Your baby is just beginning to learn about the world. The most important lesson she needs to learn now is that when she calls, you will be there— even at 3 A.M., and even when she's up for

the fourth time in six hours. "Crying it out" has its place in helping a baby figure out how to fall asleep by herself, but not for several months yet—not until she begins to feel more secure and more in control of her environment.

If you're breastfeeding, trying to institute a sleeping schedule now could also interfere with establishing a good milk supply—and with your baby's growth. Breast-fed newborns need to eat more frequently than bottle-fed babies, often every two hours, which generally prevents them from sleeping through the night until somewhere between the third and sixth months. Like the time-honored four-hour feeding schedule, the belief that babies should sleep through the night by two months is based on the developmental behavior of bottle-fed infants, and is often unrealistic for those who are nursing.

So, as your mother advises, do think ahead about building some discipline into your child's sleeping habits, but don't let her cry it out just yet.

NOISE WHEN BABY IS SLEEPING

"I have a friend who turns off the phone when her son is sleeping, has a note on the door asking people to knock instead of ring, and tiptoes around the apartment at nap time. Isn't this a little extreme?"

Your friend is programming her child to be unable to sleep except under controlled environmental conditions, conditions that she will find virtually impossible to maintain on a permanent basis—unless her baby's bedroom is a padded cell.

And what's more, her efforts will probably be counterproductive. Though a sudden loud sound may waken some babies, others can sleep through fireworks, wailing sirens, and barking dogs. For most, however, a steady hum of background noise—from a TV or stereo, a fan or air conditioner, a musical toy or one that imitates uterine sounds, or from a white-noise machine—appears to be more conducive to restful sleep than perfect silence, particularly if the baby has fallen asleep to the beat of such sounds.

Just how much noise, as well as what kinds of noise, a baby can sleep through depends in part on the sounds he became accustomed to before birth and partly on individual temperament. So parents have to take their cues from their babies in determining how far they must go to protect them from unnecessary interruptions to sleep during naps and at night. If a baby turns out to be especially sound sensitive during sleep, it's probably wise to turn the phone down to low, to change the doorbell to a less abrasive ring, and to play the radio or TV more softly. Such tactics are unnecessary, however, if a baby sleeps through everything.

By attempting to turn off all the sound in her baby's life, your friend is very likely going to make it difficult for her child to get a good night's sleep later on, when he has to sleep in the real world.

PACIFIER

"My baby has crying jags in the afternoon. Should I give him a pacifier to comfort him?"

In the long run, it's probably best for babies to learn, to some extent, to comfort themselves rather than to rely on artificial aids such as a pacifier. A thumb (or a fist) can do the job of providing extra sucking for comfort as well as a pacifier, but it's in the baby's control, not the parents'. It's there whenever he needs it; can be plucked out when he wants to smile, coo, cry, or otherwise express himself; and it won't cause nipple confusion, as a pacifier can in young infants just learning to suckle at the breast.

Because of nipple confusion, it's not a good idea to introduce a breastfeeding baby to the pacifier until lactation is well established. It shouldn't be used at all for a baby who isn't gaining weight at an adequate clip or one who is a poor nurser, because it may give him so much sucking satisfaction that he loses interest in suckling at the breast.

Occasionally a pacifier may be warranted temporarily for a baby who cries a lot and is soothed by nothing else, or for one who wants more sucking satisfaction but hasn't yet figured out how to get his fingers to his mouth. But be aware that pacifier use easily slips into pacifier abuse. What starts out as the baby's crutch can easily become the mother's. There is the ever-present temptation to use the pacifier as a convenient substitute for the attention she herself should be providing to her child. The well-meaning mother who offers the pacifier to make sure her baby has adequate sucking experience may soon find herself popping in a pacifier the moment he becomes fussy, instead of trying to determine the reason for the fussing or if there might be other ways of placating him. She may use it to get the baby off to sleep instead of reading him a story, to ensure quiet while she's on the phone intead of picking him up and consoling him while she's chatting, to buy his silence while she's picking out a pair of new shoes instead of involving him in the interaction. The result is often a baby who can only be happy with something in his mouth, and who is unable to comfort himself, entertain himself, or get himself to sleep.

Used at night, a pacifier can interfere with a baby's learning to fall asleep by himself, and can also interrupt his sleep when he loses it in the middle of the night and can't get back to dreamland without it—and who do you think will have to rise to put it back in his mouth?

Another drawback, albeit a temporary one: as with thumb sucking, sucking on a pacifier can distort the mouth, but this distortion self corrects if the habit is abandoned before the permanent teeth appear.

If you feel you must use a pacifier occasionally for your baby, do so wisely.

Be sure the pacifier you buy has air holes and is all one piece, so a part won't break off and become a choking hazard. (Those made of silicone are softer than those made of rubber, are long lasting, dishwasher safe, and don't become sticky.) *Never* attach a pacifier to the crib, carriage, playpen, or stroller, or hang it around your baby's neck or wrist with a ribbon, string, or cord of any kind—babies have been strangled this way. To avoid development of a strong habit, begin withdrawal from the pacifier by the time your baby is three months old. Until then, each time you consider plugging it in, ask yourself first whether it's the pacifier or you the baby needs.

CHECKING BABY'S BREATHING

"Everybody always jokes about sneaking into the baby's room to hear if he's breathing. Well, now I find myself doing just that—even in the middle of the night. Sometimes you can hardly hear his breathing, other times it's very noisy."

A new parent neurotically checking a baby's breathing does seem like good grist for a joke mill—until you become a new parent. And then it's no laughing matter. You wake in a cold sweat to complete silence after putting baby to bed five hours earlier. Could something be wrong? Why didn't he wake up? Or you pass his crib and he seems so silent and still that you have to shake him gingerly to be sure he's still alive. Or he's grunting and snorting so hard you're sure he's having trouble breathing. You—and millions of other new parents.

Not only are your concerns normal, but your baby's varied breathing patterns when he snoozes are, too. A major part of a newborn's sleep is spent in REM (rapid eye movement) sleep, a time when he breathes irregularly, grunts and snorts and twitches a lot—you can even see his eyes moving

under the lids. The rest of his slumber is spent in quiet sleep, when he breathes very deeply and quietly and seems very still, except for occasional sucking motions or startling. As he gets older he will experience less REM sleep, and the quiet sleep will become more like the non-REM sleep of adults. You will eventually become less panicky about whether or not he's going to wake up in the morning, and more comfortable with both you and him sleeping eight hours at a stretch.

Still, you may never totally be able to abandon the habit of checking on your child's breathing (at least once in a while) until he's off to college and sleeping in a dorm—out of sight, though not out of mind.

MIXING UP OF NIGHT AND DAY

"My three-week-old sleeps most of the day and wants to stay up all night. How can I get her to reverse her schedule so my husband and I can get some rest?"

Babies who work (or play) the night shift, getting most of their sleep by day, can turn normally active, alert parents into barely functioning zombies. Happily, this blissful ignorance of the difference between day and night isn't a permanent condition. The newborn who, before her arrival in the world of daytime light and nighttime darkness, was kept in the dark for nine months just needs a little time to adjust.

Chances are your baby will stop mixing up her days and nights within the next few weeks on her own. If you'd like to help speed the process, try limiting her daytime naps to no more than three or four hours each. Although waking a sleeping infant— except when you don't want to—can be tricky, it's usually possible. Try holding her upright, eliciting a burp, stripping off her clothes, rubbing under her chin, or tickling her feet. Once she's somewhat alert, try to further stimulate her: talk to her, sing lively

BETTER SLEEP FOR BABY

Whether a good sleeper or a poor one, your baby can be helped to sleep to potential with some or all of the following sleep enhancers, many of which help re-create some of the comforts of home in the womb:

Cozy sleeping space. A crib is a great modern invention—but in the early weeks many newborns somehow sense its vastness and balk when sentenced to solitude, smack in the center of its mattress, so clearly removed from its distant walls. If your baby seems uncomfortable in the crib, an old-fashioned cradle, a bassinet, or a baby carriage can be used for the first few months to provide a snugger fit that's closer to the nine-month-long embrace in the uterus. For added security swaddle baby, tuck bedding in snugly, and use a gown that ties at the bottom, or a baby sleeping bag instead of a blanket.

Controlled temperature. Being too warm or too cold can disturb a baby's sleep. For tips on keeping baby comfortable in warm weather, see page 385; for tips in cold weather, see page 393.

Soothing movement. In the uterus, babies are most active when their mothers are at rest; when their mothers are up and on the go they slow down, lulled by the motion. Out of the womb, movement still has a soothing effect. Rocking, swaying, and patting will all contribute to contentment—and sleep.

Soothing sound. For many months your heartbeat, the gurgling of your tummy, and your voice entertained and comforted your baby. Now sleeping may be difficult without some background noise. Try the hum of a fan or an air cleaner, the soft strains of music from a radio or stereo, the tinkling of a music box or musical mobile, or one of those baby soothers that imitate uterine or auto sounds.

Isolation. Babies sleep better when they are in a room of their own. At this stage it's not so much that they're disturbed by your presence, but that you're more likely to pick them up at the least little whimper, breaking up their sleep unnecessarily. You should, however, be close enough to hear your baby's cries before they turn into frantic ear-piercing wails—or install an intercom between baby's room and yours.

Routine. Since your newborn will fall asleep most of the time while nursing or bottle feeding, a bedtime routine might seem unnecessary. But it's never too early to begin such a routine, and certainly by the age of six months it should top off every evening. The ritual of a warm bath, followed by being dressed in night clothes, a little quiet playtime on your bed, a sing-song story or nursery rhyme from a picture book, can be soothing and soporific for even the youngest babies. The breast or bottle can be last on the agenda for babies who still fall asleep that way, but can come earlier for those who have already learned to go to bed on their own.

Adequate daytime rest. Some mothers try to solve the nighttime sleeping problems of their babies by keeping them awake during the day, even at times when their baby wants to sleep. This is a big mistake (though it's all right to limit the length of daytime naps a little in order to maintain the contrast between day and night) because an overtired baby sleeps more fitfully than a well-rested one.

---

songs, dangle a toy within her range of vision, which is about 8 to 14 inches. (For other tips on keeping baby awake, see page 60.) Don't, however, try to keep her from napping at all during the day, with the hope that she'll sleep at night. An overtired, and perhaps overstimulated, baby is not likely to sleep well at night.

Making a clear distinction between day and night may help. During the day have baby sleep in a carriage or stroller, perhaps out of doors. If she naps in her room, avoid darkening it or trying to keep the noise level down. When she wakens, ply her with stimulating activities. At night, do the opposite. Put your baby to bed in her crib or bassinet and strive for darkness (use room-darkening shades), relative quiet, and inactivity. No matter how tempting it may be, don't play with or talk to her when she wakens; don't turn on the lights or the TV while you're feeding her; keep communications to a whisper or softly sung lullabies; and be certain when she's back in her bed that sleeping conditions are ideal (see Better Sleep for Baby, page 119).

Although it may seem like a dubious blessing, consider yourself lucky that your baby sleeps for long stretches—even if it is during the day. It's a good sign that she's capable of sleeping well and that once she's got her internal clock set correctly, she will sleep well at night.

SLEEPING POSITIONS

"We were told our first baby should sleep on his tummy. Now the doctor says our new baby should sleep on her back. I'm confused."

It's getting harder and harder to keep up with the pendulum swings. For years the experts advised putting newborns to sleep on their tummies (prone) rather than on their backs to avoid the risk of their choking on spit up. But recent research indicates that the back (supine) position is safer. While there is no evidence that inhaling vomit is a major problem when infants sleep on their backs, it is clear that there is a sharp reduction in crib deaths (SIDS) in that position. This research has prompted the Back to Sleep campaign of the American Academy of Pediatrics, which recommends that all healthy, full term infants be put to sleep on their backs. There are some exceptions, however, such as infants with respiratory problems, those who spit up a lot, or those with upper airway malformations.

Ideally, you should start your baby sleeping on her back right away—so that she will get used to and feel comfortable that way. If she seems to fuss a lot in that position, try propping her on her side, against the crib bumpers, with her lower arm brought out from under her body at a right angle to stabilize her. This is not quite as safe as back sleeping, but safer than tummy sleeping. If she has trouble falling asleep on her back, let her go to sleep on her tummy and try turning her over about fifteen minutes later. If she is always *very* unhappy on her back or side, talk to her doctor about letting her sleep prone on a firm surface.

You will probably find that your baby startles more often lying on her back, which may lead to slightly more frequent wakings. It is also possible that she will develop a flat or bald spot from always facing in the same direction—usually because she is focusing on the same spot (often a window)—while lying on her back. To minimize this problem, alternate her position (head at one end of the crib one night, the other the next). If in spite of your efforts her head flattens or a bald spot develops, don't worry. These problems will gradually correct themselves as she gets older. Severe cases can be corrected with a special headband or helmet.

Putting her on her tummy to play when she's awake (and watched) will also minimize head malformations and is important for normal muscle development. Remember: *back to sleep, tummy to play.*

MOVING A SLEEPING BABY TO BED

"I'm a nervous wreck when I try to put my sleeping baby down in her crib. I'm always afraid she'll wake up—and she usually does."

She's finally asleep—after what seems like

hours of nursing on sore breasts, rocking in aching arms, lullabying in an increasingly hoarse voice. You rise ever so slowly from the armchair and edge cautiously to the crib, holding your breath and moving only the muscles that are absolutely necessary. Then, with a silent but fervent prayer, you lift her over the edge of the crib and begin the perilous descent to the mattress below. Finally you release her, but a split second too soon. She's down—then she's up. Turning her head from side to side, sniffing and whimpering softly, then sobbing loudly. Ready to cry yourself, you pick her up and start all over.

The scenario's the same in almost every home with an infant. If you're having trouble keeping a good baby down, wait ten minutes until she's in deep sleep, then try:

A high mattress. If you were a gorilla, you might be able to set your baby down in a crib with a low mattress without having to scale the rail or, alternatively, drop her the last 6 inches. Since you're only human, you will find it much easier if you set the mattress at the highest possible level (but at least 4 inches from the top of the rail), but be sure to lower it by the time your baby is old enough to sit up. Or, for the first few weeks, use a crib substitute such as carriage, bassinet, or cradle, all of which may be easier to lift a baby into and out of. Often these offer the important plus of being rockable, so the rocking motion that started in your arms can continue after you bed baby down.

The right light. Though it's a good idea to get baby to sleep in a darkened room, be sure there's enough light (a night-light will do) for you to see your way to the crib without bumping into a dresser or tripping over a toy—which is sure to jar you.

Close quarters. The longer the distance between the place where baby falls asleep and the place where you are going to put her down, the more opportunity for her to awaken on the way. So feed or rock her as close to the cradle or crib as possible.

A seat you can get out of. Always feed or rock your baby in a chair or sofa that you can rise from smoothly, without disturbing her.

A ready bed. Prepare the landing site before bedtime, unless you're coordinated enough to turn down the bed or extract a teddy with your toes. Baby will be less likely to stay asleep if you have to do a lot of juggling in order to clear the way for touchdown.

A warm bed. The shock of cold sheets on warm cheeks can rouse the best of little sleepers. Warm the sheets on cold nights with a warm hot-water bottle or a heating pad set on low, but be sure to remove it and check the bedding temperature before putting baby down. Or use flannel or knit sheets, which stay more comfortable than a flat weave.

The right side. Or the left. Feed or rock baby in whichever arm will allow you to put her in the crib without first having to turn her around. If she falls asleep prematurely on the wrong side, gently switch sides and rock or feed some more before attempting to put her down. Alternatively, position her crib away from the wall or arrange the bedding so that you can put your sleeping angel down from either side.

Constant contact. When baby is comfortable and secure in your arms, suddenly being dropped into open space, even for an inch or two, startles—and awakens. Cradle baby all the way down back first (see page 120 for information on sleep positions), easing your bottom hand out from under just before you reach the mattress. Maintain a hands-on pose for a few moments longer, gently patting if she starts to stir.

A lulling tune. Hypnotize your baby to sleep with a traditional lullaby (she won't object if you're off key) or an improvised one with a monotonous beat (aah-ah aah-ah ba-by, aah-ah aah-ah ba-by). Continue as you carry her to her crib, while you're putting her down, and for a few moments afterward. If she begins to toss, croon some more, until she's fully quieted.

CRYING

"We congratulated ourselves in the hospital on having such a good baby. We were home hardly 24 hours when she started howling."

If one- and two-day-old babies cried as much as they were destined to a couple of weeks later, new parents would doubtless think twice about checking out of the hospital with their newborns. Once they're safely ensconced at home, babies don't seem to hesitate to show their true-blue colors, with all doing some crying, and many doing a considerable amount. Crying is, after all, the only way infants have of communicating their needs and feelings—their very first baby talk. Your baby can't tell you that she's lonely, hungry, wet, tired, uncomfortable, too warm, too cold, or frustrated any other way. And though it may seem impossible now, you will soon be able (at least part of the time) to decode your baby's different cries and know what she's asking for.

Some newborn crying, however, seems entirely unrelated to basic needs. Four out of every 5 babies (some studies indicate 9 out of 10), in fact, have daily crying sessions of from 15 minutes to an hour that are not easily explained. These crying spells, like those associated with colic, a more severe and persistent form of unexplained crying, most often occur in the evening. It may be that this is the most hectic time of day in the home, with dinner being prepared, father coming home from work, parents trying to eat, other children, if any, vying for attention, and that the hustle-bustle is more than the baby can tolerate. Or that after a busy day of taking in and processing all the sights, sounds, smells, and other stimuli in her environment, a baby just needs to unwind with a good cry.

Some perfectly happy babies seem to need to cry themselves to sleep, possibly because of fatigue. If your baby cries for five or ten minutes before going off, don't be concerned. She will eventually outgrow this, and picking her up to calm her or providing a pacifier will only make it more difficult for her to get to sleep on her own when she's older. What may help is a regular prebedtime ritual and enough rest during the day so she isn't overtired at night.

Meanwhile, hang in there. Though you'll be drying some tears for the next eighteen years or so, these probably tearless newborn crying spells are likely to be a thing of the past by the time your baby is three months old. As she becomes a more effective communicator and a more self-reliant individual, and as you become more proficient at understanding her, she will cry less often, for shorter periods, and will be more easily comforted when she does cry.

A sudden bout of crying, however, in a baby who hasn't cried a lot before could signal illness or early teething. Check for fever and other signs that baby isn't well or might be teething, and call the doctor if you note anything out of the ordinary.

COLIC

"My husband and I haven't had dinner together since our baby was three weeks old. We have to take turns gulping our food and carrying him around while he cries for hours every evening."

For the parents of a colicky baby, even a steak dinner becomes fast food, choked down to the accompaniment of indigestion-provoking screams. That the doctor promises baby will outgrow colic offers little consolation for their misery.

And if misery likes company, parents of colicky babies have plenty of it. It's estimated that 1 in 5 babies has crying spells, usually beginning in late afternoon and sometimes lasting until bedtime, that are severe enough to be labeled colic. Colic differs from ordinary crying (see above) in that the baby seems inconsolable, crying

PRESCRIPTION FOR COLIC

The desperate parent of a colicky baby often turns to the physician for a magic potion to cure the crying. Unfortunately, there is no medicine that is known to completely cure colic in all infants, and because all prescription medications have side effects, most doctors prefer not to pick up their prescription pad when treating these chronic criers. There is, however, one medicine, widely used to treat colic in Europe, that is sold over-the-counter here for gas and that does seem to help reduce or alleviate symptoms in many colicky infants. Its active ingredient is simethicone,

the same anti-gas ingredient found in many adult preparations. Though there is no agreement that gas is the cause of infant colic, it is recognized that many colicky infants do seem gassy (whether this is a cause of the crying or an effect isn't clear), and studies show that reducing the gas seems to reduce the discomfort for many. Because the product isn't absorbed by the body, it is completely safe and has no side effects. If your colicky baby seems gassy, ask the doctor about simethicone drops. They are available under such brand names as Mylicon® and Phazyme®.

turns to screaming, and the ordeal lasts for two or three hours, sometimes much longer, occasionally nearly round-the-clock. Most often colicky periods recur daily, though some babies take an occasional night off.

The baby with a textbook case of colic pulls his knees up, clenches his fists, and generally increases his activity. He closes eyes tightly or opens them wide, furrows his brow, even holds his breath briefly. Bowel activity increases and he passes gas. Eating and sleeping patterns are upset by the crying—the baby frantically seeks a nipple only to reject it once sucking is begun, or dozes for a few moments only to awaken screaming. But few infants follow the textbook description exactly. No two babies experience exactly the same pattern and intensity of crying and associated behavior, and no two parents respond in exactly the same way.

Colic generally begins during the second or third week of life (later in preterm infants), and usually gets as bad as it's going to get by six weeks. For a while the nightmare seems as though it will stretch on interminably, but by twelve weeks the problem usually begins to diminish, and at three months (again, later in preterm babies) most colicky infants appear miraculously cured—with just a few continuing

their problem crying through the fourth or fifth month. The colic may abate suddenly or gradually, with some good and some bad days, until they are all good.

Though these daily screaming periods, whether marathon or of more manageable duration, are usually dubbed "colic," there is not a clear definition of exactly what colic is or how it differs, if it does, from other types of problem crying, such as paroxysmal or periodic irritable crying. Definitions and differences, however, matter very little to parents who are desperately trying to calm their infant.

What causes colic remains a mystery. Theories, however, abound. Many of the following now have been totally or partially rejected: colicky babies cry to exercise their lungs (there is no medical evidence of this); they cry because of gastric discomfort triggered by allergy or sensitivity to something in their mothers' diet if they are breastfeeding or in their formula if they are bottle-fed; (this is only occasionally a cause of colic); they cry because of parental inexperience (colic is no less common in second or subsequent babies, though parents may handle the crying with more aplomb); colic is hereditary (it does not appear to run in families); colic is more common in babies whose mothers had complications in pregnancy or childbirth (statistics don't bear this out); exposure to fresh air stirs up colic (in practice, many parents find that fresh air is the only way they can quiet their crying babies).

The theory that babies are colicky because their mothers are tense is a more controversial one. Though many experts believe it's more likely that it's the baby's crying that makes a mother tense, some insist that a mother who is very anxious may unconsciously communicate this to her baby, making him cry. It may be that although maternal anxiety doesn't cause colic, it can make it worse.

One current theory is that crying is merely a normal manifestation of a newborn's physiological immaturity: all babies cry, and colic is just an extreme form of this normal behavior. Another suggests that the immature digestive tract contracts violently when gas is passed, causing the pain of colic. A third, that painful intestinal spasms occur because of progesterone withdrawal as the level of maternal hormones in an infant's body drops off. Still another explanation: the baby's immature nervous system has not yet learned to inhibit unwanted behavior, such as crying.

Perhaps most plausible of all is the theory that newborns, who don't usually cry a lot, have a built-in blocking mechanism that shuts out stimuli, allowing them to sleep and eat without giving much attention to their surroundings. Around the end of the first month (when colic usually begins), this mechanism disappears, leaving them more alert and interested in the world around them. Bombarded with sensations (sounds, sights, and smells) all day long, and unable to tune them out when overload begins, they reach the early evening hours overstimulated and overwhelmed. The result: unexplained crying, and in extreme cases, colic. By the time the baby reaches three or four months, or occasionally five, the theory continues, these babies have acquired the ability to tune out the environment before overload occurs, and bouts of colic end.

One environmental factor that does seem to contribute to an increase in colicky behavior, though the reason for it isn't clear, is tobacco smoke in the home. And the more smokers in a household, the greater the likelihood of colic and the worse the colic will be.

What's reassuring about colic and paroxysmal crying is that babies who have these crying spells do not seem to be any the worse for the wear (though the same can't always be said for their parents), either emotionally or physically—they thrive, usually gaining as well as or better than babies who cry very little, and display no more behavioral problems than other children later on. Children who cry vigorously as infants appear, in fact, more likely to be vigorous and active problem solvers as toddlers than those with limp cries. And most reassuring of all is the certainty that the condition won't last forever. In the meantime, the tips on pages 126 and 127 should help you deal with the problem.

HELPING SIBLINGS LIVE WITH COLIC

"Our new baby's constant crying seems to really upset our three-year-old daughter. What can I do?"

If there's an innocent victim in a household with a colicky newborn, it's an older sibling. Here's this baby she probably didn't ask for, and is likely to be feeling somewhat threatened and replaced by, making a terrible racket during what was once one of her favorite times of the day—dinner with mommy and daddy. Not only is the crying unbearable for her, so is the upheaval that comes with it. Instead of being a time for eating, sharing, and quiet play, early evening turns into a time of disrupted meals, frantic pacing and rocking, and distracted parents. Worst of all, perhaps, is the helplessness the little victim feels. While the adults are able to at least take some action against the colic (though it may not help) and commiserate with each other about it, she can only sit by, powerless.

You can't make colic easy on your older child any more than you can make it easy on yourself. But you can help her cope better, if you:

Talk it out. Explain, on your older child's level, what colic is. Reassure her that it won't last, that once the baby gets used to being in his new and strange world, most of the crying will stop. If she, too, was a colicky infant, tell her—this should make it easier for her to believe that these screaming monsters actually do grow up to be nice, and relatively quiet, children.

Let her know it's not her fault. Little children tend to blame themselves for everything that goes wrong in a household, from mommy and daddy's arguing to great-grandfather's dying to a new baby's crying. They need to be reassured that no one is at fault here, least of all them.

Show and tell her you love her. Dealing with a colicky baby can be so distracting, and taking care of the basic food, clothing, and shelter needs of the rest of the family so time consuming, that you may

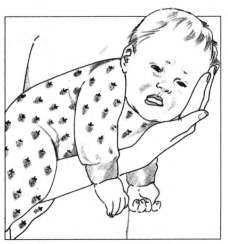

The colic carry. *Some colicky babies are soothed by the pressure applied to their abdomen when they are carried in this position.*

forget to do those special little things that show a toddler or older child you care. So make a point of doing at least one of those things (fix her hair a new way, play "swimming" in the bath, bake muffins with her, help her paint a mural on an extra-large piece of paper) every day—and of course remember to tell her several times a day how terrific she is and how much you love her.

Save some time for her alone. Even if it's only half an hour, try to find some time every day to spend with your older child without baby sibling tagging along. Snatch the time when the baby is napping (this is more important than catching up with the dusting), when your husband is walking the floor with him, when your mother comes by to visit—or, if you're able to afford it—when you have a sitter for the baby.

SURVIVING COLIC

"This is our first baby and she cries all the time. What are we doing wrong?"

Relax. You're not guilty. The theory that colic in a baby is somehow the fault of the parents just hasn't held up. And in fact, the situation would probably be just the same if you were doing everything right (of course no parent does; and what's right varies from baby to baby and parent to parent). And it probably wouldn't be much worse if you were doing a lot of things wrong (no parent does *everything* wrong). Colic, the latest research indicates, has to do with baby's development and not yours.

The "rightest" thing you can do is to try to cope with your baby's crying as calmly and rationally as possible. As anyone who's had a colicky baby knows, that's not easy, but the tips below should be helpful. Though you're not responsible for baby's crying, remaining calm may help her to calm down too.

COPING WITH CRYING

No medication, pharmaceutical or herbal remedy, or treatment approach is a sure cure for a baby's crying, and some may actually worsen it. But there are a number of things parents can do about their baby's crying; none will work all of the time, some won't work at all, sometimes none will work, but all are worth trying.

Try prevention. In societies where babies are carried papoose style, long periods of crying or fussiness in healthy children are unknown. A recent U.S. study showed that babies who were carried, in the arms or in a baby carrier, for at least three hours every day cried much less than those who were carried less. Not only does carrying give a baby the pleasure of physical closeness to mother (something that was enjoyed in the uterus), but it may help a mother tune in better to her baby's needs.

Respond. Crying is your baby's only way of wielding any control over a vast and bewildering new environment, of making things happen: "When I call, someone answers." If you regularly fail to respond, the baby may feel not only powerless, but worthless ("I'm so unimportant that no one comes when I call"). Though it may sometimes seem that you're responding in vain because no matter what you do, nothing helps, responding to your baby's calls promptly will eventually reduce crying. And, in fact, studies show that babies whose mothers responded to them promptly in infancy cry less as toddlers. In addition, crying that's been left to intensify for more than a few minutes becomes harder to interpret—the baby becomes so upset, even he or she doesn't remember what started all the fuss in the first place. And the longer baby cries, the longer it takes to stop the crying. Of course, you needn't drop everything to answer baby's call if you're in the middle of taking a shower, draining the spaghetti, or answering the doorbell. Baby's being left to cry for a couple of extra minutes now and then won't prove detrimental—as long as the infant can't get into trouble while waiting for you.

Don't worry about spoiling your baby by responding promptly. You can't spoil a young infant. And babies who get a lot of attention in the early months are more precocious. Those who don't hang on to dependency and become more demanding.

For particularly difficult cases of inconsolable crying, some experts suggest setting up a routine where you let baby cry for ten or fifteen minutes in a safe place like his crib, pick him up and try to soothe him for another fifteen minutes, then put him down and repeat. If you're comfortable with this, it apparently won't cause any long-term problems.

Assess the situation. Before deciding your baby is crying just for crying's sake, determine if there's a simple and remediable underlying cause. If you think it may be hunger, try breast or bottle, but don't make the mistake of invariably responding to tears with food. Even at this tender age, food should be a response to a need for food, not attention. If you suspect fatigue, try rocking baby to sleep—in your arms, a carriage, a cradle, or a baby carrier. If a wet diaper may be triggering the crying, change it (of course, if you use diaper pins, check for an open one). If baby seems too warm (perspiration is a clue), take off a layer or two of clothing, open the window, or turn on a fan or air conditioner. If cold may be the problem (neck, arms or body feel cold to the touch), add a layer or turn up the heat. If baby began to cry when clothes were stripped off for a bath (most newborns dislike being naked), quickly cover him with a towel or blanket. If you think his being in the same position for a while may be causing discomfort, reposition baby. If he's been staring at the same view for the last half hour, try changing it.

Ritualism. For babies who thrive on routine, having as regular a schedule as possible (feeding, bathing, changing, outing, and so on up to bedtime ritual) may reduce crying. Be consistent even to the method you use for soothing baby or reducing crying—don't go for a walk one day, ride around in the car the next, and use a baby swing the third. Once you find what works, stick with it most of the time.

Try a little comfort. Sometimes this is all a baby needs and is crying for: being separated from your mommy after nine months of constant contact can be a lonely business. Try the techniques in the box on page 128, Comforting the Crier.

Sucking satisfaction. Babies often need sucking for its own sake, rather than simply for nourishment. Some babies appreciate your help in getting their fingers (particularly their thumbs) to their mouths for their sucking enjoyment. Others prefer grown-up pinkies—but with clean nails, please, carefully and closely clipped. Still others find pleasure in a pacifier, but be sure it's safe (see page 40); that you *never* attach a string to it (which could wrap around baby's neck); that you give it only to calm baby after you've attended to other needs; and use it only as long as the colic continues.

A fresh face and a new set of arms. A parent who's been struggling for an hour to soothe a sobbing newborn will almost invariably start to show signs of stress and fatigue, which the infant is certain to sense and respond to with more crying. Hand baby over to someone else—the other parent, a relative or friend, a sitter—and the crying may cease.

Fresh air. A change to an outdoor locale will often change a baby's mood miraculously. Try a trip in the car, the baby carrier, or the stroller. Even if it's dark out, baby's sure to find distraction in the twinkling of street and car lights.

Air control. A lot of newborn discomfort is caused by swallowing air. Babies will swallow less of it if you keep them upright as much as possible during feeding and burping. The right-size nipple hole on a bottle will also reduce air intake; be sure it isn't too large (which promotes gulping of air with formula) or too small (struggling for formula also promotes air swallowing). Hold the bottle so that no air enters the nipple (see page 58), and be sure the formula is neither too hot or too cold (though most babies do fine with unheated formula, a few seem disturbed

by it). Be sure to burp baby frequently during feedings to expel swallowed air. One suggested pattern for burping: every half-ounce or every ounce when bottle feeding, every five minutes when breastfeeding, and in both cases, after feeding.

Less excitement. Having a new baby can be a fun time—everyone wants to see the baby, and you want to take him or her everywhere to be seen. You want to expose baby to new experiences, to stimulating environments. That's fine for some babies, *too* stimulating for others. If your baby is colicky, limit excitement, visitors, and stimulation, particularly in the late afternoon and evening.

A diet check. Some babies cry a lot because they aren't getting enough to eat. If your bottle baby isn't gaining well, you should talk to the doctor about increasing the amount of formula you are offering. If your breastfed baby seems underweight, see page 99 for tips on assessing and dealing with failure to thrive. Don't, however, add solids, since this isn't a technique that works or is good for a very young baby. Occasionally, allergy or sensitivity to something in formula or breast milk may trigger discomfort and crying, but usually there are other symptoms as well.

Live entertainment. In the early months, some infants are content to sit and watch the world go by, while others cry out of frustration and boredom because there is, as yet, so little they are able to do on their own. Toting them around and explaining what you're doing as you go about your business, and making an extra effort to find toys and other objects in the environment for them to look at and later swat at and play with, may help keep them busy.

Outside relief. This is one time it doesn't make sense to say, "I'd rather do it myself." Take advantage of any and every possibility for sharing the burden (see page 16).

Acceptance. Have the wisdom to accept what you can't change. You can't cure your baby's colic and, very often, you may not even be able to quiet the screaming at all. Your only other choice, and perhaps not an easy one to accept: live with it.

COMFORTING THE CRIER

Comfort for a newborn comes in many packages, and what may be soothing to one baby may increase squalling in another. Use one method at a time, being careful to give each a fair trial before switching to another, or you may find you are trying, trying, trying and baby is crying, crying, crying. Switching back and forth or using several methods at the same time could overstimulate and increase misery, though you can usually combine soft crooning with rocking or another motion activity. Try the following steps:

■ Rhythmic rocking, in your arms, a carriage, a cradle, or an automatic baby swing (but not before the baby is six weeks old). Some babies respond better to fast rocking than to slow—but don't rock or shake your baby vigorously, since this can cause serious whiplash injury. For some babies rocking side to side tends to stimulate, rocking up and down to calm. Test your baby's response to different types of rocking.

■ A ride in a stroller, carriage, or the family car. An alternative, recently devised: an FDA-approved device that makes the crib feel like an automobile going 55 miles an hour, complete with wind sounds as a soothing accompaniment. According to studies the product, SleepTight, works. (Ask your baby's doctor; order from Ross Laboratories, 1-800-NO-COLIC.)

■ Walking the floor with baby in a carrier or sling or simply in your arms. Tried and true, it's tiring but it often works.

■ Swaddling baby. Being tightly wrapped is very comforting to some young infants.

■ Cuddling in your arms. Like swaddling, cuddling gives many babies a sense of security; hold baby pressed close to your chest, encircled snugly by your arms. Patting is optional.

■ A warm water bath. But only if your baby likes the bath; some babies will scream more as soon as they hit the water.

■ Singing. Learn whether your baby is soothed by soft lullabies, sprightly nursery rhymes, or pop tunes, and whether a light, high-pitched voice or a deep, strong one is more pleasing. If you hit on a tune your baby likes, don't hesitate to sing it over and over—most babies love repetition.

■ Rhythmic sounds. Many babies are calmed, for example, by the hum of a fan or vacuum cleaner, a tape recording of uterine gurglings, or a record that plays soothing nature sounds, such as waves breaking on the beach or wind blowing through trees.

■ Laying on the hands. For babies who like to be stroked, massage can be very calming; but it can cause increased screaming in those who don't. Invest in a baby massage book if you want to perfect your technique, or simply try rubbing your baby's back, belly, arms, and legs in a firm but gentle, loving way. But be careful not to be so gentle you tickle. You may find it relaxing to both of you to administer the massage lying on your back, baby face-down on your chest.

■ Pressure tactics. Lying across an adult lap, tummy down, back being patted, is a favorite position for many colicky babies and one that often makes them more comfortable. Some prefer being upright on the shoulder, but again with pressure on their abdomens and their backs being patted or rubbed.

"Sometimes when I'm rocking the baby through his third hour of colic, and he won't stop screaming, I have this terrible urge to throw him out the window. Of course I don't—but what kind of mother am I to even think such a thing?"

You're a perfectly normal mother. Even those otherwise qualified for sainthood couldn't survive the agony and frustration of living with a baby who won't stop crying without experiencing some feelings of anger—even momentary hatred—toward him. And though few would admit it freely, many parents of chronic criers have to regularly fight off the same kinds of horrifying

WHEN TO CHECK CRYING WITH THE DOCTOR

Odds are your baby's daily screaming sessions are due to normal colic or paroxysmal crying. But just in case there might be some medical problem underlying them, be sure to mention the crying, its duration, intensity, pattern, and, especially, any variations from what has been your baby's norm, to the doctor. As the medical community learns more about crying, they are finding that certain aspects of crying (pitch, for example) may provide clues to illness.

An occasional baby does cry because of something his mother is eating or because of allergy to formula. If there is a family history of allergy, ask your baby's doctor about this possibility. He or she may suggest eliminating a food in your diet (often milk products) if you're breastfeeding, or changing the formula if you're bottle feeding. If a change reduces the colic significantly, then it's possible that allergy may be the cause. To prove it more conclusively (if you've got iron nerves and a scientific bent), you could reintroduce the offending food or formula and see if crying resumes. Crying that persists beyond three months may also point to allergy. And sudden sustained crying, in a baby who hasn't cried a lot previously, could indicate illness or pain. Check with the doctor.

impulses you've been feeling. If you find such feelings are more than momentary, and/or if you're afraid that you might really hurt your baby, get help immediately.

There's no question that parents get the worst of colic. Though it can safely be said that the crying doesn't seem to hurt baby, it certainly does leave its mark on mom and dad. Listening to a crying baby is irritating and anxiety provoking. Objective studies show that everyone, even a child, responds to the constant crying of a young infant with a rise in blood pressure, a speeding up of the heartbeat, and changes in blood flow to the skin. If the baby was born prematurely, was poorly nourished in the uterus, or if the mother had toxemia (preeclampsia/eclampsia), the pitch of his cry may be unusually high and particularly hard to tolerate.[5]

In order to survive with some semblance of sanity the two or three months of colicky behavior try the following:

Take a break. If you're the only one that has to cope with your baby seven nights a week at colic time, the strain is going to take its toll not only on your mothering, but on your health and your relationship with your husband as well. So take a break at least once a week, daily if possible, during your baby's crying time, relying on paid help if you can afford it, or imposing on grandma or other relatives or friends if you can't. (But avoid friends or relatives who drop direct or indirect hints that the crying is your fault—it's not.)

If you and your husband never have a peaceful dinner thanks to your little screamer, then have dinner out once in a while. It's not difficult to squeeze dinner in between baby's feedings, though more extensive outings may be tough if you're breastfeeding. If dinner out isn't practical, try going for a walk, visiting a friend (preferably one who doesn't have a tiny baby), playing tennis, or getting a massage.

Give baby a break. Sure, it's important to respond to baby's crying. But once you've met all his needs (feeding, burping, changing, comforting, and so on) without perceptibly altering his level of screaming, you can give him a break from you—by putting him down in his crib or bassinet for a while. It won't hurt him to cry in his bed instead of your arms for ten or fifteen min-

---

5. If a baby's cry is inexplicably high pitched, check with the doctor; such a cry could indicate illness.

utes while you do something relaxing, such as lying down, washing the dishes, baking some muffins, watching television, or reading a few pages of a book. In fact, it will do him good to have a mother who is refreshed rather than ragged.

Tune out. To lessen the impact of your baby's wails, use earplugs—they won't block out the sound entirely, just dull it so it will be more tolerable. Tucked in your ears, they can help you relax during a break from baby, or even while you're walking the floor with him.

Get physical. Exercise is a great way to work off tension, something you've got plenty of. Work out at home with baby early in the day (see page 525), swim or exercise at a health club (wallop a punching bag if they have one) that has child-care services, or take the baby for a brisk walk out of doors in his carriage when he's fussy (which may help calm him while it calms you).

Call for help. Since the main burden of baby care may fall on you if you are on maternity leave or have elected to stay home while your husband goes about business as usual, you may soon want to give up mothering as a bad job unless you get some help. The first line of assistance should be your spouse. Most fathers are very good at quieting a baby if they just give themselves a chance—though a minority can't deal with a crying baby at all. If you're lucky enough to have other relatives nearby, call on them, too. Many grandmothers, thanks to years of experience, seem to have a magic touch with babies—though as with fathers, a few may have trouble with a squaller. A sister, sister-in-law, or good friend can also make a fine relief person. If she has children of her own she can bring, at the least, experience to the task. If she has none she can bring enthusiasm, excitement, and freshness to it.

If you can't get willing volunteers, you will have to turn to paid help—an experienced baby-sitter or baby nurse, for instance, who can take over walking your crying baby for an hour or so once a week, or more. A teenager who is comfortable with babies is often an inexpensive yet effective helper who can take your baby out in the stroller, or carry him around the house while you shower and prepare dinner or even while you eat.

Talk about it. Do a little crying yourself—on any willing shoulder: your husband's, the baby's doctor's, your family doctor's, a cleric's, a family member's, a friend's. Talking about it may not cure the colic but you may feel a little better after sharing your sorry story. Most beneficial may be discussing your situation with other parents of colicky babies, particularly those who have weathered the storm successfully and are now sailing on clear waters.

If you really feel violent, get help. Almost everyone is irritated by a constantly crying baby. But for some people, such crying finally becomes more than they can bear. The result is sometimes child abuse. If your thoughts of throwing baby out the window are more than fleeting, if you feel about to give in to the urge to strike or shake your baby or harm him in any way, get help *immediately*. Go to a neighbor's, if you can, and hand the baby over until you can collect yourself. Then call someone who can help you—your husband, your mother or mother-in-law, a close friend, the baby's doctor or your own, or the local child-abuse hotline (the number should be listed inside the cover of your local classified directory). Even if your powerful feelings don't lead to child abuse, they can start eroding your relationship with your baby and your confidence in yourself as a mother unless you get counseling quickly.

SPOILING BABY

"We always pick our baby up when she cries. Are we spoiling her?"

Not sparing the comfort won't spoil the baby, at least not until she's at least six months old. In fact, studies show pouring on the comfort now—by picking her up within a couple of minutes whenever she cries and catering to all her needs—not only won't turn out a spoiled brat, it will turn out a happy, more self-reliant child who in the long run will cry less and demand less attention. She will also have a closer attachment to you (or to whoever it is who responds to her), and be more trusting. An additional plus: since she'll come to breast or bottle calm, without a bellyful of air swallowed while screaming, she will have better feeding sessions.

Of course, all isn't lost if once in a while you can't pick your baby up immediately—you might be in the bathroom, on the phone, or taking the casserole out of the oven. There's no harm done as long as you get to her as soon as possible. Nor will the results be catastrophic if you periodically take 15-minute breaks from a colicky baby.

BLOOD IN SPITUP

"When my two-week-old spit up today, there were some reddish streaks in with the curdled milk. I'm really worried about her."

Any blood that seems to be coming from a two-week-old baby, particularly when it's found in her spitup, is bound to be alarming. But before you panic, try to determine if it's your blood, which it most likely is, or the baby's. If you're breastfeeding and your nipples are cracked, even very slightly, your baby could be sucking in some blood along with the milk each time she nurses. And since what goes into a baby must come out—sometimes in the form of spitup—such a situation could definitely account for the blood you've noticed.

If your nipples aren't obviously the cause (they may be, even if you can't see the tiny cracks), then call your pediatrician to help you solve the mystery.

CHANGING YOUR MIND ABOUT BREASTFEEDING

"I had decided not to breastfeed my daughter, and I let my milk dry out. Now, seeing other mothers nursing their babies makes me have second thoughts. Is it too late to get my milk back?"

Nature allows for a change of heart—at least most of the time. This early in the game, particularly when their babies are between four and seven weeks old, women who want to breastfeed after allowing their milk to dry up (or women who've weaned their babies only to have regrets a few weeks later) can be reasonably successful at relactating.

Before you consider trying, however, be sure your change of heart is wholehearted. Success won't come easily and you'll need to be at least doubly dedicated in order to achieve it. You can expect that for the first several weeks relactation will take a great deal of time (you'll need to nurse your baby very frequently at first) and effort (you may also have to engage in some manual or mechanical expression of milk), and will produce a great deal of stress for both you and your baby (who may initially resist this new form of feeding). Even if you succeed in producing milk, you may not be able to supply all your baby's nutritional needs, and formula supplementation may be necessary.

If you decide breastfeeding is something you really want to try, or give another try to, switch to the Best-Odds Breastfeeding Diet (page 534) and follow the suggestions for inducing lactation on page 503. For many women—and their babies—the results are well worth the effort.

"I've been breastfeeding my son for three weeks, and I'm just not enjoying it. I'd like to switch to a bottle, but I feel so guilty."

There's no reason to feel guilty about your

decision, or even to regret it—as long as you're sure you've made it for the right reasons. Beginning breastfeeding is usually a series of trials and errors. As far as enjoyment goes, it can be elusive on both sides of the breasts in this early adjustment period. If you're certain that your dissatisfaction with breastfeeding isn't just the result of a bumpy start (which almost always turns into a smooth ride by the middle of the second month), and that you've given nursing your all in both time and effort, continuing is not likely to be a positive experience. But do try to wait it out until your baby is six weeks old (two months would be even better), by which time he will have received the most important health benefits of breastfeeding. Then, if you're still not enjoying nursing, feel free—and free of remorse—to wean him.

PHOTO FLASHES

"I've noticed that our baby blinks when the flash from our camera goes off. Could it be hurting his eyes?"

Only the most sought-after celebrities are as hounded by the popping of flashbulbs as a newborn baby whose paparazzi parents are determined to capture in pictures every detail of his first days of life. But unlike celebrities, infants can't hide behind dark glasses when the bulbs start flashing. To protect your baby's eyes against the possibility of injury from a flashbulb exploding near him and from too intense and too close exposure to the camera lights, it's a good idea to take a few precautions during photo sessions. Try to keep the camera at least 40 inches from baby, and use a diffusion screen over the flash unit to keep glare to a safe minimum. If your photographic equipment allows, bounce the light off a wall or ceiling instead of in baby's face. If you failed to take such precautions during previous shoots, don't worry. The risk of damage is exceedingly small.

LOUD MUSIC

"My husband likes to play loud rock music on the stereo. I'm afraid that it might damage our daughter's ears."

All ears, young and old, have a lot to lose when they're exposed for long periods of time to loud music (whether rock, classical, or any other type)—namely, a certain amount of their hearing capacity. Though some ears are more naturally sensitive and prone to damage than others, in general the hearing of babies and small children is most susceptible to the harmful effects of overly loud sound. Damage to the ears can be either temporary or permanent, depending on the noise level and the duration and frequency of exposure.

How loud is dangerously loud? While a baby's crying might signal that music (or another noise) is too loud for her, don't wait for her protests before turning the volume down; a baby's ears don't have to be "bothered" to suffer damage. According to the workplace standards set by the Occupational Safety and Health Administration (OSHA), the maximum noise level that is safe for adults is 90 decibels—a level that can easily be exceeded by a stereo set. If you don't have the equipment to measure the decibels your stereo is putting out when your husband plays his rock music, you can set the volume safely by maintaining a level that can be easily talked over—if you have to shout, it's too loud.

VITAMIN SUPPLEMENTS

"Everybody we talk to has a different opinion on vitamins for babies. We can't decide whether or not to give them to our new son."

Your great-grandmother probably never heard of vitamin supplements when she was a young mother, or even of vitamins (they weren't given that name until 1912); your grandmother was probably told to give her children cod liver oil "for its vitamins"; your mother may not have been told to give you any supplements at all. With the science of nutrition still in its infancy, you can expect that the recommendations will continue to change as new information is uncovered. Considering the constant state of flux in the scientific community, it isn't surprising that there's a lot of confusion among lay people as to just what makes sense.

Current research indicates that healthy newborns usually do not need a multivitamin supplement. They get most of the vitamins and minerals they are believed to need from breast milk if their mothers are eating a good diet and taking a pregnancy-lactation supplement daily; or from formula if it is a medically approved commercial brand and not a home brew. Exceptions are those babies who have health problems that compromise their nutritional status (those who are not able to absorb certain nutrients well from their foods and/or are on restricted diets, for example) and babies of breastfeeding vegetarians who eat no animal products and take no supplements themselves. The latter should receive, at the very least, vitamin B_{12}, which may be totally absent in their mother's milk, and probably folic acid as well; but a complete vitamin-mineral supplement with iron is probably a good idea.

Whether a supplement is necessary for a baby who is a few months old is less clear. A commercial formula with iron will continue to supply all the nutrients a baby is known to need—everything that might be in the drops and more. Breast milk, on the other hand, is variable and much less easy to analyze; its nutrient makeup depends partly on the mother's diet, partly on her health, and partly on factors we don't even understand.

Once solids are introduced, a baby's diet becomes even less easy to evaluate and control. One day he takes a big bowl of nutrition-packed cereal for breakfast, a couple of tablespoons of yogurt for lunch, then turns down his nighttime carrots and peas. The next, he may reject anything but his bottle. The following day the oatmeal ends up on the floor, most of the yogurt appears to be smeared on the high chair tray, and the evening offering of baby meat is tentatively tasted, then spit out.

So though it's true that some of the vitamins you drop carefully in baby's mouth may on some days be excreted in his urine (it's been said that Americans have the world's healthiest urine, thanks to the vast quantities of vitamin supplements they take), some physicians nevertheless recommend giving the drops daily, as health insurance. Others claim this is unnecessary. If yours is one who insists, "All babies need is a balanced diet," but you'd feel more comfortable knowing your baby is nutritionally "insured" against day-to-day dietary lapses, there's no harm, and probably some good, in giving an over-the-counter supplement that supplies *no more* than the recommended daily allowance of vitamins and minerals for your baby.

There are some individual nutrients, however, that it is widely agreed do need to be supplemented:

Vitamin D. At least thirty minutes of sunshine per week, just over four minutes a day, while clad in only a diaper, or two hours a week, about seventeen minutes daily, fully clothed but hatless, is the estimated amount of sunshine an infant would need to prevent rickets. But because getting adequate vitamin D this way is not only chancy (a run of nasty weather can block out the sun for a week, and letting baby go hatless in very hot or cold weather is not possible) but also potentially dangerous (see the risks of sunning an infant on page 306), the American Academy of Pediatrics (AAP) recommends vitamin D supplementation for babies beginning at two to four weeks of age. Such supplementation is found in commercial baby formulas (and in the fortified whole cow's milk your baby will graduate to later), but it's unclear whether or not there is adequate vitamin D in breast milk, even if the mother takes a supplement. So if you are breastfeeding, it is likely your pediatrician will recommend supplementation via vitamin drops. Do *not* give a baby (or anyone else, for that matter) more than the RDA for this vitamin (400 IU)—it is very toxic at levels not much above this level. A baby getting a formula containing vitamin D should *not* get additional supplementation.

Iron. Since iron deficiency during the first eighteen months of life can cause serious developmental and behavioral problems, mothers should make certain that iron intake is adequate. Your newborn, unless premature or having low birth weight, probably arrived with a considerable iron reserve, but this will be depleted by somewhere between four and six months of age.

The AAP recommends that some source of iron be introduced into the infant's diet at four months of age. Iron-fortified formula (but not ordinary cow's milk) will fill the bill for bottle-fed babies, but for those on breast alone, another source will be needed. An option, once solids are begun, is iron-enriched cereals, but the doctor may also suggest an iron supplement (ferrous sulfate in doses based on your child's weight is cheap and effective), either alone or as part of a baby vitamin-mineral supplement.

Adequate vitamin C intake will improve iron absorption, and once your baby begins taking a lot of solids, it's a good idea to give a vitamin C food at each meal so that the benefits of any iron taken are maximized (see page 359). In spite of what you may hear, clinical studies show that iron supplements don't cause stomach upset in babies. But remember that the mineral can be toxic in large doses. To be safe, you may want to keep no more than a one-month supply in your home at any time and store it well out of the reach of babies and children.

Fluoride. This mineral provides excellent protection against tooth decay, and the American Academy of Pediatrics recommends the following fluoride supplementation: When local water fluoride levels are under 0.3 parts per million (ppm), 0.25 mg for children six months to three years; 0.50 mg for three to six year olds. When levels are between 0.3 and 0.5 ppm, no supplement for those under three; 0.25 mg for three- to six-year-olds. When levels are 0.6 ppm or above, no supplement is needed for any child.

If you're uncertain of the fluoride levels in your tap water, your baby's doctor may be able to advise you. Or you can call your local health department. If your water is from a well or other private source, you can have its fluoride content checked by a lab (ask the health department how to have this done).

If your tap water turns out to be adequately fluoridated (0.3 parts per million is the minimum recommended for protection), try any of the following after six months to ensure your baby's intake.

■ Prepare liquid or powdered ready-to-mix (*not* ready-to-serve which should not be diluted) formula with the tap water. When you give juice, dilute it with tap water.
■ After six months, get your baby in the habit of drinking water daily, preferably from a cup.
■ Ask the doctor about prescribing fluoride or vitamin-mineral drops with fluoride if your baby doesn't get tap water in any form.

Once the teeth emerge, topical supplementation with rinses and toothpastes can also be used. The does will be tailored to the percentage of fluoride in your area's water supply.

With fluoride, as with most good things, too much can be bad. Excessive intake while the teeth are developing in the gums, such as might occur when a baby drinks heavily fluoridated water *and* takes a supplement, can cause "fluorosis," or mottling. The lesser forms of mottling (white striations) are not noticeable or aesthetically unattractive. More serious mottling, however, is not only disfiguring, but the pitting can predispose the teeth to decay.

Babies and children, because of their small size and because their teeth are still developing, and are particularly susceptible to fluorosis. So be wary of overdose. Before you give fluoride supplementation, be sure your water supply is not already adequately fluoridated. Once brushing is started, don't use toothpaste unless your baby insists (and then use a thin smear of unfluoridated baby toothpaste). Cap the paste when it's not in use, and put it out of baby's reach—some babies love to eat the stuff.

Although giving your baby a vitamin-mineral supplement that provides no more than the RDA for infants once he's no longer solely dependent on breast milk or formula may be a good idea, it's not a good idea to give any additional vitamins or mineral supplements in any form. A "nutritionist" should *not* prescribe vitamins, minerals, or herbs for your baby without the doctor's approval. Severe illness has been reported in children overdosed with vitamins or given herbal medicines by caring parents who thought they were doing good.

If your baby is one who hates the daily dose of liquid drops, try the tips for helping the medicine go down on page 411.

CIRCUMCISION CARE

"My son was circumcised yesterday and there seems to be oozing around the area today. Is this normal?"

A body can't lose a part—even a small and largely unnecessary flap of skin such as the foreskin of the penis—without reacting to the loss. In this case there is usually soreness, sometimes a little bleeding, and oozing at the site of the surgery after circumcision has been performed—a sign the body's healing fluids are rushing to the area.

Using double diapers for the first day will help to cushion the penis and also to keep the baby's thighs from pressing against it; this isn't usually necessary later. Usually the penis will be wrapped in gauze by the doctor or mohel (a ritual circumciser of the Jewish faith). You'll be asked to put a fresh gauze pad, dabbed with petroleum jelly or other ointment, on the penis with each diaper change and to avoid getting the penis wet in a bath (you probably won't be dunking your baby yet anyway, because the umbilical cord is not likely to have fallen off at this point) until healing is complete.

SWOLLEN SCROTUM

"It almost looks as though our new son has three testicles."

Your son's testicles are encased in a protective pouch called the scrotum, which is filled with a bit of fluid to cushion them. Sometimes a child is born with an excessive amount of fluid in the scrotal sac, making it appear swollen. Called hydrocele, this condition is nothing to worry about since it gradually resolves during the first year, almost always without any treatment.

You should, however, point out the swelling to your son's doctor to be sure what you see isn't an inguinal hernia (more likely if there is also tenderness, redness, and discoloration; see page 154), which can either resemble a hydrocele or occur along with it. By illuminating the scrotum, the doctor can determine if the scrotal swelling is due to excess fluid or if there is a hernia involved.

HYPOSPADIAS

"We were very disturbed to learn that the outlet in our son's penis is in the middle instead of the end."

Every so often, something goes awry during prenatal development of the urethra and the penis. In your son's case, instead of the urethra (the tube that carries both urine and semen, but not at the same time) running all the way to the glans, or tip, of the penis, it opens elsewhere. This abnormality is called hypospadias and is found in an estimated 1 to 3 in 1,000 boys born in the

KEEPING BABY SAFE

Babies are, despite their fragile appearance, pretty hardy sorts. They don't "break" when you pick them up, their heads don't snap off when you forget to support them, and they weather most falls without major injury. But they can be vulnerable. Even very young ones, who seem too innocent to get into trouble, do—sometimes the very first time they turn over or reach for something. To protect your baby from accidents that don't have to happen, be sure to follow *all* of these safety tips *all* of the time:

■ Always use a car seat for your baby when you go for a drive. Wear a seat belt yourself, and make sure whoever's doing the driving does, too; no one's safe unless the driver is. And never drink and drive, or let baby ride with anyone who does.

■ If you bathe baby in a large tub, put a small towel or cloth at the bottom to prevent slipping. Always keep one hand on baby during the bath.

■ Never leave your baby unattended on a changing table, bed, chair, or couch—not for a moment. Even a newborn who can't roll over can suddenly extend his or her body and fall off. If you don't have safety straps on your changing table, you should always keep one hand on your baby.

■ Never put baby in an infant (or car) seat or carrier on a table, counter, or any elevated surface; never leave baby unattended in a seat on *any* surface, even the middle of a soft bed—suffocation is a risk.

■ Never leave a baby alone with a pet, even a very well-behaved one.

■ Never leave baby alone in a room with a sibling who is under five years old. A game of peekaboo affectionately played by a preschooler could result in tragic suffocation for an infant. A loving but overly enthusiastic bear hug could crack a rib.

■ Don't leave the baby alone with a sitter who is younger than fourteen, whom you don't know well, or whose references you haven't checked. All sitters should be trained in infant safety and CPR.

■ Never jiggle or shake your baby vigorously or throw him or her up into the air.

■ Never leave baby alone at home, even while you go for the mail, move the car, or check the laundry in the apartment building basement; it takes only seconds for a fire to blaze.

■ Never leave a baby or child alone in an automobile. In hot weather even keeping the windows down might not prevent the baby from succumbing to heat stroke. In any weather the brakes might slip, sending the baby careening off, or a child-snatcher on the prowl could quickly make off with the car's precious cargo.

■ Never take your eyes off your baby when you're shopping, going for a walk, or sitting at the playground. A stroller or carriage makes an especially easy target for a child-snatcher.

■ Avoid using any kind of chain or string on baby or on any of baby's toys or belongings—that means no necklaces, strings for pacifiers or rattles, no religious medals on chains, no ribbons longer than 5 inches on cribs or cradles. Make sure the ends of strings in hoods, gowns, and pants are knotted so they can't slip through, and never leave cords, string, ropes, or chains of any kind around where baby might get to them. Be sure, too, that baby's crib, playpen, and changing table are not within reach of electric cords (which present double danger), telephone cords, or venetian blind or drapery cords. All of these items can cause accidental strangulation.

■ To prevent accidental suffocation, don't place filmy plastics, such as those used by dry cleaners, on mattresses or anywhere baby can get at them. Don't leave an unattended infant (awake or asleep) within reach of pillows, stuffed toys, or other plush items. Don't let a baby sleep with them or on a sheepskin, plush-top mattress, beanbag, waterbed, or a bed wedged up against the wall.

■ Do not place a baby on any surface next to an unguarded window, even for a second, and even asleep.

■ Use smoke detectors in your home and install them according to the recommendations of your local fire department. Keep them maintained.

U.S. First-degree hypospadias, where the urethral opening is at the end of the penis but not in exactly the right place, is considered a minor defect and requires no treatment. Second-degree hypospadias, where the opening is along the underside of the shaft of the penis, can be corrected with reconstructive surgery. Third-degree hypospadias, where the opening is near the scrotum, can usually be corrected, but in such cases two operations are often needed.

Because the foreskin may be used for the reconstruction, circumcision, even ritual circumcision, is not performed on a baby with hypospadias.

Occasionally, a girl is born with hypospadias, with the urethra opening into the vagina. This, too, is usually correctable with surgery.

SUPPLEMENTARY WATER

"A neighbor keeps suggesting that I give our daughter bottles of water instead of nursing her so often."

Though a bottle-fed baby may require a little extra water (up to four ounces in 24 hours) during very hot weather, healthy infants who are fed exclusively on breast milk or formula do not need additional water under ordinary circumstances. Too much water, especially commercially bottled water, can cause a drop in sodium levels in the blood, which can lead to seizures. Giving an older infant small sips of water from a cup, however, is okay. Children on solids can handle more water.

WHAT IT'S IMPORTANT TO KNOW: Babies Develop Differently

From the day a baby's born, the race is on—and it's a sure bet that most parents, rooting their offspring on from the starting line, will be disappointed if their entry doesn't make a good showing. If the child-development chart shows that some babies start turning over at ten weeks, why hasn't their baby accomplished it by twelve weeks? If the baby in the next stroller at the park grabbed an object at three and a half months, why hasn't their baby done it by then? If grandmother insists all of her children sat up by five months, why is theirs still slumping pathetically at six?

But in this race, the child who comes in first in mastering early developmental skills doesn't necessarily finish in the money, while the one who moseys along developmentally doesn't necessarily finish out of it. Though the very alert baby may indeed turn out to be a bright child and a successful adult, attempts to measure infant intelligence and correlate it with intelligence in later years have not been fruitful. The baby who seems to be a little slow, it appears, can also turn out to be bright and successful. Studies have shown, in fact, that 1 in 7 children gains 40 IQ points from the middle of the third year to the age of 17. That means an "average" toddler can become a "gifted" teenager.

Part of the difficulty, of course, is that we don't know how intelligence manifests itself in infancy, or even if it does. And even if we did know, it would be difficult to test for it because infants are nonverbal. We can't ask questions and expect answers, we can't assign a passage for reading and then test for comprehension, we can't present a problem to assess reasoning power. About all we can do is evaluate motor and social skills—and these just aren't equatable with what we later think of as intelligence. Even when we evaluate early developmental skills, our results are often in question; we never know whether a baby is not performing because of inability, lack of opportunity, or a momentary lapse in interest.

Anyone who's spent any time at all around more than one baby knows that children develop at different rates. Probably these differences are due more to nature than to nurture. Each individual seems to be born programmed to smile, lift his or her head, sit up, and take first steps at a particular age. Studies show that there is little we can do to speed up the developmental timetable, though we can slow it down by not providing an adequate environment for development, by lack of stimulation, by poor diet, by poor health care (certain medical or emotional problems can hamper development), and by simply not giving enough love.

Infant development is usually divided into four areas:

Social. How readily your baby learns to smile, coo, and respond to the human face and voice tells you something about him or her as a social being. A serious delay in this area could indicate a problem with vision or hearing, or with emotional or intellectual development.

Language. The child who has a large vocabulary at an early age or who speaks in phrases and sentences before the usual time is probably going to have a way with words. But the child who makes requests with grunts and gestures into the second year may catch up and do just as well or even better later on. Since receptive language development (how well baby understands what is said) is a better gauge of progress than expressive language development (how well baby actually speaks), the child who "understands everything" but says very little is not likely to be experiencing developmental delay. Again, very slow development in this area occasionally

indicates a vision or hearing problem and should be evaluated.

Large motor development. Some babies seem physically active from the first kicks in the womb; once born, they hold their heads up early, sit, pull up, and walk early, and may turn out to be more athletic than most. But there are slow starters who end up excelling on the football field or tennis court, too. Very slow starters, however, should be evaluated to be certain there are no physical or health impediments to normal development.

Small motor development. Early eye-hand coordination, and reaching for, grasping, and manipulating objects before the average age *may* predict a person will be good with his or her hands. However, the baby who takes longer to become skilled in this area is not necessarily going to be "all thumbs" later on.

Most indicators of intellectual development—creativity, sense of humor, and problem-solving skills, for example—don't usually become apparent until toward the end of the first year at the earliest. But eventually, given plenty of opportunity, encouragement, and reinforcement, a child's various inborn abilities will combine to create the adult who is a talented painter, a resourceful mechanic, an effective fundraiser, a savvy stockbroker, a sensitive teacher, an all-star pitcher.

The rate of development in the various areas is usually uneven. One child may smile at six weeks but not reach for a toy until six months, while another may walk at eight months but not talk until a year and a half. When an occasional child does develop evenly in all areas, this may provide a clearer clue to future potential. A child who does everything early, for instance, is likely to be brighter than average; the child who seems extremely slow in every area may have a serious developmental or health problem, in which case professional assessment and intervention is necessary.[6]

Though children develop at different rates, each child's development—assuming no environmental or physical barriers exist—follows the same three basic patterns. First, the child develops from the top down, from head to toes. Babies lift their heads up before they can hold their backs up to sit, and hold their backs up before they can hold their backs up to sit, and hold their backs up before they can stand, on their legs. Second, they develop from the trunk outward to the limbs. Children use their arms before they use their hands, and their hands before they use their fingers. Development moves, not surprisingly, from the simple to the complex.

---

6. The Denver Developmental Screening Test is often used to assess infant development. If a child isn't able to accomplish a particular skill by the age at which 90% of other children do, there is a development delay in that area. If there is a delay in two or more areas, it's probably time to seek the underlying cause and to take remedial action. Early intervention can sometimes make a remarkable difference in the future lives of children who are developing slowly.

Another aspect of infant learning is the deep concentration directed toward learning a particular skill. A child may not be interested in beginning to babble while practicing to pull up. Once a skill is mastered another moves to center stage, and the baby may seem to forget the old, at least for a while, so involved is he or she in the new. Eventually your baby will be able to integrate all the various skills and use each spontaneously and appropriately. But in the meantime, don't despair when he or she seems to forget what was recently learned or looks at you blankly when called on to perform the most recently acquired skill.

No matter what your child's rate of development, what is accomplished in the first year is remarkable—never again will so much be learned so quickly. Enjoy this time and let your baby know you're enjoying it. By accepting your baby's timetable as okay, you will be letting your child know that he or she is okay, too. Avoid comparing your child with other babies (yours or anyone else's) or with norms on developmental charts. Babies should be compared only to themselves, a week earlier or a month ago.

CHAPTER FIVE

The Second Month

WHAT YOUR BABY MAY BE DOING

**By the end of this month, your baby
...should be able to (see Note):**

■ smile in response to your smile
■ follow an object in an arc about 6 inches above the face to the midline (straight ahead)
■ respond to a bell in some way, such as startling, crying, quieting (by 1½ months)
■ vocalize in ways other than crying (e.g. cooing)

Note: If your baby seems not to have reached one or more of these milestones, check with the doctor. In rare instances the delay could indicate a problem, though in most cases it will turn out to be normal for your baby. Premature infants generally reach milestones later than others of the same birth age, often achieving them closer to their adjusted age (the age they would be if they had been born at term), and sometimes later.

...will probably be able to:

■ on stomach, lift head 45 degrees

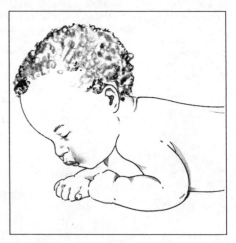

By the end of this month, most babies are able to lift their head to a 45° angle.

■ follow an object in an arc about 6 inches above the face *past* the midline (straight ahead)

...may even be able to:

■ hold head steady when upright

- on stomach, raise chest, supported by arms
- roll over (one way)
- grasp a rattle held to backs or tips of fingers
- pay attention to a raisin or other very small object
- reach for an object
- say ah-goo or similar vowel-consonant combination

...may possibly be able to:

- smile spontaneously
- bring both hands together (2⅔ months)
- on stomach, lift head 90 degrees (2¼ months)
- laugh out loud
- squeal in delight (2¼ months)
- follow an object in an arc about 6 inches above the face for 180 degrees (from one side to the other)

WHAT YOU CAN EXPECT AT THIS MONTH'S CHECKUP

Each doctor or nurse-practitioner will have a personal approach to well-baby checkups. The overall organization of the physical exam, as well as the number and type of assessment techniques used and procedures performed, will also vary with the individual needs of the child. But in general, you can expect the following at a checkup when your baby is about two months old.

- Questions about how you and baby and the rest of the family are doing at home, and about baby's eating, sleeping, and general progress. About child care, if you are planning to return to work.
- Measurement of baby's weight, length, and head circumference, and plotting of progress since birth.
- Physical exam, including a recheck of any previous problems.
- Developmental assessment. The examiner may actually put baby through a series of "tests" to evaluate head control, hand use, vision, hearing, and social interaction or may simply rely on observation plus your reports on what baby is doing.
- First round of immunizations, if baby is in good health and there are no other

contraindications. See recommendations, page 153.
- Guidance about what to expect in the next month in relation to such topics as feeding, sleeping, and development, and advice about infant safety.
- Recommendations about fluoride supplementation if needed in your area, and vitamin D supplementation if your baby is breastfed. Recommendations about iron supplementation for babies not on iron-fortified formula.

Questions you may want to ask, if the doctor hasn't already answered them:

- What reactions can you expect baby to have to the immunizations? How should you treat them? Which reactions should you call about?

Also raise concerns that have arisen over the past month about baby's health, feeding problems, or family adjustment. Jot down information and instructions from the doctor. Record all pertinent information (baby's weight, length, head circumference, birthmarks, immunizations, illnesses, medications given, test results, and so on) in a permanent health record.

FEEDING YOUR BABY THIS MONTH:
Supplementary Bottles

The kangaroo mommy doesn't have much choice. Her baby emerges from the birth canal, climbs into her pouch, latches onto a breast, starts suckling, and continues as needed until it's ready for weaning. The system is much the same in many primitive cultures; babies are slung in a carrier of some sort next to their mothers' breasts and suckle as often as they wish. There's never a need for supplementary feedings. In our society, where we revere independence, even young babies are often apart from their mothers at a long enough distance and for a long enough time to require one or more supplementary feedings. With more and more mothers of infants reentering the work force early, such supplementation is becoming increasingly common; but thanks to the development of good infant formulas and easy-to-use breast pumps, providing these feedings is becoming increasingly easier.

WHY SUPPLEMENT?

A breastfeeding mother may begin supplementary feedings for one or more of a variety of reasons:

■ Plans to return to employment or to school while her baby is young.
■ Plans to wean before her baby is able to get needed milk from a cup (usually eight or nine months at the earliest).
■ The desire to be able to have an occasional afternoon or evening out without baby (alone, or with spouse, friend, or another child), keep appointments (with doctor, dentist, clients, and so on), or attend meetings or classes without taking the child along.
■ The wish to be prepared in case of emergency—you become ill and can't nurse, you get stuck at a meeting and can't get home in time for a regular nursing, you

have to leave town for a day or two.

Mothers who decide not to supplement are more tied down than those who do, but most find it possible, on occasion, to go out to dinner between feedings, or to a movie after baby is bedded down for the night. Among the reasons for not supplementing:

■ Fear that if baby becomes dependent on a bottle, weaning will have to be accomplished twice: first from the breast, then from the bottle. These mothers usually start their babies on a cup as soon as they can sit supported, and use a cup for supplementary feedings of formula or breast milk.
■ The desire not to interfere in any way with the breast milk supply.
■ Having a baby who rejects the bottle. Mothers who see no real need for insisting on it may decide not to press the issue.

HOW TO SUPPLEMENT

When to begin. Some babies have no difficulty switching from breast to bottle and back again right from the start, but most do best with both if the bottle isn't introduced until five or six weeks. Earlier than this, supplementary feedings may interfere with the successful establishment of breastfeeding, and babies may experience nipple confusion because dining at breast and bottle call for different sucking techniques. Much later than this, many babies reject rubber nipples in favor of their beloved mamma's familiar fleshy ones.

What to use. Since cow's milk isn't appropriate fare for a young baby, the two options available to mothers who want to supplement are breast milk and formula.

■ Breast milk. This has the advantage of being free after the purchase of pumping

EMERGENCY CACHE

Even if you don't plan on giving supplementary bottles, it may be a good idea to express and freeze enough breast milk to fill six bottles—just in case. This will give you a backup supply if you become sick, you're temporarily taking medication that might pass into your milk, or you're called out of town unexpectedly. Even if your baby has never taken a bottle, it will be easier for him or her to accept one if it's filled with familiar breast milk rather than with unfamiliar formula.

paraphernalia (which can range from nominal for most hand pumps to very high for electric models). But a great deal of time must often be invested in expressing breast milk (as much as 45 minutes to an hour at first, perhaps 15 minutes to half an hour later, though some women manage to empty both breasts in under 10 minutes once they become experienced). Breast milk has the advantage, of course, of offering optimum nutrition and disease resistance; though an occasional bottle of formula won't detract from that, frequent bottles of formula could.

■ Formula. Expenditure of time and money will vary depending on the type of formula you choose. Ready-to-use formula is costly, but it takes virtually no time to prepare; it's often favored by those who give supplementary formula only occasionally. Formula that requires mixing is less expensive, but requires more time to prepare. Formula is less perfect nutritionally than breast milk, but is certainly an adequate supplement.[1]

Whether you choose to supplement with breast milk or formula, you should keep in mind that it will probably be necessary for you to express milk if you will be away

from your baby for more than three or four hours, to help prevent clogging of milk ducts, leaking, and a diminishing milk supply. The milk can be either collected and saved for future feedings or disposed of. If you're planning to use formula at all, give it in the introductory bottles to accustom baby to its taste.

How much to use. One of the beauties of breastfeeding is that you need never worry about how much or how little your baby is taking. As soon as you start using a bottle, it's easy to succumb to the numbers game. Resist. Tell your baby's caretaker to give your baby only as much as he or she wants, with no prodding or pushing to finish any particular amount. The average 9-pounder may take as much as 6 ounces at a feeding, or less than 2. Remind her, too, that you will be fitting in a couple of extra breastfeedings when you're at home so that she needn't feel obligated to overfeed, which could lead to an overweight baby— or one who doesn't want to nurse when the opportunity presents itself.

Winning baby over. Wait until your baby is both hungry (but not frantically so) and in a good mood before attempting to initiate the bottle. The first few bottles are more likely to be accepted if the nipples have been brought to body temperature under warm tap water and if they are offered by someone other than you—preferably when you're not in the same room for baby to complain to. The substitute feeder should cuddle and talk to the baby during the feeding, just as you would when nursing. If

---

1. Very rarely a baby who was sensitized to milk in the uterus or when he was given it unwittingly in the hospital nursery has a bad reaction to the first sips of cow's milk (in formula or straight). If your baby cries as if in pain, or if you notice swelling of the lips, tongue, and mucous membranes of the mouth, or wheezing within minutes of having milk, call the doctor immediately. Call 911 if you notice the baby is having difficulty breathing. If you give formula only occasionally, do not use the iron-fortified type.

you have to do it yourself, it may help to keep your breasts well camouflaged (don't bottle feed braless or in a low cut blouse) and to distract the baby with background music, a toy, or another form of entertainment. Too much distraction, however, and your baby may want to play, not drink. If your baby tries out the nipple, then drops it with seeming disapproval, try a different type of nipple the next time. For a baby who uses a pacifier, a nipple that is similar in shape may work.

Getting down to a regular schedule. If your schedule will require your regularly missing two feedings during the day, switch to the bottle one feeding at a time, starting at least two weeks before you plan to go back to work or school. Give your baby a full week to get used to one bottle feeding before going on to two. This will help not only baby adjust gradually, but your body as well, if you are planning to supplement with formula rather than breast milk. The wonderful supply and demand mechanism that controls milk production will cut back as you do, making you more comfortable when you're finally back on the job.

Dealing with the occasional bottle. If you plan to give a bottle only occasionally,

nursing fully on both breasts before going out will make fullness and leakage less of a problem. (But do insert breast pads in your bra, just in case.) Be sure your baby won't be fed too close to your return (less than two hours is probably too close) so that, if you are uncomfortably full, you can nurse as soon as you get home.

SUPPLEMENTING WHEN BABY ISN'T THRIVING

Occasionally, formula supplementation is recommended because baby isn't doing well on breast milk alone. This often leaves a mother feeling unsure of what to do. On the one hand, she hears that giving a bottle in such a situation may totally wipe out her chances of breastfeeding successfully; on the other, she is told by the doctor that if she doesn't start supplementing her baby's diet with formula, the health consequences could be serious. The best solution in many such cases is the supplemental nutrition system, shown on page 101, which provides a baby with formula while stimulating mom's breasts to produce more breast milk.

WHAT YOU MAY BE CONCERNED ABOUT

CRADLE CAP

"I wash my daughter's hair every day, but I still can't seem to get rid of the flakes on her scalp."

Don't pack away those dark-shouldered outfits yet. Cradle cap, a seborrheic dermatitis of the scalp common in young infants, doesn't doom your daughter to a lifetime of dandruff. Mild cradle cap, in which greasy surface scales appear on the scalp, often responds well to a brisk massage with mineral oil or petroleum jelly to loosen the

scales, followed by a thorough shampoo to remove them and the oil. Tough cases, in which flaking is heavy and/or brownish patches and yellow crustiness are present, may benefit from the daily use of an antiseborrheic shampoo and/or ointment that contains sulfur salicylates (make sure you keep it out of baby's eyes) after the oil treatment. (Some cases are aggravated by the use of such preparations. If your baby's is, discontinue use and discuss this with the doctor.) Since cradle cap usually worsens when the scalp sweats, keeping it cool and dry may also help—so don't put a hat on baby unless absolutely necessary, and then remove it when you're indoors or in a heated car.

When cradle cap is severe, the seborrheic rash may spread to the face, neck, or buttocks. If this occurs, your baby's doctor will probably prescribe a topical ointment.

Occasionally, cradle cap will persist through the first year—and in a few instances, long after a child has graduated from the cradle. Since the condition causes no discomfort and is therefore considered only a cosmetic problem, aggressive therapy (such as use of topical cortisone, which can contain the flaking for a period of time) isn't usually recommended, but is certainly worth discussing with your child's doctor as a last resort.

SMILING

"My son is five weeks old, and I thought he would be smiling real smiles by now, but he doesn't seem to be."

Cheer up. Even some of the happiest babies don't start true social smiling until six or seven weeks of age. And once they start smiling, some are just naturally more smiley than others. You'll be able to distinguish the first real smile from those tentative practice ones by the way the baby uses his whole face—not just his mouth. Though babies don't smile until they're ready, they're ready faster when they're talked to, played with, and cuddled a lot. So smile at your baby and talk to him often, and very soon he'll be smiling back.

COOING

"My six-week-old baby makes a lot of breathy vowel sounds, but no consonants at all. Does this mean she might have a speech defect?"

With young babies, the "ayes"—and the a's, e's, o's, and u's—have it. It's the vowel sounds they make first, somewhere between the first few weeks and the end of the second month. At first the breathy, melodic (and adorable) cooing and throaty gurgles seem totally random, and then you'll begin to notice they're directed at you when you talk to your baby, at a stuffed animal who's sharing her playpen, at a mobile up above that's caught her eye, or even at a flower on the sofa upholstery. These vocal exercises are often practiced as much for her own pleasure as for yours; babies actually seem to love listening to their own voices. They are also educational; baby is discovering which combinations of throat, tongue, and mouth actions make what sounds.

For mommy and daddy, cooing is a welcome step up from crying on the communication ladder. And it's just the beginning. Within a few weeks to a few months baby will begin adding laughing out loud (usually by three and a half months), squealing (by four and a half months), and a few consonants to her repertoire. The range for initiating consonant vocalizations is very broad—some make a few consonant-like sounds in the third month, others not until five or six months, though four months is about average.

When babies begin experimenting with consonants, they usually discover one or two at a time, and repeat the same single combination (ba or ga or da) over and over and over. The next week, they may move on to a new combination, seeming to have forgotten the first. They haven't, but since their powers of concentration are limited, they usually work on mastering one thing at a time.

Following the two-syllable, one-consonant sounds (a-ga, a-ba, a-da), come sing-song strings of consonants (da-da-da-da-da-da) called "babble," at six months on the average. By eight months, many babies can produce word-like double consonants (da-da, ma-ma, ba-ba), usually without associating any meaning with them until two or three months later. (To fathers' delight, da-da generally comes before mama.) Mastery of *all* the consonants doesn't come until much later, often not until four or five years of age. A few perfectly normal youngsters have difficulty with certain consonants (often l's or s's) into their school years.

"Our baby doesn't seem to make the same kind of cooing sounds that his older brother made at six weeks. Should we be concerned?"

Some normal babies develop language skills earlier than average, some later. About 10% of babies start cooing before the end of the first month and another 10% don't start until nearly three months. Some start with strings of consonants before the 4½-month mark; others don't string consonants until past eight months. The early verbalizers may end up very strong in language skills (though the evidence isn't that clear); those who lag far behind, in the lowest 10%, may have a physical or developmental problem, but this isn't clear either. Certainly, it's too early to be concerned that this might be the case with your baby, since he's still probably well within the norm.

If it seems to you over the next several months that your baby consistently, in spite of your encouragement, falls far below the monthly milestones in each chapter, speak to his doctor about your concerns. A hearing evaluation or other tests may be in order. It may turn out that you are so busy that you aren't really noticing your baby's vocal achievements (this sometimes happens with second children). In the less likely case that there actually is a problem, early attention may be able to remedy it.

CROOKED FEET

"Our son's feet seem to fold inward. Will they straighten out on their own?"

The answer is almost certainly yes. Most babies appear bowlegged and pigeon-toed. This is because of the normal rotational curve in the legs of a newborn and because the cramped quarters in the uterus often force one or both feet into odd positions. When he emerges at birth, after spending several months in that position, the feet are still bent or seem to turn inward.

In the months ahead, as your baby's feet enjoy their freedom and as he learns to pull up, crawl, and then walk, his feet will begin straightening out. They almost always do without the early casting or special shoes and bars that were once routine treatment. Which is probably why these treatments, most of which are now deemed to be completely ineffective, usually appeared to "cure" the problem.

Just to be sure that an abnormality isn't the cause of your baby's foot problems, express your concerns at his next well-baby visit. The doctor probably has already checked your baby's feet for abnormalities, but another check won't hurt. The doctor will also want to keep an eye on the progress of the feet as your baby grows. If your baby's feet don't appear to be straightening out on their own, casting or special shoes may be required at a later date. At just what point this becomes necessary will depend on the type of problem and on the doctor's point of view.

COMPARING BABIES

"I get together regularly with a group of other new mothers, and inevitably they all start comparing what their babies have been doing. It makes me crazy— and worried about whether my daughter is developing normally."

If there's anything more anxiety-provoking than a roomful of pregnant women comparing bellies, it's a roomful of recently delivered women comparing babies. Just as no two pregnant bellies are exactly alike, neither are any two babies. Developmental norms (such as those found in each chapter in this book) are useful for comparing your baby to a broad range of normal infants in order to assess her progress and identify any lags. But comparing your baby with someone else's child, or with an older one of your own, can only result in a lot of unnecessary fears and frustrations. Two perfectly "normal" babies can develop in different areas at completely different clips—one may forge ahead in vocalizing and socializing, another in physical feats, such as turning over. Differences between babies become even more marked as the first year progresses—one baby may crawl very early but not walk until fifteen months, another may never learn to crawl at all but suddenly start taking steps at ten months. Then, too, a mother's assessment of her baby's progress is highly subjective—and not always completely accurate. One mother may not even recognize her baby's frequent coos as the beginnings of language, while another may hear one coo and swear, "She said 'mama'!"

All of this said, it's easier to intellectualize that comparing babies isn't a good idea than to actually stop doing it or avoid those who do. Many compulsive comparers can't sit within ten feet of another mother-with-baby on a bus, in a doctor's waiting room, or at the park without assaulting her with outwardly innocent queries that lead to the inevitable comparisons ("What an adorable baby! She's sitting already? How old is she?"). The best advice, if you can't completely manage to "mind your own baby," is to keep in mind how meaningless these comparisons really are. Your baby, like your belly before her, is one of a kind.

USING A BABY CARRIER

"We usually carry our son around in a baby carrier. Is this a good idea?"

Although baby carriers—cloth sacks that harness infants to their caregivers—have become popular only recently in the U.S., they have, in one form or another, been helping transport babies in other cultures since prehistoric times. There are at least three good reasons. First, babies are usually happy riding in a carrier; they enjoy the steady gentle movement and the closeness to a warm body. Second, babies tend to cry less during the rest of the day if they are carried around a lot, something made easier by the use of a carrier. And third, carriers provide mothers, dads, and other caregivers with the freedom to attend to their daily chores while carrying baby.

But if baby carriers are a boon to today's parents, they can also be a bane. If you elect to continue using one, keep these risks in mind:

Overheating. On a very warm day, even a scantily clothed baby can simmer in a baby carrier—particularly one that encloses the baby's legs, feet, and head or is made from a heavy fabric such as corduroy. Such overheating can lead to prickly heat and even heat stroke. If you use a carrier in warm weather or in overheated rooms or vehicles, check your baby frequently to be sure he isn't sweating and his body doesn't feel warmer than yours. If he does appear to be overheated, remove some clothing or take him out of the carrier completely.

Understimulation. A baby who's always cooped up in a baby carrier, with his visual perspective limited to a chest, and if he looks up, a face, doesn't have the opportunity he needs to see the world. This is not a major problem in the first few weeks of life, when a baby's interest is usually limited to the most basic creature comforts, but it can be now, when he's ready to expand his horizons. Look for a convertible carrier in which baby can face in for a nap or out for viewing the world, or limit baby's sojourns to times when he will be sleeping or will be pacified only by being carried and you need your arms for other purposes. At other times, use a stroller or baby seat.

Too much sleeping. Babies who are toted in baby carriers tend to sleep a lot— often a lot more than they need to. With two less-than-desirable results. First, they get used to catnapping (fifteen minutes when you run out to the grocery store, twenty when you walk the dog) rather than taking longer naps in their cribs. Second, they may become so well rested during the day that they don't rest much at night. If your baby immediately falls asleep when placed in a carrier, use it only at naptime, and for the duration of the nap.

Risk of injury. A young infant's neck isn't strong enough yet to support his head when he's jiggled and jostled a lot. Though securing your baby in a baby carrier while you jog may seem like an ideal way of getting your exercise and keeping your baby happy too, the bouncing could be risky. Instead, strap him in a stroller when you go for a jog. Also be careful to bend at the knees, *not the waist,* when wearing the carrier—or your toddler could slip out.

While judicious use of a baby carrier can work well at this age, your baby won't be ready for a back carrier until he can sit by himself.

IMMUNIZATION

"My baby's pediatrician says that immunization is perfectly safe. But I've heard a lot of horror stories about serious— even fatal—reactions, and I worry about letting him give my daughter the shots."

We live in a society that considers good news to be no news. A story on the positive effects of immunizations cannot compete with one on the extremely rare instances of fatal complications associated with them. So it is likely that today's parents have heard more about the risks of immunization than the benefits. And yet, as your pediatrician has doubtless told you, for most infants those benefits continue to far outweigh the risks.

Not too many years ago, in the U.S., the most common causes of infant death were infectious diseases, such as diphtheria, typhoid, and smallpox. Measles and whooping cough were so common that all children were expected to get them, and thousands, especially infants, died or were permanently handicapped by these illnesses. Parents dreaded the coming of summer and the infantile paralysis (polio) epidemics that seemed invariably to arrive with it, killing or disabling thousands of infants and children. Today, smallpox has been virtually eliminated, and diphtheria and typhoid are extremely rare. Only a small percentage of children are stricken with measles or whooping cough each year, and infantile paralysis is a disease young mothers are not only no longer afraid of, but often aren't even familiar with. An American baby is now much more likely to die because of not being strapped into a car seat than from a communicable disease. And immunization is the reason.

Immunization is based on the fact that exposure to weakened or dead disease-producing microorganisms (in the form of vaccines) or to the poisons (toxins) they produce, rendered harmless by heat or chemical treatment (then called toxoids), will cause an individual to produce the same antibodies that would develop if the person had actually contracted the disease. Armed with the special memory that is unique to the immune system, these antibodies will "recognize" the specific microorganisms, should they attack in the future, and destroy them.

Even the ancients recognized that when someone survived a particular disease, they weren't likely to contract it again; those who had recovered from the plague were sometimes used to care for new victims. Although some societies attempted crude forms of immunization, it wasn't until Edward Jenner, a Scottish physician, decided to test the old belief that a person who contracted the lesser disease cowpox would never get smallpox, that modern immunization was born. In 1796, Jenner smeared pus from the sores of a milkmaid infected with cowpox on two small cuts in the arm of a healthy eight-year-old boy. The child developed a slight fever a week later, then a couple of small scabs on his arm. Subsequently, he was exposed to smallpox and remained healthy. He had become immune.

Today, immunization saves thousands of lives each year in this country. But it's not perfect. Though most children have only a mild reaction to immunization, some become ill, a very few seriously so. Some types of vaccine have been suspected of causing, on rare occasions, permanent damage, even death. But as the benefits of crossing the street or going for a ride in the family car outweigh the very real risks involved in these activities, so do the benefits of protection from serious disease outweigh the risks of the immunization for all but high-risk children (see page 151). And as you take precautions to decrease risks when crossing the street (by crossing with the light and looking both ways) or riding in an auto (by driving carefully and using car seats and seat belts), so should you take precautions when having your child vaccinated (by watching for and reporting side effects and being sure your child is in good health before being given a shot).

The first widely administered type of immunization, the smallpox vaccination, was so successful that it is no longer necessary. The disease seems to have been eradicated from the entire globe. It's hoped that immunization will someday wipe out other serious scourges as well. In the meantime, except as noted, your baby will probably receive the following immunizations, beginning at two months and continuing throughout childhood.

Diptheria, Tetanus, Pertussis vaccine (DTaP). Immunization against diphtheria, tetanus, and pertussis (whooping cough) is crucial. The preferred vaccine is the newer DTaP, which contains diphtheria and tetanus toxoids and an acellular pertussis vaccine, although the original DTP vaccine (with a whole-cell pertussis vaccine) is an acceptable alternative. While reactions to either of the toxoids are extremely rare, the whole-cell form of the pertussis component has sometimes caused severe reactions. Reactions to the acellular pertussis vaccine are much less common and much milder. Though there were rare reports of a link between the old vaccine and brain damage (which were unsubstantiated), there have been no such reports with the new one.

DtaP, preferably, (or DTP) is recommended at two, four, and six months, 15 to 18 months, and between four and six years. As minimal as the risk is, it's still wise to take the following steps to make certain your baby is safely vaccinated:

■ Be sure the doctor gives your baby a thorough checkup before a DTP inoculation to be certain no illness is developing that is not yet apparent.

■ Observe your baby carefully for 72 hours after the vaccination (especially during the first 48), and report any severe reactions (see page 150) to the doctor *immediately*. Also report any very unusual behavior during the first seven days that might be signs of brain inflammation.

■ Ask the doctor to enter the vaccine manufacturer's name and the vaccine lot/ batch number in your child's records, along with any reactions you report. Ask for a copy of the information for your own records. Severe reactions should be reported by the doctor to the Centers for Disease control in Atlanta.

■ When the next DTP is scheduled, remind your baby's doctor about *any* previous reactions to the vaccine.

■ If you have any fears about vaccine safety, discuss them with your baby's doctor.

Taking any possible precautions when your child is being immunized makes sense, but panicking and refusing to have your low-risk child immunized against diphtheria, tetanus, and pertussis clearly doesn't.

WHAT YOU SHOULD KNOW ABOUT DTP

COMMON REACTIONS TO DTP

The following reactions to DTP are listed in order of frequency, with the first three most common, occurring in about half of immunized children. All usually last only a day or two.

- Pain at the injection site
- Mild to moderate fever (100° to 104°F, rectally)
- Fussiness
- Swelling at the site
- Redness at the site
- Drowsiness
- Loss of appetite
- Vomiting

Baby acetaminophen can be given for fever and pain—administered right after the immunization as a prophylactic measure, it appears to significantly reduce reactions. Warm compresses on the injection site may also help to reduce baby's discomfort. Fever and local soreness may be more of a problem with each subsequent dose of DTP, but fussiness and vomiting may be less frequent.

WHEN TO CALL THE DOCTOR

If your baby exhibits any of the following within 48 hours of a DTP injection, call the doctor's office, not just for your baby's sake, but also so that the doctor can report the response to the Monitoring System for Adverse Events Following Immunization at the Centers for Disease Control. The more information that's collected for scientific evaluation, the more likely the risk of immunization will eventually be reduced.

- High-pitched persistent crying for more than three hours
- Excessive sleepiness (baby may be difficult to wake)
- Unusual limpness or paleness
- Rectal temperature of 104°F or higher
- Convulsions

Symptoms of brain inflammation, such as convulsions or changes in consciousness, may not occur until as long as a week after the immunization. (A recent study indicated that even such a severe reaction is unlikely to cause significant permanent neurological damage.)

Polio Vaccine (IPV or OPV). Immunization has virtually eliminated polio, once a dreaded disease, from the U.S. There are two types of polio vaccine: OPV, a live vaccine given by mouth, and IPV, an inactivated vaccine given by injection directly into the bloodstream. Both are effective and there are three acceptable schedules for administering polio vaccine: IPV at two and four months and OPV twelve to eighteen months and four to six years *or* IPV at two, four, and twelve to eighteen months, and four to six years *or* OPV at two, four, and six to eighteen months, and four to six years.

The vaccine has proven to be quite safe and children rarely have any reactions following a dose. But there is a minuscule risk (about 1 in 8.7 million) of paralysis and a slightly greater (about 1 in 5 million) risk that a susceptible parent or other household member might contract polio from a child immunized with OPV. For that reason, IPV, which doesn't enter the digestive tract, is recommended when either the child or a family member has cancer or has an immune system depressed either by illness or medical treatment.

When the live oral polio vaccine (OPV) is used, meticulous care should be taken when cleaning up the recently vaccinated child after a bowel movement; careful hand washing is also essential.

WHEN TO OMIT THE PERTUSSIS VACCINE

The American Academy of Pediatrics (AAP) recommends that the pertussis component of the DTP be omitted (and that DT, containing just the diphtheria and tetanus components, be substituted) for children:

■ With a past history of convulsions or seizures, unless or until neurological disease has been ruled out.

■ With confirmed or suspected neurological disease, such as epilepsy.

■ Who have had a severe allergic reaction within hours of a previous DTP shot, or convulsions within 3 days, a fever of 104.9°F or more within 2 days, or serious brain problems within 7 days.

■ Who, on a case-by-case basis, reacted to a previous shot with unusually high-pitched crying, uncharacteristically persistent crying for more than three hours, excessive sleepiness, limpness, unusual paleness. Discuss the significance of such reactions with your baby's doctor.

■ With confirmed or suspected neurological disease, such as epilepsy, unless or until such disease is ruled out or well controlled. (Children with stable neurological conditions, such as cerebral palsy, may be vaccinated.)

Policies for the administration of DTP vary slightly from doctor to doctor, and you should ask your baby's doctor about his or hers. Most will postpone the shot for a baby who has a fever, and some will do so even for a mild cold. Many wait as much as a month following a fever to administer the DTP. Vaccination is generally not postponed if a child suffers from frequent allergy-caused nasal congestion that has been traced to allergy rather than infection.

During an epidemic even high-risk children are generally immunized, since the danger from whooping cough itself, which kills 1 in 100 infected children under six months of age, is much more serious than the danger from the vaccine.

It's usually recommended that booster shots given after age seven not contain pertussis vaccine, since the disease is both less risky and less common after this age and the danger of the vaccine is greater. A reduced dose of diphtheria vaccine is also suggested after this age, when reactions tend to be more severe. The combined vaccine for older children is labeled Td, and boosters are recommended every seven to ten years throughout life.

Measles, Mumps, Rubella (MMR). You may not have been immunized against these common childhood diseases in your infancy, but your baby almost certainly will be—usually with a combination vaccine at twelve to fifteen months of age, because it is less effective earlier.[2] Measles, though often joked about, is in reality a serious disease with sometimes serious, potentially fatal, complications. Rubella, also known as German measles, on the other hand, is often so mild that its symptoms are missed. But because it can cause birth defects in the fetus of an in-

fected pregnant woman, immunization in early childhood is recommended—both to protect the future fetuses of girl babies and to reduce the risk of infected children exposing their pregnant mommies. Mumps rarely presents a serious problem in childhood, but because it can have severe consequences (such as sterility or deafness) in adulthood, early immunization is recommended.

Reactions to the MMR vaccine are fairly common, but are generally very mild and usually don't occur until a week or two after the shot. About 1 in 5 children will get a rash or slight fever lasting a few days from the measles component. About 1 in 7 will get a rash or some swelling of the neck glands, and 1 in 20,

---

2. Children under a year of age usually do not develop complete immunity to measles, mumps, and rubella when immunized; for this reason, MMR is not given earlier.

aching or swelling of the joints from the rubella component, sometimes as long as three weeks after the shot. Occasionally, there may be swelling of the salivary glands from the mumps component. Much less common are tingling, numbness, or pain in the hands and feet, all difficult to discern in infants, and allergic reactions. It is also possible (but experts aren't sure) that the MMR vaccine may be responsible for encephalitis (inflammation of the brain), convulsions with fever, or nerve deafness in very rare cases.

Caution should be taken in administering MMR to a child sick with anything but a mild cold, one with an impaired immune system (from medication, cancer, or another condition), or one who has had gamma globulin in the preceding three months or RSV-IVIG in the previous nine months.

Varicella zoster vaccine (VZV). Varicella, or chicken pox, is usually a mild disease without serious side effects. There can be complications, however, such as Reye's syndrome and bacterial infections; and the disease can be fatal to high-risk children, such as those with leukemia or immune deficiencies, or whose mothers were infected just prior to their birth. A varicella vaccine has been licensed by the FDA for use in healthy children over one year of age who have not had a confirmed case of chicken pox and in nonimmune adolescents and adults. It's not clear whether a booster shot will be needed later.

Hemophilus b vaccines. These vaccines are aimed at thwarting the deadly hemophilus influenzae b (Hib) bacteria that are the cause of a wide range of very serious infections in infants and young children. Hib is responsible for about 12,000 cases of meningitis in children in the United States annually (5% of them fatal) and for nearly all epiglottitis (a potentially fatal infection that obstructs the airways). It is also the leading cause of septicemia (blood infection), cellulitis (skin and connective tissue infection), osteomyelitis (bone infection), pericarditis (heart membrane infection) in young children.

A conjugate Hib vaccine approved in 1990 appears to have few, if any, side effects. The AAP recommends the vaccine be given at two, four, and six months, with a fourth dose at 12 to 15 months.

As with other vaccines, Hib vaccines should not be given to a child who is ill with anything more than a mild cold, or who might be allergic to any of their components (check with the doctor). Though adverse reactions are rare, a very small percentage of children may have fever, redness and/or tenderness on the site of the shot, diarrhea, vomiting, and crying after receiving the conjugate Hib vaccine.

Hepatitis b vaccine. Since programs to immunize adults against this serious infection have failed, it is now recommended that everyone be vaccinated against hepatitis B in childhood.

Preferably, all newborns should be given their first dose of HBV vaccine at birth. Such immunization is imperative for infants of infected mothers within 12 hours of birth. Additional doses are recommended at two to four months, and six to 18 months. Children who have not been vaccinated earlier, should also be immunized, no matter their ages. The vaccine has shown no serious side effects.

HbOC-DTP. A combination vaccine, which protects against Hib as well as diphtheria, tetanus, and pertussis, is now available, and can be used at 2, 4, 6, and 15 months, or just for the first three shots, with DTaP being substituted for the fourth. The plus: fewer bouts with a hypodermic needle.

If for some reason any of your baby's vaccinations are postponed, there's no cause for concern. Immunization can pick up where it left off; starting over isn't necessary.

RECOMMENDED IMMUNIZATION SCHEDULE

AGE	DTaP[1]	Td	Polio[2]	MMR	Hib[1]	Hep–B[3]	VZV[4]
Birth to 2 months						x	
2 months	x		x		x		
1 to 4 months						x	
4 months	x		x		x		
6 months	x				x[5]		
6 to 18 months						x	
12 to 15 months[8]				x	x		
12 to 18 months			x[9]				x
15 to 18 months	x[6]						x
4 to 6 years	x		x	x or			
11 to 12 years				x			
11 to 16 years		x[7]					

1. DTP or DTaP. DTaP is preferred. DTaP and Hib may be combined into 1 dose. 2. Oral (OPV) or inactivated (IPV) acceptable. 3. Infants of women positive for Hep-B, should receive 2nd dose at 1 to 2 months and the 3rd at six months. 4. Varicella zoster (chicken pox) vaccine is now approved for use in healthy children. 5. Children who have received Pedvax HIB do not require this dose. 6. The fourth dose of DTP/DTaP should be given at least 6 months after the third. 7. Given every 10 years throughout life. 8. Vaccines recommended at 12 to 15 months may all be given at one visit or divided between two. 9. Six to 12 months with OPV.

FLU IMMUNIZATION

"Everybody's talking about a big influenza epidemic. Should my two-month-old son get shots?"

Generally, influenza is a mild disease, with few serious complications in healthy people, and one that doesn't attack everyone, even during an epidemic. Because of this, flu shots are recommended only for children who are highly susceptible: those with serious heart or lung disease, those with depressed immune systems, and those with sickle-cell anemia or similar blood diseases. Though newborns are particularly susceptible to influenza, immunization against it isn't presently recommended for them because little is known about the benefits and risks of giving flu shots to children under six months of age.

If your doctor does suggest your baby be immunized against flu, only the "split-virus" form of the vaccine should be used.[1] A spray vaccine, now under study, may make flu immunization easier in the future.

---

3. Flu vaccine should not be given to anyone who has had a severe allergic reaction to eggs. High-risk children may, instead, be given antiviral medications to prevent development of influenza.

Don't confuse a flu (or influenza) shot with immunization for hemophilus influenzae type b (Hib), which is routinely recommended.

UNDESCENDED TESTICLES

"My son was born with undescended testicles. The doctor said that they would probably descend from the abdomen by the time he was a month or two old, but they haven't yet."

The abdomen may seem a bizarre location for testicles, but it isn't. The testicles (or testes) in males and the ovaries in females both develop in the fetal abdomen from the same embryonic tissue. The ovaries, of course, stay put. The testes are scheduled to descend down through the inguinal canals in the groin, into the scrotal sac at the base of the penis, somewhere around the eighth month of gestation. But in 3 to 4% of full-term boys and about one third of those that are preterm, they don't make the trip before birth. The result: undescended testicles.

Because of the migratory habits of testicles, it's not always easy to determine that one hasn't descended. Normally, the testicles hang away from the body when they are in danger of overheating (protecting the sperm-producing mechanism from temperatures that are too high). But they slip back up into the body when they are chilled (protecting the sperm-producing mechanism from temperatures that are too low) or when they are handled (again protective, to avoid injury). In some boys the testes are particularly sensitive and spend a lot of time sheltered in the body. In most, the left testicle hangs lower than the right, possibly making the right seem undescended (and making a lot of young boys worry). The diagnosis of undescended testicle or testicles is therefore made only when one or both have never been observed to be in the scrotum, not even when the

baby is in a warm bath.

An undescended testicle causes no pain or difficulty with urinating, and as your doctor assured you, usually descends on its own. By age one, only 3 or 4 boys in 1,000 still have undescended testicles. In the rare cases that remain stubbornly in the abdomen by age five, surgery is recommended and is generally successful.

HERNIA

"I was very upset when the pediatrician said that my twin boys have inguinal hernias and will have to have surgery."

A hernia is often thought of as something that occurs in a grown man who has lifted too heavy a load. But hernias are not unusual in newborns, particularly boys, and especially those born prematurely (as twins often are).

In an inguinal hernia, a part of the intestines slips through one of the inguinal canals (the same channels through which the testes descend into the scrotum) and bulge into the groin. The defect is often first noted as a lump in one of the creases where the thigh joins the abdomen, particularly when a baby is crying or very active; it often retracts when he is quiet. When the section of the intestines slips all the way down into the scrotum, it can be seen as an enlargement or swelling in the scrotum, and may be referred to as scrotal hernia.

Though most of the time an inguinal hernia causes no problems, occasionally it becomes "strangulated." The herniated section becomes pinched by the muscular lining of the inguinal canal, obstructing blood flow and digestion in the intestines. Vomiting, severe pain, even shock can result. For this reason, any parent who notices a lump or swelling in their baby's groin or scrotum should report the finding to the doctor as soon as possible. Since strangulation of an inguinal hernia is most common in babies under six months of age, doctors usually advise repair as soon as the hernia is diagnosed—assuming the baby is fit for surgery. Such surgery is usually simple and successful, with a very short (sometimes one-day) hospitalization. Only very rarely does an inguinal hernia recur following surgery, though in some children a hernia occurs on the opposite side at a later date.

Because of the usually prompt treatment of diagnosed infant inguinal hernia, most cases of strangulated hernia turn up in babies whose hernias haven't been previously diagnosed. So parents who note a baby suddenly crying in pain, vomiting, and not having bowel movements should check for a lump in the groin. If one is found, an immediate call to the doctor is necessary. If the doctor can't be reached, the baby should be taken to the nearest emergency room. Elevating the baby's bottom slightly and applying an ice pack while en route to the ER may help the intestine to retract, but don't try to push it back in by hand. And don't offer a breast or bottle to comfort the baby, since surgery will probably be necessary and an empty digestive tract will be best.

INVERTED NIPPLES

"One of my daughter's nipples sinks in instead of standing out. What's wrong with it?"

This sounds like her nipple is inverted, not at all uncommon in infants. Often, a nipple that is inverted at birth corrects itself spontaneously later. If it doesn't, it poses no functional problem until she's ready to nurse her own baby, at which point there will be steps she can take to draw the nipple out.

REJECTION OF THE BREAST

"My baby was doing very well at the breast—now suddenly, he's refused to nurse for the past eight hours. Could something be wrong with my milk?"

Something is probably wrong—though not necessarily with your milk. Temporary rejection of the breast is not unusual, and almost always has a specific cause, the most common of which are:

Mother's diet. Have you been indulging in pasta al pesto or another dish redolent with garlic? Feasting your chops and chopsticks on General Tso's chicken? Honoring St. Patrick with corned beef and cabbage? If so, your baby may simply be protesting the spicy and/or strong flavors your diet is imparting to his milk. If you figure out what turns your baby off, avoid eating it until after you've weaned him.

A cold. Babies who can't breathe through stuffy noses can't nurse and breathe through their mouths at the same time; understandably, they opt for breathing. Use a cool mist vaporizer, gently suction nostrils with an infant nasal aspirator, or ask your baby's doctor about nose drops.

Teething. Though most babies don't begin the struggle with teeth until at least five or six months, a few babies begin teething much earlier, and a very occasional two-month-old actually sprouts a tooth or two. Nursing often puts pressure on swollen gums, making suckling painful. When teeth are the cause of breast rejection, a baby usually starts nursing eagerly, only to pull away in pain.

An earache. Because ear pain can radiate to the jaw, the sucking motions of nursing can make discomfort worse. See page 423 for other clues to ear infection.

Thrush. If your baby has this fungal infection in his mouth, nursing may be painful. Be sure the condition is treated so that the infection isn't passed on to you through cracked nipples, or spread elsewhere on the baby (see page 69).

Slow let-down. A very hungry baby may grow impatient when milk doesn't flow immediately (in some women let-down may take as long as five minutes to occur), and may push away the nipple in a fury before let-down begins. To avoid this problem, express a little milk before you pick him up, so that he'll get something for his efforts the moment he starts to suck.

A hormonal change in you. A new pregnancy (very unlikely now if you're nursing exclusively, more possible if you've started your baby on solids and/or numerous supplemental formula feedings) can produce hormones that change the taste of the breast milk, causing baby to reject the breast. So can the return of menstruation, which again isn't usually an issue until partial weaning begins.

Tension in you. If you're worried or upset you may be communicating your tension to your baby, making him too agitated to nurse. Relax.

Readiness for weaning. An older baby who rejects the breast may be saying, "Mommy, I've had it with nursing. I'm ready to move on." Ironically, babies seem to do this when their mothers are not the least bit interested in weaning, rather than when mother is ready to quit nursing.

Once in a while, there appears to be no obvious explanation for a baby's turning down the breast. Like an adult, a baby can be "off his feed" for a meal or two. Fortunately, this kind of hiatus is usually temporary. If disinterest in nursing continues, or if it occurs in connection with other signs of illness, speak to his doctor.

FAVORING ONE BREAST

"My little girl hardly ever wants to nurse on my left breast and it's shrunken to be considerably smaller than the right."

Some babies play favorites. Why a baby prefers one breast over another isn't certain. It could be that she's more comfortable cradled in her mother's favored, and probably stronger, arm, so she develops a taste for the breast on that side. Or that her right-handed mother tends to place her on the left breast, so that the right hand is free for eating, holding a book or the phone, or handling other chores, leaving the right to dwindle in size and production. Perhaps one breast is the better provider, due to the mother or baby favoring one side early on in the nursing relationship, for reasons as diverse as the location of the pain from a cesarean incision and the location of the TV set in your bedroom.

Whatever the reason, preferring one breast over the other is a fact of nursing for some babies, and lopsidedness a fact of life for their mothers. Though you might try to increase production on the less favored side by pumping daily and/or starting every feeding with it (if your baby will cooperate), these efforts may not do the trick. In many cases, mothers go through the entire nursing experience with one breast larger than the other. The lopsidedness will diminish after weaning, though a slightly greater-than-normal difference may continue. The only sure solution in the interim: stuffing the roomier bra cup to make the breasts look even and clothes fit better.

Very rarely the baby rejects a breast because it harbors a developing malignancy. So do mention your baby's penchant to your doctor.

DIFFICULT BABY

"Our little girl is adorable, but she seems to cry for the least little reason. If it's too noisy, or too bright, or even if she's a little wet. My husband and I are going crazy. Are we doing something wrong?"

No parent expects to have a difficult baby. Pregnant daydreams are pink-and-blue collages of a contented infant who coos, smiles, sleeps peacefully, cries only when she's hungry, and grows into a sweet-tempered cooperative youngster. Bawling, inconsolable babies and kicking, screaming toddlers belong to others—parents who did it all wrong and are paying the price.

And then, for parents like you, just

weeks after your perfect baby is born, reality shatters the fantasy. Suddenly, it's your baby who's crying all the time, who won't sleep, or who seems perpetually unhappy and dissatisfied. Why shouldn't you wonder, "What did I do wrong?"

The answer is probably nothing, except perhaps pass on some unfortunate genes to your offspring, for a baby's temperament appears to have much more to do with heredity than environment. How the childhood environment is structured, however, can make a difference as to how inborn temperament affects future development. With more attention to stimulation, for example, difficult children often turn out to have higher IQs than average. And the child who, with help from mommy and daddy, learns to direct and develop inborn personality traits, transforming them from liabilities into assets, can go from impossible problem infant to successful adult.[4]

The parental role in this metamorphosis is critical. The first step is to identify which of several different types of personalities that have been linked to difficult behavior your own baby displays (some display a combination). Your baby seems to be a what is known as a low-sensory threshold baby. A wet diaper, a starched dress, a high neckline, a bright light, a staticky radio, a scratchy blanket, a cold crib—any or all of these may unduly upset a baby who seems to be extra sensitive to sensory stimulation. In some children, all five senses—hearing, vision, taste, touch, and smell—are very easily overloaded; in others, just one or two. Dealing with the low-sensory-threshold child requires keeping the general level of sensory stimulation down, as well as avoiding those specific things that you notice bother baby, such as:

▪ Sound sensitivity. Lower the sound level in your home by keeping the radio, stereo, and TV low or off, adjusting your tele-phone ring to low, asking people to knock instead of ringing the doorbell, and installing carpeting and draperies, where possible, to absorb sound. Speak or sing to your baby softly and have others do the same. Be sure any musical or other sound-producing devices aren't disturbing to baby. If outside noises seem to be a problem, try a white-noise machine or air cleaner in baby's room to block them out.

▪ Light or visual sensitivity. Use room darkening shades or drapes so baby can sleep later in the morning and nap during the day, and avoid very bright lights in rooms she frequents. Don't expose her to too much visual stimulation at once—hang just one toy in the crib, or put just a couple in the playpen at a time. Select toys that are soft and subtle in color and design rather than bright and busy.

▪ Taste sensitivity. If your baby is breastfed and has a bad day after you eat garlic or onions, consider that the unfamiliar taste of your milk may be the cause; if she's bottlefed and seems cranky a lot, try a formula with a different taste. When you introduce solids, recognize the fact that your baby may not relish every taste sensation and may reject some entirely.

▪ Touch sensitivity. Some babies lose their composure as soon as they wet their diapers, become frantic when they're too warm or dressed in rough fabrics, scream when they're dunked in the tub or put down on a too-cold mattress, or, later, when you buckle their shoes over wrinkled socks. So keep clothing comfortable (cotton knits with smooth seams and buttons, snaps, labels, and collars that won't irritate because of size, shape, or location are ideal), bath water and room temperatures at levels she seems happiest at, and diapers changed frequently (absorbent disposables may be better accepted than cloth diapers).

A small percentage of babies are so oversensitive to touch that they resist being held and cuddled. Don't overhandle such a baby; do a lot of your caressing and interacting with words and eye contact rather than actual physical touching. When you

4. For valuable help in dealing with a difficult baby, see *The Difficult Child* (Bantam) by Stanley Turecki, M.D.

DO YOU HAVE A DIFFICULT BABY?

The active baby. Babies often send the first clue that they're going to be more active than most right from the uterus; suspicions are confirmed soon after birth when coverings are kicked off, diapering and dressing sessions become wrestling matches, and baby always ends up at the opposite end of the crib after a nap. Active babies are a constant challenge (they sleep less than most, become restless when feeding, and are always at risk of hurting themselves), but they can also be a joy (they're usually very alert, interested and interesting, and quick to accomplish). While you don't want to squelch such a baby's enthusiasm and adventurous nature, you will want to take special protective precautions as well as learn ways to quiet him or her for eating and sleeping. The following tips should help:

■ Use a blanket sleeper in cold weather, lightweight sleepers in cool weather, for a baby who kicks off the covers.

■ Be especially careful never to leave an active baby on a bed, changing table, or any other elevated spot even for a second—they often figure out how to turn over very early, and sometimes just when you least expect it. A restraining strap on the changing table is useful, but should not be relied upon if you're more than a step away.

■ Adjust the crib mattress to its lowest level as soon as the active baby starts to sit alone for even a few seconds—the next step may be pulling up and over the sides of the crib. Keep all objects a baby might climb on out of crib and playpen.

■ Don't leave an active baby in an infant seat except in the middle of a double (or larger) bed or on the floor—they are often capable of overturning the seat. And of course, baby should always be strapped in.

■ Learn what slows down your active baby—soft music (either your own singing or a record or tape), a warm bath (but never leave him or her alone in it), or looking at a picture book (though active children may not be ready for this as early as quieter children). Build such quieting activities into your baby's schedule before feeding and sleeping times.

The irregular baby. At about six to twelve weeks, just when other babies seem to be settling into a schedule and become more predictable, these babies seem to become more erratic. Not only don't they fall into schedules on their own, they aren't interested in any you may have to offer.

Instead of following such a baby's lead and letting chaos take over your home life, or taking the reins yourself and imposing a very rigid schedule that is contrary to the infant's nature, try to find a middle ground. For both your sakes, it's necessary to put at least a modicum of order in your lives, but try as much as possible to build a schedule around any natural tendencies your baby seems to exhibit. You may have to keep a diary to uncover any hints of a recurring time frame in your child's days, such as hunger around 11 AM every morning or fussiness after 7 PM every evening.

Try to counter any unpredictability with predictability. That means trying, as much as possible, to do things at the same times and in the same ways every day. Nurse in the same chair when possible, give baths at the same time each day, always soothe by the same method (rocking or singing or whatever works best). Try scheduling feedings at roughly the same times each day, even if your baby doesn't seem hungry, and try to stick to the schedule even if he or she is hungry between meals, offering a small snack if necessary. Ease rather than force your baby into more of a structured day. And don't expect true regularity, just a little less chaos.

Nights with an irregular baby can be torture, mostly because the baby doesn't usually differentiate them from days. You can try the tips for dealing with sleep problems (page 119) and night-day differentiation problems (page 118), but it's very possible they won't work for your baby, who may want to stay up throughout the night. To survive, mommy and daddy may have to alternate night duty or share split shifts until things get better, which they eventually will if you are persistent and stay cool. In extreme situations, the doctor may recommend a sedative (for the baby, not for you) to calm your child enough to allow you to work on establishing some sort of sleeping routine.

The poor-adaptibility or initial-withdrawal baby. These babies consistently reject the unfamiliar—new objects, people, foods. Some are upset by change of any kind, even familiar change such as going from the house to the car. If this sounds like your baby, try setting up a daily schedule with few surprises. Feedings, baths, and naps should take place at the same times and in the same places, with as few departures from routine as possible. Introduce new toys and people (and foods, when baby is ready for them) very gradually. For example, hang a new mobile over the crib for just a minute or two. Remove it and bring it out again in a short while, leaving it up for a few minutes longer. Continue increasing the time of exposure until baby seems ready to accept and enjoy the mobile. Introduce other new toys and objects in the same way. Have new people spend a lot of time just being in the same room with your baby, then talking at a distance, then communicating close up, before they make an attempt at physical contact. Later, when you introduce solids, add new foods very gradually, starting with tiny amounts, and increasing portion size over the span of a week or two. Don't add another food until the last is well accepted. Try to avoid unnecessary changes when making purchases—a new feeding bottle with a different shape or color, a new gadget on the stroller, a new blanket on the crib. If an item wears out or breaks, try to replace it with an identical or similar model.

The high intensity baby. You probably noticed it right at the beginning—your baby cried louder than any other child in the hospital nursery. The loud crying and screaming, the kind that can frazzle even the steadiest of nerves, continued when you got home. Unfortunately you can't flip a switch and turn down the volume on your baby—but turning down the volume of noise and activity in the environment may help tone your child down a bit. Also, you will want to take some purely practical measures to keep the noise from bothering family and neighbors. If possible, soundproof your baby's room by insulating the walls with insulating board or padding, adding carpeting, curtains, and anything else that will absorb the sound. You can try earplugs, a white-noise machine, a fan or air conditioner to reduce the wear and tear on your ears and nerves without totally blocking out your baby's cries. As crying lessens in the months ahead, so will this problem, but your child will probably always be louder and more intense than most.

The negative or "unhappy" baby. Instead of smiling and cooing, some babies just seem miserable all the time. This is no reflection on the parents (unless, of course, they've been neglectful), but it can have a profound impact on them. They often find it difficult to love their unhappy babies, and sometimes they even reject them. If nothing seems to satisfy your baby (and no medical explanation is uncovered), then do your best to be loving and caring anyway, secure in the knowledge that one of these days, when your baby learns other ways of expression, the crying and general unhappiness will diminish, though he or she may always be the "serious" type.

HOW DO YOU TALK TO A BABY?

The roads to communication with a baby are endless, and each parent travels some more than others. Here are some you may want to take, now or in the months ahead:

Do a running commentary. Don't make a move, at least when you're around your baby, without talking about it. Narrate the dressing process: "Now I'm putting on your diaper ...here goes the T-shirt over your head... now I'm buttoning your overalls." In the kitchen, describe the washing of the dishes, or the process of seasoning the spaghetti sauce. During the bath, explain about soap and rinsing, and that a shampoo makes the hair shiny and clean. It doesn't matter that your baby hasn't the slightest inkling of what you're talking about. Blow-by-blow descriptions help get you talking, and get baby listening—thereby starting him or her on the path to understanding.

Ask a lot. Don't wait until your baby starts having answers to start asking questions. Think of yourself as a reporter, your baby as an intriguing interviewee. The questions can be as varied as your day: "Would you like to wear the red pants or the green overalls?" "Isn't the sky a beautiful blue today?" "Should I buy string beans for dinner or broccoli?" Pause for an answer (one day your baby will surprise you with one), and then supply the answer yourself, out loud ("Broccoli? Good choice.").

Give baby a chance. Studies show that infants whose parents talk *with* them rather than *at* them learn to talk earlier. Give your baby a chance to get a coo, a gurgle, or a giggle in edgewise. In your running commentaries, be sure to leave some openings for baby's comments.

Keep it simple—some of the time. Though right now your baby would probably derive listening pleasure from a dramatic recitation of the Gettysburg Address or an animated assessment of the economy, as he or she gets a bit older, you'll want to make it easier to pick out individual words. So at least part of the time, make a conscious effort to use simple sentences and phrases: "See the light," "Bye-bye," "Baby's fingers, baby's toes," and "Nice doggie."

Put aside pronouns. It's difficult for a young baby to grasp that "I" or "me" or "you" can be mommy, or daddy, or grandma, or even baby—depending on who's talking. So most of the time, refer to yourself

---

do hold your baby, learn which way seems least annoying (tight or loose, for example).

■ **Smell sensitivity.** Unusual odors aren't likely to bother a very young infant, but some children begin to show a negative reaction to certain odors before the end of the first year. The aroma of frying onions, the smell of a diaper rash medicine, the fragrance of mother's new perfume or father's new after-shave lotion, can all make such a baby restless and unhappy. If your baby seems sensitive to smells, limit strong odors when you can.

■ **Stimulation sensitivity.** Too much stim-

ulation of any kind seems to trigger trouble for some infants. These babies need to be handled gently and slowly. Loud talk, hurried movements, too many playthings, too many people around, too much activity in a day—these can all be upsetting. To help such a baby sleep better, avoid active play just before bedtime, substituting a soothing, warm bath followed by quiet storytelling or lullabies. Soft recorded music can often help such a baby to settle down, too.

Living with a difficult baby isn't easy, but with plenty of love, patience, and under-

as "mommy" (or "daddy" or "grandma") and to your baby by name: "Now mommy is going to change Jason's diaper."

Raise your pitch. Most babies prefer a high-pitched voice, which may be why women's voices are usually naturally higher-pitched than men's, and why most mothers' voices climb an octave or two when addressing their infants. Try raising your pitch when talking directly to your baby, and watch the reaction. (A few infants prefer a lower pitch; experiment to see which appeals to yours.)

Stick to the here and now. Though you can muse about almost anything to your baby, there won't be any noticeable comprehension for a while. As comprension does develop, you will want to stick more to what the baby can see or is experiencing at the moment. A young baby doesn't have a memory for the past or a concept of the future.

Imitate. Babies love the flattery that comes with imitation. When baby coos, coo back; when he or she utters an "ahh," utter one, too. Imitation will quickly become a game that you'll both enjoy, and which will set the foundation for baby's imitating your language.

Set it to music. Don't worry if you can't carry a tune—little babies are notoriously undiscriminating when it comes to music. They'll love what you sing to them whether it's an old show standard, a new Top-40 hit, or just some nonsense you've set to a familiar tune. If your sensibilities (or your neighbors') prohibit a song, then sing-song will do. Most nursery rhymes entrance even young infants (invest in an edition of Mother Goose if your memory fails you). And accompanying hand gestures, if you know some or can make some up, double the delight. Your baby will quickly let you know which are favorites, and which you'll be expected to sing over and over—and over—again.

Read aloud. Though at first the words will have no meaning, it's never too early to begin reading some simple children's rhymes to your baby. When you aren't in the mood for baby talk and crave some adult-level stimulation, share your love of literature (or recipes or gossip or politics) with your little one by reading what you like to read, aloud.

Take your cues from baby. Incessant chatter and song can be tiresome for anyone, even an infant. When your baby becomes inattentive to your word play, closes or averts his or her eyes, becomes fussy or cranky, or otherwise indicates the saturation point has been reached, give it a rest.

standing it is possible, and in the long run it can even be rewarding. Before you decide your baby is one of the difficult ones, however, you should be sure that there isn't some underlying physical cause of his or her troubling behavior. Describe it to the doctor so that any possible medical explanation—illness or allergy, for example—can be ruled out. Sometimes a baby who seems to be difficult is simply allergic to her formula, is teething, or is ill. For descriptions of other types of difficult babies, see the box on page 158.

A SECOND LANGUAGE

"My husband is French, and he wants to speak French to our baby exclusively; I speak English. I think it would be wonderful for her to speak a second language, but wouldn't it be confusing at this age?"

Because fluency in another language isn't necessary to function and succeed in most parts of our country (as it is elsewhere), Americans are sadly lagging behind the rest of the world in the ability to converse in anything other than their own native tongue. It's generally agreed that teaching a child a second language gives her an invaluable skill, may help her to think in different ways, and may even improve her self-image. If the language is one that her forebears spoke, it also gives her a significant link with her roots.

There is less agreement on just when to introduce the second language, however. Some experts suggest beginning as soon as a baby is born, but others believe that this puts the child at a disadvantage in both languages—though probably for only a while. They generally recommend waiting until a child is two and a half or three before putting on the Berlitz. By this time she usually has a pretty good grasp of English but is still able to pick up a new language easily and naturally. It is generally agreed that waiting to introduce the second language until after a child can read will impede her fluency in it.

Whether you start now or in a couple of years, there are several approaches to encouraging a child to pick up a second language. One parent can speak English and the other the foreign tongue (as your husband suggests), or both parents can speak the foreign language (with the expectation the child will pick up English in school and elsewhere), or a grandparent, sitter, or *au pair* girl can speak the foreign language and the parents English (usually the least successful of the methods). None of the methods of teaching a second language is particularly successful if the "teacher" isn't fluent in the language.

Experts recommend you forget about "teaching" a second language and instead immerse your child in it—play games in it, read books in it (many popular children's books have been translated from English into other languages, including *The Cat in the Hat,* Spot books, and Sesame Street books), sing songs in it, listen to tapes and watch videos in it, visit with friends who are fluent in it, and if possible, visit places where the language is spoken. Whoever is speaking the second language should speak it exclusively to the child, resisting the temptation to resort to English or to translate if the child seems to be struggling with comprehension. During the school years, the child should be taught to read and write in the second language in order for it to take on greater usefulness and significance. If classes aren't available at school, tutoring or computer-programmed learning may be a good idea.

BABY TALK

"Other mothers seem to know how to talk to their babies. But I don't know what to say to my six-week-old son, and when I try, I feel like an absolute idiot. I'm afraid that my inhibitions will slow down his language development."

They're tiny. They're passive. They can't talk back. And yet, for many novice mothers and fathers, newborn babies are the most intimidating audience they'll ever face. The undignified, high-pitched baby talk that seems to come naturally to other parents eludes them, leaving them tongue-tied—and feeling guilty over the awkward silence that envelops the nursery.

Though your baby will learn your language even if you never learn his, his speech will develop faster and better if you make a conscious effort at early communication. Babies who aren't communicated with at all suffer not just in language development but in all areas of growth. But that rarely happens. Even the mother who is bashful about baby talk communicates with her baby all day long—when she cuddles him, responds to his crying, sings him a lullaby, says "It's time for a walk," or mutters "Oh, not the phone again," just as she's settled down to nurse. Parents teach language when they talk to each other as well as when they talk to their baby; babies pick up almost as much from second hand dialogue as they do when they're part of a conversation.

So although it's not likely that your baby is going to spend the next year in the company of a silent mommy, there are ways to expand your baby-word power, even if you're the kind of adult to whom baby talk doesn't come naturally. The trick is to start practicing in private, so the embarrassment of gurgling and babbling to your baby in front of other adults won't cramp your conversation style. If you don't know where to begin, use the tips on page 160 as a guideline. As you grow more comfortable with baby talk, you'll likely find yourself slipping into it unawares, even in public.

WHAT IT'S IMPORTANT TO KNOW: Stimulating Your Baby in the Early Months

In our achievement-oriented society, many parents worry about turning out babies that can compete—and they begin worrying early. They worry that if he doesn't smile by the time he's three weeks old, he may not get into the right preschool program. They worry that if she hasn't turned over by two months, she may not make the prep-school tennis team. And then they worry that unless they do everything right they won't be successful in turning the basically unresponsive lump they brought home from the hospital into a candidate for Princeton.

Actually, they have little reason to worry. Babies—even those destined for that Ivy League sheepskin—develop at different rates, and those who get off to a somewhat slower start often excel later. And parents—even those who are chronically insecure—usually do a thoroughly competent job of stimulating their offspring, often without making a conscious effort.

Yet, as comforting as this knowledge should be, it doesn't always stop the worry. For many parents, there is the nagging fear that doing what comes naturally when it comes to parenting may not be quite enough. If you'd like to check what you've already been doing instinctively to see if you're on the right track, the following tips for creating the right atmosphere for learning and for supplying sensory stimulation should be helpful to you.

CREATING A GOOD ENVIRONMENT

Love your baby. Nothing helps a baby grow and thrive as much as being loved. A close relationship with a parent, or parents, and/or a substitute parent is crucial for normal development.

Relate to your baby. Take every opportunity to talk, sing, or coo to your baby—while you're changing a diaper, giving a bath, shopping for groceries, or driving the car. These casual but stimulating exchanges go further in making a brighter baby than forcing flash cards. And even the best toys in the world are useless if baby doesn't have you to play with part of the time. Your goal isn't to "teach" your baby, but to be involved with him or her.

Get to know your baby. Learn what makes your baby happy or miserable, excited or bored, soothed or stimulated, paying more attention to what you learn from your baby than from any book or adviser. Gear attempts at stimulation to your unique baby, rather than to some typical textbook child. If loud noises and/or roughhousing upset your child, then entertain with soft sounds and gentle play. If too much excitement makes your baby frantic, limit the length of playtimes and the intensity of activity.

Take the pressure off—and have fun.
Neither you nor your baby will benefit from
your preoccupation with his or her level of
performance. Learning and development
aren't hastened by pressure, and they may
be hindered. Harmful to baby's self-esteem
is the message—no matter how carefully
camouflaged—that you're not satisfied with
his or her progress up the developmental
ladder. Instead of thinking of the times you
spend stimulating your baby as intensive
cramming sessions, relax and enjoy—for
both your sakes.

Give your baby space. Adequate attention is vital; too much can be suffocating.
Though children need to know that help is
available when they need it, they also need
to learn how to seek it out. Your constant
hovering will also deprive your baby of the
chance to look for and find diversion elsewhere—in the friendly looking teddy bear
who's sharing the crib, in the pattern of
light cast by the venetian blinds, in his or
her own fingers and toes, in the sound of an
airplane overhead, a fire engine down the
street, the dog barking next door. It may
also hamper your baby's ability to play and
learn independently later on—and a dependent baby will make it difficult for you
to turn your attention to anything else. By
all means, play with your child and spend
quality time, but sometimes just get baby
and toy together and then move off while
they get acquainted.

Follow the leader. And make sure your
baby, not you, is in the lead. If he or she is
fascinated by the mobile, don't bring out
the activity board; instead, focus on the
mobile together. Allowing baby to take the
wheel once in a while not only enhances
learning by taking advantage of the "teach-
able moment," but also reinforces baby's
budding sense of self-esteem by communicating that his or her interests are worthy
of mommy's attention.

Let your baby take the lead, too, in
deciding when to end a play session—even
if it's before the rattle is grasped. Your baby
will tell you, "I've had enough," by turning
away, fussing, crying, or otherwise showing
disinterest or displeasure. Ignoring the
message and pressing on deprives a baby of
a sense of control, turns off interest in the
subject (at least for a while), and ultimately
makes playtime a whole lot less fun for
both of you.

Time it right. A baby is always in one
of six states of consciousness: (1) deep, or
quiet, sleep; (2) light, or active, sleep; (3)
drowsiness; (4) active wakefulness with interest in physical activity; (5) fussiness and
crying; and (6) quiet wakefulness. It's during active wakefulness that you can most
effectively encourage physical development, and during quiet wakefulness that
you can best foster other types of learning.
Also keep in mind that infants have very
short attention spans. A baby who turns you
off after two minutes of looking at a book
isn't rejecting intellectual pursuits, but has
simply run out of concentration.

Provide positive reinforcement. When
your baby starts achieving (when he or she
smiles, swats at a rattle, lifts shoulders and
arms off the mattress, turns over, or grasps
a toy successfully) show your approbation.
Do it with hugs, cheers, applause—whatever is comfortable for you and gets the
message across to your baby: "I think
you're terrific."

PRACTICAL TIPS FOR LEARNING AND PLAYING

Some parents, without ever reading a book
about or taking a course in infant stimulation, seem to have an easier time than others initiating learning-playing activities
with their babies. And some babies, because they are unusually responsive, are
easier to engage in such activities. But any
parent-baby team can be successful at
learning-playing with a little guidance.

The areas to nourish and encourage are:

The sense of taste. Right now you don't have to go out of your way to stimulate this sense. Your baby's taste buds are titillated at every meal on breast or bottle. But as baby gets older, "tasting" will become a way of exploring, and everything within reach will end up being mouthed. Resist the temptation to discourage this, except, of course, when what goes into the mouth is poisonous, sharp, or small enough to swallow or choke on.

The sense of smell. In most environments, the keen smelling apparatus of infants gets plenty of exercise. There's breast milk, mom's perfume, Rover scampering nearby, the roasting chicken. Unless your baby shows signs of being overly sensitive to odors, think of the various scents as additional opportunities for your baby to learn about the environment.

The sense of sight. Though we once believed that babies were sightless at birth, we now know that they can not only see, but begin learning from what they see. Through their sense of sight, they learn very quickly to differentiate between objects and human beings (and between one object or human being and another), to interpret body language and other nonverbal cues, and to understand a little bit more every day about the world around them.

Decorate your baby's room or corner with the goal of supplying stimulating visual surroundings, rather than satisfying your own tastes. When selecting wallpaper, quilts, wall hangings, toys, or books, keep in mind that babies like sharp contrasts, and that designs that are bold and bright rather than soft and delicate are more appealing (black-and-white patterns are favored for the first six weeks or so, bright colors later). Limit playthings in the crib, carriage, playpen, and baby seat to one or two at a time—too many can lead to confusion and overstimulation.

Many objects, toys among them, can stimulate baby visually:

■ Mobiles. Figures on a mobile should be fully visible from below (the baby's perspective), rather than from the side (the adult's perspective). A mobile should be no more than 12 to 15 inches over the baby's face, and should be hung to one side or the other of the child's line of vision, rather than straight above (most children prefer to gaze toward the right, but observe your child to discover a preference).

■ Other things that move. You can move a rattle or other bright toy across baby's line of vision to encourage tracking of moving objects. Take a field trip to a pet shop and position baby in front of a fish tank or bird cage to view the action. Or blow bubbles for baby.

■ Stationary objects. Babies spend a lot of time just looking at things. This isn't idle time, but learning time. Geometric patterns or simple faces in black-and-white, hand drawn or store bought, are early favorites. Bright colors and sharp contrasts are preferred over pale, more delicate designs.

■ Mirrors. Mirrors give baby an ever-changing view and most love them. Be sure to use safe metal baby mirrors rather than glass ones; hang them on the crib, in the carriage, over the changing table.

■ People. Babies delight in looking at faces close up, so you and other family members should spend plenty of time in close proximity to baby. You can also show baby family portraits, pointing out who's who.

■ Books. Show baby simple pictures of babies, children, animals, or toys and identify them. The drawings should be clear and sharply defined without a lot of extra (for a baby) detail.

■ The world. Very soon your baby is going to take an interest in seeing beyond his or her nose. Provide plenty of opportunity to see the world—from the stroller, carriage, car seat, or by carrying your baby face forward. Now and then point out cars, trees, people, and so on. But don't ramble on non-stop during every outing; you'll become bored, and baby will start tuning you out.

The sense of hearing. It's through hearing that infants learn about language, about rhythm, about danger, about emotions and feelings—and about so much else that goes on around them. Auditory stimulation can come from almost any source.

■ The human voice. This, of course, is the most significant type of sound in a new infant's life, so use yours—talk, sing, and babble to your baby. Try lullabies, nursery rhymes, nonsense ditties you create yourself. Imitate animal sounds, especially ones your baby regularly hears, such as the barking of a dog or the meowing of a cat. Most importantly, play back for your baby the sounds he or she makes.

■ Household sounds. Many young babies are captivated by either soft or lively background music, the hum of the vacuum or the blender, the whistle of the tea kettle or the splash of running water, the crinkling of paper (but don't offer newspaper for crinkling, since the newsprint could be poisonous), or the tinkling of a bell or wind chime—though they may become fearful of many such sounds later in the first year.

■ Rattles and other toys that make gentle sounds. You don't have to wait until your baby is able to shake a rattle independently. In the early months, either do the shaking yourself, put the rattle in baby's hand and help shake it, or attach a wrist rattle. Coordination between vision and hearing will develop as baby learns to turn toward sound.

■ Music boxes. You'll be surprised at how quickly your baby will learn to recognize a tune; especially nice are music boxes that have visual appeal, but if one is placed within reach, be sure it doesn't have small pieces that can be broken off and mouthed by your baby.

■ Musical toys. Be sure that keys or other parts are child-safe. Toys that make music and also provide visual stimulation and practice with small motor skills (such as a bunny that moves and makes music when baby pulls a string) are particularly good. Avoid toys that make loud noises that can damage hearing, and don't place even moderately noisy ones right by baby's ear.

■ Children's records and tapes. Try to give them a spin before buying to be sure they're good listening. Infancy is also an ideal time to start exposing your child to classical music (play it softly during playtime in the crib, or during dinner or bathtime), although many babies seem to prefer the livelier rhythms of rock or country music. Always watch your baby for reactions to music; if he or she seems disturbed by what you're playing, turn it off.

The sense of touch. Touch, though often underrated, is actually one of a baby's most valuable tools for exploring and learning about the world. It's through touch that a baby learns the softness of mommy, the relative hardness of daddy, that rubbing a teddy bear feels wonderful, that rubbing a stiff brush doesn't feel that good, and most important of all, that those who take care of him are loving—a message you send every time you bathe, diaper, feed, or rock your baby.

You can provide more varied touching experiences for your baby with:

■ A loving hand. Try to learn how your baby likes to be handled—firmly or lightly, quickly or slowly. Most babies love to be caressed and kissed, to have their tummies tickled or razzed by your lips, to have you blow gently on their fingers or toes. They love the difference between mommy's touch and daddy's, the rough way a sibling hugs or tickles them and the expert ease with which grandma rocks them.

■ Massage. Premies who are massaged for at least twenty minutes daily gain weight faster and do better overall than those who aren't (whether it's the massage or the fact that they're handled more is unclear); babies who aren't touched at all don't grow at a normal pace. Discover the kind of strokes your baby enjoys most, and avoid those that seem to annoy.

■ Textures. Try rubbing a baby's skin with different textures (satin, terry, velvet, wool, fur, or absorbent cotton) so he or she can get to know how each feels; later encourage independent exploration. Let baby lie face down on surfaces with different textures: the living room carpet, a terry towel, grandma's fur coat, your corduroy skirt, dad's wool sweater, the marble-topped coffee table—the possibilities are limitless.

■ Playthings with texture. Offer toys that have interesting textures to baby. A plush teddy bear and a coarse-haired doggy; hard wooden blocks and soft stuffed ones; a rough wooden spoon and a smooth metal bowl; a silky pillow and a nubby one.

Social development. Your baby becomes a social being through watching you, through interacting with you and the rest of the family, and later with others. This isn't the time to begin teaching your baby how to throw a successful party or make interesting small talk over the onion dip, but it is time to begin teaching by example how people should behave toward one another. A few years from now, when your growing child talks to friends, teachers, neighbors, or begins "playing house," you'll often hear your example echoed in that tiny voice; hopefully, you'll be pleased (and not shocked or disappointed) by what you hear.

Toys that help babies with social development are stuffed animals, animal mobiles, and dolls. Though it will be many months before they'll be able to hug them and play with them, even at this point they can and do begin to socialize with them— just watch an infant converse with animals prancing on the crib bumpers or revolving on a mobile. Later, books and opportunities for make-believe and dress-up play will also help children to develop social skills.

Small motor development. Right now your baby's hand movements are totally random, but in a couple of months, those tiny hands will move with more purpose and control. You can aid in the development of purposeful movement by giving your baby's hands plenty of freedom; don't keep them swaddled or tucked under a blanket (except outdoors in cold weather). Provide a variety of objects that are easy

for small hands to pick up and manipulate, that don't require fine dexterity. And since young babies usually won't grasp objects that are directly in front of them, offer these objects from the side.

Give your baby ample opportunity for "hands-on" experience with the following:

■ Rattles that fit small hands comfortably. Those with two handles or grasping surfaces allow a baby to pass the rattle from hand to hand, an important skill, and those that baby can mouth will help bring relief when teething begins.

■ Cradle gyms (they fit across carriage, playpen, or crib) that have a variety of parts for baby to grab hold of, spin, pull, and poke. Beware of those, however, with strings more than 6 inches long, and take any gym down once your baby is able to sit up.

■ Activity boards that require a wide range of hand movements to operate, many of which your baby won't be able to intentionally maneuver for a while, but some of which even a young infant can set in motion accidentally with a swipe of a hand or foot. Besides the spinning, dialing, pushing, and pressing skills these toys encourage, they also teach the concept of cause and effect.

Gross motor development. Putting your baby through the paces of an infant exercise video won't increase muscular strength or speed motor development. Good motor skills, well-developed bodies, and physical fitness for infants depend instead on the following: good nutrition; good health care (both well-baby and sick-baby); and plenty of opportunity for self-motivated physical activity. Babies kept cooped up in a swing or baby seat, harnessed in a carriage or stroller, or swaddled in a blanket or bunting will have little opportunity to learn about how their bodies work. Those who are never put down on the tummy will be slow to learn to lift their head and shoulders or turn over front to back. Change your baby's position often during the day (propping him up in a sitting position, placing her sometimes on stomach and other times on back) to maximize the opportunities for physical activity.

Encourage physical development by pulling your baby to a sitting position, letting him or her "fly" (allowing exercise of arms and legs) or "ride," (lying face down, lengthwise on your shins). Motivate rolling over by putting an interesting object to one side as baby lies on his or her back; if baby turns a bit, then give a little help in going all the way. Encourage creeping by letting baby push off against your hands when lying belly down.

Intellectual development. Encouraging the development of all the senses, as well as small and large motor control, will contribute to your baby's intellectual growth. Talk to your infant a lot, right from the start. Give names to objects, animals, and people your baby sees, point out body parts, explain what you're doing. Read nursery rhymes and simple stories, showing your baby the illustrations as you go. Expose your child to a variety of settings (the supermarket, your church or synagogue, a department store, the museum). Travel on buses, in cars, in taxicabs. Even at home, vary your baby's point of view: place the baby seat by a window (but *only* if it has a window guard) or in front of a mirror, lay baby in the middle of the living room carpet to survey the action or in the middle of the bed to watch you fold the laundry, or park the bassinet or stroller in the kitchen while you prepare dinner.

Whatever you do, however, don't put yourself or your baby under pressure to perform. The play's the thing, and it should be fun—the learning that comes with it is a bonus, though an important one.

CHAPTER SIX

The Third Month

WHAT YOUR BABY MAY BE DOING

**By the end of this month, your baby
...should be able to (see Note):**

■ on stomach, lift head up 45 degrees (2⅔ months)
■ follow an object in an arc about 6 inches above the face past the midline (straight ahead) (by 2½ months)

Note: If your baby seems not to have reached one or more of these milestones, check with the doctor. In rare instances the delay could indicate a problem, though in most cases it will turn out to be normal for your baby. Premature infants generally reach milestones later than others of the same birth age, often achieving them closer to their adjusted age (the age they would be if they had been born at term), and sometimes later.

...will probably be able to:

■ laugh out loud
■ on stomach, lift head up 90 degrees

■ squeal in delight
■ bring both hands together
■ smile spontaneously
■ follow an object in an arc about 6 inches above the face for 180 degrees—from one side to the other (3¼ months)

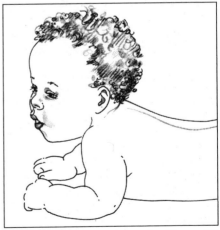

Many, but not all, three-month-olds can lift their head to a 90° angle.

...may possibly be able to:

- hold head steady when upright
- on stomach, raise chest, supported by arms
- roll over (one way)
- grasp a rattle held to backs or tips of fingers (3⅓ months)
- pay attention to a raisin or other very small object (3⅓ months)

...may even be able to:

- bear some weight on legs when held upright
- reach for an object (3⅔ months)
- keep head level with body when pulled to sitting
- turn in the direction of a voice, particularly mommy's
- say ah-goo or similar vowel-consonant combination
- razz (make a wet razzing sound)

WHAT YOU CAN EXPECT AT THIS MONTH'S CHECKUP

Most doctors do not schedule regular well-baby checkups this month. Do call the doctor if there are any concerns that can't wait until next month's visit.

FEEDING YOUR BABY THIS MONTH: Nursing While Working Outside the Home

There's an added responsibility that's not included in any job description, but which many employed mothers are electing to take on. It's time consuming, and it can be arduous, even tedious. It cuts into coffee breaks and lunch hours, and makes the hectic times before and after work even more hectic. And yet most of the women who've added nursing to their workday are glad they have—and they'd do it again.

The reasons are powerful. First of all, employed mothers who nurse can continue to give their babies many of the physical benefits of breastfeeding (fewer illnesses, decreased risk of allergy), and all of them if no supplementary formula is given. Second, they can feel less guilty about leaving their babies during the day because they know they are doing something important for them even while they are away. Third, because employed nursing mothers must nurse before going to work and again when they get home, they have the opportunity to spend time in close contact with their babies at least twice a day. No matter how busy, they can't prop a bottle or have someone else give it while they shower or get dinner ready. And finally, and perhaps most importantly, mothers who continue to nurse when they go back to their jobs can, along with their babies, enjoy the emotional benefits of breastfeeding for a longer time.

MAKING NURSING AND EMPLOYMENT WORK

As with everything else that's related to going back to work when you have a young infant, plenty of forethought is necessary. To make nursing and employment work, keep the following in mind:

■ Don't start giving bottles until your milk supply is well established. It's tempting to start very early so the bottle won't be rejected. But starting too early can lead to both nipple confusion (see page 101) and an inadequate milk supply. Wait to introduce the bottle until you've worked out any problems with nursing (such as sore nipples) and feel confident about the adequacy of your milk supply. For most women, that's somewhere around six weeks—though some women find things going smoothly a bit sooner or later.

■ Introduce the bottle well in advance of return-to-the-job day. Though you won't want to bring on the bottle much before six weeks, don't wait much longer either, even if you won't be returning to your job for a while. The older and smarter babies get, the less easy it is to persuade them to take a bottle. Work toward getting your baby used to taking at least one supplementary bottle a day—preferably at a time of day when you'll usually be working—by the time you are ready to start collecting paychecks. Use formula or breast milk, depending on which you plan to use later.

■ If you intend to supplement with breast milk rather than formula, become proficient at expressing your milk well before you return to work. Freeze a few bottles of excess milk so you'll have an emergency stash for those first frenzied days back on the job. If you plan on using formula, you will probably still have to learn to pump your breasts, since it will probably be necessary to express milk at work to avoid clogged milk ducts and a diminishing milk supply.

■ Wait, if possible, until your baby is at least sixteen weeks old before you return to work outside your home. In general, the older a baby is when a mother takes this step, the more successful the continuation of breastfeeding—probably because both breastfeeding and mother-baby relationships have had more time to become well established.

■ Work part-time if you can, at least at first. More hours with your baby will strengthen breastfeeding links. Working four or five half-days is more practical than two or three full ones for several reasons. Working half-days, you may in some cases not have to miss any feedings, and certainly no more than one daily. You will have little trouble with leakage and probably won't have to pump milk at work at all. And you will spend most of each day with your baby, which many experts believe is more beneficial. Working nights is another option that interferes very little with breastfeeding, especially if baby is sleeping through the night, but it can interfere with both rest and romance.

■ Stay faithful to your Best-Odds Breastfeeding Diet; you'll need it not only for milk production, but also to keep your energy up and your emotions on an even keel.

■ Enlist support at your workplace. If your employer and/or coworkers don't understand and support your decision to continue nursing while you work, your odds of success will drop dramatically. Try to arrange in advance a time and place for expressing milk, and for refrigeration for storage if you'll need it. If you have no way to store and/or transport what you pump, you will have to discard it and depend on breast milk pumped and stored while you are at home mornings, nights, and weekends, or on formula, for feedings.[1]

---

1. Recent studies indicate that breast milk can remain fresh for as long as six hours at room temperature; but to be extra safe, store your milk in sterilized bottles or containers and refrigerate, if possible.

■ When you arrange for a caretaker for your baby, be sure it is a person who understands and supports your plan to continue breastfeeding. If not, you may find your baby recently fed and fully satiated when you arrive home eager to nurse. Give the baby-sitter a quick course in the whys and ways of breastfeeding and breastfed babies, if she's unfamiliar with them; explain the differences in feeding schedules and bowel movements, as well as the importance of frequent nursing to keep the milk supply up. Leave strict instructions not to give bottles of milk (or juice or water) for at least two hours before you're expected home to nurse.

■ Enlist support from your husband, too. He'll have to share some of the household burdens so that you will be able to spend the necessary time nursing when you're at home.

■ Keep your priorities straight. You won't be able to do everything and do everything well. Keep your baby and your relationship with your spouse (and any other children you have) at the top of the list, and cut corners everywhere else—except, of course, at your job if it means a lot to you, either financially, emotionally, or professionally.

■ Stay flexible. A calm and happy mother is more valuable to your baby's well-being than a diet made up exclusively of breast milk. Though it's entirely possible you'll be able to continue providing all of your baby's milk (if that's what you want to do), it's also possible that you won't be able to. Sometimes the physical and emotional stresses of holding a job and nursing curtail a woman's milk supply. If your baby isn't thriving on breast milk alone, try nursing more frequently when you're at home and, if it's feasible, returning home during your lunch break to breastfeed and help rebuild your milk supply. If this doesn't work, it will probably be necessary to supplement with formula.

■ Dress for breastfeeding success. To keep leakage from being visible and from staining your best outfits, wear loose blouses or shirts in colorful prints on easy-care opaque cottons or blends. Avoid pale colors, clingy fabrics, and sheers, as well as tight tops that might either trigger let-down (by rubbing against your nipples) or inhibit it (by acting as a binder). Be sure your top can be lifted or opened easily from the front for pumping at work, and that it won't be stretched out of shape or badly wrinkled by being pulled up. Line your nursing bra with breast pads to further protect your clothing, and carry an extra supply of pads in your bag as replacements for wet ones.

■ Do a couple of trial runs. Rehearse your workday game plan, doing everything as you would if you were really going to work (including expressing milk away from home), but leave the house for just a couple of hours the first time, longer the next. Note what problems arise, and figure out how they can be handled.

If you're going back to a full-time job, you might also try returning on a Thursday or Friday to give yourself a chance to get started, see how things go, and evaluate the situation over the weekend. It will also be a little less overwhelming than starting out with five days ahead of you.

■ Arrange your schedule to maximize the number of nursings. Squeeze in two feedings before you go to work, if possible, and two or three (or more) in the evening. If you work near home and can either return during lunchtime for nursing or have the sitter meet you somewhere with the baby, consider doing this. If you leave your baby at the sitter's house, nurse when you arrive there, or in your car before you go in, if that works better. Also try nursing your baby at pickup time, instead of waiting until you get home.

■ Try taking home any work that can be done out of the office or shop (with your employer's blessing, of course). This will give you more flexibility and allow you to be home more of your baby's waking hours. Though you will probably have to relegate most of baby's care to a sitter when you're home working, you should be able to nurse as needed.

■ If your job entails travel, try to avoid trips that take you away from home for more than a day until your baby is weaned; if you must travel, do try to express and freeze enough milk for the duration of your trip in advance or get your baby accustomed to formula before you plan to go. For your own comfort and to keep up your milk supply, take along a breast pump (or rent one where you'll be) and express milk every three or four hours. When you get home you may find your milk supply somewhat diminished, but more-frequent-than-usual nursings, along with extra special attention to diet and rest, may replenish it. If it doesn't you will probably have to use formula, at least for the work-time feedings.

■ If, to ensure your baby gets the proper nutrition needed for growth and development, you must use formula supplements for home feedings, breastfeed before giving the formula feedings rather than after, so as to interfere as little as possible with what milk you are producing.

■ Do what works and seems right for you and your baby, whether it's supplementing with formula or feeding your baby exclusively on breast milk, working part-time or full-time, giving up nursing altogether—or even giving up your job.

WHAT YOU MAY BE CONCERNED ABOUT

ESTABLISHING A REGULAR SCHEDULE

"I know that the old idea of fitting a baby into a schedule is frowned upon. But I'm exhausted trying to fit into my baby's schedule. He demands and I nurse nearly every hour, all day long."

Women of this generation are vocal in demanding their rights in the workplace, but they sometimes forget that they also have rights where their children are concerned. And as your baby gets older, you can begin demanding yours from him.

Before you do, however, be certain his seemingly gluttonous nursing pattern isn't his way of trying to get adequate nourishment—either because you're not producing enough milk or because he's unusually active or going through a growth spurt. Does he seem to be growing as he should? Is his body filling out nicely? Is he outgrowing his newborn sleepers? If not, see page 100 for tips on improving your breast milk supply. If they don't work, talk to the doctor about supplementing your baby's diet with formula.

Once you've determined that your baby is thriving, and that it isn't hunger that's motivating his frequent pleas of "Please, mom, can I have some more," then it's time to start making some changes to ensure that you thrive, too. Hourly nursing sessions are too much of a strain on you, both physically and emotionally, are likely to cause sore nipples, and may understandably result in your feeling resentment toward your baby for taking up so much of your day and night with his greedy habit. As for your baby, overnursing isn't only unnecessary—it's unhealthy. It interferes with his sleep, which he needs in longer stretches now, and with his development while he's awake. Having a breast in his mouth all day long doesn't give him a chance to do much of anything else.

By three months, many babies will have established a pretty regular daily rhythm. Typically, it's something like this: he wakes about the same time each morning, feeds, perhaps stays awake for a short period, takes a nap, wakes again for lunch, follows with another nap, feeds, then perhaps has a fairly long period of wakefulness late in the afternoon, capped off by a meal and a nap in the early evening. If this nap tends to run past the parents' bedtimes, they may wake him to eat before they retire, maybe about 11 P.M. At this point he may go back to sleep again until early morning, since babies this age can often sleep six hours at a stretch, and sometimes more.

Some babies have a more idiosyncratic schedule. One, for example, may wake up at 6 A.M., feed, and go back to sleep for an hour or two. Upon awakening, he may be content to play for a while before nursing, but once he starts nursing, he wants to do so nonstop for the next three hours. After a twenty-minute nap, however, he wakes up ready to play happily all afternoon with just one nursing period and another five-minute nap. He nurses again at about 6:00 and by 7:00 is sound asleep, and he stays that way until mom wakes him for a nightcap before she retires. His isn't the traditional four-hour schedule, but it is one a mother can plan her day around.

Many babies, unfortunately, don't fall smoothly into any schedule at all, even past three months. They wake, eat, and sleep in a totally random pattern, eating frequently or infrequently, sometimes combining the two unpredictably. If your baby is one of these, it's up to you to take the initiative by trying to make the parts of his life you do have some control over as organized as possible. Baths, outings, and bedtime should come at roughly the same times every day. Try to stretch the periods between feedings by talking to, singing to, or playing with your baby before putting him to the breast or bottle. Put him in a baby swing for a few minutes, or in his crib with his musical mobile or cradle gym for entertainment—anything that he enjoys and that will successfully keep him from getting his next meal as early as he'd like. Be sure, too, that he has enough to do between feedings. His frequent nursings may have more to do with boredom than with anything else. He's no longer a newborn and needs a more active lifestyle (see page 163 for tips on stimulating him).

Once you've successfully cut down on nursings and developed some sort of daily routine, you will have more time for your own life and more control over your baby's.

"People think I'm strange or remiss when they hear I don't have any particular schedule for my baby—no special bedtime or eating times or bath time for her. But that's the way I'm comfortable."

Though much of our society is run on schedules—train schedules, work schedules, class schedules, alternate-side-of-the-street parking schedules—there are those of us who function perfectly well without them. And if baby doesn't have any serious sleep problems at night and seems perfectly contented, active, and interested by day, a laissez-faire attitude toward scheduling may be fine for the time being.

There are, however, certain pitfalls to raising children in an unstructured environment. Watch out for these problems if you choose such a lifestyle:

■ Some babies crave schedules right from the start. They become cranky when feedings are late or overtired when naps and bedtimes are delayed. If your baby reacts unhappily to your unscheduled days and nights, it may be that she needs a little more structure, even if you don't.

■ Schedules become increasingly important to family stability and to a baby's well-being as time goes by. Many children seem to do perfectly well without a schedule in early infancy, when they're extremely portable and can fall asleep or be fed anywhere. Later they often begin to respond to irregular mealtimes and sleep times with regular crying and crankiness.

■ Without a regular bedtime for their babies, parents often find they never spend any time alone. They enjoy their threesome so much in the evening, they often forget the fun two can—and should—have.

■ Families that omit regular sleep and mealtimes sometimes shortchange their babies by unthinkingly also omitting the sleep and mealtime rituals that most babies seem to need.

■ For mothers who plan to go back to a paid job sometime within the first two years of their baby's life, not having a schedule for a child-care provider to work with will mean their baby not only won't have mommy around all day, but also won't have a familiar routine to cling to that would help with adjustment.

■ For all babies, the absence of structure in their lives early on can interfere with their developing, and then exercising, self-discipline later in life. Getting to school on time, completing homework, and getting papers in on schedule can be inordinately difficult for children who have never been exposed to any kind of structure previously.

In spite of the pitfalls babies can, and do, thrive in families where a schedule, even a loose one, is nonexistent. And in fact, an extremely strict schedule can be as stifling as a too-lax one can be disorienting. How much structure you put in your baby's life should depend on your baby's natural eating and sleeping patterns, her inborn personality (does she seem to need more structure or less), and the needs of the rest of the family. What works best for other people, as in most things, may not work best for you. If it's your baby who objects to schedules, see page 158.

PUTTING BABY TO BED

"My baby always falls asleep nursing. I've heard that this is a bad habit for her to get started on."

It's an idea that looks good in print: put a baby to bed when she's awake, not already asleep, so that later, once she's weaned, she'll be able to get to sleep on her own, without the breast or a bottle. In practice, as any mother who's tried to keep her baby from falling asleep while nursing or tried to rouse a baby who's konked out while suckling knows, it's an idea that's not necessarily compatible with reality. There's just very little you can do to keep a nursing

baby awake if she wants to sleep. And if you could wake her up, would you really want to?

Teaching your baby to fall asleep without assistance from breast (or bottle) can more practically wait until baby is older—between six and nine months—and nursing less often. And if the habit hangs on, breaking it can certainly be accomplished fairly quickly after your baby has been weaned.

Whenever the opportunity presents itself, however, do try to put your baby down for a nap or at bedtime awake—not so awake that sleep will be elusive, but in a state of drowsy readiness. A little rocking, nursing, or lullabying can usually bring a baby to this state (but try not to prolong the comforting action to the point of sound sleep).

NOT SLEEPING THROUGH THE NIGHT

"My friend's baby has been sleeping through the night since he got home from the hospital, but mine is still waking up and eating as often as he did when he was first born."

Babies are creatures of habit. Create a habit for them and they're likely to cling to it, particularly if it's one that gets them food and attention.

In young infants, the habit of feeding frequently at night is often a nutritionally necessary one. Though some babies, such as your friend's, no longer need night feedings by the third month (and sometimes sooner), most two- or three-month-old babies, particularly breastfed ones, still need to eat once or twice during the night. If the night-waking habit continues into the fifth or sixth month, however, you can begin to suspect that your baby is waking not because he *needs* to eat during the night, but because he's become *accustomed* to eating then; a stomach that's used to being filled at regular intervals around the clock will cry "empty" even when it's sufficiently full to last a lot longer.

Although it may be legitimate for your baby to get one middle-of-the-night feeding, he certainly doesn't need three or four of them. You'll need to gradually reduce the number of late-show feedings he's getting now as a first step in preparing him to sleep through the night later. Here's how:

■ Increase the size of the bedtime feeding. Many sleepy babies nod off before they've totally filled their tanks for the night; restart yours with a burp or a jiggle or some other ploy, and continue feeding until you feel he's had enough. In a month or two, when baby is ready for solids, you may want to build up the evening feeding further with cereal or another food—though it isn't scientifically proven that this helps babies sleep through the night, it does sometimes work.

■ Wake your baby up to feed him before you retire at night; this may fill him enough to last him through your own six or eight hours of sleep. Unfortunately, some babies are too sleepy when they are awakened to take a lot, but sometimes even a small late-night feeding will hold them one or two hours longer than would have been the case with none at all. (Of course, if your baby begins waking more often once you've instituted this procedure, discontinue it. It could be that being awakened by you makes him more prone to waking himself.)

■ Be certain your baby is getting enough to eat all day long. If he isn't, he may be using those night feedings to catch up on calories. If you think this is so, consider nursing more frequently during the day to stimulate milk production (also check the tips on page 99). If your baby's on the bottle, increase the amount of formula you give at each feeding. Be aware, however, that for some babies feeding every couple of hours during the day sets up a pattern of eating every two hours, a pattern they continue around the clock.

■ If he's waking and demanding food every two hours (maybe necessary for a newborn, but not for a thriving two- or three-month-old), try to stretch the time between feedings, adding half an hour each night or every other night. Instead of jumping to get him at the first whimper, give him a chance to try to fall asleep again by himself—he may surprise you. If he doesn't, and fussing turns to screaming, try to soothe him without picking him up—pat or rub his back, sing a soft monotonous lullaby, or turn on a musical crib toy. If the crying doesn't stop after a reasonable time (give it a good fifteen minutes at this age), pick him up and try soothing him in your arms by rocking, swaying, cuddling, or singing. If you're breastfeeding, the soothing tactics have a better chance of success if dad's in charge; a breastfeeding infant who sees, hears, or smells his source is not easily distracted from eating. Keep the room dark, and avoid a lot of conversation or stimulation.

If, after all your efforts, baby doesn't fall back to sleep and still demands feeding, feed him—but by now you've probably stretched the interval between feedings by at least half an hour from the previous plateau. The hope is that baby will reach a new plateau within the next few nights and sleep half an hour longer between feedings. Gradually try to extend the time between meals until baby is down to one nighttime feeding, which he may continue to need for another two or three months.

■ Cut down the amounts at the nighttime feedings you want to eliminate. Reduce the number of ounces in your baby's bottle by one or the number of minutes he nurses by a couple. Continue cutting back a little more each night or every other night. With a bottle-fed baby it may work to dilute the formula, gradually adding a little more water and a little less formula each night until you're down to all water at the unwanted feedings. At that point, some babies will decide that getting up for a bottle of water isn't worth the effort, and will choose to sleep instead. Most, however, will prefer water to no bottle at all, and will continue to waken for this bottle. But since a baby's hunger can't be satisfied with water, you will at least have eliminated the hunger-feeding cycle, making it easier to eventually drop the feeding entirely. (Check with your baby's doctor before diluting the formula to be sure you won't be cutting out needed calories.)

■ Increase the amount offered at the night feeding you are most likely to continue. If your baby is getting up at midnight, two, and four, for example, you may want to cut out the first and last of these feedings. This will be easier to do if you increase the amount your baby takes at the middle one, either from bottle or breast. A nip from the breast or a couple of ounces from the bottle is not likely to knock him out for long. See the tips for keeping a sleepy baby awake for feeding on page 60.

■ Don't diaper your baby during the night unless it's absolutely necessary—a quick sniff can usually tell you when it is. (Of course, the fewer midnight snacks you indulge him in, the less necessary nighttime diapering will become). If he wears cloth diapers (which become very soggy and uncomfortable), consider using paper diaper liners at bedtime, or switching to super absorbent disposables at night. If your baby is between sizes, using the next larger size, snugly wrapped to prevent leakage (unless he's prone to diaper rash), will provide extra surface area for absorption. Also consider that if you do have to change him, it will be swifter and less disruptive to fasten on a fresh disposable than to fuss with a cloth set.

■ If you're sharing a room with your baby, now's a good time to think about splitting up (see page 185). Your nearness may be the reason he's waking so often and why you're picking him up so often.

STILL USING A PACIFIER

"I was planning to let my daughter use a pacifier only until she was three months old, but she seems so dependent on it, I'm not sure I can take it away now."

Babies are also creatures of comfort. The comfort they crave can come in a number of packages—a mother's breast, a bottle, a soothing lullaby, or a pacifier. And the more accustomed they become to a particular source of comfort, the more difficult it becomes for them to do without it. If you don't want to run into the problems that may later be associated with pacifier use, now is an ideal time to make a break. For one thing, at this age her memory is short and she will easily forget the pacifier when it disappears from her life. For another, she is more open to change than an older baby —more likely to accept an alternative route to pacification. A toddler not only won't forget her pacifier, but will probably demand it with a storm of will and temper. And of course a habit of three months is easier to break than one that has been building for a year or more.

To comfort your baby without a pacifier, try rocking, singing, a clean knuckle for sucking (or help her to find her own fingers), or some of the other techniques listed on page 128. Admittedly, all of these take more time and effort on your part than tucking a pacifier in her mouth, but they'll be better for baby in the long run, especially if they are gradually eliminated in favor of letting baby learn to comfort herself. (See page 71 for the pros and cons of using a pacifier.)

SPASTIC MOVEMENTS

"When my son tries to reach for something he doesn't succeed, and his movements seem so spastic I'm worried that there's something wrong with his nervous system."

There's probably nothing wrong with his nervous system—it's just very young and inexperienced. Though it has come a long way from the days when you felt little twitches in your uterus, your baby's nervous system still hasn't worked out all the kinks. When his arm whips out at a toy that's caught his eye but doesn't land anywhere near its target, the lack of coordination may be worrisome to a new parent, but it's actually a normal stage in infant motor development. Soon he will gain more control, and the purposeful, clumsy batting will be replaced with skillful reaching movements. And once he gets to the stage when nothing within that cunning reach is safe again, you may look back fondly on a time when he looked, but wasn't able to touch.

If you'd like some additional reassurance, check with your baby's doctor at his next checkup.

GIVING BABY COW'S MILK

"I'm breastfeeding and would like to give my baby a supplement, but I don't want to use formula. Can I give him cow's milk?"

Cow's milk is a great drink for little cows—but it just doesn't have the right mix of nutrients for human babies. It contains more salt (much more) and protein than breast milk or commercial formula, and these excesses put a strain on young kidneys. It is also lacking in iron. Babies who are fed cow's milk exclusively, as well as those who receive iron-poor formulas, require iron supplementation in the form of vitamin-mineral drops (later, iron-fortified cereal can also supply iron needs). The composition of cow's milk also varies from that of breast milk in a variety of other ways. In addition, it causes mild intestinal bleeding in a small percentage of infants. Though the blood lost in the stool is generally not visible to the naked eye, the bleed-

ing is significant because it can lead to anemia.

So if you're planning to supplement your breastfeeding, it's best to use expressed breast milk or a formula recommended by the doctor—preferably until your baby is a year old. Easiest are ready-to-use formulas, which require no preparation other than the screwing on of a clean nipple. If, once you start solids, using a bit of formula or breast milk for such purposes as mixing baby cereal is cumbersome, ask your baby's doctor about using small amounts of whole cow's milk.

DIAPER RASH

"I change my baby frequently, but she still gets diaper rash—and I have trouble getting rid of it."

There's a good reason why your baby (and 7 to 35% of her comrades-in-diapers) isn't sitting on a pretty bottom. Exposed as it is in the diaper area to high moisture, little air, a variety of chemical irritants and infectious organisms in urine and feces, and oftentimes the rubbing of diapers and clothing, it's an easy target for a wide variety of problems. Diaper rash can remain a problem as long as a baby is in diapers, but incidence usually peaks between seven and nine months when a more varied diet is reflected in the more irritating nature of her stools, and then starts to diminish as baby skin toughens.

Unfortunately, diaper rash tends to repeat in some babies—perhaps because of an inborn susceptibility, allergic tendencies, an abnormal stool pH (an imbalance between acidity and alkalinity), excessive ammonia in the urine, or simply because once skin becomes irritated, it is more susceptible to further irritation.

The exact mechanism responsible for diaper rash isn't known, but it is believed that it probably begins when a baby's delicate skin becomes irritated by chronic moisture. When the skin is further weakened by friction from a diaper or clothing, or by irritating substances in stool or urine, it is left open to attack by germs on the skin or in the urine or stool. Aggressive and frequent cleansing of the diaper area with detergents or soaps can increase the susceptibility of an infant's skin, as can very tight diapers or rubber pants, which keep air out and moisture in. The ammonia in urine, once thought to be the major culprit in diaper rash, doesn't appear to be a primary cause, but can irritate already damaged skin. But the rashes do tend to start where urine concentrates in the diaper, toward the bottom with girls and the front with boys.

The term "diaper rash" describes a number of different skin conditions in the diaper area. Just what distinguishes one diaper rash from another is not widely agreed on in the medical community (maybe the subject just hasn't aroused enough interest to stimulate serious study and clearer definitions), but they are often described this way:

Perianal dermatitis. Redness around the anus usually is caused by the alkaline stools of a bottle-fed baby and does not usually occur in breastfed infants until after solids have been introduced.

Chafing dermatitis. This is the most common form of diaper rash and is seen as redness where friction is greatest, but not in a baby's skin folds. It generally comes and goes, causing little discomfort if not complicated by a secondary infection.

Atopic dermatitis. This diaper rash is itchy, and may turn up in other parts of the body first. It usually begins to spread to the diaper area between six and 12 months.

Seborrheic dermatitis. This deep red rash, often with yellowish scales, usually starts on the scalp as cradle cap, though it sometimes begins in the diaper region and spreads upward. Like most diaper rashes, it's usually more bothersome to parents than to baby.

Candidal dermatitis. Bright red and tender, this uncomfortable rash appears in the inguinal folds (the creases between the abdomen and the thighs), with satellite pustules spreading from that point. Diaper rashes that last more than 72 hours often become infected with candida albicans, the same yeast infection responsible for thrush. This type of rash may also develop in a baby on antibiotics.

Impetigo. Caused by bacteria (streptococci or staphylococci), impetigo in the diaper area occurs in two different forms: bullous, with large, thin-walled blisters that burst and leave a thin yellow-brown crust, or non-bullous, with thick, yellow, crusted scabs and a lot of surrounding redness. It can cover thighs, buttocks, and lower abdomen, and spread to other parts of the body as well.

Intertrigo. This type of rash, which manifests itself as a poorly defined reddened area, occurs as a result of the rubbing of skin on skin. In infants it is usually found in the deep inguinal folds between the thighs and the lower abdomen, and often in the armpits. Intertrigo rash may sometimes ooze white to yellowish matter, and may burn when urine touches it, causing baby to cry.

Tidemark dermatitis. This is an irritation precipitated by friction from the edge of a diaper rubbing against the skin.

The best cure for diaper rash is prevention—though it isn't always possible. Keeping the diaper area dry and clean is one of the most important principles of prevention. See page 77 for diapering practices that will help you to do this. If preventive measures don't work, the following may help eliminate your baby's simple diaper rash, and will be helpful in warding off recurrences:

Less moisture. To reduce moisture on the skin, change the diaper often, even in the middle of the night if your baby's awake. Put any plans to train her to sleep through the night on hold until the diaper rash has cleared up. For persistent diaper rash, change baby as soon as you're aware that she's wet or had a bowel movement. Less superfluous liquid should go into baby, too. Drinking bottle after bottle of juice leads to excessive urination and more diaper rash. Better, use a cup only for juice, to avoid overdosing.

More air. Keep baby's bottom bare part of the time, placing her on a couple of folded cloth diapers or receiving blankets over a plastic or waterproof pad or sheet to protect the surface below. If necessary let her sleep the same way, but be sure the room is warm enough so she won't be chilly. If she's in cloth diapers, use diaper wraps instead of rubber pants, or leave the pants off altogether and put her on a water-proof pad. If she's wearing disposables, poke a few holes in the waterproof outer cover. This will allow some air in, and it will also allow some moisture to seep out—which will encourage more frequent diaper changes.

Fewer irritants. You can't limit the natural irritants such as urine and stool except by changing diapers frequently, but you can limit those that you apply to baby's bottom. Soap can dry and irritate the skin, so use it only once daily. Dove and Johnson's baby soap are generally recommended for babies (most so-called "gentle" soaps aren't), or ask the doctor for a suggestion. For diaper changes when the infant has had a bowel movement, wash skin thoroughly (for about thirty seconds to one minute) with warm water and cotton balls instead of "wipes." Wipes may contain substances that irritate your baby's skin (different babies are sensitive to different substances); those that contain alcohol are particularly drying. If the ones you're using seem to cause a problem, switch—but don't use wipes at all when your baby has a rash. A really messy movement may be best cleaned by a dip in the tub or sink, when that's convenient. Be careful to pat baby dry

thoroughly after washing. A baby who is merely wet needn't be cleaned up at all—just changed.

Different diapers. If your baby has a recurrent diaper rash, consider switching to another type of diaper (from cloth to disposables or vice versa, from one type of disposable to another) to see if the change makes a difference. If you home-launder diapers, rinse them with ½ cup of vinegar or a special diaper rinse, and if necessary, boil them in a large pot for ten minutes.

Blocking tactics. Spreading a thick protective layer of ointment (A & D, Desitin, zinc oxide, Lassar's paste, Eucerin, Nivea, teat balm, or whatever your baby's doctor recommends) on baby's bottom after washing it at changing time will prevent urine from reaching it. If you buy these products in the largest sizes, you'll save money and be more likely to use them liberally—which is best. But don't use the ointment when you're airing baby's bottom.

Do not use boric acid or talc when treating the rash. Though boric acid may help relieve simple diaper rash, it is very toxic when taken internally and most doctors suggest not using it around infants, or even having it in the house. The talc may also help by absorbing moisture and keeping baby drier, but it can be inhaled by an infant and cause pneumonia, and it is also carcinogenic. Cornstarch is an effective and safer substitute. And don't use medications around the house that have been prescribed for other family members; some combination ointments (those that contain steroids and antibacterial or antifungal agents) are a major cause of allergic skin reactions, and you could sensitize your baby by using them.

If your baby's diaper rash doesn't clear up or improve in a day or two, or if blisters or pustules appear, call her doctor, who will try to uncover its cause and then treat it. For seborrheic dermatitis, a steroid cream may be necessary (but it should not be used long-term); for impetigo, antibiotics given by mouth; for intertrigo, careful cleansing plus a hydrocortisone cream and protective ointments; and for candida, the most common diaper infection, a good topical antifungal ointment or cream. Ask how long it should take for the rash to clear, and then report back to the doctor if it isn't better by then or if the treatment seems to make it worse. If the rash persists, the doctor may check for dietary or other factors that may be contributing to it. In rare cases, the expertise of a pediatric dermatologist may be needed to unravel the mystery of a baby's diaper rash.

PENIS SORE

"I'm very concerned about a red raw area at the tip of my son's penis."

What you see is very likely nothing more than a localized diaper rash. It is common and can sometimes cause enough swelling to prevent a baby from urinating. Because spread to the urethra could eventually cause scarring, you should do everything you can to get rid of the rash as soon as possible. If you've been using home-laundered diapers, switch to a diaper service or disposables until the problem has resolved, and follow the other tips for treating diaper rash given above, adding warm soaks if your baby is having trouble urinating. If the rash persists after two or three days of home treatment, call the doctor.

If you return to using home-laundered diapers, be sure to use a special diaper rinse to sanitize them.

SUDDEN INFANT DEATH SYNDROME

"Since a neighbor's baby died of crib death, I'm so nervous that I've been waking my baby up several times a night to make sure she's okay. Would it be a good idea to ask my doctor about a monitoring machine?"

The fear that a baby might die suddenly in the middle of the night has plagued mothers probably from the beginning of time— long before such deaths were given a medical name: Sudden Infant Death Syndrome (SIDS). Ancient writings mention such deaths; the baby described in the Book of Kings as being "overlaid" by his mother was very likely a victim of crib death.

But unless your baby has experienced an actual life-threatening episode in which she stopped breathing and needed to be revived (in which case, see page 183), the chances of her actually succumbing to SIDS are less than 2 in 1,000. And preoccupation with the idea that your child will be one of the two is more harmful than helpful—to both of you.

For most mothers, no reassurance will totally obviate the need they feel to check their baby's breathing occasionally at night. Many, in fact, don't breathe easily themselves until their babies have passed the one-year mark, the age when infants seem to outgrow the problems that cause SIDS. And that's okay as long as you don't let worry pervade your every activity.

Though investing in a monitor, an apparatus that can signal if your baby suddenly stops breathing, may seem like an ideal (if expensive) way of easing your fears, monitoring a normal baby can cause more problems than it solves. It upsets family dynamics and often adversely affects the way a mother and child interact. And the false alarms that are common with monitors result more in worry than relief. Monitors are recommended only for babies who have had life-threatening episodes of apnea (cessation of breathing), who have heart and lung problems that make them particularly susceptible to SIDS, or who have two or more siblings who died of SIDS or had near misses.

What can make you (and every other mother) feel more secure is learning infant CPR, and being sure that dad, baby-sitters, housekeepers, and anyone else who spends time alone with your baby also knows this lifesaving technique—so that if your baby

WHAT IS SIDS?

SIDS, or Sudden Infant Death Syndrome, is defined as the sudden death of an infant that is unexplained either by the baby's history, a postmortem exam, or the examination of the scene of death. It's the major cause of infant death between the ages of two weeks and twelve months, claiming more than 6,000 lives a year in the U.S. alone. Though it was once believed that victims were "perfectly healthy" babies stricken suddenly without reason, researchers are now convinced that SIDS babies only *appear* healthy, and actually have some underlying defect—one that hasn't as yet been identified—that predisposes them to sudden death.

The risk of the average baby dying of SIDS is very small—about 1.7 in 1,000. It's even lower for the majority of healthy babies. But it is higher for certain small groups of infants. At high risk are those who have survived a very serious life-threatening event unrelated to injury or accident during which they stopped breathing, turned blue, and required resuscitation. (Babies who have had brief spells of apnea lasting under twenty seconds appear not to be at increased risk.) At lesser risk, but still more susceptible than "normal" babies, are small and/or premature infants, and those from multiple births. SIDS strikes males more often than females.

The theory that the root of the problem may go back to prenatal fetal development is supported by the fact that babies of women who had poor prenatal care or who smoked during pregnancy, and possibly of smokers who had severe anemia during pregnancy, are also at somewhat increased risk. Babies of young mothers (under twenty) are, too, but this may be as much (or more) because of the poor prenatal care as because of age.

Suspicion that heredity is a major factor in SIDS hasn't been borne out by research, but there does seem to be a very slight increase in risk among siblings of SIDS victims, possibly because the same factors that contributed to the first event—poor medical care or maternal smoking, for example—are present during both pregnancies. Racial differences—SIDS occurs more often among blacks than whites, most often among Native Americans and least often among Asians—seem to point to a genetic factor. But it isn't clear whether these differences are partly or entirely due to economic inequalities and/or cultural differences, since SIDS is more common among the poor.

There does *not* seem to be a correlation between SIDS and the use of anesthesia or pain medication in labor, the length of first or second stages of labor, cesarean deliveries, urinary tract infections, vaginitis, or STDs in the mother. Letting baby sleep in parents' bed doesn't reduce risk.

A great deal of research is being done to try to determine just what it is that causes SIDS; it may turn out that there is more than one type of SIDS, each with a different cause, or that several factors combine to cause the syndrome. A leading theory is that delay in maturation of the brain stem predisposes a baby to SIDS. Another suggests an occasional case may be related to child abuse. Recent studies abroad point to sleeping prone (face down), particularly on a soft surface in which recesses can form, as a major factor. A mild cold or other infection, swaddling, and overheating may compound the risk when an infant sleeps tummy down. Information is being collected on the characteristics that SIDS babies have in common (which include certain types of tissue changes and signs of unexplained asphyxiation) and on other common factors in the deaths (they are most likely to occur between the second and fourth months of life, at home, in the crib, more often in cold weather, and mostly between midnight and 8 A.M.).

ever does stop breathing, for whatever reason, resuscitation can be attempted immediately (see page 448). If gnawing fears continue to plague you, you might talk to your baby's doctor about doing an evaluation of his lung and heart functions—usually reserved for cases where there have been previous indications of a problem—to give you some reassurance. If an evaluation shows your baby not to be at high risk for SIDS, relax. If you can't relax, talk to a therapist who is familiar with SIDS and can help to allay your fears.

"Yesterday afternoon I went in to check on my baby, who seemed to be taking a very long nap. He was lying in the crib absolutely still and blue. Frantic, I picked him up and shook him and he was okay. Now his doctor wants to put him in the hospital for tests and I'm terrified."

As terrifying as the experience may have been for you, you can actually consider yourself very lucky that it occurred. Not only did your baby survive, but he gave you a very good warning that this kind of event might happen again (though it usually doesn't), and that you should get medical help to prevent a more serious recurrence.

Your doctor's suggestion that your baby, who experienced what is called "apnea of infancy," be hospitalized is a good one. This kind of episode does put an infant at increased risk for SIDS, though the chances are 99 to 1 on his side. A brief stay at the hospital will enable the staff to evaluate your baby's health through a complete health history and physical exam, diagnostic testing, and possibly, monitoring for further spells of prolonged apnea (when a baby stops breathing for more than twenty seconds), in order to try to find an underlying cause for the event. Sometimes it's something fairly simple—such as an infection, a seizure disorder, or an airway obstruction—that can be treated, eliminating the risk of future problems.

Unfortunately, no test will always accurately predict the infant at risk for SIDS. But a comprehensive evaluation will tell the doctor whether or not a baby should be monitored at home or possibly put on medication.

This kind of evaluation may also be done on an infant who has no history of apnea, but who has had two or more siblings who succumbed to SIDS or one who died and others who suffered apparent life-threatening events (ALTE), and possibly, on one with cousins who were SIDS victims.

If tests at a local hospital are inconclusive, the doctor may recommend referral to a major SIDS center. For information on the center nearest you or for more information on SIDS, call the National SIDS Alliance (1-800-222-SIDS) or the American SIDS Institute (1-800-232-SIDS, or 1-800-447-SIDS if you are calling from Georgia).

If it is discovered that an illness caused your baby's apnea, it will be treated. If the cause is undetermined, or if heart or lung problems that put him at high risk for sudden death are discovered, the doctor may recommend putting your baby on a device that monitors breathing and/or heartbeat at home. The monitor is usually attached to the baby with electrodes, or is embedded in his crib, playpen, or bassinet mattress. You, and anyone else who cares for your baby, will be trained in connecting the monitor as well as in responding to an emergency with CPR. The monitor won't give your baby absolute protection against SIDS, but it will help your doctor learn more about his condition and help you feel you are doing something, rather than sitting helplessly by waiting for the worst to happen.

Don't, however, let your baby's problem and his monitor become the focus of your life. Doing so could be very destructive, turning your probably normal baby into an invalid, interfering with his growth and development, and damaging your relationship with him and others in the family. Seek help from your doctor or a qualified counselor if a monitor seems to add to family tension rather than reduce it.

Though criteria may vary from doctor to doctor and community to community, babies who've had no critical episodes since their first usually come off a monitor when they have been free of events requiring prolonged and vigorous stimulation or rescue for two months. More stringent requirements for going off the monitor are usually set for those who have had a second critical episode. Though babies are rarely removed from the monitor until they pass six months, when the peak period for SIDS is over, a total of 90% are off their monitors by the time they reach one year.

"My premature baby had occasional periods of apnea for the first few weeks of her life, but her doctor says that I shouldn't worry, that she doesn't need to be monitored."

Apnea is very common in premature babies; in fact, about 50% of those born before 32 weeks gestation experience it. But this "apnea of prematurity," when it occurs before the baby's original due date, appears totally unrelated to SIDS; there is no increased risk of SIDS or of apnea, itself, later. So unless your baby has serious apneic episodes after her original due date, there's no cause for concern or follow-up.

Even in full-term babies, brief lapses in breathing without any blueness or limpness or need for resuscitation are not believed by most experts to be a predictor of SIDS risk; few babies with such apnea are lost to SIDS, and most babies who do die of SIDS weren't observed to experience apnea previously.

"I've heard that DTP immunizations can cause SIDS, and I'm really worried about having my baby immunized."

The theory has been put forth that SIDS may be related to DTP injections—though of course, even if this were so, it would only be one cause, since sudden infant death considerably predates the use of immunization. But to date, the only large controlled case study found no relationship between SIDS and DTP. It isn't surprising, of course, that some babies who get DTP shots also die of SIDS, since these shots are routinely administered at two and four months of age, and SIDS is at its peak between two and four months. But if you're still concerned, talk to your baby's doctor. His or her reassurance will doubtless make you more comfortable about going ahead with DTP shots.

REPORTING BREATHING EMERGENCIES TO YOUR DOCTOR

Though very brief (under twenty seconds) periods of breathing lapse can be normal, longer periods, or short periods accompanied by the baby turning pale or blue or limp and having a very slowed heartbeat, require medical attention. If you have to take steps to revive your baby, call the doctor or emergency squad immediately. If you can't revive your baby by gentle shaking, try CPR (see page 448), and call or have someone else call 911. Try to note the following to report to the doctor:

■ Did the breathing lapse occur when baby was asleep or awake?

■ Was baby sleeping, feeding, crying, spitting, gagging, or coughing when the event occurred?

■ Did baby experience any color changes; was he or she pale, blue, or red in the face?

■ Were there any changes in baby's crying (higher pitch, for example)?

■ Did baby seem limp or stiff or was he or she moving normally?

■ Does your baby often have noisy breathing (see the discussion of stridor on page 416); does he or she snore?

■ Did baby need resuscitation? How did you revive him or her, and how long did it take?

EARLY WEANING

"I'm going back to work full-time at the end of the month, and I'd like to give up nursing my daughter. Will it be hard on her?"

A three-month-old is, in general, a pretty agreeable and adaptable sort. Though well past the newborn-as-blob stage, with a budding personality all her own, she's still far from the opinionated (and sometimes tyrannical) toddler she'll eventually turn into. So if you're going to pick a time for weaning from the breast that's going to be easiest for her, this may be it. Though she may thoroughly enjoy nursing, she probably won't cling to it as stubbornly as a six-month-old who's never had a bottle and is suddenly subjected to weaning. All in all, you'll probably find that weaning at three months is less difficult for your baby than it is for you.

Ideally, mothers who want to wean their babies early should begin giving supplementary bottles, using either expressed milk or formula, by around five or six weeks so the infants become adjusted to suckling on the bottle as well as on the breast. If you haven't, your first step is to get baby acclimated to an artificial nipple; silicone may be more appealing than rubber, and you may have to try several different styles to find one your baby likes. At this point it would be best to use formula, so that your present breast milk supply will begin to diminish. Be persistent, but don't force the nipple. Try giving the bottle before the breast; if your baby rejects the bottle the first time, try again at the next feeding. Bottles may be more acceptable to baby if someone other than the mother gives them. (See page 143 for more tips on introducing the bottle.)

Keep trying until she takes at least an ounce or two from the bottle. Once she does, substitute a meal of formula for a nursing at a midday feeding. A few days later, replace another daytime breastfeeding with formula. Making the switch gradually, one feeding at a time, will give your breasts a chance to adjust without uncomfortable engorgement. Eliminate the evening breastfeeding last, as this will give you and your baby a quiet and relaxing time together when you get home from work. If you like, you may—assuming your milk supply doesn't dry up entirely, and assuming your baby is still interested—be able to continue this once-a-day feeding for a while, postponing total weaning until a later date, or until your milk is gone.

SHARING A ROOM WITH BABY

"Our ten-week-old has been sharing our room since birth. When should we move him to his own room?"

In the first weeks of life, when baby's at the breast or bottle as much as he's in bed, and nights are a blur of feedings, diaper changes, and rocking sessions interrupted only occasionally by snatches of sleep, having him within a weary arm's reach makes sense. Once he outgrows the physiological need for frequent feedings during the night (anywhere from about two weeks to three months, or sometimes later), having your baby for a roommate raises a number of serious problems:

Less sleep for parents. Being in the same room with your baby all night, you're tempted to pick him up every time he whimpers. And even if you resist picking him up, you're sure to lie awake waiting for the whimper to turn to a howl. You may also lose a few good nights' sleep over his tossing and turning; babies are notoriously restless sleepers.

Less sleep for baby. The fact that you pick him up more often at night if he's in your room not only means less sleep for you, but for him, too. In addition, during his lighter phases of sleep, your son is likely to be wakened by your activity, even if you tiptoe around in soft slippers and climb silently into bed.

Less lovemaking. Sure, you know (or at least you hope) your baby is sleeping when you start to make love. But how uninhibited can you really be in your ardor when you've got company (breathing loudly, tossing his head back and forth, moaning softly in his sleep) so close by?

More problems adjusting later. In societies where whole families sleep in one room, there's no need to socialize children to sleep alone. But in our culture, where most children are expected to do so, having your baby in your room for a lengthy period will make it more difficult when you finally do move him to a room of his own.

Of course, "a room of his own" isn't possible in every household. If you live in a one-bedroom apartment or a small house with several children, there may be no option but for your baby to share. If that's the case, consider a divider—either a screen, or a heavy drape hung from a ceiling track (the drape is also a good sound insulator). Or give your bedroom up to the baby and invest in a sleep sofa in the living room for you. Or partition off a corner of the living room for the baby and do your late night TV watching or talking in the bedroom.

If your baby will have to share with another child, how well the sleeping arrangement will work out will depend on how well the two sleep. If either one or both are light sleepers with a tendency to awaken during the night, you may all be in for a difficult period of adjustment until each has learned to sleep through the other's wakings. Again, a partition or drape may help muffle the sounds, while providing the older child with privacy.

SHARING A BED

"I've heard a lot about the benefits of children sharing a bed with their parents. And with all the night waking our *daughter has been doing, it seems like such an arrangement would mean more sleep for everyone."*

Co-sleeping, parents and children sharing a bed at night, does work well—but chiefly, it seems, in other societies. In a society like ours, which stresses the development of independence and the importance of privacy, co-sleeping is associated with a wide range of problems:

Sleep problems. Probably most significant for overtired parents is the fact that bed sharing seems to increase the incidence of sleep disorders in children. One study of those six months to four years of age showed that sleep problems were present in 50% of co-sleepers, compared with only 15% of those who slept in their own beds; another showed that 35% of toddlers who slept with parents had sleep problems compared to 7% of those who slept alone. It's theorized that co-sleeping deprives children of the chance to learn how to fall asleep on their own—an important lifelong skill.

Dental problems. It appears that co-sleeping encourages, rather than discourages, the chronic nighttime feeder's greedy habit. And for the nursing baby who is allowed to use the co-sleeping arrangement for convenient nipping and napping all night long, dental caries (the decay is caused, as in baby-bottle mouth, by milk that stays in baby's mouth while she sleeps) can be an unfortunate result—particularly if nighttime nursing continues past the first birthday.

Developmental problems. Though more research is required to analyze the effects of co-sleeping on a child's emotional development, some experts have speculated that the arrangement may interfere with a child developing a strong sense of being a separate person, a feeling of independence, and a sense of privacy. It may also lead to separation anxiety lasting longer than normal; a child may feel lonely and insecure whenever she's without her parents.

Peer problems. If co-sleeping continues into the school years, children who share a bed with their parents may be ridiculed by friends.

Marital problems. If sleeping in the same room with a baby is inhibiting to the parents' sexual relationship, having a baby in the same bed can be fatal to it. And though there's no evidence that a very young baby can be emotionally scarred if she accidentally wakes up and views her parents making love, that may not be true for an older child.

Safety problems. Potential risks include: plush mattresses, pillows, comforters, waterbeds; a crevice between bed and wall; a bed that doesn't meet crib safety standards; a sound sleeping or drug or alcohol impaired parent who rolls over on the infant.

Drawing-the-line problems. It's one thing to have an infant, or even a toddler, in bed with you—but where do you draw the line? And when you do, how will you teach a child who has always slept with you to suddenly sleep in her own bed? And is it fair to accustom a child to having a warm body beside her at night, only to suddenly banish her to a cold and lonely bed? Even if you deem it fair, you may find it next to impossible. A child who's formed a habit of sleeping with parents will return as surely as a swallow to Capistrano.

Though the evidence seems stacked in favor of separate beds and bedrooms for babies once they've passed the three-month birthday (when excessive nighttime crying has usually subsided), the issue is still a personal one. It's true that co-sleeping has worked in countless societies for countless generations, and that children do experience a special warmth and comfort when they sleep with their parents. Some families will decide that they don't want to give in to social pressures, and will opt for the "family bed." That's fine, as long as they are aware of the possible risks. And those who elect to sleep alone can achieve some family togetherness by bringing baby into bed, some mornings or every morning, for a feeding or some cuddling.

ROUGHHOUSING

"My husband loves to roughhouse with our twelve-week-old, and she loves when he does it. But I've heard that shaking an infant too much, even in fun, can cause injury."

Watching the glee in a young baby's face as she's tossed up in the air by her adoring dad, it's hard to imagine that such fun could end in tragedy. And yet it could. There are two kinds of damage that can occur during such roughhousing. The first is a detached retina, which can cause serious vision problems or even blindness. The second is whiplash, which in an infant, whose neck is very unsteady, could lead to serious brain damage, and in rare cases, even to death.

Such injuries occur most often when a baby is being shaken in anger, but they can happen at play. So avoid roughhousing that vigorously shakes or jostles your baby's unsupported head or neck. Also avoid jogging or other "bouncing" activities with a young infant in a baby carrier (do your running while pushing baby in a stroller, instead). That doesn't mean no fun at all—babies love a good, smooth "fly" through the air supported by a pair of strong hands, and other non-jarring physical games.

Although roughhousing should be avoided in the future, don't worry about any your baby has been treated to in the past. If damage had been done, it would have been apparent.

FEWER BOWEL MOVEMENTS

"I'm concerned that my breastfed baby may be constipated. She always had six or eight bowel movements a day, and now she rarely has more than one, and sometimes even misses a day."

Don't be concerned—be grateful. This slowdown in production is not only normal, but will send you to the changing table less often. Definitely a change for the better.

It's normal for many breastfed babies like yours to start having fewer bowel movements somewhere between one and three months of age. Some will even go several days between movements. Others will continue their prodigious production rates as long as they are nursing. That's normal, too.

Constipation is rarely a problem for breastfed babies, and infrequency isn't a sign of it; hard, difficult-to-pass stools are (see page 113).

LEAVING BABY WITH A SITTER

"We'd love a night out alone, but we're afraid of leaving our daughter with a sitter when she's so young."

Go to town—and soon. Assuming you're going to want to spend some time alone together (or just alone) during the next eighteen years, getting your baby used to being cared for occasionally by a non-parent will be an important part of her development. And in this case, the earlier she starts making the adjustment, the better. Infants two and three months old may recognize their mothers, but out-of-sight usually means out-of-mind. And as long as their needs are being met, young babies are generally happy with any attentive person. By the time babies reach nine months (much sooner in some babies), most begin experiencing what is called separation or stranger anxiety—not only are they unhappy being separated from mother or father, they're also very wary of new people.

At first you'll probably want to take only short outings, especially if you're nursing and have to squeeze your dinner in between baby's meals. What shouldn't be short, however, is the time you spend choosing and preparing the sitter, to ensure your baby

will be well cared for. The first night, have the sitter come at least half an hour early so you can fully acclimate him or her to the eccentricities of your child's needs and habits and so baby and sitter can meet. (See the Baby-Sitter Checklist, page 189 and What It's Important to Know, page 190.)

"We almost always take our baby with us when we go out; we only leave her with a sitter when she's asleep, and then only for a few hours. Friends say this will make her too dependent."

A lot of people today seem more concerned about the child whose mother or father never leaves her than the one whose parents regularly do. But there's no evidence to support such concern. Though there are some advantages to getting your baby adjusted to a sitter now (before stranger anxiety rears its unfriendly head), and to not feeling so tied down yourself, a baby whose mommy is always around doesn't necessarily become overly dependent. Often, in fact, the child who spends a majority of the time in early infancy with one or both parents turns out to be very secure and trusting. She has unswerving faith that she is loved, that any sitter her parents leave her with will take good care of her, and that when her parents go out they will return when they say they will.

So do what makes you most comfortable, not what will satisfy your friends.

BEING TIED DOWN BY A NURSING BABY

"I was happy with my decision not to give our little boy supplementary bottles until I realized it's almost impossible to have a long evening out.

Nothing's perfect, not even the decision to breastfeed exclusively. It has its advantages, of course, but there are occasions when it can bring regrets. Many women, however, have survived the decision and managed to retain some semblance of a social life in

BABY-SITTER CHECK LIST

Even the best baby-sitter needs instructions. Before you leave your baby with anyone, make certain that he or she is familiar with the following:

■ How your baby is most easily calmed (rocking, a special song, a favorite mobile, a ride in the baby carrier)
■ What your baby's favorite toy is
■ How your baby likes to sleep (on back, side, or tummy)—for most infants, back is best (see page 120)
■ How your baby is best burped (over the shoulder, on the lap, after feeding, during feeding)
■ How to diaper and clean baby (Do you use wipes or cotton balls? A double diaper or single? Rubber pants? An ointment for diaper rash?) and where diapers and supplies are kept
■ Where extra clothing is kept in case those baby is wearing get soiled
■ How to give the bottle, if your baby is bottle fed or is to get a supplement of formula or expressed milk
■ What your baby can and can't eat or drink (making it clear that no food, drink or medicine should be given to your baby without your okay, or the doctor's)
■ The setup of your kitchen, the baby's room, and so on, and any other pertinent facts about your house or apartment (such as a burglar alarm that might go off, and where fire exits are located)
■ Any habits or characteristics of your baby that the sitter might not expect (spits up a lot, has a lot of bowel movements, cries when wet, falls asleep only with a light on, can roll off the changing table)
■ The habits of any pets you may have that the sitter should be aware of, and rules concerning your baby and pets
■ Where the first aid kit (or individual items) is located

■ Baby safety rules (see page 136); you might want to photocopy rules and post them in an obvious place for the sitter
■ Where a flashlight (or candles) is located
■ What to do in case the fire alarm goes off or smoke or fire is observed, or if someone who hasn't been cleared by you rings the doorbell
■ Who is cleared by you to visit when you are not at home, and what your policy is on a sitter's having visitors

You should also leave the following for the sitter:

■ Important phone numbers (the baby's doctor, where you can be reached, a neighbor who will be home, your parents, the hospital emergency room, the poison control center, the building superintendent, a plumber or handyman), and a pad and pencil for taking messages
■ The address of the nearest emergency room and the best way to get there
■ Cab fare in case of an unexpected emergency (such as the need to take the baby to the emergency room or the doctor's office), and the number to call for a cab
■ A signed consent form authorizing medical care within specific limits, if you cannot be reached (this should be worked out in advance with baby's doctor)

It's helpful to combine all the information necessary for caring for your baby—phone numbers, safety and health tips, and whatever else you deem necessary—in a small loose-leaf binder. Information can easily be changed or added as required, and everything is always at close hand for the sitter. The "mad money" can be stashed in an envelope taped to the cover of the binder.

spite of it. First of all, though it may be difficult to get out now, it will get easier once your baby begins to go to sleep for the night at 8 or 9 P.M., allowing you to head out for a late night on the town. Also, once

solids are introduced, a sitter will have something to offer your baby should he awaken hungry. And finally, once you've introduced the cup, your baby will even be able to have a drink if he's thirsty.

In the meantime, if you have a special event you'd like to attend that will keep you from home for more than a couple of hours, try these:

- Take baby and sitter along, if there's some place for them to stay, such as a lobby. It may be cumbersome, but it will allow baby to nap in a stroller or carriage while you enjoy the affair. Should he awaken, the sitter can notify you and you can slip out and nurse in the ladies' room or another suitable area.

- If the event is out of town, take the family along. Either bring your own sitter or hire one where you will be staying. If the place where you are staying is near enough to the reception, you can pop in at feeding time.

- Adjust baby's bedtime, if possible. If your baby usually doesn't go to bed until after nine, and you need to leave at seven try to get him to skip his afternoon nap and put him to bed a couple of hours early. Be sure to give him a full nursing before you leave, and plan on feeding him again when you return home, if necessary.

- Leave a bottle of expressed milk or water and hope for the best. If your baby wakes up and is really hungry, he may take the bottle. At this stage nipple confusion won't interfere with his nursing, so you needn't worry on that score. If he doesn't take it, he may scream for a while, but will very likely fall back to sleep eventually. When you get home, feed him if necessary. Of course, if the sitter feels he is so upset that you should return, you should be ready to do so.

WHAT IT'S IMPORTANT TO KNOW:
The Right Caretakers for Baby

Leaving your child with a sitter for the first time is traumatic enough without worrying about whether you're leaving him or her with the right person in the right place. And finding child care that you're confident about is no longer as easy—at least, not for most—as picking up the phone and enlisting grandma or the grandmotherly next-door neighbor. With extended family often extending beyond city and state limits, and many grandmothers working themselves, the mother who needs a sitter usually must depend on a stranger.

When grandmother was the sitter, a mother's biggest worry was whether her child would be plied with too many cookies. Turning your baby over to a stranger (or group of strangers) raises a great many more concerns. Will she be responsible and reliable? Attentive and responsive to your baby's needs? Capable of providing your baby with the kind of play-learning stimulation that will help develop mind and body to their fullest potential? Will her child-care philosophies mesh comfortably with yours, and will she accept your ideas and respect your wishes? Will she be warm and loving enough to act as mother substitute without presuming to take your place as a mother?

Separating from your baby—whether for a 9-to-5 job or a Saturday night dinner and a show—will never be easy, especially not the first few times. But separating satisfied that you've left your baby in the best possible hands will help ease both your anxiety and your guilt.

IN-HOME CARE

Most experts agree that if a mother can't be with her baby all of the time (because of work, school, or other commitments), the next best option is a mother substitute (a nanny, sitter, au pair) who cares for the child at home.

The advantages are many. Baby is in familiar surroundings, with his or her own crib, high chair, and toys; is not exposed to a lot of other babies' germs; and doesn't have to be transported to and fro. He or she also has the complete attention of the caregiver, assuming she hasn't been assigned a multitude of other tasks, and there is a good chance for a strong relationship to develop between baby and caregiver.

There are some disadvantages, however. If the caregiver is sick, unable to come to work for other reasons, or suddenly quits, there is no automatic backup person. A strong attachment between sitter and baby can lead to a crisis if the sitter leaves suddenly, or if the mother develops more than a mild case of envy. For some parents, the loss of privacy if the caregiver lives in is an added complication. And home care can be costly, probably more so if you choose a professionally trained nanny, probably less so if you choose a college student, an au pair, or someone with little experience.

Starting the Search

Finding the ideal caretaker can be a time-consuming process, so allow as much as two months for the search. There are several trails you can take to track her down:

The baby's doctor. Probably no one else you know knows as many babies—and their mothers and fathers—as your baby's doctor. Ask him or her for recommendations, check the office bulletin board for notices put up by care providers seeking employment (some pediatricians require that references be left at the reception desk when such notices are posted), or put up a notice of your own. Ask around the waiting room, too.

Other parents. Don't pass one by—at the playground, at a baby exercise class, at cocktail parties and business meetings—without asking if they've heard of, or have employed, a good caregiver.

Your church or synagogue. Here, too, the bulletin board can be an invaluable resource. So can your minister, priest, or rabbi, who may know of congregants who would be interested in caring for your child.

Teachers of nursery-age children. Nursery school teachers often know of, or employ part-time in their programs, experienced child-care workers. They sometimes are available themselves evenings and weekends.

The Parent's League. In New York City, this organization can provide to members listings of experienced caregivers. Membership fees are nominal, and also entitle parents to information on schools, birthday party services, and almost everything else related to child rearing. Ask around, or check your phone book (under "parents") to see if there are similar organizations in your city or area.

Nursing agencies and registries. Trained and licensed (and usually expensive) child-care workers and nannies are available through these services; selecting a caregiver this way eliminates a lot of guess-work and legwork. (But check references yourself, anyway.)

Baby-sitting services. Screened baby-sitters are available through these services, listed in your local classified phone book, for full-time, part-time, or occasional work.

A local hospital. Some hospitals offer baby-sitting referral services. Generally, all sitters referred have taken a baby-sitting course offered by the hospital, which includes baby CPR and other first-aid procedures. At other hospitals and nursing schools, nursing students may be available for baby-sitting jobs.

Local newspapers. Check daily papers and specialized parent papers for ads run by caregivers seeking employment and/or run an ad yourself.

College employment offices. Part-time or full-time, year-round or summer help may be found through local colleges.

Senior citizen organizations. Lively seniors can make terrific sitters—and surrogate grandparents at the same time.

Au pair or nanny organizations. These services can provide families with a live-in au pair, usually a young woman from a foreign country who wants to visit or study in the U.S. for a year or so, or with a well-trained nanny.

Sifting Through the Possibilities

You won't want to spend endless days interviewing obviously unsatisfactory candidates, so sift them out either through résumés that have come in the mail or phone conversations. Before you begin talking to people, develop a detailed job description so you know just what you are looking for. This may include such things as marketing and laundry responsibilities, but be wary of overloading with activities that will distract a sitter's attention from your baby. In a preliminary phone interview, ask the person's name, address, telephone number, age, education, experience (this is actually less important than some other qualities, such as enthusiasm and natural ability), salary requirements (check beforehand to see what the going rate is in your area), and why she wants the job. Explain what the position will entail, and see if she is still interested. Set up a personal interview with those applicants who sound promising.

During interviews, look for clues in a candidate's questions and comments ("Does the baby cry a lot?" might reflect impatience with normal infant behavior) as well as in her silence (the woman who never says anything about liking kids and never comments on yours may be telling you something) to learn what she's like. To learn more, ask questions such as the following, phrasing them so that they require more than a yes or no answer (it doesn't mean much when you get a "yes" to "Do you like babies?"):

- Why do you want this job?
- What was your last job, and why did you leave it?
- What do you think a baby my child's age needs most?
- How do you see yourself spending the day with a baby this age?
- How do you see your role in my baby's life?
- What is your position on breastfeeding? (This is important, of course, only if you are breastfeeding and intend to continue—which will require her support.)
- When my baby starts getting more active and getting into trouble, how will you handle it? How do you discipline young children?
- How will you get to work in inclement weather?
- Do you have a driver's license and feel comfortable behind the wheel? (If driving will be necessary on the job.)
- How long do you envision staying with this job? (The sitter who leaves as soon as your baby becomes adjusted to her can create a multitude of problems for your entire family.)
- Do you have children of your own? Will their needs interfere with your work? (Allowing a caregiver to bring her children along has some benefits and some drawbacks. On the one hand, it gives your child the chance to be exposed to the companionship of other youngsters on a daily basis. On the other hand, it gives your child more of a chance to be exposed to all of the youngsters' germs on a daily basis; and having other children to care for may also affect the quality and quantity of attention the caregiver can give your own baby. It may also result in greater wear and tear on your home.)

■ Do you cook or do housework? (Having some of these chores taken care of by someone else will give you more time to spend with your baby when you're at home. But if the caregiver spends a lot of time with these chores, your baby may be neglected.)

■ Are you in good health? Ask for evidence of a complete physical exam and a recent negative TB test, as well as about smoking habits (she should be a nonsmoker), alcohol and drug use. This last information will probably not be forthcoming from a drug abuser, but be alert for clues, such as restlessness, talkativeness, nervousness, agitation, dilated pupils, poor appetite (stimulants, such as amphetamines or cocaine); slurred speech, staggering, disorientation, poor concentration, and other signs of drunkenness with or without the odor of alcohol (alcohol, barbiturates and other "downers"); pinpoint pupils and craving for sweets (early heroin addiction); euphoria, relaxed inhibitions, increased appetite, loss of memory, possibly dilated pupils and bloodshot eyes, even paranoia (marijuana). A sitter who is trying not to use drugs or alcohol at work may exhibit signs of withdrawal of the abused substance, such as watery, runny eyes, yawning, irritability, anxiety, tremors, chills and sweating. Of course, many of these symptoms can be signs of illness (mental or physical) rather than drug abuse. In either case, should they show up in a child-care worker, they should concern you. You will also want to avoid someone with a medical condition that could interfere with regular attendance at work.

■ Have you recently had, or are you willing to take, CPR and baby first-aid training?

Though you'll be asking the questions, the job applicant shouldn't be the only one answering them. Ask these questions of yourself, based on your observations of each candidate, and answer them honestly:

■ Did the candidate arrive for the interview well groomed and neatly dressed? Though you may not require a freshly starched nanny's uniform on the job, soiled clothes, unwashed hair, and dirty fingernails are all a bad sign.

■ Does she seem to have a sense of orderliness that's compatible with your own? If she has to rummage through her handbag for five minutes for her references and you're a stickler for organization, you'll probably clash. On the other hand, if she seems compulsively neat and you're compulsively messy, you probably won't get along either.

■ Does she seem reliable? If she's late for the interview, watch out. She may be late every time she's due to work. Check this out with previous employers.

■ Is she physically capable of handling the job? A frail older woman may not be able to carry your baby around all day now, or chase your toddler later.

■ Does she seem good with children? The interview isn't complete until the applicant spends some time with your baby so that you can observe the interaction, or lack thereof. Does she seem patient, kind, interested, really attentive and sensitive to your baby's needs? Find out more about her aptitude for child care from previous employers.

■ Does she seem intelligent? You'll want someone who can teach and entertain your child the way you would yourself, and who will show good judgment in difficult situations.

■ Are you comfortable with her? Almost as important as the rapport the candidate has with your baby is the rapport she has with you. For your baby's sake, there needs to be constant, open, comfortable communication between a chosen caregiver and you; be certain this will be not only possible, but easy.

If the first series of interviews doesn't turn up any candidates you feel good about, don't settle—try again. If it does, the next step in narrowing down your selection is to check references. Don't take the word of a candidate's friends or family on her abilities and reliability; insist on the names of previous employers, if any, or if work experience is limited or nonexistent, those of teachers, clergy, or other more objective judges of character.

Getting Acquainted

You'd probably be very unhappy left to spend the day with a perfect stranger. You can expect your baby, who will experience the added stress of missing mommy, to be unhappy, too. To minimize the misery, introduce baby and sitter in advance. If it's a sitter-for-the-evening, have her come at least half an hour earlier the first time (an hour if your baby is more than five months old), so that your baby will have some time to adjust. Make the introduction gradually, starting baby off in your arms, moving him or her next to an infant seat or swing, so the sitter can approach on neutral territory then, finally, as baby becomes more comfortable with the newcomer, into the sitter's arms. Then, once the initial adjustment has been made, stay away for just an hour or two. The next time, have the sitter arrive half an hour ahead of your departure once again, and stay out a little longer. By the third time, a fifteen-minute period with you still at home should suffice, and after that sitter and charge should be bosom buddies. (If they aren't, consider whether you've chosen the right sitter.)

The daily sitter needs an even greater introduction period. She should spend at least a full day with you and the baby, becoming familiar not only with your baby, but also with your home, your child-care style, and your household routines. That will give you a chance to make suggestions, and her a chance to ask questions. It will also give you a chance to see the sitter in action—and a chance to change your mind about her if you don't like what you see. (Don't judge the sitter on baby's reaction, but rather on how the sitter responds to it. No matter how good a sitter is, children— even very young children—often protest being with one as long as mommy is around.)

Your baby, incidentally, will probably adjust to a new caregiver most easily before the age of six months, before stranger anxiety appears on the scene.

The Trial Period

Always hire a child-care person on a trial basis so that you can evaluate her performance before deciding whether you want to keep her on for the long term. It's fairer to her and to you if you make clear in advance that the first two weeks or month on the job (or any specified period) will be probationary. During this time, observe your baby. Does he or she seem happy, clean, alert when you come home? Or more tired than usual, and more cranky? Does it seem a diaper change has been made fairly recently? Important, too, is the caregiver's frame of mind at day's end. Is she relaxed and comfortable? Or tense and irritable, obviously happy to be relieved of her charge? Is she eager to tell you about her day with the baby, reporting the infant's latest achievements, as well as any problems she's noted, or does she routinely tell you only how long the baby slept and how many ounces of the bottle were emptied— or worse, how long the baby cried? Does she keep in mind that this is still *your* baby, and accept the idea that you make the major decisions about her care? Or does she seem to feel that she's in charge now?

If your evaluation shows the new caregiver is less than the best, start looking anew. If you're not certain, you might try arriving home early and unannounced to get a look at what's really happening in your absence. Or you could ask friends or neighbors who might see the sitter in the park, at the supermarket, or walking down the street how she seems to be doing. If a neighbor reports your usually happy baby is doing a lot of crying while you're away, that should be a red flag.

If, from your point of view, the right full-time sitter seems not to have been born yet, perhaps you should reconsider your decision to go back to work rather than subject your baby to a series of incompetent or uncaring caregivers.

GROUP DAY CARE

Though it's not considered the ideal situation for infants, some mothers nevertheless turn to group day care because they have no other choice.

A good day-care program can, however, offer some significant advantages. In the best of them, trained personnel provide a well-organized program specifically geared to a baby's development and growth, as well as opportunities for play and learning with other babies and children. Because such facilities are not dependent on one person, as in-home care is, there is generally no crisis if a teacher is sick or leaves, though the baby may have to adjust to a new one. And, in communities where day-care services are licensed, there may be safety, health, and in some cases, even educational monitoring of the program.

The disadvantages for babies can also be significant. First of all, not all programs are created equally good. Even in a good one, care is less individualized than it is in a baby's own home, there are more children per caregiver, and teacher turnover may be high. There is less flexibility in scheduling than in a more informal setting, and if the center follows a public school calendar, it may be closed on holidays when you're working. The cost is usually fairly high, unless subsidized by government or private sources, but may be less expensive than good in-home care. Possibly the greatest disadvantage is the increased rate of infection among children in day-care situations. Since many employed mothers don't have another option when their children have colds and other minor ills, they often send them to the center anyway.

Certainly there are some excellent day-care facilities; the trick is to find such a facility that has space for your baby.

Where to Look

You can get the names of local day-care facilities (which may be non-profit, cooperative, or for profit) through recommendations from friends and acquaintances, or by calling the state regulatory agency (your state health or education department should be able to refer you to the proper agency), by asking at your church, synagogue, or local Y, or by sending a stamped, self-addressed, business-size envelope to the American Academy of Pediatrics, Dept. C, PO Box 927, Elk Grove Village, IL 60007, for a list of day-care centers. You can also check the phone book for child-care referral services or day-care centers themselves.

What to Look For

Day-care centers range in quality from top-of-the-line to bottom-of-the-barrel, with most falling in the mediocre middle. If you'll accept only the best for your baby, you'll have to examine every aspect of each possibility. Look for:

Licensing. Most states license day-care facilities, checking them for sanitation and safety, but *not* for the quality of care. Some states, however, don't even have adequate fire and sanitation regulations. (Check with your local fire and health departments if you have any questions.) Still, a license does provide some safeguards.

A trained and experienced staff. The "head" teachers, at least, should have degrees in early childhood education; the entire staff should be experienced in caring for infants. Too often, because of the low pay, day-care workers are people who are in the job because they are qualified for nothing else; in that case, it's likely they aren't qualified for child care, either. The staff turnover should be low; if there are several new teachers each year, beware.

A healthy and safe staff. All child-care workers should have had complete medical checkups, including a TB test. Background checks should have ascertained that they have not previously been involved in anything unsavory.

A good teacher-to-baby ratio. There should be at least one staff person for every three infants. If there are fewer, a crying baby may have to wait until someone is free to met his or her needs.

Moderate size. A huge day-care facility might be less well supervised and operated than a smaller one—though there are exceptions to this rule. Also, the more children, the more chance for the spread of illnesses. Whatever the size of the facility, there should be adequate space for each child. Crowded rooms are a sign of an inadequate program.

Separation of age groups. Infants under one year should not be mixed with toddlers and older children.

A loving atmosphere. The staff should seem to genuinely like children and caring for them. Children should look happy, alert, and clean. Be sure to visit the facility unannounced in the middle or toward the end of the day, when you will get a more accurate picture of what the school is like than you would first thing in the morning. (Be wary of any school that does not allow unannounced parent visits.)

A stimulating atmosphere. Even a two-month-old can benefit from a stimulating atmosphere, one where there is plenty of interaction—both verbal and physical—with caregivers, and where age-appropriate toys are available. As children become older and able to handle objects more effectively, there should be plenty of opportunity for manipulation of toys, as well as exposure to books and music and the out-of-doors. The best programs include occasional "field trips": three to six children along with one or two teachers go to the supermarket, the dry cleaners, or other places a baby might go with a stay-at-home mother.

Parent involvement. Are parents invited to participate in the program in some way; is there a parent board that makes policy?

A compatible philosophy. Are you comfortable with the day-care center's philosophy—educationally, religiously, ideologically?

Adequate opportunities for rest. Most infants, in day care or at home, still take a lot of naps. There should be a quiet area for such napping in individual cribs, and children should be able to nap according to their own schedules—not the school's.

Strict health and sanitation rules. In your own home, you needn't be concerned with your baby putting everything in his or her mouth; in a day-care center, with a convergence of children, each with his or her own set of germs, you should be. Day-care centers can become a focus for the spread of many intestinal and upper respiratory illnesses. To minimize germ spreading and safeguard the health of the children, a well-run day-care center will have a medical consultant and a written policy that includes:

- Caregivers must wash hands (with liquid soap) thoroughly after changing diapers or helping children use the toilet, wiping runny noses or handling children with colds, and before feedings.
- Diapering and food preparation areas must be entirely separate, and each should be cleaned after every use.
- Diapers should be disposed of in a covered container, out of reach of children.
- Toys must be rinsed with a sanitizing solution between handling by different children, or a separate box of toys must be kept for each child.
- Stuffed animals should not be shared and should be machine-washed frequently.
- Teething rings, pacifiers, washcloths, towels, brushes, and combs should not be shared.
- Feeding utensils must be washed in a dishwasher or, better still, must be disposable (infant bottles should be labeled with their owners' names so they aren't mixed up).
- Food preparation for infants on solids must be carried out under sanitary conditions (see page 230).

■ Immunizations must be up to date for all babies.

■ Children who are moderately to severely ill, particularly with diarrhea, vomiting, high fever, and certain types of rashes, must be kept at home (this isn't necessary with colds, since the cold is most contagious before it is evident) or in a special infirmary section of the facility.

■ Medication for attending children should be administered according to a written policy of the school.

■ When a baby has a contagious disease, all the parents of children in the center must be notified by the center; in cases of hemophilus influenzae, immunization or medication may be given to prevent spread of the disease.[2]

Also check with the local health department to be sure there are no outstanding complaints or violations against the center.

Strict safety rules. Injuries, mostly minor, are not uncommon in day-care facilities. The top hazards are climbers, slides, hand toys and blocks, other playground equipment, doors, and indoor floor surfaces. Even a crawling baby can get into trouble with these; all babies can get into trouble with small objects (that can be choked on or swallowed), sharp objects, poisonous materials, and so on. A child-care center should meet the safety requirements you maintain in your own home. Particular attention should be paid to open stairways, doors that can slam on little fingers or can open on little faces, windows

above ground level (they shouldn't be able to be opened more than 6 inches and/or should have window guards), radiators and other heating devices, electrical outlets, cleaning materials and medications (often teachers have to dispense medication for several recovering children or those with chronic health problems), and to floors (they should not be littered with toys, which can trip a caregiver carrying an infant). Materials used by older children (paints, clay, and so on, as well as toys with small or sharp parts) should be kept out of reach of babies. Smoke detectors, clearly marked fire escape routes, fire extinguishers, and other fire safety precautions should be in evidence. Staff should be trained in CPR and first aid, and a fully equipped first-aid kit should be readily available.

Careful attention to nutrition. All meals and snacks should be healthful, safe, and appropriate for the ages of the children being served. Parental instructions regarding formula (or breast milk), foods, and feeding schedules should be followed. Bottles should never be propped.

HOME DAY CARE

Many parents feel more comfortable leaving a baby in a family situation in a private home with just a few other children than in a more "sterile" day-care center; and for those who can't arrange for a sitter in their own homes, home day care is often the choice.

There are many advantages to such care. Family day care can often provide a warm, homelike environment at a lower cost than other forms of care. Because there are fewer children than in a day-care center, there is less exposure to infection and more potential for stimulation and individualized care (though this potential is not always realized). Flexible scheduling— early drop-off or late pickup when that's necessary—is often possible.

The disadvantages vary from situation

---

2. A particular problem for mothers who are planning to become pregnant again shortly is the possibility of the transmission of cytomegalovirus (CMV), spread easily among babies because of the more frequent contact with virus-laden urine and saliva. In an expectant mother who is not immune, the CMV poses a risk to her unborn child. CMV, which studies show spreads to 1 in 5 parents without immunity, usually causes no symptoms in adults or children. Because of the risk to the unborn, women who are considering another pregnancy and who are not immune might want to consider another type of child care.

YOUR CHILD AS A BAROMETER OF CHILD CARE

No matter which child-care alternative you select for your baby, be alert to signs of discontent: sudden changes in personality or mood, clinginess, fretfulness that doesn't seem attributable to anything else. If your baby seems unhappy, check into your child-care situation; it may need altering.

to situation. Such day-care facilities are often unlicensed, giving little protection in the way of health and safety. The care provider is often untrained, lacking in professional child-care experience, and may have a child-rearing philosophy that differs from the parents'. If she or one of her children is ill, there may be no backup. And though the risk may be lower than in a larger day-care facility, there is always the possibility of germs spreading from child to child, especially if sanitation is lax.

CORPORATE DAY CARE

A common option in European countries for many years, day-care facilities in or adjacent to a parent's place of work are too rarely offered in the U.S. It's an option many parents would choose if they had it.

The advantages are attractive. Your child is near you in case of emergency; you can visit during your lunch hour or coffee break, even breastfeed; and since you commute with your child, you spend more time together. Such facilities are usually staffed by professionals and very well equipped. Knowing your child is nearby and well cared for allows you to give fuller attention to your work. The cost for such care, if any, is usually low.

There are some possible disadvantages. If your commute is a difficult one, it may be hard on your child. In some cases, seeing you during the day, if that's part of the program, may make each parting more difficult for your baby, especially during times of stress. And visiting may take your mind

from your work.

Corporate day care, of course, should meet all the educational, health, and safety standards of any child-care facility. If the one set up by your employer doesn't, then speak to those responsible for the facility about what can be done to rectify the deficiencies.

BABIES ON THE JOB

Very occasionally, a mother is able to take her baby to work with her even when no day care is provided. And very occasionally, it works. It works best before a baby is mobile and if colic is not a problem—and of course, when the mother has the space for a portable crib and other baby paraphernalia near her work area and the support of her employer and those who work around her. Ideally, she also has a baby-sitter on the spot, at least part of the time. This kind of situation is perfect for the nursing mom, or for any mom who wants her job and her baby, too.

WHEN YOUR CHILD IS SICK

No mother likes to see her baby sick, but the working mother particularly dreads that first sign of fever or upset stomach. She knows that caring for her sick baby may present a great many problems, the central ones being who will take care of the baby, and where?

Ideally, either you or your spouse should be able to get sick leave when your child is ill so that you can administer care yourself at home. Next best is having a trusted and familiar sitter or another family member you can call upon to stay with your baby at home. Some day-care centers have a sick-child infirmary or satellite, where a child is in familiar surroundings with familiar faces. There are also special sick-child day-care facilities, both in homes and in larger freestanding centers sprouting up to meet this need; but in these, of course, the child has to adjust to being cared for by strangers in a strange environment when he's least able to handle change. Some corporations, in order to keep parents on the job, actually pay for sick-child care, such as space in a sick-child day-care center or a sick-baby nurse to stay with the child at home (which will also require adjustment to an unfamiliar caregiver).

These options are better than no care at all, of course. But as anyone who's ever been a sick child knows, there's nothing quite the same as having your mommy to hold your hot little hand, wipe your feverish brow, and administer specially prescribed doses of love and attention. And because of a sick child's special needs, the American Academy of Pediatrics recommends that there should be more liberal parental leave for parents of sick children, so that they can have parental care during illness.

SAFE SLEEPING

If you are leaving a young infant with a caregiver, be sure the caregiver is aware of the back-to-sleep tummy-to-play policy of the American Academy of Pediatrics. All children should nap on their backs (unless a medical condition dictates otherwise) and should spend some wakeful time on their tummies (but only under constant supervision).

CHAPTER SEVEN

The Fourth Month

Wʜᴀᴛ ʏᴏᴜʀ ʙᴀʙʏ ᴍᴀʏ ʙᴇ ᴅᴏɪɴɢ

By the end of this month, your baby ...should be able to (see Note):

- on stomach, lift head up 90 degrees
- laugh out loud (3⅔ months)
- follow an object in an arc about 6 inches above the face for 180 degrees (from one side to the other)

Note: If your baby seems not to have reached one or more of these milestones, check with the doctor. In rare instances the delay could indicate a problem, though in most cases it will turn out to be normal for your baby. Premature infants generally reach milestones later than others of the same birth age, often achieving them closer to their adjusted age (the age they would be if they had been born at term), and sometimes later.

...will probably be able to:

- hold head steady when upright
- on stomach, raise chest, supported by arms

- roll over (one way)
- grasp a rattle held to backs or tips of fingers
- pay attention to a raisin or other very small object (4¼ months)

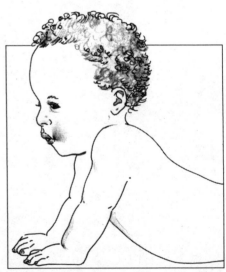

Many, but not all, four-month-olds can raise their body on their arms.

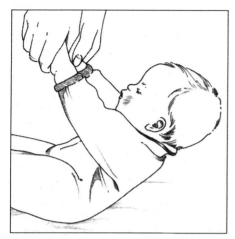 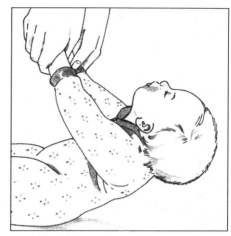

At the end of the fourth month, most babies still cannot keep their head level with their body when they are pulled to a sitting position (left). Their head usually falls backward (right).

- reach for an object
- squeal in delight

- razz (make a wet razzing sound by 4½ months)

...may possibly be able to:

- keep head level with body when pulled to sitting (4¼ months)
- turn in the direction of a voice, particularly mommy's
- say ah-goo or similar vowel-consonant combinations

...may even be able to:

- bear some weight on legs when held upright
- sit without support
- object if you try to take a toy away
- turn in the direction of a voice

WHAT YOU CAN EXPECT AT THIS MONTH'S CHECKUP

Each doctor or nurse-practitioner will have a personal approach to well-baby checkups. The overall organization of the physical exam, as well as the number and type of assessment techniques used and procedures performed will also vary with the individual needs of the child. But in general, you can expect the following at a checkup when your baby is about four months old.

- Questions about how you and baby and the rest of the family are doing at home, and about baby's eating, sleeping, and general progress. About child care, if you are working.
- Measurement of baby's weight, length, and head circumference, and plotting of progress since birth.
- Physical exam, including a recheck of any previous problems. The posterior fon-

tanel, on the back of the head, may have closed by now; the anterior, on the top of the head, may have grown since last visit.

■ Developmental assessment. The examiner may actually put baby through a series of tests to evaluate head control, hand use, vision, hearing, and social interaction, or may simply rely on observation plus your reports on what baby is doing.

■ Second round of immunizations, if baby is in good health and there are no other contraindications. See recommended schedule on page 153. Be sure to discuss any reactions to the first round of immunizations beforehand.

■ Guidance about what to expect in the next month in relation to such topics as feeding, sleeping, development, and infant safety.

■ Recommendations about fluoride supplementation if needed in your area, and vitamin D supplementation if your baby is breastfed. Recommendations about iron supplementation for babies not on iron-fortified formula.

Questions you may want to ask, if the doctor hasn't already answered them:

■ What reactions can you expect baby to have to the second round of immunizations? How should you treat them? Which reactions should you call about?

■ When is it suggested that you introduce your baby to solids?

Also raise concerns that have arisen over the past month. Jot down information and instructions from the doctor (you're sure to forget them, otherwise). Record all pertinent information (baby's weight, length, head circumference, birthmarks, immunizations, illnesses, medications given, test results, and so on) in a permanent health record.

FEEDING YOUR BABY THIS MONTH: Thinking About Solids

The messages that today's new mother receives about when to start feeding solids are many and confusing. Her mother declares, "I started *you* at two weeks. What are you waiting for?" Buttressing her argument, she points to the obvious: "*You're* healthy, aren't you?" The pediatrician gives instructions to wait until her baby is five or six months old. For corroboration, he points to what little research there's been in the area. A well-meaning friend insists that starting solids earlier will help any baby sleep through the night. Her proof positive: a baby who's slept through since his first spoonful of cereal.

Whom do you listen to? Does mother know best? Or doctor? Or friends? Actually, your baby does—nobody can tell you when to start giving solids better than he or she can. And recent research indicates that an infant's individual development, rather than arbitrary age parameters, should be the deciding factor in promoting a baby to a more varied diet.

Very early introduction to solids (fashionable when your mother was mothering, and still common in Europe) isn't believed to be physically harmful in most cases. But medical research indicates that a very young baby's digestive system—from a tongue that pushes out any foreign substance placed on it, to intestines lacking many digestive enzymes—is developmentally unready for solids. It does not appear, however, to support the idea that because solid foods interfere with some of the beneficial aspects of breast milk and with the absorption of iron, they should be postponed for most children until the end of the first year.

Picking the right time to introduce foods—neither too early nor too late—is important. Extremely early introduction of solids isn't harmful physically, but it can undermine future eating habits. When the infant who isn't ready for solids rejects them, frustration on both sides of the cereal bowl can set the stage for mealtime hassles later in childhood. Yet, waiting too long to introduce food (until late into the second half of the first year) can also lead to difficulties. An older baby may resist being taught the new tricks of chewing and swallowing solids if he or she has been too long accustomed to getting nourishment and oral satisfaction from nursing. And like habits, tastes may be tough to change at this point; unlike the more malleable four- to six-month-old, the year-old child may not be open to new gastronomic experiences.

To decide if your baby is ready for the big step into the world of solid foods (most will be between four and six months), look for the following clues, then consult the doctor:

■ Your baby can hold his or her head up well. Even strained baby foods should not be offered until a baby holds his head up well when propped to sit; chunkier foods should wait until a baby can sit well alone, usually not until seven months.

■ The tongue thrust reflex has disappeared. This is a reflex that causes young infants to push foreign matter out of their mouths (an inborn mechanism that protects them from choking on foreign bodies). Try this test: place a tiny bit of infant rice cereal thinned with breast milk or formula in your baby's mouth from the tip of a demitasse or baby spoon, or your finger. If the food comes right back out again with the tongue, and continues to after several tries, the thrust is still present and baby isn't ready for spoon feeding.

■ Baby reaches for and otherwise shows an interest in table foods. The baby who grabs the fork out of your hand or snares the bread from your plate, who watches intently and exhibits excitement with every bite you take, is telling you he's eager to try more grown-up fare.

■ The ability to execute back-and-forth movements with the tongue, as well as up-and-down ones, is present. You can discover this by observation.

■ Baby is able to draw the lower lip in so that food can be taken from a spoon.

There are instances, however, when even a baby who seems developmentally ready for solids may have to wait—most often because there is a strong history of allergy in the family. Until more is known about the development of allergies, it is generally recommended that children in such families be breastfed exclusively for most of the first year, with solids added very cautiously, one at a time, thereafter.

WHAT YOU MAY BE CONCERNED ABOUT

WRIGGLING AT CHANGING TIME

"My daughter won't lie still when I'm changing her—she's always trying to turn over. How can I get her to cooperate?"

As far as cooperation when changing your daughter is concerned, you can expect to receive less and less as the months go by and her physical development continues to spurt ahead of her moral development. The indignity of diapering, teamed with the turtle-on-its-back frustration of being temporarily immobilized, will set off a battle with each change. The trick: be quick (have all the diapering paraphernalia ready and waiting before you lay baby on the table), and provide distractions (a mobile above the changing table, a music box, preferably one that's also visually tempting, a rattle or other toy to occupy her hands, and hopefully, her interest).

PROPPING BABY

"I had my baby propped up in his stroller and I was scolded by two older women who insisted he was too young to sit up."

If your baby wasn't old enough to sit up, he'd tell you so. Not in so many words, of course, but by slumping down or sliding off to one side when you tried to prop him. Though you shouldn't attempt to prop a younger infant whose neck and back need more support than he would get with propping, a three- or four-month-old who holds his head up well and doesn't crumble when propped up is ready for such a position. (Specially designed head supports are

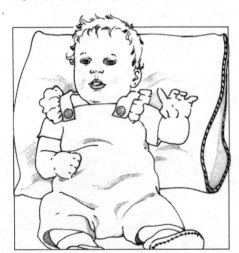

Propping baby up to a sitting position will not only offer him or her a welcome change of perspective, but it will also help build the muscles and experience needed for unassisted sitting.

available to keep babies' heads upright when propped.) Babies will usually signal when they've had enough of sitting by complaining or beginning to slump.

Besides providing a welcome change of position, sitting allows a baby an expanded view of the world. Instead of just the sky, the inside of the stroller, or a carriage mattress, an upright baby can see passersby (including those who are sure to upbraid you), stores and homes, trees, dogs, other babies in strollers, children walking home from school, buses, cars—and all the other marvelous things that inhabit his growing universe. He's also likely to stay happy longer than he would lying down, which will make outings more pleasant for both of you.

BABY'S STANDING

"My baby likes to 'stand' on my lap. She cries if I make her sit down. But my grandmother insists that letting her stand so early will make her bowlegged."

Babies usually know what they're ready for even better than their great-grandmothers do. And many babies of your daughter's age are ready, and eager, for supported lap "standing." It's fun, it's good exercise, it's an exciting change from lying on her back or slumping in an infant seat—and it most assuredly does not cause bowleggedness.

On the other hand, any baby who doesn't seem to want to stand shouldn't be pushed into doing so until she's ready. A baby who's allowed to set her own developmental pace will be happier and healthier than one whose parents try to set it for her.

THUMB SUCKING

"My son has taken to sucking his thumb. At first I was happy because it was helping him sleep better, but now I'm afraid it's going to become a habit I won't be able to break him of later on."

It isn't easy being a baby. Every time you latch on to something that gives you the comfort and satisfaction you're searching for, somebody wants to take it away from you. Sometimes without good reason.

Virtually all babies suck on their fingers at some time during the first year of life; many even begin the habit in the uterus. That's not surprising. The mouth in the infant is an important organ not just for eating, but for exploration and pleasure, too (as you will soon discover, to your dismay, when everything baby picks up goes into his mouth, whether it's a rattle or a long-deceased insect he's unearthed at the bottom of a closet). But even before a baby can reach for objects, he discovers his hands—and how natural to put the newly discovered hands into that wonderful sensory cavity, the mouth. The first time the hands may make it to the mouth by random chance, but the baby quickly learns that the fingers in the mouth provide a pleasurable sensation. Soon he's mouthing his fingers regularly. Eventually, many babies decide that the thumb is the most efficient and satisfying finger to suck on (maybe it's the most succulent) and switch from finger mouthing to thumb sucking. Some stick with one or two fingers, or even a whole fist.

At first you may think the habit is cute, or even be grateful that your baby has found a way to pacify himself without your intervention. Then, as the weeks pass and the habit intensifies, you begin to worry, envisioning your little boy trooping off to school with his thumb firmly implanted in his mouth, ridiculed by his classmates, reprimanded by his teachers. Will you have to paint his thumbnails with bitter solutions to make them unpalatable, then nag and plead when that doesn't work? Will you have to make monthly trips to the orthodontist for the work necessary to straighten the bite deformed by thumb sucking, or worse, weekly trips to the therapist to try to uncover the underlying emotional problems that made him suck on his thumb in the first place?

Well, stop worrying and start letting your baby indulge himself. There is no evidence that thumb sucking is in itself "dangerous" or a sign of emotional illness. Nor, if it ceases by age five, does it appear to do damage to the alignment of permanent teeth; any distortion of the mouth that does occur before that time returns to normal when the habit is ended. Most experts agree that, since it is a developmental behavior that usually is put aside as a child gets older anyway, attempts to wean a child from the thumb shouldn't begin before age four.

Some studies show that nearly half of all children do some thumb or finger sucking past infancy. The behavior peaks on average between 18 and 21 months, though some have already abandoned the habit by then. Nearly 80% give it up by age five, and 95% by age six, usually on their own. Those who use it to help themselves get off to sleep hang on to the habit longer than those to whom it is simply a form of oral gratification.

As the child nears the time for permanent teeth to come in, a time when thumb sucking could hinder proper development of the mouth and lead to deformity, he is also mature enough to take an active part in eliminating the habit. And since most thumb sucking is not the result of emotional disturbance, thumb suckers are more likely to be weaned from their habit with specially designed dental appliances than through psychological counseling. (A few children do seem to suck their thumbs for emotional support and can benefit from counseling.)

In the meantime, let your baby suck away. Be sure, however, that if he is breast-fed, he isn't sucking his thumb to compensate for suckling he isn't getting at the breast; if he seems to want to nurse a little longer at each feeding, let him (he won't get too much milk because the breast will have been emptied, or nearly so, at this point). And if thumb sucking seems to become the focus of his daily activities, preventing him from using his hands for other explorations, occasionally remove his finger from its station long enough to distract him with toys, with finger or hand games ("this little piggy," "patty-cake," or "so big," for instance), or by holding his hands and letting him stand, if he likes that.

If your baby does continue to suck his thumb into toddlerhood, you can expect some unfavorable comments, particularly from your parents' generation—many of whom have been thoroughly programmed to demonstrate disdain for thumb sucking. If you feel obliged to, explain to them that recent research indicates that thumb sucking is not harmful and doesn't mean a child is emotionally deprived.

If you yourself are disturbed by the thumb sucking because of prior programming, try to psych yourself out of it. If that doesn't work, you might want to substitute a pacifier for your baby's thumb temporarily—assuming you don't also have an aversion to that. But, of course, that will leave you with a new habit to break.

CHUBBY BABY

"Everybody admires my chubby little daughter. But I am secretly afraid she's getting too fat. She's so round, she can hardly move."

With dimples on her knees and her elbows, a belly to rival any Buddha's, several chins to chuck, and an endearing amount of pinchable flesh on her cheeks, she's the picture of baby cuteness from head to chubby toes. Yet is the plump baby also the picture of health? Her grandparents probably think so. Her mother, on the other hand, convinced that slim is in, is likely to be concerned that her plump baby is on the way to being an unhappy fat child and a miserable obese adult. Most doctors, however, take a position somewhere in between. They agree that fat is not fit, but are less concerned with chubbiness in babies since it became clear that an increase in fat cells in infancy doesn't necessarily lead to obesity later. Only 1 in 5 fat babies are

destined, in fact, to become fat adults.

Still there are disadvantages to extreme chubbiness early on. The baby who is too plump to budge may become a victim to a vicious cycle of inactivity and overweight. The less she moves, the fatter she gets; the fatter she gets, the less she can move. Her inability to move makes her frustrated and fussy, which may lead her mother to overfeed her to keep her happy. If she stays overweight through age four, a problem that is becoming more and more common among American children, the odds that she will be an overweight adult increase.

Before you make a reservation at the fat farm for your baby, however, be certain she is indeed overweight and not just nicely rounded (remember, since babies haven't yet developed much in the way of muscle, even a slim one will sport a certain amount of soft padding). Compare her growth with the curve on the height-weight chart on page 650. If her weight seems consistently to be moving upward faster than her height, discuss this with her doctor.

Unlike the prescription for a fat adult, the prescription for a fat baby is not usually a diet. Instead of trying to get an overweight baby to lose weight, the goal is to slow down the rate of gain. Then as she grows taller, she will slim down—something many babies do without intervention as they become more active. Some of the following tips may help not only if your baby is already overweight, but also if you're afraid she's on her way:

■ Use feeding only to assuage hunger, not to meet other needs. A baby who's fed for all the wrong reasons (when she's hurt or unhappy, when her mother's too busy to play with her, when she's bored in the stroller) will continue to demand food for the wrong reasons, and as an adult, will eat for the same wrong reasons. Instead of nursing her every time she cries, comfort her with a hug or a soothing song. Instead of propping her up with a bottle, prop her in front of a mobile or a music box when you're too busy to play with her, or let her watch what you're doing (slice the carrots or fold the laundry on the floor beside her infant seat). Instead of always plying her with teething biscuits to quiet her in the supermarket, attach a toy to her stroller to keep her occupied while you shop. In spite of what your mother may have believed, constantly pushing food on your baby is not a sign of love.

■ Make dietary adjustments, if necessary. One reason that breastfed babies are less likely to become overweight is that breast milk automatically adjusts to a baby's needs. The lower-fat, lower-calorie "fore" milk, which comes at the beginning of a feeding, encourages the hungry baby to suckle. The higher-fat, higher-calorie "hind" milk, which comes at the end of a feeding, tends to dampen the appetite, sending the message, "You're feeling full." If that isn't discouragement enough, and baby continues to nurse away, the breast is eventually emptied. Suckling for suckling's sake can go on without an excess of calories being consumed. Though baby formulas aren't customized in the same way, if your baby is gaining weight too quickly and is extremely overweight, her doctor may recommend switching to a lower-calorie formula. Before you make such a switch, however, be certain you are not underdiluting the ready-to-mix formula you are presently using—which could increase its calorie count per ounce considerably. Don't decide to overdilute it, either, without the doctor's okay. Or to switch to skim or low-fat milk. Babies, even overweight ones, need the cholesterol and fat in breast milk and formula (or when they're older, in whole cow's milk).

■ Try water, the ultimate calorie-free beverage. Most of us tend to drink too little water. Infant diets (because they are entirely, or almost entirely, liquid) don't absolutely require supplementation with water. But water can be very useful for the overweight baby who wants to keep sucking after her hunger is satisfied, or who is thirsty rather than hungry in hot weather. Instead of breast or formula, offer a bottle or cup of plain tap water (with no sugar or other sweetening added) when your baby seems to be looking for a nibble between meals—that is, within an hour or two of a previous feeding. (Getting your baby used to the taste, or rather the non-taste, of water early on will make it more likely that she'll have the healthy habit of drinking water later.)

■ Don't give solids prematurely as a way to encourage sleeping through the night—it rarely works and may lead to overweight. (Instead, try the tips for helping baby to sleep through the night on page 175.)

■ Evaluate your baby's diet. If you've already started your baby on solids (on your own, or on your doctor's recommendation) and she's taking more than just a few spoonfuls of cereal, check to see if she seems to be drinking as much breast milk or formula as before. If she is, this is probably the reason for excessive weight gain. Cut back on solids if you've started them prematurely, or cut them out entirely for a month or two (most experts recommend not beginning solids until four to six months anyway). A young infant does not need the nutrients in solid foods (except for iron, which can come from a supplement). Later, as more solids are added, the amount of breast milk or formula should usually be gradually reduced and the emphasis placed on solids such as vegetables, yogurt, fruits, cereals, and breads. If baby is taking juices, dilute them half-and-half with water. And don't put thin cereal or other solids in a bottle for feeding—babies take too much that way.

■ Get your baby moving. If your baby can "hardly move," encourage activity. When you change her diaper, touch her right knee to her left elbow several times, then the reverse. With her grasping your thumbs and your other fingers holding her forearms, let her "pull up" to a sitting position. Let her stand on your lap—and bounce, if she likes. (See page 167 for other tips on getting your baby moving.)

THIN
BABY

"My friends' babies are all roly-poly; mine is long and thin—the 75th percentile in height and the 25th in weight. The doctor says he's doing just fine and I shouldn't worry, but I do."

Thin continues to be in—everywhere but in the nursery. While the lean look is favored on adults, plumpness is what many look for and love in babies. And yet, though they might not win as many diaper commercial roles as their roly-poly peers,

slender babies are usually as healthy.

In general, if your baby is alert, active, and basically content, is gaining weight steadily, and if his weight, though on the low side of average, continues to keep pace with his height, there is, as the doctor has pointed out, no cause for concern. There are often factors that affect a baby's size about which you can do very little. Genetic factors, for example—if you and/or your husband are thin and small boned, your baby is likely to be, too. And activity factors—the baby-on-the-go is usually thinner than the inactive one.

There are, however, a few reasons for

HOW DOES
YOUR
BABY GROW?

How does a baby grow? Quite contrary to the fears of nervous parents who scan weight and height charts frantically for signs that all is not well, usually in a pattern that's normal for him or her.

A baby's future height and weight are to a great extent preprogrammed at conception. And assuming prenatal conditions are adequate, and neither love nor nutrition is lacking after birth, most babies will eventually realize that genetic potential.

The programming for height is based primarily on the midpoint between the father's height and the mother's. Studies show that, in general, boys seem to grow up to be somewhat taller than this midpoint, girls somewhat shorter.

Weight also seems to be preprogrammed. A baby is usually born with the genes to be slim, stocky, or a happy medium. But the eating habits learned in infancy can help a baby to fulfill this destiny or defeat it.

Growth charts, like the one in the Ready Reference section in the back of this book, shouldn't become a source of anxiety

for parents—it's too easy to misread or misinterpret them. But they are useful in telling parents and doctors when a baby's growth is departing from the norm, and when an evaluation, taking into account parental size, nutritional status, and general health, is necessary. Since growth often comes in spurts during the first year, one measurement that seems to show too little growth or too much may not be significant. It should, however, be viewed as a red flag. A two-month halt to weight gain may indicate only that baby is slowing down because he or she is genetically destined to be small (particularly if growth in the height department is also easing off), but it can also indicate that baby is being underfed or is ill. A weight gain that is double what is normal during the same two months (if it is not accompanied by a similar jump in height) may just be baby's way of catching up if birth weight was low or weight gain has been slow so far, but it can also be a sign that baby is on the way to creeping obesity later in life.

thinness that do need remedying. A major one is underfeeding. If a baby's weight curve keeps dropping off for a couple of months, and if the loss isn't compensated for by a jump the following month, the doctor often will consider the possibility that the child is not getting enough to eat. If you're breastfeeding and this is the case, the tips on page 99 should help get baby gaining again. If you're bottle feeding, you can supplement baby's diet with solids *if* the doctor okays them, or you can try diluting the formula a little less—again with the doctor's approval.

And don't underfeed intentionally. Some parents, eager to get their babies started on the path toward a future of slimness and good health, limit calories and fat in infancy. This is a very *dangerous* practice, since infants need both for normal growth and development. You can start them on the road to good eating habits without depriving them of the nourishment they need now.

Be sure, too, that your baby isn't one who is either so sleepy or so busy that he forgets to demand his meals regularly. Between three and four months old, an infant should be eating at least every four hours during the day (usually at least five feedings), though he may sleep through the night without waking to eat. Some breast-fed babies may still be taking more feedings, but fewer feedings could mean your baby isn't eating enough. If your baby's the kind who doesn't make a fuss when he's not fed, take the initiative yourself and offer meals to him more often—even if it means cutting short a daytime nap or interrupting a fascinating encounter with his crib gym.

Rarely, a baby's poor weight gain is related to the inability to absorb certain nutrients, a metabolic rate that is out of kilter, or an infectious or chronic disease. Such illness, of course, requires prompt medical attention.

HEART MURMUR

"The doctor says my baby has a heart murmur, but that it doesn't mean anything. Still, it's scary."

Anytime the word "heart" is part of a diagnosis, it's scary. After all, the heart is the organ that sustains life; any possibility of a defect is frightening, particularly to the parents of an infant whose life is just beginning. But in the case of a heart murmur there is, in the vast majority of cases, really nothing to worry about.

When the doctor tells you your baby has a heart murmur, it means that on examination abnormal heart sounds, caused by the turbulence of the flow of blood through the heart, are heard. The doctor can often tell just what kind of abnormality is responsible for the murmur by the loudness of the sounds (from barely audible to almost loud enough to drown out normal heart sounds), by their location, and by the type of sound (musical or vibratory, a twang, a click, or a rumble, for example).

Most of the time, as is likely in your baby's case, the murmur is the result of irregularities in the shape of the heart as it grows. This kind of murmur is called "innocent" or "functional," and can usually be diagnosed by the baby's doctor by simple office examination with a stethescope. No further tests or treatments or limitations of activities are necessary. But the existence of the murmur will be noted on your baby's record so other doctors who examine him at a later date will know it has always existed. Very often, when the heart is fully grown, the murmur will disappear.

There are, however, heart murmurs that do require follow-up. Some will cure themselves, but others may require surgical or medical treatment, and a few may become worse. If your baby's murmur is a problem, the doctor will tell you so and recommend a course of therapy. In most cases children with murmurs can—and should—maintain regular activities. The exceptions are those who become breathless or turn blue on exercising, or who are not growing well.

If you're worried no matter what anyone says, you can ask your baby's doctor to tell you exactly what type of murmur your baby has and whether or not it can be expected to cause any problems, now or in the future, and to explain just why you have nothing to worry about. If the answers aren't reassuring enough, ask for referral to a pediatric cardiologist for consultation.

BLACK STOOL

"My daughter's last diaper was filled with a black stool. Could she be having a digestive problem?"

More likely she's been having an iron supplement. In some children, the reaction between the normal bacteria of the gastrointestinal tract and the iron sulfate in a supplement causes the stool to turn dark brown, greenish, or black. There's no medical significance in this change, no need to be concerned by it, and no need to discontinue the iron. Studies show that the iron doesn't increase digestive discomfort or fussiness. If your baby has black stools and isn't taking a supplement or a formula with iron, check with her doctor.

BABY MASSAGE

"I've heard that massage is good for babies. Is this true?"

Yes, indeed. Massage is no longer for adults only. Several years ago, it was discovered that premature newborns do better with therapeutic massage—they grow faster, sleep and breathe better, and are more alert. Now it appears that massage also benefits healthy infants—and healthy children, as well.

We know that being held, hugged, and kissed by a parent helps a baby thrive and enhances parent-child bonding. But the therapeutic touch of massage may do even more, possibly strengthening the immune system, improving muscle development, stimulating growth, even easing colic.

If you'd like to try massage, get a book or video or take a class with a massage therapist familiar with baby massage. The touch you use should not be too light (it will tickle) or too strong (it will hurt) and you should stop when your baby isn't enjoying it.

EXERCISE

"I've heard a lot about the importance of exercising your baby. Is it really necessary for me to take my little girl to an exercise class?"

Americans tend to be extremists. Either they're totally sedentary, getting all their exercise turning on the TV and reaching for a beer, or they embark on a overly rigorous jogging program that lands them in the sports specialist's office with aches and pains. And either they confine their babies to a stationary life in high chairs, strollers, and playpens, or they rush out and enroll them in exercise classes the moment they can lift their heads, in hopes of creating a fit-for-life infant athlete.

But extremism in the pursuit of good health tends to be ineffective, and is usually doomed to failure. Moderation is a much better goal to aim for, in your lifestyle and your baby's. So instead of ignoring your baby's physical development or pushing her beyond her abilities, take the following steps to start her on the road to fitness:

Stimulate body as well as mind. We tend to like to teach our children intellectual matter from the cradle, but often figure the physical will take care of itself. And, for the most part, it will—but paying a little extra attention to it will remind both you and your baby of its importance. Try to spend some part of your playtime with your baby in physical activity. At this stage, it may be nothing more than pulling her to a sitting position (or a standing one, when she's ready), gently raising her hands over her head, bending her knees up to meet her elbows in a rhythmic way, or holding her up in the air with your hands around her middle, making her flex her arms and legs.

Make the physical fun. You want her to feel good about her body and about physical activity, so be sure she enjoys these little sessions—and certainly don't be grim about them yourself. Talk or sing to her and tell her what you're doing. She'll come to identify little rhythmic ditties (such as "exercise, exercise, how I love my exercise") with the fun of physical activity.

Don't fence her in. A baby who's always strapped safely into a stroller or an infant seat or snuggled into a baby carrier, without opportunity for physical explorations, is well on her way to becoming a sedentary—and unfit—child. Even an infant who's too little to crawl can benefit from the freedom to move that a blanket on the floor or the center of a large bed (with constant supervision, of course) can offer. On their backs in such a position, many three- and four-month-olds will spend great stretches of time attempting to turn over (help them practice by slowly turning them over and back again). On their bellies, many will inch around, exploring with their hands and mouths, pushing their bottoms up in the air, raising their heads and shoulders. All of this activity naturally exercises tiny arms and legs—and is impossible to duplicate in a confined space.

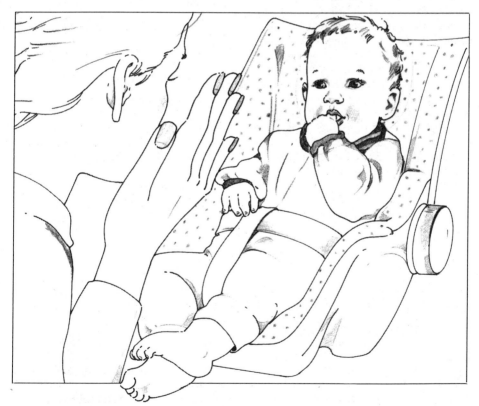

For a baby, playtime is learning time. Not only will a game of peekaboo elicit delighted giggles from a three- or four-month-old, it will help teach the important lesson of object permanence: when mommy or daddy hides their face behind their hands, they're still there.

Keep it informal. Exercise classes or taped programs for infants are not necessary for good physical development, and in fact can be detrimental. Babies, given the opportunity, get all the exercise they need. Classes or tapes that have parents doing exercises to children will not, in spite of what you may have heard, speed development, improve muscle tone, or teach children to love exercise. Their basic value is that they encourage your playing with your child and, if in class form, provide exposure to other children. If you do choose to take your baby to an exercise program, check the program first for the following:

■ Do teachers have good credentials? Is the program pediatrician approved? (Though this can sometimes be misleading; an uninformed pediatrician can attach his or her name to a program that isn't the best.) Any program that encourages exercises that jostle or shake babies is a dangerous one (see page 187). Beware, too, of classes that are high pressure, rather than fun, encouraging competition instead of individual growth.
■ Do babies seem to be having fun? If an infant isn't smiling or laughing while exercising, she isn't enjoying it. Beware especially if the babies seem confused or frightened, or pressured to do things that make them uncomfortable.
■ Is there a lot of age-appropriate equipment for your baby to play with—things like carpeted steps, miniature slides, and rockers?

■ Are babies given plenty of opportunity for free play—explorations made on their own and with you? Most of the class should be devoted to this, rather than structured group activities.
■ Is music an integral part of the program? Babies like music and rhythmic activities, such as rocking and singing, and the two go together well in an exercise program.

Let baby set her pace. Pushing a baby to exercise, or to do anything else she isn't ready for or in the mood for, can set up very negative attitudes. Begin exercise with your baby only when she seems receptive, and stop when she tells you, by her disinterest or fussiness, that she's had enough.

Keep her energized. Good nutrition is as important to your baby's good physical development as exercise. Once solids are introduced (with the doctor's permission, of course), start her on the Best-Odds Diet for Beginners (page 220) so that she has the energy needed for fun and games and the nutrients for optimal development.

Don't be an unfit mother. Teach by example; the family that exercises together stays fit together. If your child grows up watching you walking half a mile to the market instead of driving, doing daily aerobics in front of the TV instead of munching chips, swimming laps in the pool instead of sunbathing alongside it, she'll enter adulthood with good feelings about fitness that she can pass on to her own offspring.

WHAT IT'S IMPORTANT TO KNOW: Playthings for Baby

Walking into a toy store is like walking into a carnival in full swing. With every aisle vying for attention with its selection of eye-catching wares, bombarding the senses and sensibilities with an endless array of colorful boxes and displays, it's hard to know where to start. And though such trips can bring out the child in any adult, for parents several responsibilities come along with the joys of choosing toys.

To make sure you don't succumb to the prettiest packages and the most alluring gimmicks the toy industry has to offer, and end up with a vast selection of the wrong toys for your baby, consider these questions when contemplating a purchase—or when deciding whether to keep out, shelve, or return to the store playthings that have come as gifts:

Is it age appropriate? The most obvious reason for making sure a toy you purchase is age appropriate is so that your baby will appreciate it and enjoy it fully now. A less apparent reason, though, is just as important. Even an advanced baby who might be interested in a toy that's classified as appropriate for older children, and who might even manage to play with it on a primitive level, could be harmed by it since age appropriateness also takes safety into consideration. Giving your baby toys before he or she is ready for them has another disadvantage, as well; it's possible that by the time baby is ready for them, he or she will also be bored by them.

How can you tell if a toy is appropriate for your baby? One way is the age range listed on the packaging, though your baby may be able to appreciate a particular toy a little earlier or a little later than average. Another is to observe your child with the toy—if you have the toy already or can try it out at a friend's house or the store. Is he or she interested in it? Does he or she play with it the way it's meant to be played with? The right toy will help your baby to perfect skills already learned or promote the development of new ones just about to be tackled. It will be neither too easy (which encourages boredom), nor too difficult (which promotes failure).

Is it stimulating? Every toy doesn't have to bring your baby one step closer to that Harvard acceptance letter; babyhood (and childhood) are times for just plain fun, too. But your baby will have more fun with a toy if it's stimulating to the sense of sight (a mirror or a mobile), hearing (a music box or a clown with a bell in his belly), touch (a cradle gym or activity board), or

taste (a teething ring, or anything else that's mouthable) than if it's merely cute or pretty. As your baby grows, you will want toys that help a child learn eye-hand coordination, large and small motor control, the concept of cause and effect, color and shape identification and matching, auditory discrimination, spatial relationships, and that stimulate social and language development, imagination, and creativity.

Is it safe? This is perhaps the most significant question of all, since toys (not including bikes, sleds, skates, and skateboards, which cause hundreds of thousands of injuries of their own) are responsible for over 100,000 injuries a year. In selecting playthings for your baby, look for the following:

- Sturdiness. Toys that will break or fall apart easily can often cause injury to a young child.
- Safe finish. Be sure that the paint or other finish isn't toxic.
- Safe construction. Toys with small pieces, sharp edges, or breakable parts are usually unsafe for babies.
- Washability. Toys that can't be washed can become breeding places for germs—a problem with infants who put everything in their mouths.
- Safe size. Toys that are tiny enough to be swallowed (smaller than baby's fist), or have removable or breakable parts that are that small, present a serious hazard.
- No strings attached. Toys (or anything else) with strings, cords, or ribbons longer than six inches should never be left anywhere near a baby because of the strangulation risk. Toys can be attached to cribs, playpens, and elsewhere with plastic links that are not only safe, but bright and attractive playthings in themselves.
- Safe sound. Loud sounds, such as those from toy guns, model planes, and motorized vehicles, can damage baby's hearing, so look for toys that have musical or gentle sounds rather than sharp, loud, or squeaky ones.

Do you approve of it philosophically? This is less of a problem in infant toys than it will be later, but it's not too early to think about the subliminal message a toy is sending, and to consider whether that message agrees with your values. Don't let society— at least the part of society that creates some of the TV toy mayhem for children—decide what values will be passed on to your child. Even in infant toys, you will find some junk, and before you know it your innocent babe will be begging for a popular toy that you should not buy unless you truly approve. And should your child end up with a toy you wouldn't have bought (it happens), then explain to him or her what your feelings about that toy are. If, for example, you're uncomfortable with the tyke-size machine gun Uncle Bill gave your child for a birthday gift, explain when your baby is old enough to understand that it's a toy, that real guns are dangerous, that they hurt people.

CHAPTER EIGHT

The Fifth Month

WHAT YOUR BABY MAY BE DOING:

By the end of this month, your baby ...should be able to (see Note):

■ hold head steady when upright (by 4¼ months)
■ on stomach, raise chest, supported by arms (by 4⅓ months)
■ roll over (one way)
■ pay attention to a raisin or other very small object
■ squeal in delight (4⅔ months)
■ reach for an object
■ smile spontaneously
■ grasp a rattle held to backs or tips of fingers

Note: If your baby seems not to have reached one or more of these milestones, check with the doctor. In rare instances the delay could indicate a problem, though in most cases it will turn out to be normal for your baby. Premature infants generally reach milestones later than others of the same birth age, often achieving them closer to their adjusted age (the age they would be

if they had been born at term), and sometimes later.

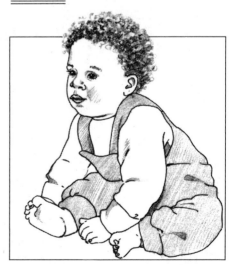

By the month's end, a few babies will be able to manage unassisted sitting when propped up by their hands, but most will still tumble forward in this position.

...will probably be able to:

- bear some weight on legs (5¼ months)
- keep head level with body when pulled to sitting
- say ah-goo or similar vowel-consonant combinations
- razz (make a wet razzing sound)

...may possibly be able to:

- sit without support (5½ months)
- turn in the direction of a voice

...may even be able to:

- pull up to standing position from sitting
- stand holding on to someone or some-thing
- feed himself or herself a cracker
- object if you try to take a toy away
- work to get to a toy out of reach
- pass a cube or other object from one hand to the other
- look for dropped object
- rake a raisin and pick it up in fist
- babble, combining vowels and con-sonants such as ga-ga-ga-ga, ba-ba-ba-ba, ma-ma-ma-ma, da-da-da-da

WHAT YOU CAN EXPECT AT THIS MONTH'S CHECKUP

Most doctors do not schedule regular well-baby checkups this month. Do call the doctor if there are any concerns that can't wait until next month's visit.

FEEDING YOUR BABY THIS MONTH: Starting Solids

It's the moment you've been waiting for, and you're giddy with anticipation. As daddy stands by with the video camera, ready to capture the momentous event, baby is decked out in party clothes and freshly laundered bib, propped up and se-cured in that spanking new high chair. As the camera rolls, baby's first bite of solid food—heaped on the engraved sterling sil-ver spoon from Great-Aunt Alice—is lifted from the bowl to baby's mouth. Baby's mouth opens, then, as the food makes its bizarre first impression on inex-perienced tastebuds, screws itself into a knot of displeasure, and spews the un-familiar offering onto chin, bib, and high chair tray. Cut!

The challenge to get your child to eat (or at least, eat what you'd like him or her to eat), a challenge that's likely to continue as long as you share the same dining table, has begun. But it's more than a matter of pro-moting good nutrition; it's one of instilling healthy attitudes toward mealtimes and snack times. As important as ensuring that the food that goes into your baby's mouth is wholesome is ensuring that the atmosphere in which the food is eaten is pleasant and noncombative.

In the first few months of solid feedings, the actual quantity of food consumed is not of great significance as long as breast or bottle feeding is continued. Eating at first is less a matter of gaining sustenance than of gaining experience—with eating techniques, with different flavors and varying textures, with the social aspects of dining.

OPENING NIGHT— AND BEYOND

Getting the video equipment set up isn't the only preparatory step you'll have to take to ensure a memorable first eating experience. You'll also want to pay attention to the timing, setting, and props to make the most of this feeding—and future ones.

Time it right. If you're breastfeeding, the show should go on when your milk supply is at its lowest (in most women this is late in the afternoon or early in the evening). Evening is also a good choice if your baby awakens at night hungry and might be sustained longer by a more substantial evening meal. If, on the other hand, your baby seems hungriest in the morning, you might offer solids then. Don't worry if the menu is cereal and the serving time is 6 P.M.—baby will hardly be expecting steak.

Humor your headliner. You've slotted a 5:00 performance only to find that the star is cranky and overtired. Postpone the show. You can't introduce your baby to anything new, food included, when he or she is in this condition. Schedule meals for times when your baby is usually alert and happy.

Don't open to a full tummy. Whet baby's appetite before offering the solids, but don't drown it. Start off with an appetizer of a small amount of formula or breast milk. That way your baby won't be too ravenous to put up with the new experience, and won't be so satiated that the next course will have no appeal. Of course, babies with small appetites may do better starting solids hungry; you'll have to see which works best for yours.

Be ready for a long production. Don't try to schedule baby's meals in five-minute segments between other chores. Baby feeding is a time-consuming process, so be sure to leave plenty of time for it.

Set the stage. Holding a squirming baby on your lap while trying to deposit an unfamiliar substance into an unreceptive mouth is a perfect script for disaster. Set up a sturdy high chair or feeding seat (see page 235) several days before the first feeding experience and allow your baby to become comfortable in it. If your baby slides around or slumps in it, pad it with a small blanket, quilt, or some towels. Fasten the restraining straps for baby's safety and your peace of mind. If your baby can't sit up at all in such a chair or seat, it's probably a good idea to postpone solids for a bit longer.

Also be sure you have the right kind of spoon. It doesn't have to be a family heirloom or baby spoon, but it should have a small bowl (perhaps a demitasse or iced-tea spoon) and, possibly, a plastic coating, which is easier on baby's gums. Giving baby a spoon of his or her own to hold and attempt to maneuver discourages a tug-of-war over each bite, and also gives your budding individualist a sense of independence. A long handle is good for your feeding baby, but choose a short one with a curved handle for baby's use to avoid unintended pokes in the eye. If your young gourmand insists on "helping" you with your feeding spoon, let a little hand hold on to the spoon as you firmly guide it to the target—most of the time you'll get there.

Finally, use a big, easy-to-clean, easy-to-remove, comfortable bib. Depending on your preference, it can be firm or soft plastic that can be wiped or rinsed off, cloth or plastic that can be tossed into the wash, or a paper disposable. You may not be concerned about your baby getting cereal stains on almost-outgrown sleepers now, but if the bib habit isn't instilled early, it is often difficult (if not impossible) to instill later. And don't forget to roll up long

sleeves. An at-home alternative (room temperature permitting) to the bib is to let baby
eat topless. You'll still have to do some
wiping off, but stains won't be a problem.

Play a supporting role. If you give your
baby a chance to run the show, your odds of
succeeding at feeding are much improved.
Before even trying to bring the spoon to
baby's mouth, put a dab of the food on the
table or high chair tray and give your child a
chance to examine it, squish it, mash it, rub
it, maybe even taste it. That way, when you
do approach with the spoon, what you're
offering won't be totally foreign. Though
offering new food in a bottle (with a large-
holed nipple) might seem like a good way to
give baby a chance to self-feed, it's not
recommended for several reasons. First, it
can cause a baby to choke. Second, it reinforces the bottle habit and doesn't teach a
baby how to eat like the rest of us, which
after all is what early feedings are all about.
And third, because babies tend to eat too
much this way, it can lead to overweight.

Start with coming attractions. The
first several meals won't be real meals at all,
but simply introductions for those to come.
Start with a quarter to a full teaspoon of the
selected food. Slip just the tiniest bit of it
between baby's lips and allow some time
for baby to react. If the morsel finds favor,
the mouth will probably open more for the
next bite, which you can place farther back
for easier swallowing. Even if baby seems
receptive, the first few tries may come sliding right back out of the mouth; in fact the
first few meals may seem like total wash-
outs. But a baby who is ready for solids will
quickly start taking in more than he or she
is spitting out. If the food continues to slide
out, baby is probably not developmentally
prepared for the big time yet. You can
continue wasting time, effort, and food at
this fruitless pursuit—or wait a week or
two, then try again.

Know when to end the show. Never
continue a meal when your baby has lost
interest. The signals will be clear, though
they may vary from baby to baby and meal
to meal: fussiness, a head turned away, a
mouth clamped shut, food spit out, or food
thrown around.

If your baby rejects a previously enjoyed
food, taste it to be sure it hasn't gone bad.
Of course there may be another reason for
the rejection. Maybe your baby's tastes have
changed (babies are very fickle about food),
or maybe he or she is out of sorts or just not
hungry. Whatever the reason, don't force
the issue or the food. Try another selection,
and if that doesn't go over, bring down the
curtain.

FOODS TO PREMIERE WITH

Though everyone agrees that the perfect
first liquid for baby is mother's milk, there
is not total agreement—even among pediatricians—about what the perfect first solid
is. The reason is that there is little substantial scientific evidence that points to any
single, best first solid food, and babies
seem to do as well on one as on another
(assuming it's appropriate fare for an infant). If your baby's doctor has no specific
recommendations, try one of the following.
Keep in mind that you won't be able to
accurately assess baby's reaction to first-
time foods by his or her expression—most
babies will initially screw up their mouths
with shock no matter how pleased they are
with the offering, particularly if the taste is
tart. Instead go by whether baby opens up
for a refill.

Rice cereal. Because it is easily thinned
to a texture not much thicker than milk, is
very easily digested by most infants, is not
likely to trigger an allergic reaction, and
provides needed iron, iron-enriched baby
rice cereal is probably the most commonly
recommended first food and the first choice
of the American Academy of Pediatrics.
Mix it with formula, breast milk, water, or
whole cow's milk (once your baby's doctor
approves; many will allow small amounts

GOOD EARLY FOODS TO OFFER BABY

All of the following are usually enjoyed and tolerated well by young babies. But before introducing the selections from the sweeter fruit list, do try getting your baby acclimated to several foods from the first three categories. Meat and poultry are usually introduced later—somewhere around seven or eight months. The foods, which can be prepared at home or purchased ready to use, should at first be very smooth in texture—strained, puréed, or finely mashed, and thinned with liquid if necessary to the consistency of thick cream. The texture should continue to be smooth until the sixth or seventh month, becoming progressively thicker as baby becomes a more experienced eater. Babies usually take less than half a teaspoon at first, but many work up to 2 to 3 tablespoons, sometimes more, in a short time. Food can be served at room temperature (which most babies prefer) or slightly warmed, though heating is usually done more for the adult's taste than the baby's.

Rice cereals	*Squash*	*Yogurt (unsweetened)*	*Applesauce*	*Beef*
Barley cereals	*Sweet potato*	*Kefir (unsweetened)*	*Bananas*	*Chicken*
Oat cereals	*Carrots*		*Peaches*	*Turkey*
	Green beans		*Pears*	*Lamb*
	Peas			
	Avocado			

Note: Spinach, which is very high in oxalic acid, is often not recommended until a baby is older.

---

of cow's milk before six months for mixing in cereal). Resist the temptation to stir in mashed bananas, applesauce, or fruit juices, or to buy ready-prepared cereal with fruit, or your baby will quickly come to accept only sweet foods, rejecting all else.

A food similar to milk. On the theory that a baby will most easily accept something familiar, a food that is close to milk in consistency and/or taste (such as plain, unsweetened, whole milk yogurt or kefir) is a popular starter. Whether you give yogurt first or add it later, don't serve it with fruit or sugar to make it what you deem more palatable; most babies will lap it up straight, and many will develop a taste for the tart and unsweetened that will serve them well later on. Babies who are allergic to or intolerant of milk products, of course, should begin with something else.

Something sweet. Many babies are started off on finely mashed or strained banana (thinned with a bit of formula or breast milk if necessary) or applesauce.

True, most take to these foods eagerly, but they also then tend to refuse less sweet foods, such as vegetables and unsweetened cereals, when they are offered later. This is not usually an ideal choice.

Vegetables. Vegetables are, in theory, a good first food—nutritious and not sweet. But their strong, distinctive flavors make them less appealing to many babies than cereal or yogurt, so they may not create a positive attitude toward the gastronomic experience. It's wise, however, to introduce them before fruit, while baby's palate is more receptive to new tastes. The "yellows," such as sweet potatoes and carrots, are usually more palatable (as well as more nutritious) than such "greens" as peas or green beans.

EXPANDING BABY'S REPERTOIRE

Even if your baby devours her very first serving of breakfast cereal, don't plan on presenting her with a lunch of yogurt and string beans and a dinner of strained meats and sweet potatoes. Each new food you introduce to your baby, from the first one on, should be offered alone (or with foods that have already passed muster) so that if there's a sensitivity or allergy to it, you will recognize it. If you're starting with cereal, for example, give it exclusively, at least for the next three or four days (some doctors recommend five days). If your baby has no adverse reactions to it (excessive bloating or gassiness; diarrhea or mucus in the stool; vomiting; a rough rash on the face, particularly around the mouth, or around the anus; a runny nose and/or watery eyes or wheezing that doesn't seem to be associated with a cold; unusual night wakefulness or daytime crankiness), you can assume he or she tolerates the food well.

If you spot what you think is a reaction, wait a week or so and try the food again. The same reaction two or three times is a good indication that your baby has a sensitivity to the food. Wait several months before introducing it again, and in the meantime try the same procedure with a different new food. If your baby seems to have a reaction to several foods or if there is a history of allergy in your family, wait a full week between new foods. If every food you try appears to cause a problem, talk to the baby's doctor about waiting a few months before reintroducing solids.

Introduce each new food in the same cautious manner, keeping a record of the food, the approximate amounts taken, and any reactions (memory can fail). Be sure to begin with single foods—just strained carrots or strained peas, for example. Most baby food companies make special single-food beginner lines for this purpose (which also come in small jars to avoid waste). Once a baby has taken both peas and carrots without any ill effects, it's fine to serve them up as a combo. Later, as baby's repertoire expands, a new food that isn't packaged solo (tomato, for example) can be introduced in a medley along with already accepted vegetables.

Some foods, because they are more allergenic than others, are introduced later. Wheat, for example, is usually added to the infant diet after rice, oats, and barley have been well accepted. Occasionally this happens as late as the eighth month, although the okay is usually given earlier for babies with no signs and no family history of food allergy. Citrus juices and fruits and introduced after other fruits and juices, seafood after meat and poultry. Egg yolks (scrambled, or hard cooked and mashed) usually aren't given until at least the eighth month; the whites, which are much more likely to provoke an allergic reaction are often not given until near the end of the year. Chocolate and nuts are not only highly allergenic, but inappropriate infant fare and aren't usually given at all during the first year.

BEST-ODDS DIET FOR BEGINNERS

Right now your baby is only dabbling in solids; he or she is still getting most nutritional requirements from breast milk or formula. But from the sixth month on, breast milk or formula alone won't be enough to meet all your baby's needs, and by the end of the year, most of baby's nutrition will come from other sources. So it's not too early to start thinking in terms of the Nine Basic Principles of Good Nutrition (page 357) when planning your baby's meals now, and a simplified Daily Dozen (below) once your baby begins taking a variety of foods—usually at about eight or nine months. Since a prudent diet is the best prevention for heart disease and many forms of cancer, the eating habits you help your baby develop in the high chair now may be life-saving later in life. Optimum nutrition started early will optimize your child's physical, emotional, intellectual, and social development. It will help make him or her a better student and a happier person.

NO HONEY FOR YOUR LITTLE HONEY

Honey not only offers little more than empty calories, it also poses a health risk in the first year. It may contain the spores of *Clostridium botulinum*, which in this form is harmless to adults but can cause botulism (with constipation, weakened sucking, poor appetite, and lethargy) in babies. This serious though rarely fatal illness can lead to pneumonia and dehydration. Some doctors okay honey at eight months; others recommend waiting till year's end. Because corn syrup may also contain these spores, it too should not be given to babies. It's safe, however, in infant formulas.

Over the next few months, you can start introducing the Infant Daily Dozen, gradually adding new foods and increasing quantities to those below. As baby's first birthday approaches, the Toddler Daily Dozen will be more appropriate. Additional Daily Dozen choices are listed beginning on page 359.

THE INFANT DAILY DOZEN

Calories. You don't need to count your baby's calories to tell if he or she is getting enough—or too many. Is he or she unpleasingly plump? Too many calories are the likely reason. Or is your baby very thin or growing too slowly? Then caloric intake is probably insufficient. Right now most of the calories that keep baby thriving come from breast milk or formula; gradually more and more of them will come from solid foods.

Protein. Two or three tablespoons a day of egg yolk (once it has been approved), meat, chicken, fish, cottage cheese, or yogurt, or an ounce of cheese or two of tofu will do while the greater share of protein is still received from formula or breast milk.

Calcium foods. Breast milk and/or formula supplies adequate calcium for an infant, but as these are decreased and solids increased, other calcium foods such as hard cheeses, yogurt, whole milk, and tofu coagulated with calcium nigari should be added to the diet. The total requirement can be met with about two cups of whole milk or the equivalent in breast milk, formula, other milk products, or other calcium foods, until baby reaches a year (see page 360 for equivalents).

Whole grains and other concentrated complex carbohydrates. Two to four servings of grain foods, legumes, or dried peas a day will add essential vitamins and minerals, as well as some protein, to baby's diet. One serving equals ¼ cup baby cereal, a half-slice of whole-grain bread, or ¼ cup of cooked whole-grain cereal or pasta, ½ cup of dry whole-grain cereal, or ¼ cup puréed lentils, beans, or peas, but don't expect this intake for months.

Green leafy and yellow vegetables and yellow fruits. Two or three tablespoons of winter squash, sweet potato, carrots, broccoli, kale, apricots, yellow peaches (puréed at first, chunky later) or ¼ cup ripe cantaloupe, mango, or peach cubes, when baby moves on to finger foods, will provide adequate vitamin A.

Vitamin C foods. Just ¼ cup of baby fruit juice fortified with vitamin C or orange or grapefruit juice (which are usually not introduced until after the eighth month) will provide enough vitamin C. So will ¼ cup cantaloupe or mango cubes, or ¼ cup puréed broccoli or cauliflower.

DOUBLE-DUTY
JARS

Use empty baby food jars, thoroughly washed in a dishwasher or by hand with detergent in very hot water, for heating and/or serving small portions of baby foods. Heat by placing the open jar in a small amount of hot water rather than in the microwave oven (it may heat foods unevenly).

Other fruits and vegetables. If your baby has room for more food in his or her diet, add one of the following daily: one or two tablespoons of applesauce, mashed banana, puréed peas or green beans, or mashed potatoes.

High fat foods. The baby on formula or breast milk entirely gets all the fat and cholesterol needed. But as the switch to a more varied diet takes place and a baby spends less time at bottle or breast, it's important to be sure that fat and cholesterol intake remains adequate. Most dairy products served should be full-fat or made from whole milk. If you add instant nonfat dry milk to foods as part of your baby's protein and calcium allowance, add 2 tablespoons of half-and-half to each ⅓ cup dry milk to replace the fat. If you use low-fat cottage cheese for the rest of the family, you can use the same for baby if you add a bit of sweet or sour cream, or be sure baby also gets some full-fat hard cheese (such as Swiss or Cheddar, preferably low in sodium), which is very high in fat, daily. Though it's important not to remove dairy fats from the diet, it's equally important not to load a baby's diet with large quantities of other fats or fried foods, which can add unneeded pounds, be difficult to digest, and set up poor eating habits.

Iron foods or supplementation. To help prevent iron-deficiency anemia, your baby should have one of the following daily: iron-fortified cereal or formula, or a vitamin supplement with iron. Additional iron can come from such iron-rich foods as meat, egg yolks, wheat germ, whole-grain breads and cereals, and dried peas and other legumes, as they are introduced into the diet.

Salty foods. Since a baby's kidneys can't handle large quantities of sodium, and because developing a taste for salt early in life can lead to problems with hypertension later on, baby's foods should not have added salt. Most foods contain some sodium naturally, particularly dairy foods and many vegetables, so baby can't possibly come up short even if you don't add salt to the menu.

Fluids. During the first four or five months of life virtually all of a baby's fluids come from bottle or breast. Now small amounts will come from other sources, such as juices, milk from a cup, and fruits and vegetables. As the quantity of formula or breast milk taken begins to decrease, it's important to be sure that the total fluid intake doesn't. In hot weather it should increase, so offer water and fruit juices diluted with water when temperatures soar.

Vitamin supplement. As a simple nutrition insurance policy, give vitamin and mineral drops especially formulated for infants. These drops should contain iron, if your baby does not take an iron-fortified formula, and no more than the Recommended Daily Allowance of vitamins and minerals for babies. Do not give any other vitamin or mineral supplements without the doctor's approval.

WHAT YOU MAY BE CONCERNED ABOUT

TEETHING

"How can I tell if my baby's teething? She's biting on her hands a lot, but I don't see anything on her gums."

When the teething fairy visits, there's no telling how extended or how unpleasant her stay will be. For one child it may be a long, drawn-out, painful affair. For another it may seem to pass with a single wave of the wand in the middle of a restful night. Sometimes a lump or a ridge seems visible in the gum for weeks or months; sometimes there seems to be no visible clue at all until the tooth itself appears.

On the average the first tooth arrives sometime during the seventh month, although it can rear its pearly white head as early as three months, as late as twelve, or in rare instances, even earlier or later. Tooth eruption often follows hereditary patterns, so if you or your husband teethed early or late, your baby may do likewise. Symptoms of teething, however, often precede the tooth itself by as much as two or three months. These symptoms vary from child to child, and opinions as to exactly what these symptoms are and how painful teething actually is vary from physician to physician. But it's commonly accepted that a teething baby may experience any or all of the following:

Drooling. For a lot of babies, starting at anywhere from about ten weeks to three or four months of age, the faucet's on. Teething stimulates drooling, more in some babies than in others.

Chin or face rash. In a prolific drooler, it's not unusual for a dry skin rash or chapping to develop on the chin and around the mouth because of irritation from constant contact with saliva. To help prevent this, gently wipe the drool periodically during the daytime, and place a towel under the crib sheet to absorb the excess while your baby sleeps. Should a patch of dry skin appear, keep it well lubricated with a mild skin cream (ask the doctor for a recommendation).

A little cough. The excess saliva can cause baby to gag or cough occasionally. This is nothing to worry about, as long as your baby seems otherwise free of cold, flu, or allergy symptoms. Often babies will continue the cough as an attention getter or because they find it an interesting addition to their vocalization repertoires.

Biting. In this case, taking a nip is not a sign of hostility. A teething baby will gum down on anything she can get her mouth on —from her own tiny hand, to the breast that feeds her, to a perfect stranger's unsuspecting thumb—the counterpressure from any of which will help relieve the pressure from under the gums.

Pain. Inflammation is the protective response of the tender gum tissue to the impending tooth, which it considers an intruder to fend off. It causes seemingly unbearable pain in some babies, but almost none in others. Discomfort is often worst with the first teeth (apparently most babies become accustomed to the sensations of teething and learn to live with them) and with the molars (which, because of their greater size, seem to be more painful, but which, fortunately, you won't have to worry about until sometime after baby's first birthday).

Irritability. As inflammation increases and a sharp little tooth rises closer to the surface, threatening to erupt, the ache in baby's gum may become more constant. Like anyone with chronic pain, she may be cranky, out of sorts, not "herself." Again, some babies (and their parents) will suffer more than others, with irritability lasting weeks instead of days or hours.

Refusal to feed. A teething baby may appear fickle when it comes to nursing. While she craves the comfort of something in her mouth—and may seem to want to "nurse all the time"—once she begins to suck, and the suction created increases her discomfort, she may reject the breast or bottle she so passionately desired only moments before. With each repetition of this scenario (and some babies repeat it all day long when they're teething), she (and mother) becomes more frustrated and more out of sorts. A baby who's started solids may lose interest in them for the time being; this needn't be a source of concern, since your baby is still getting almost all of her necessary nutrition and needed fluids from nursing or formula, and her appetite will pick up where it left off once the tooth comes through. Of course, if your baby refuses more than a couple of feedings or seems to be taking very little for several days, a call to the doctor is in order.

Diarrhea. Whether this symptom actually has a relationship to teething or not depends on whom you ask. Some mothers insist that every time their babies teethe, they have loose bowel movements. Some doctors admit that there appears to be a connection—perhaps because the excess saliva swallowed loosens the stool. Other doctors refuse to acknowledge this link, at least for the record—probably not because they are entirely sure it doesn't exist, but because they fear that legitimizing the theory could cause mothers to overlook possibly significant gastrointestinal symptoms, attributing them to teething. So though it may be that your baby will have looser movements with teething, you should report actual diarrhea that lasts more than two bowel movements to her doctor whenever it occurs.

Low-grade fever. Fever, like diarrhea, is a symptom that doctors are hesitant to link to teething. Still, some acknowledge that a low-grade fever (under 101°F, rectally) can occasionally accompany teething as a result of inflammation of the gums. To play it safe, treat fever with teething as you would low-grade fever at any other time, calling the doctor if it persists for three days.

Wakefulness. Babies don't teethe only during the daylight hours. The discomfort that has her fussing during the day can keep her awake at night. Even the baby who has been sleeping through the night may suddenly begin night waking again. To avoid her lapsing back into old habits, don't rush to comfort or feed her. Instead, see if she can settle back down herself. Night waking, like many other teething problems, is more common with first teeth and with molars.

Gum hematoma. Occasionally, teething initiates some bleeding under the gums, which may appear as a bluish lump. Such hematomas are nothing to worry about, and most doctors recommend allowing them to resolve on their own without medical intervention. Cold compresses may lessen discomfort and speed the resolution of gum hematomas.

Ear pulling; cheek rubbing. Pain in the gums may travel to the ears and cheeks along nerve pathways they share, particularly when the molars begin pushing their way in. That's why some babies, when they are teething, pull at an ear or rub a cheek or the chin. But keep in mind that babies also tug at their ears when they have ear infections. If you suspect an ear infection (see page 423), teething or no, check with the doctor.

There are probably as many home-tested treatments for teething discomfort as there are grandmothers. Some work, some don't. Among the best that old wives and new medicine have to offer are:

Something to chew on. This is not for nutritive benefits, but for the relief that comes from counterpressure against the gums—which is enhanced when the object being chewed is icy cold and numbing. A frozen bagel, a frozen banana (albeit messy), a clean washcloth with an ice cube tightly wrapped and secured inside with a rubber band, a chilled carrot with the thin end sliced off (but don't use carrots once teeth are actually in and can chip off chokable bits), a bumpy rubber teething ring or other teething toy, even the plastic railing of a crib or playpen will all provide a wholesome chew. Health food stores sell nutritious teething biscuits that are fine before the teeth erupt, but afterward, with their high carbohydrate content, could cause a decay problem if kept constantly in the mouth. Whatever food you use to soothe a teething baby, she should have it only in a sitting position and while under adult supervision.

Something to rub against. Many babies appreciate a grownup finger rubbed firmly on the gum. Some will protest the intrusion at first, since the rubbing seems to hurt at the start, and then calm down as the counterpressure begins to bring relief.

Something cold to drink. Offer your baby a bottle of icy cold water. If she doesn't take a bottle or is bothered by the sucking, offer the soothing liquid in a cup—but remove any ice cubes first. This will also augment the teething baby's fluid intake, important if she is losing fluids through drooling and/or loose movements.

Something cold to eat. Applesauce, puréed peaches, or yogurt, chilled in the freezer, may be more appealing to a teething baby than warm or room-temperature foods, and they offer more nutrition than a chilled teething ring.

Something to relieve the pain. When nothing else spells relief, acetaminophen should do the trick. Check with your doctor for the right dose, or see page 628 if he or she is not available. Avoid giving any other medication by mouth or rubbing anything on baby's gums unless recommended by the doctor. This caveat includes brandy or any other alcoholic beverage. Alcohol is a dangerous poison to infants—and even a touch could encourage your baby to develop a taste for it.

CHRONIC COUGH

"For the last three weeks my baby has had a little cough. He doesn't seem sick, and he almost seems to be coughing on purpose. Is this possible?"

Even as early as the fifth month, many babies have begun to realize that all the world's a stage, and that nothing beats an admiring audience. So when a baby discovers that a little cough—either triggered by excess saliva or stumbled upon in the ordinary course of vocal experimentation—gets a lot of attention, he often continues this affectation purely for its effect. As long as he's otherwise healthy, and seems in control of the cough rather than

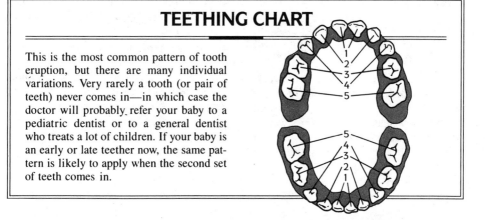

TEETHING CHART

This is the most common pattern of tooth eruption, but there are many individual variations. Very rarely a tooth (or pair of teeth) never comes in—in which case the doctor will probably refer your baby to a pediatric dentist or to a general dentist who treats a lot of children. If your baby is an early or late teether now, the same pattern is likely to apply when the second set of teeth comes in.

vice versa, ignore it. And though your little Olivier-in-training may never lose his flair for the dramatic, he will probably give up this attention-getter as he (or his audience) becomes bored with it.

EAR PULLING

"My daughter has been pulling at her ear a lot. She doesn't seem to be in any pain, but I'm worried that she might have an ear infection."

Babies have a lot of territory to conquer—some of it on their own bodies. The fingers and hands, the toes and feet, the penis or vagina, and another curious appendage, the ear, will all be subjects of exploration at one time or another. Unless your baby's pulling and tugging at her ear is also accompanied by crying or obvious discomfort, fever, and/or other signs of illness (see page 423 if it is), it's very likely that it's only a manifestation of her curiosity, not a symptom of an ear infection. Some babies may also fuss with their ears when teething. Redness on the outside of the ear isn't a sign of infection, just a result of constant manipulation. If you suspect a problem, do check with the doctor.

Peculiar mannerisms such as ear pulling are common and fairly short-lived; they are replaced by newer and more exciting ones once baby outgrows or grows tired of them.

NAPS

"My baby is awake more during the day now and I'm not sure—and I don't think he is either—how many naps he needs."

It's inevitable. The first couple of weeks home from the hospital the proud mom and dad, eager to begin active parenting, stand forlornly over their new baby's crib, waiting for him to wake from what seems like endless slumber. Then, as he spends more time awake, they begin to wonder, "Why doesn't he ever sleep?"

Though the typical baby in the fifth month takes three or four pretty regular naps of an hour or so each during the day, some babies thrive on five or six naps of about twenty minutes each, and others on two longer ones of an hour and a half or two. The number and length of naps your baby takes, however, are less important than the total amount of shut-eye he gets (about 14½ hours a day on average during the fifth month, with wide variations). Longer naps are more practical for you because they allow you longer stretches in which to get things done. In addition, the baby who gets into catnapping during the day may follow the same pattern during the night, waking up frequently.

You can try to encourage longer naps by:

■ Offering a comfortable place to nap. Letting baby sleep on your shoulder will not only result in a stiff shoulder for you, but also in a shorter nap for him. A crib, stroller, carriage, or even a sofa (with a chair or a low table padded with pillows alongside in case baby inches toward the edge) is preferable.

■ Keeping the room temperature comfortable, neither too hot nor too cold, and coverings appropriate. But remember that we all need a little extra covering during sleep, when we're inactive.

■ Not letting your baby fall asleep just before mealtime (when his empty stomach is likely to rouse him prematurely), when his diaper needs changing (he won't sleep as long if his bottom's drenched), when company (and noise) is expected, or any other time when you know the nap is destined not to last.

■ Avoiding predictable disturbances. You will quickly learn what disturbs your baby's sleep. Maybe it's wheeling his stroller into the supermarket. Or moving him from car seat to crib. Or the dog's shrill bark. Or the telephone in the hallway near his room. By trying to control the circumstances under which your baby sleeps, you may be able to eliminate these disturbances.

■ Keeping baby awake for longer periods between naps. Your baby should now be able to stay awake for about three and a half hours at a stretch. If he does, he's more likely to take a longer nap. Try any of the infant-stimulating ideas on pages 165 and 263 to increase stay-awake time.

Though many babies regulate themselves pretty well when it comes to getting their quota of sleep, not every baby gets as much as he needs to. It may be that yours isn't napping enough or getting enough total sleep if he frequently seems cranky. If you believe your baby needs more sleep, you will have to intervene to increase sleeping time. But if your baby sleeps very little and seems perfectly happy, you will have to accept the fact that he's one of those babies who doesn't need a lot of shut-eye.

ECZEMA

"Just after I weaned my baby from breast to bottle, she began to break out in a red rash on her cheeks. It must be itchy, because she keeps trying to scratch it and is making the skin raw."

This sounds like a classic case of infantile eczema, also known as atopic dermatitis. A skin disorder that sometimes arises when a baby is put on solids or switched from breast milk to formula or from formula to cow's milk, eczema is believed to be a type of allergic reaction. It's rare in babies who are breastfed exclusively, and more common in those with family histories of eczema, asthma, or hay fever. In formula-fed babies, the rash usually first appears around three months of age.

A bright red scaly rash commonly starts on the cheeks and often spreads elsewhere, most frequently to the area behind the ears, to the neck, arms, and legs. (It usually doesn't spread to the diaper area until between six and eight months.) Small papules, or pimples, develop and fill with fluid, then ooze and crust over. The severe itching causes children to scratch, which can lead to infection. Except for the very mildest, self-limiting cases, eczema re-

quires medical treatment to prevent complications. It clears by eighteen months in about half the cases, and usually becomes less severe by age three in the others. Approximately 1 in 3 children with eczema, however, will develop asthma or other allergies later.

The following are all-important in the handling of eczema:

Clip nails. Keep your baby's fingernails as short as possible to minimize the damage caused by scratching her rash. You may be able to prevent her from scratching by covering her hands with a pair of socks or mittens, particularly while she's sleeping, but she may still rub her face against the bedsheets to get relief.

Curtail bathing. Since contact with soap and water increases skin dryness, limit baths to no more than 10 or 15 minutes, three times a week. Though no soap should be used on affected areas, you can use an extra mild soap (Dove or liquid baby soap, for example) on dirty hands and knees and diaper area. Use the same soap, rather than shampoo, for hair washing. And keep your baby out of chlorinated pools and salt water, though fresh-water dips are okay.

Lubricate lavishly. Spread plenty of rich skin cream (one that her doctor recommends) on affected areas after baths while the skin is still wet. Do not use vegetable fats or oils or petroleum jelly (such as Vaseline).

Control the environment. Since excessive heat, cold, or dry air can worsen eczema, try to avoid taking your baby out of doors in extremes of weather; keep your home neither too warm nor too cold, and use a cold-mist humidifier to keep the air moist. (But be sure the humidifier is cleaned regularly; see page 629.)

Keep it cotton. Since perspiration can make eczema worse, avoid synthetics, wool, and overdressing. Also avoid itchy fabrics and clothing with rough seams or trim, all of which can exacerbate the condition. Soft cotton clothing, loosely layered, will be most comfortable and least irritating. When your baby plays on carpeting, which can irritate the skin, too, place a cotton sheet under her.

Institute a limited quarantine. Not to protect other children from your baby (eczema isn't contagious), but to protect your baby from other children who might pass a virus (particularly herpes) or other illness that could lead to a serious secondary infection of the skin, which is open and vulnerable.[1]

Control diet. Under the doctor's supervision, eliminate any food that seems to trigger a flare-up or a worsening of the rash.

Get medical treatment. Eczema that comes and goes in infancy usually leaves no lasting effects. But if the condition continues into childhood, affected skin can become thickened, depigmented, and cracked. Therefore treatment—which will usually include a steroid cream to spread on the affected areas, antihistamines to reduce the itching, and antibiotics if a secondary infection develops—is essential.

USING A BACK CARRIER

"Our baby is getting too big to lug around in a front baby carrier. Is it safe to use a back carrier?"

Once your baby can sit independently, even briefly, he's ready to graduate to a back carrier—assuming it suits you both. Some parents find the conveyance a comfortable and convenient way to carry their babies, others find it awkward and a strain on the muscles. Some babies are thrilled by the

height and view a back carrier affords them, others are frightened by the precarious perch. To find out whether a back carrier is right for you and your baby, take him for a test ride in a friend's or in a store floor sample before buying.

If you do use a back carrier, always be certain baby is fastened in securely. Also be aware that the position allows a baby to do a lot more behind your back than sightseeing—including pulling cans off the shelves in the supermarket, knocking over a vase in the gift shop, plucking (and then eating) leaves of shrubs in the park. Keep in mind, too, that acquiring this appendage will require you to judge distances differently—when you back into a crowded elevator or go through a low doorway, for example.

GRATUITOUS ADVICE

"Every time I go out with my son, I have to listen to at least a dozen strangers tell me that he's not dressed warmly enough, what I should do for his teething, or how I could make him stop crying. How am I supposed to handle all this unwanted advice?"

Although it's true that if you're very discriminating you can occasionally benefit from the voices of experience that chorus around the stroller every time you leave your home, most of what you'll hear from these well-meaning strangers is best passed swiftly, without processing, in one ear and out the other.

You could come back with a smart retort or spend fifteen frustrating and fruitless minutes trying to persuade advice givers of the wisdom of your ways. But wiser in most situations is to plaster on a smile, extend a perfunctory thank you, and move on as speedily as possible. By letting them speak their piece without letting what they have to say get under your skin, you'll make their day without ruining yours.

---

1. Though it is highly unlikely that your child will come into contact with anyone who has recently had a smallpox vaccination, you should be aware that such contact—or actual smallpox vaccination—is very risky for a child with eczema.

If the advice that's been proffered seems as if it might have some validity, but you're not sure, check it out with your baby's doctor or with another reliable source.

STARTING THE CUP

"I don't give my baby a bottle, but the doctor said I can give her juice now. Is it too early to start her on the cup?"

Whether she is started on the cup in the fifth month, the tenth month, or the eighteenth month, there's certainty in the fact that your baby will eventually get all of her fluids from one. But teaching her to drink from a cup early offers certain important advantages. For one, she learns that there's a route to liquid refreshment other than the breast or bottle, an alternative that will make it easier to wean her from either or both. For another, it provides an additional way to give fluids (water, juice, and after six months, milk) when a mother can't or doesn't want to nurse or isn't available, or when a bottle isn't handy.

Another advantage of early cup training: a five-month-old infant is markedly malleable. But wait until your baby's first birthday to introduce a cup, and you'll likely encounter considerable resistance. Not only will she be stubbornly set in her ways, but she's apt to sense that giving in to a cup will lead to her having to give up her bottle or breast. And even if she accepts the cup, it may be a while before she becomes skilled at using it, which means that it could be weeks or months before she will be able to drink significant amounts from it—hence, weeks or months before you can wean her.

To ease your baby into using the cup early and successfully:

Wait until she can sit supported. Babies as young as two months can be started on the cup, but gagging will be less of a problem once a baby can sit up with support.

Choose a safe cup. Even if you're holding the cup, baby may knock it down or swat at it impatiently when she doesn't want any more, so be sure the cups you use are unbreakable. A cup that is weighted at the bottom will not tip over easily. A paper or plastic cup, though unbreakable, won't work for training because—much to baby's delight—it's crushable.

Choose a compatible cup. The type of cup preferred differs from child to child, so you may have to experiment with several to find one your child really likes. Some children favor a cup with one or two handles they can grip; others prefer a cup without handles. (If such a cup tends to slip from baby's wet little hands, wrap a couple of strips of adhesive tape around it, changing the tape when it becomes ratty.) A cup with a spouted lid theoretically offers a nice transition from sucking to sipping (probably more so for babies who've taken a bottle than for those who are used to a human nipple), but some children just don't like it—perhaps because they find the liquid more difficult to extract from it, perhaps because they want to drink from a cup that's just like mommy's or daddy's. And though there will be fewer major spills at the start with a spouted lid, baby will eventually have to face the hurdle of learning to do without its protection—which may result in more spills later on.

Protect all concerned. Teaching your baby to drink from a cup won't be a neat affair; for quite some time you can expect more to drip down her chin than down her gullet. So until she becomes proficient, keep her covered with a large absorbent or waterproof bib during drinking lessons. If you are feeding her on your lap, protect it with a waterproof square or apron.

Get baby comfortable. Seat her so she feels secure—on your lap, in an infant seat, or propped up in a high chair.

Fill the cup with the right contents. It's easiest and least damaging to start with water. You can then also try expressed

FEEDING BABY SAFELY

With an estimated 10 million cases occurring each year, food poisoning is one of the most common illnesses in the United States. And it's also one of the most easily prevented. Other hazards that originate at the feeding table (glass splinters, passing of cold germs) can also be avoided. To make sure you do everything you can to make eating safe for your baby, take the following precautions every time you prepare food:

■ Always wash your hands with soap and water before feeding baby; if you touch raw meat, poultry, fish, or eggs (all of which harbor bacteria) during the feeding, wash them again. Wash your hands, too, if you blow your nose or touch your mouth. If you have an open cut on your hand, cover it with an adhesive strip before feeding your baby.

■ Store dry baby cereals and unopened baby food jars in a cool dry place away from extremes of heat (over the stove, for example) or cold (as in an unheated cellar).

■ Wipe the tops of baby food jars with a clean cloth or run them under the tap to remove dust before opening.

■ If a jar is hard to open, run warm tap water over the neck or pry the side of the lid open with a bottle opener until you hear a pop;

don't tap the top as this may splinter glass into the contents.

■ Don't feed baby directly out of a baby food jar unless it's the last meal from that jar, and don't save a bowl of food baby's eaten from for the next meal, since enzymes and bacteria from baby's saliva will begin "digesting" the food, turning it watery and causing it to spoil more quickly.

■ Make sure the button is down on safety lids before opening a jar for first time; when opening listen for the "pop" to make sure the seal was intact. Discard or return to the store any jar that has a raised button or that doesn't pop. If you use ordinary canned foods for an older baby (or anyone else), discard cans that are swollen or leaky. Don't use foods in which a liquid that should be clear has turned cloudy or milky.[2]

■ Whenever you use a can opener, make sure it's clean (wash it after each use, scrubbing gears with a toothbrush set aside for this purpose), and discard it when it begins to look rusty or you can't get it clean.

■ Remove one serving at a time from a jar of baby food with a clean spoon. If baby wants a refill, use a fresh spoon to scoop it out.

breast milk or formula (but not regular cow's milk until your doctor has okayed it), or diluted juice; some children will initially accept only juice in a cup and not milk, others only take milk.

Use the sip-at-a-time technique: Put just a small amount of fluid in the cup. Hold the cup to baby's lips and pour a few drops into her mouth. Then take the cup away, giving her a chance to swallow without gagging. Stop each session when your baby signals she's had enough by turning her head, pushing the cup away, or starting to fuss.

Even with this technique, you can still expect that almost as much liquid will exit your baby's mouth as enters it. Eventually, with plenty of practice, patience, and perseverance, more will make its mark than escape it.

Encourage participation. Your baby may try to grab the cup from you, with an "I'd rather do it myself" attitude. Let her try. A very few babies can manage a cup

2. Canned foods are less nutritious than frozen or fresh and often are high in salt and/or sugar, so use them sparingly, if at all, for baby.

■ After you've taken a serving out of a jar, recap the remainder and refrigerate until it's needed again; if it hasn't been used within three days for juices and fruits, and two days for everything else, discard it.

■ It's not necessary to heat baby food (adults may have a preference for warm meats and vegetables, but babies have developed no such gustatory bias), but if you do, heat only enough for one meal and discard any unused heated portion. Do not heat baby's food in a microwave oven; though the container may stay cool, the inside continues cooking for a few minutes after you take it out, and may get hot enough to burn baby's mouth. Heat instead in an electric feeding dish or in a heat-resistant glass bowl over simmering water (hot water feeding dishes won't heat foods, but will keep them warm). When testing the temperature, stir up the food, then splash a drop on the inside of your wrist rather than taking a taste from baby's spoon; if you taste, use a fresh spoon for baby.

■ When preparing fresh baby foods, be certain utensils and work surfaces are clean. Keep cold foods cold and warm foods warm; foods spoil fastest between 60° and 120°F, so don't keep baby's food at those temperatures for more than an hour. (For adults, the safe period is closer to two or three hours.)

■ When the doctor okays egg whites for your baby, cook them well before serving. Raw whites can harbor salmonella. Do not give baby unpasteurized juice or cheese.

■ When tasting during food preparation, use a fresh spoon each time you taste, or wash the spoon between tastings.

■ *When in doubt* about the freshness of a food, *throw it out.*

■ On an outing, take unopened jars or dehydrated baby food (to which you can add fresh water). Carry any open jars or containers of anything that needs refrigeration in an insulated bag packed with ice or an ice pack, if it will be more than an hour before you serve it. Once the food no longer feels cool, don't feed it to the baby.

Another source of danger in baby's foodstuffs is chemical contamination—pesticides on fruits and vegetables, additives in prepared foods, accidental or incidental contaminants in meat, poultry, and fish (see page 241). Though for the most part, avoiding these chemicals means not buying foods containing them, you can also get rid of some of them in the kitchen:

■ Peel vegetables and fruit, when possible, unless they are certified organically grown.

■ Wash all fruits and vegetables that you don't peel in dish detergent and water, scrubbing with a stiff brush when practical. Rinse well to remove all traces of detergent.

even at this early age. Don't worry if she spills it all—that's part of the learning process. She can also learn by sharing the job, holding the cup along with you.

Take no for an answer. If your baby resists the cup, even after a few tries, and even after you've tried several different liquids and several different types of cups, don't pressure her to accept it. Instead, shelve the project for a couple of weeks. When you try again, use a new cup and a little fanfare ("Look what mommy has for you!") to try to generate excitement. Or you might try letting your conscientious objector handle an empty cup as a toy for a while.

FOOD ALLERGIES

"Both my husband and I have a lot of allergies. I'm worried that our son may have them, too."

Unfortunately, it isn't just the better traits—lustrous locks, long legs, musical ability, mechanical aptitude—that are inheritable. The less desirable ones are, too, and having two parents with allergies does make a baby much more likely to develop them than if he has two allergy-free parents. But that doesn't mean your baby is doomed to a lifetime of hives and sneezing. It does mean you should discuss your concerns with your baby's doctor, and if necessary with a specialist in pediatric allergies.

A baby becomes allergic to a substance when his immune system becomes sensitized to it by producing antibodies. Sensitization can take place the first time his body encounters a substance or the hundreth time. But once it does, antibodies rev into action whenever the substance is encountered, causing any one of a wide range of physical reactions, including runny nose and eyes, headache, wheezing, eczema, hives, diarrhea, abdominal pain or discomfort, violent vomiting, and in severe cases, anaphylactic shock. There is even some evidence that allergy may also manifest itself through behavioral symptoms, such as crankiness.

The most common food offenders include milk, eggs, peanuts, wheat, corn, fish, shellfish, berries, true nuts, peas and beans, chocolate, and some spices. In some cases even a tiny amount of a food causes a severe reaction; in others, small amounts don't seem to cause a problem at all. Children often outgrow food allergies, but later develop hypersensitivities to other substances in the environment, such as household dusts, pollens, and animal dander.

Not every adverse reaction to a food or other substance, however, is an allergy. In fact in some studies of children, specialists were able to confirm allergy in fewer than half the subjects—all of whom had been previously diagnosed as "allergic." What appears to be an allergy may sometimes be an enzyme deficiency. Children with insufficient levels of the enzyme lactase, for example, are unable to digest the milk sugar lactose, and thus react badly to milk and milk products. And those with celiac disease are unable to digest gluten, a substance found in many grains, and thus appear to be allergic to those grains. The workings of an immature digestive system or such common infant problems as colic

may also be misdiagnosed as allergy.

For infants in families with a history of allergy, doctors generally recommend the following precautions:

Breastfeeding. Bottle-fed babies are more likely to develop allergies than breastfed infants—probably because cow's milk is a relatively common cause of allergic reaction. If you are nursing your baby, continue, if possible, for the entire first year. The later cow's milk becomes a mainstay of his diet, the better. Using a soy-based formula when a supplement is needed is often suggested in allergic families, but some babies turn out to be allergic to soy, too.[3] For those babies, a protein hydrolysate formula will be needed.

Delaying solids. It's now believed that the later a baby is exposed to a potential allergen, the less likely it is that sensitization will take place. So most doctors recommend postponing solids in allergic families—starting no earlier than five months, often not until six, and sometimes later.

More gradual introduction of new foods. It's always wise to introduce new foods to a baby one at a time, but this is especially important in allergic families. It may be recommended that you give each new food every day for an entire week before starting another. If there is any kind of adverse reaction—looser movements, gassiness, rash (including diaper rash), excessive spitting up, wheezing, or runny nose—it's generally advised that the food be discontinued immediately and not be resumed for several weeks at least—at which time it may be accepted without distress.

Introduction of less allergenic foods first. Baby rice cereal, the least likely to cause allergy, is usually recommended as a

3. Occasionally, recent research indicates, babies can have an allergic reaction to egg or cow's milk protein in their mothers' milk. More study is needed to confirm this.

starter food. Barley and oats are less allergenic than, and are generally given before, wheat and corn. Most fruits and vegetables cause no problems, but parents are often advised to hold off on introducing berries and tomatoes. Shellfish and peas and beans can also wait. Most of the other highly allergenic foods (nuts, peanuts, spices, and chocolate) are not appropriate for babies anyway and can be introduced after two years of age.

Elimination diets and special liquid diets can be used to diagnose allergy, but they are complicated and time-consuming. Skin tests for food allergies are not highly accurate; a person can have a positive skin test to a particular food, yet have no reaction at all when he eats it. "Food sensitivity" screening tests that claim to diagnose allergies from blood samples are even less accurate, extremely expensive, and have not been approved by either the FDA or the American Academy of Pediatrics.

Happily, many childhood allergies are outgrown. So even if your baby is hypersensitive to milk or wheat now, he may no longer be in a few years—or even less.

For more on allergies and allergy testing, see page 413.

WALKERS

"My daughter seems very frustrated that she can't get around yet. She's not content to lie in her crib or sit in her infant seat, but I can't carry her all day. Can I put her in a walker yet?"

Both the baby (who is all revved up with no place to go) and the parent (because the only options seem to be either to carry baby around or listen to her cry) are frustrated in a situation like yours. Such frustrations are often at a peak from the time a baby begins to sit fairly well until she can get around on her own (by crawling, cruising, or whatever method she's devised). The obvious solution, until recently, was to get a walker—a seat set inside a table framework, on four wheeled legs. But because walkers are the cause annually of about 24,000 infant injuries that require medical treatment, and thousands more that are kissed-and-made-better at home, they are no longer recommended. Safer choices: a stationary walker or one that only goes around in circles; these give a certain amount of flexibility, though with less true freedom of movement than a walker.

If you nevertheless elect to use an ambulatory walker, keep in mind that it doesn't grant *you* freedom of movement—you must stay nearby and supervise closely. You should also see page 43 for tips on selecting a safe walker and:

Take your baby for a test drive. The best way to assess your baby's readiness for a walker is to let her try one out. If you don't have a friend whose baby has one, go to a store and let your baby try out a floor model. As long as she seems happy and doesn't slump pitifully in it, she's ready for a walker. Don't expect her to be able to go far yet; she may not go anywhere at first, and she's likely to take many steps backward before she takes one forward.

Don't walk out while she's "walking." Your baby should *never* be left unsupervised for even a moment when she's in a walker, even if she hasn't yet demonstrated any great mobility in it. A push off the wall and a couple of quick strides, and she could end up at the other end of the room—and out the door or down the stairs.

Do your childproofing early. Most any trouble a crawling or walking baby can get into, a baby in a walker can get into, too. So even if your baby can't get around without the help of a walker, she should be considered as hazardous to her own health as a mobile baby. Read "Making Home Safe for Baby" (page 292), and make all necessary adjustments before you let baby loose in her walker.

Keep dangers out of walker's way. The most potentially dangerous place for a baby in a walker to be is at the top of a flight of stairs; don't let your baby roam freely near a stairway in her walker, even if it is protected with a closed safety gate. Although most walker/stairway accidents occur on staircases where there is no safety gate or where a gate is left open, some do take place when a gate is not fastened to the wall securely. It's best, therefore, when your baby is in her walker, to block off entirely—with chairs or other heavy obstacles—areas leading to staircases. Other hazards to the walker-walking baby, which should be removed or blocked off before letting her loose, include room thresholds, changes in grade (as from carpet to linoleum or blacktop to grass), toys left on the floor, loose area rugs, and other low obstructions that can topple the walker.

Don't let her walk around the clock. Limit baby's time in the walker to thirty minutes per session. The walker gives a baby an artificial means of mobility, which might make her lazy about achieving mobility on her own. Every baby needs to spend some time on the floor, practicing skills that will eventually help her to crawl, such as lifting her belly off the ground while on all fours. She needs the opportunity to pull up on coffee tables and kitchen chairs in preparation for standing, and later, walking. She needs more chances to explore and handle safe objects in her environment than a walker allows. And, too, she needs the interaction with you and others that free play requires and allows.

Don't wait until she can walk before you take away the walker. As soon as your baby can get around some other way—crawling or cruising, for instance—put away the walker. Its purpose, you remember, was to ease your baby's frustration at being immobile. Keeping her in the walker not only won't help her to walk sooner, but its constant use may cause "walking confusion" (much as giving a baby a bottle before she's learned to suck at the breast can cause nipple confusion) because walking in a walker and walking solo require different body movements. The

walker doesn't require learning to balance or learning how to fall, both absolute necessities for walking independently. And traveling in it is, after all, easier, more fruitful, and less risky than those first few unassisted steps will be.

JUMPERS

"We received a jumping device, which hangs in the doorway, as a gift for our baby. He seems to enjoy it, but we're not sure if it's safe."

Most babies are ready and eager for vigorous exercise long before they're independently mobile. Which is why many enjoy the acrobatics they can perform in a baby jumper. But there are potential problems associated with the use of such devices. Some pediatric orthopedic specialists warn that certain kinds of injuries to the bones and joints can occur to babies using a jumper. In addition, baby's exhilaration with the freedom of movement afforded by the jumper can quickly turn to frustration as he discovers that no matter how or how much he moves his arms and legs, he's destined to stay put in the doorway.

If you do opt to use the jumper, check with the doctor about safety considerations. As with any baby-busying device (a walker, a swing, a pacifier, for example), be sure that you use it to meet your baby's needs, not yours; if he's unhappy in it, take him out immediately. And never leave your baby, even thoroughly contented, unattended in the jumper—even for a moment.

FEEDING CHAIRS

"So far I've been feeding my baby on my lap, but it's getting very messy. When can I put her in a high chair?"

Though there's no perfectly neat way to feed a baby (both of you will need washable wardrobes for some time to come),

SAFETY TIPS
FOR FEEDING CHAIRS

Feeding baby safely doesn't just mean introducing new foods gradually and being scrupulous about avoiding contamination from spoilage. In fact, feeding baby safely begins even before the first spoon is filled—when baby's placed in a feeding chair. To help make sure every mealtime passes safely, follow these rules:

All Feeding Chairs
■ Never leave a young baby unattended in a feeding chair; have the food, bib, napkins, utensils, and anything else necessary for the meal ready so that you don't have to leave your child alone while you fetch them.
■ Always secure the safety or restraining straps, even if your baby seems too young to climb out. Be sure to fasten the strap at the groin to prevent him or her from slipping out the bottom.
■ Keep all chair and eating surfaces clean (wash with detergent or soapy water and rinse thoroughly); babies have no compunctions about picking up a decaying morsel from a previous meal and munching on it.

High Chairs and Low Feeding Tables
■ Always be certain slide-off trays are safely snapped into place; an unsecured one could allow a lunging and unbelted baby to go flying out headfirst.
■ Check to be sure that a folding-type chair is safely locked into the open position and won't suddenly fold up with baby in it.

■ Place the chair away from any tables, counters, walls, or other surfaces that baby could possibly kick off from—causing the chair to tumble.
■ To protect baby's fingers, check their whereabouts before attaching or detaching the tray.

Hook-On Seats
■ Use the seat only on a stable wooden or metal table; do not use on glass-topped or loose-topped tables, tables with the support in the center (baby's weight could topple it), card tables, aluminum folding tables, or on a table leaf.
■ If a baby in a hook-on seat can rock the table, the table isn't stable enough; don't attach the seat to it.
■ Avoid using placemats or tablecloths, which can interfere with the gripping power of the seat.
■ Be certain any locks, clamps, or snap-together parts are securely fastened before putting your baby in the seat; always take your baby out of the seat before releasing or unfastening them. Be sure the clamps are always clean and functioning properly.
■ Don't put a chair or other object under the seat as a safeguard should baby fall, or position the seat opposite a table brace or leg; a baby can push off against such surfaces, dislodging the seat. And don't allow a large dog or older child under the seat while baby is in it, because they might also dislodge it from below.

using a feeding chair of some sort does minimize the mess while maximizing the efficiency of the feeding process. While a baby still needs support to sit, an infant seat (with baby strapped in and under your *constant* supervision) can double as a feeding seat. Once she can sit up fairly well by herself, it's time to change to a high chair or other type of feeding table.

Most babies will slip, slide, and slump in their new seat at first. Small pillows, rolled towels, or a baby quilt or blanket can be used to wedge a novice sitter in snugly, and fastening the safety belt or tether (which should be fastened in any case) should help, too.

WHAT IT'S IMPORTANT TO KNOW: Environmental Hazards and Your Baby

What effect does growing up in a world of questionable safety, filled with contaminants and pollutants and suspected and proven carcinogens (things that cause cancer) and mutagens (things that cause changes in the genes), have on the young and vulnerable bodies of babies? How vigilant do parents have to be to protect their children from such dangers?

Fortunately life is not quite as perilous as many mothers fear or many journalists suggest. And, as during pregnancy, there are far more factors influencing a child's long-term health that are within a mother's control than are not. Ensuring adequate well-baby and sick-baby care from birth. Getting her baby off to the best nutritional start possible. Encouraging healthy lifestyle habits, such as exercise, and discouraging unhealthy ones, such as smoking and alcohol abuse, through example.

But there are some hazards in our environment that we control only partially or indirectly. And though they are believed to present a smaller risk than those things we can control, they do pose some perils. They are of particular concern to parents of young children because children are more susceptible to damage by the environment than adults. One reason is their smaller body size—the same dose of a hazardous substance could do considerably more damage. Another is the fact that their organs are still in the process of maturation, and thus are more vulnerable to insults of various kinds. Still another is the longer life span a child is looking forward to; since the damage often takes many years to develop, it has more time to develop in a child. Clearly then, it makes sense to know what the potential risks are and what, if anything, you can do about them.

But it is also important to keep in mind that there is no possibility of a risk-free world, only a less risky one. We are constantly in the position of having to weigh risks against benefits: penicillin saves millions of lives but in a rare instance takes a life (the benefit is clearly worth the risk); tobacco gives a great deal of pleasure to smokers, but is responsible for hundreds of thousands of premature deaths annually (most would agree the benefit is not worth the risks); tens of thousands of people die in auto accidents annually in the U.S., but the auto provides the benefit of needed transportation for billions of passenger miles (here, most seem to agree that the benefits outweigh the risks).

We can't eliminate all risks, but we can reduce them to a greater or lesser extent in most instances. In the case of penicillin, for example, we can reduce risks by not giving the drug to anyone who has shown an adverse reaction to it previously. In the case of tobacco use, smokers can somewhat reduce their risks by not inhaling (though they increase the risks of those around them that way), or by using low-tar or low-nicotine cigarettes (though smokers often smoke more to compensate for the lost chemicals) or by smoking fewer cigarettes (though they then often smoke more of each one). And in the case of auto use, we can cut risks tremendously by careful and sober driving, avoiding excessive speeds, choosing safer cars, and using such safety equipment as infant car seats and seat belts.

All of the following present both risks and benefits, but reducing the risks is almost always possible.

HOUSEHOLD PESTICIDES

Household pests carry and transmit disease, are aesthetically unappealing, and, in the case of rodents, can inflict painful and dangerous bites. But most home pesticides are dangerous poisons, particularly in the hands (or mouths) of infants and toddlers. You can minimize the risk while achieving the benefits of keeping home and hearth free of infestation with the following:

Blocking tactics. Use window screens and screen or otherwise close off entry points for insects and vermin.

Sticky insect or rodent traps. Not dependent on killer chemicals, these trap crawling insects in enclosed boxes (roach traps) or containers (ant traps), flies on old-fashioned fly paper, mice on sticky rectangles. Because human skin can stick to these surfaces (often the separation can be painful), these traps, when open, must still be kept out of the reach of children or put out after they are in bed at night and taken up before they are up and around in the morning. And they have the disadvantage of prolonging the death of rodents.

Box traps. The tenderhearted can catch rodents in box traps and then let the victims loose in fields or woods far from residential areas, though this isn't always easy. Because these rodents can bite, the traps should be kept out of the reach of children or put out when children are not around.

Safe use of chemical pesticides. Virtually all, including the much-touted boric acid, are highly toxic not just to pests but to humans as well. If you opt to use them, *do not* spread them (or store them) where babies or children can get to them or on surfaces where food is prepared. Always use the least toxic substance (check with your local EPA or health department). If you use a spray, keep the children out of the house while spraying and for the rest of the day, at least. Better still, have the spraying done while you're on vacation, visiting grandma, or otherwise away from home. When you return, open all the windows to air out the house or apartment.

LEAD

For years it has been known that large doses of lead could cause severe brain damage in children. Now it is also recognized that even in relatively small doses, lead can reduce IQ, alter enzyme function, retard growth, damage the kidneys, as well as cause learning and behavior problems, hearing and attention deficiencies. It may even have negative effects on the immune system.

It makes sense, then, for parents to know what the sources of lead are in their baby's environment and what can be done to minimize exposure.

Lead paint. In spite of legislation prohibiting its use, lead paint continues to be the major source of lead exposure in children. Many older homes still harbor lead paint, often containing very high concentrations of lead beneath layers of newer applications. As paint cracks or flakes, microscopic lead-containing particles are shed. These end up on baby's hands, toys, clothing—and eventually in the mouth. If there is the possibility of lead in your housepaint, have all the paint professionally removed—while the family, especially children and any pregnant women, are out. And be certain that any painted object— toy, crib, or anything else your baby comes in contact with—is lead free. Be particularly wary of items that are imported or were purchased outside the U.S.

Gasoline emissions. Until federal regulations were passed that resulted in the elimination of most of the lead in automotive fuel, this was a major source of lead in our environment. Thanks to the legislation, lead levels in the air and in exposed individuals have been dramatically reduced.

Drinking water. The EPA estimates that the water in tens of millions of American homes is probably contaminated with lead. The lead usually leaches into the water in buildings where there are lead

---

EPA HOTLINE

Call toll-free 1-800-426-4791

---

pipes or where pipes are soldered with lead, especially where the water is particularly corrosive. Since most of the contamination occurs once the water has entered individual buildings rather than in the public water supply, most communities haven't made major efforts to correct the problem. If you fear your drinking water may be contaminated by lead (or other hazardous substance), have it tested by the local water department, department of health, or EPA, if they do such testing, or by a state certified private testing agency. If lead is found, you can install a reverse osmosis filter (which removes not only lead but beneficial fluorides as well) on your kitchen sink. Or you can let the tap water run for at least three minutes before using for drinking or cooking. Avoid using water from the hot tap for cooking, since it leaches more lead, and don't boil water for more than five minutes, which concentrates lead in the water.

Soil. Lead housepaint that flakes off, industrial residue, dust from the demolition of houses that have been painted with lead can all end up contaminating the soil. Though you needn't be fanatic, do try to keep your baby from ingesting fistfuls of the stuff.

Newspapers and magazines. Because of the high level of lead in printing inks, particularly those used in four-color illustrations, these reading materials should not be a regular part of your baby's diet. When baby stops skimming headlines and starts mouthing, it's time for a change of activity.

In addition to keeping your child away from known sources of lead, you should also try to increase his or her resistance to

lead poisoning with good nutrition, particularly adequate levels of iron and calcium. And ask the doctor about screening tests for lead, particularly if you live in a possibly high risk area.

OTHERWISE CONTAMINATED WATER

Most water in the U.S. is fit to drink, but a small percentage (about 2%) of community water supplies contain substances that pose significant health risks. Water systems purified with activated charcoal rather than chlorine are believed to provide safer water, but only a few water districts presently use this type of purification. If you suspect your water is not safe, check with your local EPA about how to have it tested. Should it turn out to be contaminated, a water purifier can often make it safe to drink. Which type of purifier will be best for your home will depend on the contaminants in your water and how much you can spend.

POLLUTED INDOOR AIR

Most babies spend a great deal of time indoors, so the quality of the air they breathe there is extremely significant. Because the air in a home can, on occasion, be as polluted as that on a busy highway, be alert for the following indoor air risks:

Nonstick cookware fumes. Apparently safe for cooking purposes, the fumes given off by Teflon or Silverstone coatings when they are overheated or burning can be extremely toxic. There have been numerous reports of birds dying from exposure to such fumes and of adults coming down with "polymer fume fever." The long-term effects of Teflon toxicosis are unknown, but may include such potentially serious changes in the lungs as fibrosis and scarring. Nor are the effects on children known. To prevent any possible problems in your home, never use nonstick drip pans on your range (they overheat rapidly), never use any nonstick cookware at high temperature settings (on range top or in oven, especially to catch drips on the oven bottom), and never leave such cookware unattended (so that liquids could cook out, allowing burning of the surface).

Carbon monoxide. This colorless, odorless, tasteless, but treacherous gas (it can cause lung ailments, impair vision and brain functioning, and is fatal in high doses) that results from the burning of fuel can seep into your home from many sources: improperly vented wood stoves or kerosene heaters (have the fire department check venting); slow-burning wood stoves (speed up burning by keeping the damper open); poorly adjusted or unvented gas stoves or other appliances (have adjustment checked periodically—the flame should be blue—and install an exhaust fan to the outside to remove fumes); gas ranges each time they are turned on (an electric ignition reduces the amount of combustion gases released); fireplaces with residue-blocked chimneys (fires should never be left to smolder, and chimneys should be cleaned regularly); an attached garage (never leave a car idling, even briefly, in a garage that shares a wall or ceiling with your home, since the fumes can seep through).

Benzopyrenes. A long list of respiratory illnesses (from eye, nose, and throat irritation to asthma and bronchitis to emphysema and cancer) can be attributed to presence of the tarlike organic particles that result from the incomplete combustion of tobacco or wood. To prevent your baby's exposure, allow no tobacco smoking in your home (let smoking guests step out to light up), be sure the flue that vents smoke from a wood fire does not leak, vent combustion appliances (such as driers) to the outdoors, change air filters on various appliances regularly, and increase ventilation in your home. Tight weatherstripping will keep heat in more efficiently, but will also trap potentially dangerous fumes.

Particulate matter. A wide variety of particles, invisible to the naked eye, can fill the air in our homes and present a hazard to our children. They come from such sources as household dust (which can trigger allergies in susceptible children), tobacco smoke, wood smoke, unvented gas appliances, kerosene heaters, and asbestos construction materials (which contribute to a wide variety of diseases including some

UNSAFE PLAY SAND

Bad news for tiny sand lovers. Recent evidence indicates that an occasional batch of play sand may be contaminated with a type of asbestos called tremolite. The tremolite fibers float in the air, and if breathed can cause serious illness. The problem is more severe indoors, where sand tends to be dry and dusty, than outdoors, where it is often damp. Though it's virtually impossible for you to learn if the sand your baby digs in (at home or at a daycare center or in the playground) is contaminated, you can determine if it is dusty, and possibly risky to breathe. Return or get rid of the sand if it makes a cloud of dust when you dump a pailful, or if when you mix a spoonful in a glass of water the water remains cloudy once the sand settles. Find another source, preferably ordinary beach sand (a lot of play sand is ground up stone or marble).

cancers and heart disease). The same pre-cautions (no smoking, proper venting, filter changing) discussed above can minimize this threat. Air filter units can often remove many of these particles and are particularly useful if someone in the family has al-lergies. If you find asbestos in your home that may need removal, get professional assistance in dealing with it before particles begin to fly.

Miscellaneous fumes. Fumes from cleaning fluids, from some aerosol sprays (if they contain fluorocarbons, they can also be hazardous to the environment), and from turpentine and other painting-related materials can be highly toxic. If you use these substances at all, always use the least toxic product (water-based paints, beeswax floor waxes, paint thinners made from plant oils), use it in a well-ventilated area (even better, out of doors), and never use it when infants or children are nearby. Store these, like all other household products, safely out of reach of curious little hands. They are best stored in outdoor storage areas where, if they begin to evaporate, fumes won't seep into living areas.

Formaldehyde. With so many products in our modern world containing for-maldehyde (from the resins in particle-board furniture to the sizing in decorator fabrics, and the adhesives in carpeting), it isn't surprising that the gas, which has been found to cause nasal cancer in animals and respiratory problems, rashes, nausea, and other symptoms in humans, is everywhere. The levels of formaldehyde gas released are highest when an item is new, but the gases can continue to be released for years. To minimize the potential damage, look for products that are formaldehyde-free when building or furnishing your home. To re-duce the effects of formaldehyde already in your home, seal such materials as particle-board with an epoxy sealer, or even simpler and nicer, invest in a small indoor garden. Fifteen or twenty houseplants can appar-ently absorb the formaldehyde gas in an average-size house. If you suspect high lev-els of formaldehyde in your home, contact the 3-M Corporation in St. Paul, Min-nesota, which produces a testing device.

Radon. This colorless, odorless, radio-active gas, a naturally occurring product of the decay of uranium in rocks and soil, is the second leading cause of lung cancer in the U.S. Breathed in by unsuspecting resi-dents of homes in which it has accumu-lated, it bombards the lungs with radiation. Such exposure over many years can lead to cancer.

Accumulation occurs when the gas seeps into a home from decaying rocks and soil beneath it and is retained because of poor ventilation in the structure. Taking the following precautions can help prevent the serious consequences of radon:

▢ Before you buy a home, especially in a high-radon area, have it tested for radon contamination. Your local or state EPA can give you information on where to turn for testing.
▢ If you live in a high-radon area, or sus-pect your home may be contaminated, have it tested. Ideally testing should take place over a several month period to obtain an average. Levels are usually higher in seasons when windows are closed.
▢ If your home turns out to have high levels of radon, consult the EPA for help in locating a radon abatement company in your community and ask them for any written material they might have on the subject of radon reduction. The first step will probably be to seal cracks and other openings in the foundation walls and floors. More important will be in-creasing ventilation by opening win-dows, installing vents in crawl spaces, attics, and other closed spaces, and eliminating airtight weatherstripping and air-to-air heat exchangers. In some cases, a special house-wide ventilation system may be needed.

CONTAMINANTS IN FOOD

In this world of mass production, manufacturers have learned to use chemicals of various sorts to make the foods they produce look better, feel better, taste better (or at least more like the real thing), and last longer. But even foods that haven't passed through a manufacturing plant are often contaminated—by pesticides or other chemicals used in growing or storing, or picked up incidentally from water or soil. In many cases, the risks from such chemi-

cals to humans is either unknown or believed to be small, sometimes smaller than the risks from "natural" foods such as coconut oil (which can contribute to heart disease) or spoiled peanuts (the aflatoxins in them can cause cancer). Nevertheless, it's prudent to protect your baby by following these basic rules when selecting and preparing foods:

■ Don't buy processed foods with a lot of chemical additives. Such foods, in addition to their chemical content, are usually less nutritious than fresh, and thus make poor

---

WHAT TO KEEP OUT OF THE MOUTHS OF BABES

■ Smoked or cured meats, such as hot dogs, bologna, and bacon. Usually high in fat and cholesterol as well as in nitrates and other chemicals, and sometimes containing bone meal (which can be contaminated with lead and other substances), these should be served to babies rarely, if at all.

■ Smoked fish, such as smoked salmon or whitefish. Usually cured with nitrites to protect freshness, they are not ideal infant foods.

■ Fish from contaminated waters. Your local department of health should be able to give you information on which fish are safe and which aren't at any particular time in your community, and which can be served only occasionally. Or call 800-FDA-4010.

■ Foods or beverages such as coffee, tea, cocoa, and chocolate that contain caffeine or related compounds. Caffeine can make a baby jittery or worse, can interfere with absorption of calcium, and can replace worthwhile dietary items.

■ Imitation foods, such as nondairy creamers (full of fat, sugar, and chemicals), frozen tofu desserts (ditto), citrus or other fruit drinks or beverages (contain unneeded sugar and, sometimes, chemicals). Feed food, not chemical cocktails, to your baby.

■ Herbal teas. These often contain questionable substances (comfrey tea, for ex-

ample, contains a carcinogen) and frequently have unwanted, even dangerous, effects on the body.

■ Vitamin supplements, other than those designed for infants (and given as directed). Excessive vitamins can be particularly harmful to babies, whose bodies don't process them as quickly as adult bodies do. The acid in chewable vitamin C can damage tooth enamel and should be avoided by both adults and children.

■ Raw fish, such as in sushi. Young children don't chew well enough to destroy the parasites that might dwell therein and that could cause serious illness.

■ Alcoholic beverages. No one would put this on a baby's regular diet, but some folks do think it's fun to give a baby a sip—a dangerous game, both because alcohol can be poisonous for a baby and because it can give the infant a taste for the stuff.

■ Tap water that is contaminated with lead, PCBs, or any other hazardous material. Check with your local EPA or water department, or have your water tested privately if you suspect contamination.

■ Fruits or vegetables known to be contaminated. When news stories announce that a particular fruit or vegetable may be hazardous, avoid buying it until its name has been cleared or until you can buy an uncontaminated variety.

■ Unpasteurized apple juice or cider.

FOOD HAZARDS IN PERSPECTIVE

Though it makes sense to limit chemicals in your family's diet when you can, fear of additives and chemicals can so limit the variety of foods your family eats that it can interfere with good nutrition. It's important to remember that a well-balanced nutritious diet, high in whole grains and fruits and vegetables (especially cruciferous ones like broccoli, cauliflower, and Brussels sprouts, and those high in vitamin A, such as green leafies and deep yellows) will not only provide the nutrients needed for growth and good health, but will also help to counteract the effects of possible carcinogens in the environment. So limit chemical intake when practical, but don't drive yourself and your family crazy in the process.

choices for a child's diet. Though many common food additives are believed to be safe, there are also many of questionable safety. Be particularly wary of foods containing any of the following: brominated vegetable oils (BVO), butylated hydroxyanisole (BHA), butylated hydroxytoluene (BHT), caffeine, monosodium glutamate (MSG), propyl gallate, quinine, saccharin, sodium nitrate and sodium nitrite, sulfites, and artificial colors and flavors, all of which are on the "avoid" list of the Center for Science in the Public Interest. Questionable are carrageenan, hyptyl paraben, phosphoric acid and other phosphorus compounds (not because phosphorus is dangerous, but because excesses could cause dietary imbalance, particularly of calcium).

■ Don't give your baby foods containing artificial sweeteners. Saccharin has been shown to cause cancer in animals and remains on the market only because it is believed to be a valuable weight control aid. Since infants do not need—and should not be put on—calorie-restricted diets, the sweetener doesn't belong in a baby's diet. And though the sweetener aspartame (Equal, Nutrasweet) does appear to be safe for normal individuals,[4] and may even be for infants (extensive testing has not taken place in the very young), it doesn't belong in a baby's diet either, again because calorie restriction is inappropriate.

■ Buy fruits and vegetables that are free of chemicals, when possible. (But don't worry when it's not possible, since risks from such chemicals are believed by many scientists to be small.) Locally grown produce in season tends to be safest, since large quantities of chemicals aren't needed to preserve it during shipping or storage. Also safer are foods with heavy protective husks, leaves, or skin (such as corn, cauliflower, and bananas) that keep out pesticides. Food that doesn't look perfect (has blemishes and black spots) may also be safer, since it's usually chemical protection that keeps foods looking beautiful. In most instances, U.S. produce is less contaminated than imported (though the reverse is true with grapefruit, pears, spinach, onions, and sweet and white potatoes at the present time). Buying foods that are labeled "organically grown" may help, but it isn't always a guarantee of freedom from chemicals (see page 243).

■ Peel fruits and vegetables before using (particularly those with a waxy finish), or wash with water and dish detergent, scrubbing with a stiff brush when feasible. Don't try the brush on lettuce or strawberries; do use it on apples and zucchini. This, unfortunately, won't remove systemic chemical residues, but does offer some protection.

---

4. Aspartame should not be used by those with Phenylketonuria (PKU) or anyone else who has difficulty metabolizing phenylalanine, one of the constituents of the sweetener.

■ Keep baby's diet as varied as possible once a wide-range of foods have been introduced. Variety adds more than spice to life—it adds a measure of safety (not to mention better nutrition by providing a wide range of vitamins and minerals from different sources). Instead of always offering apple juice, vary the juices from day to day (apple one day, orange the next, apricot the third, and pear the fourth). Vary the protein foods, cereals and breads, and fruits and vegetables you serve, too. Though this won't always be easy—many children fall into, and won't budge from, food ruts—it's important to make the effort.

■ Limit your baby's intake of animal fat (other than that in milk or formula) because the fat is where chemicals (antibiotics, pesticides, and so on) are stored.

Cook with oil or margarine instead of butter (better for the heart, too), trim fats from meat, trim fat and skin from poultry. And keep portions of beef, pork, and chicken small. When possible, choose meat and poultry labeled as having been raised without chemicals or antibiotics.

■ Never feed your baby fish caught in possibly contaminated waters (see page 241).

■ Don't use foods of questionable freshness. Some of the greatest dangers in the food supply are from spoiled foods. Not only can they cause food poisoning (see page 230 for prevention of this problem), but certain ones, such as spoiled peanuts, corn, or other grains on which aflatoxins have formed, can actually contribute to the development of cancer.

■ Keep abreast of the latest in food safety through reading your local newspapers,

ORGANIC FOODS—GROWING AVAILABILITY

Organically grown foods are appearing more often in health food stores and even in some supermarkets. But for most of us it still isn't possible to fill our shopping carts with nothing but the purest organic foods. Not enough of them are being produced, and what is available is expensive. But as demand grows and as farmers discover that organic farming is not only better for their customers, their environment, and themselves, as well as the fact that it can also be lucrative, more acreage will be plowed and planted without the use of chemicals. And we will continue to find a growing supply of organics at the grocery.

At present, unfortunately, there are no federal standards, so not everything labeled "organic" was grown without herbicides, pesticides, or other chemicals. Look for certification by a state or private agency.

Fortunately for young children and their parents, more and more jarred organic baby foods—preparations that are untainted by chemicals, as well as having no added sugar or salt—are turning up at the supermarket as well as at health food stores. Everything a fledgling eater can desire can be found in an organic line, from beginner cereals and strained fruits, vegetables and meats, to combination main courses. Toddler foods will also be available soon.

Buying organic, when you can find what you need and can afford the often higher prices, serves a couple of purposes. One, of course, is protecting your family from unwanted chemicals. Though there is no hard evidence linking chemically treated foods with illness in humans, there certainly has not been enough study to prove beyond a doubt that there aren't any long term effects. The second purpose is to encourage markets to stock organic products. If organic foods are not available in your neighborhood, ask your supermarket or produce store to carry them; consumer interest will help bring the supply up and the prices down. And, again, don't worry if you can't find or can't afford organic produce—the risks involved with serving up other produce are small.

subscribing to a sensible, non-alarmist food-health newsletter such as the *Nutrition Action Healthletter* of the Center for Science in the Public Interest (1501 16th Street NW, Washington, DC 20036-1499), and adjusting your family's diet accordingly.

- Feed foods that are believed to have an anti-cancer effect, such as cruciferous vegetables (broccoli, Brussels sprouts, cauliflower, cabbage), dried peas and beans, foods rich in beta carotene (carrots, pumpkin, sweet potatoes, broccoli, cantaloupe), and those high in fiber (whole grains, fresh fruits and vegetables).

- Remember that while it's sensible to be cautious, hysteria is unwarranted. Even by the most pessimistic estimates, only a small percentage of cancers are caused by chemical contamination of foods. The risks to your child's health from tobacco, alcohol, poor diet, lack of immunization, or ignoring such safety precautions as seat belts are considerably greater.

YOUR ROLE AS A CONSUMER

Taking all the precautions we can in safeguarding our children against environmental threats isn't enough. To protect their future, and the future of their children, we need to reach out and put pressure on those who control those things we don't have total control of: the outdoor air, the food we eat, the water we drink—and the government that regulates them. In the long run, making your appeal heard may be one of the most important things you can do for your baby. Pressure your representatives—local, state and federal—to legislate stricter regulations of chemicals used in growing and processing foods, and clear labeling of foods containing chemical residues (such as antibiotics in chickens, Alar on apples). Also write the FDA and EPA to express your concern about the proliferation of chemicals in foods. For more information, write the Center for Science in the Public Interest, 1501 16th Street, N.W., Washington, D.C., 20036

AN APPLE A DAY—BACK IN STYLE

The furor raised about the use of Alar (daminozide) in the late 1980s is an example of how, on the one hand, extremist pronouncements can confuse consumers and, on the other hand, of how public pressure can affect public policy. Used to hasten the ripening of fruit (mostly apples, grapes, and peanuts), Alar raised concern because some studies showed it might be a cancer threat, particularly for small children, who tend to consume gallons of apple juice weekly. There was so much fear raised in the minds of concerned parents, that many banned apples and all apple products from their homes and their children's diets. Some even began to limit fruits and vegetables of all kinds. This extremism was unwarranted, and may have deprived children temporarily of needed vitamins and minerals. But the fact that consumers did raise their voices, did refuse to buy Alar-tainted products, and did question store managers and manufacturers, helped to bring about an immediate drop in the use of the chemical and subsequent legislation to ban it from the orchards entirely. The moral: Don't panic in the face of food threats, but do make your voice heard.

CHAPTER NINE

The Sixth Month

WHAT YOUR BABY MAY BE DOING

By the end of this month, your baby ...should be able to (see Note):

■ keep head level with body when pulled to sitting (6⅓ months)
■ say ah-goo or similar vowel-consonant combinations

Note: If your baby seems not to have reached one or more of these milestones, check with the doctor. In rare instances the delay could indicate a problem, though in most cases it will turn out to be normal for your baby. Premature infants generally reach milestones later than others of the same birth age, often achieving them closer to their adjusted age (the age they would be if they had been born at term) or sometimes later.

...will probably be able to:

■ bear some weight on legs when held upright
■ sit without support (by 6½ months)

...may possibly be able to:

■ stand holding on to someone or something
■ feed self a cracker (5⅓ months)
■ object if you try to take a toy away

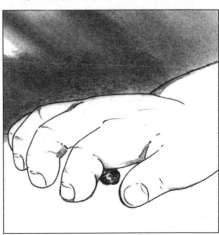

Some babies can pick up small and possibly dangerous objects with their fists — so be wary of leaving such things within reach.

- work to get to a toy out of reach
- pass a cube or other object from one hand to the other
- look for dropped object
- rake a raisin and pick it up in fist (5½ months)
- turn in the direction of a voice
- babble, combining vowels and consonants such as ga-ga-ga, ba-ba-ba, ma-ma-ma, da-da-da (by 6⅓ months)

...may even be able to:

- pull up to standing position from sitting
- get into a sitting position from stomach
- pick up tiny object with any part of thumb and finger
- say mama or dada indiscriminately

WHAT YOU CAN EXPECT AT THIS MONTH'S CHECKUP

Each doctor or nurse practitioner will have a personal approach to well-baby checkups. The overall organization of the physical exam, as well as the number and type of assessment techniques used and procedures performed will also vary with the individual needs of the child. But, in general, you can expect the following at a checkup when your baby is about six months old.

- Questions about how you and baby and the rest of the family are doing at home, and about baby's eating, sleeping, and general progress, and about child care, if you are working.
- Measurement of baby's weight, length, and head circumference, and plotting of progress since birth.
- Physical exam, including a recheck of any previous problems. Mouth will probably be checked now and at future visits for the arrival, or imminent arrival, of teeth. The posterior fontanel, on the back of the head, will have closed by now; the anterior fontanel, on the top of the head, will probably now begin to grow smaller.
- Developmental assessment. The examiner may rely on observation plus your reports on what baby is doing, or may actually put baby through a series of evaluation "tests," such as head control when pulled to sitting; vision; hearing; ability to reach for and grasp objects, to rake at tiny objects, to roll over and bear some weight on legs; and social interaction and vocalization.

- Third round of immunizations, if baby is in good health and there are no other contraindications. See page 153 for recommended schedule, which may vary depending on situation. Be sure to discuss any reactions to previous immunizations beforehand.
- Possibly, a hemoglobin or hematocrit test to check for anemia (usually by means of a pin prick on the finger), particularly for low-birth-weight babies.
- Guidance about what to expect in the next month in relation to such topics as feeding, sleeping, development, and safety.
- Recommendations about fluoride supplementation if needed in your area, and vitamin D supplementation if your baby is breastfed. Recommendations about iron supplementation for babies not on iron-fortified formula.

Questions you may want to ask, if the doctor hasn't already answered them:

- What reactions can you expect baby to have on the third round of immunizations? How should you treat them? Which reactions should you call about?

■ What foods can be introduced to baby now? Can baby get milk in a cup?

Also raise concerns that have arisen over the past month. Jot down information and instructions from the doctor (you're sure to forget them, otherwise). Record all pertinent information (baby's weight, length, head circumference, immunizations, illnesses, medications given, foods that can now be introduced, and so on) in a permanent health record.

FEEDING YOUR BABY THIS MONTH: Commercial or Home-Prepared Baby Foods

When baby foods made their debut on supermarket shelves in the 1930s, they were met gratefully by harried and weary mothers eager to stow away their food mills, proud to enter the age of modern convenience. Today, still at least as harried and weary and even more short on time, many mothers are shunning the commercial baby food products and returning instead to shifts at the food mill (or, more likely, the blender or food processor). And those who do opt for convenience often do so with embarrassment.

Do commercial baby foods deserve the bad label they've been plastered with lately? Are they any less wholesome than homemade? Is homemade more nutritious—and safer? Read on before you decide.

COMMERCIAL BABY FOOD

The turn-around in attitudes toward commercial baby foods came about in the 1970s when it was discovered that the foods mothers were buying because they thought they were especially good for their babies might be especially harmful. They contained added sugar and salt, non-nutritive fillers and thickeners, and questionable additives such as MSG. With this discovery came improvements in commercial baby food formulations, partly due to pressure from consumers and the medical community, and partly due to the industry's desire to improve both its product and its image.

Today's commercial baby foods usually contain no added salt or chemicals, and sugar and fillers are rarely added to single-ingredient varieties. The convenience that was always a plus still is; foods come in ready-to-serve, baby-portion jars, reclosable for refrigerated storage of leftovers. But there are many other pluses as well. Since the fruits and vegetables are cooked and packed soon after picking, they retain a reliably high proportion of their nutrients. The foods are consistent in texture and taste, and are safe and sanitary. They are also relatively economical, particularly if the time you save by using them is valuable to you, and when you consider that less food is likely to be wasted than when you prepare large batches.

The advantages of using commercial baby foods are greatest in the early months of feeding solids. The strained varieties are the perfect consistency for beginners, and single-ingredient starter foods make it easy to screen for allergies. Although major manufacturers do offer graduated textures for use as babies are ready for them, many families dispense with commercially prepared foods as soon as their young are able to handle softly cooked, mashed, coarsely chopped, or flaked foods from the family menu. They may still find ready-to-eat convenient for travel, however, and good to have on hand for emergencies or when they're going to be eating out.

Of course, not everything sold as "baby food" is good for babies. Read labels, and avoid such ingredients as sugar or corn syrup, salt, modified food starch and other thickeners, partially or completely hydrogenated shortening or fat, monosodium glutamate (MSG), artificial flavors or colors, and preservatives. The sugar added to some cereals, fruits, and other desserts is just not necessary for an infant, whose taste buds are unspoiled and completely content with the natural sweetness of such foods. (If you want to occasionally treat junior to something extra sweet, use the recipes beginning on page 618 or purchase products sweetened only with fruit juice concentrates.) A few custards and puddings contain eggs; if your baby hasn't been introduced to them yet, avoid these desserts.

"Instant," or dehydrated, baby foods offer great convenience because they're lightweight, don't need refrigeration after opening, and can be mixed with liquids other than water to increase nutritive value. But they have some drawbacks: first of all, some of them contain partially hydrogenated or saturated vegetable oils and/or starchy fillers, ingredients your baby doesn't need. Second, the nutritive value of the instant as compared to the jarred foods is sometimes lower. Finally, the taste of a rehydrated dehydrated food is unavoidably different from the fresh, possibly confusing baby's taste buds when he or she moves on to table foods. So while dehydrated baby foods may be extremely handy on a trip, they probably aren't the best for your baby all of the time.

"Organic" baby foods are new on the market, but are expensive and not widely available. These offerings are safe and provide good nutrition, but don't worry if you can't find or afford them. Commercial varieties, while not organic, are usually free of known potential hazards (such as MSG, Alar, preservatives, and colorings) and present no risk to your baby.

HOME-PREPARED BABY FOODS

If you have the time, the energy, and the motivation, there's nothing wrong, of course, with making your own baby foods—assuming you follow these rules:

- When introducing a new food, prepare and serve it without any other ingredients.
- Don't add sugar or salt. If you're cooking for the whole family, remove baby's portion before adding salt and spices.
- Don't add fat to baby's food, either in cooking or at the table.
- Don't cook in copper pots, as this may destroy vitamin C.
- Don't cook acidic foods (such as tomatoes) in aluminum, since this can cause small quantities of aluminum to dissolve and be absorbed into the food.
- Steam, pressure cook, or waterless-cook vegetables, exposing them to a minimum of light, air, heat, and water.
- Boil, microwave, or bake potatoes in their skins and peel after cooking.
- Never add baking soda; it may preserve color, but it depletes vitamins and minerals.
- Don't soak or boil dried legumes (peas or beans) overnight; bring to a *full* boil, boil them for two minutes, then let them stand for an hour, and cook in the soaking water.
- Follow the principles of safe food preparation in Feeding Baby Safely on page 230.

For the first several weeks of feeding solids or at least until baby is six months old, the food you serve should be finely puréed, and strained or sieved (though you can mash bananas and thin with liquid). For convenience, you can prepare a batch of carrots, peas, or other vegetables, then freeze in ice cube trays. Keep individual cubes stored in airtight freezer bags. Before using, thaw in the refrigerator, in a double boiler, in a microwave (at defrost, not cooking, settings), or under cold water (still in the plastic bag)—not at room temperature.

WHAT YOU MAY BE CONCERNED ABOUT

CHANGES IN BOWEL MOVEMENTS

"Since I started my breastfed baby on solids last week, his bowel movements have been more solid—which I would expect—but they are also darker and smellier. Is this normal?"

Alas, the time when everything that passed through your baby came out sweet and innocent is past. For the breastfeeding mother, the change from soft, mustardy, nonoffensive stools to thick, dark, smelly ones can be something of a shock. But, though the change may not be aesthetically pleasing, it is normal. Expect your baby's stools to become increasingly adult-like as his diet does—though a breastfed baby's may remain somewhat softer than a bottlefed's up until weaning.

"I just gave my baby carrots for the first time, and his next bowel movement was bright orange."

What goes in must come out. And in babies, with their immature digestive systems, it sometimes doesn't change very much in the process. Once they start solids, stools seem to vary movement to movement, often reflecting the most recent meal in color or texture. Later, foods not chewed thoroughly, especially those that are harder to digest, may come out whole or nearly so. As long as bowel movements don't also contain mucus and aren't unusually loose, which might signal gastrointestinal irritation (and the need to withhold the offending food for a few weeks), you can continue his newly varied diet without concern.

BOTTLE REJECTION

"I'd like to give my baby an occasional supplementary bottle of expressed milk to free me up a little, but she refuses to drink it. What can I do?"

Your baby wasn't born yesterday. And unlike a relative newcomer she's developed a strong sense of what she wants, what she doesn't want, and how she can best go about getting things her way. What she wants: your nice, soft, warm breasts. What she doesn't want: a fabricated rubber or plastic nipple. How she can best go about getting things her way: crying for the former, and rejecting the latter.

Waiting this long to introduce a bottle into your baby's life has turned the odds against you; the introduction is better made at about six weeks (see page 143). But it's still possible that you'll be able to win her over by following these tips:

Feed her on an empty stomach. Many babies will be more receptive to the bottle as a source of nourishment when they're in the market for something nourishing. So try offering the bottle when your baby is really hungry.

Or, feed her on a full stomach. With some babies, offering a bottle when they are looking for a breast makes them feel hostile toward the imposter and perhaps a little betrayed by the bottle giver. If this is the case with your baby (and you'll only find out through trial and rejection), don't offer the bottle when she's at her hungriest; instead, offer it casually between nursings—when she may be more in the mood to experiment and be ready for a snack.

Feign indifference. Instead of acting as though there's a lot at stake when you give her the bottle (even if there is), remain nonchalant no matter what her response.

Let her play before she eats. Before attempting to get down to business, let her play with the bottle. If she's had a chance to explore it on her own, she may be more likely to let it into her life and, hopefully, into her mouth. She may even put it there herself—as she does everything else.

Banish your breast. And the rest of you, when the bottle is launched. A breast-fed baby is more likely to accept a bottle given by father, grandma, or another care-taker when mother is well out of smelling distance. At least until supplementary feed-ing is well established, even the sound of your voice may spoil baby's appetite for a bottle.

Try a favorite fluid. It's possible it's not the bottle baby's objecting to, but the fluid inside it. Some infants will take to a bottle better if it's filled with familiar breast milk, but others, reminded of breast milk's orig-inal source, are more comfortable with an-other drink. Try formula or diluted apple juice instead.

Sneak it in during sleep. Have your bottle giver pick up your sleeping baby and try to give the bottle then. In a few weeks the bottle may be accepted awake.

Know when to surrender—temporar-ily. Don't let the bottle become the object of a battle, or your side doesn't stand a chance of winning the war. As soon as your baby raises objections to the bottle, take it away and try again another day. Perseverance—while retaining your non-chalant attitude—may be all that's neces-sary. Try the bottle once every few days for at least a couple of weeks before you con-sider admitting defeat.

Should defeat become a reality, however, don't give up hope. There's another alter-native to your breasts: the cup. Most babies enjoy drinking from a cup, even at four or five months of age, and happily take sup-plementary feedings from it (see page 229); many become proficient enough cup drink-ers by the end of the first year (sometimes as early as eight or nine months) to be weaned directly from the breast to the cup—which saves their mothers the extra step of weaning from the bottle.

SHOES FOR BABY

"My baby's not walking yet, of course, but I don't feel she's completely dressed without shoes."

Although socks or booties or, weather per-mitting, bare feet are best for your baby at this stage of development, there's nothing wrong with outfitting her little tootsies in snappy footwear on special occasions—as long as it's the right kind. Since your baby's feet aren't made for walking (at least not yet), the shoes you buy shouldn't be, either. Shoes for infants should be lightweight, made of a breathable material (leather or cloth, but not plastic), with soles so flexible that you can feel baby's toes through them (hard soles are absolutely out). Shoes with stiff ankle support (high-tops) are not only unnecessary and unhealthy for feet now, but will be when baby starts walking, too. And considering how quickly first shoes will be outgrown, it makes sense that they also be inexpensive.

To check for proper length, press down on the toe of each shoe with your thumb. If there is a full thumb's width between your baby's longest toe (usually the big toe, but sometimes the next one) and the end of the shoe, the length is right and there is room for growth. To check width, try to pinch a bit of shoe at the widest part of the foot. If you can, there's enough room. Do not put shoes on your baby that are too small—now or later.

BATHING IN THE BIG TUB

"My son's far too big now for his infant tub, but I'm afraid of washing him in our bathtub."

Taking the plunge into the family bathtub may seem a frightening prospect for both you and the baby; he is, after all, such a little—and slippery—fish for such a big pond. But if care is taken both to prevent accidents and to alleviate baby's fears, the big tub can turn into a veritable water wonderland for the six-month-old, and bathtime into a favorite, if wet, family ritual. To ensure a happy water baby, see the basic tips on bathtub bathing in the Baby-Care Primer, page 73, and try the following:

Wait until he's a sitting duck. You'll both be more comfortable with big-tub bathing if your baby's capable of sitting alone, or with only minimal support.

Ensure safe seating. A wet baby is a slippery baby, and even a baby who sits well (even an adult, for that matter) can slip in the tub. If he should go under the water momentarily, it won't be hazardous, but the scare could create a long-term fear of baths. (Of course, if he slips and you're not there, the consequences could be much more serious.) Fortunately, today's parents have an alternative to having to keep one hand on baby at all times during bathing: the bath seat with rubber suction cups that attach it securely to the bottom of the tub. The seat can be as simple as a ring for baby to sit within, or as elaborate as a large plastic seahorse for him to sit on. Some seats have foam pads to place under baby so he won't slide around. If yours doesn't, put a clean washcloth or small towel under baby's bottom to achieve the same effect. Rinse, squeeze, and hang the cloth to dry, or use a fresh one each bathtime to prevent the multiplication of germs in the damp material. If the seat has a foam pad, dry it in the dryer between uses for the same reason.

Let your baby test the waters in a familiar boat. For a few nights before he graduates from it, bathe him in his baby tub placed in the empty grownup tub. This way the new tub won't seem quite so formidable when it's filled with water—and him.

No swimming after eating. Whether your mother's ubiquitous summer chant was medically sound is debatable. But it may make sense not to bathe your baby directly after meals, because the increase in handling and activity could cause spitting up.

Avoid the big chill. Babies dislike being cold, and if they associate being chilled with being bathed, they may rebel against bathing. So be sure that the bathroom is comfortably warm. If your bathroom isn't adequately heated, you might want to warm the room with a small space heater or a heating unit in the ceiling (heed safety precautions, page 295). Don't remove baby's clothes until the tub is filled and you are ready to slip him into it. Have a large, soft towel, preferably with a hood, ready to wrap him in as soon as you lift him from the water. In cold weather, warming the towel on a radiator is a nice touch, but be sure the towel doesn't get too hot. Dry baby thoroughly, being sure to get into the creases, before unwrapping and dressing him.

Be prepared. Towel, washcloth, soap, shampoo, tub toys, and anything else you'll need for baby's bath should be on hand *before* you put baby in the tub. If you do forget something and you have to get it yourself, *bundle baby in a towel and take him with you.* Also prepare by removing everything from tubside that's potentially dangerous, such as soap, razors, and shampoo.

Do the elbow test. Your hands are much more tolerant of hot water than is a baby's sensitive skin. To make sure the temperature of the water you're running is just right, test it with your elbow or wrist before dunking baby. While it should be comfortably warm, it should not be hot. Turn the hot water tap off first, so that any drips from the faucet will be cold and baby won't be scalded. A safety cover on the tub spout will protect baby from burns and bumps.

Be there. Your baby needs adult super-vision every moment of every bath—and will continue to for his first five years of bathing. *Never leave him in the tub unattended,* even in a baby seat (he could slip out or climb out), even for a second.

Have entertainment on hand. Make the tub a floating playpen for your baby so that he'll be diverted while you tend to the more serious task of washing him. Specially designed tub toys (particularly those that bob atop the water) and plastic books are great, but so are plastic containers of all shapes and sizes. To avoid mildew buildup on tub toys, towel off after use and store in a dry container.

Let baby make a splash. But don't make one yourself. For most babies, splashing is a large part of bathtime fun, and the wetter a baby can make you, the happier he'll be (wear a plastic apron if you mind getting very wet). But while he almost certainly will like to make a splash, he may not like to be the target of one. Many a baby has been turned off to baths with a single playful splash.

Don't pull the stopper until baby is out of the tub. Not only can it be a physically chilling experience to be in an emptying tub, it can be a psychologically chilling one, too. The gurgling sound can frighten even a young infant, and an older baby who sees the water rushing down the drain may fear that he's going down next.

BATH FEARS

"My daughter is so terrified of being bathed in the bathtub that she screams irrationally and we have to force her to stay in the tub."

Though it may seem irrational to an adult who's taken countless baths, a baby's fear of the bath is very real, looming larger than the tub itself at every bathtime. And forcing your baby to face the source of her fear won't help her to overcome it. Your goal should be to gradually, with patience and understanding, reverse her feelings about bathing—to make the tub a friendly place to visit and water a friendly companion within it.

Take well-traveled roads to clean. Until your baby's completely willing to take a tub bath, don't force her to. Continue

bathing her in her familiar infant tub, or if she's wary of that, too, or has outgrown it entirely, give her sponge baths instead.

Try a dry run. If she's willing, put her in the tub (on a large bath towel or a bath seat to minimize slipping) without water and with a pile of toys, so she can become accustomed to the scenery and discover she can have fun playing in that locale. If the room is nice and warm and she's a baby who's comfortable being naked, let her play in there unclothed. Otherwise, keep her clothes on. As in any bathtub situation, don't leave her side for a moment.

Use a stand-in. While someone else holds your baby, give a demonstration bath to a washable doll or stuffed animal in the bathtub, with a running commentary each step of the way. When your baby is old enough, let her help with the bath if she likes, or bathe her "baby" in a small basin as she sits in the dry tub.

Try some good wet fun. For the sitting baby, fill a plastic tub (you can use her infant tub or a dish basin) with warm water and bubbles made with liquid baby soap, and a couple of water toys. Put it in a towel-lined empty bathtub, or on the kitchen or bathroom floor if your baby refuses to get into the tub at all. Place your baby, clothed or unclothed, next to it and let her explore under your constant supervision. For the baby who's not sitting well yet, fill a smaller basin or bowl and put it on the tray of her feeding chair or walker for water play.

Dressed or not, she may try to climb into the smaller tub herself—a clue that she's ready to try a bath again. If she doesn't, you'll have to take the lead, dunking her toys and fingers in the water in the hope that she will follow. If she doesn't, give her a little more time.

Use the buddy system. Some babies are more amenable to a bath if they've got company. Try bathing with your baby, but at bath temperatures geared to her comfort. Once she becomes adjusted to these duet baths you can try her solo.

Be patient. Eventually your baby will take to the tub again. But she'll do it faster if she's allowed to do it at her own pace, and without parental pressure.

BRUSHING BABY'S TEETH

"My daughter just got her first tooth. A neighbor said I should start brushing it now, but that seems silly."

Those tiny pearls that bring so much pain before they arrive and so much excitement when they first break through the gums are destined for extinction. They can all be expected to fall out during the early and mid school years, to be replaced by permanent teeth. So why take good care of them now?

There are several reasons: first of all, since they hold a place for the permanent teeth, decay and loss of these first teeth can deform the mouth permanently. Then, too, your baby will need these primary teeth for biting and chewing for many years; bad teeth could interfere with nutrition. And healthy teeth are also important for the development of normal speech and appearance—both important to a child's self-confidence. The child who can't speak clearly because of faulty teeth, or who keeps her mouth shut to hide rotten or missing teeth, doesn't feel good about herself. Finally, if you start your child brushing early, she is likely to develop good dental habits.

The first teeth can be wiped with a clean damp gauze pad or washcloth or brushed with a very soft, tiny (with no more than three rows of bristles) infant toothbrush moistened with water, after meals and at bedtime. Ask your dentist or pharmacist to recommend a brush. The gauze pad will probably do a more thorough job until the molars come in, but using the brush will get baby into the habit of brushing, so a combination of the two is probably best.[1] But be gentle—baby teeth are soft. Lightly brush or wipe the tongue, too, since it harbors germs.

No toothpaste is necessary for baby's teeth, though you can flavor the brush with a tiny bit of toothpaste if it makes her more interested in brushing. But don't use more than a pea-size dab until she can spit it out—most babies like to eat the stuff and could overdose on the fluorides, especially if the water is fluoridated. Most babies are eager to "do it themselves." Once she has the dexterity, which won't be for several months yet, you can let your baby brush on her own after meals, adding a more thorough cleaning with a gauze pad yourself before she goes to bed as part of the bedtime ritual. Also let her watch you care for your own teeth. If mommy and daddy set a good dental-care example, she's more likely to be meticulous about brushing and, later, flossing.

Though brushing and flossing will continue to be important throughout your baby's life, proper nutrition will have equal impact on her dental health, starting now (actually, it started before she was born). Ensuring the adequate intake of calcium, phosphorus, fluoride, and other minerals and vitamins (particularly vitamin C, which helps to maintain the health of gums) and limiting foods high in refined sugars (including commercial teething biscuits) or sticky natural sugar (such as dried fruit, even raisins) can help prevent the miseries that accompany a mouthful of decaying teeth and bleeding gums. Ideally, limit sweets (even healthy ones) to once or twice a day, since the more sugar intake is spread out over the day, the greater the risk to the teeth. Serve them with meals, when they do less damage to the teeth, rather than between meals. Or brush baby's teeth right after the sweets are eaten.

When your baby does have sweets or snacks high in carbohydrates between meals and a brush isn't available, follow them with a piece of cheese (such as Swiss

---

1. A pediatric dentist may be able to tell you where you can purchase disposable cloth finger slips that are even more effective for cleaning tiny teeth than a gauze pad.

BABY'S FIRST TOOTHBRUSH

Bristles should be soft, and when they become ragged, it's time for a change. Even a toothbrush that still looks new should be changed after six or eight weeks (some recommend as frequently as every three weeks) because over time bacteria from the mouth accumulate on the brush. Favorite Sesame Street or Disney character toothbrushes make brushing more appealing, but check their quality with your dentist.

or Cheddar), which seems to be able to block the action of tooth-decaying acids produced by the bacteria in plaque. For further tooth insurance, get your baby used to drinking juice from a cup now, and never let her go to sleep with a bottle.

In addition to good home care and good nutrition, your baby will need good professional dental care to ensure healthy teeth in healthy gums. Now, before an emergency arises, ask your baby's doctor to recommend a reliable pediatric dentist or a general dentist who treats a lot of children and is good with them. If you have a question about your baby's teeth, call or make an appointment as soon as it comes up. If not, you won't need to arrange for a checkup until somewhere between her second and third birthdays. Some infant dental problems, such as a bad bite or the decay caused by baby-bottle mouth, need to be corrected early. Others, such as widely spaced teeth, which usually move closer later, are rarely a cause for early intervention.

GIVING BABY COW'S MILK

"I'm breastfeeding, and want to wean my baby. I don't want to start with formula —can I give him cow's milk?"

Though small amounts of cow's milk are not likely to be a problem for a child in the first year of life, it is now becoming clear that weaning a breast- or formula-fed baby entirely to cow's milk before the first birthday is not a good idea. The American Academy of Pediatrics now recommends that when possible, continue breastfeeding until the end of the first year. When that isn't possible, an *iron-fortified* infant formula should be the choice. There are several reasons. First of all, cow's milk contains inadequate stores of iron, linoleic acid, and vitamin E, and excessive levels of sodium, potassium, and protein. Secondly, the composition of cow's milk may also interfere with a baby's absorption of iron from other foods, such as cereals. And thirdly, cow's milk can cause intestinal bleeding in some babies.

Because the nutritional needs of a six month old differ from those of a newborn, ask the doctor about the possibility of weaning your child to one of the formulas designed for older babies.

When you switch to cow's milk at a year, be sure you use whole milk, rather than skim (nonfat) or low-fat. Whole milk is usually recommended until age two, though some doctors okay using 2% milk after 18 months.

BABY-BOTTLE MOUTH

"I have a friend whose baby's front teeth had to be pulled because of baby-bottle mouth. How can I prevent this from happening to my little boy?"

There's nothing cuter than a first-grader whose grin reveals a charming space where his two front teeth used to be. But there's nothing cute about a toddler whose two front teeth have been lost years before their time to baby-bottle mouth. And yet this becomes the fate of a large number of babies every year.

Fortunately, baby-bottle mouth is completely preventable. It occurs most often in the first two years of life, when teeth are most vulnerable, and most frequently as a result of a baby's falling asleep regularly with a bottle in his mouth. The sugars in whatever beverage he's imbibing (cow's milk, breast milk, formula, fruit juice, or sugar drinks) combine with bacteria in his mouth to decay the teeth. The dirty work is abetted during sleep when the production of saliva, which ordinarily dilutes food and drink and promotes the swallowing reflex, slows dramatically. With little swallowing occurring, the last sips baby takes before falling asleep pool in his mouth and remain in contact with his teeth for hours.

To avoid baby-bottle mouth:

■ Never give glucose (sugar) water, even before baby's teeth come in, so that he won't become "addicted." The same applies to such sugary drinks as cranberry juice cocktail, fruit punches, fruit drinks, or fruit-juice drinks.

■ Once your baby's teeth come in, don't put him to bed for the night or down for a nap with a bottle of milk or juice. An occasional lapse won't cause a problem, but repeated lapses will. If you must give him a bottle to take to bed, make it a bottle of plain tap water, which will not harm the teeth and if it is fluoridated will help strengthen them.

■ Don't let your baby use a bottle of milk or juice as a pacifier, to crawl or lie around with and suck on at will. All-day nipping can be as harmful to the teeth as night time sucking. Bottles should be considered part of a meal or snack and like these should routinely be given in the appropriate setting (your arms, a baby seat, and later, a high chair) and at appropriate times.

■ Don't allow a baby who sleeps in your bed to remain at your breast all night and nurse on and off. Breast milk can cause decay this way, particularly after the twelfth month.

■ Wean your baby from breast or bottle at about 12 months.

ANEMIA

"I don't understand why the doctor wants to test my son for anemia at the next visit. He was premature, but is very healthy and active now."

At one time many children became anemic somewhere between six and twelve months of age, and many in poor families still do. Screenings for anemia became routine because babies with mild anemia usually seem to be healthy and active, not exhibiting the kinds of symptoms that often appear in adults,[2] and the only way to uncover their problem is with a test to determine the proportion of hemoglobin in the blood. When hemoglobin (the protein in red blood cells that performs the important function of distributing oxygen) is in low supply, anemia is diagnosed.

Today, thanks to more attention to iron supplementation, only 2 or 3 in 100 middle-class infants become anemic, and a routine screening is no longer deemed absolutely necessary. Still, many physicians continue to perform the test (between six and nine months for low-birthweight infants and between nine and twelve months for others) as a precaution.

Babies are occasionally born anemic, usually because of a loss of red blood cells due to bleeding, destruction of cells due to a blood incompatibility problem, or an inherited illness such as sickle-cell disease or thalassemia (see pages 493 and 497). They may become anemic later in infancy because of hidden bleeding (such as might develop from drinking cow's milk at too early an age) or because of an infestation of parasites (often hookworms). Anemia may strike, too, because an inadequate intake of folic acid or vitamin B_{12}, both of which are insufficient in the breast milk of strict vegetarian moms, or of vitamin C is interfering

---

2. Symptoms of anemia in adults or older children include: initially, paleness, irritability, weakness, lack of appetite, little interest in their surroundings; and later, waxiness and sallowness of the skin, and susceptibility to infection.

with the production of hemoglobin.

But it's iron that's the most essential building block of hemoglobin, and iron deficiency is the most common reason for babies to develop anemia. Full-term babies are generally born with stores of iron built up during the last few months of pregnancy that carry them for the first few months. After that, as babies continue to require the mineral in large quantities to help expand their blood volume to meet the demands of rapid growth, they need a source of iron in the diet, such as a vitamin and mineral supplement with iron, iron-fortified baby cereal, or iron-fortified formula (for bottle-fed babies).[3] And though breastfeeding exclusively for the first four to six months is generally considered the best way to nourish your baby, and the iron in breast milk is very well absorbed, breastfeeding does not ensure adequate iron intake once his prenatal iron stores have been depleted.

Iron-deficiency anemia is most common in babies born with poor iron stores, such as premature infants who didn't have time before birth to lay down sufficient reserves and those whose mothers didn't have enough iron during pregnancy. It often develops later in infants with intestinal problems (such as diarrhea) or metabolic problems (such as celiac disease) that interfere with the absorption of iron. But anemia can also develop in babies without absorption problems who start out with good iron stores but who don't receive any form of supplementary iron when their stores run out.

Just when iron supplementation should begin is a matter of medical opinion, and you should rely on your baby's doctor for a recommendation.

Typically, the baby who develops iron-deficiency anemia is one who depends mainly on breast or cow's milk or iron-

poor formula for nourishment, and takes very few solids. Because the anemia tends to slacken his appetite for solids, his sole source of iron, a cycle of less iron/less food/less iron/less food is set up, worsening matters. Prescribed iron drops usually corrects the situation.

To help prevent iron-deficiency anemia in your baby, try the following:

- Be sure that if bottle-fed, your baby is getting a formula fortified with iron.
- Be sure that if breastfed, your baby is getting iron in some supplementary form, such as an iron-fortified cereal or vitamin drops containing iron. And feed a vitamin C food (see page 359) at the same time, when possible, to improve iron absorption.
- As your baby increases his intake of solids, be sure to include foods rich in iron.
- Avoid feeding bran to your baby, since it can interfere with iron absorption.

VEGETARIAN DIET

"We're vegans—strict vegetarians—and plan to raise our daughter the same way. Can vegetarianism provide enough nutrition for her?"

There are millions of vegetarians who raise their children as vegetarians with little or no effect, except slightly lower childhood weights. But there are risks to limiting all animal products, both for children and for adults. What's good for the goose and gander can be good for the gosling, if you:

- Breastfeed your baby. Since soy milk formulas are an imperfect substitute for breast milk, the vegan mother who can breastfeed should do so, to ensure her infant gets all the necessary nutrients for the first six months and most of them for the first year—assuming she's getting all the nutrients she needs (including folic acid and vitamin B_{12} in a supplement) to produce high-quality breast milk. If she can't breastfeed, she should be certain that the soy formula she uses is one recommended by her baby's doctor.

---

3. Phytates in the grains, which normally bind iron, making it unusable by the body, once made iron fortification in infant cereal ineffective. This problem has been overcome with new production methods, however, and these cereals are now a good source of iron.

■ Give your breastfed baby an infant vitamin-mineral supplement that contains iron, vitamin D (other than sunshine, the only major source is milk, to which vitamin D is routinely added), folic acid and vitamin B_{12} (found only in animal products). (See page 132 for more on vitamin supplements.) Give a supplement, too, when your baby is weaned from formula or breast milk.

■ Serve only whole-grain beans and cereals once your baby graduates from beginner baby cereals. These will provide more of the vitamins, minerals, and protein ordinarily obtained from animal products than would their refined counterparts.

■ Use tofu and other soy-based products to provide added protein when your baby moves on to solids. Near the end of the first year, brown rice cooked fairly soft, mashed chickpeas or other legumes (beans and peas), and high-protein or whole-grain pastas can also be added to the diet as sources of protein. (See page 361 for a more complete list of vegetable proteins.)

■ Once you wean your baby, be sure that she gets adequate calcium in her diet to promote strong and healthy bones and teeth. Good vegetarian sources include tofu prepared with calcium (but beware the many soybean beverages and frozen desserts that contain little or no calcium), broccoli and other green leafies, and finely ground almonds and pine nuts (ground so baby won't choke on them). Since these foods are not standard favorites with infants, you may also have to add a calcium supplement to your daughter's diet if you prefer not to give her milk. Check with her doctor.

Vegetarians who do use milk products have a much easier time ensuring good nutrition for their babies and children than those who don't. Dairy products provide the protein and calcium needed for growth and good health, as well as adequate amounts of vitamins A, B_{12}, and D. If egg yolks are also part of the diet, they provide an additional source of iron—but, as for most children, iron supplementation may still be a good idea. (And, of course, as your baby gets older, eggs shouldn't be an everyday food.) Again, check with the doctor.

SALT INTAKE

"I'm pretty careful about how much salt my husband and I get. But how careful do I have to be about the salt in my daughter's diet?"

Infants, like all of us, do need some salt. But also like the rest of us, they don't need a lot of salt. In fact, their kidneys cannot handle large quantities of sodium, which is probably why Mother Nature made breast milk a very low-sodium drink (with only 5 milligrams of sodium per cup, as compared to 120 milligrams per cup of cow's milk). And there is growing evidence that too much salt too soon, especially when there is a family history of hypertension, can set the stage for high blood pressure in adulthood. Studies also show that babies do not have an inherent preference for things salty, but may develop a preference for them if they are fed a diet high in sodium—a preference that can prove deadly later in life.

In response to the mounting evidence that an excess of sodium is not good for babies, major baby food manufacturers have eliminated salt from their recipes. Mothers who prepare their own baby foods should do likewise. Don't assume that string beans or mashed potatoes won't appeal to your child unless they've been sprinkled with salt just because you like them that way. Give her taste buds a chance to learn what foods taste like when not adulterated with salt, and she'll develop a taste for food au naturel that'll last a lifetime.

To be sure that your baby doesn't pick up the high-salt habit and to help the rest of the family reduce salt intake, read labels routinely. You'll find large amounts of sodium in the most unlikely products, including cottage cheese and hard cheeses (choose the low-sodium varieties), breads and

SODIUM CONTENT OF FOODS FED TO BABIES

FOOD	AMOUNT	MG OF SODIUM
Breast milk	1 cup	5 mg
Formula	1 cup	Varies, but usually approximates breast milk
Whole cow's milk	1 cup	120 mg
Baby cereal	¼ cup	0 mg
Baby fruits (range)	½ jar	2–10 mg
Baby sweet potatoes	½ jar	20 mg
Baby carrots	½ jar	35 mg
Baby peas	½ jar	7 mg
Whole milk yogurt	2 tbl.	20 mg
Whole milk cottage cheese	2 tbl.	110 mg
Cottage cheese, unsalted*	2 tbl.	15 mg
Whole-wheat bread	½ slice	90 mg
Whole-wheat bread, unsalted	½ slice	5 mg
Rice cakes	1 whole	28 mg
Rice cakes, unsalted	1 whole	0 mg

*If you use unsalted cottage cheese, which is usually available only in low-fat varieties, be sure baby gets adequate fat from other sources such as breast milk, formula, hard cheese, and plain yogurt. Or add a tablespoon of light sweet or sour cream to each ¼ cup of cottage cheese.

breakfast cereals, cakes and cookies. Since a baby between the ages of six months and one year requires no more than 250 to 750 milligrams of sodium a day, foods that contain 300 or more milligrams per serving will quickly push the intake over this level. When buying for baby, opt for foods with under 50 milligrams per serving most of the time.

THE WHOLE-GRAIN HABIT

"I know that whole-wheat bread is best for my baby, but I don't like it and I don't think she will either. Isn't it better for her to eat her white bread than not to eat her whole wheat?"

What was the first bread your mom gave you in the high chair? What kind of toast did you have with your eggs when you were growing up? What kind of bread sandwiched the tuna salad in your lunch box? It's a pretty good bet the answer to all three questions is "white"—and it isn't any wonder that you prefer it. The food preferences we develop early stay with us for life (unless we make a concerted effort to change them), and that's exactly why it's important to give your baby *only* whole grains now and throughout childhood. If you do, not only will she grow up liking whole grains, but she'll prefer them—with white bread tasting bland and pasty by comparison. If the rest of the family jumps on the whole-wheat wagon with her, it won't be long before you all favor the darker and healthier loaves.

EARLY RISING

"At first we were grateful that our daughter was sleeping through the night. But with her waking up like clockwork at 5:00 every morning, we almost wish she'd wake up in the middle of the night instead."

With a night waker, at least there's the promise of another few hours of sleep once baby beds down again. But with a baby who greets her parents with infuriating alertness and energy, ready and eager to start every day when even the roosters are still snoozing, there's no hope of further rest until night falls once more. And yet this rude awakening is faced daily by countless parents.

Often, parents have no choice but to learn to live with this problem. But in some cases, it is possible to reset such a wayward little alarm:

Keep out the dawn's early light. Some babies (like some adults) are particularly sensitive to light when they're sleeping. Especially when the days are longer and it becomes light earlier, keeping baby's room

dark can help her stay asleep longer. Invest in room-darkening shades or lined draperies, or hang a heavy blanket over the window at night.

Keep the traffic out. If your baby's window faces a street that carries a lot of traffic in the early morning hours, the noise could be waking her prematurely. Try keeping her window closed, hanging a heavy blanket or curtains at the window to help muffle sound, or moving her, if possible, to an off-street room. Or use a fan or a white-noise machine to drown out street noises.

Keep baby up later at night. It's possible that your baby is getting up earlier than she should because she's going to bed too early. Try putting her to bed ten minutes later each night until you've gradually postponed her bedtime an hour or more. To make this work, it will probably help to move her naps and meals forward simultaneously and at the same pace.

Keep baby up later during the day. Some early risers are ready to go back to sleep in an hour or two. To discourage this, postpone her return to the crib by ten minutes more each morning until she's napping an hour or so later, which may eventually help her to extend her night's sleep.

Keep daytime sleeping down. A baby needs only so much total sleep—an average of 14½ hours at this age, with wide variations in individual babies. Maybe yours is getting too much sleep during the day and thus needs less at night. Limit daytime naps, cutting one out or shortening all of them. But not to the point of your baby's being fatigued by the end of the day.

Keep her waiting. Don't rush to greet her at the first call from the crib. Gradually lengthen the time before you go to her, starting with five minutes—unless of course, she's screaming. If you're lucky, she may roll over and go back to sleep, or at least amuse herself for a while.

Keep a stash of toys in the crib. If keeping the room dark doesn't help, try letting the light seep through and keeping a supply of safe toys (activity centers attached to the side of the crib, stuffed but not plushy animals, which might pose a suffocation risk, and other crib-safe toys) around for your baby to play with before you rise.

Keep her waiting for breakfast. If she's used to eating at 5:30, hunger will regularly call at that time. Even if you're getting up with her then, don't feed her right away. Gradually postpone breakfast, so that she's less likely to wake up early for it.

All these efforts may, unfortunately, be in vain. Some babies just need less total sleep than others, and if yours turns out to be one of them, you may have to rise and shine early until she's old enough to get up and make her own breakfast. Until then, turning in earlier yourselves, and sharing the pre-dawn burden by taking turns getting up with your baby (this will work only if mommy's presence isn't required for nursing), may be your best survival technique.

STILL NOT SLEEPING THROUGH THE NIGHT

"My baby's still getting up twice a night, and she won't go back to sleep without nursing no matter how much we rock her or soothe her. Will we ever get any sleep?"

Your baby will continue to awaken several times a night for the rest of her life, as we all do. But until she learns how to fall back to sleep on her own, neither you nor she will be able to get a good night's sleep.

Helping her to fall back to sleep—with a breast, a bottle, a pacifier, rocking, patting, rubbing, singing, sleep tapes—will only postpone her learning how to do it herself. But the inevitable moment will come when it will no longer be practical or possible for you to be her sandman. If you make that moment now, not only will you get more sleep, so will she.

Your first step should be to review the tips on page 175 for reducing the number of night wakings and for cutting down daytime naps. Then pick one of the following approaches to getting your baby started on the road to sleeping independence:

Cold turkey. If your baby generally wakes for a feeding once or twice a night, don't respond—let her cry it out.

Gradual withdrawal. If your baby is in the habit of waking three or four times a night, or more, or if you are just uncomfortable with cold-turkey tactics, move more slowly. Respond when she calls, but not by feeding her. Instead attempt to help her get back to sleep some other way (patting, singing, rocking). Once she can do without night feedings, start a gradual program of letting her cry it out.

If, in spite of your elaborate machinations, your baby still doesn't sleep through the night, the problem probably lies with how she falls asleep at the beginning of a nap or at night. While some babies can drift off at the bottle or breast at naptime and bedtime and still manage to go back to sleep without these aids in the middle of the night, others can't. If your child is one of these, you will also have to change her going-to-bed patterns. Give feedings well before an intended nap or bedtime and then, later, when she seems sleepy, try to put her into her carriage or crib drowsy but awake. Most babies will have trouble getting to sleep this way at first, but almost all will succeed after a few chances to cry it out.

Sounds sensible—but is it possible? What if your baby invariably falls asleep feeding, whether you plan it that way or not? Under these circumstances, it probably makes more sense to postpone your crusade rather than to try to rouse your babe in arms after every meal so she can fall asleep again on her own. Fortunately, as babies get older they are less likely to doze off while feeding, and you will have more opportunities to put your baby down awake.

Take the opportunity whenever it comes up and eventually you will have a baby who knows how to get herself to sleep.

There are some breastfed babies who continue waking and feeding at night well into toddlerhood, not because they need the food, but because night after night they're presented with an offer they can't refuse: the comfort of nursing. And they usually continue to awaken nights as long as the offer stands. Their mothers are usually willing to sacrifice unbroken sleep to serve as round-the-clock milk dispensers until their children are weaned (at which time they apparently begin sleeping through the night, as if by magic), but it's not clear whether prolonged nighttime nursing is of any benefit to children. The babies most likely to have night waking problems are those breastfeeders who sleep with their mothers—a practice more common than most of us realize and one which can contribute, through frequent night feedings once teeth appear, to tooth decay.

CRYING IT OUT

"Everyone is urging me to let my baby cry it out when he wakes in the night. But it seems so cruel."

To a caring parent, programmed to respond to her baby's every need, "crying it out" may indeed seem cruel and inhuman punishment, especially when his only crime is wanting mommy or daddy in the middle of the night. But it is actually the best way, sleep experts tell us, to respond to a baby's need to learn how to fall asleep on his own. Still, if you're philosophically opposed to the idea, don't try it. You probably won't stick to the game plan and the mixed signals you send will only confuse your baby, not help him sleep. Instead, let him use a back-to-sleep crutch (preferably one other than midnight snacking) for as long as necessary.

For hardier—or more desperate—souls, letting baby cry it out almost invariably works. You can use one of two approaches:

Crying it out all the way. If you can tolerate an hour or more of vigorous crying and screaming, don't go to baby, soothe him, feed him, or talk to him when he wakes up in the middle of the night. Just let him cry until he's exhausted himself—and the possibility, in his mind, that he's going to get anywhere, or anyone, by crying—and has fallen back to sleep. The next night do the same; the crying will almost certainly last a shorter time. Its duration

---

ANOTHER ROUTE TO SLEEPING THROUGH THE NIGHT?

If you're among the softhearted or weak-nerved parents who just can't or won't listen to their babies crying it out, you may have another choice besides sleepless nights. A recent study showed that a program called "systematic awakening" may work as well as crying it out, though perhaps a bit more slowly. There are still a great many unanswered questions about systematic awakening—chief among them is why it works. Still, it's certainly worth a try.

Here's how: keep a diary of your baby's nighttime awakenings for a week so you will have an idea of the usual times. Then, set your alarm clock for about half an hour before you expect the first howl. At the alarm, get up, wake the baby, and proceed with what you usually do when the waking is spontaneous (diaper, feed, rock, or whatever). Anticipate each usual waking in the same way. Gradually expand the time between these systematic wakings and then begin to eliminate them. Within a few weeks you should be able to begin phasing them out entirely.

should continue to diminish even further over the following few nights, until finally it ends completely. Your baby will have learned something that neither you nor he would have believed before: that he can go back to sleep without a nipple in his mouth or a pair of arms to rock him.

Until the dawn of that momentous morning when you awaken at 6:00 and realize you've slept through the night and that your baby seems to have, too, your nerves will probably be screaming as frantically as your baby. You may find that earplugs, the whir of the fan, or the hum of voices or music on the radio or TV can take the edge off the crying without blocking it out entirely. If you have an intercom from baby's room, the magnified crying may be particularly grating. You can reduce that problem by turning it off when the crying starts. If baby is truly hysterical, you may hear him anyway. If you can't hear him at all, set a minute timer for twenty minutes. When the buzzer rings, turn the intercom back on to see if he's still at it. Repeat this every twenty minutes until the crying stops.

If at any time your baby's crying changes and he sounds as though he might be in trouble, do check to be sure he isn't tangled in his covers or hasn't pulled up and found himself stranded, unable to get down. If he does have a problem, make him comfortable again, give him a loving pat and a few gentle words, and leave.

Crying it out, a little at a time. If you don't have the constitution to tolerate an hour's worth of heartrending pleas, let your baby cry for a few minutes (or as long as you can stand it), then go to him (or, if you're the feeding connection, have daddy go to him), reassure him with a pat and a whispered "I love you" (without picking him up), and leave him again. Don't stay with him long enough for him to fall asleep while you're calming him. Repeat the pro-

cess, extending the time you leave him alone by five minutes or more each time, until he falls asleep. The next night, extend the periods he spends by himself by a few more minutes, and continue extending them over several nights until he falls asleep after the very first period. There is a problem, however, with this approach: some babies may be unsettled by the parental visits and actually be stimulated to cry more heartily, increasing the time it will take them to fall back to sleep.

Unhappily for their parents, a few babies will not learn to fall back to sleep on their own, even when a program of crying it out is followed with stalwart determination. Some may not be getting enough food during the day and wake up because they're really hungry in the middle of the night. For these babies, increased daytime feedings, particularly late in the day, may help. (Remember, if your baby was premature or small for gestational age, he may continue to need night feedings longer than other babies.) Others may be suffering from allergy or illness. For these babies, and any for whom night waking seems an insoluble problem, a consultation with the doctor is a must. Still others may be hypersensitive, disturbed by stimuli other babies wouldn't even notice at the normal wakings, and unable to fall back to sleep. For these babies, a carefully controlled environment—with noise, light, temperature, and clothing all comfortable and conducive to sleep—can often do the trick. Others just don't need a lot of sleep and find 2 A.M. a great time to play. With these babies, parents can only hope that soon their offspring will be able to enjoy their middle-of-the-night play sessions alone.

An occasional baby always cries for a few minutes before falling asleep and also when waking at night. That's nothing to be concerned about—unless it invariably awakens you.

WHAT IT'S IMPORTANT TO KNOW:
Stimulating Your Older Baby

If stimulating a baby in the first few months of life takes ingenuity, stimulating a baby who's approaching the half-year mark takes sophistication. No longer is baby physical, emotional, and intellectual putty in your hands. Now he or she is ready and able to take an active role in the learning process and to coordinate the senses—seeing what's being touched, looking for what's being heard, touching what's being tasted.

The same basic guidelines discussed in Stimulating Your Baby in the Early Months (page 163) will continue to apply as you approach the second half of baby's first year, but the kinds of activities you can provide are greatly expanded. Basically, they will be directed at these areas of development:

Large motor skills. The best way to help baby develop the large motor strength and coordination necessary for sitting, crawling, walking, throwing a ball, and

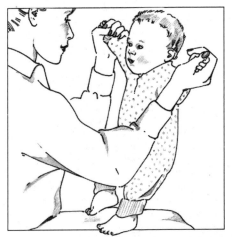

Babies love a lap to stand on. Pulling baby up to this position not only entertains, but also helps develop the leg muscles baby will need to pull up, and later stand, unassisted.

riding a tricycle is to provide plenty of opportunity. Frequently change your baby's position—from tummy to back, from propped up to prone, from the crib to the floor—to provide the chance to practice feats of physical prowess. As your baby seems ready (which you may not know until you try), provide the opportunity to do the following:

- Stand on your lap and bounce
- Pull to sitting
- Sit in a "frog" position
- Sit upright, propped with pillows if necessary
- Pull to standing, holding on to your fingers
- Pull to standing in a crib or playpen, or on other furniture
- Lift up on all fours
- "Fly" through the air

Small motor skills. Developing the dexterity of baby's little fingers and hands will eventually lead to the mastering of many essential skills, such as self-feeding, drawing, writing, brushing teeth, tying shoelaces, buttoning a shirt, turning a key in a lock, and so much more. Proficiency develops more quickly if babies are given ample opportunity to use their hands, to manipulate objects of all kinds, to touch, explore, and experiment. The following will help hone small motor skills:

- Activity boards—a variety of activities give baby plenty of practice with small motor skills, though it will be months before most babies can conquer them all.
- Blocks—simple cubes of wood, plastic, or cloth, large or small, are appropriate at this age.
- Soft dolls and stuffed animals—handling them builds dexterity.
- Real or toy household objects—babies usually love real or toy telephones (with cords removed), mixing spoons, measuring

HOW DO YOU SPEAK TO YOUR BABY NOW?

Now that your baby hovers on the brink of language development, what you say to him or her takes on new meaning. It will provide the foundation for learning language, both receptive (understanding what is heard), which comes earlier, and expressive (speaking), which is slower to evolve. You can help your baby develop both kinds of language in the following ways:

Slow down. When your baby is starting to try to decode our confusing jargon, fast talk will slow his or her efforts. To give baby the chance to begin picking out words, you must speak more slowly, more clearly, and more simply most of the time.

Focus on single words. Continue your running commentaries, but begin emphasizing individual words. Follow "Now we're going to change your diaper," with "Diaper—this is your diaper," as you hold it up. At feeding time, when you say "I'm putting juice in the cup," hold up the juice and add "Juice, here is the juice," and the cup, and say "Cup." In general, keep your phrasing shorter and less complex and focus primarily on words commonly used in baby's everyday life. Always pause to give baby plenty of time to decipher your words before going on to say more.

Continue to downplay pronouns. Pronouns are still confusing for your baby, so stick to "This is mommy's book," and "That is Jamie's doll."

Emphasize imitation. Now that the number of sounds your baby makes is growing, so is the fun you can have imitating each other. Whole conversations can be built around a few consonants and vowels. Baby says, "Ba-ba-ba-ba," and you come back with a profound, "Ba-ba-ba-ba." Baby replies, "Da-da-da-da," and you respond, "Da-da-da-da." You can continue such stimulating dialogue for as long as you're both enjoying it. If baby seems receptive, you can try offering some new syllables ("Ga-ga-ga-ga," for example), encouraging imitation. But if the role reversal seems to turn baby off, switch back again. In not too many months, you'll find your baby will begin trying to imitate your words—without prompting.

Build a repertoire of songs and rhymes. You may find it tedious having to repeat the same nursery rhyme or little ditty a dozen times a day every day. Your baby, however, will not only love the repetition, but learn from it. Whether you lean on Mother Goose, Dr. Seuss, or your own creativity matters not; what counts is consistency. Now is also the time to expand the variety of music baby listens to on a record or tape player.

Use books. Baby's not ready for listening to stories yet, but simple rhymes in books with vivid pictures often catch even a young infant's attention. Do plenty of pointing out of single objects, animals, or people. Start asking, "Where is the dog?" and eventually baby will surprise you by placing a pudgy finger right on Spot.

Wait for a response. Though baby may not be talking yet, he or she is starting to process information, and often will have a response to what you say—even if it's just an excited squeal (when you've proposed a walk in the stroller) or a pouty whimper (when you've announced it's time to come off the swing).

Be commanding. It's important for your baby to learn to follow simple commands such as "Kiss grandma," or "Wave bye-bye," or "Give mommy the dolly" (add "please" if you want the word to come naturally with your baby's own requests). It won't happen right away, but don't show disappointment when baby doesn't perform. Instead, help your child to act out your request, and eventually he or she will catch on. Once that happens, beware of treating your baby like a trained seal, demanding performances of the latest "trick" whenever there's an audience.

cups, strainers, pots and pans, paper cups, empty boxes.

■ Balls—of varying sizes and textures, to hold, to squeeze; they are especially fun once baby is able to sit up and roll them or crawl after them.

■ Finger games—at first you'll be the one to play clap hands, patty-cake, the itsy bitsy spider, and similar games, but before you know it baby will be performing some of them independently. After you do a demonstration or two, assist baby with the finger play while you sing along.

Social skills. The middle of the first year is a very sociable time for most babies. They smile, laugh, squeal, and communicate in a variety of other ways and are willing to share their friendliness with all comers—most haven't yet developed "stranger anxiety." So this is a perfect time to encourage socialization, to expose your child to a variety of people of different ages—from other babies to elderly people. You can do this at church or synagogue, while shopping, when having friends over or while visiting them, even by having baby fraternize with his or her image in the mirror. Teach a simple greeting like "hi" and some of the other basic social graces, such as waving bye-bye, blowing a kiss, and saying thank you.

Intellectual and language skills. Comprehension is beginning to dawn. Names (mommy's, daddy's, sibling's) are recognized first, followed by basic words ("no," "bottle," "bye-bye," for example), and soon thereafter, simple, often heard sentences ("Do you want to nurse?" or "Make nice to the doggy"). This receptive language (understanding what you say) will come before spoken language. Other types of intellectual development are also on the horizon. Though it won't seem so at first, your baby is taking the first steps toward acquiring the skills of rudimentary problem solving, observation, and memorization. You can help by doing the following:

■ Play games that stimulate the intellect (see page 318), that help baby observe cause and effect (fill a cup with water in the tub and let baby turn it over), that explain object permanence (cover a favorite toy with a cloth and then have baby look for it, or play peekaboo).

■ Continue sharpening baby's auditory perception. When a plane goes by overhead or a fire engine speeds down the street, sirens screaming, point them out to baby: "Is that an airplane?" or "Do you hear the fire engine?" will help tune your child in to the world of sounds. Emphasizing and repeating the key words (airplane, fire engine) will also help with word recognition. Do the same when you turn on the vacuum or the water in the bathtub, when the tea kettle whistles or the doorbell or phone rings. And don't overlook those favorite funny noises— razzes on baby's belly or arm, clicks with your tongue, and whistles are all educational, too, encouraging imitation, which in turn encourages language development.

■ Introduce concepts. This teddy is soft, that coffee is hot, the car goes fast, you got up early, the ball is under the table. The broom is for sweeping, the water is for washing and drinking, the towel is for drying, the soap is for washing. At first your words will be meaningless to baby, but eventually, with lots of repetition, you will get the ideas across.

■ Encourage curiosity and creativity. If your child wants to use a toy in an unusual way, don't be discouraging or disparaging. (Where would we be today if the parents of Edison, Einstein, and Marie Curie had objected to their children's doing things differently?) Give your child a chance to experiment and explore—whether that means pulling up tufts of grass in the garden or squeezing out a wet sponge in the tub. A baby will learn much more through experience than through being told.

■ Encourage a love of learning. Though teaching specific facts and concepts to your child is important, equally important is teaching how to learn and imparting a love of learning.

CHAPTER TEN

The Seventh Month

WHAT YOUR BABY MAY BE DOING

By the end of this month, your baby ...should be able to (see Note):

- sit without support
- feed self a cracker (6¼ months)
- razz (make a wet razzing sound by 6½ months)

Note: If your baby seems not to have reached one or more of these milestones, check with the doctor. In rare instances the delay could indicate a problem, though in most cases it will turn out to be normal for your baby. Premature infants generally reach milestones later than others of the same birth age, often achieving them closer to their adjusted age (the age they would be if they had been born at term) or sometimes later.

...will probably be able to:

- bear some weight on legs when held upright
- object if you try to take a toy away
- work to get a toy out of reach

- pass a cube or other object from one hand to the other
- look for dropped object
- rake a raisin and pick it up in fist
- turn in the direction of a voice (by 7⅓ months)
- babble, combining vowels and consonants such as ga-ga-ga-ga, ba-ba-ba-ba, ma-ma-ma-ma, da-da-da-da
- play peekaboo (by 7¼ months)

...may possibly be able to:

- stand holding on to someone or something

...may even be able to:

- pull up to standing position from sitting
- get into a sitting position from stomach
- play patty-cake (clap hands) or wave bye-bye
- pick up tiny object with any part of thumb and finger
- walk holding on to furniture (cruise)
- say mama or dada indiscriminately

WHAT YOU CAN EXPECT AT THIS MONTH'S CHECKUP

Most doctors do not schedule regular well-baby checkups this month. Do call the doctor if there are any concerns that can't wait until next month's visit.

FEEDING YOUR BABY THIS MONTH: Moving Up From Strained Foods

Whether baby's passage to solids has been smooth sailing or bumpy and fraught with mishaps so far, another channel awaits crossing: between strained foods and coarser textures. And whether baby has proven to be an eager and adventurous gourmand or a hard-to-please, fussy eater, whether he or she is a veteran solids feeder or a newcomer to the high chair, that crossing is better made now than later on in the first year, when new experiences are more likely to encounter obstreperous rebuffs.

But the time has not yet arrived for a family junket to your favorite steak house. Even when the first couple of teeth are in place, babies continue to chew with their gums—which are no match for a hunk of meat. For now, coarsely puréed or mashed foods, which have just a touch more texture than strained, will fill the bill of baby's fare.

You can use the commercial "junior" or "stage 2" foods, or mash baby's meals from what you serve the family, as long as they have been prepared without added salt or sugar. You can try homemade oatmeal thinned with milk (but remember, unlike baby oatmeal, it usually has no added iron); mashed small-curd cottage cheese (preferably unsalted, see footnote on page 258); scraped apple or pear (scrape tiny bits of fruit into a dish with a knife); mashed or coarsely puréed cooked fruit (such as apples, apricots, peaches, plums); and vegetables (such as carrots, sweet and white

potatoes, cauliflower, squash). By seven months, you can usually add meat and skinless poultry (puréed, ground, or minced very fine) and small flakes of soft fish. When the doctor okays starting egg yolk (it will probably be suggested you wait on the white, which is very allergenic), serve it hard-cooked and mashed, scrambled, or in French toast or pancakes, and serve it at the same meal as a vitamin C food, such as orange juice, to facilitate iron absorption. Watch out for strings from fruits (such as bananas and mangos), vegetables (such as broccoli, string beans, and kale), and meats. And be sure to check fish very carefully for bones that might be left after mashing.

Some babies can also handle bread and crackers by seven months, but make your selections carefully. They should be whole grain, prepared without added sugar or salt, and have a melt-in-the-mouth texture. Ideal starters are whole-wheat bagels that have been frozen (they're hard, but whatever baby manages to scrape off will be mushy) and unsalted rice cakes (they crumble easily but dissolve on the tongue, and though not very tasty are loved by most babies). Once these are handled well, baby is ready for whole-grain breads. To decrease the risk of choking, remove crusts and serve sliced bread in cubes, and rolls or loaves in hunks; avoid commercial white breads, which tend to turn pasty when wet and can cause gagging or choking. Give bread and crackers—and all finger foods—only when your baby is seated and only under your supervision. And be sure you know how to deal with a choking incident (see page 454).

WHAT YOU MAY BE CONCERNED ABOUT

BITING NIPPLES

"My daughter now has two teeth and seems to think it's fun to use them for biting my nipples during nursing."

There's no need to let your baby have her fun at your expense. Since a baby can't bite while actively nursing (her tongue comes between teeth and breast), biting usually signals that she's had enough milk and is now just toying with you. It's possible the fun began when she accidentally bit down on your nipple, you let out a yelp, she giggled, you couldn't help laughing, and she continued the game—biting you, watching for a reaction, smirking at your mock "no," and seeing through your feeble attempts to keep a straight face.

So resist the temptation to laugh, and let her know that her biting you is not acceptable by issuing a firm but not harsh "no!" and by removing her from the breast. If she tries to hang on to your nipple, use your finger to break her grip. After a few such episodes, she'll catch on and give up.

It is important to nip the biting habit now, to avoid more serious biting problems later. It's not too soon for her to learn that while teeth are made for biting, there are things that are appropriate to clamp down on (a teething ring, a piece of bread, a banana) and things that are not (mother's breast, brother's finger, daddy's shoulder).

SPOILING BABY

"I pick my baby up the minute he cries, and end up carrying him around with me much of the day. Am I spoiling him?"

Though sparing the rod won't spoil your child (in fact, experts recommend that it be spared almost without exception), carrying him around with you all day at this age may. By the seventh month babies are already expert mommy manipulators; mothers who play "baby taxi"—picking their little ones up the moment they are hailed by a pathetic wave of the arm—can count on being "on duty" throughout their baby's waking hours.

There are societies where babies are carried around, usually strapped to mommy, round the clock, but ours is not one of them. Here, a baby is expected to gain some measure of independence early on—through learning to entertain himself for at least short periods of time. This not only gives his mother a chance to attend to her own needs or other responsibilities, but also increases a baby's self-esteem by reinforcing the idea that he is good company. It also begins to teach him that other people have rights and needs, another important concept to grasp early on.

Assuming you don't want to spoil your baby, or that you want to unspoil him, now's the time to start a little manipulating of your own. Try the following, staying casually cool throughout. If your baby senses that you expect this to be an anxiety-provoking experience, he will try all the harder to fulfill your prophecy:

■ First of all, determine if your baby is nagging to be carried because he really isn't getting quality attention. Have you actually sat down to play with him several times during the day—to read a book, play with an activity toy, or practice pulling up—or has most of your interaction consisted of dropping him in the playpen with a toy, strapping him in the car seat and driving to the market, leaving him in the baby swing while you start dinner, picking him up in response to his crying and carting him around while you go about your business? If so, your baby has probably come to the conclusion that being carried around all day by you, while not very stimulating, is better than getting no attention at all.

■ Next, see if your baby has physical needs. Is his diaper soiled? Is it time for lunch? Is he thirsty? Tired? If so, satisfy his needs, then go on to the next step.

■ Move him to a new location: the playpen, if he was in the crib; the walker, if he was in the playpen; the floor, if he was in the walker. This may satisfy his wanderlust.

■ Be sure he has toys or objects to entertain him—pots and pans, a cuddly stuffed animal, or an activity board—you know what he likes. Since his attention span is short, have two or three playthings within reach; too many toys at his disposal, however, will overwhelm and frustrate him. Provide a fresh selection when he seems to be getting restless.

■ If he continues to complain, try distracting him, getting down on his level for a moment, but not picking him up. Show him how to bang on a pot with the wooden spoon, point out "eyes-nose-mouth" on the stuffed animal, spin the cylinder and turn the dial on the busy box to get him started, and challenge him to do the same.

■ If he's momentarily diverted, and even if he's still voicing halfhearted objections, tell him you have work to do and move off to do it without hesitation. Stay within view, chatting or singing to him if it seems to help; but move out of eyeshot (but not earshot and only if he's in a safe playpen or crib) if your presence increases his dissatisfaction. Before you do, poke your head around a corner, playing peekaboo, to show him that when you disappear, you return.

■ Leave him to his own devices a little longer each time, letting him object a little longer if necessary. But always return to his side before he starts screaming, to reassure him, and start the process over. Postpone picking him up for as long as you can, but don't get into a battle of wills—he'll almost always win. If you wait until he's screaming to pick him up, he'll conclude that that's the way to get attention.

■ Don't feel guilty or anxious about not picking him up or playing with him every minute of the day. If you do, you'll be transmitting the message that playing alone is punishment and can't be fun, that there's something wrong with solitude. As long as you do spend plenty of time playing with him, some time apart will actually benefit both of you.

BABY'S STILL NOT SLEEPING THROUGH THE NIGHT

"My baby seems to be the only one on the block who's not sleeping through the night yet. Will she ever?"

All babies wake up during the night, and most, by this time, have acquired the ability to fall back to sleep on their own. Unfortunately, this is not something you can teach your daughter to do, the way you teach her to play peekaboo or wave bye-bye; it's something she must learn by herself. And the only way she'll be able to learn is if you give her the chance. That means not nursing her, giving her a bottle, rocking her, or using any other method to help her get back to sleep when she wakes up crying at night, but letting her struggle to fall back to sleep without your help. It may take her a few nights, even a week, to learn this skill—but rarely more than that.

If you've never tried the tips for helping baby sleep through the night on page 260, or if you tried them earlier and they didn't work or you caved in before baby did, now is the time to try or try again. The odds are very good that if you do, you'll all be sleeping as soundly as the rest of the block very soon.

GRANDPARENTS SPOILING BABY

"My parents live nearby and see my daughter several times a week. When they do, they stuff her with sweets and give in to her every whim. I love them, but I don't love the way they spoil her."

Grandparents have the best of all worlds: they can have the joy of spoiling a baby without the misery of living with the consequences. They can watch with pleasure as their grandchild relishes the sugary cookies they've plied her with, but don't have to struggle with a fussy—and unhungry—baby come mealtime. They can keep her up through her naptime, so they'll have more time to play, but don't have to deal with her crankiness afterward.

Is it an inalienable right of grandparents to spoil their grandchildren? To some extent, yes. They've paid their dues as the heavies during your childhood, weaning you from your precious bottle, cajoling you to eat the spinach you despised, battling with you over curfews. Now that it's your turn to play the heavy, they've earned the cushy job of spoilers. There should, however, be some sensible guidelines agreed upon by all:

▪ **Wider latitude can be given to grandparents whose longitude is distant from yours.** Occasional grandparents—those who see your baby only two or three times a year, on holidays or special occasions—can't possibly spoil her, but should be given almost every opportunity to try. If baby misses a nap or stays up past her bedtime when your folks are on a one-day, half-birthday visit, or if she is toted around royally much more than you'd prefer while visiting them for the holidays, don't worry. Let everyone enjoy these infrequent lapses, and rest assured that your daughter will quickly return to her normal routine afterward.

▪ **Grandparents who live near Rome should do as the Romans do**—most of the time. It is possible for grandparents who live in the same town, and especially for those who live in the same house, to spoil a baby, making life miserable not only for the baby's parents, but for baby as well. Mixed signals—mother won't pick her up at every whimper, grandmother will—make for a confused and unhappy baby. On the other hand, a baby will readily learn that the ground rules can vary with the territory: she can mush the food all over the table at grandma's, but not at home. So some leeway, in areas of lesser consequence, needs to be allowed even close-by grandparents.

▪ **Certain parental rules must be inviolate.** Since it's the parents who live with their child on a 24-hour-a-day basis, it's the parents who must lay down the law on more significant issues—and it's the grandparents, near or far, who must abide by those rules, even if they don't necessarily agree with them. In one family, a bone of contention may be the bedtime hour; in another, sugar and junk foods in the diet; in yet another, what the children are permitted to watch on TV (not an issue yet with a seven-month-old but one that will enter the picture soon enough). Of course, if the parents wish to stand firm on every issue, then the grandparents should be allowed to negotiate on occasion.

▪ **Certain grandparental rights must be inviolate.** The right to give gifts, for example, that the parents might not have chosen—either because they're very expensive, or frivolous, or, in the parents' opinion, tasteless. And to give them more often than mommy and daddy might. (Though gifts that are unsafe should be taboo and those that violate parental values should be negotiated prior to purchase.) In general, to indulge (yes, spoil) their grandchildren with a little extra of everything—love, time, material things. But not to the point where this spoiling regularly violates parental rules.

What if grandparents overstep the boundaries of fair grandparenting? What if they ignore or openly flout all the rules you have so thoughtfully set up and try consistently to follow? Then it's time to open an honest dialogue. Keep the exchange on a loving and light level—but if any of your differences center on life-and-death issues (your father refuses to recognize the importance of using the car seat to go around the corner, your mother-in-law smokes while holding the baby in her arms), emphasize the seriousness of the problem. Explain (even if you have before) how much you want them to spend time with the baby, but how their breaking the rules you've established is confusing her and upsetting her schedule and the family equilibrium. Tell them you are willing to be flexible on certain issues, but that on others they will have to do the bending. If that doesn't work, leave this book, open to "Grandparents Spoiling Baby," in a place where they can't miss it.

IS MY BABY GIFTED?

"I don't want to be a pushy mother. But I don't want to neglect my daughter's talents if she's gifted. How can you tell an ordinary bright baby from a gifted one?"

Every child is gifted in some way. Musically. Socially. Athletically. Artistically. Mechanically. And whatever talent emerges in a child, it's important for parents to encourage its development, to praise the child for it, and not to wish it could be a talent they valued more. This encouragement should come as soon as the gift becomes apparent—which might even be in the first year. But encouraging is very different from demanding and pushing, neither of which is good for your child.

When most people talk about the "gifted" child, however, they mean a child who excels intellectually. Even among those who are blessed with exceptional intellectual ability, there are differences. Some children are good with numbers, others with spatial relations, still others with words. Some are creative; others are great at organization. Many, but not all, of these talents can later be measured by intel-

ligence testing, but all are difficult to recognize in infancy. Tests of motor development, most often used to evaluate IQ in the first year, do not correlate well with a child's IQ later on. Tests that evaluate a baby's ability to process information and manipulate the environment do correlate, but are not widely available. Still, there are clues to intelligence in the first year that you can look for in your own baby:

Uniformly advanced development. A baby who does everything "early"—smiles, sits, walks, talks, picks up objects with a pincer grasp, and so on—is probably going to continue to develop at an advanced clip, and may turn out to be truly gifted. Though early language ability, particularly the use of unusual words before the end of the first year, is the trait noted most frequently by parents in their gifted children, and is probably indicative of high intelligence, some gifted children are not verbal until fairly late.

Good memory and powers of observation. Gifted children often amaze their parents with the things they remember, often long before most babies have exhibited much memory at all. And when things differ from what they recollect (mommy's gotten her hair cut, daddy's wearing a new coat, grandpa's wearing a patch on his eye after surgery), they notice immediately.

Creativity and originality. Though most babies under a year are not competent problem solvers, the gifted child may surprise parents by being able to figure out a way to get to a toy that's stuck behind a chair, reach a high shelf in the bookcase (pile up books from lower shelves to climb on, perhaps), or use sign language for a word that's beyond their linguistic abilities (such as pointing to her own nose to indicate that the animal in the book is an elephant, or to her ears if it's a rabbit). The baby on the way to being a gifted child may also be creative in play, using toys in unusual ways, using non-toys creatively as playthings, enjoying playing "pretend."

Sense of humor. Even in the first year, a bright child will notice and laugh at the incongruities in life: grandma wearing her glasses on top of her head or daddy tripping over the dog and spilling his glass of juice, for example.

Curiosity and concentration. While all babies are intensely curious, the very gifted are not only curious, but have the persistence and concentration to explore what it is they are curious about.

Ability to make connections. The gifted child, more so and earlier than other children, will see relationships between things and will be able to apply old knowledge to new situations. A baby nine or ten months old may see in the store a book that daddy's been reading at home and say, "Dada." Or, accustomed to pushing the button for the elevator in her apartment house, she sees an elevator in a store and looks for the button.

Rich imagination. Before a year, the gifted child may be able to pretend (to drink a cup of coffee or to rock a baby) and soon after that may become heavily involved in making up stories, games, pretend friends, and so on.

Difficulty sleeping. Gifted children may be so involved in observing and learning that they have trouble tuning out the world so they sleep—a trait that can exasperate parents.

Perceptiveness and sensitivity. Very early the gifted child may notice when mommy is sad or angry, may note that daddy has a boo-boo (because he's wearing a band-aid on his finger), may try to cheer up a crying sibling.

Even if your baby displays many or all of these traits, it's much too early to tag her with the "gifted" label. What she needs now is not to be labeled, but to be loved. You can, of course, encourage her growth and development by being certain you raise her in a stimulating environment. Read to her, talk to her, play with her. But don't just pay attention to the talents you would like to see her develop—linguistic or musical, perhaps. Rather concern yourself with her overall development—physical and social as well as intellectual. As she grows, let her know that you love her not because of her special gifts, but because she's your child, and that you would never withdraw that love if she stopped being "smart." Encourage her to be kind and caring and to appreciate others, including those with fewer or different gifts.

SNACKING

"My baby seems to want to eat all the time. How much snacking is good for her?"

With their own mothers' pronouncements about snacking ("Not before dinner, dear—it'll spoil your appetite!") still ringing in their ears, today's mothers are often reluctant to dole out between-meal goodies to their children on demand, even as they themselves choose to graze through their day's nutritional requirements. Yet snacks, in moderation, do play an important role in the lives of babies and children.

Snacks are a learning experience. At mealtimes, baby usually is spoon-fed from a bowl; at snacktime she has the opportunity to pick up a piece of bread or cracker with her fingers and get it to and into her mouth herself—no small accomplishment considering how tiny her mouth is and how primitive her coordination.

Snacks fill a void. Babies have small stomachs that fill quickly and empty quickly, and can rarely last from meal to meal, as adults can, without a snack in between. And as solids become the most significant part of your baby's diet, snacks will be needed to round out nutritional requirements. You'll find it almost impossible to give baby her Daily Dozen in just three meals a day.

Snacks give baby a break. Like most of us, babies need a break from the tedium of work or play (their play *is* their work), and a snack provides this breather.

Snacks provide oral gratification. Babies are still very orally oriented—everything they pick up goes right to the mouth. Snacking gives them a welcome chance to put things in their mouths without being chastised.

Snacks smooth the way for weaning. If you didn't offer your baby a snack in the form of solids, the odds are good she would insist on one in the form of a breast or a bottle. Snacks will lessen the need to nurse frequently, and eventually help to make weaning a reality.

For all its virtues, however, snacking can have some drawbacks. To reap the benefits of snacking without stumbling into the pitfalls, remember these pointers:

Snacks by the clock. Mom was right— snacks that come too close to mealtime can interfere with a baby's appetite for meals. Make an attempt to schedule snacks about midway between meals to avoid this problem. Non-stop snacking gets baby accustomed to having something in her mouth all the time, a habit that could be hazardous to the waistline should it be perpetuated into childhood and adulthood. And having the mouth continuously full of food can also lead to tooth decay—even a healthy starch like whole-wheat bread turns to sugar when exposed to saliva in the mouth. One snack in the morning, one in the afternoon, and if there's a long span between dinner and bedtime, one in the evening should suffice. Make an exception, of course, if a meal is going to be delayed longer than usual.

Snack for the right reasons. There are good reasons to snack (as discussed above) and not-so-good reasons. Avoid offering snacks if baby's bored (distract her with a toy), hurt (soothe her with a hug and a

song), or has accomplished something that should be rewarded (try verbal praise and an enthusiastic round of applause).

Snack in place. Snacking should be treated pretty much as seriously as mealtime eating. For reasons of safety (a baby eating lying on her back, crawling around, or walking can choke too easily), etiquette (good table manners are best learned at the table), and consideration to the housekeeper (you, or whoever does the cleaning, will appreciate not finding crumbs and spills in every nook and cranny), snacks should be given while baby is sitting, preferably in her feeding chair. Of course, if you're out and baby is in her stroller or car seat at snacktime, you can serve it up there. But don't give her the idea that a snack is her compensation for serving time in these confining quarters; getting into stroller or car should not be a signal to bring on the crackers.

GRAZING

"I've heard that grazing is the healthiest way for anyone to eat, particularly a young child. Should I feed my son this way?"

Long before grazing became fashionable among adults, it was the preferred way of gastronomic life for young children. Presented with the option, many babies would choose to snack the day away, nibbling crackers and sipping juice as they play, and never actually sitting down to a square meal. But though some experts propose that this is a healthier choice than the conventional one of three substantial meals supplemented by light snacks, others disagree. Consider the following:

Grazing interferes with proper nutrition. A heifer who grazes in fields of clover gets most of the nourishment she needs that way. But while it's possible that a baby who does nothing but graze all day on favorite finger foods will get his Daily

Dozen, it's not likely. Nutritional requirements are filled much more efficiently when meals are taken, along with two or three nutritious snacks.

Grazing interferes with play. Always having a cracker or breadstick in hand (like always having a bottle) limits the amount and kind of playing and exploring a baby can do. And as baby becomes mobile, crawling or toddling around with food becomes dangerous because of the risk of choking.

Grazing interferes with sociability. A baby who's always got food in his mouth can't practice his social skills or his language skills, and also misses out on the social experience of mealtime.

Grazing interferes with the development of good table manners. Children won't learn table manners munching a cookie on the sofa, sipping milk on the bed, or savoring cheese on the carpet.

NOT SITTING YET

"My baby hasn't started sitting up yet, and I'm worried that she's slow for her age."

Because normal babies accomplish different developmental feats at different ages, there's a wide range of "normal" for every milestone. Though the "average" baby sits unsupported somewhere around six and a half months, some normal babies sit as early as four months, others not until nine. And since your child has a long way to go before she reaches the outer limits of that range, you certainly needn't worry about her lagging behind.

A child is programmed by genetic factors to sit, and to accomplish other major developmental skills, at a certain age. Though there may not be much a parent can do to speed up the timetable, there are ways to avoid slowing it down. A baby who is propped up often at an early age, in either an infant seat, a stroller, or a high chair, gets a lot of practice in a sitting position before she's able to support herself, and may sit sooner. On the other hand, a baby who spends a majority of her time lying on her back or harnessed in a baby carrier, and is rarely propped to sit, may sit very late. In fact, babies in primitive countries who are carried constantly in baby carriers at their mothers' breast often stand before they sit, so accustomed are they to the upright position. Another factor that might interfere with the development of early sitting (and other large motor skills) is overweight. A roly-poly baby is more likely than a leaner child to roll over when attempting a sitting position.

As long as you're giving your baby plenty of opportunity to reach her goal, chances are she will sometime during the next two months. If she doesn't, and/or if you feel she's developing slowly in several other ways, consult her doctor.

TOOTH STAINS

"My daughter's two teeth seem to be stained a grayish color. Could they be decaying already?"

Chances are what's keeping your baby's pearly whites a dismal gray isn't decay, but iron. Some children who take a liquid vitamin and mineral supplement that contains iron develop staining on their teeth. This doesn't harm the teeth in any way and will disappear when your child stops taking liquid and begins taking chewable vitamins. In the meantime, brushing your baby's teeth or cleaning them with gauze (see page 253) right after giving her supplement will help minimize staining.

If your baby hasn't been taking a liquid supplement, and especially if she's been doing a lot of sucking on a bottle of formula or juice at bedtime, the discoloration might suggest either decay, trauma, or a congenital defect in the tooth enamel. Discuss this with her doctor or a pediatric dentist as soon as possible.

BABY'S MISBEHAVING WITH YOU

"The baby sitter tells me that my baby is just wonderful with her, but he always starts to act up the minute I walk in the door after work. I feel like I must be a terrible mother."

Like most babies his age, your baby's already learning how to be manipulative. And like most good mommies, you're falling right into his trap. Even at this tender stage, albeit at a very fundamental level, your baby is shrewd enough to see that playing the abandoned and neglected victim is the best way to guarantee that he'll get an extra dose of love and attention when you arrive home. He plays on your insecurities, instills the guilt, and gets what he wants—which is probably what you'd give him anyway, but he's not taking any chances.

The fact that most babies and toddlers, and even older children, are more likely to act up with their parents than with other caretakers is a sign that they are more comfortable and secure with their parents. They know they can let their emotions show without risking loss of love. But this acting up isn't always random—it often has a purpose. Not only does it get and keep parental attention, but it also is a way of testing limits: "How far can I go before mommy (or daddy) explodes or gives in?" The baby who cries for a middle-of-the-night feeding is doing that. So is the one who smears the mashed carrots in his hair, or keeps dropping toys out of his playpen. And the one who repeatedly maneuvers his walker to the brink of the stairway—the one area he's forbidden to explore.

A certain amount of manipulation is not only normal, it's probably healthy, giving a child a chance to exercise some control over his environment. But when it gets out of hand, it can be detrimental to emotional growth. So go along with your baby when it seems to make sense—when he really needs your attention and he's letting you know you're not giving it. But do set the limits you think are important for his health and safety and for your sanity, and stick to them.

WHAT IT'S IMPORTANT TO KNOW: Raising a Superbaby

We've seen their photographs on the covers of major magazines and watched them perform on television talk shows. With an odd mixture of curiosity, disapproval, and envy we've listened as their proud parents described their incredible accomplishments: reading words at six months, books at a year, *The New York Times* at two. We wonder how anyone could push their baby so intensely. And we wonder whether we should be doing the same with our own.

The Superbaby concept has undeniably made a significant splash in the media, even a few waves among the general public, and in some communities has reached tidal proportions. Programs and books that dedicate themselves to the raising of these tiniest of wunderkinds have proliferated—there is even an institute devoted to this purpose. But among the most reliable experts in the field of child development, the proposition that babies and children should be pushed to achieve way beyond their normal rate of development has yet to make a ripple. That's because scientifically there's no evidence that such programs are beneficial, or even that they work. Though it's possible to teach an infant a wide variety of skills long before they are ordinarily learned, including how to recognize words, there is no proven consistent method for doing so. Nor is there any evidence that intense early learning actually provides a long-term advantage over more traditional learning patterns. Studies of extremely successful adults in such vastly different fields as music, athletics, and medicine have shown that not only did their acquisition of skills in their fields not begin early in childhood, but when it did begin, it was more likely to have taken the form of play than serious, high-pressured activity.

Babies have lots to learn in the first year of life—more, in fact, than they'll be expected to learn in the first year of school. During these twelve busy months, their agenda will include building attachments to others (mommy, daddy, siblings, sitters, and so on), learning to trust ("When I'm in trouble, I can depend on mommy or daddy to help me"), and grasping the concept of object permanence ("When mommy hides behind the chair, she's still there, even though I don't see her"). They'll also need to learn to use their bodies (to sit, stand, walk), their hands (to pick up and drop, as well as to manipulate), and their minds (solving problems such as how-to-get-that-truck-from-the-shelf-I-can't-reach); the meanings of hundreds of words and how to reproduce them using a complicated combination of voice box, lips, and tongue; and something about who they are ("What kind of person am I, what do I like, what don't I like, what makes me happy or sad?"). With such a heavy course load lined up already, it's probable that adding supplementary learning material would force one or more of these critical scheduled developmental areas to be neglected.

Though few parents would force a child to stand before he appeared ready and eager, many wouldn't hesitate to push a mental accomplishment such as reading. Why? Maybe because it's easier to imagine injury to a leg pushed too far than injury to an overworked mind. Or maybe because, in some homes, more value is placed on intellectual than on physical achievement.

Parents who are tempted to try to produce a superbaby, in spite of the clear stack of sentiment against early learning programs in the child development community, should ask themselves the following questions:

■ What's my goal? To make my child feel superior to other children? (Will such a feeling serve him or her well through life?) To provide early access to education—college at ten, grad school at twelve? (And then what? What of the emotional impact and psychological stigma of being a child in college?) There is no evidence that the lives of child prodigies are richer and more fulfilling than those of children who are not pushed (in fact, there have been instances where the lives of child "geniuses" have been disastrous). Even early on, parents and others tend to judge these superbabies by their success at learning what they are taught rather than for who they are as individuals.

■ Am I motivated by fear that my child will not do well in today's highly competitive academic world without such early preparation? While it's true that children who learn to read before starting school often continue to read ahead of grade level, a child with a rich reading preparation background (exposure to the alphabet, songs and stories, and a variety of enriching experiences), who doesn't start deciphering words until formal education begins, can catch up quickly and do equally well.

■ Am I uncomfortable with babies and children? Some people, unable to bring themselves down to the level of their babies (because they don't have the knack for baby talk, for example), want to bring their children up to their own level as soon as possible. But babies need their babyhood, and with some effort, it may be fairer for you to meet them down where they are than to drag them up to you.

■ How would pushing one area of my child's development—language, for example, through reading—impact on other areas? Will you have time to help your child develop socially (through play groups or at the playground) and physically (with opportunities to climb a slide, throw a ball, jump down a step), and to encourage his or her growing curiosity (about everything from a dust ball on the floor to clouds in the sky)? Not every adult is "well-rounded" or needs to be—but children need to understand their strengths and weaknesses, to uncover and explore every possible avenue to personal fulfillment, before sorting out those dimensions of self they most want to develop. This is a selection that should be made by the child, not the parents, and certainly not in the first year.

Even the parent who decides not to try to create a superbaby can produce a pretty terrific child, one who reaches his or her maximum potential at a rate that's personally appropriate, by offering ample stimulation and assistance in the ordinary tasks of infancy; by exposing him or her to a variety of settings (stores, zoos, museums, gas stations, parks, and so on); by talking about people you see ("That lady is very old," "That man has to ride around in a chair because he has a boo-boo on his leg," "Those children are going to school"); and by describing how things work ("See, I turn on the faucet and water comes out of the tap"), what they are used for ("This is a chair—you sit in a chair"), and how they differ ("The horse has a long flowing tail and the pig has a little curly one"). It's more important for your baby to know that a dog barks, eats, can bite, has four legs, and has hair all over than to be able to recognize that the letters d-o-g spell dog.

If your baby does show an interest in words, letters, or numbers, by all means nurture that interest. But don't suddenly forsake trips to the playground so you and baby can spend all your time with flashcards. Learning—whether it's how to recognize a letter or how to throw a ball—should be fun. But there is little fun for either of you in a pressured environment in which you're faced with a never-ending list of goals that must be met. Take your cues from your baby, let him or her set the pace, and if your little scholar seems unhappy at any activity, it's time to switch gears.

Children gain confidence from learning what is important to them, not what's important to their parents. The message that what mommy (or daddy) wants me to do is more important than what I want to do can deal a major blow to self-respect. So can failure to perform up to mommy's or daddy's expectations, realistic or not. In the long run, whether children learn to like and respect themselves is much more important than whether they learn to read or play piano in toddlerhood.

CHAPTER ELEVEN

The Eighth Month

WHAT YOUR BABY MAY BE DOING

By the end of this month, your baby …should be able to (see Note):

- bear some weight on legs when held upright
- feed self a cracker
- pass a cube or other object from one hand to the other (usually by 8½ months)
- rake a raisin and pick it up in fist
- turn in the direction of a voice (by 8⅓ months)
- look for a dropped object

…will probably be able to:

- stand holding on to someone or something (8½ months)
- object if you try to take at toy away
- work to get a toy out of reach
- play peekaboo
- get into a sitting position from stomach

Note: If your baby seems not to have reached one or more of these milestones, check with the doctor. In rare instances the delay could indicate a problem, though in most cases it will turn out to be normal for your baby. Premature infants generally reach milestones later than others of the same birth age, often achieving them closer to their adjusted age (the age they would be if they had been born at term) or sometimes later.

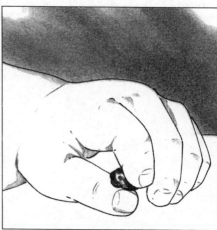

By the eighth month, a few babies can pick up small objects using the thumb and forefinger.

...may possibly be able to:

- pull up to standing position from sitting
- pick up tiny object with any part of thumb and finger
- say mama or dada indiscriminately

...may even be able to:

- play patty-cake (clap hands) or wave bye-bye
- walk holding on to furniture
- stand alone momentarily
- understand the word no (but not always obey it)

WHAT YOU CAN EXPECT AT THIS MONTH'S CHECKUP

Most doctors do not schedule regular well-baby checkups this month. Do call the doctor if there are any concerns that can't wait until next month's visit.

FEEDING YOUR BABY THIS MONTH: Finally—Finger Foods

For most mothers, the novelty of feeding their babies soon wears as thin as the rice cereal they've been struggling to direct into those little mouths. The lips clenched willfully, the head turned away just at the critical moment (splat!), the pudgy hand grabbing the spoon and overturning it just before it reaches its destination, and the sheer tedium of repeating this messy ritual three times a day, every day, makes these mothers ready to relinquish the role they couldn't wait to take on a few months earlier. Fortunately, the opportunity to do so presents itself fairly quickly. Most babies are not only eager but able to begin finger foods by the time they are seven months old, some even earlier.

The transition is more sudden than gradual. Once babies discover they can get food into their mouths independently, the number of foods that they can expertly express to the mouth increases rapidly. At first, most babies hold the rice cake or piece of bread in the fist and munch on it that way, not having learned yet to coordinate individual fingers for pickup and transport. When the problem of how to get that last piece of food wrapped tightly in the palm into the mouth arises, they may demonstrate their frustration with a tearful outburst. The solution for some is to open the hand flat against the mouth, for others to put the food down and pick it up again with more of it exposed.

The ability to position an object between thumb and forefinger in the pincer grip doesn't develop in most babies until between nine and twelve months of age—though some perfect their pincers earlier and others later. Once this skill is mastered, it allows a baby to pick up very small objects, such as peas and pennies, and bring them to the mouth, considerably expanding the dining repertoire—and the risk of choking.

Learning to handle finger foods is usually the first step on the road to dinner-table independence. At first, finger foods merely supplement a young child's diet; as facility with self-feeding grows, a large proportion of the daily intake will be delivered by baby's own hand. Some will learn to wield a spoon respectably well by the middle of the second year or even sooner, and will switch to this more civilized style of eating; others will continue to get most of their meals to their mouths (even such dubious finger fare as cereal and cottage cheese) via the fingers for a long time to come. A few, usually those who were never allowed to "do it themselves" because of the time or mess involved, will insist on being fed long after they are capable of feeding themselves.

The foods that qualify for first finger-food honors are those that baby can gum to swallowable consistency or that will dissolve in the mouth without chewing, and that have been well received in puréed form on earlier tries. Most of these foods should be cut into manageable cubes or chunks—pea-size for firmer items, marble-size for softer foods. Good choices include a whole-wheat bagel, whole-grain bread or toast, rice cakes or other crackers that become mushy in the mouth; oat circle cereals (best are the varieties made without added salt or sugar, found in health-food stores), corn and wheat puffs; tiny cubes of natural cheese, such as baby Swiss, Cheddar, Edam, Havarti; chunks of ripe banana, very ripe pear, peach, apricot, cantaloupe, honeydew, or mango; small chunks of cooked-to-very-tender carrot, white or sweet potato, yam, broccoli or cauliflower (flowerets only), peas (cut in half or crushed); flakes of broiled, baked, or poached fish (but screen *carefully* for bones); soft meatballs (cook in sauce or soup so they don't get crusty); well-cooked pasta of various sizes and shapes (break up before or cut after cooking, as necessary) if they contain no ingredients that baby isn't allowed yet; scrambled or hard-cooked egg yolk, and whole eggs once baby can have the whites; cubes of soft-cooked French toast or whole-wheat pancakes (again,

made at first with yolk only, then as whites are introduced, with whole eggs). About the same time you add finger foods, you can add more texture to the other foods baby is eating by using commercial toddler foods, or table foods that are chopped or mashed but that contain small, soft chunks baby can gum.

To serve finger foods, scatter four or five pieces onto an unbreakable plate or directly onto baby's feeding tray, and replace as baby eats them. Beginning eaters, confronted by too much food, especially all in one spot, may respond either by trying to stuff all of it in their mouth at once or by sending it all to the floor with one deft swipe. As with other foods, finger foods should be fed only to a baby who is seated, and not to one who is crawling, cruising, or toddling around.

Because of the danger of choking, don't give your baby foods that won't dissolve in the mouth, can't be mashed with the gums, or can be easily sucked into the windpipe—such as uncooked raisins, popcorn, nuts, whole peas, raw firm-fleshed vegetables (carrots, bell peppers) or fruits (apples, unripe pears), chunks of meat or poultry, or hot dogs (which, with their high sodium and additive content, aren't meant for babies anyway).

Once the molars come in (the first teeth are for biting, and don't improve your child's ability to chew), somewhere around the end of the year for early teethers, some foods that require real chewing can be added, such as raw apples and other firm-fleshed raw fruits and vegetables, small slices of meat and poultry (cut across the grain), uncooked raisins (soft and fresh, squashed at first), and seedless or seeded grapes (skinned and halved). But hold off for many months on such frequent troublemakers as carrots, popcorn, nuts, and hot dogs. Introduce them only when your baby is chewing well.

No matter what the texture, there are some types of food that should not be introduced to your baby at all, now or later: junk foods that offer no nutrition, foods prepared with added sugar or salt, and refined breads or cereals. They will certainly be introduced eventually outside the home, but by then your child will know they aren't acceptable everyday fare.

WHAT YOU MAY BE CONCERNED ABOUT

BABY'S FIRST WORDS

"My baby has started saying 'ma-ma' a lot. We were all excited until my neighbor said that she's just making sounds without understanding their meaning. Is she right?"

Only your baby knows for sure, and she isn't telling, at least not yet. Just when a baby makes the transition from sounds that mimic real words but have no meaning to meaningful speech is difficult to pinpoint exactly. Your baby may just be practicing her "m" sounds now, or she may be calling for mommy, but it really doesn't matter which. The important thing is that she's vocalizing and attempting to imitate sounds she hears. Many babies, of course, say "da-da" first—not a sign of favoritism, just a reflection of the consonant a baby has found easiest to pronounce initially.

In many languages the informal words for male and female parents sound very similar. Daddy, pappa, papa, abba. Mommy, mama, mummy, imma. It's a good bet that they all developed from babies' earliest mouthing of syllables, picked up on by eager parents trying to recognize their baby's first word. When, long ago, a young Spanish baby uttered her first "maa-maa," complaining in the fashion typical of babies, her proud mother probably was certain she was calling "madre." And when an early Hebrew infant first vocalized "ah-ba," his father probably puffed up his chest and said, "He's trying to say av."

When the first real word is spoken varies a great deal—and is, of course, subject to less-than-objective parental interpretation. According to the experts, the average baby can be expected to say what she means and mean what she says for the first time anywhere between ten and fourteen months. A small percentage of children start a couple of months earlier and some perfectly normal babies don't utter a single recognizable word until midway through their second year, at least as far as anyone can tell. Often, however, a baby may already be using syllables, alone and in combination, to represent objects ("ba" for bottle, "ba-ba" for bye-bye, or "daw" for dog), but her parents may not be tuned in enough to notice until the enunciation becomes clearer. A child who is very busy developing motor skills—one who, perhaps, crawls and walks early, is involved in learning to climb stairs and ride a fire engine—may be slower than less active babies in starting to vocalize. This is nothing to worry about as long as it's clear from her behavior that she understands a lot of the familiar words she hears.

Long before your baby utters her first word, she will be developing her linguistic skills. First, by learning to understand what is said. This receptive language starts developing at birth, with the first words your baby hears. Gradually, she begins to sort out individual words from the jumble of language around her, and then one day, about the middle of the first year, you say her name and she turns around. She's recognized a word. Pretty soon thereafter she should begin to understand the names of other people and objects she sees daily, such as mommy, daddy, bottle, juice, bread. In a few months, or even earlier, she may begin to follow simple commands, such as "Give me a bite," or "Wave bye-bye" or "Kiss mommy." This comprehension moves ahead at a much faster pace than speech itself and is an important forerunner to it. You can encourage both receptive and spoken language development every day in many ways (see page 264).

BABY'S NOT CRAWLING YET

"My friend's baby started crawling at six months. My son's almost eight months, and he hasn't shown any interest in crawling. Is he delayed developmentally?"

When it comes to crawling, a baby's prowess shouldn't be compared to that of other babies. Crawling is not a skill that babies accomplish by a certain age and by which we can gauge their overall development. Moving about on the belly, or creeping, is usually a precursor to moving about on the hands and knees, or crawling. Some babies crawl as early as six months, but 7½ to nine months is more typical. A few babies never crawl at all—they just pull up, start cruising (from chair to coffee table to sofa), and then take off and walk. Because crawling, unlike sitting or pulling up, is not a predictable part of the developmental pattern, it isn't included on most assessment scales.

Even among babies who do crawl, styles vary. Many begin crawling backward or sideways, and don't get the hang of going forward for weeks. Some scoot on one knee or on their bottom, and others travel on hands and feet, a stage that many babies reach just before walking. The method a baby chooses to get from one point to another is much less important than the fact that he's making an effort to achieve independent locomotion.

Before a baby can crawl, he has to be able to sit well. Whether or when he begins to crawl after that is an individual matter and not one for concern unless he's behind in at least a couple of developmental areas (social, large or small mo-

tor, language, and so on) or if he does not seem to be using both sides of his body (arms and legs) equally—in which case, check with his doctor. Good crawlers are often late walkers, while children who never take to crawling may walk early.

Some babies don't crawl because they haven't been given the chance. A baby who passes most of his day confined in a crib, stroller, baby carrier, playpen, and/or walker won't learn how to raise himself on all fours or put his hands and knees in motion. Be sure your baby spends plenty of supervised time on the floor (don't worry about dirt as long as the floor has been swept or vacuumed free of small particles and cleared of dangerous objects). To encourage him to move forward, try putting a favorite toy or interesting object a short distance ahead of him. Do cover his knees, however, since bare knees on a cold, hard floor or a scratchy carpet can be uncomfortable and might even discourage your baby from attempting to crawl. Wean him from the walker if he's using one, and limit playpen exile to times when you can't supervise him.

One way or another, in the next few months your baby will be taking off—and

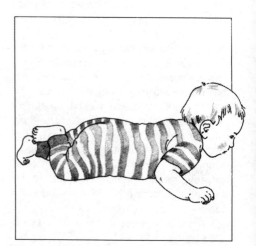

Some babies start off dragging themselves around on their belly. While many graduate to hands-and-knees crawling, a few will cling to creeping until they're up on their feet.

off into trouble—and you'll be left wondering, "Why was I in such a hurry?"

SCOOTING

"Our little girl scoots around on her bottom instead of crawling. She gets around, but looks strange."

For a baby eager and determined to get from one place to another, form and grace are of little consequence. And they should be to you, too. As long as your baby is attempting to get around independently, it doesn't matter how. You need only be concerned if your baby seems unable to coordinate both sides of her body, can't move her arms and legs in sync. This could be a sign of a learning disability, for which early treatment can be very helpful.

MESSY HOUSE

"Now that my son is crawling around and pulling up on everything, I can't keep up with the mess he makes. Should I try to control him—and the mess—better, or give up?"

Clutter may be your worst enemy, but it's an adventurous baby's best friend. A home that is kept compulsively tidy provides about as much interest and challenge to a baby who's newly mobile as a wading pool would to Christopher Columbus or a suburban parking lot to Lewis and Clark. Within the parameters of reason (you needn't let baby dismantle your checkbook or reorganize your Rolodex) and safety, your child needs to flex and extend his curiosity as he exercises his muscles. Letting him roam—and mess—freely is as important to his intellectual growth as it is to his physical development. Accepting this reality is important to your mental health; parents of young children who fight it, struggling to keep the house as neat as it was pre-baby, are in for a disappointment—as well as overwhelming frustration and anxiety.

You can, however, take some steps to make coping with the reality easier:

Start with a safe house. While it may be okay for him to scatter underwear on the bedroom floor or build a house of napkins

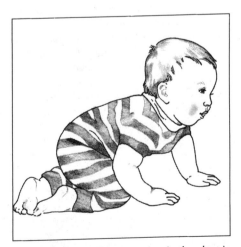

Hands-and-knees locomotion is the classic crawling technique. Some babies are so content zipping around this way that they don't bother with walking for months to come.

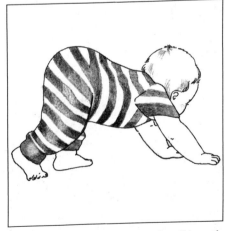

A cross between crawling and walking, the hands-and-feet posture may be one that baby settles on at first and sticks with, or one that he or she evolves into as a precursor of walking.

on the kitchen linoleum, it isn't okay for him to clang liquor bottles together to see what happens or to empty the chlorine cleanser on the rug. So before you let your baby loose, be sure to make the house safe for him and from him (see page 292).

Contain the chaos. The compulsive side of you will be a lot happier if you try to confine the mess to one or two rooms or areas in the home. That means letting your baby have free run only in his own room and perhaps the kitchen, family room, or living room—wherever you and he spend the most time together. Use closed doors or baby-safe gates to define the areas. If you have a small apartment, of course, you may not be able to place such restrictions on your baby; instead, you may have to resign yourself to daily messes and nightly cleanups.

Also reduce the potential for mess by wedging books in tightly on shelves accessible to your baby, leaving a few of his indestructible books where he can reach them and take them out easily; sealing some of the more vulnerable cabinets and drawers (especially those that contain breakables, valuables, or hazards) with childproof safety locks; keeping most knickknacks off low tables, leaving only a few you don't mind his playing with. Set aside a special drawer or cabinet for him to call his own, and fill it with such fun items as paper cups and plates, wooden spoons, a metal cup or pot, empty boxes, and plastic hair curlers.

Don't feel guilty about not letting your baby adorn the bathroom with your lipstick, tear the pages out of your favorite books, empty boxes of cereal all over the kitchen floor, and generally redecorate your home as he pleases. Setting limits will not only help save your sanity but also help your baby's development—children really do thrive when limits are set for them— and teach him the important lesson that other people, even parents, have rights too.

Restrain yourself. Don't follow your baby around as he wreaks havoc, putting away everything he takes out. This will frustrate him, giving him the sense that everything he does is not only unacceptable but totally in vain. And it will frustrate you if he immediately redoes the damage you've just undone. Instead, do the serious cleaning up twice a day, once at the end of his morning play period while he's napping or in his playpen or high chair, and once at the end of the afternoon or after he's in bed.

Teach him a lesson in neatness—over and over again. Don't do your intensive cleanups with him around. But do pick up a couple of things with him at the end of each play session, making a point (even if he's not old enough to get the point) of saying, "Now, can you help mommy pick this toy up and put it away?" Hand him one of the blocks to put back into the toy chest, give him a pot to return to the cabinet or some crumpled paper to throw into the wastebasket, and applaud each effort. Though he will be messing up a lot more often than he'll be cleaning up for years to come, these early lessons will help him to understand— eventually—that what comes out must go back in.

Let him make a mess in peace. Don't deliver continuous monologues of exasperated criticisms to your baby ("Oh, what a bad boy you are. I'll never get that crayon off the wall!"). Don't make him feel that expressing his natural and healthy curiosity ("If I turn this cup of milk over, what will happen?" "If I take all these clothes out of the drawer, what will I find underneath?") is bad or means that he is bad. If it was something you would rather not see happen again, let him know—but as a teacher, not a judge.

You can't beat him, but don't join him. Don't decide that since you're fighting a losing battle anyway, you might as well let the mess mount and learn to ignore it. Living that way won't help your morale and will be of no benefit to your baby. Though it's healthy for a baby to be allowed to make a mess, it isn't healthy for him to always be surrounded by disorder. It will give him a sense of security to know that even though he leaves an untidy world at bedtime, it will be returned to order come morning. And it will also make making a mess more fun and more fulfilling—what challenge is there, after all, in messing up a room that's already a mess?

Set aside a sanctuary. You won't always be able to keep up with damage left behind by your junior hurricane, but do try to preserve a place of calm in the midst of the storm—your bedroom or the den or living room, for instance—either by not permitting baby to play there or by making sure that it invariably gets picked up in the afternoon or evening. Then at the end of every day, you and your husband will have a haven to escape to.

Play it safe. The exception to a laissez-faire attitude toward disorder is when it presents a threat to safety. If baby spills his juice or empties the dog's water bowl, wipe it up immediately—fresh spills turn an uncarpeted floor into a skating rink where falls are inevitable. Also pick up sheets of paper and magazines as soon as baby is through with them, and keep traffic lanes (stairways especially) clear of toys, especially those with wheels, at all times.

EATING OFF THE FLOOR

"My baby's always dropping her cracker on the floor and then picking it up and eating it. It seems so unsanitary—is it safe?"

Even if you don't keep your floors "clean enough to eat off," it's safe for your baby to picnic on them. There are germs on the floor, but not in significant numbers. And for the most part, they're germs your baby has been exposed to before, particularly if she frequently plays on the floor. The same is generally true of floors in other people's homes, supermarkets, and department stores, although if your child's recycling a cracker off a foreign floor offends your aesthetic sense, there's nothing wrong with throwing it in the trash and replacing it with a fresh one.

There are exceptions, however. Although bacteria don't have a chance to multiply much on dry surfaces, they can multiply very rapidly on those that are damp or wet. If you have the choice, don't let her eat food that's been dropped in the bathroom, in puddles, or on other damp or wet surfaces. Moisture on food itself can also be a problem. A cracker or any food that's been mouthed for a time, then left (even in a clean place) for a few hours while bacteria multiply, isn't fit for consumption. So don't leave wet discards lying around where your baby can pick them up again. You won't always have the choice, of course; babies often reclaim long-lost foodstuffs and thrust them in their mouths before you can stop them. Fortunately, they rarely become ill as a result.

Out-of-doors, too, you need to be vigilant. Though many a baby has dropped a bottle in the street and then returned it to her mouth without ill effect, there is certainly more risk of picking up nasty germs where dogs defecate and urinate and thoughtless people expectorate. Replace or rinse any food, bottle, pacifier, or toy that has fallen into the street, especially if the ground is damp. Use wipes to clean a nipple or toy when running water is not available. In playgrounds, where dogs aren't allowed and where adults usually have more sense than to spit, there's probably less to worry about as long as the ground isn't wet—a quick brush-off of surface dirt should suffice. But even there, puddles can harbor dangerous disease-causing germs, and babies as well as their toys and snacks should be kept away from them. To avoid having to choose between appeasing a screaming baby and playing it safe by discarding a snack that you aren't sure is sanitary, always carry extras.

EATING DIRT—
AND WORSE

"My son puts everything in his mouth. Now that he plays on the floor so much, I have less control over what goes in. What's safe and what isn't?"

Into the mouths of babes goes anything and everything that fits: dirt, sand, dog food, roaches and other insects, cigarette butts, rotten food, even the contents of a soiled diaper. Though it's obviously best to avoid his sampling from such a smorgasbord, it's not always possible. Few babies get through the creepy-crawly stage without at least one oral encounter with something his parents consider revolting; some can't even get through a single morning.

But you've got a lot less to fear from what's unsanitary than from what's used to sanitize. A mouthful of dirt rarely hurts anyone, but even a lick of some cleansers can cause serious damage. You can't keep everything out of baby's inquisitive grasp, so concentrate on substances with the most harmful potential (see page 294 for a list), and concern yourself less with the occasional bug or clump of dog hair that finds its way into his mouth. If you do catch him with the cat-that-is-about-to-swallow-a-canary look, squeeze his cheeks with the thumb and forefinger of one hand to open his mouth, and sweep the object out with a hooked finger.

Of most concern—in addition to obviously toxic substances—are foods that are in the process of spoiling. Illness-causing bacteria or other microorganisms can multiply rapidly at room temperature, so be sure to keep food that's gone bad or is about to—which can most often be found in pet feeding bowls, in the kitchen garbage, and on an unswept kitchen or dining room floor—out of baby's reach.

You should also be very careful not to let your baby mouth items small enough to swallow or choke on—buttons, bottle caps, paper clips, safety pins, coins, and so on. Before you put your baby down to play, survey the floor for anything that's less than 1⅜ inches in diameter and remove it. Also put out of reach items that are potentially toxic, such as newspapers and lead-painted furniture. See Making Home Safe for Baby, (page 292) for additional tips on what should be kept away from baby.

ERECTIONS

"When I'm diapering my baby, he sometimes gets an erection. Am I handling his penis too much?"

As long as you're handling his penis only as much as it needs to be handled to be cleansed at diaper changes and bathtimes, you're not handling it too much. Your son's erections are the normal reaction to touch of a sensitive sexual organ—as are a little girl's clitoral erections, which are less noticeable but probably as common. A baby may also have an erection when his diaper rubs against his penis, when he's nursing, or when you're washing him in the bathtub. All baby boys have erections sometimes (though their mothers may not be aware of them), but some have them more often than others. Such erections require no particular notice on your part.

DISCOVERING
GENITALS

"My daughter has recently started playing with her genitals whenever her diaper is off. Is this normal at such an early age?"

If it feels good, humans do it. Which is what Mother Nature banked on when she created genitals; if she made them pleasurable to touch, they would be touched, at first by their owner and eventually, when the time was ripe, by a member of the opposite sex—thereby ensuring the perpetuation of the species.

Babies are sexual beings from birth, or more accurately, from before birth—male fetuses have been observed having erections in the uterus. Some, like your baby, begin fledgling explorations into their sexuality in the middle of the first year, others not until year's end. This interest is as inevitable and healthy a part of a baby's development as fascination with fingers and toes was earlier. Trying to stifle such curiosity (as generations past have felt obliged to do) is as misguided as stifling her interest in fingers and toes.

No matter what anyone may tell you, there is no harm—either physical or psychological—in babies or children handling their own genitals (this play can't be called masturbation until a later age). Making a baby or child feel that she's "dirty" or "bad" for engaging in such play, however, can be harmful and have a negative effect on future sexuality and self-esteem. Making self-stimulation taboo can also make it more inviting.

The fear that fingers that touch their genitals aren't clean enough to go into their mouths is also unfounded; all the germs that are in a baby's genital area are her own and pose no threat. If, however, you see your little girl probing with very dirty hands, it would be a good idea to wash them, to avoid the possibility of infection. A boy's genitals are not susceptible in the same way, but both boys and girls should have their hands washed after they've touched a soiled diaper area.

When your baby gets old enough to understand, you will want to explain that this part of her body is private, and that though it's okay for her to touch it, it isn't okay for her to touch it in public or to let anyone else touch it.

GETTING DIRTY

"My daughter would love to crawl around at the playground if I let her. But the ground is so dirty...."

Break out the all-fabric bleach, and break down your resistance to letting your daugh-

ter get down and dirty. Babies who are forced to watch from the sidelines when they'd really like to be in the scrimmage are likely to stay spotless but unsatisfied. Children are eminently washable. The most obvious soil can be removed with diaper wipes or premoistened towelettes while you're still at the playground or in the backyard, and ground-in dirt will come off later in the bath. Even the dirt that ends up in their mouths—babies who spend any amount of time outdoors will inevitably consume some soil and sand—won't be harmful; you may get sick from watching her eat dirt, but she's not likely to. So ignore the slight to your sensibilities and, checking first to be sure there's no broken glass or dog droppings in her path, allow your little sport a carefully supervised crawl around. If she gets into something really dirty, give her hands a once-over with a diaper wipe and send her on her way again.

Not all babies enjoy getting dirty; some would rather be spectators than players. If yours is one of these, be sure she isn't hesitating because she thinks you don't want her to get dirty. Encourage her to gradually become more active, but don't force her.

Soft shoes or sneakers will protect her feet when she's crawling on concrete; on grass in warm weather, bare feet are fine. It will be easier on her knees (but a challenge to your laundering skills) if she wears pants or overalls during these excursions. If you take pride in her looking fresh and clean in public, keep a set of playclothes in your diaper bag and change her into them before handing her her traveling papers; then wash her up and put her back into clean clothes before you set off again.

ROUGH PLAY

"My brother-in-law likes to roughhouse with our son, throwing him in the air and catching him, and that sort of thing. The baby seems to love it, but we wonder if it's safe."

It isn't. In most cases you can trust your baby to tell you when his body's not ready for something—starting solids, for instance, or standing. but not when it comes to this kind of roughhousing. Many babies enjoy the sensation of being whirled through the air or tossed up and caught (though some are terrified of it), but such handling—whether in fun or in anger—can be extremely dangerous for children under two years of age.[1]

There are several types of injuries that can result from throwing a baby in the air or shaking or vigorously bouncing him (as when jogging with him in a front or back baby carrier). One is a whiplash type of insult (such as an adult can get when rear-ended in an auto accident). Because the baby's head is heavy in proportion to the rest of his body and his neck muscles are not fully developed, support for the head is poor. When the baby is shaken roughly, the head whipping back and forth can cause the brain to rebound again and again against the skull. Bruising of the brain can cause swelling, bleeding, pressure, and possibly, permanent neurological damage with mental or physical disability. Another possible injury is trauma to the delicate infant eye. If detachment or scarring of the retina or damage to the optic nerve occurs, lasting visual problems, even blindness, can result. The risk of damage is compounded if a baby is crying or being held upside down during the shaking, because both increase blood pressure in the head, making fragile blood vessels more likely to rupture. Such injuries are relatively rare, but the damage can be so severe that the risk is certainly not worth taking.

Don't spend time worrying about past

roughhousing sessions. If your child hasn't exhibited any symptoms of injury, he's probably escaped unscathed thus far. If you have any concerns, consult your baby's doctor.

Some other kinds of roughhousing are also unsafe at this age. Because of a baby's (or even a young child's) still rather loose joints, don't swing him by the hands or suddenly twist or tug an arm (to get him moving when he's recalcitrant). The result could be a very painful (if easy-to-repair) dislocated elbow or shoulder.

This doesn't rule out roughhousing completely; it only dictates more careful rough play. Many babies love "flying" as they are held securely midtrunk and glided gently through the air, participating in ticklefests (though stop when baby is winded) and "wrestling" matches, and being chased when they are old enough to crawl. There are some babies, however, both male and female, who dislike any kind of rough handling, and they have the right to more gentle treatment—even from exuberant uncles and grandpas.

PLAYPEN USE

"When we bought our playpen a couple of months ago, our baby couldn't seem to get enough time in it. Now he screams to get out after only five minutes."

A couple of months ago, the playpen didn't seem confining to your baby; on the contrary, it seemed his own personal amusement park. Now he's beginning to realize that there's a whole world—or at least a living room—out there, and he's game to take it on. The four walls that once enclosed his paradise now represent frustrating barriers to him, keeping him on the inside looking out.

Take your baby's hint and start using the playpen for emergency duty only, for those times when he needs to be penned in for his own safety or, briefly and infrequently,

---

1. Some parents shake rather than spank a baby when they are angry because it seems the preferable way of disciplining, or they shake a baby to let off steam and frustration, assuming it won't hurt. Neither assumption is true; any parent who feels compelled to "punish" an infant needs help dealing with his or her feelings and caring for a child.

for your convenience—while you mop the kitchen floor, put something in the oven, answer the phone, go to the bathroom, or straighten up for last-minute company. Limit the time he's sentenced to the pen to no more than five to fifteen minutes at a stretch, which is about as long as an active eight-month-old will tolerate it. Vary the company he has to keep, rotating his stock of toys frequently so he won't become bored prematurely. If he prefers to be able to see and hear you as he plays, keep the pen near you; if he seems contented longer when you're out of sight, keep it in the next room (but check him frequently). If he protests before he's done his time, try giving him some novel playthings—a few pots and pans, perhaps, or an empty plastic soda bottle or two (without the cap)—anything he doesn't usually play with in this setting. If that doesn't work, parole him as soon as you reasonably can.

Be alert to the possibility of a jailbreak. The extremely agile and resourceful baby may be able to escape by climbing on large toys—so keep them out of the playpen. Also avoid hanging toys across the top.

"My daughter could stay in the playpen all day if I let her, but I'm not sure I should."

Some placid babies seem perfectly happy to stay in the playpen for hours on end, even late into the first year. Maybe they just don't know what they're missing, or perhaps they're not assertive enough to demand their freedom. But though such a situation lets a mother accomplish much, it prevents a baby from accomplishing enough, intellectually or physically. So encourage your baby to see the world from a new perspective. She may be hesitant at first to leave the playpen, a little uneasy about losing the security of its four walls. Sitting with her on the wide-open floor, playing with her, giving her a favorite toy or a favorite blanket, or cheering on her attempts at crawling will make the transition easier.

READING TO BABY

"I'd like my son to develop an interest in reading. Is it too early to start reading to him?"

In an age when television seduces children away from books easily and early, it's probably never too soon to start reading to a child. Some believe there's value to reading to a baby still in the uterus, and many begin their babies on books shortly after birth. But it isn't until about some time in the second half of the first year that a baby becomes an active participant in the reading process—at first, by chewing on the corners of the book. Soon he begins to pay attention to the words as you read them (at this point, to the rhythm and sounds of the words rather than their meanings) and to the illustrations (enjoying the color and patterns, but not necessarily relating the pictures to known objects).

To make sure your baby catches the book worm early, use the following strategies:

Read to yourself. Reading to your baby will have less impact if you yourself spend more time in front of the TV than behind a book (or newspaper, or magazine). Though it's hard for parents of young children to find a spare moment for a quiet read, it's worth the effort; as with any behavior, desirable or undesirable, children are much more likely to do as you do than to do as you say. Read a few pages from a propped-up book while you nurse or give your baby a bottle, read a book in his room while he plays, keep a book on your nightstand for reading before you fall asleep and for showing your baby ("this is mommy's book").

Start a juvenile collection. There are thousands of children's books on the shelves of bookstores, but only a limited number are appropriate for a beginner. Look for the following:

■ Sturdy construction that defies destruction. Sturdiest are books with laminated cardboard pages with rounded edges, which can be mouthed without disintegrating and turned without tearing. Laminated cloth books are good, too, but books of soft cloth, though indestructible, are pretty useless—they don't lie flat, babies can't turn their pages, and they bear little resemblance to real books. A spiral binding on a board book is a plus, since not only does it allow a book to lie flat when open, but baby can play with the fascinating spiral design. Vinyl books are good for bathtime, one of the few times some children sit still long enough for a reading session. To keep these free of mildew, dry thoroughly after each bath, and store in a dry place.

■ Illustrations that include bold, bright, realistic pictures of familiar subjects, particularly animals, vehicles, toys, and children. The pictures shouldn't be cluttered, so that baby won't be overwhelmed at a glance.

■ Text that is not too complicated. Rhymes have the best chance of holding a baby's attention when you're reading to him since he's listening largely for ear appeal, not comprehension, and it'll be many months before he'll be able to follow a story line. One-word-on-a-page books are good, too, since they help him to increase his comprehension vocabulary, and eventually his spoken vocabulary.

■ Activity tie-ins. Books that stimulate games like peekaboo, touch-and-feel books that encourage learning about textures, and books that have surprises hidden under little flaps encourage audience participation.

■ Discardable reading matter. Babies also like to handle and look at magazines with a lot of full-color illustrations, so instead of discarding old ones, keep a rainy-day collection for your baby. Of course, when he's through with them, you'll have to discard them.[2]

2. Be sure, however, that your baby doesn't mouth the pages of a magazine or newspaper. Both can contain high levels of lead, and frequent ingestion could result in dangerous levels for your baby. (Burning will also release lead into the air, so don't use newspapers or magazines for kindling.)

Learn to read parent-style. If you passed second-grade reading, you know how to pick up a volume of Mother Goose and read it aloud. But there's more to reading to a baby. Tone and inflection are important; read slowly, with a lilting singsong and exaggerated emphasis in the right places. Stop at each page to stress salient points ("Look at the little boy falling down the hill," or "See the baby doggie laughing?") or to show him animals or people ("That's a cow—a cow says 'moo,'" or "There's a baby in a cradle—the baby's going 'rockabye baby'").

Make reading a habit. Build reading into baby's agenda—a few minutes at least twice a day, when he's quiet but alert, and when he's already been fed. Before naptime, after lunch, after bath, and before bed are all good reading times. But keep to the schedule only if baby's receptive; don't push a book on him when he's in the mood to practice crawling or to make music with two pot covers.

Keep the library open. Store precious, destructible books on a high shelf for parent-supervised reading sessions, but keep a small (to prevent baby from being overwhelmed), rotating (to prevent baby from becoming bored) library of baby-proof books where he can reach and enjoy them. Sometimes a baby who resists being sat down for a reading session with mommy or daddy will be happy to "read" to himself, turning pages and looking at pictures at his own pace.

LEFT- OR RIGHT-HANDEDNESS

"I've noticed that my baby picks up and reaches for toys with either hand. Should I try to encourage him to use his right?"

We live in a world that treats minorities unequally; the left-handed, a minority of about 10%, are no exception. Most doors, irons, potato peelers, scissors, and table settings are designed for righties. And lefties are destined to bump elbows at the dinner table and to shake with what to them is the "wrong" hand. Many parents, reluctant to relegate their children to this minority status, try to force right-handedness onto lefty-prone offspring.

Experts once believed that such parental pressure to change what is thought to be a genetically determined trait led to stuttering and a variety of learning disabilities. Now, though they still don't recommend trying to change a child's natural-handedness, they suspect that several traits—both positive and negative—are genetically intertwined with left-handedness. Many of these appear to be related to differences between lefties and righties with respect to development in the right and left hemispheres of the brain. In lefties the right side of the brain is dominant, making them excel in such areas as spatial relations, which may be why they are overrepresented in such fields as sports, architecture, and art. Since more boys than girls are left-handed, it is also theorized that levels of testosterone, a male hormone, somehow affect brain development and handedness. Much more study is needed before we fully understand what makes a person left- or right-handed and just how handedness affects various areas of one's life.

Most babies use both hands equally at first; some show a preference for one hand or the other within a few months, others not until they reach their first birthdays. Some seem to favor one hand at first, and then switch. What's important is letting baby use the hand he's most comfortable with, not the one you would like him to use. Since about 70% of the population is strongly right-handed (the other 20% is ambidextrous), you can assume, until he demonstrates otherwise, that your baby will be, too. Offer things to his right hand. If he reaches over and grabs them with his left, or takes them with his right and then passes them to his left, he may be on his way to winning twenty games for the Mets or to

designing the world's tallest building.

CHILDPROOFING YOUR HOME

"I always said that a baby wasn't going to change the way we live. But with our daughter's crawling around, many of the valuable things we've collected over the years are at risk. Should I pack them away, or try to teach her to stay away from them?"

Many china shops would be as happy to host a bull as a seven- or eight-month-old baby. And indeed, your breakable valuables might stand as much of a chance of surviving in a living room with your baby as they would in a ring with El Toro.

So if you don't want to see the Baccarat bowl you picked up in Paris or the Wedgwood vase your best friend gave you for a wedding gift shattered at your baby's feet, put them well out of reach until she's old enough and responsible enough to treat them with respect—which may not be for a couple of years. Do likewise with objects (of art or otherwise) that are heavy enough to hurt her should she pull them down.

Still, your family shouldn't spend the next years in a house stripped bare of ornamentation—for your child's sake as much as for yours. If you want her to learn to live with the fine and fragile things in life, she should be exposed to some even at this age. Leave a few of the sturdier and less valuable pieces in your collection within your baby's reach. When she reaches, sternly tell her, "No, don't touch that. That's mommy and daddy's." Hand her a toy and explain that it is *hers*. If she persists in reaching for the forbidden object, take it away (too many no's begin to lose their effect) and put it out another day. Though you can't count on compliance now (young babies have short memories), eventually your child will understand—and you can bring on the Baccarat and Wedgwood.

WHAT IT'S IMPORTANT TO KNOW: Making Home Safe for Baby

Put a fragile day-old baby next to a sturdy seven-month-old and the newborn will seem, in comparison, so helpless, so much more vulnerable to harm. But in reality, it's the older baby who's more vulnerable. Newly acquired skills unmatched by good judgment, in fact, make babies in the second half of their first year extremely hazardous to their own health.

Once a baby is able to get around alone (or is getting around in a walker), the average home becomes a wonderland as dangerous as it is exciting, replete with potential booby traps capable of causing injury or even death. Newborn or toddler, the only protection for your baby during what the Metropolitan Life Insurance Company has called the "risky first year of life" is your good sense, foresight, and eternal vigilance.

It usually takes a combination of factors to trigger an accident, including a dangerous object or substance (in the case of a baby, perhaps a staircase or drug), a susceptible victim (your baby), and possibly, environmental conditions (ungated steps, an unlocked medicine chest) that allow victim and danger to come together. In the case of baby accidents, it may also hinge on the faltering vigilance—sometimes only for a moment—of a parent or caretaker.

To minimize the possibility of an accident, all of these factors must be modified in some way. Dangerous objects and substances must be removed from reach, the susceptible baby has to be made less susceptible by gradual safety training, the hazardous environment must be modified (with gates on stairs, locks on cabinets), and, possibly most important of all, caretakers must be ever on the alert, especially at times of stress, when most accidents occur. Because a great many accidents occur at the homes of others—particularly the homes of grandmas and grandpas—you should extend many of these safety measures to homes baby visits often and offer this chapter as reading material to those who frequently care for your child.

Here's how to modify the factors that contribute to accidents.

Change Your Ways

Since modifying baby's behavior will be a long, slow educational process, which can begin now but won't be complete for many years, it's your behavior that will have the most impact on the safety of your child at this stage.

■ Be eternally vigilant. No matter how carefully you attempt to childproof your house, remember that you can't make it completely accident-proof. Your attention, or that of another caretaker, must be continuous, especially if yours is a particularly resourceful child.

■ Don't let your attention be diverted in mid-activity when using household cleaning products, medicines, electrical appliances, power tools, or any other hazardous object or substance when your baby is on the loose. It takes no more than a second for baby to get into serious trouble.

■ Be particularly alert during times of stress and stressful times of day. It's when you're distracted that you're likely to forget to take the knife off the table, strap baby into the high chair, or close the stair gate.

■ Do not leave baby alone in your house or apartment at any time, nor alone in a room except in a playpen, crib, or other safe enclosure—and then only for a few minutes, unless he or she is sleeping. Do not leave a baby alone, even "safely" enclosed in a crib or playpen, awake or asleep, with a preschooler (they often don't know their own strength or realize the possible consequences of their actions) or with a pet (even a docile one).

■ Make baby less susceptible with appropriate clothing. Use only flame-retardant sleepwear (and wash it properly); be sure that pajama feet aren't too floppy, pants cuffs too long, or socks or slippers too slippery for a baby who is pulling up or starting to walk. Avoid long scarves or sashes that can trip baby up, and always shun strings that can strangle (those over 12 inches long).

■ Become familiar, if you aren't already, with emergency and first-aid procedures (see page 434). You can't always prevent accidents, but knowing what to do if a serious one occurs can save lives and limbs.

■ Give your baby plenty of freedom. Once you've made your baby's environment as safe as possible, avoid hovering. Though you want your child to be safety conscious, you don't want to discourage the normal experimentation of childhood. Children, like the rest of us, learn from their mistakes; never allowing them to make a mistake can prevent growth. And a child who is afraid to run, climb, or try new things misses out not only on the education that comes through free play, but on a lot of the fun of childhood as well.

Change Your Baby's Surroundings

Until now, your baby has seen the world—and your home—mostly from your arms, at your eye level. Now that he or she is beginning to get a look at it from down on all fours, you will have to begin looking at it from that perspective, too. One way to do this is to actually get down on the floor yourself; from there, you will see a multitude of dangers you may not have even realized existed. Another way is to examine everything that is within three feet above the floor—the usual range of a baby's reach.

Changes throughout the home. As you tour your home, these are the things you should look at and alter as necessary:

■ Windows. If they are above ground level, install window guards according to manufacturer's directions; or adjust them so they can't open more than 6 inches.

■ Cords to blinds or draperies. Tie them up so baby can't become entangled in them; do not place a crib or playpen, or a chair or bed baby can climb on, within reach.

■ Electrical cords. Move them out of reach, behind furniture so that baby won't mouth them, risking electric shock, or tug at them, pulling lamps or other heavy items down.

■ Electrical outlets. Cover with caps or shields or place heavy furniture in front of them to prevent baby from inserting something (such as a hairpin) or probing with a drooly finger and getting a shock.

■ Unstable furnishings. Put rickety or unstable chairs, tables, or other furniture that might topple if baby pulls on it out of the way for the time being; securely fasten to the wall bookcases or other structures that baby could pull down.

■ Dresser drawers. Keep them closed so baby won't climb in them and pull the dresser down; if the dresser isn't stable, consider fastening it to the wall.

■ Painted surfaces within baby's reach. Be sure they are lead free; if they aren't or if you aren't sure, repaint or wallpaper. If testing shows lead in the paint, it is best to remove it entirely.

■ Ash trays. Put them out of reach so baby won't touch a hot butt or sample a handful of ashes and butts; better still, for your baby's health as well as safety, banish tobacco from your home entirely.

■ Houseplants. Keep them out of baby's reach, where baby can't pull them down on him- or herself or nibble on them; be especially wary of poisonous plants (see page 301).

■ Loose knobs on furniture or cabinets. Remove or secure any that are small enough to be swallowed (smaller than baby's fist) or cause choking.

POISON CONTROL

Every year some 130,000 children in the U.S. are victims of accidental ingestion of hazardous substances. That's sad, but not surprising. Children, particularly very young ones, do a lot of their discovery of the world orally. Virtually anything they pick up will go right to the mouth. They haven't yet learned to categorize substances or objects as "safe" or "unsafe"—everything is merely "interesting." Nor are their tastebuds sophisticated enough to warn them, as ours do, that a substance is dangerous because it tastes terrible.

To protect your innocents from perils, follow these rules without fail:

- Lock all potentially poisonous substances out of reach and out of sight of your baby—even crawlers can climb up on low chairs and stools or cushions.
- Follow all safety rules for administering or taking medicines (see page 410).
- Avoid buying brightly colored or attractively packaged household cleansers, laundry detergents, and other substances. They will attract your baby. If necessary, cover illustrations with black tape (but don't cover instructions or warnings). Also avoid toxic substances with attractive food fragrances (such as mint, lemon, or apricot).
- Purchase products with childproof packaging, when possible.
- Make it a habit to return hazardous items to safe storage immediately after each use; don't put a spray can of furniture polish or a box of mothballs down "just for a minute" while you answer the phone.
- Store food and non-food items separately and never put nonedibles in empty food containers (bleach in an apple juice bottle, for example, or lubricating oil in a jelly jar). Babies learn very early to identify where their food comes from, and won't understand why they can't drink what's in the juice bottle or lick what's in the jelly jar.
- Avoid using non-foods that look like foods (such as wax fruit).
- When discarding potentially poisonous substances, empty them down the drain, rinsing the containers before discarding unless the label instructs otherwise, and putting them out in a tightly closed trash can immediately. *Never* dump them in a wastebasket or kitchen garbage can.
- Choose the less hazardous product over the one with a long list of warnings when possible. Among those household products generally considered less hazardous: non-chlorine bleaches, vinegar, Bon Ami, borax, washing soda, lemon oil, beeswax, olive oil (for furniture), non-chemical fly-paper, Elmer's glue, mineral oil (for lubrication, not internal use), compressed air drain openers (rather than corrosive liquids or granules).
- To help you think "poison" whenever you see one, put "poison" labels on all possibly poisonous products. If you can't locate such labels, simply put an "X" of black tape on each product (but don't cover instructions or warnings). Eventually your child will also come to recognize that these products are unsafe.
- Think of all of the following as potentially perilous:
Alcoholic beverages
Ammoniated mercury (not useful medicinally)
Aspirin
Boric acid (not useful medicinally)
Camphorated oil (not useful medicinally)
Chlorine bleach
Cosmetics
Dishwasher detergents
Drain cleaners
Furniture polish
Insect or rodent poisons
Iron pills (even baby's own)
Kerosene
Lye (better not to have in the home at all)
Medicines of all kinds
Mothballs
Turpentine (not useful)
Oil of wintergreen (not useful medicinally)
Sleeping pills
Tranquilizers
Weed killers

■ Radiators. Put barriers around them or radiator covers over them during the heating season.

■ Stairs. Put a gate at the top and another three steps up from the bottom.

■ Bannisters and railings. Be sure the gap between upright posts on stairs or balconies is less than 5 inches, and that none are loose.

■ Fireplaces, heaters, stoves, floor furnaces. Put up protective grills or other barriers to keep small fingers from hot surfaces (even the grill on a floor furnace can get hot enough to cause second-degree burns) as well as fire. Unplug space heaters when not in use, and whenever possible store them where children can't get at them. (For information on the environmental risks of space heaters, see page 239.)

■ Tablecloths. If they hang over the side of the table and are not well anchored, remove them until your baby knows not to pull up on them or, alternatively, keep baby off the floor when you have a cloth on the table.

■ Glass-topped tables. Either cover with a heavy table pad or put them out of reach temporarily.

■ Sharp edges or corners on tables, chests, and so on. If baby can bump into them, cover them with homemade or purchased cushioned strips and corner guards.

■ Scatter rugs. Be sure they have nonskid backings; don't place them at the top of stairs or allow them to remain rumpled.

■ Floor tiles and carpets. Repair all loose areas to prevent tripping.

■ Heavy knickknacks and bookends. Place them where baby can't reach out and pull them over; babies have more strength than you may think.

■ Toy chests. These should have lightweight lids with safety closing mechanisms (or no lids at all), as well as ventilation holes (in case baby should become locked in). In general, open shelves are safer for toy storage.

■ Crib. Once your baby starts showing interest in pulling up (don't wait until the feat has been achieved), adjust the mattress to its lowest position and remove bulky toys, pillows, bumper pads, and anything else that can be used as a stepping stone to freedom—and disaster. When your baby is 35 inches tall, it's time for a bed.

■ Floor clutter. Try to keep it out of traffic lanes to prevent tripping. Wipe up spills and pick up papers immediately.

■ Garage, basement, and hobby areas. Lock securely and keep children out, since these areas usually contain a variety of hazardous implements and/or poisonous substances.

■ Other areas with hazardous or breakable objects, such as a living room housing a collection of fine teacups. Put up a gate or other barrier to keep baby out.

Also be alert to the host of hazardous items found in the typical home and see that they are safely stored, generally in childproof drawers, cabinets, or chests or on absolutely out-of-reach shelves (you'd be surprised at how high some babies can manage to climb). When you're using such items, be sure baby can't get at them when you turn your back, and always be sure to put them away as soon as you've finished with them or as soon as you spot one that has been left out. Be particularly careful with:

■ Sharp implements such as scissors, knives, letter openers, razors (don't leave these on the side of the tub), and blades.

■ Swallowable notions such as marbles, coins, safety pins, and anything else smaller than 1⅜ inches in diameter.

■ Pens, pencils, and other writing implements (substitute chunky non-toxic crayons).[3]

■ Sewing and knitting supplies, particularly pins and needles, thimbles, scissors, and buttons.

---

3. Some children enjoy using pencils or pens just like mommy and daddy; if your baby does, allow such use only when he or she is safely seated and you can supervise closely.

SAFETY EQUIPMENT

Cabinet locks (to keep kitchen cabinets and drawers safe from prying fingers)
Cabinet latches (to do likewise)
Stove guards
Doorknob guards (to make it difficult for little ones to open doors)
Clear plastic corner cushioning (to soften corners of tables)
Edge cushions (to do same for sharp edges)

Outlet plugs or covers (in addition to snap-in caps, there are hinged shields that can be used even when appliances are plugged in)
Tub spout safety cover
Non-skid decorations for bathtub bottoms
Skid-resistant step stool (when baby walks)
Kid-proof patio door locks
Potty proofer (suction cups or latch to keep lid down when not in use)

■ Lightweight plastic bags such as produce bags, dry cleaning bags, and packaging on new clothing (babies can suffocate if such a bag is placed over the face).

■ Incendiary articles such as matches and matchbooks, lighters, and hot cigarette butts.

■ Tools of your trade or hobbies—paints and thinners, if there's an artist in the house; pins and needles if there's a dress-maker; woodworking equipment if there's a carpenter; and so on.

■ Toys (if they belong to older siblings, they generally should not be played with by babies or toddlers under three; this includes building sets with small pieces, trikes and scooters, miniature cars and trucks, and anything with sharp corners, small pieces, removable or breakable small parts, or electrical connections).

■ Button batteries—the disc-shaped type used in watches, calculators, hearing aids, cameras, and so on (they are easy to swallow, and can release hazardous contents into baby's esophagus or stomach).

■ Food fakes of wax, papier-mâché, rubber, or any other substance that isn't safe for a baby or child to mouth (a wax apple, a candle that smells and looks like an ice-cream sundae, a child's eraser that smells and looks like a ripe strawberry).

■ Cleaning materials.

■ Glass, china, or other breakables.

■ Light bulb, especially small ones, such as those in night lights, that a baby can mouth and break.

■ Jewelry, particularly beads, which can be pulled apart; and small items such as rings (all are attractive to baby and easily swallowed).

■ Mothballs (they're poisonous).

■ Shoe polish (besides making a mess, it can make baby sick).

■ Perfumes and all cosmetics (they are potentially toxic); vitamins and medicines.

■ Toy whistles (baby can choke on them, and on the small ball inside should it come loose).

■ Balloons (uninflated or burst, they can be inhaled and cause choking).

■ Small, hard finger foods, such as nuts or raisins, popcorn or hard candies that may be left around in candy dishes (baby can choke on them).

■ Guns (if you must have them in the home).

■ Lye and acid (better not to have these in your home at all).

■ Alcoholic beverages (an amount that merely relaxes you could make your baby deathly ill).

■ Strings, cords, cradle gyms, tape cassettes, or anything else that could get tangled around a baby's neck and cause strangulation. (Babies shouldn't sleep with dolls or stuffed animals that hold audio tapes.)

■ Anything else in your home that would

be dangerous if mouthed or swallowed by a baby. See list of poisons, page 294.

Fire-safety changes. Hearing that a child or children perished in a fire is distressing enough. To know that the fire could have been prevented, or could have been discovered before it spread to fatal proportions, is even more disturbing. Check every corner of your home for possible fire hazards to be sure "it can't happen here":

■ If smoking is permitted in your home (and everyone will be better off if it isn't), dispose of all cigar or cigarette butts, ashes, pipe ashes, and used matches carefully and never leave them where a baby can get at them. Any smokers in your home should make a habit of disposing of butts immediately, and you should empty ashtrays promptly when you have smoking guests.

■ Do not permit anyone (visitors included) to smoke in bed.

■ Keep matches and lighters out of the reach of children and babies.

■ Do not allow rubbish to accumulate (especially combustibles such as paint or paint rags).

■ Avoid using flammable liquids, kerosene as well as commercial products, for spot removal on clothing.

■ Don't wear (or let anyone else who is cooking or working near a fireplace, wood stove, or space heater wear) clothing with long sleeves, dragging scarves, or hanging shirttails, any of which could accidentally catch fire.

■ Be sure your baby's sleepwear meets federal standards for flame resistance.

■ Have your heating system checked annually, be careful not to overload electrical circuits, always remove plugs from sockets properly (don't jerk the cord), and check electric appliances and cords regularly for wear and/or loose connections. Use only 15-amp fuses for lighting; never substitute anything else for a fuse.

■ If you use space heaters, be sure they turn off automatically if toppled or if something is placed against them.

■ Place extinguishers in areas where fire risk is greatest, such as in the kitchen or furnace room, and near the fireplace or wood stove. In an emergency, bicarbonate of soda can be used for putting out kitchen fires. Try to put out a fire only if it is small and contained (such as in your oven, a frying pan, or a wastebasket). If it is not contained, get out of the house instead.

■ Install fire and smoke detectors as recommended by your local fire department, if you haven't already. Check periodically to see that they are in good working order and that batteries haven't run down.

■ Install chair and rope ladders at selected upper floor windows to facilitate escape; teach older children and adults how to use them. Practice getting down holding a baby doll.

■ Hold fire drills periodically so that everyone who lives or works in your household will know how to get out safely and quickly in an emergency and know where to meet other family members. Assign parents and other adults to evacuate specific children. Be sure everyone (including baby-sitters) knows that the priority in case of fire is to evacuate the premises immediately—without worrying about dressing, saving valuables, or putting out the fire.[4] Most deaths occur from suffocation or burns due to hot fumes and smoke, not from direct flame. The fire department should be called as soon as possible from a street phone or a neighbor's house.

Changes in the kitchen. Make a special tour of the kitchen, one of the most intriguing places in the house to your newly mobile baby—and also one of the most dangerous. You can make it safer by taking the following steps:

■ Attach child-guard latches to drawers or cabinets that contain anything off limits to

---

4. The only exception is a well-contained fire that can be put out with a fire extinguisher.

little ones, such as breakable glass items, sharp implements, hazardous cleaning compounds, medicines, or dangerous food-stuffs (such as peanuts, peanut butter—on which a baby could choke—and hot peppers). If your baby figures out how to un-latch the safety latches (some very wily ones do), you will have to relegate all dangerous items to out-of-reach storage areas or just keep your baby out of the kitchen entirely with a gate or other barrier. What is truly out of reach will change as your baby gets older, so your storage arrangement may have to as well.

■ Set aside at least one cabinet (baby is less likely to catch his or her fingers in a cabinet than in a drawer) for your little explorer to enjoy freely. Some sturdy pots and pans, wooden spoons, strainers, dish towels, plastic bowls, and so on can provide hours of entertainment and may satisfy your baby's curiosity enough to keep him or her out of forbidden places.

■ Keep the handles of pots and pans that are on the stove turned toward the rear and out of baby's reach. If controls are on the front of the range, erect some sort of barrier to keep them untouchable or snap on stove knob covers. An appliance latch will keep conventional and microwave ovens inaccessible.

■ Don't sit baby on a countertop near electrical appliances, the stove, or anything else that might be hazardous—or you may find him or her with fingers in the toaster, hands on a hot pot, or a knife heading for an open mouth the moment you turn your back.

■ Don't carry baby and hot coffee—or any hot liquid—at the same time. It's just too easy for the baby to suddenly bolt and spill it, possibly burning you both. Also be sure not to leave a hot beverage or a bowl of soup at the edge of a table where your baby can reach it.

■ Keep garbage in a tightly covered container that baby can't open or under the sink behind a securely latched door. Children love to rummage through garbage, and the dangers—from spoiled foods to broken glass—are numerous.

■ Clean up all spills promptly—they make for slippery floors.

■ Follow the safety rules for selecting, using, and storing kitchen detergents, scouring powders, silver polishes, and all other kitchen supplies (see page 294).

Changes in the bath. Nearly as alluring to a baby as the kitchen, and equally dangerous, is the bathroom. One way to keep it off limits is to put a hook and eye or other latch high up on the door, and to keep it latched when not in use. Baby-safe the bathroom by taking the following precautions:

■ Keep all medications (including over-the-counter ones such as antacids), mouth-washes, toothpaste, vitamin pills, hair preparations and sprays, skin lotions, and cosmetics safely stored out of baby's reach. (Actually, medicines and vitamins are better kept in the bedroom, where there is less exposure to moisture, than in the bathroom.)

■ Don't leave a sunlamp or heater where baby can turn it on; if you can't store it out of the way, remove sunlamp bulb and un-plug the lamp when it is not being used.

■ Don't use, or let anyone else use, a hair dryer near your baby when he or she is in the bath or playing with water.

■ Never leave small electrical appliances plugged in when you aren't using them. A baby could dunk a hair dryer in the toilet and get a fatal electric shock, switch on a razor and get cut, or get burned on a curling iron. Unplugging appliances won't be enough if your child has good manual dexterity (those little whizzes often figure out how to plug in an appliance, with possibly disastrous results) or if the appliance is a pre-October 1987 hair dryer (which can cause shocks even when not connected to a power source). Better not to leave these appliances out at all.

■ Keep water temperature in your home set at between 120° and 125°F to avoid accidental scalding, and always turn off the hot water faucet before the cold. Routinely test bath water temperature with your elbow before putting baby in the tub. If your tub doesn't have a nonskid finish, add some skidproof stick-ons.

■ When not in use, keep the toilet lid closed with suction cups or another device made expressly for this purpose. Most babies see the toilet as a private little swimming pool, and love to play in it any chance they get. Not only is this unsanitary, but an energetic toddler could topple in headfirst, with catastrophic results.

■ Invest in a protective cover for the tub spout to prevent bumps or burns should baby fall against it.

■ Do not leave your baby in the tub unattended, even once he's sitting well, and even in a special tub seat. This rule should be in force until your child is five years old.

■ Never leave water in the tub when it's not in use; a small child may topple into the tub at play, and a drowning can occur in as little as *an inch* of water.

Changes for a safer out-of-doors. Though the home is the most dangerous environment for a baby, serious accidents can also occur in your own backyard—or someone else's—as well as in the local streets and the community playground. Many of these accidents are relatively easy to prevent:

■ Never let an infant or toddler play out-of-doors alone. Even a baby in a safety harness, napping in a carriage or stroller, needs to be watched almost constantly—he or she could suddenly wake and become tangled in the harness while struggling to be free. A sleeping baby who is not strapped in needs to be under someone's watchful eye full-time.

■ Keep swimming or wading pools and any other water catchments (even if filled with only an inch of water) inaccessible to babies and toddlers—whether they are crawling, walking independently, or navigating in a walker. If you have a swimming pool, fence it in and keep gates or doors to the pool locked at all times; empty and turn wading pools upside down, and drain any other areas where water can accumulate before allowing baby to play nearby.

■ Check public play areas before letting your baby loose. Though it's fairly easy to keep your backyard free of dog droppings (they can harbor worms), broken glass, and other dangerous debris, park attendants may find it more difficult to do so.

■ It's not enough to beseech: "Please don't eat the daisies!" You've got to be sure that your baby knows it's not okay to eat *any* plants, indoors or out. Avoid planting, or at least fence in, poisonous plants (see box, page 301).

■ Be sure that outdoor play equipment is safe. It should be sturdily constructed, correctly assembled, firmly anchored, and installed at least 6 feet from fences or walls. Cap all screws and bolts to prevent injuries from rough or sharp edges, and check for loose ones periodically. Avoid S-type hooks for swings (the chains can swing out of them), and rings anywhere on the equipment that are between 5 and 10 inches in diameter, since a child's head might become entrapped. Swings should be of soft materials (such as leather or canvas rather than wood or metal) to prevent serious head injuries. The best surfaces for outdoor play areas are sand, sawdust, wood chips, bark, rubber composition, grass, or other shock-absorbent material.

Change Your Baby

Accidents are much more likely to happen to those who are susceptible to them—and of course, babies easily fall into that category. But it isn't too early to begin accident-proofing your baby even as you accident-proof your home. Teach your baby about the dangers. Pretend to touch the point of a needle, for example, saying "Ouch," and pulling your finger away quickly in mock pain. Build and use a vocabulary of warning words ("Ouch," "Boo-boo," "Hot," "Sharp") and phrases ("Don't touch," "That's dangerous," "Be careful," "That's an ouch," "That will give you a boo-boo"), so that your baby will automatically come to associate them with dangerous objects, substances, and situations. At first your little dramatizations will seem to be going right over your little one's head—and they will be. But gradually the brain will begin storing the information, and one day it will be apparent that your lessons have taken hold. Begin teaching your baby now about the following:

Sharp or pointy implements. Whenever you use a knife, scissors, razor, or letter opener in front of your baby, be sure to mention that it is sharp, that it's not a toy, that only mommy and daddy or other grownups can touch it. As your child becomes older and gains better small motor control, teach cutting with a child's safety scissors and a butter knife. Finally, advance to supervised use of the "adult" versions of these implements.

Hot stuff. Even a seven- or eight-month-old will begin to catch on when you consistently warn that your coffee (or the stove, a lit match or candle, a radiator or heater, a fireplace) is hot and shouldn't be touched. Very soon the word "hot" will automatically signal "Don't touch" to your baby. Illustrate your point by letting him or her touch something hot, but not hot enough to burn—the very warm outside of your coffee cup, for example. When a child is old enough to strike a match or carry a cup of coffee, he or she should be taught the safe way to do so.

Steps. Parents are often advised to put up safety gates at stairways in homes where there are babies who are beginning to be mobile—either independently or in walkers. On the one hand, this is an important safety precaution and one that too few families take. On the other hand, the baby who knows nothing about steps save that they are off limits is the one who is at greatest risk of accident the first time an open stairway is discovered. So put a gate at the top of every stairway of more than three steps

in your home—getting down is much trickier, and thus much more hazardous, for a baby than getting up. But also put a gate three steps up from the bottom so that baby can practice going up and down under safe conditions. When he or she becomes proficient, open the gate occasionally to let baby tackle the full flight as you stand or crouch a step or two below, ready to lend support if a little foot or hand slips. Once going up is mastered, teach baby how to come down safely—a much more challenging task and one that may take several months to achieve. Children who know how to climb up and down steps are much safer should they happen upon an unprotected stairway, which every child does now and then, than those with no climbing experience. But continue to keep the gates in place, fastening them when you're not around to supervise, until your child is a very reliable step climber (somewhere around two years of age).

Electrical hazards. Electrical outlets, electric cords, and electrically operated appliances all have great appeal for curious little minds and hands. It's not enough to distract a baby on the way to probing an unprotected outlet or to hide all the visible cords in your home; it's also necessary to repeatedly remind the baby of their dangerous potential ("ouch!"), and to teach older children respectful use of electricity and the risks of mixing it with water.

Tubs, pools, and other watery attractions. Water play is fun and educational; encourage it. But also teach a baby not to get into the tub, a pool, a pond, or any other body of water without mommy or daddy or another grownup—and that includes babies and children who have gone through swimming classes. You can't sufficiently "waterproof" a young child, so you can never leave one alone near water—but you can begin to teach some water safety rules.

Poisonous substances. You're always careful about locking away household

RED LIGHT ON GREENERY

Many common house and garden plants are poisonous when eaten. Since plant leaves and flowers are no exception to a baby's everything-in-the-mouth-that-fits rule, poisonous varieties must be off limits for babies. Place houseplants high up, where leaves or flowers can't fall on the floor below, and where baby can't get to them by pulling up, crawling, or climbing. Better still, give poisonous houseplants to childless friends. Label with the accurate botanical name any houseplant you do keep, so that if your baby accidentally ingests some leaves or flowers, you will be able to supply the accurate information to the poison center or your baby's doctor. Place all plants, even nonpoisonous ones, where they can't be toppled with a tug.

The following houseplants are poisonous, some in very small doses:

Dumb cane, English ivy, foxglove, hyacinth bulbs (and leaves and flowers in quantity), hydrangea, iris rootstalk and rhizome, lily of the valley, philodendron, Jerusalem cherry.

Outdoor plants that are poisonous include:

Azalea, rhododendron, caladium, daffodil and narcissus bulbs, daphne, English ivy, foxglove, holly, hyacinth bulbs (and leaves and flowers in quantity), hydrangea, iris rootstalk and rhizome, Japanese yew seeds and leaves, larkspur, laurel, lily of the valley, morning glory seeds, oleander, privet, rhubarb leaves, sweet peas (especially the "peas," which are the seeds), tomato plant leaves, wisteria pods and seeds, yews.

Holiday favorites holly and mistletoe, and to a lesser extent poinsettia, are also on the danger list.

---

cleansers, medicines, and so on. But your parents are visiting and your dad leaves his heart medicine on a living room table. Or you're at your single sister's house, and she has chlorine bleach and dishwasher detergent under the kitchen sink. You're asking for trouble if you haven't begun to teach your baby the rules of substance safety. Repeat these messages over and over again:

■ Don't eat or drink anything unless mommy or daddy or another grownup you know gives it to you (this is a difficult concept for a baby, but an important one for all children to learn eventually).

■ Medicine and vitamin pills are *not* candy, though they are sometimes flavored to taste that way. Don't eat or drink them unless mommy or daddy or another grownup you know gives them to you.

■ Don't put anything in your mouth if you don't know what it is.

■ Only mommy or daddy or another grownup can use aspirin, scouring powder,

spray wax, or any other potentially poisonous substance. Repeat this every time you take or give a medication, scrub the tub, polish the furniture, and so on.

There are dangers outside your home, too, that your baby needs to be prepared for:

Street hazards. Begin teaching street smarts now. Every time you cross a street with your baby, explain about listening and watching for cars, about crossing at the green and not in between, and waiting for the Walk light. If there are driveways in your neighborhood, then you should explain that it's necessary to "stop, look, and listen" at them, too. Once your child is walking, teach him never to cross without holding on to an adult's hand—even if there's no traffic. It's a good idea to hold hands on the sidewalk, too, but many toddlers love the freedom of walking on their own. If you permit this (and you probably will have to at least some of the time), you will have to keep an eye on your child literally every second—that's all it takes for a child to dart into the path of an oncoming car. Infractions of the don't-go-in-the-street-alone rule deserve a sharp reprimand.

Be sure, too, that your baby knows not to leave the house or apartment without you or another adult. Every once in a while a toddler toddles alone out the front door and into trouble.

Auto safety. Be certain that your baby not only becomes accustomed to sitting in a car seat, but understands the reason why it's essential. Also explain other auto safety rules, such as no throwing toys around, no grabbing the steering wheel, and no playing with door locks or window buttons. Teach older children how to open the locks, in case they should become locked in alone.

Playground safety. Even a baby can begin learning playground safety rules. Teach yours not to twist a swing (when they or someone else is on it, or even if it's empty), push an empty swing, or walk in front of a moving one. Observe these rules yourself, and regularly mention them to your baby. Also explain that it's necessary to wait until the child ahead of you is off the slide before going down, and that it is unsafe to climb up from the bottom.

The best way you can teach your baby about safe living is to practice it. You can't expect a child to be happy about being strapped into a car seat when you don't buckle up yourself, to obey traffic signals if you dash across the street in spite of a Don't Walk light, or to respect fire if you leave the fireplace unscreened and burning cigarette butts all over the house.

CHAPTER TWELVE

The Ninth Month

WHAT YOUR BABY MAY BE DOING

By the end of this month, your baby ...should be able to (see Note):

- work to get to a toy out of reach
- look for dropped object

Note: If your baby seems not to have reached one or more of these milestones, check with the doctor. In rare instances the delay could indicate a problem, though in most cases it will turn out to be normal for your baby. Premature infants generally reach milestones later than others of the same birth age, often achieving them closer to their adjusted age (the age they would be if they had been born at term) or sometimes later.

...will probably be able to:

- pull up to standing position from sitting (by 9½ months)
- get into a sitting position from stomach (by 9⅓ months)
- object if you try to take a toy away

- stand holding on to someone or something
- pick up tiny object with any part of thumb and finger (by 9¼ months)
- say mama or dada indiscriminately
- play peekaboo

...may possibly be able to:

- play patty-cake (clap hands) or wave bye-bye
- walk holding on to furniture (cruise)
- understand word "no" (but not always obey it)

...may even be able to:

- "play ball" (roll ball back to you)
- drink from a cup independently
- pick up a tiny object neatly with tips of thumb and forefinger
- stand alone momentarily
- stand alone well

- say dada or mama discriminately
- say one word other than mama or dada
- respond to a one-step command with gestures (give that to me—with hand out)

WHAT YOU CAN EXPECT AT THIS MONTH'S CHECKUP

Each doctor or nurse-practitioner will have a personal approach to well-baby checkups. The overall organization of the physical exam, as well as the number and type of assessment techniques used and procedures performed will also vary with the individual needs of the child. But in general, you can expect the following at a checkup when your baby is about nine months old:

- Questions about how you and baby and the rest of the family are doing at home, and about baby's eating, sleeping, and general progress. Questions about child care, if you are working.
- Measurement of baby's weight, length, and head circumference, and plotting of progress since birth.
- Physical exam, including a recheck of any previous problems. The fontanel on top of baby's head is smaller now, and may even have closed.
- Developmental assessment. The examiner may actually put baby through a series of "tests" to evaluate baby's ability to sit independently, to pull up with or without help, to reach for and grasp objects, to rake at and pick up tiny objects, to look for a dropped or hidden object, to respond to his or her name, to recognize such words as mommy, daddy, bye-bye, and no-no, and to enjoy social games such as patty-cake and peekaboo, or may simply rely on observation plus your reports on what baby is doing.
- Immunizations, if not given before and if baby is in good health and there are no other contraindications. Be sure to discuss previous reactions, if any, beforehand. Tuberculin skin test may be administered now

in high-risk areas, or may wait until fifteen months. It may be given prior to, or at the time of, the MMR (measles/mumps/rubella) immunization.
- Possibly, hemoglobin or hematocrit test to check for anemia (usually by means of a pinprick on the finger).
- Guidance about what to expect in the next month in relation to such topics as feeding, sleeping, development, and infant safety.
- Recommendations about fluoride, iron, and vitamin D, or other supplementation, as needed.

Questions you may want to ask, if the doctor hasn't already answered them:

- What are positive and negative reactions to the tuberculin test, if one was administered? When should you call if there is a positive reaction?
- What new foods can be introduced to baby now? Can baby have milk in a cup? When can citrus, fish, meats, egg whites, be introduced, if they haven't been already?
- When should you consider weaning from the bottle, if your baby is bottle fed, or from the breast, if you haven't already weaned to cup or bottle?

Also raise concerns that have arisen over the past month. Jot down information and instructions from the doctor (you're sure to forget them, otherwise). Record all pertinent information (baby's weight, length, head circumference, immunizations, foods introduced, test results, illnesses, medications given, and so on) in a permanent health record.

FEEDING YOUR BABY THIS MONTH:
Establishing Good Habits Now

We've all met her. The mother of a preschooler who moans when her child gorges on ice cream, cake, and candy at a party, howls for French fries instead of a sensible lunch in a restaurant, or insists on a soft drink instead of juice at dinner. Who groans when he refuses the sandwich on whole wheat offered at a friend's house and rolls her eyes when the teacher reports that he won't drink milk at snacktime. She talks a lot about how she wishes she could get him to eat more nutritiously, but deep down inside she's convinced she'd be fighting a losing battle. Aren't kids, after all, born with a preference for junk foods?

The answer, though our well-meaning but misguided mom might be astonished to hear it, is no. A child's palate is born a clean slate; the tastes that develop depend on the foods introduced—even in those first months of eating. A Szechuan child, after all, doesn't favor cold noodles with sesame sauce, or an Indian child raita, or an English child kidney pie because of genetic fate, but because of what he's exposed to at the dinner table. And how your child will eat—whether he or she will choose sandwiches on white bread or whole wheat, find snack satisfaction in a bag of carrot chips or a box of chocolate chip cookies, clamor for plain dried apricots or candied ones—will be primarily influenced by the foods you set on his or her high chair tray now.

So that you don't end up bemoaning your child's eating habits later, start feeding your baby right, right from the start.

Keep white out of sight. A disdain for white bread, rolls, pancakes, cookies, cakes, and crackers is a form of color discrimination that's actually good to teach young children. A child who never develops a taste for bland, refined baked goods will never balk at the whole-grain varieties. Select only whole-grain products at the supermarket, bake with only whole-grain flours at home, and order only whole-grain breads, when possible, in restaurants.

Don't cut that sweet tooth yet. The longer you hold off on introducing really sweet foods, the better. Don't assume that baby won't eat cottage cheese or plain yogurt unless it's been mixed with mashed ripe banana, or cereal unless it's been sweetened with applesauce or strained peaches; babies whose taste buds haven't been corrupted will not only accept such foods "straight," they'll learn to love them. Limit fruits, serving them only after your baby's had something that isn't sweet, and serve vegetables often, early on. Although it's okay to gradually introduce fruit-juice-sweetened cookies, cake, and jams as treats, don't get into the habit of doling out the cookies instead of fresh fruit in the afternoon, topping off every meal with a sweet, or spreading jam on every cracker you hand your baby. When there is no older sibling, the introductions can often wait until baby's first birthday or later.

Keep baby sugar-free. Banning sugar from your baby's diet entirely—at least for the first year, and preferably for the first two—is actually a lot easier than trying to moderate sugar intake. If you allow sugar-sweetened sweets from the start, it will be difficult to restrict them later. It's better to forbid all such dubious treats until your baby understands such concepts as "just one" and "special occasion." Such a restriction will have two important benefits. First, it will modify his or her taste for sugar later—studies show babies who were exposed to sugar early developed a significantly stronger taste for it than those who weren't. And second, it will provide the chance for developing a taste for treats that are nutritionally sound.

Expose your child to germs. The germ of the wheat, that is. Not only will sprinkling wheat germ on your baby's cereal, yogurt, cottage cheese, applesauce, or pasta supply a whopping measure of vitamins and minerals and extra protein found together in few other foods, it will help to nurture a taste for this versatile staple. In not too many months, you may find your toddler banging on the table demanding "more wheat germ" on breakfast cereal while your neighbor's child is demanding another spoonful of sugar. In later years, when you no longer select what your child eats, this preference may help ensure good nutrition.

Eschew the mashed. Even a completely toothless baby needs something to sink his or her gums into. By now, strained foods should be a thing of the past, with coarsely mashed and finger foods having taken their place in baby's diet (see page 267). Babies who continue too long on strained foods tend to reject lumpier textures when they are finally offered, and become very lazy about chewing. This pattern could severely hamper their getting a nutritionally adequate variety of foods later.

Serve the milk straight. When the doctor okays cow's milk—sometimes only in small amounts at this age—give it to your baby unadulterated. Not only does chocolate milk contain lots of sugar, but the chocolate somewhat diminishes the absorption of the calcium in milk (though recent studies indicate this may not be to a significant degree) and can also trigger allergic reaction in some children. In addition, any time you disguise the flavor of milk (even if it's in a juice-sweetened shake), you'll be sabotaging your baby's taste for the pure thing. Save such techniques for the inevitable "I don't want my milk" rebellion of the preschool years.

Save the salt. Babies don't need salt in their foods beyond what is found there naturally. Don't salt food you prepare for baby and be particularly careful not to serve up salty snacks, which can give your child an unhealthy taste for foods high in sodium.[1]

Spice baby's diet with variety. It's not surprising that so many children turn their noses up when confronted with an unfamiliar food. In most cases, their parents have served up the same cereal every morning for breakfast and the same varieties of baby food for lunch and dinner day in and day out, never offering a change of pace or a chance to taste anything different. Be adventurous in feeding your baby—without, of course, overstepping any boundaries set by the doctor or mandated by your baby's age. Try different types of whole-grain cereals, hot and cold; varieties of whole-grain breads (oatmeal and rye, as well as wheat) in different forms (rolls, bagels, loaves, crackers, and later pitas); different shapes of whole-wheat or high-protein pastas; dairy products in different forms (yogurt, cottage cheese, kefir, pot cheese, such hard cheeses as Swiss and cheddar, lower-fat cream cheese); vegetables and fruits beyond carrots, peas, and bananas (sweet potato cubes, kale creamed with evaporated milk, ripe cantaloupe and mango slivers, split fresh blueberries, and so on).

Variety now is no guarantee that your child won't go through a peanut-butter-and-jelly-only phase—most children do at one time or another. But a familiarity with a wider range of foods will make for a broader diet base and, in the long run, better nutrition.

Brainwash. Don't just practice good nutrition in your home, preach it as well. Even a very young child can learn that sugar is "bad," white bread isn't good, whole wheat is best. That doesn't mean, of course, that your toddler will never ask for sugar or

---

1. Some older children like to shake salt on their palms and then lick it off. Check with your doctor if your child does this. Though in most cases it's no more than a habit, there is a very small possibility that the craving for salt is related to a metabolic disorder.

white bread and will always insist on whole wheat. Children test their parents, and yours is sure to test you by asking for a taste of such forbidden fruit. Don't buckle under. If you're wishy-washy once, then your baby will be even more persistent the next time, anticipating your giving in once again.

Make exceptions. If junk food is totally forbidden, your baby will come to crave it. Instead of a permanent ban, allow such foods as treats once in a while, when your baby is old enough to understand the idea of treats for special occasions. Of course, if you've gotten his or her taste buds properly acclimated, these treats may not taste as good as expected.

Do it yourself. All the above efforts are doomed to failure if the preacher is lax in her own practices. If you breakfast on Danish, lunch on white bread and bologna, and nibble the rest of the day away on chips and candy, you can't expect more from your child, now or ever. So if you haven't already switched to the Best-Odds Diet (see page 534), now is the time for you—and everyone else in your household, young and old —to do so.

Don't cave in to guilt. The reason most mothers end up giving their babies the kinds of things they know aren't good for them is guilt. Reluctant to deprive their children of what they themselves consider to be the just desserts (and chocolate milk, and hot dogs) of childhood, they give in, and give up. If you think you might find yourself doing just that, consider these two points: First, at a tender age, a baby doesn't really know what he or she is missing. If you're at a party and ice cream and cake is being served up, your baby will probably be just as happy if you pull out a fruit-juice-sweetened cookie for him or her to munch on. And second, though you are very likely to begin hearing complaints once the age of enlightenment dawns (so cottage cheese isn't the same as ice cream after all?), and can be sure your child will try very hard to stir up your guilt when you limit the goodies at a birthday party or treats at Halloween, in the long run your child will thank you. If you must feel guilty, better to feel it now than when the dentist announces your child has a mouthful of cavities, or when your teenager has a weight problem, or when, as an adult, blood pressure is high as a result of poor dietary habits.

WHAT YOU MAY BE CONCERNED ABOUT

FEEDING BABY AT THE TABLE

"We've been feeding our son separately, and putting him in the playpen while we eat. When should he start eating with us?"

Feeding themselves and their babies at the same time is a juggling feat most parents can't master—at least not gracefully, or without having to pop a couple of antacid tablets after every meal. So until your baby is a competent self-feeder, continue to give him his meals separately. But that doesn't mean he shouldn't begin to sit in on adult meals (as long as your schedules permit) for practice in table manners and sociability. Whenever it's practical and desirable, draw his high chair up to the table at your mealtime, or set him up in a hook-on dining seat, give him his own place setting (non-breakable dishes and a spoon only) and some finger foods, and include him in the table conversation. On the other hand, do reserve some late dinners for adults only in order to keep (or put back) the romance in your lives.

WALKING TOO EARLY

"Our daughter wants to walk all the time, holding on to the hands of any willing adult. Several relatives have warned that we shouldn't let her, saying walking before she's ready will damage her legs."

It's more likely to damage your backs than her legs. If your daughter's legs weren't ready for this kind of pre-walking activity, she wouldn't be clamoring for it. Like early standing, early walking (assisted or unassisted) can't cause bowleggedness (actually a normal characteristic of babies under two) or any other physical problem. In fact, both these activities are beneficial, as they exercise and strengthen some of the muscles used in walking solo. And if she's barefoot, they will help strengthen her feet as well. So as long as your backs hold out, let her walk to her legs' content.

A baby who doesn't want to walk at this stage, of course, shouldn't be pushed into it. As with other aspects of development, just follow your half-pint-size leader.

PULLING UP

"Our baby just learned to pull up. He seems to love it for a few minutes but then starts screaming. Could standing be hurting his legs?"

If your child's legs weren't ready to hold him, he wouldn't be pulling up. He's screaming out of frustration, not pain. Like most babies who've just learned to stand, he's stranded in this unfamiliar position until he falls, collapses, or is helped down. And that's where you come in. As soon as you notice frustration setting in, gently help him down to a sitting position. Slowly does it—so that he can get the idea of how to do it himself, which should take a few days, or at most, a few weeks. In the meantime, expect to spend a lot of time coming to the rescue of your baby-in-distress.

"My baby is trying to pull up on everything in the house. Should I keep her in the playpen for safety?"

The more our children learn to do, the more nervous we become—and rightly so. As they learn to pull up, then cruise, and finally walk, they enter a stage when they have more brawn than their brains can be responsible for—and are at high risk of accidental injury. But banishment to the playpen (except for brief periods when no one is available to closely supervise) is not the solution. Nerve-racking as it may be to you, your almost-toddler needs plenty of opportunity to explore the world outside the playpen. And you need to make that world as safe as possible.

Be especially certain now that anything she might attempt to pull up on (get down on her level if necessary to determine what that might be) is secure. Unstable tables, bookcases, chairs, and floor lamps should be put away or out of reach for the time being. Corners and sharp edges on remaining coffee or end tables should be cushioned in case baby falls against them (she probably will, and often). Be sure that breakable or dangerous knickknacks she couldn't reach before are put away. If you have a dishwasher, don't leave it open when she's on the loose. To prevent slips and trips, be sure that electrical cords are out of the way, that papers are not left lying around on the floor, and that spills on smooth-surfaced floors are wiped up quickly. And to be sure her feet won't sabotage her, keep her barefoot or in skid-proof socks or slippers, rather than in smooth-soled shoes.

When a child begins pulling up, cruising around the room—from chair to table to wall to sofa to daddy's legs, for example—can't be far behind. Which means that if you put her down in one spot in the room, you should be prepared to see her move to a totally different spot, or even to another room. So every corner of every room in your home (except those behind always-closed doors) has to be baby-proofed. If you didn't attend to this when your baby began crawling, or if she never crawled, see page 292 for tips on making home safe for baby.

FEAR OF STRANGERS

"Our little girl has always been friendly and outgoing. But when my in-laws—with whom she always loved to play—came in from out of town yesterday, she broke into tears every time they came near her. What's come over her?"

Maturity—of a very immature sort. Though she'll show a definite preference for her mother and father after the first couple of months, a baby under six months or so will generally respond positively to almost any grownup. Whether they are familiar adults or strangers, she lumps them pretty much into the category of people who are capable of taking care of her needs. Often, as a baby approaches eight or nine months (though "stranger anxiety," the official term for this phenomenon, can begin at six months or even earlier), she begins to realize which side her zwieback is really buttered on; that mother and father, and possibly another familiar person or two, are her primary caretakers; and that she ought to stick close to them and steer clear of anyone who might try to separate her from them (strangers). During this time, even once-beloved grandmothers and baby-sitters may be suddenly rejected, as baby clings desperately to her parents (particularly the parent who provides the most care).

Wariness of strangers may disappear quickly or not peak until somewhat past a year; in about 2 in 10 babies it never develops at all (possibly because these babies adjust easily to new situations of all kinds) or passes so quickly it isn't noticed. If your baby does exhibit stranger anxiety, don't pressure her to be sociable—she'll come around eventually, and it's best that she does on her own terms. In the meantime,

warn friends and family that she's going through a shy stage (which they shouldn't take personally) and that quick advances will frighten her. Suggest that instead of trying to hug her or pick her up immediately, they try to break down her resistance slowly—by smiling at her, talking to her, offering her a plaything—while she sits securely on your lap. Eventually she may warm up, and even if she doesn't, at least there won't have been any tears and bad feelings along the way.

If it's a longtime baby-sitter your child suddenly doesn't want to go to, the odds are that once you leave the house—no matter how hysterical she may be in your presence—she will quiet down. If it's a new sitter, you may have to spend some additional orientation time before your baby will be willing to stay with the newcomer. If your baby is truly inconsolable when left with a sitter, new or old, then it's time to reevaluate your child-care situation. Maybe the sitter is not giving your baby the kind of attention and love she needs, even if she seems caring when you're around. Or it may simply be a case of extreme stranger anxiety. Some infants, particularly those who are breastfed, can cry for hours when mommy is gone, even when daddy or grandma is the baby-sitter. In such a case, you may have to limit time away from your child, if possible, until this "missing-mommy" phase has passed.

SECURITY OBJECTS

"For the last couple of months our baby has become more and more attached to his blanket. He even drags it around when he's crawling. Does this mean he's insecure?"

He is a little insecure, and with good reason. In the last couple of months he's discovered he's a separate person, not an extension of his parents. The discovery is undeniably exciting (so many challenges!), yet more than a little frightening (so many risks!). Many babies, when they realize that mommy and daddy may not always be available to lean on from now on, become attached to a transitional comfort object (a soft blanket, a cuddly stuffed animal, a bottle, a pacifier) as a sort of stand-in. Like parents, the object offers comfort—particularly appealing when a baby is frustrated, sick, or tired—but unlike parents, it's under the infant's control. For the baby who has trouble separating from his parents, taking the security object to bed makes going to sleep alone easier.

Sometimes a baby who hasn't become attached to a security object earlier will do so suddenly when confronted with a new and unsettling situation (a new sitter, a day-care center, moving to a new home, and so on). The transitional comfort object is usually given up sometime between the ages of two and five (about the same time that thumb sucking is abandoned), but often not until it is lost, disintegrates, or in some other way becomes unavailable. Some children mourn for a day or two, but then get on with their lives; others hardly note the passing of their old friend.

Though parents (or other caregivers) should never tease or scold a baby or child about a security object or pressure him to give it up, it is often possible to set some limits early on that will make the habit less objectionable and help to prepare a baby for the inevitable separation:

■ If the habit is in its early stages and is not yet deeply entrenched, try to head off future hassles by limiting its use to home or to bedtime. But don't forget to take it along on overnights and vacations.
■ Before the object begins to take on a grubbiness that your baby can smell, wash it. Otherwise, he may become attached as much to the odor as to the object itself, and complain strenuously if it returns from the wash smelling like springtime. If you can't get it away from him during waking hours, wash it while he's asleep.
■ If the object is a toy, you might want to invest in a duplicate. This will give you a ready replacement in case of loss, let you wash them alternately, and allow you to rotate the items so that neither becomes too grimy. If it's a blanket, you might consider cutting it into several sections so that lost or thread-worn pieces can be replaced as needed.
■ Though the less said about the object, the better, you can remind your child now and then that when he's more grownup he won't need his blanket (or other object) anymore.
■ Although an empty bottle or a bottle of water is acceptable, don't let your baby use a bottle of juice or milk as a comfort object. Sucking on such liquids for long periods at a time—particularly at night—can cause dental decay and interfere with a baby's getting adequate solids.
■ Make sure your baby is getting the comfort (and love and attention) he needs from you, including plenty of hugs and kisses, if he enjoys them, and frequent talking and playing sessions in which you give him your undivided attention.

Though attachment to a comfort object is a normal developmental step for many infants, a baby who becomes so obsessed with the object that he doesn't spend enough time interacting with people, playing with toys, or practicing physical feats may have some emotional needs that aren't being met. If this seems to be the case with your baby, check with his doctor.

FLAT FEET

"My baby's arches look totally flat when he stands up. Could he have flat feet?"

In babies, flatness is the rule, not the exception. And it's a rule that you're not likely to find an exception to. There are several reasons: first of all, since young babies don't do much walking, the muscles in their feet haven't been exercised enough to fully develop the arches. Second, a pad of fat fills the arch, making it difficult to discern, particularly in chubby babies. And when babies begin to walk, they stand with feet apart to achieve balance, putting more weight on the arch and giving the foot a flatter appearance.

In most children, the flat-footed look will slowly diminish over the years, and by the time full growth is attained, the arch will be well formed. In only a small percentage will the feet remain flat (not a serious problem, anyway), but that's something that can't be predicted now.

NO TEETH

"Our baby is almost nine months old and still doesn't have a single tooth. What could be holding her teething up?"

Enjoy those toothless grins while you can, and be reassured that there are many nine-month-olds who are all gums—even a few who finish their first year without a single tooth with which to bite into their birthday cake—but that teeth come to every baby eventually. Though the average baby cuts a first tooth at seven months, the range is from two months (occasionally earlier) to twelve (sometimes later). Late teething is usually hereditary, and is no reflection on your baby's intelligence or development. (Second teeth will come in later, too.) Toothlessness needn't interfere, incidentally, with a baby's moving on to chunkier foods; the gums are used for chewing in toothed and toothless babies alike until molars arrive in the middle of the second year.

STILL HAIRLESS

"Our daughter was born bald, and still has little more than peach fuzz. When will she get some hair?"

To a mother tired of hearing "Oh, what a cute little boy" whenever she's out with her daughter, and eager to make a definitive gender statement with barrettes and bows, baldness or near baldness that persists well into the second half of the first year can be frustrating. But, like toothlessness, hair-lessness at this age is not unusual—and not permanent. The problem is most common among fair babies with light hair and is not a forecast of baldness later in life. In time your daughter's hair will come in (though perhaps not in quantity until sometime late in the second year). For now, be thankful that you don't have to wrestle with a tangled headful of hair during shampoos and comb-outs.

LOSS OF INTEREST IN NURSING

"Whenever I sit down to breastfeed my son, he seems to want to do something else—play with my buttons, pull up on my hair, look at the television screen, anything but nurse."

In the early months, when a breastfeeding baby's whole world seems to revolve around his mother's breasts, it seems implausible that a time will ever come when he will be disinterested in nursing. And yet, though some babies remain passionate about nursing until weaning, many display waning interest and concentration somewhere around the ninth month. Some simply begin to refuse the breast entirely; others nurse seriously for a minute or two, and then pull away; still others are easily distracted during nursing, either by what's going on around them or by their desire to practice their new-found physical prowess. Sometimes the boycott is just transient. Maybe baby is going through a readjustment in his nutritional needs, or perhaps he's put off by the altered taste of your breast milk brought on by hormonal changes during your menstrual period or from the garlicky *pasta al pesto* you dined on the previous night. Or maybe he's lost his appetite to a virus or a bout of teething.

But if your baby regularly rejects the breast, it's possible he's telling you he's ready for weaning, because he either has a decreased need for sucking, is taking more solids and milk from a cup or bottle, or doesn't like being held and/or lying still for lengthy feedings. Before you decide, however, that weaning is imminent, be sure the problem isn't a feeding environment that is so distracting your baby can't concentrate on the task at hand. To rule out this possibility, try nursing in a quiet room with lights dimmed, no television or radio blaring, no older children playing, and no adult conversation being carried on. If your baby still seems lackadaisical about nursing, he may truly be on the verge of giving up the breast. Of course, *you* may not be ready for this—but as many mothers before you have learned, you can lead a baby to the breast, but you can't make him drink.

Still, you should try to keep the weaning gradual—for your baby's health as well as your own comfort. Gradual weaning will allow baby time to increase his intake of a nutritional replacement, such as cow's milk or formula, before he gives breast milk up entirely. And it will give your breasts the chance to reduce production slowly to avoid painful engorgement. (See page 342 for tips on weaning; if your baby absolutely refuses to take any breastfeedings, see page 344 for making abrupt weaning easier.)

Ask his doctor if you should give your baby whole cow's milk (not skim or low-fat) now, or if you should stick with formula until he's a year old. If he's been taking a bottle, it's likely he will be able to get enough milk from this source—unless, as sometimes happens, he is no longer interested in sucking on a bottle nipple either. In that case, or if he's never accepted a bottle at all, or if you'd rather not face the task of weaning him from the bottle later, milk from a cup is the alternative. Babies who were started on the cup earlier are often very proficient by this age; those who weren't often catch on quickly. Plain whole-milk yogurt or hard cheeses can be given as a calcium supplement for children who won't drink enough milk or formula straight.

FUSSY EATING HABITS

"When I first introduced solids, my daughter seemed to love everything I gave her. But lately, she won't eat anything but bread."

To hear their parents tell it, some children (up until adolescence, when a week's worth of groceries lasts three days) live on nothing but air, love, and the occasional crust of bread. But in spite of parental concerns, even picky eaters manage to drink, nibble, and nosh enough during the day to thrive. Children are programmed to eat what they need to live and grow— unless something happens to alter that programming early in their eating history.

At this stage of development, most babies are still getting a major portion of their needed nutrition from breast milk, formula, or whole milk and this is usually rounded out sufficiently by whatever bits of solid foods they get during the day. Vitamin drops with iron provide added insurance. But at nine months, nutritional requirements are beginning to increase and the need for milk begins to decrease. To be sure that your baby's intake continues to meet her requirements, incorporate the following into your feeding strategy:

Let them eat bread... Or cereal, or bananas, or whatever food they favor. Many babies and toddlers seem to be on a food-of-the-week (or -month) plan, refusing to eat anything but a single selection during that time. And it's best to respect their dietary preferences and aversions, even when taken to extremes: cereal for breakfast, lunch, and dinner, for example. Eventually, if given a chance to do so on her own, a child will expand her repertoire of tastes.

...but make sure it's whole wheat. Of course, if your baby's eating only one or two foods (and actually, even if she's eating a variety), make sure that they provide high-quality nourishment. So if it's bread, bagels, crackers, or cereal she craves, give her only whole-grain varieties. If it's fruit or fruit juice, be sure it's unsweetened and try to encourage the more nutritious types, such as apricots, yellow peaches, cantaloupes, mangos, and oranges.

Add on when you can. While you shouldn't push food on your baby, there's nothing wrong with trying to sneak it by her. Spread the bread with whipped or thinned cream cheese,[2] mashed banana, puréed pumpkin sweetened with apple juice concentrate and cinnamon, or cottage cheese, or melt some Swiss cheese on it. Or turn it into French toast, or "eggie bread," served whole or cut into small pieces. Or try baking and buying breads that incorporate other Best-Odds requirements, such as pumpkin, carrot, cheese, or fruit. If it's cereal your baby craves, sprinkle cereal with wheat germ, and slip in a serving of fruit in the form of a diced banana, applesauce, cooked diced peaches or other fruit, or some iron in the form of diced cooked dried fruit. If bananas are her sole passion, try dipping slices in milk and rolling in wheat germ, serving them conspicuously with a small amount of cereal or cottage cheese, or mashing them on bread.

Omit the mush. Your baby's recent rebellion may simply be her way of telling you that she's had it with the mushed and the mashed and is ready for more grownup fare. Changing to chunky foods and finger foods that are soft enough for her to manage but intriguing enough in taste and texture to satisfy her maturing palate may turn her into the epicure you seek.

Vary the menu. Maybe your baby's just tired of the same old meals; a change may be what she needs to spark her appetite. If she lacks interest in cereal at breakfast,

offer yogurt and toast instead. If cottage cheese with mashed baby peas and carrots for lunch seems to bore her, toss some buttered noodles with finely minced cooked cauliflower and broccoli and grated or shredded Cheddar. If minced meat and mashed potatoes doesn't appeal at dinner, try poached fish and baked yams. (See Best-Odds listings for additional ideas, page 359.) Also consider, when you plan your baby's menus, that she may enjoy eating what everyone else is eating rather than being an outcast. (If you are introducing new foods your baby hasn't had before, see page 219.)

Turn the tables. Perhaps it's just a newly emerging streak of stubborn independence that's keeping her mouth clenched at mealtime. Hand her the responsibility of feeding, and she may open her mouth eagerly to a wide range of food experiences she would never take from the spoon you offer. (For appropriate choices for the self-feeding baby, see page 279.)

Don't drown her appetite. Many babies (and toddlers) eat very little because they're drinking too much juice, formula, or breast milk. Your baby should have no more than two Best-Odds fruit servings in the form of juice (preferably one of juice and one of whole fruit) and no more than three of formula (or later, milk) a day. If she wants to drink more than that, give her water or watered-down juice, spreading the servings out over the day. If you're breastfeeding, you don't know exactly how much milk she's taking, but you can be pretty sure that nursing her more than three or four times a day will interfere with her appetite; cut back.

Attack snacks. What does mom do when baby refuses breakfast? Plies her with snacks all morning, of course, which means she isn't likely to have any appetite for lunch. And what happens after lunch is missed? Baby's hungry again in the afternoon, snacking continues, and there's no

---

2. Fat-reduced cream cheeses have more protein than the regular varieties, and are thus more nutritious for baby. But read labels to be sure of what you're buying.

room for dinner. Avoid this cycle, depressing to both baby's appetite and your spirit, by strictly limiting snacks to one midmorning and one midafternoon, no matter how little your child eats at mealtimes. You can, however, increase the amount fed at snacktime by a bit in order to tide baby over from a light or skipped meal to the next feeding time.

Keep smiling. The easiest way for you to lay the foundation for a permanent feeding problem is to frown with displeasure when your baby turns her head away from the oncoming spoon, to comment unhappily when she comes out of the high chair as empty of food as when she went in, or to spend half an hour trying to get a couple of spoonfuls of pablum into her closed mouth with cajoling, pleading, or tricks ("here comes the choo choo train into the tunnel"). She needs to feel she's eating because she's hungry, not because you want her to. So at all costs—even at the cost of some missed meals—don't make eating (or not eating) an issue. If she clearly doesn't want any more, or doesn't want to eat at all, remove the dish and end the meal without further ado.

Short-term appetite loss, of course, can accompany colds and other acute illnesses, particularly when fever is present. Rarely, a baby will show a chronic lack of appetite due to anemia (see page 255) or malnutrition (both uncommon among middle-class American babies) or other illness. If your baby's loss of appetite is accompanied by lack of energy, lack of interest in her environment, a slowdown in development, insufficient weight gain, or a marked change in personality (sudden irritability or nervousness, for instance), check with her doctor.

SELF-FEEDING

"Every time the spoon comes near my baby, she grabs for it. If her bowl is near enough, she dips her fingers in and makes a mess trying to feed herself. She's getting nothing to eat and I'm getting frustrated."

It's clearly time to pass the spoon to a new generation. Your baby is expressing her desire to be independent, at least at the table. Encourage rather than discourage her. But to minimize the mess and keep her from going hungry until she can pass muster with Miss Manners, pass the responsibility on gradually—if possible.

Begin by giving her a spoon of her own while you continue feeding her. She may not be able to do much more than wave it around at first, and when she does fill it and get it to her mouth it will usually be upside down. Still, wielding a spoon may keep her content enough to let you take care of most of the meal, at least for a while. The next step is to provide finger foods that she can feed herself while you spoon feed her. The combination of finger foods and a personal spoon (and/or a covered cup to take swigs from) usually keeps a baby occupied and happy enough for mom or dad to get the rest of the meal into her, but not always. Some babies insist on doing it all themselves; if this is the only way your baby will eat, let her. Mealtimes will take longer and be messier at first, but the experience will make your child a more proficient self-feeder sooner. (Spreading newspaper on the floor beneath baby's chair will at least make cleanup easier.)

Whatever you do, don't let mealtime become battle time, or you'll risk setting her up for permanent eating problems. When self-feeding degenerates into all play and no eating (some play is normal), you can try picking up the spoon and taking over the feeding yourself. If your baby balks, it's time to wipe the carrots off the chin and the cottage cheese from between the fingers and call it quits until the next meal.

CHANGES IN SLEEP PATTERNS

"Suddenly my daughter doesn't want to nap in the morning. Is one nap a day enough for her?"

Though one nap a day may not be enough for the exhausted parents, it is all many babies need as they approach their first birthday. A few babies even try to give up both naps at this time. Most often it is the morning nap that goes first, but occasionally it's the after-lunch siesta. The babies of some lucky parents continue to nap twice a day well into the second year, and this is perfectly normal, too, as long as it doesn't seem to be interfering with a good night's sleep. If it does seem to be, baby should be weaned down to one nap (see page 226).

How much a baby sleeps is of less consequence than how well she functions on the sleep she's getting. If your baby refuses to go down for a nap or naps but seems cranky and overtired by dinnertime, it may be that she needs the extra sleep but is protesting because she doesn't want to waste precious time—that she could use for activity and exploration—on sleep. Not getting needed naps makes for a less happy, less cooperative baby during the day, and often one who goes to bed less easily and sleeps less well at night; being overtired and overcharged, she has a difficult time settling down and staying down.

If your baby doesn't seem to be getting the naps she needs, make a special effort to encourage her. Try putting her down—fed, changed, and relaxed by a little quiet play and quiet music—in a dark room with no distractions. If that doesn't work, you may need to resort to walking her in the stroller or driving around with her in the car. (Many city babies do all their napping in the stroller, suburban babies in the car.) If necessary, try letting your baby "cry it out" before giving up on getting her to nap, but not for as long as you would at night. More that twenty minutes of crying, and there goes her naptime.

"We thought we'd done everything right. Our baby always went to sleep without a fuss. Now he seems to want to stay up and play all night."

It's something like making a sudden move from a small town in Nebraska to New York City. A couple of months ago, there wasn't much to keep your baby up at night. Now, with so many discoveries to make, toys to play with, people to interact with, and physical accomplishments to fine-tune (who wants to lie down when you're just learning to stand up?), your baby doesn't want to take time out to sleep.

Unfortunately, in this case baby doesn't know what's good for him. As with not sleeping enough during the day, going to sleep too late at night can make him overtired, which, in turn, can keep him from settling down well at all. Children who aren't getting adequate sleep are more likely to have trouble falling asleep and to wake up during the night. They may also be cranky during the day and more prone to accidents.

If your baby isn't going to sleep readily at night, be sure he's napping sufficiently during the day (see page 226). Next, establish a bedtime routine—or if you've already established one but have been adhering to it halfheartedly, enforce it. If baby-sitter or grandparents will be putting baby to bed occasionally, make sure they are familiar with the rituals.

If you aren't certain what to include in a bedtime routine, you can try some or all of the following:

A bath. After a day of cleaning the floor with his knees, massaging his scalp with mashed banana, and rolling in the sandbox, a baby needs a bath. But the evening bath does more than get a baby clean—it relaxes him. Warm, soothing waters wield magical, sleep-inducing powers; don't waste them by giving baby his bath earlier in the day.

A sleep-inducing atmosphere. Dim the lights, turn the TV off, send older children from the room, and keep other distractions to a minimum.

A story, a song, a cuddle. After your baby's been diapered and pajama-ed, settle down together into a comfortable chair or sofa, or on baby's bed once he's graduated to one. Read him a simple story, if he will sit still for one, in a soft monotone rather than a lively, animated voice. Or if he prefers, let him look at some picture books himself. Sing quiet songs and lullabies, hug a little, but save rougher fun (such as wrestling matches and tickling sessions) for other times. Once baby's motor is turned on, it's hard to turn off.

A light for the wary. Some babies are afraid of the dark. If yours is one of them, give him a night light to keep him company.

Goodbyes. Put a favorite toy or animal to bed. Encourage your baby to wave bye-bye to it, as well as to stuffed animals, siblings, mommy and daddy. Share good-night kisses all around, tuck baby into his crib and make your departure.

If he cries when you leave the room, return for a moment to be sure he's okay, kiss him again, then leave. If he continues crying, you will probably have to resort to letting him cry it out. The tried-and-usually-true technique, described on page 261 is likely to work, but it may be harder on you now that he's not only older but wiser. At this age, he will probably know how to get you back into the room, or at least how to make you feel guilty if you don't return. He may repeatedly pull up and scream until you help him to get down again. Or he may start calling "ma-ma" or "da-da," making it difficult for you not to respond. And rather than being calmed by a visit, as a younger baby might, he will probably be all the angrier when you leave him again. Your best bet with such a little wise guy is to try to stay away entirely while he gets himself back into the habit of going to sleep on his own.

"We haven't been able to set up a bed-time routine for our baby because he always falls asleep nursing before we start."

If your baby routinely falls asleep with the last nursing of the evening, go through the entire go-to-bed routine—including the good-nights—before settling down to nurse. Or, if you'd like to try to break him of the nursing-to-sleep habit, try nursing him before his bath under conditions not conducive to sleep—with plenty of noise, light, and activity, and the promise of a bath and story ahead. If he falls asleep in spite of all your efforts, try waking him for the bath. If that doesn't work, go back to nursing after the bedtime rituals and try again in a couple of weeks.

"I think my baby's having trouble sleeping because she's cutting teeth. Even though there's nothing I can do for her, I feel guilty letting her cry at night."

Better guilty now than sleepless from now on. As parents know all too well, there's very little you can do to comfort a baby who's experiencing severe teething pain. And in the middle of the night, there's no use trying. Stay up with her during these teething bouts, and you'll get her so used to having your presence at night that she'll demand it long after the new tooth (or teeth) comes through. Teething pain usually keeps a baby up sporadically, for only a few nights at a time; knowing that a parent will appear when she cries can keep her up indefinitely. So resist the temptation to go to her, and let her settle back down by herself—though you might want to peek in to be sure she hasn't pulled up and stranded herself, unable to get back down again, become uncovered, or otherwise gotten into trouble. If it makes either or both of you happier, go to her, pat her for a minute or two, tell her to go back to sleep, and then leave.

If she seems inconsolable, ask her doctor about the possibility of giving her a dose of baby acetaminophen before she goes to bed. Do be sure, however, that your baby's night waking isn't prompted by illness—an ear infection, for example, the pain of which often worsens at night—which such pain medication could mask.

SLOW DEVELOPMENT

"We're worried because our baby has begun only recently to sit well by himself—much later than our friends' babies."

Each baby's rate of development is predetermined primarily by his genes, which determine how quickly his nervous system develops. He is programmed to sit, pull up, stand, walk, smile his first smile and say his first word at a certain age. Few develop at a uniform rate in all areas; most are faster in some and slower in others. One baby might, for example, be quick to smile and talk (social and language skills), but not pull up until nearly a year (a gross motor skill). Another might walk (a gross motor skill) at eight months, yet not exhibit a pincer grasp (a fine motor skill) until after his first birthday. The rate at which motor skills develop is in no way related to intelligence.

Doing even most things later than other children, as long as development falls within the wide range considered normal and progresses from one step to the next, is not usually a matter for concern. When a child routinely reaches developmental milestones long after other children, however, a consultation with his doctor is in order. In most cases, such a consultation will put a parent's fears to rest. Some children mature slowly, yet are perfectly normal. Occasionally, further workups will be necessary to determine whether or not a problem really exists, which of course it sometimes does.

Once in a great while, the baby's doctor is not concerned but the parents have some lingering doubts in spite of every reassurance. Their best route to peace of mind: a referral to a developmental specialist. Sometimes the baby's doctor, who sees him

only for brief evaluations, misses signs of poor development that a parent sees or senses, and that an expert doing a lengthier workup can pick up. The consultation serves a dual purpose. First, if parental concern turns out to be truly unnecessary, worry, at least about development, can be cast aside. Second, if there does turn out to be a problem, early intervention may improve the child's chances of living up to his full potential.

STRANGE STOOLS

"When I changed my baby's diaper today I was really puzzled. Her stool seemed to be filled with grains of sand. But she never plays in a sandbox."

Just when you're getting bored with changing diapers, another surprise turns up in one. Sometimes it's easy to figure out what went into baby to produce the change in her stools. Frightening red color? Usually innocent beets or beet juice. Black specks or strands? Bananas. Small dark foreign objects? Maybe blueberries or raisins. Light green pellets? Perhaps peas. Yellow ones? Corn. Seeds? Very likely tomatoes, cucumbers, or melon from which the seeds were not completely removed.

Because babies don't chew thoroughly and their digestive tracts are not fully mature, what goes in often comes out largely unchanged in color and texture.[3] Sandy stools, such as those in your baby's diaper, are fairly common, not because babies snack from the sandbox (though they do), but because certain foods—particularly Cheerios and similar oat cereals, and pears—often appear sandy once they've passed through the digestive tract.

Odd changes in the stool come not just from natural items in your baby's diet, but also from those synthesized in the food lab (most of which aren't appropriate for

3. Squashing, mashing, or splitting raisins, berries, peas, and corn kernels will make them not only easier to digest but safer.

babies, but nevertheless sometimes find their way into small tummies). Such products have been known to color stools such dramatic hues as fluorescent green (from a grape-flavored beverage) and shocking pinkish red (from berry-flavored cereal).

So before you panic at the sight of what's filling your baby's diaper, think about what's been filling her. If you're still puzzled, show a sample to the doctor.

BABY AND BIKING

"My husband and I are ardent bike riders. Is it safe to take our baby along?"

Biking may seem like the perfect way to combine quality family time and exercise, but child-safety experts now believe that bike riding with a baby involves too many risks. So if you really want to play safe, do your biking solo.

If, in spite of this warning, you decide to hit the bike trails with your child, faithfully observe these vital rules:

■ Don't even consider taking your baby along unless your child is at least a year old, you're a very competent biker, and your bike is in perfect condition.
■ Never bicycle unless you are both wearing

approved and appropriate safety helmets.
■ Have your child ride in an approved child bicycle seat that protects her feet and hands from becoming caught in the spokes and minimizes both the impact of a fall and the risk of injury should you take a tumble. Be sure the seat is properly installed and that your child is securely belted before you start off.
■ Or use a bicycle "trailer" to pull your child behind you. The advantage is that even if you and your bike take a spill, the trailer and your baby will remain upright. The disadvantage: Because it is below windshield level of most vehicles, it may leave your child more vulnerable in traffic. So it's probably safest to use such a trailer only on bike paths.
■ Restrict your bike trips to safe areas, such as parks, bicycle trails, quiet streets or roads. Avoid busy thoroughfares; snowy, icy, or wet roads; and roads strewn with wet leaves. Walk your bike when you come to a downhill grade—on a slope, dangerous speeds can be reached without even trying, and braking becomes surprisingly difficult.

Better yet, hire a sitter, take turns biking, or wait until your child is old enough to ride alongside you.

WHAT IT'S IMPORTANT TO KNOW: Games Babies Play

When it comes to baby care, a lot has changed since our mothers' mothers were mothers. The trend is now toward breastfeeding, instead of away from it. Dirty diapers are tossed into the trash instead of scrubbed and boiled on the stove for reuse. Schedules are less by the book and more by the baby. Yet with all the changes, some things have remained the same. The sterling silver teething ring too precious to allow baby to teethe on it. The

handmade cradle that has helped rock three generations to sleep. And the games that babies love.

Time-honored as any heirloom, the peekaboos and this-little-piggies that brought squeals of delight to your grandmother's baby are guaranteed to do the same for yours. But such games do more than entertain; they improve socialization skills, teach such concepts as object permanence (peekaboo), coordination of words and actions (the itsy-bitsy spider), counting skills (one, two, buckle my shoe), and language skills (eyes, nose, mouth).

Chances are that even if you haven't heard a nursery game in decades, many your mother played with you will come back to you now that you're in her shoes. If they don't, ask your mother for a replay of her favorites (a mother never forgets). Tap, too, the resources of other relatives, particularly any who came from "the old country," for venerable folk songs, nursery rhymes, and games that might otherwise be lost, and your husband's side of the family for their favorites.

Refresh your memory or learn a few new games from the list below.

Peekaboo. Cover your face (with your hands, the corner of a blanket, a piece of clothing, a menu in a restaurant, or by hiding behind a curtain or the foot of the crib) and say, "Where's mommy?" (or daddy). Then uncover your face and say, "Peekaboo, I see you!" Be ready to repeat and repeat until you collapse; most babies have a voracious appetite for this game. Or say "Peekaboo" when you cover your face, "I see you" when you uncover it.

Clap hands. While you sing—"Clap hands, clap hands, till daddy comes home, 'cause daddy has money and mommy has none" is the traditional verse—take your baby's hands and show him or her how to clap. At first, your baby's hands will probably not open wide, but the ability to hold the hands flat will finally come, though maybe not until the end of the year; don't push it. It may also be a while before your baby can clap independently, but that, too, will come. During the interim, he or she may enjoy holding your hands and patting them together.

You can modernize the ditty, if you like: "Clap hands, clap hands, till mommy comes home, 'cause mommy has money and baby has none." Or you can try clapping feet, for a change of pace. Or you can use this rhyme: "Patty-cake, patty-cake, baker's man, bake me a cake as fast as you can. Mix it, and pat it, and mark it with a 'B,' and put it in the oven for baby and me."

The itsy bitsy spider. Use your fingers—the thumb of one hand to the pointer finger of the other—to simulate a spider climbing up an invisible web, and sing: "The itsy bitsy spider went up the water spout." Then, use your fingers to imitate rain falling, and continue: "Down came the rain and washed the spider out." Throw your arms up and out for "Out came the sun and dried up all the rain." And then back to square one, the spider goes back up the web and you end with, "And the itsy bitsy spider went up the spout again."

This little piggy went to market. Take baby's thumb or big toe and start with, "This little piggy went to market." Move on to the next finger or toe, "This little piggy stayed home." And the next, "This little piggy had roast beef" (or if you're a vegetarian, "pizza"), fourth finger, "This little piggy had none." As you sing the final line, "This little piggy cried wee, wee, wee, all the way home," run your fingers up baby's arm or leg to under the arms or neck, tickling all the way.

So big. Ask, "How big is baby?" (or use child's name, the dog's name, or a sibling's name), help your child to spread his or her arms as wide as possible, and exclaim, "So big!"

Eyes, nose, mouth. Take both baby's hands in yours, touch one to each of your eyes, then both to your nose, then to your mouth (where you end with a kiss), naming each feature as you move along: "Eyes, nose, mouth, smooch." Nothing teaches these body parts faster.

Ring-a-round the rosies. Try this one once your baby is walking. Hold hands with him or her (invite a sibling, playmate, or other adult to join the circle, when possible) and walk around in a circle, singing,

"Ring-a-round the rosies, a pocket full of posies, ashes, ashes, we all fall down"—at which point you all collapse down on the floor. One variation is to substitute "hopscotch, hopscotch" for "ashes, ashes," and to jump up at each one.

One, two, buckle my shoe. When climbing stairs or counting fingers, sing: "One, two, buckle my shoe. Three, four, close the door. Five, six, pick up sticks. Seven, eight, close the gate. Nine, ten, start again."

Pop goes the weasel. You can turn slowly in a circle with baby if you're standing, or rock him or her back and forth if you're seated, as you sing, "All around the mulberry bush, the monkey chased the weasel. The monkey thought it was all in fun...." Then, "Pop goes the weasel!" as you bounce baby with the pop. Once baby is familiar with the song, wait a moment before bouncing to give him or her a chance to do the popping.

CHAPTER THIRTEEN

The Tenth Month

WHAT YOUR BABY MAY BE DOING

By the end of this month, your baby ...should be able to (see Note):

- stand holding on to someone or something
- pull up to standing position from sitting
- object if you try to take a toy away
- say mama or dada indiscriminately
- play peekaboo

Note: If your baby seems not to have reached one or more of these milestones, check with the doctor. In rare instances the delay could indicate a problem, though in most cases it will turn out to be normal for your baby. Premature infants generally reach milestones later than others of the same birth age, often achieving them closer to their adjusted age (the age they would be if they had been born at term), or sometimes later.

...will probably be able to:

- get into a sitting position from stomach

- play patty-cake (clap hands) or wave bye-bye
- pick up tiny object with any part of thumb and finger
- walk holding on to furniture (cruise)
- understand word "no" (but not always obey it)

...may possibly be able to:

- stand alone momentarily
- say dada (by 10 months) or mama (by 11 months) discriminately

...may even be able to:

- indicate wants in ways other than crying
- "play ball" (roll ball back to you)
- drink from a cup independently
- pick up a tiny object neatly with tips of thumb and forefinger
- stand alone well
- use immature jargoning (gibberish that sounds like baby is talking in a made up

foreign language)
- say one word other than mama or dada
- respond to a one-step command with ges-

tures (give that to me—with hand out)
- walk well

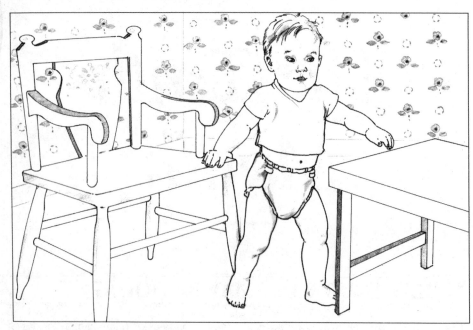

Many ten-month-olds have gained "cruise control," the last step before unassisted walking. With one hand holding cautiously onto home base, they reach first with their other hand, then with a foot, toward another piece of furniture. Ensure sure footing by letting baby cruise only around steady chairs and tables.

WHAT YOU CAN EXPECT AT THIS MONTH'S CHECKUP

Most doctors do not schedule regular well-baby checkups this month. Do call the doctor if there are any concerns that can't wait until next month's visit.

FEEDING YOUR BABY THIS MONTH: Thinking About Weaning

In most of the rest of the breastfeeding world, definite cultural norms—for either early or late weaning—have evolved. But in the United States, where breastfeeding is in its own infancy after a recent rebirth, no such patterns exist. Some women breastfeed for six weeks, some six months, some three years or longer. The intended time of weaning may be set long before a baby is born, based on a scheduled return to work or simply a notion of what seems right. Or it may be spurred by the moment, when baby or mother suddenly loses interest in nursing, for example.

When deciding how long you are going to breastfeed, you will probably want to consider many personal factors, as well as the few scientific ones available.

The facts. We have already stated that nursing even for just a few weeks is beneficial to an infant, since it's at this time that babies receive important antibodies to fight disease. But babies thrive better—with less illness and fewer allergies—if they are on breast milk for the first six months. And in fact, though it's acceptable to begin solids once a baby is four months old, breastfed babies can usually live quite well by breast milk alone during their first six months of life. Beyond the half-year mark, breast milk can continue to be the major source of a breastfed baby's nutrition (as formula can be for a bottle-fed infant), but it becomes necessary to augment it with solids.

By the end of the first year, however, scientists tell us that breast milk ceases to be adequate—not only is its protein content insufficient for the older baby, but it suffers from a decline in several vital nutrients including zinc, copper, and potassium. In the second year, infants require the nutrients in cow's milk, and the mother who is still breastfeeding should recognize that although both she and her baby may still be enjoying the experience, breast milk can't be considered a major source of nutrition for her baby. Nor do babies past a year appear to need the sucking breastfeeding provides.

In spite of much speculation, there's no solid evidence that nursing past the first year—or even well into the second or third or beyond—hinders a child's emotional development. But it does seem that prolonged breastfeeding, like prolonged bottle feeding, can lead to dental decay because during sucking (from breast *or* bottle) there is steady pooling of milk in the mouth that doesn't occur with drinking from a cup, which encourages a sip-and-swallow pattern. Another possible drawback to continuing either breast or bottle feeding much past the end of the first year is the increased risk of ear infection from feeding lying down, which many children do while suckling, especially just before bedtime.

Your feelings. Are you still enjoying breastfeeding, or are you starting to grow weary of hauling your breasts in and out of your shirt all day (and perhaps all night) long? Are you beginning to yearn for some of the freedom and flexibility that seem unattainable while you're still nursing? Are you uncomfortable about the prospect of nursing an older child? If your feelings about your breastfeeding relationship have soured, your baby's radar will certainly pick this up. He or she may even take it as a personal rejection, rather than a rejection of the nursing experience. So weaning is probably in order.

Your baby's feelings. Some babies are self-weaners. Through their actions and reactions (restlessness and indifference at the breast, nursing that is erratic and brief) they show that they're ready to move on to other ways of obtaining nourishment. Be aware, however, that it's possible to misinterpret a baby's signals. At five months, disinterest in nursing may be only a sign of your baby's growing interest in the environment; at seven months, it may suggest a craving for physical activity that outweighs any craving for food; at nine months or later, it often signifies growing independence and maturity. At any age, it could be a response to illness or teething. At no age should it be construed as a rejection of you, only of the milk you provide.

A baby is most likely to self-wean somewhere between nine and twelve months. If your baby's attachment to the breast doesn't show any signs of letting up by the age of eighteen months (and this is not uncommon), it's not likely that he or she will ever be the one to take the initiative in weaning.

Your situation. Even mothers who at first thrive on nursing often begin to find breastfeeding onerous as inconveniences multiply, and as it begins to interfere more and more with work, school, sports, love-making, or other activities (be they necessities or luxuries) in their lives. When that happens, their negative feelings are easily transmitted to their babies, making nursing more problem than pleasure for both. Weaning is an appropriate step in such cases, but be wary of attempting it concurrently with other major changes in your lives. When possible, give yourself and your baby a chance to adjust to each change separately. Illness or the need for travel may also call for weaning, sometimes even sudden weaning.

Your baby's situation. The best time to wean a baby is when all's quiet on the home front. Sickness, teething, moving, traveling, your return to work, a change of sitters, or any other kind of change or stress in a baby's life suggests putting weaning on hold, so that an additional strain won't be imposed.

Your health. If you're perpetually exhausted and there seems to be no explanation other than the physical and emotional demands of nursing, you may want to discuss with your doctor the advisability of weaning so that you can recoup your strength. Before you do, however, be sure that it isn't some easily remedied problem, such as inadequate nourishment and/or insufficient rest, that's kayoing you.

Your baby's health. Sometimes the supply of breast milk seems to diminish excessively as a baby gets older. If your baby is gaining weight poorly, is lethargic, irritable, or shows other signs of failure to thrive (see page 99), your breast milk may not be meeting all of his or her nutritional needs. Consider adding solids, supplementing with formula, or weaning completely.

Often a weaned baby takes a sudden interest in other forms of nourishment that didn't appeal when the breast was available, and begins to thrive anew.

Your baby's other sources of nourishment. If your baby has been accepting bottles all along, weaning to a bottle at any point will be relatively easy. Likewise, if your baby has learned to take fluids from a cup with fair skill, weaning directly to a cup will be possible—though not usually until about nine or ten months. If, on the other hand, your baby won't take milk from any source but your breast, weaning will have to be postponed until either bottle or cup is mastered.

Your baby's age. Even if they don't take the initiative, most babies are weanable sometime between nine and twelve months —they're less interested in and have less need for sucking, resist being held or sitting still for feedings (some even prefer to nurse standing up), and are generally more independent. They are also less attached to the breast at this age than they seem to be later on, and less opinionated, making them easier to wean than they will be when they become toddlers.

Making the decision to wean is only a step in the long process of switching a baby from the breast to other sources of nourishment, which begins with the first sip from the bottle or the first spoonful of solids. For some women the decision is easier than the weaning; for others it's the decision that causes the most turmoil. Whenever and however it comes, weaning is a time of mixed emotions for many women. They're relieved to no longer be completely tied down by their babies' needs, and they're proud that their offspring have achieved a new step on the road to growing up. But, at the same time, they're saddened by the loosening ties and by the fact that their babies don't depend on them as much as they did—and never will again.

Whether early or late, weaning is an inevitable step in a child's development.

Babies (even the really ardent nursers) rarely end up missing it for more than a brief time, and mothers do survive—though they may experience pangs when they watch other mothers nurse, even years later.

WHAT YOU MAY BE CONCERNED ABOUT

MESSY EATING HABITS

"My son doesn't eat anything until he's smushed it, smashed it, and rubbed it into his hair. Shouldn't we try to teach him some table manners?"

Eating with the average ten-month-old is enough to make anyone lose her appetite. There's as much playing with the food as eating it, and it's not unusual for more of it to end up *on* baby (and his clothes, his high chair, and the family dog who's waiting eagerly below) than *in* him.

But that's because mealtimes are no longer just for nourishment, but for exploring and discovering as well. As in the sandbox and the bathtub, he's finding out about cause and effect, about textures, about temperature differences. When he squeezes yogurt in his fist, mashes sweet potatoes into the table, slings a glob of oatmeal from his high chair tray, rubs banana into his T-shirt, blows bubbles in his cup of juice, crumbles crackers with his fingers—it's a mess for you, but a learning experience for him.

Expect the mealtime mayhem, and your need for paper towels by the caseful, to continue for months to come until your child has learned everything he can about the fascinating physical properties of food and is ready to move on to something else. That doesn't mean you have to grin (if you can) and bear it without taking some steps in defense of your sensibilities and your home and preparing your baby for a future of respectable (well, at least somewhat respectable) table manners:

Use coverups. An ounce of protection is worth a pound of paper towels. Use all the protective measures available to you: newspaper spread all around the base of the high chair or table, to be dumped after the meal; a wipe-clean bib that covers baby's front and shoulders, but which is comfortable enough so that he won't balk at wearing it; sleeves rolled up past the elbow to keep them dry and relatively clean. (Room temperature permitting, it may be more sensible to feed baby seriously messy foods in a diaper only.)

Thwart unwanted advances. You don't want to inhibit your baby's experimentation, but you also don't want to make it too easy for him to make a mess. So give him his food in a bowl, rather than a flat plate from which food can be pushed off easily. Or put it directly on his high chair tray (making sure that it's completely clean). Using a bowl that attaches to table or tray with suction gives additional protection, but will work only on a non-porous surface such as plastic. To minimize spills, give beverages in a tumbler or cup with a snap-on lid if your baby will drink from such a spout. If he won't, put just an ounce or so of liquid in a regular cup, and hand it to him whenever he's ready for a drink, but keep it out of reach between sips. Don't offer more than one bowl of food at a time, and don't serve more than two or three items in the bowl—babies tend to be overwhelmed by too many choices and react by playing and tossing instead of eating. All utensils and dishes should be nonbreakable, for both safety and economy.

Remain neutral. As you have probably

already learned, babies are natural-born performers. If you respond by laughing at their antics in the high chair, you'll only encourage more of the same. They also don't take well to criticism. So scoldings and warnings to "stop that now!" not only won't curb the behavior—they will increase it. The best policy: don't comment on poor manners. If, however, your baby does take a few neat bites, with either the spoon or his fingers, praise him generously. Let him know whenever possible that neatness counts.

Retaliate with silverware. Even though he may do nothing with it but wave it through the air (while he continues to use his other hand for the transport of food), put a spoon in your baby's hand at the beginning of the meal, and also periodically during the proceedings. Eventually he'll get the idea of actually using it to eat with.

Don't resort to a hostile takeover. Desperate mothers tend to take desperate actions—in this case taking the feeding, and thus the ability to mess, completely out of their baby's control. But while such a takeover will result in neater mealtimes, it will also result in a baby who's delayed in learning how to feed himself and who, as a result, is also slow to develop polite table manners and good eating habits.

Be a model leader. It's not lectures and warnings that will teach your baby good table manners in the long run, but what he observes at family meals. If other family members eat with their fingers, shovel food in without a breath, chew loudly, reach for food instead of asking for it to be passed— if everyone talks with their mouths full, or worse, no one talks at all during the meal— your baby will cultivate these habits instead of the ones you hope to instill.

Know when to call a cease-fire. When the amount of time spent playing with the food begins to significantly outweigh the time spent eating it, it's time to call it a meal. Clear the table and remove your baby

from his high chair as soon as this moment arrives. It's unlikely that baby will protest (boredom with mealtime has prompted this behavior in the first place), but if he does, distract him with a toy or activity.

HEAD BANGING, ROCKING, AND ROLLING

"My son has taken to banging his head on the wall or the side of his crib. Though it's painful for me to watch him, he doesn't seem to be in pain at all—in fact, he seems quite happy."

It sounds as though your son has discovered that he's got rhythm, and this is his way of expressing it—at least until he takes to dancing or playing his Fisher-Price drum set. Head banging (like head rolling, rocking, and bouncing, all of which are also common at this age) is a rhythmic movement, and rhythmic movements, especially of their own making, are fascinating to babies. Though most infant rock 'n' rollers rock when they hear music during waking hours, there seems to be more to such pursuits than simple fun. It's suspected that some of these children may be trying to reproduce the feeling of being rocked by mommy or daddy. Or that teething infants may be trying to cope with the pain—in which case rocking continues only as long as the teething, unless by that time it has become a habit. For those who bang, rock, or roll at naptime, bedtime, and when they awaken in the middle of the night, these activities appear to be an aid to sleep, and perhaps may be a way of releasing tensions built up during the day. The behavior is sometimes triggered, or increased, by stress (weaning, learning to walk, getting a new sitter, and so on) in a child's life. Though boys and girls are equally likely to rock or roll, head banging is much more common in boys.

Rocking usually begins somewhere around six months, banging usually not until about nine months. These habits can last a few weeks or months, or a year or more. But most children abandon them by the time they are three years old without parental intervention. Scolding, teasing, or otherwise drawing attention to the behavior not only does no good, it may make the problem worse.

Though it may be hard to believe, rocking, rolling, and even head banging are not ordinarily hazardous to your baby's health. Neither are they, in a normally developing child, associated with neurological or psychological disorders. If your baby seems otherwise happy, isn't banging his head in anger, and isn't constantly bruising himself (an occasional black-and-blue mark isn't a cause for concern), there is nothing to worry about. But if these activities are taking up a good deal of your baby's time, if he seems to display other unusual behavior, is developing slowly, or seems unhappy most of the time, do talk to his doctor about the problem.

You can't force a baby to give up one of these habits before he's ready, but the following tips may make it easier for both you and your baby to live with the habit and to eventually ease him out of it:

■ Give your baby extra love, attention, cuddling, and rocking during the day and at bedtime.
■ Supply other—and to you, more acceptable—rhythmic activities for your baby during the day. Possibilities include: rocking in a rocking chair with him or showing him how to rock in a child-size one of his own; giving him one or more toy instruments, or just a spoon and pot, from which to elicit sounds; pushing him on a swing; and playing patty-cake or other finger or hand games, especially to music.
■ Allow your baby plenty of time for active play during the day and ample opportunity to wind down before bedtime.
■ Establish a regular, soothing presleep routine that includes quiet games, hugging, and perhaps some rocking (though not to the point of sleep).

■ If your baby does most of his head banging in the crib, don't put him down until he's sleepy.
■ If your baby rocks or bangs in his crib, minimize the danger to furniture and walls (which is usually much more serious than any damage to baby) by setting the crib on a thick rug and removing the casters so the crib won't bounce across the floor. Place the crib as far from the wall or other furniture as possible, and if necessary, pad the sides of the crib to soften the impact.
■ You can try to protect your baby's head by placing bumper pads in the crib and a mat on the floor where he likes to bang if it isn't already carpeted—but the odds are good he won't be satisfied with the cushioned blows and will make his way to a harder surface.

BLINKING

"For the last couple of weeks, my daughter has been blinking a lot. She doesn't seem to be in any discomfort, and she doesn't seem to have trouble seeing, but I can't help worrying that there's something wrong with her eyes."

It's probably more likely that there's something right with her curiosity. She knows what the world looks like through open eyes, but what if she closes her eyes partially, or if she opens and shuts them quickly? The results of her experimentation may be so intriguing that she may keep the "blinking" up until the novelty wears off. (When she gets older, somewhere around age two, she will probably try similar experiments with her ears, putting her fingers in them or covering them with her hands to see what happens to sound.)

Of course, if your baby seems to have difficulty recognizing people and objects, or to have trouble focusing, call her doctor immediately. If not, and if the mannerism hasn't run its course by the time your baby goes for her next checkup, mention it to the examiner.

Squinting is another temporary habit that some babies cultivate, also for the change of scenery. Again, it shouldn't concern you unless it's accompanied by other symptoms or is persistent. In which case, check with her doctor.

HAIR ROLLING AND PULLING

"When my daughter is sleepy or cranky, she pulls at a lock of her hair."

Hair stroking or pulling is another way that a baby or a young child releases tension or tries to re-create the soothing comfort she received as an infant during nursing or bottle feeding, when she would stroke her mother's breast or cheek or pull at her hair. Since she's more likely to crave this comfort during times of stress, especially when she's overtired or cranky, she's more likely to indulge in such a mannerism during those times.

Occasional hair twirling, stroking, or pulling, which is often accompanied by thumb sucking, is common, and can linger into childhood without ill effect. Continuous or vigorous tugging at the hair, or hair pulling that results in lost patches of hair should, obviously, be stopped. These tips may help:

- Provide your child with more comfort and attention, especially at times of increased stress.
- Get her hair cut in a short style, so she won't be able to get a good grip on it.
- Give her something else to pull on—a long-haired stuffed animal, for instance.
- Engage her in other activities that keep her hands occupied.

If all else fails, seek advice from her doctor.

TEETH GRINDING

"I often hear my son grinding his teeth when he's down for a nap. Is this harmful in any way?"

Like head banging or rolling, hair pulling, or thumb sucking, teeth grinding is a way some babies discharge tension. To minimize grinding, reduce the tension in your baby's life when possible, and be sure that he has plenty of other outlets for releasing it—such as physical activity and toys that encourage banging. Lots of love and attention before nap or bedtime can also decrease the need for teeth grinding by helping a baby unwind. In most cases the habit is relinquished as a baby's coping skills improve, and before any damage is done to the teeth.

Tension isn't always the cause of teeth grinding. Sometimes a baby accidentally discovers the mannerism when experimenting with his new teeth, enjoys the sensation and sound of it, and adds it to his growing repertoire of skills. But before long, the thrill is gone and he loses interest in his dental orchestra.

If you find that your baby's teeth grinding is becoming more frequent, rather than diminishing, and you fear that he might begin to do damage to his teeth, consult his doctor or a pediatric dentist.

BREATH HOLDING

"Recently my baby has started holding his breath during crying spells. Today he held it so long he actually passed out. Could this be dangerous?"

Invariably it's the parents who suffer most when a child holds his breath. While the adult witnessing the ordeal is likely to remain shaky for hours, even a baby who turns blue and passes out during a breath-holding session recovers quickly and completely, as automatic respiratory mechanisms click into place and breathing resumes.

The breath holding is usually precipitated by anger, frustration, or pain. The crying, instead of letting up, becomes more and more hysterical, baby begins to hyper-ventilate, then finally stops breathing. In mild events, the lips turn blue. In more severe instances, baby turns blue all over and then loses consciousness. While un-conscious, his body may stiffen or even twitch. The episode is usually over in less than a minute—long before any brain dam-age can occur.

About 1 in 5 infants holds his breath at one time or another. Some have only occa-sional episodes, others may have one or two a day. Breath holding tends to run in families and is most common between six months and four years, though it can occa-sionally begin earlier or run later. It can usually be distinguished from epilepsy (to which it is in no way related) by the fact that it is preceded by crying and the fact that baby turns blue before losing con-sciousness. In epilepsy, there is usually no precipitating factor and the child doesn't ordinarily turn blue before a seizure.

No treatment is necessary for a child who has passed out due to breath holding. And though there's no cure for the habit—other than the passing of years—it is possi-ble to head off some of the temper tantrums that result in these tactics:

■ Be sure your baby gets enough rest. A baby who is overtired or overstimulated is more susceptible than a well-rested one.
■ Don't make every issue a battleground. There's no question that you're the authority figure, and that you're bigger and wiser; you don't have to prove it constantly.
■ Try to calm baby before hysteria sets in, using music, toys, or other distractions (but not food, which will create another bad habit).
■ Try to reduce the tension around baby—yours and everyone else's—if this is at all possible.
■ Respond calmly to breath-holding spells; your anxiety can make them worse.
■ Don't cave in after a spell. If your baby knows he can get what he wants by holding his breath, he will repeat the behavior frequently.

If your baby's breath-holding spells are se-vere, last more than a minute, are unrelated to crying, or have you worried for any other reason, do discuss them with his doctor as soon as possible.

TOILET TRAINING

"My mother insists my sister and I were toilet trained at ten months. Today, I see children in diapers at three years of age. When's the right age to start training my son?"

From the stories we hear from our moth-ers, it would seem that babies thirty years ago—all fully toilet trained before the first birthday, or at least soon after—were a more precocious breed than today's tots. But it wasn't the babies who were trained—it was their mothers. It is possible to achieve early bowel training with a baby who is very regular (has a movement every morning after breakfast, for instance) or who gives clear warning of an impending movement (by squatting, for example). It's much harder to predict urination, though an occasional baby does cry before wetting his diaper. But "catching" a baby this way is but a small victory, as the cooperation is purely reflexive and the baby has little or no understanding of what he's doing and why. And it often turns into a defeat later, when the baby who seemed trained sud-denly balks at even going near the potty, or holds back when put on the seat and be-comes constipated.

Training is far more successful, is ac-complished much more quickly, and is far less taxing on the trainer and far less trau-matic for the trainee when the following signs of readiness are exhibited: the child becomes aware of elimination (first, that he's just had a bowel movement, then that he's having one, and finally that he's about to have one); he can stay dry for two or three hours at a stretch; he can dress and undress himself for toileting; and he is able to understand and follow directions.

But just because your baby isn't ready for potty training doesn't mean he can't start becoming familiar with potty protocol right now:

Let him know what he's doing. It's often very obvious that a baby's having a bowel movement; he may stop what he's doing, squat, grunt, strain, get red in the face, or simply turn very serious suddenly. When you catch your baby in the act, tell him what he's doing, using the same word or phrase to describe his efforts and their yield each time (BM, doodoo, or whatever's your family's traditional favorite). Then use the full diaper as a visual aid when you're cleaning him up.

It's virtually impossible to know when your baby's urinating, of course, unless he's bare bottomed. But when the opportunity presents itself—when he releases a stream in the bathtub, while you're changing his diaper, or when he's romping naked in the backyard—do point out what is happening. Again, use the same term each time (pee-pee, wee-wee, urine, or whatever you're comfortable with). And when you change his wet diaper, explain to him why it's wet.

Let him see what you're doing. Children are great imitators, particularly of people they look up to, such as parents or older siblings. So instead of barring baby from the bathroom while you use the toilet, invite him in for a live demonstration, accompanied by a running commentary on the goings-on. If you have an older child willing to admit an audience (some will demand privacy), encourage baby to attend some of these performances, too. Explain to your baby that mommies and daddies, and big boys and girls, go on the potty and that when he is big, he will too. If the sound doesn't frighten him and he can manage the handle, let him flush; then, together, watch the contents swirling down and out. If he seems eager to sit on the toilet himself, buy a potty that fits on the regular seat or a separate children's potty (which is safer, more comfortable, less intimidating, and easier to push on), and let him try it

out. But *don't* leave him unattended, and take him off as soon as he tires of the position. Becoming comfortable on the potty now—as long as it's his idea and not yours—may make it a less fearful place later on.

Make him feel good about the products of elimination. Positive self-image is very important to the success of any kind of training. So don't make baby feel that what comes out of him is offensive ("Oh, what a smelly mess!"), even if you find it so. Resist making faces and unfavorable remarks when you clean up his diapers. Instead, be positive and matter-of-fact in demeanor and comments.

While the end of the first year, when a baby is curious and still fairly malleable, is a good time to familiarize him with the potty, don't push your child at any age to perform on the potty. Encourage him, enlighten him, but wait until he's fully ready—probably somewhere around his second birthday, but possibly not until he's closer to his third—before beginning serious training.[1]

STARTING CLASSES

"I see so many advertisements for classes for babies that I feel as if I'm depriving my daughter if I don't enroll her in at least one."

You probably didn't take a class until you went to kindergarten, unless you were one of the few in your generation who went to nursery school at three or four. You cer-

1. One reason why the new generation is becoming trained so late is the disposable diaper. These modern miracles absorb urine so well and keep it away from baby's skin so successfully that children hardly notice when they are wet. It's no wonder that they are in no hurry to be trained—unlike previous generations of children who were perpetually uncomfortable in sopping wet cloth diapers.

tainly didn't study art, music, or swimming before you could walk or talk—and you probably don't consider yourself deprived. And in spite of the enthusiasm of today's parents for getting their children involved in organized activities as early as possible, your baby won't be deprived if she isn't signed up for classes soon, either.

In fact, formal classes are not only unnecessary for infants, they can sometimes be harmful. What babies need to develop well is plenty of time to explore the world on their own and to learn about it at their own pace, with just a little help from their adult friends. Being required to explore or learn at a predetermined time, place, and pace, as in a classroom, can dampen a child's natural enthusiasm for new experiences and damage her self-esteem. This doesn't mean that you should automatically reject all opportunities for group activities for your baby. It's nice for your child to play near other children—she probably isn't yet ready to play *with* them—and to spend time with and get to know other adults. It's even nicer for you to have a chance to talk to other mothers, sharing common concerns and experiences and picking up some new ideas for playing with your child.

There are some ways for you to reap group benefits for your baby without premature matriculation:

- Take her to a local playground. Even if she isn't walking, she will enjoy the baby swings, small slides, and the sandbox—and she will especially enjoy watching other children.
- Start or join a play group. If you don't know other mothers with babies your daughter's age, post recruitment notices in the pediatrician's office, in your church or synagogue, even in the supermarket. Play groups, which usually meet weekly in homes or at playgrounds, are often very informal, have frequent turnover, and provide an ideal introduction to group activities.
- Enroll her in an informal baby exercise class, observing the guidelines on page 212.

SHOES FOR WALKING

"Our daughter has just taken her first steps. What kind of shoes does she need now?"

The best shoes for a new walker are no shoes. Doctors have discovered that the feet, like hands, develop best when they are bare, not covered and confined; walking barefoot helps build arches and strengthen ankles. And just as your baby's hands don't need gloves in warm weather, her feet don't need shoes indoors and on safe surfaces outdoors, except when it's cold. Even walking on uneven surfaces, such as sand, is good for her feet since it makes the muscles work harder.

But for safety and sanitation (you wouldn't want her to step on broken glass or in dog droppings) as well as appearance, your baby will need shoes for most excursions, as well as for special occasions (what's a party dress without Mary Janes?). Choose shoes that are closest to no shoes at all by looking for the following:

Flexible soles. Shoes that bend fairly easily when the toe is bent up will interfere least with the foot's natural motion. Many doctors recommend sneakers for their flexibility, but some maintain that traditional first-walker shoes are even more flexible and babies are therefore less likely to fall in them. Ask your baby's doctor for a recommendation, and test those available at your local store before making your selection.

Low cut. Don't buy the high-top shoes your mother probably bought for you when you started stepping out. Even though such shoes may stay put better than low ones, most experts believe they are too confining and interfere with ankle movement. They certainly shouldn't be used to prop up a baby who is not yet ready to walk.

Porous and flexible uppers. To stay healthy, feet need to breathe and to get plenty of exercise. They breathe best, and have the most freedom of movement, in shoes of leather, cloth, or canvas. Plastic or imitation leather is usually stifling and sometimes stiff, and tends to cause the feet to sweat excessively. Avoid "running" shoes with wide bands of rubber around them since they can also increase sweating. If you purchase rain shoes or boots that are made of plastic or rubber for your baby, use them only when needed and take them off as soon as she is indoors.

Flat, non-skid bottoms with no heels. A beginner walker has enough difficulty maintaining her balance without having to contend with slippery soles. Rubber or composition soles, particularly when they are grooved, usually provide a less slippery surface than leather, unless it is scored or grooved. If an otherwise appropriate pair of shoes is too slippery, rough up the soles a bit with sandpaper or a few strips of adhesive tape.

Firm counters. The back of the shoe (behind the heel) should be firm, not flimsy. It's best if the top edge is padded or bound, and the back seam smooth with no irregularities that could cause irritation to the back of your baby's heel.

Roomy fit. Shoes are better too large than too small, but of course "just right" is best of all. Though shoes can't provide as much foot freedom as going bare, too-tight shoes provide no freedom at all. If shoes are to be worn with thick socks, be sure to try shoes on with such socks. Have feet measured and test new shoes (both of them) for size when the baby is standing with her full weight on her feet. The top of the shoe shouldn't gap open while she's standing (though it's okay if it does when she walks), nor should her heels slip up and down with each step. To check the width, try to pinch the shoe at its widest point. If you can grasp a tiny bit of it between your fingers, the width is fine; if you can pinch a good piece of shoe, it's too wide; and if you can pinch none at all, it's too narrow. To check the length, press your thumb down between your baby's toes and the end of the shoe. If there's a thumb's width (or about

half an inch), the length is right. There should also be room for your pinky at the back of the shoe. Once you've purchased a pair of shoes for your baby, check the fit every few weeks since babies outgrow shoes quickly, sometimes within six weeks, often within three months. When that distance at the toe shrinks to less than half a thumb's width, start to think about new shoes. Reddened areas on baby's toes or feet when shoes are removed are also a sign of poor fit.

Standard shapes. Unusual styles— such as cowboy boots or pointy-toed party shoes—can distort the foot as it grows. Look instead for a shoe with a broad instep and toe and a flat pancake heel.

Durability is not a requirement in children's shoes because they are rapidly outgrown. Though the temptation is great—because of the high price of children's shoes and their brief life span with each child—to pass shoes on from child to child, resist. Shoes mold to the shape of the wearer's foot, and wearing shoes molded by someone else is not good for little feet. Make an exception only for those shoes (such as dress-up shoes) that are no more than lightly worn, have held their shape, and aren't run down at the heels.

A good shoe is only as good as the sock in it. Socks, like shoes, should fit well and be of a material (such as cotton or Orlon) that allows feet to breathe. Socks that are too tight can cramp foot growth; those that are too long can wrinkle and cause irritations or blisters, though neatly folding up the tip of a too long sock before putting on the shoe can often solve the problem of wrinkling. Stretch-to-fit socks usually do fit well, but be alert for the point at which they become too small and begin squeezing, usually indicated by marks left on baby's feet.

BITING

"My baby has started biting us play-

fully—on the shoulder, the cheek, any soft, vulnerable area. At first we thought it was cute. Now we're beginning to worry that he's developing a bad habit— and besides, it hurts!"

It's only natural for your baby to want to test his new set of chompers on every possible surface, you included. But it's also only natural for you not to want to be bitten— and only fair that you be allowed to put a stop to the biting, which can become a bad habit and, as more teeth come in, increasingly painful for its victims.

The biting at first is playful and experimental; baby has absolutely no idea he's hurting anyone with it. After all, he's bitten down on many a teething ring, sucked on many a stuffed toy, and chewed on many a crib rail with nary a complaint. But then, when he gets a human reaction, he's often encouraged to continue in order to elicit more reactions. He finds the expression on mommy's face when he bites down on her shoulder funny, the startled look and mock "Ouch!" from daddy hilarious, and the "Isn't that cute, he's biting me," from grandma a definite sign of approval. Oddly enough, even an angry "Ouch!" or stern reprimand can reinforce the biting habit, because the baby either finds it amusing or sees it as a challenge to his emerging sense of independence, or both. And biting him back can make matters worse; not only is it cruel, but there's the not so subtle implication that what's good for the goose is fair play for him. For the same reason, love bites from parents or grandparents can also trigger biting.

The most effective way to respond is to remove the little biter calmly and matter-of-factly from the part he's biting, with a firm "No biting." Then quickly divert his attention with a song, a toy, or other distraction. Do this each time he bites and he will eventually get the message.

HAIR CARE

"Our daughter was born with a headful

of hair and it's gotten quite straggly and hard to manage."

To the parents of countless hairless nine-month-olds, yours would seem an enviable problem. But handling an unruly head of superfine hair, particularly when it belongs to a squirming, uncooperative baby, could make even Vidal Sassoon want to throw in his comb. Things will probably get worse before they get much better; for some toddlers and preschoolers, every shampoo and comb-out is an excuse for a tantrum. But short of resorting to a short haircut (which, if you're brave enough, may be the best way to go), you can best minimize the travail while keeping your baby's hair healthy and well groomed by using the following tips:

■ Untangle hair before beginning to shampoo to prevent even worse tangles afterward.

■ Use a baby conditioner after shampoos if your baby will sit still for this double procedure. If not, use a combination shampoo-conditioner, or a spray-on cream rinse that doesn't need to be rinsed out. This will make comb-outs much easier.

■ Use a wide-tooth comb or a brush that has bristles with plastic-coated tips for comb-outs on wet hair. A fine-tooth comb tends to tear the ends and also pulls more.

■ Untangle from the ends up, keeping one hand firmly on the roots as you work to minimize the pulling on baby's scalp and the pain that comes with it.

■ If you must use a blow dryer, use a low or cool setting to avoid damaging baby's delicate hair or burning her sensitive scalp.

■ Don't braid baby's hair or pull it tightly into a ponytail or pigtails, since these styles can lead to patches of baldness or thinning of hair. If you do make ponytails or pigtails, make them loose and tie them with special protective clips or coated bands rather than with regular rubber bands or barrettes, both of which can pull out and damage hair.

■ Trim hair (or have it trimmed at a salon that specializes in children's cuts) at least every two months, for healthier growth.

Trim bangs when they reach the brows.
■ If your baby has a part in her hair, change it every few days to avoid the hair thinning around it.
■ Plan hair grooming for a time when your baby isn't tired, hungry, or cranky. Make it more pleasant by getting her occupied with a toy before beginning, possibly a doll and a comb. Or set her up in front of a mirror so she can watch you work on her hair; eventually she may learn to appreciate the end result, making the sessions more tolerable.

FEARS

"My baby used to love to watch me turn on the vacuum cleaner; now he's suddenly terrified of it—and anything else that makes a loud noise."

When he was younger your baby wasn't frightened by loud noises—though they may have momentarily startled him—because he didn't perceive the possibility they might present a danger. Now, as his understanding of the world grows, it's likely, especially if he's gotten a few "boo-boos," that he's beginning to realize the perils and the potential for injury that surround him.

There are any number of things in a baby's everyday life that, though innocuous to you, can cause debilitating fear in him: sounds, such as the roar of a vacuum cleaner, the whir of a blender, the barking of a dog, the whine of a siren, the flushing of a toilet, the gurgle of water draining from the bathtub; having a shirt pulled over his head; being lifted high in the air (especially if he's begun to climb, pull up, or otherwise develop depth perception); being plunked down in a bath; the motion of a wind-up or mechanical toy.

Probably all babies experience fears at some point, though some overcome them so quickly their parents are never aware of them. Children who live in a lively, active environment, particularly when there are older siblings, tend to experience these fears earlier.

Sooner or later, most children leave the fears of late babyhood behind and burst forth as brash, and sometimes foolishly brave, toddlers. Till then, you can help your baby deal with his fears in these ways:

Don't force. Making your baby come nose to nozzle with the vacuum cleaner not only won't help, it may intensify his fear. Though his phobia may seem irrational to you, it's very legitimate to him. He needs to wait and confront the noisy beast on his own terms and in his own time, when he feels it's safe.

Don't resort to ridicule. Making fun of your child's fears, calling them silly or laughing at them, will only serve to undermine his self-confidence and his ability to deal with them. Take his fears seriously—he does.

Do accept and sympathize. By accepting your baby's fears as real, and comforting him when his personal demons are about, you will lessen his burden and help him to cope. If he wails when you switch on the vacuum cleaner (or flush the toilet, or turn on the blender) be quick to pick him up and give him a great, big, reassuring hug. But don't overdo the sympathy or you may reinforce the idea that there is something to be afraid of.

Do reassure and support, then build confidence and skills. Though you should sympathize with his fears, your ultimate goal is to help him overcome them. He can only do this by becoming familiar with the things he fears, learning what they do and how they work, and gaining some sense of control over them. Let him touch or even play with the vacuum when it's turned off and unplugged—he is probably as fascinated with the machine as he is afraid of it.

Once he becomes comfortable playing with the vacuum when it's off, try holding him securely in one arm while you vacuum with the other—if this doesn't upset him. Then show him how to turn the machine on himself, with a little help from you if the switch is tricky. If it's the toilet's flush he fears, have him throw some paper in and encourage him to flush it down himself when he feels ready. If it's the draining tub, let him watch the water drain when he is safely out of it, fully dressed, and if need be, in your arms. If dogs are his nemesis, try playing with one while your baby watches from a distance—perhaps from daddy's lap. When he's finally willing to approach a dog, encourage your baby (while you hold him) to make "nice doggy" to a dog you know is gentle and won't suddenly snap.

WHAT IT'S IMPORTANT TO KNOW: The Beginnings of Discipline

You applauded wildly your baby's first successful attempt at pulling up, and cheered proudly from the sidelines as creeping finally became crawling. Now you're wondering what all the celebration was about. Along with the new mobility has come a talent for getting into trouble to rival Dennis the Menace. If your baby's not adroitly turning off the VCR while your favorite show is being taped, he or she is triumphantly removing the tablecloth (along with the fruit bowl atop it) from the dining room table, gleefully unraveling whole rolls of toilet paper into the toilet, or industriously emptying the contents of drawers, cabinets, and bookshelves onto the floor. Before, all you had to do to keep both baby and home from harm was to deposit your child in a safe spot; now, no such haven exists.

For the first time, you're likely to be upset by rather than proud of your offspring's exploits. And for the first time the question of discipline has probably come up in your home. The timing is right. Waiting to introduce discipline into a child's life much later than ten months could make the task much more difficult; trying to have done so much earlier, before memory was developed, would have been futile.

Why discipline a baby? First of all, to instill a concept of right and wrong. Though it'll be a long time before your child will fully grasp it, it's now that you should begin to teach right from wrong by both example and guidance. Second, to plant the seeds of self-control. They won't take root for a while, but unless they do eventually, your child won't be able to function effectively. Third, to teach respect for the rights and feelings of others, so that a child will grow from a normally self-centered baby into a sensitive and caring child and adult. And finally, to protect your baby, your home, and your sanity—now and in the months of mischief ahead.

As you embark on a program of child discipline, keep the following in mind:

■ Though the word "discipline" is associated with structure, rules, and punishment in many minds, it actually comes from the Latin word for "teaching."

■ Every child is different, every family is different, each situation is different. But there are universal rules of behavior that apply to everyone, at all times.

■ Until infants understand what is safe and what is not, or at least which actions are permissible and which are not, their parents have total responsibility for keeping the environment safe, as well as for safeguarding their own belongings and those of others.

■ Withdrawal of parental love threatens a child's self-esteem. It's important to let children know that they are still loved, even when their behavior is disapproved of.

■ The most effective discipline is neither uncompromisingly rigid nor overly permissive. Strict discipline that relies entirely on parental policing rather than encouraging the development of self-control usually turns out children who are totally submissive to their parents but totally uncontrollable once out of reach of parental or other adult authority. But overly permissive parents aren't likely to turn out well-behaved children, capable of coping in the real world, either. Their overindulged children are often selfish, rude, and unpleasant, quick to argue, slow to comply.

Both extremes of discipline can leave a child feeling unloved. Strict parents may seem cruel, and thus unloving; permissive parents may seem uncaring. A more nurturing brand of discipline falls somewhere in between—it sets limits that are fair, and enforces them firmly but lovingly.

That's not to say that there aren't normal variations in discipline styles. Some parents are simply more relaxed and some more rigid. That's okay as long as neither goes to the extreme.

■ Effective discipline is individualized. If you have more than one child, you almost certainly noticed differences in personality from birth. Such differences will affect how each child is best disciplined. One, for instance, will refrain from playing with an electric outlet after a gentle remonstrance. Another won't take your warning seriously unless there is a toughness—or perhaps fear—in your voice. A third may need to be physically removed from the source of danger. Tailor your style to your child.

■ Circumstances can alter a child's response to discipline. A child who ordinarily requires strong admonitions may be crushed if scolded when tired or teething. Switch gears, if need be, to meet your child's immediate needs.

■ Children need limits. They often can't control themselves or their impulses and become frightened at the loss of control. Limits, set by parents and lovingly enforced, provide a comforting tether to keep children secure and steady while they explore and grow. Stretching those limits be-

cause he or she's "just a baby" isn't fair to your child or to those whose rights are being violated. Tender age—at least after ten months—shouldn't guarantee carte blanche to pull a sibling's hair or tear up mommy's magazine before she's read it.

Just which limits you set depends on your priorities. In some homes, keeping shoes off the sofa and not eating in the living room are paramount issues. In others, staying out of mommy's or daddy's desk is of vital importance. In most families, common courtesy and simple etiquette—using "please" and "thank you," sharing, respecting other people's feelings—are primary expectations. Set rules you will enforce carefully and limit their numbers.

Learning to live with limits from an early age can help calm some of the turmoil of the terrible twos. It will also be necessary for survival in a society that is full of limits—at school, work, and play.

It's easier, of course, to talk about setting limits for babies than to actually enforce them. It's tempting to give in to an adorable kid who gives you an impish smile when you say "no!" or to a sweet, sensitive one who breaks into tears at the very sound of the word. But steel yourself and remember it's for your child's own good. It may not seem vital now to stop your baby from taking the crackers into the living room, but if he or she doesn't learn to follow at least a few rules now, it will be harder to handle the many that will be faced later. You can continue to expect protestations, but gradually you will find that more and more, your child will accept limits matter-of-factly.

■ A baby who gets into trouble isn't "bad." Babies and young toddlers don't know right from wrong, so their follies can't be considered wicked. They learn about their world by experimenting, observing cause and effect, and testing the adults in it. What happens when I turn over a glass of juice? Will it happen again? And again? Or what's inside the kitchen drawers, and what will happen if I take it all out? What will mommy's reaction be?

Repeatedly telling your child that he or she is bad can damage the ego and interfere with self-confidence and achievement down the road. And the child who hears "You're bad!" over and over may fulfill the prophecy in later years ("If they say I'm bad, I must be bad"). Criticize your baby's actions, but not your baby ("Biting is bad," not "You're bad").

■ Consistency is important. If shoes on the sofa are forbidden today but permitted tomorrow, or if hand washing before dinner was compulsory yesterday but overlooked today, the only lesson learned is that the world is confusing and rules are meaningless. If you fail to be consistent, you lose credibility.

■ Follow-through is crucial. Looking up from your book long enough to mutter "no" to a baby who's tugging at the television wires but not long enough to make sure that he or she stops is not effective discipline. If your actions don't speak at least as loud as your words, your admonitions will lose their impact. When the first "no" is ineffective, take immediate action, especially in such a dangerous situation. Put down your book, pick up your baby, and move him or her away from the tempting TV wires—preferably far away, into another room. Then take your baby's mind off the television with a favorite plaything. For most babies, what's been taken out of sight is quickly out of mind—though a few may try to return to the scene of the crime, in which case you may have to block it off. Distraction, when it works, also allows a baby who feels that "no" is a challenge to his or her ego to save face.

■ Babies and young toddlers have limited memories. You can't expect them to learn a lesson the first time it's taught, and you can expect them to repeat an undesirable action over and over again. Be patient, and be prepared to repeat the same message— "Don't touch the VCR" or "Don't eat the dog food"—every day for weeks before it finally sinks in or the fascination is lost.

■ Babies enjoy the "no game." Most babies love the challenge of a parent's "No!" as much as the challenge of climbing a flight of stairs or fitting a circle into a shape sorter. So no matter how your baby goads you, don't let your "No!" deteriorate into a game or a fit of laughter. Your baby won't take you seriously.

■ Too many "No's" lose their effectiveness and are demoralizing. You wouldn't want to live in a world ruled by an unforgiving dictator whose three favorite words were "No! No! No!" And neither should you want your baby to live in one. Limit the no's to those things in which baby's well-being or that of another person or of your home is threatened. Remember that not every issue is worth a fight. Fewer no's will be needed if you create a childproof environment (see page 292) in your home, with plenty of opportunities for exploration under safe conditions.

Along with each "No," always offer a "Yes" in the form of an alternative: "No, you can't play with daddy's book, but you can look at this one," or "You can't empty the cereal cabinet, but you can empty the pots and pans shelves." Instead of "No, don't touch those papers in mommy's desk" to the baby who already has emptied several items on the floor, try "Let's see if you can put those papers back in mommy's drawer and close the drawer." This face-saving approach gets the message across without making your baby feel "bad."

Once in a while, when the stakes aren't high or when you realize you've made a mistake, let baby win—an occasional victory will help make up for the many losses he or she must take each day.

■ Children need to be allowed to make some mistakes, and to learn from them. If you make it impossible for your child to slip up (stashing away all knickknacks, for instance), you won't have to say no very often, but you will also miss important chances to teach. Allow room for errors (though you'll want to avoid those that are dangerous and/or expensive through prudent childproofing), so that your baby can learn from them.

■ Correction and reward work better than punishment. Punishment, always of questionable value, is particularly useless for young children since they don't understand why they're being punished. A baby is too young to associate being "grounded" in the playpen with having just dumped the salt out of the salt shaker, or to understand that a bottle is being withheld because he or she bit a sibling. Instead of punishing misbehavior, catch your baby being good. Positive reinforcement, rewarding and praising good behavior, works much better. It builds, rather than smashes, self-confidence and reinforces good behavior. Another productive approach, one that teaches that actions have consequences, is to have the perpetrator help remedy the results of the crime—wipe up the spilt milk, pick up the scattered dish towels, hand you the books to put back on the shelf.

■ Anger triggers anger. Indulge in an angry outburst when your baby breaks a favorite candy dish by tossing it like a ball across the room, and he or she's likely to follow in fury, rather than respond with remorse. If necessary, take a few moments to calm down before addressing the guilty party—leave the scene of the crime briefly, if that will help you temper your temper. Once your cool is collected, explain to your baby that what he or she did was wrong, and why. ("That wasn't a toy, it was mommy's dish. You broke it and now mommy's sad.") This is important to do even if the explanation seems to be sailing clear over your baby's head, or if distraction has already set in.

Try to remember at moments of high anxiety (it won't always be easy) that your long-term goal is to teach right behavior, and that screaming or swatting will teach wrong behavior, setting poor examples of what's appropriate when one is angry.

Don't worry if you occasionally find it impossible to put the brakes on your anger. As a human mother, you're allowed your share of frailties, and your baby needs to know that. As long as your tirades are relatively few, far between, and short-lived,

they won't interfere with effective parenting. When they occur, be sure to apologize: "I'm sorry I yelled at you, but I was very angry." Adding "I love you" will not only be reassuring, but will let your baby know that sometimes we get angry at people we love and that such feelings are okay.

■ Discipline can be a laughing matter. Humor is the leavening of life—and a surprisingly effective disciplinary tool. Use it liberally in situations that would otherwise lead you to exasperation—for instance, when baby refuses to allow you to put a snowsuit on him. Instead of doing fruitless combat over shrill screams of protest, head off the tantrum and the struggle with some unexpected silliness. Suggest, perhaps, that you put the snowsuit on the dog (or the cat, or the dolly, or on mommy), and then pretend to do so. The incongruity of what you are proposing will probably take your baby's mind off objections to wearing the garment long enough for you to accomplish your goal.

Humor can be brought into a variety of disciplinary situations. Give orders while pretending you're a dog or a lion, Big Bird, or another of your child's favorites; perform unpopular chores with silly-song accompaniments ("This is the way we wash the face, wash the face..."; carry baby to the dreaded changing table upside down; make silly faces in the mirror with baby instead of chiding, "Don't cry, don't cry." Taking each other less seriously more often will add sunshine to your days, particularly as the stormy second year approaches. Stay serious, however, when a dangerous situation is involved, since then even a smile can be fatal to the effectiveness of the lesson you are trying to impart.

■ Accidents require different treatment from intentional wrongdoings. Remember, everyone's entitled to mistakes, but babies, because of their emotional, physical, and intellectual immaturity, are entitled to a great many more of them. When yours knocks over a glass of milk while reaching for a slice of bread, "Oops, the milk spilled.

Try to be more careful, honey" is an appropriate response. But when the cup is up-ended intentionally, "Milk is to drink, not to spill. Spilling makes a mess and wastes the milk—see, now there's no more" is more fitting. In either case, it also helps to hand baby a paper towel to help in the cleanup, to fill cups with only small amounts of liquids in the future, and to be sure that your baby has plenty of opportunity to pursue his or her experiments with pouring fluids in the tub or other acceptable surroundings.

■ Parents have to be the adults in the family. If you expect your child to act responsibly, you'll have to, too: You promised baby a trip to the playground, but then would rather watch the afternoon soaps. A mature

mommy would keep her promise, anyway. If you expect your child to admit mistakes comfortably, you'll have to lead the way: You made baby cry over spilled milk and learn later that it was daddy who spilled it. A mature mommy would apologize, and try to avoid jumping to conclusions next time. If you often find yourself getting down to your baby's level, following his or her tantrum, for example, with one of your own, or demanding things your way when they could just as easily be done your baby's way, it may be time to reevaluate your own behavior.

■ Children are worthy of respect. Instead of treating your baby as an object, a possession, or even "just a baby," treat him or her

TO SPANK OR NOT TO SPANK

Though spanking has been passed on from generation to generation in many families, most experts agree that it is not, and never has been, an effective way to discipline a child. Children who are spanked may refrain from repeating a misdemeanor rather than risk another spanking, but they obey only as long as the risk is there. They often don't like or respect the people who hit them and frequently don't learn to differentiate right from wrong (only what they get spanked for and what they don't get spanked for)—a prime goal of discipline.

Spanking also has many negative aspects. For one, it teaches violence. Child beaters and wife beaters are almost always former victims of beatings themselves, and many a child who whacks a peer and is asked, "Where did you learn that?" will respond with "From my mommy (or daddy)." For another, spanking teaches children that the best way to settle disputes is with force, and denies them the chance to learn alternative, less hurtful, routes to dealing with anger and frustration. It also represents an abuse of power by a very large, strong party against a very small, weak one. And it can lead to serious injury of a child, often unintentionally, particu-

larly when it is done in anger. Spanking after the anger is cooled, though it may do less physical damage, seems even more questionable than lashing out in the heat of the moment. It is certainly more cruelly calculated, and it is even less effective in correcting behavior.

If it's inadvisable for a parent to spank a child, it is even more inadvisable for another person to do so. Though with a parent a child is usually secure in the knowledge that the spanking is being administered by someone who cares; with another person there's generally no such security. Sitters, teachers, and others who tend to your child should be instructed *never* to strike him or her or administer any form of physical punishment.

Most experts (and parents) would agree that a sound smack on the hand or the bottom may be warranted in a dangerous situation to get a serious message across to a child too young to understand words— for example, when a toddler wanders out into the street or approaches a hot stove and a stern reprimand doesn't do the trick. Once comprehension is established, however, physical force is no longer justifiable.

with the respect you would accord any other person. Be polite (say please, thank you, and excuse me), offer explanations (even if you don't think they'll be understood) when you forbid something, be understanding of and sympathetic to your baby's wants and feelings (even if you can't permit acting them out), avoid embarrassing your baby (by scolding in front of strangers), and listen to what he or she is saying. In this preverbal stage, when grunts and pointing are the main modes of communication, listening is a challenge, and it continues to be so until speech becomes clear and language is well developed (somewhere around four or five)—but making that effort is important. Remember, it's frustrating for baby, too.

▪ There should be a fair distribution of rights between parents and child (or children). It's easy, when a baby is young, for inexperienced parents to err in this area, going to one extreme or the other. Some abrogate all their rights in favor of their child—they base their lives on the baby's schedule, never go out, forget the value of adult friends. Others live their lives as though they were still childless, heedless of their infant's needs—they drag an overtired baby to parties, skip baby baths in favor of a football game, and miss pediatrician appointments because of a big sale at a favorite store. The latter abuse their power (and it's tremendous when you compare it to that of an infant); the former don't use theirs at all. A balance is what's needed.

▪ Nobody's perfect—and nobody should be expected to be. Avoid setting unattainable standards for your baby. Children need all the years childhood provides to develop to the point at which they can behave as adults. And they need to know that you don't expect perfection. Praise particular achievements rather than make sweeping pronouncements about your child's nature: "You were very good today" rather than "You're the best baby in the world." Since no one can be "good" all the time, such overlavish praise on a regular basis can make a child fear that your expectations can't possibly be lived up to.

Neither should you expect perfection from yourself. Parents who never lose their temper, never yell, and never even have the remotest desire to slug a difficult toddler don't exist; even the father of that early television series didn't always know best. And letting it out and clearing the air once in a while may be better than keeping your anger and frustration bottled up inside. Bottled-up anger has a way of bursting out inappropriately, often far out of proportion to the crime of the moment.

If, however, you find yourself losing your temper at your baby too often, try to determine the underlying cause. Are you angry about being responsible for all the child-care chores? Are you really angry at yourself or someone else, and taking it out on the most convenient and defenseless target, your baby? Have you set too many limits or provided too many opportunities for baby to get into trouble? If so, try to remedy the situation.

▪ Children need to know they have some control over their lives. For good mental health, everyone—even a baby—needs to feel as though he or she calls at least some of the shots. It won't always be possible for baby to have his or her way, but when it is, allow it. Give your baby a chance to make choices—the cracker or the piece of bread, the swing or the baby slide, the bib with the elephant or the one with the clown.

CHAPTER FOURTEEN

The Eleventh Month

WHAT YOUR BABY MAY BE DOING

By the end of this month, your baby ...should be able to (see Note):

- get into a sitting position from stomach
- pick up tiny object with any part of thumb and finger (by 10½ months)
- understand word "no" (but not always obey it)

Note: If your baby seems not to have reached one or more of these milestones, check with the doctor. In rare instances the delay could indicate a problem, though in most cases it will turn out to be normal for your baby. Premature infants generally reach milestones later than others of the same birth age, often achieving them closer to their adjusted age (the age they would be if they had been born at term), or sometimes later.

...will probably by able to:

- play patty-cake (clap hands) or wave bye-bye
- walk holding on to furniture (cruise)

...may possibly be able to:

- pick up a tiny object neatly with tips of thumb and forefinger
- stand alone momentarily
- say dada or mama discriminately
- say one word other than mama or dada

...may even be able to:

- stand alone well
- indicate wants in ways other than crying
- "play ball" (roll ball back to you)
- drink from a cup independently
- use immature jargoning (gibberish that sounds like baby is talking a foreign language)
- say three or more words other than mama or dada
- respond to a one-step command without gestures (give that to me—without hand out)
- walk well

WHAT YOU CAN EXPECT AT THIS MONTH'S CHECKUP

Most doctors do not schedule regular well-baby checkups this month. Do call the doctor if there are any concerns that can't wait until next month's visit.

FEEDING YOUR BABY THIS MONTH:
Weaning Your Baby From the Breast

As the task of weaning your baby looms as large as any child-care challenge you've faced so far, it may be comforting to know that you've probably already begun the process. The first time that you offered your baby a sip from a cup, a nip from a bottle, or a nibble from a spoon, you took a step toward weaning.

Weaning is basically a two-phase process:

Phase One: Getting baby accustomed to taking milk or formula from a source other than your breasts. Since it can take a breastfeeding baby a while to catch on to drinking from a bottle or a cup, and some a considerable time to be willing to even try such alternative methods of feeding, it's best to introduce them well before you hope to complete weaning.[1]

If you don't introduce either bottle or cup early on, weaning may be slower and more difficult. In some cases, it may even be necessary temporarily to "starve" your baby into submission by skipping one breastfeeding each day for three or four days, and offering only your chosen alternative. Though a stubborn baby may reject a substitute at first, all eventually switch from the breast.

Use expressed breast milk, formula, or water for bottle or cup practice before six months; after that, most doctors will okay giving small amounts of whole cow's milk, or fruit juices diluted with water. Since your baby is more likely to be receptive to receiving these feedings from daddy than from mommy, this is a great time for him to get in on the baby-feeding act.

Phase Two: Cutting back on breast-feedings. Unlike a smoker giving up cigarettes or a chocoholic giving up chocolate, cold turkey isn't the best route for a baby giving up the breast. Nor is it best for the mother whose breasts are being retired. For the baby, it's much too traumatic, physically and emotionally. For the mother, leaking, engorgement, clogged ducts, and infection are all more likely if nursing stops suddenly. So unless illness or some other event in your lives makes hurried weaning necessary, wean gradually, beginning at least several weeks before your targeted weaning completion date. Postpone the process entirely at a time of change (major or minor) in your baby's life—such as when a new baby-sitter is taking over, mommy is returning to work, or the family is moving to a new house.

The most common approach to weaning is to begin dropping feedings one at a time,

---

1. If you do decide to wean *to* a bottle, remember that it's a good idea to wean *from* the bottle by the first birthday or shortly after, in order to avoid the problems of tooth decay from baby-bottle mouth (see page 254).

KEEPING YOURSELF COMFORTABLE

Gradual weaning is likely to prevent any serious discomfort, though occasionally, especially if your baby is still very young when you wean and has been exclusively breastfed, you may suffer some engorgement. If you do, express just enough milk to relieve it; expressing too much could stimulate further milk production. Gradual weaning will also lessen the emotional impact on you, but it probably won't eliminate it entirely. Weaning, like menstruation, pregnancy, childbirth, and the postpartum period, is a time of hormonal upheaval and the result is often mild depression, irritability, and mood swings. The feelings are often exaggerated by a sense of loss and sadness over giving up this most special relationship with your baby, especially if you don't plan on having any more children. (In a few women, postweaning depression can be severe and requires immediate professional help; see page 546 for the warning signs).

A few weeks after weaning, your breasts may seem totally empty of milk. But don't be surprised if you're still able to express small amounts of milk months, even a year or more, later; this is perfectly normal. It's also normal for breasts to take time to return to close to their former size—often they end up somewhat larger or smaller, and they are frequently less firm, due as much to heredity factors and pregnancy as to nursing.

If weaning must be accomplished suddenly, especially in the early months when the milk supply is at its most copious, discomfort for the mother can be considerable. Extreme engorgement accompanied by fever and flulike symptoms may result, and the chance of infection and other complications is much greater than with gradual weaning. Hot compresses and/or hot showers plus aspirin may relieve some of the pain from engorgement, and cutting back on fluids may help decrease the milk supply. Expressing just enough milk to relieve engorgement, but not enough to stimulate renewed production, may also help. Check with your doctor if symptoms don't diminish after 24 hours.

Sudden weaning can also be stressful to a baby. If you must wean without any prior preparation, be sure to give your infant plenty of extra attention, love, and cuddling, and try to minimize other stresses in his or her life. If you have to be away from home, see that daddy, grandma, another relative, or a doting baby-sitter remembers to do likewise.

waiting at least a few days, but preferably a week, until your breasts and your baby have adjusted to that loss before imposing another. Most mothers find it's easiest to first omit the feeding baby seems least interested in and takes the least amount at, or the one that most interferes with her own day. In the case of an employed mother, that's often the midday feeding. With babies under six months, who are mostly dependent on milk for their nourishment, each breastfeeding dropped should be replaced by formula. With older babies, a snack or meal can replace the nursings, as appropriate.

If you've been breastfeeding your baby on demand, and demand has been quite erratic, you may have to become more strict, getting down to a fairly regular schedule and a reduced number of feedings before you can get serious about weaning.

No matter what a mother's schedule, the early morning and late evening feedings—which provide the most comfort and pleasure for both mother and baby—are usually the last to go. Some women, in fact, continue to give one or both of these feedings to their otherwise weaned babies for weeks or even months, just for the joy of it. (This option isn't available for everyone; some women find that their milk supply depletes rapidly once they cut nursing back that far.)

For some women, particularly those who are at home full-time, cutting back on all feedings, rather than cutting out individual feedings, is a method that works well. To start, the baby is given an ounce of milk from cup or bottle prior to each breastfeeding, and then allowed less time at the breast. Gradually, over the course of several weeks, the amount in the cup or bottle is increased and time at the breast for each feeding is decreased. Eventually the baby is taking adequate quantities of cow's milk or formula, and weaning is accomplished.

Occasionally illness, a bout of painful teething, or a disorienting change of locale or routine (such as on vacation) can lead to backsliding, with baby demanding the breast more often. Be understanding and don't worry—such a setback will only be temporary. Once baby's life is back to normal, you can begin your mission anew.

Keep in mind that nursing is only one part of your relationship with your baby. Giving it up won't weaken the bond or lessen the love between you; in fact, some women find that the relationship is enhanced as they spend less time nursing and more time actively interacting.

Your baby may take to other sources of comfort, such as the thumb or a blanket, when the breast is taken away, and this is normal and healthy. He or she may also hunger for extra attention from you; give it freely. Such attention gives young children the security they need to become independent later on.[2]

Don't be concerned that your baby might pine away indefinitely for the breast after weaning. That won't happen. Babies seem to have a built-in survival mechanism whereby even those with the best of memories appear to quickly forget the breastfeeding experience, or at least, cease to crave it.

WHAT YOU MAY BE CONCERNED ABOUT

BOWED LEGS

"My daughter just started taking steps and she seems to be terribly bowlegged."

Bowed until two, knock-kneed at four, a small child's legs certainly couldn't give Betty Grable's a run for their money. But even Betty's were probably bowed when she took her first steps. Almost all children are bowlegged (their knees don't touch when they stand with feet together) during the first two years of life. Then, as they spend more time walking, they become knock-kneed (their knees meet, but their ankles don't). Not until the teen years do the knees and ankles align and the legs appear to be shaped normally. Special shoes or orthotics (bars, braces, or other orthopedic appliances) aren't needed and won't make a difference in this normal progression.

Occasionally, a doctor will note a true abnormality in a child's legs. Perhaps just one leg is bowed, or one knee turns in, or perhaps the baby is knock-kneed (though sometimes a baby only *looks* that way because of very chubby thighs), or normal bowing becomes progressively more pronounced once walking begins. In such cases, or if there is a history of bowlegs or knock-knees in adults in the family, the baby may need further evaluation, either by the baby's doctor or by a pediatric orthopedist. Depending upon the particular

---

2. If you plan on weaning your baby after a year, and for more information on breastfeeding, see *The Complete Book of Breastfeeding* (Workman Publishing), by Dr. Marvin Eiger and Sally Wendkos Olds.

case, treatment may or may not be recommended (see page 146). Fortunately, rickets, once the most common cause of permanent bowed legs, is fairly rare in the United States today, thanks to the fortification of formula, milk, and other dairy products with vitamin D, and to vitamin D supplements for breastfed babies.

UNCLEAR SPEECH

"Our little girl says several words, but only my husband and I understand them. She seems to have trouble with a lot of consonants, says 'b' for 'f' and 'd' for 'k' and so on. Does this mean she'll need speech therapy?"

It's much too early to start thinking about sending your Eliza off to Professor Higgins. There are, after all, 21 consonants in the English language, which alone and in combination represent at least 23 different sounds, and it's usually not until well into the third or fourth year, sometimes much later, that a child learns to pronounce all of them skillfully. (Many children are still having trouble with "th" sounds in the sixth and seventh year.) Multisyllabic words are especially difficult to handle at first. Though some children speak clearly enough to be understood by adults outside the family by age two, many don't until they reach age four or five.

It's not unusual for outsiders to be completely baffled by toddler talk that is easily deciphered by a child's own parents, whose ears have become accustomed to the child's language patterns. It takes time and plenty of exposure to toddlers to be able to tune in to them, just as it takes time and plenty of exposure to a new language to be able to tune in to it.

Don't keep correcting your child when she says "frow" for throw, or "dee" for key. And don't withhold favors because of poor pronunciation, refusing to give her her bottle

if she requests a "ba-ba," or denying her a cup of water if she asks for "wa-wa." That approach will only make her hesitant about trying new words or even about saying old ones. But don't echo her words, use them when talking to her ("da-da's coming home soon"), or let her know you think her pronunciation's cute (even though it is). If she gets the idea that her mispronunciations are charming, she'll use them far longer than she would have without the encouragement.

What you can do, however, is accept and applaud her efforts, and at the same time teach correct pronunciation by example. When she points to the lamp and says "wight," respond (displaying proper parental pride, of course) with "Very good— that's the *light!*" When she asks for "bana" in her cereal, say, "Oh, you want some ba-na-na in your cereal. Here's some ba-na-na." She may not be able to say "banana" for months, or even a couple of years, but she will appreciate that you accept her present way of saying it, and she will get the subtle message that her pronunciation is not yet perfect. Of course, proud as you will be when she finally says bottle, water, daddy, light, and banana as clearly as you do, you will doubtless experience a twinge or two of regret for the loss of her adorable baby talk.

PARENTAL NUDITY

"I sometimes dress in front of my baby, but I'm a little worried that seeing me naked might be detrimental in some way to his development."

You've got some time before you'll have to start retreating behind closed doors to do your dressing and undressing. Experts agree that up until the preschool years parental nudity won't disturb a child in any way. Beyond the age of three or four, however, the consensus changes. At that point, some believe, it may be less healthy for children to see parents of the opposite sex fully undressed. Certainly, an infant under a year is too young to be stimulated by seeing his mother undressed (unless he's a breastfeeder)—and he's also too young to remember, years later, what he's seen. In fact, he's as unlikely to notice anything special about mom's birthday suit as he is about her best dress, and will probably largely ignore it.

If your baby is curious about what he views, however, and wants to touch your pubic hair or pull at your nipples, feel free to end any explorations that bother you. Be matter-of-fact, and don't overreact. His interest in the private parts of your body is, after all, no less wholesome than his interest in the public parts, such as your nose or ears. "That's mommy's" is a response that will help a baby begin to understand the concept of body privacy and help him keep his private parts private later on—but one that won't instill guilt.

FALLS

"I feel as though I'm living on the brink of disaster ever since my little boy started to walk and climb. He trips over his own feet, bangs his head on table corners, topples off chairs...."

This is an age that many parents fear neither they nor their babies will survive. Split lips, black eyes, bumps, bangs, bruises, and countless close calls for baby. Frazzled nerves and skipped heartbeats for mommy and daddy.

Yet babies keep going back for more. And a good thing, too, or they'd never learn to get around on their own—or, in fact, learn much of anything at all. Though horseback riding can be mastered, according to the old adage, with just seven falls, mastery of walking and climbing takes a good deal more—with seven or more falls not being uncommon in the space of a single morning. Some children learn caution fairly quickly; after the first topple off

the coffee table, they retreat for a few days, and then proceed more carefully. Others seem as though they will never learn caution, never know fear, never feel pain; five minutes after the tenth topple, they're back for number eleven.

Learning to walk is a matter of trial and error—or more accurately, step and fall. You can't, and shouldn't try to, interfere with the learning process. Your role, other than that of proud but nervous spectator, is to do everything possible to ensure that when your baby falls, he falls safely. While taking a tumble on the living room rug can bruise his ego, tumbling down the stairs can bruise a lot more. Bumping into the rounded edge of the sofa may draw some tears, but colliding with the sharp corner of a glass table may draw blood. To decrease the chance of serious accidents, be sure that your house is safe for your baby (see page 292). And even if you have removed the most obvious hazards from your toddler's path, remember that the most important safety feature in your home is you (or whoever else is minding your child). While your child needs plenty of freedom for exploration of the world around him, it should be permitted only under very close and *constant* adult supervision.

Even in the most conscientious of homes, however, serious accidents can happen. Be prepared for this possibility by knowing just what to do if one should occur; take a baby-resuscitation course and learn the first-aid procedures beginning on page 434.

Parental reaction often colors a baby's response to mishap. If each fall brings one or more panicked adults rushing to his rescue, chorusing "Are you okay? Are you okay?" between gasps and shudders, your fallen soldier is likely to overreact as much as those around him—shedding as many tears when he's not really hurt as when he really is—and may soon become overcautious or lose his sense of adventure, perhaps even to the point of hesitating to attempt normal physical developmental hurdles. If, on the other hand, the adult's reaction is a calm "Oops, you fell down! You're all right. Up you go," then the child is likely to turn out to be a real trooper, taking minor tumbles in stride and getting right back on his feet without missing a beat.

NOT PULLING UP YET

"Although she's been trying for some time, my baby hasn't yet pulled up to stand. I'm worried that she's not developing normally."

For babies, life's a never-ending series of physical (and emotional and intellectual) challenges. The skills that adults take for granted—rolling over, sitting up, standing—are for them major hurdles to be confronted and scaled with no small effort. And no sooner is one challenge met than another looms ahead.

As for pulling up, there will be babies who will master this skill as early as five months and those who will wait until well after the first birthday, though most will fall (or rather, stand) somewhere between the two developmental extremes. A baby's weight may have an impact on when she first pulls up; a heavier baby has more baggage to take with her than does a lighter one, and so the effort needed may be greater. On the other hand, a strong and well-coordinated baby may be able to pull up early no matter how much she weighs. The baby who's cooped up in a stroller, baby carrier, or mesh playpen much of the day won't be able to practice her pull-ups. Nor will a baby want to practice if she is surrounded by fragile furniture that buckles under her every attempt to steady herself. Slippery shoes or socks can also hamper efforts to pull up, and can cause falls that dampen enthusiasm for the activity—bare feet or slipper-socks with non-skid soles give baby a better foot to stand on. You can encourage your baby to try to

pull up by putting a favorite toy in a place where she has to stand to get to it. Also, help her to pull up in your lap frequently, which will build her leg muscles as well as her confidence.

The average age for passing the pulling-up milestone is nine months; and most, but certainly not all, children have accomplished the skill by twelve months. Of course, it's a good idea to check with the doctor if your child hasn't successfully pulled up by her first birthday, just to rule out the possibility of a physical problem. Right now, all you need to do is sit back and wait for her to stand—in her own good time. Children gain confidence from being allowed to progress at their own pace, from discovering "I can do it myself." Trying to force a child to stand or walk before she's ready could set her back rather than move her forward.

CHOLESTEROL IN BABY'S DIET

"My husband and I are very careful about cholesterol in our diets, but when we asked our pediatrician whether we should start our son on skim milk, he said no. Does this mean we don't have to worry about his cholesterol at all?"

A child in the first year of life, and probably in the second year as well, is in an enviable position—at least from the point of view of parents who miss their daily steak and eggs. Not only are fat and cholesterol not hazardous to a baby's health, they're believed to be essential for proper growth and for development of the brain and the rest of the nervous system. In addition, skim and low-fat milks are not appropriate fare for infants because their high ratio of protein to fat and high sodium levels put too great a strain on the kidneys. Most doctors recommend formula or breast milk for at least the first six months to a year, and whole milk after weaning. Some say it's okay to switch to 2% milk at fifteen months and skim at eighteen months; others hold out for whole milk until baby's second birthday.

Lack of sound scientific evidence makes it difficult to say precisely how much fat is too much or not enough in childhood. Moderation probably makes the most sense.[3]

Though it may not be necessary, or even wise, to strictly limit your baby's intake of fat and cholesterol, it is necessary to be sure that the eating habits he develops now will lay the foundation for a lifetime of healthy eating. Studies show that preschoolers in this country are already beginning to get buildups in their arteries of the atherosclerotic plaque that leads to heart disease in adulthood, and that by age four, the average American child has a blood cholesterol level as high as an adult's and much higher than levels in children in countries where heart disease is uncommon. These disturbing statistics, which don't bode well for the coronary future of America, are due largely to the typical diet consumed here. Begun in the high chair, it is high in saturated fat and cholesterol and low in fiber. In addition to cardiovascular diseases, it has been linked to several types of cancer, including some of the most pervasive: breast, colon, and rectal.

So while you should continue to include whole milk in your baby's diet for a while yet, and needn't rigidly limit eggs or hard cheese, you should take steps to reduce his future risk of premature illness or death by instilling prudent eating habits now.

Ban the butter. If your baby becomes accustomed to bread, pancakes, vegetables,

fish, and other foods without added butter now, he won't have to undergo the ordeal of trying to cut back later. And if, when he's older, he wants to butter his bread or butter-sauté his broccoli, a smidgen will doubtless satisfy.

Forgo the frying. Fried foods aren't good for anyone—little children included. Serve or order baked potato instead of fries for your baby (and the rest of your family), broil the chicken instead of frying it, pan-fry the fish in a non-stick skillet or bake it in the oven.

Be choosy with your cheese. High in protein and calcium, hard cheeses such as Swiss, Gouda, mozzarella, and Cheddar would be a balanced diet's best friend—if it weren't for their very high saturated fat and cholesterol counts, high even for babies, for whom a diet moderately high in cholesterol appears necessary. So look for the lower-fat cheeses (such as part-skim mozzarella, Emmenthaler, or other skim-milk cheese) with no more than 5 to 7 grams of fat per ounce, and use them in moderation since even they cannot truly be considered "low-fat."

Since the high sodium content of most cheeses is neither good for babies now nor for heart health later, choose cheeses that are relatively low in sodium—for example, those that contain no more than 35 milligrams per ounce.

If children develop a taste for lower-fat, low-sodium cheeses when they're very young, they may even prefer them over the higher-fat and -salt varieties when they're older.

Defat other dairy products. Though you won't be switching your baby to skim milk yet, you can start weaning to lower-fat cream cheeses, yogurts, and cottage cheese (choose salt-reduced or salt-free varieties of the latter) by the end of the first year (assuming your baby is getting adequate quantities of whole milk and/or hard cheeses and some eggs), so baby won't crave the richer kind. Because they contain large amounts of sugar as well as fat, commercial ice

3. Apparently strict limitations on fat and cholesterol for children with a hereditary tendency to produce excess cholesterol is helpful in lowering cholesterol levels and appears not to hamper growth and development. If there is such a tendency in your family, and especially if there is also a history of premature heart attack, stroke, or other vascular disease, speak to your baby's doctor about doing a blood cholesterol test soon.

RAISING A HEALTHY HEART

It's never too early to start reducing your baby's risk of heart attack later in life. The following will help:

■ Feed a diet low in saturated fat and cholesterol from the end of the second year, but introduce prudent diet habits earlier. If there is a family history of hypercholesteremia (very high cholesterol), have your child's cholesterol monitored by the doctor.

■ Feed a diet low in salt from infancy on.

■ Feed a diet high in omega-3 fatty acids, which are found in plentiful supply in oily fish (salmon, shad, and mackerel, for example). Don't use omega-3 fish-oil capsules, as their effectiveness and safety have not been proven.

■ Watch your child's weight, and take action if it begins to shoot up much faster than his or her height (see page 208). An overweight baby may become an overweight child, who will almost certainly become an overweight adult.

■ Don't smoke or permit smoking in your home. Parents who smoke are more likely than nonsmokers to have children who smoke. Educate your child from infancy about the dangers as well as the unpleasantness of tobacco, and he or she is not likely to ever light up.

■ Teach your child early on the value and pleasure of exercise and physical activity; don't be sedentary yourself, and don't let your child be.

■ If your child's blood pressure is high or borderline, follow the doctor's instructions for controlling it.

■ Keep consumption of sugar low. Sugar increases chromium needs, and it may increase the chance of diabetes developing, which is a heart attack risk factor.

---

creams and other frozen desserts (including tofu desserts, which contain little nourishment and much sugar) shouldn't be given to babies at all; for nutritious homemade frozen dessert recipes, see page 626.

Be picky with your protein. Protein in adequate amounts is important for your entire family, but it's wise to select the sources that are low in cholesterol and fat, such as: fish, skinless poultry, dried beans and peas, tofu (bean curd). If your baby learns to enjoy fish and chicken now, he's less likely to spurn "anything but hamburger" later. Serve red meat no more than three times a week, and then buy lean cuts and trim fat well. It's okay to avoid red meat entirely, but then be certain your baby has other sources of iron in his diet.

Fill out your menu with fiber. If fat increases blood cholesterol levels and the risk of heart attack, certain types of fiber, such as pectin and oat bran, decrease both. Be sure your baby's diet frequently contains pectin-rich fruits such as apples, and oats in some form.

Favor fish. Like fiber, fish in the diet seems to have the effect of lowering blood cholesterol levels, probably thanks to the omega-3 oils found in it. Introduce your baby early to a variety of fresh fish, most of which have a pleasingly mild taste and an easily chewable texture, and which are low in fat and sodium. But check very carefully for bones.

Look at the label. Most of the fat and cholesterol in the diets of both adults and children is hidden in prepared foods. Cakes and pastries are, surprisingly, the major source of dietary fat for Americans, bypassing butter and margarine. To avoid hidden fat, read labels carefully and don't buy products that contain fats from the "bad" column on the facing page. Look instead for those made either without fat or with preferred fats or oils. The farther down "fat" is on the list of ingredients, the less total fat a product contains, and the less the threat to your family's health.

Cut fat in cooking. When cooking, you can reduce the fat called for in most recipes

350   THE FIRST YEAR

without otherwise altering them. Using nonstick pans and cookware as well as vegetable cooking sprays will allow you to greatly reduce the amount of fat used in sautéing or pan-frying. When baking, reduce the fat and replace it with an equivalent amount of liquids.

Divide the eggs, and conquer cholesterol. All of the roughly 280 milligrams of an egg's cholesterol are in the yolk. Use whites for all or some of the eggs called for in recipes (two egg whites equal one whole egg) when baking and cooking for the entire family. In general, children and adults should have no more than three yolks a week; those with high cholesterol levels should have fewer. Your baby can still have an egg daily now, but start cutting back on the number of yolks he gets at about eighteen months. Remember, eggs used in cooking count in the quota.

Go on a family fast-foods fast. Most fast foods are very high not only in fat and cholesterol, but in salt as well. They are also usually lacking in many nutrients. So take the family to fast-food restaurants rarely—and then select those items that are lower in fat (pizza, baked fish, broiled chicken, plain baked potatoes, undressed vegetables from the salad bar). Though burgers at home are okay for baby, the fast-food variety are usually too high in sodium and fat, and the white-flour bun is nutritionally superfluous.

Once your baby is over two years old, he can join the rest of the family on a diet in which 50 to 55% of calories come from carbohydrates (whole-grain breads and cereals, legumes such as dried beans and peas, vegetables, fruits), 15 to 20% from protein (fish, poultry, meat, dairy products, legumes, tofu), and only 30% from fat (no more than 10% should be saturated and 10% should be in the form of polyunsaturated oils or olive oil).[4] Total daily intake of cholesterol (found in large quantities in animal products such as butter, whole milk, cheese, meat, and especially eggs), according to prudent-diet guidelines, should not exceed 100 milli-

grams per 1,000 calories consumed up to a maximum of 250 to 300 milligrams a day. Consider that one large egg contains approximately 280 milligrams of cholesterol; one pat of butter, 10 milligrams; a cup of whole milk, 33; 1 ounce of Cheddar cheese, 30; a 3-ounce hamburger, 76; and that a two-year-old consumes about 1,000 to 1,300 calories a day, a typical adult 1,800 to 2,400.

GROWTH SWINGS

"The pediatrician just told me that my son has dropped from the 90th to the 50th percentile in height. She said not to worry, but I'm afraid something might be wrong with his development."

When a doctor assesses a child's developmental progress, she looks at more than the curve of his growth chart. Are both height and weight keeping pace fairly closely? Is baby passing developmental mileposts (sitting, pulling up, etc.) at about the right time? Is he active and alert? Does he appear happy? Does he seem to relate well to mommy? Are hair and skin healthy looking? Apparently your baby's doctor found your child to be developing normally, and you should take your cue from that.

The most common reason for such a growth shift at this time is that a baby who was born on the large side is just moving closer to his genetically predestined size. If you and your husband are not very tall, you shouldn't expect your son to stay in the 90th percentile—chances are he won't. Height, however, isn't inherited through a single gene. So a child with a 6-foot father and a

---

4. This is what the American Heart Association recommends for those in good health and at low risk for a heart attack (most Americans get more). Do *not* reduce your child's intake of fat below this level without medical advice. Fats, particularly those (such as breast milk, safflower, corn, and soy oils) containing linoleic acid, an essential fatty acid, are an absolute requirement for a good diet. And a diet that is extremely low in fat is inherently deficient in certain essential nutrients.

FATS: THE GOOD, THE BEST, AND THE BAD

The oils you select when preparing food for your family will have a major impact on their health. Whenever possible, choose those from the "The Good" or "The Best" list, rather than from the "The Bad."

THE GOOD	THE BEST	THE BAD
Margarine with a polyunsaturated to saturated fat ratio of 2:1 or better	Avocado oil	Palm and palm kernel oil
Peanut oil	Olive oil	Coconut oil
Cottonseed oil (a little higher in saturated fats)	Canola oil (rapeseed)	Cocoa butter
	Safflower oil	Hydrogenated vegetable fat or shortening
	Sunflower oil	Chicken or other poultry fat
	Corn oil	Suet (beef fat)
	Soy oil	Lard (pork fat)
	Other oils high in polyunsaturates	Butter*
		Partially hydrogenated fats

*If your family prefers the taste of butter as a spread, using small amounts (no more than a pat—1 teaspoon—per person per day) will not appreciably increase cholesterol intake.

5-foot mother isn't likely to reach adulthood exactly the same height as one or the other. More likely, he will end up somewhere in between. (Each generation is, however, on the average, a little taller than the previous one.)

Occasionally a measuring error has been made, either at the present time or on a previous visit. Babies are usually measured while they're lying down, and a baby's wriggling can easily yield inaccurate results. When a child graduates to upright measurement, he may appear to lose an inch or so in height because his bones settle a little when he stands.

Do be certain, of course, that your baby is well nourished, and continues to be as he grows older. And bring any health concerns to the attention of his doctor. After that, record your baby's checkup statistics and forget about them. As you will soon realize, kids grow up too fast anyway.

WHAT IT'S IMPORTANT TO KNOW: Helping Baby to Talk

Your baby's come a long way, mommy. From a newborn whose only way of communicating was crying, and who understood nothing but his or her own primal needs; to a six-month-old who was beginning to articulate sounds, comprehend words, and express anger, frustration, and happiness; to an eight-month-old who was able to convey messages through primitive sounds and gestures; and now, to an eleven-month-old who's uttered (or will soon utter) his or her first real words. And yet with all the accomplishments already behind your baby, still more astounding growth is up ahead. In the months to come, your baby's comprehension will increase at a remarkable rate; by around a year and a half, there will be a dramatic expansion in expressive language.

Here's how you can help your baby's language development:

Label, label, label. Everything in your baby's world has a name—use it. Verbally label objects in baby's home environment (bathtub, toilet, kitchen sink, stove, crib, playpen, lamps, chair, couch, and so on); play "eyes-nose-mouth" (take baby's hand and touch your eyes, your nose, and your mouth, kissing the hand at the last stop), and point out other body parts; point to birds, dogs, trees, leaves, flowers, cars, trucks, and airplanes while you're out walking. Don't leave out people—point out mommies, daddies, babies, ladies, men, girls, boys. Or baby—use his or her name often to help develop a sense of identity.

Listen, listen, listen. As important as what you say to your baby is how much you let your baby say to you. Even if you haven't identified any real words yet, listen to the babble and respond: "Oh, that's very interesting," or, "Is that so?" When you ask a question, wait for an answer, even if it's just a smile, excited body language, or undecipherable babble. Make a concerted effort to pick out words from your baby's verbal ramblings; many "first words" are so garbled that parents don't notice them. Try to match baby's unrecognizable words with the objects they may represent; they may not even sound remotely correct, yet if the child uses the same "word" for the same object consistently, it counts. When you have trouble translating what your baby's asking for, point to possible candidates ("Do you want the ball? the bottle? the puzzle?"), giving him or her a chance to

tell you whether you've guessed right. There will be frustration on both sides until baby's requests become more intelligible, but continuing to attempt to act as interpreter will help speed language development as well as provide baby with the satisfaction of being at least somewhat understood.

Concentrate on concepts. So much of what you take for granted, baby has yet to learn. Here are just a few concepts you can help your baby develop—you can probably think of many more.

- *Hot and cold:* let baby touch the outside of your coffee cup, then an ice cube; cold water, then warm water; warm oatmeal, then cold milk.
- *Up and down:* gently lift baby up in the air, then lower to the ground; place a block up on the dresser, then put it down on the floor; take your baby up on the see-saw, then down.
- *In and out:* put blocks in a box or pail, dump them out; do the same with other objects.
- *Empty and full:* fill a container with bath water, then empty it; fill a pail with sand, then empty it.
- *Stand and sit:* hold baby's hand, stand together, then sit down together; play ring-around-the-rosies.
- *Wet and dry:* compare a wet washcloth and a dry towel; baby's just-shampooed hair with your dry hair.
- *Big and little:* set a large ball beside a small one; show baby that "mommy's big and baby's little" in the mirror.

Explain the environment and cause and effect. "The sun is bright so we have light." "The refrigerator keeps food cold so it will taste good and stay fresh." "Mommy uses a little brush to brush your teeth, a medium brush to brush your hair, and a big brush to scrub the floor." "Flip the wall switch up and the room becomes light, down and it's dark." "If you tear the book, we won't be able to read it anymore." And so on. An expanded awareness and understanding of his or her surroundings, as well as sensitivity to other people and their needs and feelings, is a far more important step toward your baby's eventual mastery of language and reading than learning to parrot a lot of meaningless words.

Become color conscious. Start identifying colors whenever it's appropriate. "See, that balloon is red, just like your shirt," or "That truck is green; your stroller is green, too," or "Look at those pretty yellow flowers."

Use double-speak. Use adult phrases, then translate them into baby shorthand: "Now you and I are going for a walk. Mommy, Amy, go bye-bye." "Oh, you've finished your snack. Baby made all gone." Talking twice as much will help baby understand twice as much.

Talk like a grown-up. Using simplified grown-up talk, rather than baby talk, will help your baby learn to speak correctly faster: "Benjy wants a bottle?" is better than "Baby wanna baba?" Forms like "doggie" or "dolly," however, are okay to use with young children—they're naturally more appealing.

Introduce pronouns. Though your baby probably won't be using pronouns correctly for a year or more, now is a good time to start developing familiarity with them by using them along with names. *"Mommy* is going to get *Josh* some breakfast—*I'm* going to get *you* something to eat." "This book is *mommy's*—it's *mine*—and that book is *Nina's*—it's *yours.*" This last also teaches the concept of ownership.

Urge baby to talk back. Use any ploy you can think of to try to get your baby to respond, in either words or gestures. Present choices: "Do you want bread or crackers?" or "Do you want to wear your Mickey Mouse pajamas or the ones with airplanes?" and then give baby a chance to point to or vocally indicate the favored selection, which you should then name. Ask questions: "Are you tired?" "Would you like a snack?" "Do you want to go on the swing?" A shake

of the head will probably precede a verbal yes or no, but it's still a legitimate response. Get baby to help you locate things (even if they aren't really lost): "Where's the ball? Can you find Raggedy Ann?" Give baby plenty of time to turn up the item, and reward with cheers and hugs. Even looking in the right direction should count—"That's right, that's Raggedy Ann!"

Don't force the issue. Encourage your baby to talk by saying "Tell mommy what you want" when he or she uses nonverbal communication (pointing, grunting) to indicate a need. If baby grunts or points again, offer a choice; for instance, "Do you want the ball or the truck?" If you still get a nonverbal response, name the item yourself, "Oh, it's the ball you want," and then hand it over. *Never* withhold something because your child can't ask for it by name or because he or she pronounces the name incorrectly. But do try to elicit the name of the item again next time—in the same patient, nondemanding way.

Keep directions simple. Most babies at this age can follow only simple commands, so give directions one step at a time. Instead of "Please pick up the spoon and give it to me," try "Please pick up the spoon," and when that's been done, add "Now, please, give the spoon to mommy." You can also help your baby enjoy early success in following commands by giving commands that he or she is about to carry out anyway. If, for example, your baby is reaching for a cracker, say "Pick up the cracker." These techniques will help develop comprehension, which must precede speech.

Correct carefully. Very rarely will a young child say even a single word perfectly, and none say everything with adult precision. Many consonants may be beyond your baby's capability for the next several years or more, and the ends of words may be omitted for at least many more months ("mo mi" may mean "more milk and "go dow" "go down"). When your baby mispronounces a word, don't correct with schoolmarmish brusqueness—too much criticism could prompt a baby to give up trying. Instead, use a more subtle approach, teaching without preaching to protect your baby's tender ego. When baby looks up at the sky and says, "moom, tar," "That's right. There's the moon and the stars." Though baby mispronunciations are adorable, your repeating them will be confusing (baby knows the way they should sound).

Expand your reading repertoire. Rhymes are still favorites with babies entering their toddler years, as are books with pictures of animals, vehicles, toys, and children. A few children are ready for very simple stories, though most won't be willing to sit still for them for several months yet. Even those who are ready usually can't handle more than three or four minutes with a book at this age—their attention span is still short. Children tolerate reading better if they can participate actively. Stop to discuss the pictures ("Look, that cat is wearing a hat!"), ask your child to point to familiar objects (naming them will come later), and name those he or she hasn't seen before or doesn't remember. Eventually (fairly soon for some children), your child will be able to fill in last words of rhymes or sentences in favorite books.

Think numerically. Counting is a long way off for baby, but the concept of one and many isn't. Comments like "Here, you can have one cookie," or "Look, see how many birds are in that tree," or "You have two kitty cats" will start to inculcate some basic mathematical concepts. Count, or recite "One, two, buckle my shoe," as you climb the stairs with your baby, particularly once he or she can walk up while you hold both hands. Sing number rhymes, such as "Baa, baa, black sheep" (when you get to the "three bags full" hold up three fingers, then bend down one finger at a time as you "distribute" the bags), "This old man, he played one, he played knickknack on my thumb," and "ten little Indians," using your fingers to indicate the numbers. Integrate counting into your baby's life: when you do your sit-ups, count them out in one through tens; when you're adding flour to the cookie dough, count out the cups one by one as you add them; when you're adding banana to your baby's cereal, count out the slices.

CHAPTER FIFTEEN

The Twelfth Month

WHAT YOUR BABY MAY BE DOING

*By the end of this month, your baby
...should be able to (see Note):*

■ walk holding on to furniture (by 12⅔ months)

Note: If your baby seems not to have reached this milestone, check with the doctor. In rare instances the delay could indicate a problem, though in most cases it will turn out to be normal for your baby. Premature infants generally reach milestones later than others of the same birth age, often achieving them closer to their adjusted age (the age they would be if they had been born at term), or sometimes later.

...will probably be able to:

■ play patty-cake (clap hands) or wave bye-bye (most children accomplish these feats by 13 months)

■ drink from a cup independently (many can't do this until 16½ months)
■ pick up a tiny object neatly with tips of thumb and forefinger (by 12¼ months; many babies do not accomplish this until nearly 15 months)
■ stand alone momentarily (many don't accomplish this until 13 months)
■ say dada or mama discriminately (most will say at least one of these by 14 months)
■ say one word other than mama or dada (many won't say their first word until 14 months or later)

...may possibly be able to:

■ indicate wants in ways other than crying (many don't reach this stage until past 14 months)
■ "play ball" (roll ball back to you; many don't accomplish this feat until 16 months)
■ stand alone well (many don't reach this point until 14 months)

- use immature jargoning (gibberish that sounds like a foreign language; half of all babies don't start jargoning until after their first birthday, and many not until they are 15 months old)
- walk well (3 out of 4 babies don't walk well until 13½ months, and many not until considerably later; good crawlers may be slower to walk; when other development is normal, late walking is rarely a cause for concern)

...may even be able to:

- say three words or more other than mama or dada (a good half of all babies won't reach this stage until 13 months, and many not until 16 months)
- respond to a one-step command without gestures (give that to me—without hand out; most children won't reach this stage until after their first birthday, many not until after 16 months).

WHAT YOU CAN EXPECT AT THIS MONTH'S CHECKUP

Each doctor or nurse-practitioner will have a personal approach to well-baby checkups. The overall organization of the physical exam, as well as the number and type of assessment techniques used and procedures performed, will also vary with the individual needs of the child. But in general, you can expect the following at a checkup when your baby is about twelve months old:

- Questions about how you and baby and the rest of the family are doing at home, and about baby's eating, sleeping, and general progress. About child care, if you are working.
- Measurement of baby's weight, length, and head circumference, and plotting of progress since birth.
- Physical exam, including a recheck of any previous problems. Now that baby can pull up, feet and legs will be checked when standing supported or unsupported, and walking if baby walks.
- A hemoglobin or hematocrit test to check for anemia (usually by means of a pinprick on the finger), if not performed earlier.
- Developmental assessment. The examiner may actually put baby through a series of "tests" to evaluate baby's ability to sit independently, to pull up and to cruise (or

even walk), to reach for and grasp objects, to pick up tiny objects with a neat pincer grasp, to look for dropped or hidden objects, to respond to his or her name, to do some self-feeding, to use a cup, to cooperate in dressing, to recognize and possibly say such words as mommy, daddy, bye-bye, and no-no, and to enjoy social games such as patty-cake and peekaboo; or he or she may simply rely on observation plus your reports on what baby is doing.

- Immunizations, if not given before and if baby is in good health and there are no contraindications. Be sure to discuss previous reactions, if any, *beforehand*. A Mantoux test for tuberculosis will be performed if your child is at high risk of having come into contact with an infected person. It may be given before, or at the same time as, the MMR.
- Guidance about what to expect in the next month in relation to such topics as feeding, sleeping, development, and infant safety.
- Recommendations about fluoride, iron, and vitamin D, or other supplementation, as needed.

You may want to ask these questions if the doctor hasn't already answered them:

■ Who will interpret the TB test, if one was administered? What is a positive reaction? (Redness during the first 24 hours is common, but redness or swelling after 48 to 72 hours is considered positive.) When should you call or come in?

■ What new foods can be introduced to baby now? Can baby get milk in a cup? When can whole milk, citrus fruits, fish, meats, and egg whites be introduced, if they haven't been already?

■ When should you consider weaning from the bottle, if your baby is bottle fed, or from the breast, if you haven't already weaned?

Also raise concerns that have arisen over the past month. Jot down information and instructions from the doctor (you're sure to forget them, otherwise). Record all pertinent information (baby's weight, length, head circumference, immunizations, test results, illnesses, medications given, and so on) in a permanent health record.

FEEDING YOUR BABY THIS MONTH: The Best-Odds Toddler Diet

With little but mashed bananas and strained sweet potatoes under his or her gastronomic belt, your toddler's palate is basically a clean plate waiting to be filled with a whole world of as yet undiscovered eating experiences. Exactly what it will be filled with now and in the next few formative years will have a great influence on what will please it in later years—which, of course, will have a significant impact on your child's future health and longevity. But good nutrition will also provide more immediate benefits. As your excellent diet prenatally gave your baby the best odds of being born alive and well, an excellent diet during early childhood will assure him or her of the best odds of staying healthy, as well as adequate energy to fuel a busy toddler's explorations.

THE BEST-ODDS NINE BASIC PRINCIPLES

The basic principles for nutritious eating are very much the same for your toddler as they are for the rest of the family, though there are slight variations because of your child's age.

Every bite counts. This was an important principle when you were feeding your baby through the placenta, and then with your milk, if you breastfed; it's likewise important now that you're doing the feeding with spoons, cups, and bowls and it's baby who's taking the bites. For young children, whose capacities and appetites are limited and whose tastes are often more so, bites wasted on non-nutritious fare are not likely to be made up. Empty treats (such as sugary cookies, cakes, and candies) should be rare—though healthful treats (such as juice-sweetened whole-grain muffins, cookies, and cakes) can be a mainstay of the diet.

All calories are not created equal. The 100 calories in a square of chocolate aren't nutritionally equivalent to the 100 calories in a small banana; plan meals and snacks accordingly.

Meal skipping is risky. Skipped meals deprive babies and young children of nutrients they need for growth and development. Not eating at regular intervals during the day zaps kids of energy, as well as making them cranky and irrational, sometimes because of low blood sugar. And because of their small capacities, toddlers usually need snacks in addition to their three squares. Of course, toddlers sometimes reject a meal or a snack—and you shouldn't push if they do. As long as you provide regular meals, you can let your baby skip a few now and then.

Efficiency is effective. Weight problems often begin in childhood. But if a toddler is gaining unwanted weight, dieting isn't in order; careful food selection is. Favor items that offer a lot of nutrition for few calories, such as fresh fruits and vegetables and whole-grain bread without butter. If a toddler is underweight or gaining too slowly, efficient food selection means choosing foods that provide bountiful nutrition in combination with a lot of calories and not too much bulk (peanut butter, bananas, avocado, cheese). Whether or not weight is an issue, selecting foods that fill more than one nutrient requirement at a time (broccoli for vitamin C and vitamin A, yogurt for protein and calcium) is always efficient and makes particularly good sense where small appetites are concerned.

Carbohydrates are a complex issue. Carbohydrates, starches and sugars, are childhood favorites, and very young children—particularly those who refuse "protein" foods such as meat or fish—often seem to live on nothing else. But there are carbohydrates, and there are *carbohydrates*. Some, known as complex carbohydrates, provide vitamins, minerals, protein, and fiber, as well as calories (whole-grain breads and cereals, brown rice, peas, beans, whole-grain or high-protein pasta, fruits and vegetables); others, known as simple sugars and refined starches, provide little or nothing else besides calories (sugar, honey, refined grains, and foods made with them). Serve the right carbohydrates at home, and allow others only rarely (at parties, when visiting, or at other times when there's no choice).

Sweet nothings are nothing but trouble. Sugar provides nothing but empty calories, and sugary foods often fill children up, leaving no room for needed nutrients. In ad-

dition, sugar contributes significantly to tooth decay, probably by encouraging the growth of the bacteria that do the dirty work. It may also be involved, indirectly, in the development of diabetes (by increasing the body's need for chromium). The jury is still not in on whether or not sugar is a cause of hyperactivity. One federally funded study found that children who ate a lot of sugar were more active than those who didn't; other studies have not linked sugar to hyperactivity.

Almost all children seem to favor the sweet over the nonsweet right from the start, but research shows that children who eat a lot of sugary foods early on are more likely to crave them later. Keep sugar (including brown sugar, raw sugar, turbinado sugar, fructose, maple syrup, corn syrup, and honey) out of your kitchen and offer sugar-sweetened foods as treats only rarely, if at all. Many mothers find it fairly easy to ban sugar entirely, at least until their children reach the age of two or begin socializing more with other children. No sugar doesn't, however, mean no sweets. Children in a sugar-free household should be able to enjoy cakes, cookies, and muffins. And they can if you supply them with such goodies, homemade or from the increasing selection commercially available, sweetened with fruit and fruit juice concentrates.

Serve foods that remember where they came from. The closer to its natural state a food is, the more likely it is to have retained the nutrients it started out with. But what is often added to processed foods—questionable chemicals, accidentally or incidentally—may be even more threatening than what might be lost. Because children process and dispose of foreign chemicals more slowly (thus retaining them longer), have smaller body sizes, and theoretically have a lot more years to live during which the chemicals can do their damage, they are more susceptible to the dangers of chemical contamination than adults. So serve foods that stay close to their roots, allowing highly processed foods rarely if at all, opting for the unrefined over the refined, choosing fresh meats and cheese over the processed varieties, and selecting fresh or fresh-frozen fruits and vegetables over heavily processed canned, frozen, or dehydrated ones. Then tamper with them as little as possible—don't overcook, store for long periods, or expose unnecessarily to air, water, or heat.

Make good eating a family affair. Junior won't eat carrots, forgo sugary sweets, or prefer whole wheat over white if dad's always leaving his carrots on his plate, mom is always breakfasting on donuts or snacking on cookies, and an older sibling lives on peanut butter on white. Having to eat virtuously alone is unfair; having company is fun. And cleaning up the family's dietary act for the sake of the youngest will benefit not only him or her, but everyone who sits at the family table.

Watch out for diet sabotage. Your toddler isn't likely to start undermining his or her diet with tobacco, excess alcohol or caffeine, or other drugs at any time soon. But excess junk food can sabotage the diet, too, by replacing more nutritious fare. And, if a child learns at home that tobacco or illegal drugs in any amount and excess amounts of alcohol and caffeine are acceptable, those kinds of diet sabotage may come sooner than you'd imagine.

THE BEST-ODDS DAILY DOZEN— FOR TODDLERS

The Daily Dozen was first developed as an easy-to-follow outline for Best-Odds prenatal nutrition. In this modified form, it is the easiest way to nourish your toddler. Since children usually take small portions, feel free to mix and match partial servings to reach the needed requirements—remembering, too, that many foods can be counted for more than one requirement, (cantaloupe for vitamin C and a yellow fruit, for instance). The amounts need not

be exact, but you may want to measure or weigh until you feel pretty comfortable judging an ounce of cheese or a half-cup of carrots with the naked eye. Routinely using measuring spoons or cups to scoop foods from containers to serving dishes is a painless way of keeping track of portions.

Calories—an average of 900 to 1,350. No calculations are necessary. You'll know if your toddler is getting the right number of calories simply by following his or her weight at checkup times. If it's staying on approximately the same curve, caloric intake is sufficient but not excessive, though there may occasionally be a jump or dip as a thin baby fills out or a chubby one slims down. The amount of food a child needs to eat to maintain that curve will depend on individual size, metabolism, and level of activity. But keep in mind that too few calories can seriously hamper a toddler's growth and development.

Protein—four toddler servings (about 25 grams). One toddler serving equals any of the following: ¾ cup milk; ¼ cup nonfat dry milk; ½ cup yogurt; 3 tablespoons cottage cheese; ¾ ounce hard cheese; 1 whole egg or 2 egg whites; ¾ to 1 ounce fish, poultry, or meat; 2 ounces tofu; 1½ tablespoons peanut butter; 1 ounce high-protein pasta; 1 toddler vegetarian protein combination (see page 361).

Vitamin C foods—two or more toddler servings.[1] Spreading out these servings over the day—giving orange juice at breakfast, a sliver of cantaloupe at lunch, and broccoli at dinner—will enhance the absorption of iron from any iron-containing foods served. One toddler serving equals any of the following: ½ small orange or ¼ medium grapefruit; ¼ cup fresh strawberries; ⅛ cantaloupe or 1/12 small honeydew; ¼ cup fresh or frozen reconstituted orange juice; ¼ large guava or ¼ cup papaya; ½ large plantain; ¼ cup broccoli or Brussels

---

1. Increase to four toddler servings when your child has a cold or flu.

MILK SENSE

If you've weaned your baby, or are about to, it's important to select the right milk to replace breast milk or formula. The American Academy of Pediatrics and most pediatricians recommend whole milk because skim milk has too much protein and sodium content for infants and toddlers, and because very young children seem to continue to need the extra fat and cholesterol for optimal brain and nervous system development at least until fifteen months. Some believe that it is advisable to then switch to 2% milk, and finally to skim milk at eighteen months. Others believe whole milk should be continued until age two. Discuss the matter with your baby's doctor.

It is also urged that the milk be pasteurized. Though it is true that pasteurization does rob milk of some of its nutritive value, experts believe the risk of illness from the drinking of raw milk is too great to warrant its use.

You may be wondering how you can be sure your baby is getting enough milk now that you've abandoned clearly calibrated baby bottles. One way is to measure out the day's requirements—2⅔ cups (adding an additional ⅓ cup to allow for spillage)—each morning, pour it into a clean jar, and refrigerate. Serve all your baby's milk (for cereal, drinking, mashing with potatoes or other vegetables) from this supply. If it's all gone at the end of the day, and baby didn't

spill or leave over a great deal, the milk requirement was probably met. If a lot is left in the jar or lost to the high-chair tray or to the floor several days in a row, fit some additional calcium in baby's diet this way:

■ If your baby has been drinking only about 1½ cups of milk a day, add ½ cup nonfat dry milk plus 1 tablespoon light cream or 2 tablespoons half-and-half to that amount of fluid milk, and use the mixture as baby's daily allotment. If baby has been drinking about 2 cups, add ⅓ cup nonfat dry milk plus 1 tablespoon light cream or 2 tablespoons half-and-half.

■ Switch to calcium-added milk, which your baby needs less of (2 cups, rather than 2⅔) to fill the calcium requirement. But add 1 tablespoon of light cream or 2 tablespoons of half-and-half to each serving.

■ Add one of the following to your baby's diet for each ⅓ cup of whole milk your baby doesn't drink: about ⅜ to ½ ounce lower-fat hard cheese (such as mozzarella); ⅔ ounce higher-fat hard cheese (such as Cheddar); about ¼ cup yogurt; 3 ounces calcium-coagulated tofu; 2 ounces calcium-enriched orange juice; or half of any other toddler calcium serving.

Don't be concerned if some days your baby misses a calcium serving or two. He or she will probably make up for it the next day.

sprouts; ½ cup cooked greens; ¼ medium green or ⅙ medium red bell pepper; 1 small tomato, skinned; ¾ cup tomato sauce or ½ cup juice; ⅜ cup vegetable juice.

Calcium foods—four toddler servings. One toddler serving equals any of the following: ⅔ cup milk; ⅓ glass milk enriched with ⅛ cup nonfat dry milk; ¼ cup nonfat dry milk; ½ cup calcium-added milk;[2] ½ cup yogurt; about ¾ to 1 ounce lower-fat hard cheese; 1⅓ ounces high-fat

cheese; 4 ounces calcium-fortified orange juice.

One-half a toddler calcium serving equals 3 ounces tofu prepared with calcium, ⅔ scant cup cooked broccoli, ½ cup cooked kale or turnip greens, 1⅓ ounces

2. Using nonfat dry or calcium-added milk is an easy way of adding calcium to your baby's diet, but don't use them frequently unless you add 1 tablespoon of light cream or 2 of half-and-half to each serving—your baby still needs the fat. Also add cream to calcium-added milk if it is less than 4% fat.

VEGETARIAN PROTEIN COMBINATIONS FOR TODDLERS

It's preferable for your child to get some of his or her protein from animal sources: meat, fish, poultry, eggs, or dairy products. If your dietary practices make this wholly impossible, or if you occasionally like to serve purely vegetarian meals, the following food combinations will each provide an adequate serving of protein.

For a full toddler protein serving (about 6 grams), combine one portion from the Legumes column with one from the Grains column.

LEGUMES*
3 tablespoons lentils, split peas or chickpeas (garbanzos), soybeans, mung, lima, or kidney beans
1/4 cup cowpeas, black-eyed peas, white, broad, or Great Northern beans
1/3 cup green peas
1 ounce tofu

GRAINS
1/2 ounce soy or high-protein pasta
1 ounce whole-wheat pasta
1 1/2 tablespoons wheat germ
1/6 cup (before cooking) oats
1/4 cup cooked wild rice
*1/3 cup cooked brown rice, bulgur, kasha (buckwheat groats), or millet***
1 slice whole-grain bread
1 small (1 ounce) whole-wheat pita
1/2 whole-wheat English muffin or bagel
3/4 tablespoon peanut butter

*Beans and peas should be split or lightly mashed so they won't be a choking hazard.
**These grains are protein poor; when serving them, routinely add 1 1/2 teaspoons wheat germ per portion.

Note: Nuts are high in protein and can also be combined with legumes to provide vegetable protein servings. But do not serve them to toddlers unless they are finely ground, since nuts are a choking hazard.

---

canned salmon with the bones (mashed), 1 ounce sardines with the bones (mashed).

Green leafy and yellow vegetables and yellow fruits—two or more toddler servings daily.[3] One toddler serving equals any of the following: 1 medium fresh apricot or 2 small dried halves; a sliver of cantaloupe, or about 1/2 cup cubed; 1/8 large mango; 1 medium nectarine, peeled; 1/2 large yellow (not white) peach, peeled; 1/2 medium plaintain; 6 asparagus spears; scant 1/2 cup cooked broccoli; 3/4 cup peas; 2 to 3 tablespoons chopped cooked greens; 1/4 small carrot; 1/2 tablespoon unsweetened pumpkin purée; 2 tablespoons cooked mashed winter squash; 1 tablespoon orange sweet potato; 1 small tomato, skinned; scant 1/2 cup cooked tomatoes or purée; 3/4 cup tomato or 3 ounces vegetable juice; 1/4 large red bell pepper.

Other fruits and vegetables—one to two, or more, toddler servings. One toddler serving equals any of the following: 1/2 apple, peeled; 1/2 pear, peeled; 1/2 white peach, peeled; 1 medium plum, peeled; 1 small banana; 1/4 cup applesauce; 1/3 cup cherries, berries, or grapes; 1 large fig; 2 dates; 3 dried peach halves; 1 dried pear half; 1/2 slice pineapple; 2 tablespoons raisins, currants, or dried apple rings; 2 or 3 asparagus spears; 1/4 medium avocado; 3/8 cup green beans; 1/2 cup beets, eggplant, or diced turnip; 1/4 cup sliced mushrooms, yellow summer squash, or zucchini; 5 okra

3. Excessive amounts of carotene, the form in which vitamin A appears in fruits and vegetables, can tint a child's skin yellow (and an adult's, at much higher doses). Don't overdo in this category—three or four carrots a day, for example, are too many.

DAIRY PROTEIN COMBINATIONS FOR TODDLERS

Combine one of the following with one portion from the Legumes or Grains list in the Vegetarian Protein Combinations for Toddlers box (see page 361) for a Dairy Protein Combination.

2 tablespoons cottage cheese
⅓ cup milk
2 tablespoons nonfat dry milk
⅙ cup evaporated milk

⅓ cup yogurt
½ egg or 1 egg white
⅓ ounce lower-fat hard cheese (such as Swiss or mozzarella)
½ ounce high-fat cheese (such as blue or Camembert)
1 tablespoon Parmesan cheese

pods; ⅓ cup peas; ½ small ear of corn. Cut corn kernels in half by slicing each row lengthwise, and peel fruit with tough skin before serving to a toddler.

Whole grains and other concentrated complex carbohydrates—six or more toddler servings. One toddler serving equals any of the following: 1 tablespoon wheat germ; ½ slice whole-grain bread; ½ small (1 ounce pita); ¼ whole-wheat bagel or English muffin; 1 toddler serving (or ½ adult serving) Best-Odds muffin or other baked good; 3 to 4 whole-wheat bread sticks or 2 to 3 whole-grain crackers; ¼ cup brown or wild rice; ½ serving whole-grain breakfast cereal, unsweetened or fruit sweetened; ½ ounce whole-wheat or high-protein pasta; ¼ cup cooked lentils, chick-peas, pinto or kidney beans (cooked until soft, and split).

Iron-rich foods—some every day. Good sources include: beef; blackstrap molasses; baked goods made with carob or soy flour; whole grains; wheat germ; dried peas and beans, including soybeans; dried fruit; liver and other organ meats (serve infrequently because they are high in cholesterol and are storehouses for the many chemical contaminants found in livestock today); sardines; spinach (serve infrequently because of high nitrate and oxalic acid levels). The iron in these foods will be better absorbed if

a vitamin C food is eaten at the same meal. If your baby doesn't eat a lot of high-iron foods, or if he or she is anemic, the doctor may recommend an iron supplement.

High-fat foods—six to seven toddler servings daily. One toddler serving equals any of the following: ½ tablespoon polyunsaturated oil, olive oil, butter, margarine, or mayonnaise; 1½ tablespoons cream cheese; 1 tablespoon peanut butter; ¼ small avocado; 1 egg; ⅔ cup whole milk; ¾ cup whole-milk yogurt; 3 tablespoons half-and-half; 1 tablespoon heavy cream; 2 tablespoons sour cream; ⅔ ounce hard cheese; 6 slices whole-grain bread or ½ cup wheat germ; 1½ ounces lean beef, lamb, or pork. This allowance provides about 30% of daily calories from fat. For the toddler who is drinking whole milk (or eating the equivalent in other listed dairy products) and eating several eggs a week, additional animal fats are unnecessary; the remainder of the high-fat food requirement should be met with those vegetable fats high in polyunsaturates (safflower or sunflower oil, for example) or monounsaturated oil (olive oil) rather than saturated fats (coconut oil or hardened vegetable shortening). A typical toddler might get fat this way: 2 cups milk; ⅔ ounce cheese; 1 egg; 3 slices whole-wheat bread; and 1½ ounces ground beef. No added fats are needed.

Salty foods—restrict added salt. All human beings require the sodium in sodium chloride (better known as salt) for survival, but most Americans, including infants and toddlers, consume much more than they need. Since sodium is found naturally in or added in preparation to most of the foods children eat (milk, cheese, eggs, carrots, bread and most other baked goods), the requirement for salt in the diet is easily met, and easily exceeded. To avoid excessive salt intake, salt foods only lightly or not at all when cooking for children, and limit the consumption of presalted foods such as salted crackers, potato chips, pretzels, pickles, green olives, and so on (nuts of any kind are not safe for toddlers unless ground first). All salt you do use should be iodized to guard against iodine deficiency.

Fluids—four to six cups daily. Your toddler will get a portion of his or her fluid requirement in food, particularly fruits and vegetables, which are 80 to 95% water. But 4 to 6 additional cups of fluid should be consumed in fruit juices (preferably diluted with seltzer or water), vegetable juices, soups, seltzer, or straight water. Milk (which is ⅓ milk solids) provides only ⅔ of a fluid serving per cup. Extra fluids are needed in hot weather or when baby has a fever, cold, or other respiratory tract infection, or diarrhea or vomiting.

Supplements. Some doctors do not believe supplements are necessary for healthy babies one year or older. But others recommend an infant vitamin-mineral supplement with iron be continued past one year as an insurance policy. Considering the bizarre and erratic eating habits of toddlers, this makes good sense. However, giving your child a vitamin tablet each day doesn't give you license to abandon your commitment to providing him or her with a good diet. And the formulation you choose should be appropriate for a toddler and *not* contain more than 100% of the RDA for your child's age. (Some vitamins are toxic in levels not much higher than the RDA). Continue a liquid preparation until your child's molars are in, then switch to sugar-free chewable tablets.

WHAT YOU MAY BE CONCERNED ABOUT

THE FIRST BIRTHDAY PARTY

"Everyone in the family is gearing up for my daughter's first birthday. I want the party to be special, but I don't want it to be too much for her."

Many parents, caught up in the excitement of planning a party for baby's first birthday, seem to lose track of the fact that baby is still a baby. And the gala they so painstakingly stage is rarely suitable for the guest of honor, who is likely to end up cracking under the pressure and spending much of her fête in tears.

To plan a first-birthday-party-to-remember, instead of one you'd rather forget, follow this strategy:

Keep the invites light. A room too crowded with even familiar faces will probably overwhelm your birthday pixie, with the undesirable but probable result of clinging and weeping. Save the long guest list for her wedding, and keep this crowd intimate, limiting it to a few family members and close friends. If she spends time with other babies her age, you may want to invite two or three; if she doesn't, the occasion of her first party probably isn't a good time to launch her social career.

Ditto the décor. A room decorated

with all that your local party store has to offer, and then some, may be your dream but your baby's nightmare. Too many balloons, streamers, banners, masks, and hats, like too many people, may prove too much for a toddler to handle. So decorate with a light hand, perhaps in a theme you know she'll appreciate (Big Bird, if he's a favorite, or Mickey Mouse, or teddy bears). And if balloons will round out your party picture, remember that tiny tots can choke on the rubber scraps left after balloons go pop.

Let her eat cake... But make sure it's not the kind of cake she shouldn't eat (one with chocolate, nuts, sugar, or honey). Instead serve up a Best-Odds carrot cake topped with unsweetened fresh whipped cream or fruit juice–sweetened cream cheese frosting—shaped like, or decorated with, a favorite character if you're feeling artistic. Serve your confection à la mode if you like, with homemade or store-bought ice cream.[4] Cut the cake at your baby's usual snacktime, if possible, keeping toddler portions small to avoid waste. And if the cake you've selected is nutritious enough to pass for a meal, it won't really matter if your child surprises you, really digs in, and is too full (or too tired) to eat much dinner later on. Finally, if you choose to put out party nibbles, choose them with safety as well as nutrition in mind. A birthday party's no time to risk a baby's choking on popcorn, peanuts, grapes, or small, chunky pretzels. Also for safety's sake, insist that all young guests do their eating sitting down.

Don't send in the clowns. Or magicians, or any other paid or volunteer entertainment that might frighten your baby or a playmate. One-year-olds are notoriously

sensitive and unpredictable; what delights them one minute may terrify them the next. Also don't try to organize the toddler set into formal party games—they're not ready for that yet. If there are several young guests, however, do have a selection of toys out for non-structured play, with enough of the same items to avoid competition. Simple, safe favors such as brightly colored rubber balls, board books, or bath toys are a fun extra and can be handed to young guests just before the gifts are opened.

Don't command a performance. It would be nice, of course, if baby would smile for the camera, take a few steps for the company, open each present with interest and coo appreciatively over it—but don't count on it. She might learn to blow out the candles if you give her enough practice during the month before the party, but don't expect complete cooperation, and don't put the pressure on. Instead, let her be herself—whether that means squirming out of your arms during that party pose, refusing even to stand on her own two feet during the step-taking exhibition, or opting to play with an empty box over the expensive gift that came in it.

Time it right. Scheduling is everything when it comes to a baby's party. Try to orchestrate the big day's activities so that baby is well rested, recently fed (don't hold off her lunch figuring she'll eat at the party), and on her usual schedule. Don't plan a morning party if she usually naps in the A.M., or an early afternoon party if she usually conks out after lunch. Inviting a tired baby to participate in the festivities is tantamount to inviting disaster. And keep the party brief—an hour and a half at the most—so she won't be a wreck when the party's over or, worse, in the middle of it all.

Record it for posterity. The party will be over much too quickly, and so will your baby's childhood. Recording the occasion in snapshots, on videotape, or on film will be well worth the effort.

---

4. The good news: ice cream sweetened with fruit juices is available in most health food stores; it's delicious and all natural. The bad news: some of it is made with heavy cream and egg yolks. So consider it special occasion, rather than daily, fare, or look for the "light" varieties.

NOT YET WALKING

"Today is my son's first birthday, and he hasn't even attempted to take his first step. Shouldn't he be walking by now?"

It may seem appropriate for a baby to take his first steps at his first birthday party (and great adult entertainment, to boot), but few babies are willing or able to oblige. Though some start walking weeks, or even months, earlier, others won't totter toward the momentous milestone until much later (sometimes when mom and dad aren't around). And while passing the first birthday without a step may be a disappointment to the relatives, and especially those who've dragged out the video equipment to capture history in the making, it in no way signals a developmental problem.

The majority of children, in fact, don't start walking until after their first birthday, with various studies placing the average age for first step–taking between thirteen and fifteen months. And the age at which a child first steps out, whether nine months, fifteen months, or even later, is no reflection on his intelligence.

When a baby walks is often related to his genetic makeup—early (or late) walking runs in families. Or to his weight and build—a wiry, muscular baby is more likely to walk earlier than a placid, plump one, and a child with short, sturdy legs before one with long, slender ones that are difficult to balance on. It may also be related to when and how well he learns to crawl. A child who is an ineffective crawler or who doesn't crawl at all sometimes walks sooner than the baby who is perfectly content racing about on all fours.

Poor nutrition or a non-stimulating environment can also delay walking. So can a negative experience—perhaps a bad fall the first time a tentative toddler let go of mommy's hand. In such a case, the child may not take a chance again until he's very steady, and then he may take off like a pro rather than with the stiff awkwardness of an amateur. The child who's been forced by overeager parents to endure walking practice sessions several times daily may rebel (particularly if he has a stubborn streak) and walk independently later than he would have if he had been allowed to do it on his own terms and at his own pace. The first steps of a baby who's had his energy zapped by an ear infection, the flu, or other illness may be delayed until he's feeling better. A child who's been virtually waltzing from room to room may suddenly regress to the two-step-and-tumble when under the weather, only to rebound just as quickly once he's feeling himself again.

A baby who's always corralled in a mesh playpen (in which he may not be able to pull up to a standing position), strapped in a stroller, or otherwise given little chance to develop his leg muscles and his confidence through standing and cruising may walk late—in fact, may develop slowly on other fronts as well. Likewise, an older baby who's in a walker a good deal of the time is likely to be delayed in his independent walking rather than given an edge. Give your baby plenty of time and space for practicing pulling up, cruising, standing, and stepping in a room that doesn't have scatter rugs or a slippery floor to slip him up, and which has plenty of safe-for-pulling-up-on furniture arranged close enough together for confident transfers or very short toddles. He'll do best if he's barefoot, since babies use their toes for gripping when they take their first steps; socks are slippery, shoes too stiff and heavy.

Though many perfectly normal, even exceptionally bright, babies don't walk until the second half of their second year, particularly if one or both parents didn't, a baby who isn't walking by eighteen months should be examined by his doctor to rule out the possibility that physical or emotional factors are interfering with walking. But even at that age—and certainly at twelve months—a child's not walking yet isn't cause for alarm.

ATTACHMENT TO THE BOTTLE

"I was hoping to wean my son from the bottle at a year, but he's so attached to it I can't even get it away from him for a minute, much less permanently."

Like a favorite teddy bear or blanket, a bottle is a source of emotional comfort and gratification for a small child. But unlike a teddy or blanket, a bottle can be harmful if used improperly or much past a baby's first birthday.

The most serious threat bottle drinking poses is to a baby's teeth, both those that have already erupted and those yet to come, including the permanent set. Baby-bottle mouth can lead to tooth loss and poor mouth development, and interfere with good eating habits. Another threat is to the ears; babies who continue on the bottle past the first year are more likely to suffer ear infections. Bottles also pose a threat to baby's nutrition. Sucking from a bottle of milk or juice all day long can satisfy his hunger and suppress his appetite for other foods, interfering with a balanced diet. And if those threats aren't sufficient to warrant a switch to a cup about now, factor in the effect the ever-present bottle can have on development. A toddler who's constantly toting a bottle has only one hand free for playing, learning, and exploring; and one who's always sucking on a bottle (or on a pacifier) has a mouth too full to speak out of.

For these reasons, many pediatricians recommend weaning from the bottle by the first birthday or soon after. And though weaning of any kind at any time is rarely easy, particularly when a strong attachment has formed, it will be easier now than later, when negativity and stubbornness become more pronounced. The weaning tips given on page 342 should ease the process further.

If you don't feel your baby is ready to give up the bottle entirely at this age, at least try to limit when, where, and how often he has it. Offer the bottle only two or three times a day, supplementing between meals with snacks and drinks from a cup. Filling the bottle with water rather than juice or milk may also reduce your child's interest in it while protecting his teeth. Don't allow your baby to take the bottle to bed, walk or crawl around with it, or suck on it casually as he plays. Instead, insist he drink from it on an adult's lap. When he wants to get down, put the bottle in the refrigerator if it isn't empty. Eventually, he should become restless enough with the lap feedings to be willing to give the bottle up. And even if that day is a long way off, restricting the use of the bottle this way will limit the amount of harm it can do in the meantime.

PUTTING THE WEANED BABY TO BED

"I've never put my daughter to bed awake—she's always been nursed to sleep. How am I going to get her to sleep at night once she's weaned to a cup?"

How easy it's always been for your baby to suck her way blissfully into dreamland. And how easy for you to nurse your way hassle-free to a peaceful evening. From now on, however, if you're serious about weaning your baby from her nightcap, bedding her down is going to take a little more effort on both sides of the crib rail.

Like an addiction to any sleep aid—from pills to late-night talk shows—an addiction to bedtime nursing can be broken. And once it is, your child will have mastered one of life's most valuable skills: the ability to fall asleep on her own. To make this goal a reality, follow this plan:

Keep the old rituals. A bedtime routine, with each item on the agenda carried out in the same order each evening, can work its soporific magic on anyone, adult or child. If you haven't instituted such a ritual yet for your baby, do so at least two weeks before you plan to wean her off the nighttime feeding. Also make sure environmental conditions are conducive to sleep: the bedroom dark unless baby prefers a nightlight, neither too warm nor too cold, and quiet; the rest of the house maintaining a business-as-usual hum that lets her know you're there if she needs you. (See page 119 for more tips on making a baby sleepy.)

Add a new twist. A few days to a week before W-Day, add a bedtime snack to your baby's ritual, one she can eat after she's in pajamas and while you're reading to her. Keep it light but satisfying (a juice-sweetened cookie and a half cup of milk, perhaps, or a piece of cheese), and let her enjoy it on your lap if she likes. Not only will the mini-meal eventually come to take the place of the nursing she'll be giving up, but the milk will have a sleep-inducing effect. Of course, if you've been brushing baby's teeth earlier in the evening, you will now have to move this part of the routine to after her snack. If she's thirsty once her teeth have been cleaned, offer her water.

Break the old addiction, but don't replace it with a new one. If there's anything a sleep-aid addict craves, it's an easy route to slumber. Supply your baby with another crutch (rocking, patting, singing, or music) to help her fall asleep and you'll only create another habit to break. Total sleeptime self-sufficiency develops only when a child is left to her own devices. So utilize cuddling, music, and such in your baby's pre-bedtime routine if you like, but not to the point of sleep. Put her down dry, happy, snug, cuddly—and drowsy but awake.

Expect some crying. And, possibly, lots of it. Chances are your baby will resist this bold new approach to bedtime—vociferously. Few babies will accept the switch without a fight. But fortunately, the crying should tone down and lessen considerably within a few nights, and soon subside altogether. (See page 261 for the cold turkey and gradual methods of letting baby cry it out.)

WAKING UP AT NIGHT

"Our baby used to sleep through the night, but suddenly he started waking up once or twice. He gets very upset when I leave him alone in his bedroom, too, so I'm reluctant to let him cry."

Separation anxiety, the familiar gremlin of the daylight hours that usually peaks between twelve and fourteen months, can also come out at night. In fact, since separating at night leaves a baby completely alone, it can become a source of even more emotional trauma than daytime separation. The result for many babies: anxious, restless nights, and sleep problems.

Nighttime separation anxiety is often worse among the children of employed mothers (the child who doesn't see much of his mother during the day may be fearful of losing her at night as well), particularly if there's a new sitter on the scene. Whether you're with your baby during the day or not, try to alleviate some of his apprehension with some pre-bedtime reassurance in the form of some extra cuddling and undivided attention (leave those dinner preparations or dishes for later). A concentrated dose of mother and/or father love before you separate for the night can help make parting easier.

If your baby is having trouble falling asleep or if he awakens fearful in the middle of the night and "crying it out" isn't working or seems too heartless, try sitting beside his crib for ten minutes or so, soothing him with a soft "Shhhh" and a gentle hand on his back. But don't stay with him until he's asleep; he'll only become dependent on your presence for falling off. Instead, leave him drowsy and, hopefully, calm—and try not to return if he cries.

If baby begins waking because of molar pain, see page 415. When all else fails, ask his doctor about a milk-free diet; milk intolerance sometimes causes sleeplessness.

SHYNESS

"My husband and I are very social, and it upsets us to see how shy our daughter is."

As sociable as you and your husband are, your daughter's shyness, if she's truly shy, comes from you. Not from the example you set, but from the genetic mold you created. Shyness, like a knack for figures or a flair for writing, is an inherited trait. Even if it's a trait parents don't display themselves, it's one that they carried to their child's conception. Though it's possible to modify shyness, it's rarely possible to eradicate it entirely. Nor should parents want to, if it's part of their child's personality.

Though many shy children retain an inner core of reserve all their lives, most turn out to be fairly gregarious adults. It's not parental prodding and pressure that brings them out of their shells, but a great deal of loving nurturing and support. Drawing attention to a child's shyness as a shortcoming will only undermine her self-confidence, which in turn will only make her more bashful. On the other hand, helping her feel more comfortable with herself will help her feel more at ease with others, and eventually diminish her shyness.

It's also possible that what seems to be shyness in your child is just a toddler's normal lack of sociability. One-year-olds and often even two-year-olds are not ready to make friends. As she approaches her third birthday, she may surprise you by her rapid progress in the art of socializing.

SOCIAL BACKWARDNESS

"We've been involved in a play group for the last few weeks, and I've noticed that my baby doesn't play with the other children. How can I get her to be more sociable?"

You can't, and you shouldn't try. A child under the age of two is not a social being, and no amount of Emily Post programming will change that. This lack of sociability wasn't an issue for previous generations, since most children were not exposed to group-play situations until at least three or four years of age, more often five. But it raises a great many concerns for today's parents, who often enroll their youngsters in play groups and group day care before their first birthdays, and nursery school by their second or third.

Though no harm (apart from a few extra colds and other viruses) can come to babies from early exposure to their peers, emotional damage can result from parental pressure to perform socially. That's because children under three just aren't ready. They are rarely capable of more than parallel play—they'll play side-by-side, but not together. It's not that they're selfish, it's just that they're not yet able to recognize that other children might be worthy of their time and attention.

Remember that your baby doesn't need or know how to handle playmates, and that her behavior is age appropriate. Pushing her to play with other children in her group will only make her withdraw from such situations altogether. For best results, you'll have to accept your baby's very normal social shortcomings and be prepared to let her set her own pace with her peers, not just now, but in the years to come as well.

SHARING

"My little boy belongs to a play group. He and the other children seem to spend most of their time fighting for the same toys. When will things get better?"

Not for a while. It's not until two, or more often three, years of age that children begin to understand the concept of sharing. Right now their own needs and desires are the only ones that matter to them—peers are treated as objects, not people. Not surprisingly, each child in the play group believes that his right to play with any and all toys whenever he wants is absolute. It will take a great deal of explaining and cajoling (never force) over the next couple of years to bring your child to the point of being able to share. And of course it's important for him to reach that point. But it's also important to keep your perspective when your two- or three-year-old refuses to let a guest so much as touch his trucks or teddy bears, won't share his cookies with a child in the park, and howls when his younger cousin is given a ride in his stroller. How often do you, after all, let a friend, much less a stranger, drive your car, have half of your hot fudge sundae, or take your place in a favorite arm chair?

HITTING

"My son is in a play group with a few children who are slightly older than he is. Some of them hit when they don't get their way, and my son has started doing it, too. How should I handle this?"

The right hook of a toddler rarely packs enough punch to do any real damage; playground shiners won't be brought home for many years to come. But just because a baby's hitting rarely harms doesn't mean it should be allowed to continue. Though a child under two may be incapable of understanding that others have feelings (he is the only little boy in his universe who does), he is capable of understanding that hitting is unacceptable.

When your child hits (or bites, or displays another form of undesirably aggressive behavior), respond immediately, firmly, and calmly. Anger is likely to put your child on the defensive and elicit more angry behavior. Slapping or spanking him will only teach him that violence is an appropriate way of expressing anger. And

overreacting to the incident will probably encourage a repeat performance in a quest for more attention. Take your child away from the scene of the crime while explaining (though the explanation may well be beyond his comprehension) that hitting is bad and that it can hurt people. Once the reprimand's over, use distraction to change the subject. Use this approach as many times as it proves necessary, and eventually he'll get the idea.

In the meantime, always make sure that play sessions with other children are carefully supervised, since there's always the chance that a child might use more than a fist to strike with, and there's much more risk of injury from a foot, a toy, a rock, or a stick.

"FORGETTING" A SKILL

"Last month my daughter was waving bye-bye all the time, but now she seems to have forgotten how. I thought she was supposed to move forward developmentally, not backwards."

She *is* moving forward developmentally, on to other skills. It's very common for a baby to practice perfecting a skill almost continuously for a while—to her delight and everyone else's—and then, once she's mastered it, to put it aside while she takes on a new challenge. Though your baby has tired of her old trick of waving bye-bye, she's more than likely excited by those she's rehearsing now, perhaps barking every time she sees a four-legged animal and playing peekaboo and patty-cake. All of which she will eventually temporarily retire once they, too, lose their attraction. Instead of worrying about what your baby seems to have forgotten, tune in to and encourage her in whatever new skills she's busy developing.

You need to be concerned only if your baby suddenly seems unable to do many things she did formerly, and if she isn't learning anything new. If that's the case, check with the doctor.

A DROP IN APPETITE

"All of a sudden, my son seems to have no interest in his meals—he only picks at his food and can't wait to get out of the high chair. Could he be sick?"

More likely Mother Nature has placed him on a maintenance diet. Because if he continued eating the way he did during the first year of life, and continued gaining at the same rate, he would soon resemble a small blimp instead of a toddler. Most babies triple their birthweight in the first year; in the second year they add only about a quarter of their weight. So a decline in appetite now is your baby's body's way of ensuring this normal decline in weight gain.

There are also other factors that may affect your baby's eating habits now. One is increased interest in the world around him. During most of his first year of life, mealtimes—whether spent in mommy's arms or in a high chair—were highlights of his existence. Now they represent an unwelcome interruption in "a day in the life of a fledging toddler," who'd rather be on the go (so many things to do, so many places to see, so much trouble to make—so little time in a day!).

Growing independence can also influence a child's reaction to the food placed in front of him. The baby in the throes of becoming a toddler may decide that he, not you, should be the arbiter of the dinner table. Wide taste swings may be the rule— peanut butter on everything one week, rejection of anything vaguely resembling it the next. And it's better to accept baby's dictatorial menu planning (as long as what he chooses is nutritious) than to fight it. Eventually, eating eccentricities will diminish.

Maybe your baby's not eating because he dislikes being exiled to the high chair; if so, try seating him at the family table in a clip-on dining chair. Or maybe he can't sit still as long as the rest of the family; in which case, don't put him in the seat until his food is served, and release him as soon as he starts to get restless.

Some babies lose their appetites temporarily during teething bouts, particularly when they're cutting their first molars. If your baby's loss of appetite is accompanied by irritability, finger chewing, and other symptoms of teething, you can be pretty sure that it will pass once the discomfort eases. If it's accompanied by signs of illness, however, such as fever, listlessness, or fatigue, check with his doctor. Also seek medical counsel if his weight gain stops altogether, if he looks very thin, if he seems weak, apathetic, and irritable, or if he has particularly dry, brittle hair and dry skin with little tone.

Though there's nothing you can do (or should do) about an appetite that's falling off as a result of your baby's normal growth slowdown, there are ways to make sure he eats what he needs to grow (see below).

BABY'S GETTING ADEQUATE NUTRITION

"I'm afraid my son's not getting enough protein or vitamins because he won't eat meat or vegetables."

It may seem to parents that a one-year-old who eats sporadically and fussily couldn't possibly get his Daily Dozen of nutrients from the dribs and drabs of food he consumes over the course of a day, but, because the nutritional requirements for a one-year-old are surprisingly small, he can quite easily. And the requirements don't just come in the most obvious packages (protein in meat and fish, vitamin A in spinach), they also come in some unexpected and unexpectedly delicious ones.

■ Protein. Your baby can get adequate protein without ever tasting meat or poultry or fish. Cottage cheese, hard cheeses, milk, milkshakes, yogurt, eggs, whole-grain cereals and breads, wheat germ, dried beans and peas, and pastas (especially high-protein brands) all provide protein. The Daily Dozen requirement for a one-year-old can be met with 2⅔ cups of milk and 2 slices of bread *or* 2 cups of milk and 1 ounce of Swiss cheese *or* 1 cup of milk, 1 cup of yogurt, 1 bowl of oatmeal, and 1 slice of whole-wheat bread *or* 1 cup of milk, ¼ cup of cottage cheese, 1 bowl of oat-circle cereal, and 2 slices of bread.

If your baby doesn't like protein foods straight, try a little sleight of hand. Make pancakes with nonfat dry milk, eggs, and wheat germ; French toast with whole-grain bread, eggs, and milk; fish pancakes with fish and eggs; high-protein pasta with grated cheese. See recipes beginning on page 618, and the toddler vegetable protein combinations on page 361.

▪ **Vegetable vitamins.** You can serve up all of the vitamins in vegetables in a variety of tempting disguises: pumpkin muffins, carrot cake, tomato-broccoli sauce on pasta, veggie pancakes, vegetables tossed with cheese sauce or in a noodle casserole. Many taste favorites, including cantaloupe, mangoes, yellow peaches, and sweet potatoes, provide the vitamins found in less-loved green leafies and yellows. See the list of green leafy and yellow vegetables and yellow fruits for more sources. And try the recipes on page 618.

Also keep the following points in mind when feeding the picky eater:

Let baby's appetite be your guide. Let him eat heartily when he's hungry, and let him pick when he's not. Never force. But do sharpen his appetite for meals by limiting snacking just before them.

Avoid the spoilers. Large amounts of apple or grape juice and even small amounts of junk foods (sugary sweets, fried foods, refined grains) can fill a baby up, leaving no room for the nutritious foods he

needs. So make foods that offer little more than a full tummy mostly off limits.

Don't give up. Just because your baby won't eat his meat (or chicken or fish) and spinach (or broccoli or carrots) today doesn't mean he won't eat them tomorrow. Make them available to him at the family table—but don't ever force him to eat them—in various forms regularly. One day he may surprise you by helping himself.

And even if he ends up eating nothing all day but orange juice, cereal with banana, pumpkin muffins, and milk, or cantaloupe, pancakes, bread with cheese, and apple juice—and he drinks some water and takes his vitamin-mineral supplement—you'll have the satisfaction of knowing that he's satisfied his Daily Dozen.

INCREASE IN APPETITE

"I thought a one-year-old's supposed to experience a drop in appetite. My daughter's has seemed to increase substantially. She's not fat, but I can't help worrying that she will be if she keeps eating at this rate."

Chances are she's eating more because she's drinking less. Babies who are either just, or just about, weaned from the breast or bottle to the cup are likely to be getting less of their total caloric intake from milk and other liquids, and may compensate by stepping up their intake of solids. Though it may seem that your daughter is taking in more calories, she probably is taking the same number or less, only in a different form. Alternatively, it could be that she's eating more because she's going through a growth spurt, or because she's become more active—possibly because she's walking a lot—and her body needs the extra calories.

Healthy babies, when allowed to eat as dictated by their appetites, hearty or not, continue to grow at a normal rate. And if your daughter's weight and height curves aren't suddenly parting company, there's no need to worry that she's overeating. Pay more attention to the quality, rather than the quantity, of her intake; and be sure that her robust appetite isn't squandered on nutritionally frivolous foods and that her diet isn't overloaded with high-fat fare (which could lead to obesity). Be aware, too, of her motivation for eating. If she seems to be eating out of boredom, for instance, instead of hunger, you can help by making sure she has plenty to keep her busy outside the kitchen between meals (see page 272 for more tips on keeping snacking under control). Or if you suspect she's eating out of a need for emotional gratification, make sure she gets enough attention and tender loving care.

REFUSING TO SELF-FEED

"I know my son is perfectly capable of feeding himself—he's done it several times. But now he absolutely refuses to hold his bottle, pick up a cup, or try a spoon."

The inner struggle between wanting to remain a baby and wanting to grow up has only just begun for your baby. For the first time he's capable of taking care of one of his needs, but he's not sure he wants to if it means giving up the secure and cushy role of baby. Instinctively, he senses that if he becomes less of a baby, you will become less of a mommy.

Don't force your baby to grow up too soon. When he wants to feed himself, let him. But when he wants to be fed, feed him. Eventually the big boy will triumph over the baby, if you let the two of them battle it out in the natural course of things—although the inner conflict will recur in every stage of his development into adulthood. In the meantime, present him with every opportunity to be self-suffi-

cient—make the bottle, the cup, and the spoon available to him without insisting he use them. Offer him finger foods often, at meals as well as snacktimes. Few children at this age are really competent with a spoon, and most will make their first ventures into self-feeding with the five-pronged utensils that are conveniently attached to their wrists.

When he does feed himself, reinforce his decision by sticking around to give him plenty of encouragement, praise, and especially, reassuring attention. He needs to know that giving up being fed by mommy doesn't have to mean giving up mommy.

UNPREDICTABILITY

"My little girl can't seem to make up her mind what she wants. One minute she's chasing me around the house, hanging on my legs while I'm trying to get work done. The next, she's trying to get away from me when I sit down to hug her."

Your daughter's not schizophrenic—she's a normal one-year-old. Like the baby who refuses to self-feed, she's split between a craving for independence and a fear of paying too high a price for that independence. When you're busy with something other than her, especially when you're moving about faster than she can follow, she worries that she's losing her hold on you and the love, sustenance, comfort, and safety that you represent, and she responds by clinging. On the other hand, when you make yourself more available, she's able to play hard-to-get and to test out her independence in the security of your presence.

As she becomes more comfortable with her independence and more secure in the fact that you'll be her mommy no matter how grown-up she becomes, she'll be less clingy. But this split in her personality will manifest itself repeatedly for years to come, probably even when she's a mom herself. (Don't you sometimes wish you could be mommy's little girl again, if only for a moment, at the same time resenting her smallest interference in your life?)

In the meantime, you can help her to strike out on her own by making her feel more secure. If you are in the kitchen peeling carrots and she's across the divider in the living room, chat with her, stop periodically and visit with her, or invite her to help you, stationing her high chair next to you at the sink, for example, and giving her some carrots and a vegetable scrub brush. Support and applaud your baby's steps toward independence, but be patient and understanding when she stumbles and rushes back to the solace of your arms.

Also be realistic in terms of the amount of time you can humanly supply in response to her demand. There will be moments when you'll have to let her hang on your feet crying while you get dinner on the table and moments when you will be able to provide only intermittent bursts of attention while you balance your checkbook. As much as it's important for her to know that you'll always love her and will meet her needs, it's important for her to know that other people—you included—have needs, too.

INCREASED SEPARATION ANXIETY

"We've left our baby with a sitter before. But now he makes a terrible fuss if he sees us getting ready to go out, and we feel very guilty."

That's exactly what he's aiming to make you feel. Next to getting you to change your mind entirely and stay home, getting you to feel guilty about going out is his primary objective. And though you should remain understanding throughout his desperate attempts at mommy and daddy manipulation, you should also try not to let him succeed at it. Heightened separation anxiety is normal at this stage of development, and is rarely a result of anything parents have or haven't done—as many parents dealing with this problem fear it might be. It's due partly to the fact that your child now has a much better memory. He recalls what your putting on your coat, picking up your handbag, and going "bye-bye" without him means, and he's able to anticipate that you will be gone for some indefinite length of time when you walk out the door. And in fact, if you haven't left him with a sitter often in the past, he may have some doubt that you'll return.

But although the guilt baby has succeeded in burdening his parents with may last the whole evening, the histrionics that created it generally subside soon after the goodbyes are over, the door is shut, and the baby realizes that further carrying on will be futile.

To minimize baby's upset and your guilt, and to maximize his adjustment to being left with a sitter, follow these steps before stepping out:

■ Make sure you're leaving your baby with a sitter who not only is reliable, but also will be understanding, patient, responsive, and loving, no matter how difficult he becomes.

■ Have the sitter arrive at least fifteen minutes before you're planning to leave (earlier if it's her first time sitting for your baby), so that the two of them can get involved in an activity (crayoning, watching Sesame Street, looking out the window, building with blocks, putting dolly to bed) while you're still bustling around. Don't worry if your baby refuses to have anything to do with the sitter while you're still home; this is a shrewd child telling his parents he won't accept substitutes. Once you've left, he'll almost certainly consent to her advances.

■ Give your baby advance notice of your departure. If you try to avoid a scene this time by sneaking out of the house while he's not looking, he may begin to fear that you'll leave without warning at any time and respond with excessive clinginess. Instead, tell him ten to fifteen minutes before you leave that you'll be going out. Give him more time than that and he might forget, less and he won't have a chance to adjust.

■ Make a happy ritual out of leaving, with a hug and kiss from both of you. But don't prolong the goodbyes, or make them overly sentimental. Keep a smile on your face, even if he's tearful—and try to look as if you're taking it all in stride. If there's a window, he can watch you leave; ask the sitter to take him there so you can wave to him.

■ If your baby is crying when you leave, be comforting. Instead of telling him to be grown-up and not to cry, tell him that you understand that he'll miss you and that you'll miss him, too.

■ Reassure him you'll be back. "See you later, alligator" is a good light phrase to use that he can begin to associate with your leaving and coming back. And one day he'll be able to respond happily with "After a while, crocodile."

If your baby screams for the entire time you're gone, consider that you may have the wrong baby-sitter, that you may not be giving your baby enough reassurance and attention when you're with him, or that you may need to give him some extra help adjusting to your going out. To do the latter, begin by leaving your baby with someone he knows well, for fifteen minutes at a time, on several occasions. Once he's confident that you will return, he may be comfortable enough with these short outings to be ready for longer ones. Increase the time you spend away by fifteen-minute increments until you can stay away for several hours at a time.

NONVERBAL LANGUAGE

"Our little girl says very few words, but seems to have developed a system of sign language. Could her hearing be bad?"

It probably isn't that your child's hearing is bad, but that her resourcefulness is good. As long as your child seems to understand what you say and tries to imitate sounds, even unsuccessfully, her hearing is almost certainly normal. Her use of sign language or other, more primitive, ways of expressing needs and thoughts (such as grunting) is merely an inventive way of coping with a temporary handicap: a limited comprehensible vocabulary. Some children simply have more difficulty forming words at this age than others; for many the difficulty continues, usually well into their preschool years and sometimes into kindergarten and first grade. They may be saying "wove" for "love" or "toof" for "tooth" when most of their age mates are speaking very clearly.

To compensate for the inability to communicate verbally, many of these children develop their own forms of language. Some, like your child, are good at talking with their hands. They point to what they want, and push away what they don't. A wave is bye-bye, a finger pointed up is up, a finger pointed down is down. They may bark to indicate a dog, point to their nose to "say" elephant or to their ears for rabbit. Some hum songs to communicate: "Rock-abye baby" when they are sleepy, "Rain Rain Go Away" when it's pouring out, the Sesame Street theme when they want to watch TV.

Since this takes a lot of creativity and a strong desire to communicate—both good qualities to cultivate—you should do your best to decipher your child's special language and to show her you do understand. But don't forget that the ultimate goal is real speech. When she hums a lullaby, say, "Do you want to go to sleep?" When she points to the milk, respond, "You'd like a glass of milk? Okay." And if she points to her ears when she sees a rabbit in her storybook, reply, "Very good. That's a rabbit. A rabbit has long ears."

If, however, she doesn't seem to hear you calling from behind her or from another room, or to understand simple commands, then you should ask the doctor about testing her hearing.

GENDER DIFFERENCES

"We're trying very hard not to raise our children in a sexist way. But we find that no matter how we try, we can't induce our eleven-month-old son to be nurturing with dolls—he prefers to throw them against a wall."

You're making the same discovery that many well-meaning parents, determined to avoid molding their offspring into home-made sexual stereotypes, make. Sexual equality is an ideal whose time has come, but sexual sameness is an idea whose time can never come—at least as long as Mother Nature continues to have some say in the matter. Boys and girls, it appears, are, for the most part, molded in the womb, not in the playroom and backyard.

The differences between the sexes, scientists now believe, begin in the uterus when sex hormones such as testosterone and estradiol begin to be produced. Male fetuses receive more of the former and females more of the latter. This apparently makes for somewhat different brain development and different strengths and approaches to life.

Though much more work needs to be done before scientists can spell out all the differences precisely, we are aware of some differences that exist from birth on. Even before they've come home from the hospital, girls may focus longer on faces, particularly talking faces. Girls react more to touch, pain, and noise; boys react more to visual stimuli. Girls are more sensitive, but are more easily soothed and comforted; boys tend to cry more and be more irritable. These differences, of course, apply for groups of boys and girls and not necessarily for individuals; some girls may have more "masculine" traits than some boys, and some boys more "feminine" traits than some girls.

It's also apparent early on that boys have more muscle mass, larger lungs and hearts, and a lower sensitivity to pain, while girls have more body fat, a different shape to their pelvises, and a different way of processing oxygen in their muscles, giving them less stamina than boys later in life. Girl babies, however, are definitely not the weaker sex—they tend from the start to be healthier and hardier than boys.

As physical development progresses, it becomes clear that most boys are more physically active than most girls. Girls generally show more interest in people, boys in things—which may be why girls like dolls and dress-up play, while boys prefer trucks and fire engines. Girls acquire language skills earlier and faster, possibly because, as a result of the hormonal environment in the uterus, both hemispheres of their brains are similar in size and function in harmony. Boys, on the other hand, are better at tasks that require spatial and mechanical skills, possibly because their right hemispheres are more developed than their left. Interestingly, though, boys are as kind as girls, even as infants, and girls are no more fearful than boys, though they may show their fears more readily—probably a learned trait.

By the time children play with others (at this age they engage in parallel play), it becomes clear that, in general, boys are much more aggressive both physically and verbally, while girls are more compliant. Boys come to like group play, girls one-on-one. In school, girls continue to excel in language areas (spelling, reading comprehension, vocabulary, creative writing) and boys in spatial skills (depth perception, solving mazes and geometric puzzles, map reading) and in math in the teen years (though it's not clear whether this is the result of nature or nurture). Girls tend to mature earlier—though there is overlap.

Psychological and emotional differences become more obvious as children grow. Boys are more vulnerable psychologically—it's they who are more likely to have difficulty handling a parental divorce. Moral development also seems to differ: boys appear to make moral judgments on the basis of justice and law, while girls make them on the basis of caring.

Does the fact that most girls dote on dolls while most boys career around with trucks mean that their destinies are preordained? Partly, yes—girls will grow up to be women and boys will grow up to be men. But much in their attitudes will depend on the attitudes their parents display and on the examples they set. You can raise children who are not "sexist" in their points of view, who have respect for both males and females, who enjoy being the gender they were born into, who will choose their future life roles not on the basis of stereotypes (of any kind), but on the basis of their own personal strengths and desires. Following these tips will help you meet those goals:

■ Remember that the fact that there are innate differences between males and females in no way means that one sex is in any way better or worse, stronger or weaker. Differences are enriching, sameness is stultifying. Pass this attitude on to your children.

■ Treat your children as individuals. While as a group men have more muscles and are more aggressive than women, there are some women who have more muscle and are more aggressive than some men. If you have a daughter who has more "male" traits or a son with more "female" ones, don't berate or belittle them. Accept, love, and support your child as he or she is.[5]

■ Modify extremes. Accepting your child as he or she is doesn't mean never using

your good sense to make some alterations. If a child is overly aggressive, you should teach him to tone the aggression down. If, on the other hand, he is overly passive, you can encourage assertiveness.

■ Select toys not because you're trying to either make or break a stereotype, but because you truly believe your child will enjoy them and benefit from them. If a child uses a toy differently from the way you expect (boys and girls will use the same toys in different ways, and even within each sex the use will vary), accept that.

■ Don't fall unconsciously into sexist traps. Don't tell your sobbing toddler not to cry because he's a big boy and then cuddle his sister when she's tearful. Don't limit your compliments to a daughter to "How pretty you look," and to a son to "Oh, how strong you are," or "What a big boy you are." Say these things, by all means, when appropriate. But also compliment a boy on his being sweet to his sister, and a girl for throwing a ball well. Do this not because you're trying to switch your children's sex roles—you're not—but because a child's personality is made up of many facets, all of which need nurturing.

■ Try to avoid making value judgments about different types of skills or roles in life. If, for example, you give your children the impression that child care is a job that commands low respect, neither boys nor girls will come to value it as adults. If you give them the idea that going to an office to work is somehow more worthwhile than working as a full-time parent or working in a non-office environment, they won't value the latter choices, either.

■ Apportion family chores according to abilities, interests, and time, rather than according to a preconceived stereotype or in order to break such a stereotype. That means the best cook should do most of the cooking (the other partner can do the dishes and clean up) and the best bookkeeper should balance the checkbook. If one parent has a less time-consuming job or no work outside the home at all, that parent should

5. Boys who display feminine traits early in childhood, like to play with dolls, and avoid rough sports are more likely to become homosexual in later life if their parents (particularly fathers) try to force them to "be a man," either through teasing, subtle pressure, withdrawal of affection, or physical punishment. These boys become estranged from their fathers and, it is speculated, may ever hunger for male love and companionship in adulthood. If a child seems truly unhappy with his or her sexual assignment and doesn't enjoy playing with children of the same sex, professional consultation may be a good idea.

spend more time with the children and the other parent should make spending time with the children, whenever possible, a priority. Jobs no one wants to do can be rotated, apportioned by agreement, or relegated on the spur of the moment ("Honey, can you take out the garbage, please?") but this latter system can fail miserably unless it's carefully monitored (as when nobody takes out the garbage).

■ Set an example. Decide which qualities in both males and females you and your husband value most and try to cultivate them in yourselves as well as in your children. Be a model of the sex roles you want to see your children adopt. Giving a little boy dolls to play with can be much less effective in teaching him to be nurturing than giving him a daddy who is nurturing himself. Having a bat and ball can be much less effective in encouraging a little girl to develop her physical aptitude than having a mother who jogs daily. Young children develop their gender identity partly through play with those of their own sex and partly through identification with the parent of the same sex; if you're unsure of what your sex role is, they may be, too.

SWITCHING TO A BED

"We're expecting a second baby in six months. When and how should we switch our son from his crib to a bed?"

Whether or not your child is ready for a bed depends more on his age and size than on whether or not there's a new sibling on the way. The generally accepted rule: if a child is 36 inches tall or can climb out of a crib on his own, he's ready for a bed. Some particularly agile children can climb out of a crib before they reach the 36-inch cutoff; others, less adventurous, may never even try.

If you feel your older child isn't yet ready for a bed, and that he may not be even once the new baby arrives, buy him a new crib that converts into a youth bed. This way you can move him to the new crib now, so he won't feel displaced by the baby later on. When he meets the criteria for the youth bed or seems mature enough for it, simply convert his crib. Be prepared for the possibility of his climbing out of bed in the middle of the night by keeping his door closed or gated and by keeping his room as child-safe by night as by day, free of such hazards as open windows and electric fans within the reach of small hands. If you are afraid you won't hear him from your own bedroom, install an intercom to signal you of activity in his room. For restless sleepers who tend to topple out of bed, a guard rail is a good precaution.

If your firstborn can understand, tell him you are going to get him a special new bed. Add a strategic, "The baby won't be able to sleep in it because it's a big-boy bed." Have him participate in its selection, if this is possible, or if you plan on transferring him to a bed you already have, let him choose new linens and blankets. Make an occasion of the move to the new bed, supplying a festively wrapped new toy or doll for company in it and perhaps a few "grown-up" decorative touches for the room, along with plenty of pomp and circumstance. Ideally, you should then take the crib down for a few weeks, not readying it until the new baby arrives or at least not much more than two weeks before the due date. This way the older child will feel less directly displaced. The new baby can sleep in a carriage, cradle, or bassinet for the first few weeks, giving your toddler even more time to adjust to the change. When it's time for the crib takeover, explain to your older child that it's time to get out the baby crib for his new brother or sister ("Remember when you were a baby, and you slept in the crib?"). Don't ask his permission to use it; if he says "no," you will have a major problem. Do ask him to help you attach some toys to the crib for the baby, and perhaps to help select some pictures or other decorations for the baby's room or corner.

WATCHING TV

"I feel very guilty because I have begun turning on Sesame Street for my baby when I start to prepare dinner. She seems to love it, but I'm concerned she'll become addicted to TV."

That's a sound concern. According to the Nielsen Index, children two to twelve years of age watch an average of 25 hours of television a week. If your daughter becomes one of these, she will have spent 15,000 hours glued to the set by the time she graduates high school—about 4,000 hours more than she will have spent in school. And if her viewing isn't carefully screened, she will, research suggests, have witnessed 18,000 murders, countless other crimes from robberies and rapes to bombings and beatings, and more casual sex than you could imagine (13.5 suggestive moments an hour). She will also have been the innocent target of 350,000 commercials trying to sell her (and through her, you) products of dubious value.

Excessive TV viewing by children has other drawbacks. It's linked to obesity and poor school performance. And because it can reduce interaction among familiy members, it can interfere with family life. Perhaps worst of all, it creates a picture of the world that is distorted and inaccurate, and confuses a child's developing value system by establishing norms of behavior and belief that are not accepted in the real world.

The TV problem for parents is compounded by the fact that television in the U.S. presents almost no decent programming for children (cartoons, usually violent, and sitcom reruns are the standard fare). Public television programming is often a notable exception, with its worthy goal of teaching such positive attributes as self-control, sharing, cooperation, racial tolerance, and kindness toward others. But even it is not usually recommended for children under 10 months, for whom a tele-vision screen is believed to be nothing more than a confusing and hypnotic montage of lights and colors; they have no inkling of what is going on.

When your toddler does seem to be ready for some television (she jumps up and down when Big Bird comes on the screen or claps her hands excitedly when she hears the Sesame Street theme, for example), limit her viewing to a single, non-commercial show of redeeming value. Even when she's older, television viewing should be limited. Such restrictions may be hard to enforce, however, if either you or someone else in the family watches TV all day long. A young child's attention span is usually very short, so she may watch only a brief segment before losing interest, or she may watch in spurts. But if the TV is on all the time, she'll think that's the way it's supposed to be and miss it when the screen is blank. Try to keep the television off during mealtimes, especially during the family dinner hour, or much time for family interaction will be lost to the monotonous, mesmerizing effect of the tube.

Resist as much as possible (realistically, you won't always be able to) the temptation to use the TV as a convenient baby-minder. Instead, watch TV with your baby and participate in the viewing by pointing out familiar objects, animals, and people, and by explaining what's going on. When your child is older, expand these explanation-and-discussion sessions. If your child's TV time is your time to get things done, try to get them done in view of the set so that you'll be able to throw in occasional comments.

Rather than relying on TV as the only audiovisual entertainment for your toddler, turn to audio tapes and records for stimulating her imagination and providing plenty of musical activity as well. And supplement with quality video tapes (Disney classics are popular during the second year and beyond), which allow you more control over when and what your child views and, like public television, are commercial-free.

HYPERACTIVITY

"My daughter is on the go all day long— crawling, walking, climbing, always moving. I'm afraid she may turn out to be hyperactive."

Observing the frenetic pace that the average toddler sets, it's easy to see why so many mothers of one-year-olds share the concern that their child is hyperactive. Yet the vast majority have nothing to worry about. What seems an abnormally high activity level to someone relatively inexperienced with toddlers is much more likely to be a normal one. After many months of frustration, the mobility your child struggled so hard to attain is finally hers. It's no wonder that she's off and running (or toddling, or crawling, or climbing) every chance she gets. As far as she's concerned, the day's too short for all the expeditions she wants to take.

True hyperactivity—officially labeled "Attention Deficit Disorder with Hyperactivity (ADD)" and ten times more common in boys than in girls—is characterized by excessive activity that is both inappropriate and unproductive, by a very brief attention span, and by impulsiveness. As any parent knows, these qualities are common among all young toddlers; but it is only when they are exaggerated to the point that they interfere with functioning that a problem is signaled.

If worrisome hyperactive behavior continues and your child's attention span doesn't grow as she does, do speak to her doctor; there are several approaches to controlling true hyperactivity that can help. Since ADD is occasionally associated with mental retardation, brain damage, hearing loss, or emotional difficulties, these problems should be ruled out before treatment begins.

In the meantime, do be sure your child gets adequate amounts of rest—an overtired child tends to speed up rather than slow down. Entice her into quiet activities (such as reading books, doing puzzles, and sorting shapes), but keep in mind her normally short attention span and remember that, at this age, such play usually requires adult participation. Try a warm bath to calm her when she seems to be getting out of control. Also be sure she is well nourished and that she's not getting a high-sugar diet—the evidence isn't conclusive, but a small percentage of children may react to sugar, and possibly some other foods, food dyes, and additives, with hyperactive behavior.

NEGATIVISM

"Ever since my son learned to shake his head and say 'No,' he's been responding negatively to everything—even to things I'm sure he wants."

Congratulations—your baby is becoming a toddler. And with this transition comes the beginning of a behavior pattern you're going to see a lot more of, with increasing intensity, in the next year or so: negativism.

As hard as it is on parents, negativism is a normal and healthy part of a young child's development. For the first time, he's able to be his own person rather than your malleable baby, to exert some power, test his limits, and challenge parental authority. Most importantly, he's able to express opinions of his very own clearly and distinctly. And the opinion, he's discovered, that has the most impact is "no!"

Fortunately, at this stage of negativism, your child isn't likely to mean "no" as fiercely as he expresses it. In fact, he's often likely not to mean it at all—as when he says "no" to the banana he was just clamoring for, or shakes his head when you offer the ride on the swing that you know he really wants. Like pulling up or taking steps, learning how to say "no" and how to shake his head are skills—and he needs to practice them, even when they're not appropriate. That babies invariably shake their heads "no" long before they shake their heads "yes" has less to do with negativism than with the fact that it's a less complex, more easily executed movement, which requires less coordination.

Negativism can sometimes be avoided with a little clever verbal manipulation on your part; if you don't want to hear a "no," don't ask a question that can be answered with one. Instead of "Do you want an apple?" try "Would you like an apple or a banana?" Instead of "Do you want to go on the slide?" ask "Would you like to go on the slide or the swing?" Be aware, however, that some children will answer even multiple-choice questions with a "no."

Occasionally, a twelve-month-old will even act out a primitive version of the "terrible-twos" tantrum. These are usually laughable, though laughing at them (or at the vigorous use of "no" and of head shaking) will only prolong the behavior and encourage repetition. Though it won't work later on (an older toddler can keep a tantrum going full steam until he—or his parent—drops), ignoring a year-old baby's tirade will usually result in his giving up the struggle and sheepishly picking himself up to go play with a toy.

The "no's" will probably have it in your household for at least another year—and they'll probably intensify before they taper off. The best way to weather this stormy period is to pay little mind to negative behavior; the more you fuss over baby's "no's," the more "no's" you'll hear. Keeping negativism in perspective while keeping your sense of humor may not help check the "no's," but it may aid your ability to cope with them.

WHAT IT'S IMPORTANT TO KNOW:
Stimulating the Toddler

First words. First steps. With these two feathers in the toddler's cap, or nearly so, the learning game becomes more exciting than ever before. The world is growing by leaps and bounds; give your toddler a chance to explore and learn about it, and promote his or her continued physical, social, intellectual, and emotional development, by offering the following:

Safe space to walk in—both indoors and out. The rookie walker usually objects to being strapped in a stroller or back pack, so use these only when absolutely necessary. Encourage baby to walk as often as possible, but keep an eagle eye out for dangers, especially near streets, roads, and driveways. For the baby who isn't quite walking yet, put some enticing objects up out of reach, to provide incentive for pulling up and/or cruising.

Safe space for supervised climbing. Babies love to climb steps (when you're not supervising, a gate is a must), clamber up a slide (stay right behind, just in case), maneuver onto a low chair or off the bed. Let them—but stand by and be ready to come to the rescue if need be.

Encouragement to be physically active. The inactive baby may need a little cajoling to become more active. You may need to get down and crawl yourself and challenge such a child to come crawling or running after you ("Try and catch me!") or feign a threatening "I'm gonna' get you" to encourage baby's moving away from you. Put toys or other favorite objects out of reach and encourage some sort of locomotion to retrieve them. The fearful baby may need some moral—and physical—support. Try to persuade such a baby to try, but don't

SAFETY REMINDER

Your baby is getting smarter all the time—but it will be a long while before judgment catches up with intelligence and motor skills. So as baby enters the second year of life, be sure to continue your constant vigilance as well as all the safety precautions you have already put into effect, and then some—taking into account the fact that your toddler can now, or will soon be able to, climb with great skill. This means that virtually nothing in your home that is not behind lock and key or safety latch is safe from tiny hands—and that baby can get into even more trouble even faster than before. So do a second safety inventory, taking stock not only of those things that your toddler can reach from the floor, but also anything he or she could conceivably get to by climbing, and remove any hazards as well as anything you want to protect from baby. And be forewarned that toddlers have been known to show great resourcefulness in getting at what they want, piling up books or pulling a chair or toy over to reach a shelf they want to get to, for example. Also be sure that anything baby might climb on—chairs, tables, shelves—is sturdy enough to hold his or her weight. Continue setting limits ("No, you can't climb on that"), but don't, just yet, depend on your young child to remember today's prohibition tomorrow.

ever force the issue or belittle him or her for not trying. Climb up and slide down the slide with a timid child until he or she is comfortable enough to go it alone. Stroll with the tentative walker, lending a hand (or two) for support. Go on a "big kid" swing together until your little kid is willing to risk the "baby" swing solo.

A varied environment. The baby who sees nothing but the inside of his or her own home, the family car, and the supermarket is going to be a very bored baby (not to mention how bored the caretaker will be). There's an exciting world outside the door, and your baby should see it daily. Even going out in the rain or snow (barring flooding or blizzard conditions) can be a learning experience. Give your baby a tour of area playgrounds, parks, museums (toddlers are usually fascinated by paintings and statues; on slow days, roomy galleries are terrific arenas for toddling or crawling), toy stores (where supervision is essential), restaurants (pick those that welcome children), pet shops, and shopping malls or other busy business areas with lots of store windows to peer into and lots of people to see.

Pull-and-push toys. Toys that need to be pushed or pulled provide practice for those who've just begun to walk, and confidence (and physical support) for those just tottering on the brink. Riding toys babies can sit astride and propel with their feet may help some children walk, though others find walking independently easier. The use of a walker at this stage, on the other hand, will hinder, not help.

Creative materials. Scribbling with crayons provides tremendous satisfaction for many year-old babies. Taping the paper to a table, the floor, or an easel will keep it from sliding all over, and confiscating the crayons as soon as they are applied where they shouldn't be or if baby decides to chew on one will help teach their proper use. Don't allow pens and pencils, except under close supervision, since the sharp points can spell disaster if baby falls on either one. Finger painting can be fun for some, while others are uncomfortable with the muddy fingers that are an occupational hazard of the art. Though hand washing demonstrates that the condition is only temporary, some children continue resisting the medium. Musical toys can be fun, too—but look for those with fairly good quality sound. Baby can also learn to improvise musically, with a wooden or metal spoon on a pot bottom, for instance, if you demonstrate first.

Putting-and-taking toys. Babies love to put things in and take them out although the latter skill develops before the former. You can buy putting-and-taking toys, or just use objects around the house such as empty boxes, wooden spoons, measuring cups, paper cups and plates, and napkins. Fill a basket with a variety of small items (but not small enough for baby to mouth and choke on) for starters. Be ready to do most of the putting in until baby becomes much more proficient. Sand (see page 239; in the house, many parents prefer to use raw rice) and water (you can limit its indoor use to the tub and baby's high chair) allow for putting in and taking out in the form of pouring—and most toddlers love both materials, but they require constant supervision.

Shape sorters. Usually long before babies can say circle, square, or triangle, they have learned to recognize these shapes and can put them in the proper opening in a shape-sorter toy. These toys also teach manual dexterity and, in some cases, colors. Be aware, however, that baby may need many demonstrations and much assistance before mastery of shape sorters is achieved.

Dexterity toys. Toys that require turning, twisting, pushing, pressing, and pulling encourage children to use their hands in a variety of ways. Many parental demonstrations may be needed before babies are able to handle some of the more complicated maneuvers, but once mastered, these toys provide hours of concentrated play.

Bath toys for water play. These teach many concepts, and allow the joy of water play without a mess all over the floor or furniture. The tub is also a good place for blowing bubbles—but you'll probably have to do the blowing yourself for a while yet.

Follow-the-leader play. Daddy starts clapping, then mommy. Baby is encouraged to follow suit. Then daddy flaps his arms, and mommy does, too. After a while, baby will follow the leader without prodding, and eventually will be able to take the lead.

Books, magazines, anything with pictures. You can't have a live horse, elephant, and lion in your living room—but you can have all of them, and more, visit your home in a book or magazine. Look at and read books with your baby several times during the day. Each session will probably be short, maybe no more than few minutes, because of your child's limited attention span, but together they will build a firm foundation for later enjoyment of reading.

Materials for pretend play. Toy dishes, kitchen equipment, pretend food, play houses, trucks and cars, hats, grown-ups' shoes, sofa cushions—almost anything can be magically transformed in an imaginative toddler's world of make-believe. This kind of play develops social skills as well as small motor coordination (putting on and taking off clothing, scrambling eggs or cooking soup), creativity, and imagination.

Patience. Though the skills babies on the brink of toddlerhood display are much advanced over what they were at six months, their attention spans haven't expanded very much. They may be able to play with some toys for extended periods, but when you try to read a story or involve them with other toys, they may not be able to sit still for much longer than five minutes. Be understanding of these limitations, and don't despair—as babies grow, so do their attention spans.

Applause. Cheer your baby on as new skills are mastered. Achievement, while satisfying, often means more when accompanied by recognition.

PART TWO

Of Special Concern

CHAPTER SIXTEEN

A Baby for All Seasons

Unless you're raising your baby in a climate-controlled plastic bubble, the vagaries of weather will have some impact on your lives. As the seasons change, and as sun, wind, heat, cold, snow, and rain come and go with them, a wide range of new questions arise in the minds of parents—particularly first-timers. Questions about feeding, dressing, and playing, about sunburn and frostbite, about window screens and fireplace screens, about swimming lessons and holiday decorations.

Feeding Your Baby: 'Round the Calendar

Your baby's nutritional needs are pretty much the same year-round, but seasonal temperature extremes do dictate some variations:

In cold weather. If your baby spends a lot of time outdoors in cold weather, extra calories are needed to fuel the body to provide extra heat. And because during the chillier months babies aren't exposed to much direct sunlight, you need to be sure enough vitamin D comes from the diet, either in the form of fortified formula, milk, and other dairy products or, for babies who are getting almost all of their milk from the breast, in a multiple vitamin supplement.[1] A switch to comfortably warm (never hot) cereals may be more satisfying than a cold breakfast on wintry mornings. Most children, however, will

---

1. Your baby's doctor may recommend year-round vitamin D supplementation, since too much exposure to the sun's rays is inadvisable, especially for infants.

still prefer drinking milk or formula cold, which is best anyway since heating destroys some of the nutrients. To keep the immune system strong, and ensure that those illnesses that do strike don't strike hard, provide your baby with plenty of vitamin A via green leafy and yellow vegetables and yellow fruits and vitamin C through vitamin C foods (see page 221).

In warm weather. In the summer, or in an ever-warm climate, your baby will sweat more and may feel like eating less. To compensate for the fluids lost through perspiration, increase fluid intake. For the very young baby, offer water frequently between feedings of breast milk (if a bottle is taken; if it isn't, nurse more frequently) or formula. For older children, add diluted fruit juices in bottles or cups, and once they've been introduced, juicy fruits such as melons, peaches, and tomatoes. Do not serve drinks that are sweetened with sugar, such as sodas, juice drinks, or punches, since they increase thirst (and are inappropriate for babies, anyway), or drinks that contain added salt (such as special athletic drinks),

since contrary to popular theory, large quantities of sodium are not only unnecessary in hot weather, they can be harmful.

To overcome a heat-dampened appetite, do not feed your baby immediately after coming inside on a hot day. Allow time to cool off first, then if possible, feed baby in a room that is air-conditioned or cooled by a fan. If solids have been introduced, serve smaller meals and larger snacks when baby doesn't seem to want to eat a lot at any one time, and stick to favorite fare. Provide foods that are nutrition dense (such as carrots, cantaloupe, mango, broccoli, cheese) and avoid empty-calorie items. Sprinkle wheat germ on cereals, desserts, and pastas, or stir it into juice or a milk shake if your baby doesn't seem to be taking enough grain foods. If milk or formula is being rejected in favor of juices, ensure calcium intake by adding nonfat dry or whole evaporated milk to cereals and desserts, serving cubes of cheese at snack time, making homemade frozen desserts (see page 626) and serving commercial juice-sweetened ice cream, which will cool, refresh, delight, and provide plenty of nutrition.

WHAT YOU MAY BE CONCERNED ABOUT IN SUMMER OR SUMMERY WEATHER

KEEPING BABY COOL

It's summertime—and the dressing is easy. Or is it? A common sight: a mother in sundress and sandals, hair lifted off her neck in a cooling pony tail, pushing a carriage holding an infant dressed for an arctic winter. What such well-intentioned mothers fail to realize is that in warm weather babies, even very new babies, needn't be dressed any more warmly than adults. Not only is adding extra clothing unnecessary, it can lead to undesirable consequences such as prickly heat and, in extreme cases, heatstroke.

Unless you've got an unreliable personal thermostat (you're always warm when everyone else is cool, or you're always cool when everyone else is warm), feel free to dress your baby as you would yourself. If you're comfortable in shorts and a tank top, your baby will be fine in the junior equivalent. If you're sweltering in a sweater, your baby will be, too. Lightweight, loose-fitting, light-colored clothing will be most comfortable when temperatures soar; a lightweight porous cap, hat, or bonnet will protect baby's head without overheating it. Materials should be absorbent to soak up perspiration, but when clothing becomes damp, it should be changed—so routinely carry along an extra set of clothes for baby. Don't use a baby carrier constructed of heavyweight fabric that totally covers baby, head to toe. Lack of ventilation in combination with your body warmth and a high outdoor temperature could add up to excessive heat within the confines of the carrier. If baby is to be in direct sun, protection from its damaging rays needs to be considered in selecting clothes.

Indoors in hot weather, your baby will enjoy the cooling effects of an air conditioner or fan as much as you do. Just be sure neither blows directly on the baby, that the room temperature doesn't drop much below 72°F, and that cooling equipment and its electrical cords are out of baby's reach. A diaper alone will do for sleeping on hot nights, but a lightweight sleeper and, possibly, a light cover may be needed if the air conditioner is running.

Cool hands or feet are not a sign that your baby is chilly; but perspiration (check the neck, head, underarms) is a sign of being too warm.

HEATSTROKE

Though mothers commonly worry about their babies being too cold, they often don't realize that being too hot can be just as dangerous. In the first year of life babies are particularly susceptible to heat because their temperature-regulatory systems aren't yet perfected and it's difficult for them to cool themselves effectively. As a result, overheating can lead to serious, even fatal, heatstroke. Heatstroke typically comes on suddenly. Signs to watch for include hot and dry (or, occasionally, moist) skin, very high fever, diarrhea, agitation or lethargy, confusion, convulsions, and loss of consciousness. Should your baby exhibit such symptoms, summon emergency medical help immediately and follow the first aid procedures on page 443.

As with most other medical emergencies, the best treatment is prevention. You can prevent heatstroke in these ways:

■ Never leave an infant or child in a parked auto in hot weather. Even with the windows open, the interior temperature can rise rapidly and dangerously. When the outdoor temperature is 96°F, for example, temperatures in the car can shoot up to more than 105°F within fifteen minutes with the windows rolled halfway down, and to nearly 150°F if the windows are closed.

■ Don't bundle up a baby who has a fever with blankets or heating pads. A child with a fever needs cooling down, not heating up. "Sweating it out" is not a recommended treatment in any type of weather.

■ Dress baby lightly in hot weather, and avoid direct sunlight. Beware of overheating in a baby carrier.

■ Always be sure that your child gets extra fluids in hot weather.

■ Limit outdoor exercise for active toddlers in very hot or humid weather to no more than thirty minutes at a stretch, preferably in the shade.

TOO MUCH SUN

There was a time when we considered youngsters who were tanned brown as berries, frolicking in the hot sun of a summer afternoon, healthy; "sickly" children were those who were pale from too much time spent indoors. The sun's rays, we believed, were as wholesome as apple pie and as restorative as chicken soup. Unfortunately, we were wrong. As we now know, nothing is more likely to cause skin cancer (including the potentially fatal melanoma), brown spots, and premature wrinkling and aging of the skin later in life. Though a tan looks "healthy," it's actually a sign of injury to the skin and is that sensitive organ's way of trying to protect itself against further damage.

Excessive exposure to the sun's rays has also been strongly linked to the development of cataracts (they are much more common in sunny climes), and has recently been found to reduce body levels of beta-carotene (a substance in the body believed to be protective against cancer). If that's not enough to make you take a dim view of bright sunshine, consider this: it can also precipitate certain other diseases, or make them worse, among them herpes simplex and some other viral skin diseases; vitiligo (white, or depigmented, spots on the skin); PKU; and photosensitive eczema. And for those taking certain antibiotics (such as tetracycline) or other medications, it can cause serious side effects. A pretty long rap sheet for an all-purpose panacea.

At least a few minutes of direct sunshine a day *was* once crucial to healthy growth and development in childhood—for it was the only available source of vitamin D, needed for building strong bones. Today, infant formulas, all milk, and many other dairy products are fortified with the vitamin, and it is also found in baby vitamin supplements; you needn't sacrifice the future of your children's skin to ensure them the required dose of vitamin D.

To be certain your baby doesn't suffer the consequences of too much sun, keep in mind the following sun-safety facts and sun-safety tips.

Sun-Safety Facts:

■ The sun's intensity is greatest, thus its rays most dangerous, between 10 A.M. and 3 P.M. (or 11 A.M. and 4 P.M. daylight savings time).

■ Fully 80% of the sun's radiation penetrates cloud cover; so protection is needed on hot, cloudy days as well as on clear ones.

■ Water and sand reflect the sun's rays, increasing the risk of skin damage and the need for protection.

■ Wet skin allows more ultraviolet rays to penetrate than dry skin—so extra protection is needed in the water.

■ The shade of sun umbrellas and trees is not reliable protection against the sun's rays, particularly at the beach.

■ Extreme heat, wind, high altitude, and closeness to the equator also accentuate dangers of the sun's rays, so take extra precautions under such conditions.

■ Snow on the ground can reflect enough of the sun's rays on a bright day to cause a sunburn.

■ Infants are particularly susceptible to sunburn because of their thin skin. A single episode of severe sunburn during infancy or childhood doubles the risk of the most deadly of skin cancers, malignant melanoma. And even seemingly innocent tanning without burning in the early years has been linked to basal cell and squamous cell carcinomas, the most common types of skin cancer, as well as to premature aging of the skin. The sun is believed responsible for at least 90% of all skin cancers, most of which could have been prevented.

■ Fair-skinned individuals with light eyes and hair are most susceptible, but no one is immune from the hazardous effects of the sun's rays.

■ There is no such thing as a safe tan, no matter how gradually acquired. Nor does a base tan protect the skin from further damage.

■ The nose, lips, and ears are the parts of the body most susceptible to sun damage.

Sun-Safety Tips:

■ Avoid exposing babies under six months to strong sunlight, particularly at the height of the sun's intensity in summer or in climates that are warm year-round. Protect these young infants with a sunshade or parasol on strollers or carriages, but do not use a sunscreen without a doctor's okay.

■ At least fifteen (but preferably thirty) minutes before exposing an older baby or young child to the sun, apply sunscreen to all areas of the body not covered by clothing—though a dark-skinned child can tolerate brief exposures without sun protection. Avoid getting sunscreen into baby's mouth or eyes, or on the eyelids. For extra protection on very sensitive areas, such as lips, nose, and ears, ask the doctor about using a sun-blocking lip balm or stick, or zinc oxide.

■ Initial exposures to the sun should be no more than a few minutes, and can gradually be increased, by a couple of minutes a day, up to twenty minutes.

■ Once your baby is six months old, carry a sunscreen in your diaper bag in case you should need it unexpectedly.

■ In the sun, all babies and children should wear light hats with brims to protect eyes and face, and shirts to protect the upper body, even when they're in the water. Clothing should be of lightweight, tightly woven fabrics. Two thin layers may protect better than one, since the sun's rays can pass through some fabrics—but be wary of overdressing.

■ During hot weather, try to schedule most outdoor activity for early morning or late afternoon. Keep children out of the midday sun whenever possible.

■ Apply waterproof sunscreen all over little ones who are cooling off under sprinklers or in wading or swimming pools. After water play, towel-dry, then reapply sunscreen.

■ Avoid artificial tanning devices such as sun lamps, since they, too, contribute to premature aging and skin cancer, and are inappropriate for babies.

■ If your child is taking any medication, be sure that it doesn't cause photosensitivity (increased sensitivity to sunlight) before allowing sun exposure.

■ Set a good example by protecting your

WHAT TO LOOK FOR IN SELECTING A SUNSCREEN

High SPF. Sunscreens are labeled with a sun protection factor, or SPF, from 2 to 30 (or rarely, as high as 50). The higher the number, the greater the protection. An SPF of at least 15 is recommended for babies and children, though a 30 is best for those with very fair or sensitive skin. Do not use tanning products on babies or children; they don't protect at all.

Effectiveness. Look for a product that contains ingredients that screen out both the short ultraviolet (UVB) rays of the sun that burn and can cause cancer as well as the longer ultraviolet (UVA) rays that tan, can cause long-term skin damage, and enhance the carcinogenic effects of the UVB rays.

Safety. Some sunscreen ingredients are irritating to or cause allergic reactions in some people, particularly infants with tender skins. Most common offenders are PABA (para-aminobenzoic acid) and forms of PABA (padimate O or octyl dimethyl PABA, for example), fragrances, and colorings. So test a product out with a 24-hour patch test before smearing it all over your baby. Apply a small amount of sunscreen to the inside of baby's arm and cover with a band-aid. Remove the band-aid 24 hours later, and expose the area to fifteen minutes of sunlight while the rest of the body is protected by a hat and clothing. If the test patch reddens or swells, try a different product. If, once you've begun using a product, your baby develops an itchy red rash or any other kind of skin reaction, or if his or her eyes seem irritated, try another product, preferably one that is designed for use by infants or is hypoallergenic.

Protection in the water. When your baby is going to be in the water, select a product that is waterproof (which means it will retain its effectiveness after four 20-minute dunkings) or water resistant (it will retain effectiveness after two such dunkings).

And remember, even with a sunscreen, exposure to the sun should be limited.

own skin from the ravages of the sun's rays.

Signs of Sunburn

Many parents assume their babies are fine in the sun as long as there is no reddening of the skin. Unfortunately, they're mistaken. You can't see sunburn when it's occurring, and when you do see it, it's too late. It's not until two to four hours following exposure that the skin becomes red, hot, and inflamed, and the color doesn't peak at lobster red until ten to fourteen hours after exposure. A bad sunburn will also blister and will be accompanied by localized pain and, in the most severe cases, headache, nausea, chills, and prostration. Redness usually starts to fade and symptoms diminish after 48 to 72 hours, at which point the skin, even in fairly mild cases, may start to peel. Occasionally, however, discomfort may continue for a week to ten days. See page 437 for tips on treating sunburn.

INSECT BITES

Though most insects are harmless, their bites and stings almost always cause pain or uncomfortable itching, and can occasionally transmit serious disease or cause a severe allergic reaction. So it makes sense to protect your baby from bugs and their bites whenever you can. (For treating insect bites, see page 435.)

Bite Protection

Bees and other stinging insects. Keep baby out of areas where bees congregate, such as clover or wildflower fields, fruit orchards, or near birdbaths. Protect baby even in your own backyard, especially on bright, warm days or after a heavy rain. If you discover a beehive or a wasp nest in or near your home, have it removed by an expert. To avoid attracting bees, dress your family for outdoor play in white or pastels rather than dark or bright colors or flowered prints. Don't use fragrant pow-

ders or lotions, cologne, or scented hair spray. Keep a light piece of fabric handy in your auto to trap insects.

Mosquitoes. They breed in water, so drain puddles, rain barrels, and other areas that collect water near your home. Keep baby indoors at night when mosquitoes swarm, and be sure windows are screened, and screens kept in good repair.

Deer ticks. Before outings in high tick areas, apply an insect repellent containing low concentrations (10% or less) of deet to clothing—*not* skin. Check family, pets, and gear frequently for the pinhead-size ticks. (They are easier to spot on light-colored clothing, and cling less to tight weaves.) To prevent Lyme disease, remove ticks promptly (see page 435).

All biting or stinging insects. Keep arms, legs, feet, and head covered in areas where such insects might be lurking. Where ticks are prevalent, tuck pants into socks.

SUMMER SAFETY

The arrival of summer signals a whole new set of accident possibilities. The following precautions will help minimize the chance that the possibilities will become realities:

■ Because warm weather often means open windows, be sure to install window guards on all windows in your home. Don't depend on screens, since they can be pushed out by a vigorous baby. If window guards aren't in place in your home, or where you're visiting, open windows no more than 6 inches (and be sure they can't be pushed open farther), or open them only from the top. Don't put furniture, or anything else a baby can climb, under windows.

■ Doors, too, are often left open in warm weather, inviting crawlers to crawl and toddlers to toddle out and into trouble. Be sure to keep all doors, including sliding doors and screens locked.

■ Out of doors, never take your eyes off the baby who can crawl or toddle, and be especially watchful around swings and other playground equipment. Be sure any equipment in your own backyard is at least 6 feet from fences or walls, and that there is protective surfacing (rubber, sand, sawdust, wood chips, or bark) under it. Always insist that your baby hold on with both hands when in a swing, sit in the center, and not try to get out unless it has stopped moving. Discourage head-first sliding down the slide, and teach your child to watch for other children at the bottom or top. Don't use metal slides in warm weather without feeling them first—in the sun they can get hot enough to cause burns.

■ Don't put baby down in deep grasses or anywhere there could possibly be poison ivy, poison oak, or poison sumac, or where he or she might get a hand on or nibble at other poisonous flowers, shrubs, or trees. When in wooded areas, be sure your baby is protected with cover-up clothing. If your baby accidentally has contact with poison ivy, oak, or sumac, remove all clothing while protecting your own hands with gloves or paper towels. Wash baby's skin thoroughly with soap (preferably yellow) and water immediately—wait five minutes and it may be too late to ward off a reaction. Anything else that might have touched the plants (clothing, stroller, even the dog) should be washed, too. Shoes should be swabbed with cleaning fluid. Should a reaction occur, apply calamine or another soothing lotion to relieve itching (see page 414).

■ Since warm weather also brings out the barbecues, take steps to protect babies from accidental burns. Keep grills out of reach of small hands; be sure there are no chairs or anything else on which a baby can climb to reach these hot attractions. Tabletop grills and hibachis should be placed only on stable surfaces. Remember that coals can stay hot for a long time. To reduce the risk of accidental burns, drench the coals with water when the cooking is complete, then dispose of them where your child can't get to them.

WATER BABIES

Parents, eager to "waterproof" their babies as well as to give them a competitive edge over their pint-size peers, are often enticed to enroll their babies in swim classes. But according to the American Academy of Pediatrics, as well as many other experts, swim classes are not a good idea for babies. Though it is easy to teach crawlers to float—young children float naturally because they have a higher proportion of body fat than adults—it isn't possible to teach them to use this skill in a life-threatening situation. Nor do infant swim lessons make children better swimmers in the long run than do lessons taken later on in childhood. There is, in fact, some question as to whether children under three can benefit at all from swimming classes. In addition, there has been some suggestion that such early exposure to public pools could increase the risk of such infections as diarrhea (because of germs swallowed along with pool water), swimmer's ear (because of water entering the ear) and swimmer's itch and other skin rashes.

That doesn't mean you shouldn't try to help your baby to feel comfortable in water—an important first step in water safety training. Before you take the plunge with your baby, however, do acquaint yourself throughly with the following points. Keep them in mind, too, if you plan on enrolling your baby in a swim class.

■ A baby should not be taken into a pool or other large body of water until good head control is achieved—that is, when the head can be lifted to a 90° angle routinely. Before this skill is mastered, usually by four or five months of age, the head might accidentally bob under the water.

■ A baby with any kind of chronic medical problem, including frequent ear infections, should have the doctor's okay before you allow him to play in water. A baby with a cold or other illness should be temporarily barred from water activities, other than in the bathtub, until recovery is complete.

■ The baby who likes and is used to water is probably less safe near it than one who is afraid of it. So don't leave a child, even one who has had "swimming" lessons, unattended near water (a pool, hot tub, bathtub, lake, ocean, puddle) for *any* period of time. Drowning can occur in less time than it takes to answer the phone—in *less than an inch* of water. If you must leave the waterside, even for a second, take baby with you.

■ All infant water activity should be on a one-to-one basis with a responsible adult. The adult should not be fearful of the water because such fear could be passed on to the infant.

■ Infant swim instructors should be qualified to teach swimming to babies and should be certified in infant CPR.

■ A baby who is fearful of the water or resistant to being dunked should not be forced to participate in water play.

■ Water in which an infant plays should be comfortably warm. In general, babies like water between 84° and 87°. Infants under six months should never be dunked in water cooler than this. Air temperature should be a least 3° warmer than water temperature, and water play should be limited to thirty-minute sessions to avoid chilling. Also, to reduce the risk of infection, pool water should be properly chlorinated and natural bodies of water should be unpolluted.

■ Infants in diapers should wear waterproof pants that have snug elastic around the leg, but undue concern about leakage is unnecessary. Since babies have tiny bladders, the amount of urine passed is negligible; the chlorine should take care of any stray germs.

■ An infant's face should not be submerged. Though babies instinctively hold their breath under water, they continue to swallow. Swallowing large quantities of water, which many babies do during water play, can dilute the blood, leading to water intoxication. This watering down of the blood can dangerously reduce the levels of sodium. The resultant swelling of the brain can cause restlessness, weakness, nausea, muscle twitching, stupor, convulsions, and even coma. Babies are much more susceptible than adults to water intoxication because of a smaller blood volume (it doesn't take a huge quantity of water to dilute it) and because they tend to swallow anything in their mouths. Water intoxication is a devious condition. Since a baby doesn't show any signs of trouble while in the water, and symptoms don't appear until three to eight hours after its ingestion, the illness is often not connected with swimming.

Submersion also increases the risk of infection, particularly of the ears and sinuses, as well as of hypothermia (dangerously low body temperatures).

■ Tubes, water wings, mattresses, or other flotation devices lend a false sense of security to a baby and the parent. It takes but a moment for a little one to slip from a tube or tumble off a float. Coast Guard–approved vests should be worn around the water by babies and young children, but even these should never replace constant adult supervision.

■ A toy bobbing in a pool can become a fatal attraction: keep all objects out of the pool when not in use.

■ A pool, wading pool, or spray with a missing drain cover should not be used until the drain is repaired. A baby or young child could be seriously injured by the force of the suction.

■ Adults supervising babies or children near water should be familiar with resuscitation techniques (see page 448), preferably through a hands-on course. Rescue equipment, such as life preservers, and a CPR-technique poster should be posted near any swimming area. A phone should be readily available for emergency calls.

WEANING IN SUMMER

Though old wives (or young mothers who've consulted with their elders) may tell

DROWNPROOFING YOUR FAMILY

The best way to "drownproof" your family is to:

1. Teach your children never to enter the water without an adult present and never to horseplay near the water. Even children who can swim well should never enter the water without a buddy around.

2. Be sure that children are *always* supervised by a responsible adult when they are around water, even a small wading pool with barely an inch of water in it.

3. Always drain kiddie pools when not in use, and turn them over so they won't fill with rainwater.

4. Make certain any pool areas (yours and your neighbors') that are accessible to your children are enclosed with high fencing they can't scale and locked securely

with a self-latching lock they can't reach.

5. Insist that children playing around pools or natural bodies of water, or on boats, wear life vests (not flotation toys) until they can swim on their own and are old enough to be responsible in the water.

6. Install a pool alarm, if you have a pool, but recognize that it doesn't provide absolute security.

7. Never use a pool with the cover partly in place—children can become entrapped in it.

8. Remember that pool covers can fill with water and become as dangerous as the pool itself.

9. Teach your children to float and to dog-paddle in the water when they are three or four years old.

---

tales to the contrary, there's no reason to hurry babies into giving up the breast or bottle before summer starts or to postpone weaning until autumn. The best time for weaning is the time that's best for you and your baby—it needn't be planned by the season or dictated by the weather report.

That fable foiled, it is true that babies need more fluids in the warm-weather months (and year-round in warm climates) than when the mercury plummets. So just make sure your baby gets enough fluids—whether from breast, bottle, cup, or foods high in water.

FOOD SPOILAGE

Food is much more likely to spoil when the sun shines and temperatures rise, so take special precautions with your baby's food in warm weather. Follow the tips on page 230 to reduce the chances of food poisoning. On outings, use an ice pack to keep formula, milk, opened jars of juice or baby food, or table foods chilled (keep several small ice packs in the freezer, ready to

go), or tote beverages in a thermos or in a jar with added ice cubes (for juice only, since formula or milk shouldn't be diluted). A soft-sided six-pack cooler gives extra protection on longer outings and is easy to carry. Don't use food or drink once it's no longer cool to the touch—at warmer temperatures bacteria might have had some time to multiply.

SWOLLEN CHEEKS

Every once in a while, both mother and doctor are confounded in the summer by the unexplained swelling of a baby's cheeks, sometimes accompanied by redness. The problem usually turns out to be "popsicle panniculitis," a seasonal diagnostic oddity caused by tissue damage from sucking on ice pops. The cure is simple: switching to another, less-chilling snack. The swelling subsides quickly, and the coloration fades within a few weeks.

WHAT YOU MAY BE CONCERNED ABOUT IN WINTER OR WINTRY WEATHER

KEEPING BABY WARM

Baby, it's cold outside. And, just as when it's warm outside, your own comfort can be your guide to dressing older babies and children. But infants under six months—because they have a greater ratio of body surface to body weight and because they can't yet shiver to generate heat—need a little more protection than you do.

Even when the weather is only slightly cool, a young baby should wear a hat to help retain heat (25% of body heat is lost via the head). When the temperature is near freezing, the hat should cover baby's ears, mittens the hands, warm socks and booties the feet, a scarf or neck warmer the neck. When the wind is biting or temperatures are very low, a scarf can be wrapped around the face or a knitted mask hat slipped over it, but be careful not to block the nose. A raincover will keep wind and snow out of a stroller or carriage, and warmth in.

But even a well-bundled baby shouldn't be out in very cold weather for long periods.

In cold weather, a lot of lightweight layers are more effective and less restrictive than a couple of heavy garments. If at least one layer is wool, baby will be warmer. Down or imitation down makes for a warm snowsuit or bunting.

The following cold weather tips will also help to keep your baby cozy and comfortable:

■ Be sure your baby has recently had a meal or snack before going out—it takes a lot of calories to maintain body heat in cold weather. A hot meal is comforting, but its warming effects don't last long.
■ If any of your baby's clothes should become wet, change them immediately.
■ A toddler should wear waterproof, lined boots when walking in wintry weather; the boots should be roomy enough to let in air, which will offer some extra insulation, to

CHANGEABLE WEATHER

If there's any kind of weather that puzzles even those who top best-dressed lists, it's that neither-here-nor-there weather so common in the spring and fall. For the inexperienced mother of a young baby, the puzzle is even more complex. How do you piece together an outfit from baby's closet when the day dawns like a lamb but is expected to roar like a lion by sundown (or vice versa)?

In general, the layered look is the key to dressing for success in changeable weather. Most practical are lightweight layers, which can be easily added or subtracted as the weather unpredictably zigzags from warm to cool and back again. An extra sweater or blanket is always a sensible take-along in case the mercury

takes a sudden sharp dip. A hat is a good idea for a young baby in almost any weather—a very light one with a sunshade when it's balmy, a warmer one on blustery days. An older baby can go hatless when temperatures are in the 60s or 70s and sun or wind isn't excessively strong. And remember, once your baby's thermostat becomes well regulated (at about six months), let your own comfort be your baby-dressing guide. A quick check of baby's arms, thighs, or nape of the neck (but not the hands or feet, which are almost always cool in young babies) will tell you if baby's comfortable. If you find these body parts are cool and/or if baby is fretful, he or she may be chilly.

circulate around stockinged feet.

■ In a car, remove your baby's hat and one or more layers of clothing, if possible to prevent overheating; if not, take care to keep the car cool. Also remove some clothing on a warm bus or train.

■ In windy weather, use a mild moisturizing lotion or cream on exposed skin to keep it from chapping.

■ Don't worry if your baby's nose runs when outdoors in cold weather. The cilia, or little hairs, that ordinarily move nasal secretions to the back of the nose instead of letting them drip out are temporarily paralyzed by the cold; once indoors, the running should stop. A little cream or Vaseline under the nose (not in it) will help prevent chapping.

FROSTBITE

While you needn't worry about your baby's nose running, you'd better be concerned if the nose (or ears, cheeks, fingers, or toes) becomes very cold, and turns white or yellowish gray. This indicates frostbite, which can cause very serious injury. Frostbitten body parts must be rewarmed immediately. See page 441 for how to do this.

After prolonged exposure to cold weather, a baby's body temperature may drop to below normal levels. This is a medical emergency—no time should be wasted in getting a baby who seems unusually cold to the touch to the nearest emergency room.

Prevent such cold weather emergencies by dressing your baby adequately, protecting exposed areas of skin, and limiting the time your baby spends outdoors in extreme weather.

SNOW BURN

It isn't just the baby tagging along to tropical beaches for the winter holidays who is in danger of suffering a sunburn in winter—a baby enjoying a white Christmas or Hanukkah is, too. Since snow re-flects up to 85% of the sun's ultraviolet rays, even a weak winter's sun can burn a baby's sensitive skin if it bounces off a snowy landscape first. So be sure to protect your baby's skin with clothing, a brimmed hat, and sunscreen whenever you'll be spending a lot of time in sun and snow.

KEEPING BABY WARM INDOORS

In cold weather, baby's room should be kept at between 68° and 72° by day, and between 60° and 65° by night. If indoor temperatures are higher than this, the arid heated air can dry the mucous membranes of the nose, making them more vulnerable to cold germs, and also the skin, making it itchy. You can prewarm your baby's sheets with a heating pad or hot-water bottle, but be sure the sheets aren't too hot at bedtime. Or use flannel sheets, which tend to stay comfortable to the touch even on cold nights. Layer light blankets for warmth and comfort. If your baby regularly kicks the blankets off, use a sleeping bag or a blanket sleeper. Keep in mind that your baby's room is cooler at night than during the day (at least it should be), and that extra covering is needed during sleep, when metabolism slows. But try not to make the common mistake of overdressing your baby for bed. And if he or she awakens in the night in a pool of perspiration, remove a layer or two of covering.

DRY SKIN

Few people, of any age, are exempt from the dry, itchy skin of winter. Though most people assume that merely protecting babies from the cruel assaults of wind and cold outdoors will keep their skin soft and supple, this isn't so. The major cause of winter dry skin is found indoors, not out. In most homes, once the heating season begins, the indoor air becomes hot and dry. And it's this hot, dry air that is a major contributor to skin dryness in winter. You can help counteract this effect in these ways:

Up the moisture in your home. Get a humidifier for your heating system, or at least a cold-mist unit (see page 629) for your baby's room. If this isn't possible, put pans of hot water on radiators (safely out of baby's reach); as the water evaporates, room air will be moisturized.

Up the moisture inside your baby. Babies (and all of us) get moisture for their skin from inside as well as out. Be sure your baby is getting enough fluids.

Up the moisture on baby's skin. Smoothing a good-quality baby lotion on baby's damp skin right after the bath will help retain the moisture. Ask the doctor to recommend a particular product, or select one that is hypoallergenic at the pharmacy .

Reduce the soap. Soap is drying. It rarely needs to be used on tiny infants—except once a day in the diaper area. Crawlers may need a sudsing on knees, feet, and hands. But in general, use very little soap; particularly avoid using bubble bath or liquid soap to make bubbles in baby's bath, since soapy water is more drying than clear water. And use a gentle soap—ask your doctor for a recommendation.

Turn down the heat. The hotter the house, the drier the air (assuming no humidity is being returned to the air as the house is heated). For babies more than a few weeks old, the home need not be warmer than 68°. If baby seems chilly at this temperature, it's better to add layers of clothing rather than degrees of heat.

FIREPLACE FIRES

Before there were televisions, there were fireplaces to draw families together on a cold winter's evening. And even today, a roaring fire can rival whatever prime time has to offer, bringing warmth to both body and spirit. The trick, however, when babies and young children are part of the family circle, is to keep them safe when 'round the fire. Keep the fireplace covered, even once the fire's out (embers can stay hot for hours), with a screen that's too heavy for even strong and persistent little hands to move. For added protection, teach your baby early on that fire is "hot!" and that touching it can cause pain. Be sure, too, that the flue is clear so fumes don't fill the room.

HOLIDAY HAZARDS

Nothing is more wondrous to a young child than a home that's been decked out for the holidays. But if proper precautions aren't taken, nothing can turn out to be more dangerous. Concealed in many idyllic Currier and Ives living-room scenes are a host of hazards. All of the following are potential threats to your baby. Some should be used with care, others shouldn't be used at all—at least until your child is older, wiser, and less vulnerable.

Mistletoe and Jerusalem cherry. Both of these can be deadly if eaten. Do not bring them into your home or let your baby play near them when visiting.

Holly. This plant is only slightly poisonous (large quantities must be consumed for a baby to suffer serious consequences), but it's wise to keep it out of baby's reach. Christmas cactus is safe, however.

Poinsettia. This holiday beauty can cause local irritation to the mouth, and more serious poisoning if large quantities are ingested. Keep out of reach.

Evergreen trees and branches. These may aggravate asthma or similar disorders, and can also be a fire hazard if not handled with care. If anyone in your home has such allergies, perhaps you should consider an artificial tree.

Pine needles. These can cause a persistent croupy cough if they lodge in the trachea (they can usually be dislodged by turning the child over and slapping the midback). Sweep them up regularly, and if possible, keep pine trees, wreaths, and branches out of reach of babies and toddlers.

Snow-scene paperweights. Despite long-circulated rumors to the contrary, the liquid inside these is not poisonous. But once broken, it can become contaminated with germs; discard if the paperweight becomes cracked.

Angel hair. This is spun glass, which can irritate skin and eyes and cause internal bleeding if swallowed; use high up and out of baby's reach, if at all.

Artificial snow spray or flocking. These can aggravate a respiratory problem; don't use if anyone in your family has one.

Tree lights. Because young children may bite these enticing ornaments and suffer internal cuts, hang them high out of reach. Be particularly careful with small blinking lights, which contain a chemical that is hazardous if ingested.

Hanukkah or other candles. Light them and keep them completely out of baby's reach—and, of course, away from curtains or other flammable materials. If you display them in a window, be sure curtains are securely tied back.

Mini decorations. Very small tree ornaments, tree lights, dreidels, or any items smaller than the diameter of baby's fist (or with parts that small that can be broken or pulled off) can cause choking. Don't use these, or use them only where you're sure baby can't get to them.

Tinsel, glass or plastic ornaments, and Styrofoam. All of these decorative items are alluring choking hazards. If a piece is bitten off, it can become stuck in the throat.

Tree preservatives. If you use one, check to see that it doesn't contain nitrates, which can cause a blood disorder if consumed. A curious baby may dip into the tree container for an unusual snack.

Gifts. These present numerous dangers.

Perfumes, colognes, and cosmetics can cause poisoning; button batteries and toys with small pieces can cause choking. And throw away wrappings and ribbons. They are also easy for babies to choke on.

Food and drink. It isn't just the things that set the scene that can be dangerous; those that set the table can be, too. Every year, hundreds of young children are rushed to hospital emergency rooms after downing a martini, beer, or cupful of eggnog or spiked punch left carelessly within their reach. Thousands more do mischief to their teeth, appetites, and eating habits with sugary holiday foods, which are too often passed into their tiny hands. So be sure that alcoholic drinks aren't left around, even briefly, on coffee or end tables where even moderately active crawlers can get to them. And indulge your baby (and your holiday guests, as well) with baked goods sweetened with fruit juice concentrates; a wide variety of such cookies and cakes are commercially available, and many more can be baked at home.

While you're adorning your home for the holidays, keep decorations where baby can't get at them, or do your decorating while baby's asleep. Just in case a mishap should occur in spite of all your precautions, prepare for the holidays by becoming familiar with first-aid and CPR techniques, if you aren't already, and by posting the number of your local poison control center where it will be handy.

SAFE GIFT GIVING

First on any parent's list when doing holiday toy shopping should be safety. As tempting as toy stores are at this time of year, resist them until you've completely familiarized yourself with the tips for buying safe and worthwhile playthings for your baby, starting on page 212. Remember, manufacturers can't always be counted on to produce what's best for your baby—particularly during the holiday season you, the buyer, must beware.

WHAT IT'S IMPORTANT TO KNOW:
The Season for Travel

In the days before parenthood, any season was the season for a trip. Summer excursions to a friend's beach house, winter holidays with parents in the Sunbelt, whirlwind ski weekends squeezed in between busy work weeks, leisurely tours of Paris in the spring, escape weekends to the Caribbean when the streets back home were covered with ice, or to the mountains when they were steaming with heat and humidity.

But now what? Considering the effort involved in taking your baby across town on a simple shopping expedition—the hours of planning, the exacting execution, and the 20 pounds worth of baby, equipment, and supplies lugged on your aching shoulders—the logistics of a two-week vacation, or even a two-day trip to grandma's, might seem too mind-boggling to consider attempting.

Yet you needn't wait until your children are old enough to carry their own luggage or are off to summer camp to satisfy your wanderlust or grandma's pleas for a visit. Though vacations with baby will rarely be restful and will always be a challenge, they can be both feasible and enjoyable.

PLANNING AHEAD

The days of spur-of-the-moment weekend getaways, when a restless spirit and a few garments and toiletries flung into an overnight bag took you where you wanted to go, ended abruptly with your baby's arrival. Now you can expect to spend more time planning a trip than taking one. Sensible preparatory steps for any trip with baby include:

Underschedule yourself. Forget itineraries that will take you through six scintillating cities in five whirlwind days. Instead, set a modest pace with plenty of unscheduled time—for an extra day on the road should you end up needing it, an extra afternoon at the beach or morning by the pool should you end up wanting it.

Update passports. You won't be able to take your baby abroad on your passport. These days every traveler, no matter what age, needs his or her own.

Take medical precautions. If you're going abroad, check with the doctor to be sure baby's immunizations are up to date. If you're heading for exotic destinations, all of you may need specific immunizations (against typhoid, for example) or prophylactic treatments (to prevent malaria or hepatitis A).

Before taking an extended trip, schedule a well-child checkup if it's been a while since the last one. In addition to providing assurance that your baby's in good health, the visit will give you an opportunity to discuss your proposed trip with the doctor and ask any questions that might otherwise plague you while you're away—when it may be impossible, or at least impractical, to pick up the phone and call the office. If your baby has had a checkup within the previous month, a telephone consultation may be all that's needed.

If your baby takes medication, be sure you have enough for the trip, plus a prescription in case the supply is lost, spilled, or otherwise meets with calamity. If a medication needs to be refrigerated, keeping it on ice continuously may be difficult, so ask the doctor if it's possible to substitute another medication that needn't be kept cold. Since a stuffy nose can make a baby miserable, interfere with sleep, and cause ear pain when flying, also ask the doctor to recommend a decongestant in case your child should come down with a cold. If you are going to a place where "traveler's stomach" might be a problem, ask for a prescription for diarrhea, too. For any medication you are taking along, be sure you know the safe dosage for a child your baby's age, as well as the conditions under which it should be administered and the possible side effects. Also useful, especially for extended trips: the name of a pediatrician at your destination or destinations.

Time your trip. What hour of the day or night you begin your journey will depend on, among other things, baby's schedule and how he or she reacts to changes in it, your mode of travel, your destination, and how long it will take to get there. If you're leaving the East Coast for the West by plane, for example, it might make sense to plan to arrive around baby's bedtime (East Coast time). Assuming a nap has been taken en route, the excitement and chaos of arrival will probably make it possible to keep baby awake a couple of hours past the usual bedtime. This may enable baby to sleep until a relatively respectable 6:00 Pacific Time rather than rising raring to go at an indecent 3:00 or 4:00 A.M. (Of course, you will also have to pray trains and planes will be on schedule.)

Consider the advantages of traveling at off-peak times, when there are more likely to be empty seats for your baby to crawl over and fewer fellow passengers who might be disturbed.

If your baby habitually falls asleep in the car and you're planning a long-distance car trip, plan, if possible, to do most of your driving when he or she would ordinarily be asleep—during nap times or at night. Otherwise, you may arrive at your destination with a baby who's slept all day and is ready to play all night. If your baby sleeps well on trains or planes but is fussy when awake in such confined quarters, coordinate nap time with travel time. But if your baby is always too excited to sleep in such environments, plan to travel after nap time to avoid crankiness during the trip.

It may seem that getting to your destination as quickly as possible makes the most sense. But it doesn't always. For an active baby, for example, a connecting flight with some time to let off steam between legs of the trip may be better than a long nonstop.

Order ahead. When flying, don't plan on feeding even an older baby from a standard airline tray; entrées are astronomically high in sodium, bread is invariably of the refined variety, desserts are routinely sugary and nutritionally worthless. Instead, plan on sharing a special order, such as a cottage cheese and fruit platter and whole-wheat bread, with your older baby. Special orders are usually just a 24-hour-in-advance phone call away, and you can often arrange for one when confirming your tickets. Even once you've put in your order, however, plan to take along a substantial stash of snacks. When flights are delayed or special orders go astray (neither unheard of these days), long waits between meals can make baby, and everyone else in the vicinity, miserable.

Some airlines, particularly on overseas flights, offer baby foods, bottles, diapers, and bassinets. Ask about these when you make your reservations.

Arrange for suitable seating. If you're traveling by air, try to reserve bulkhead seats, which will give you extra room to move around and allow baby to sleep or play at your feet. If they're not available, request seats on the aisle—you may spend a lot of time pacing up and down it. Whatever you do, don't accept seats in the middle of a wide center section, not just for your sake, but for the sake of those seated around you.

When reserving, also ask if it's possible to get a seat with an empty next to it—at least unless and until the plane is fully booked.

Though you can, and should, reserve space on many railroad trains in this country, you can't reserve specific seats. But you can reserve sleeper compartments on some long-distance runs. Such compartments give you a measure of privacy, something you may really appreciate when spending long hours or days on a train with a baby.

Book in advance. You may assume that

when traveling by road in off-peak seasons, motel reservations won't be necessary. But in this nation of travelers, many roadside establishments, especially those with lower rates, hang out "no vacancy" signs nightly. So plan ahead where you will be stopping overnight, allowing more time to get there than you could ever possibly imagine needing, and reserve a motel room with a crib.

Choose a helpful hostelry. Whenever possible, look for a hotel or motel that caters to the needs of families; many do not. One clue to what you can expect is whether or not cribs (or cots, as they're called in Great Britain and commonwealth countries) and baby-sitters are available. You will probably have an uncomfortable stay at a hotel without such amenities. And you will probably feel unwelcome, too.

Equip yourself. Getting around, especially if you're traveling without another adult or with more than one child, will be easier if you have the right equipment:

- A baby carrier, if baby is small. It will free your hands to juggle luggage—important when boarding and disembarking.
- A lightweight and very compact umbrella stroller, for an older baby. You can hang totes from the handles, but be careful not to let the stroller tip backward.
- A wrist-to-wrist "leash," for an active toddler. This may seem barbaric, but may be the only way to keep your child in tow.
- A portable baby seat—a cloth one adds almost no weight to your luggage.
- A car seat. On airplanes, if there is an empty seat next to you it can double as a safety seat, or it can be stored overhead.[2] Or if you plan on renting a car at your destination, you can rent a car seat with it—but be sure to reserve the seat at the time you reserve the car.

You can also rent or borrow other equipment, such as cribs, playpens, high chairs,

and feeding seats, at the other end. Try to make these arrangements in advance.

Don't rock the boat before you set sail. To avoid unnecessary problems on your trip, avoid unnecessary changes just before it. Don't try weaning your baby, for instance, just prior to departure—the unfamiliar surroundings and changes in routine will be hard enough to deal with without adding other stresses. Besides, no other way of feeding baby on the road is as easy for you or as comforting for baby as breastfeeding. Don't introduce solids close to departure, either—beginning to spoon-feed is enough of a challenge (for both of you) at home. If your baby is ready for finger foods, however, consider introducing them a few weeks in advance. Portable nibbles are great for keeping babies occupied and happy en route.

If your baby isn't sleeping through the night, now is not the time to try to remedy the situation. There's likely to be some regression into night waking during a trip (and for a while, upon return), and letting baby cry it out in a hotel room or at grandma's will enhance neither your vacation nor your welcome.

Don't be defensive or diffident. If you're met with less than total cooperation when making your advance requests, keep your cool. Avoid becoming demanding or unpleasant yourself, but don't buckle under unnecessarily, either. The mixed reviews you get on these calls will continue throughout your trip: some flight attendants and hotel managers won't be able to do enough for you, others won't look your way except to glare.

Confirm. The day before your departure, confirm all your reservations if they haven't already been confirmed, and call to check departure times before leaving home. You don't want to arrive at the airport to find your flight's been canceled or delayed four hours. Or at the train station to find the train is going to be late.

---

2. But be sure the seat is FAA approved—the product label will probably so specify.

PACKING WISELY

While virtually everything, including the kitchen sink (for rinsing off dropped bottles and dousing stains), might come in handy on your trip, packing it all would obviously not be advisable. Neither, however, would be starting out perilously underpacked. Instead, strive for a happy (albeit heavy) medium, taking only what you absolutely need, being as efficient as possible in your selection: sample sizes of liquid baby soap, acetaminophen, toothpaste, and the like; the extra-trim and extra-absorbent variety of disposable diapers; mix-and-match clothes in bright patterns that conceal stains well and thus hold out longer between launderings, and in lightweight fabrics that will dry fast if you need to rinse them out.

You can pack less if you'll be someplace where you can fill in the blanks, particularly if filling them in will be part of the fun—buying a couple of tiny shorts and T-shirt sets in Bermuda, for example, or a bottle of *bébé* shampoo in Paris. But if you'll be hiking in the Adirondacks or camping in Yosemite, all that you could conceivably end up needing should end up in your backpack. For the typical trip, you will probably want to pack these bags, filled as follows:

A diaper bag. It should be lightweight, plastic lined, have outside compartments for storing tissues, wipes, bottles, and other needed-in-a-hurry items, and a shoulder strap so you won't need to tie up a free hand carrying it. The items you'll want to keep handy in the bag include:

■ A light jacket (waterproof nylon with a hood is best, since it doubles as a raincoat) or sweater in case the car, train, plane, or bus is chilly.
■ Enough disposable, extra-trim, extra-absorbent diapers for the first leg of your journey, and then some, in case of a delay or an attack of traveler's tummy. Plan on buying diapers as you go rather than carrying cases with you from home, unless

you're traveling by car and have the room, or unless you won't be able to purchase them at your destination.
■ Diaper wipes for your hands (and baby's) as well as the obvious. They can also serve to sanitize the arm of the plane seat that baby seems intent on chewing or the train window that he or she is set on licking clean and to outsmart spills on clothing or upholstery before they become stains.
■ Diaper rash ointment, since unfamiliar foods, infrequent diaper changes, and warm weather can all prompt an outbreak of diaper rash.
■ A large waterproof bib, or a pack of disposable ones, to protect clothing. Just in case you accidentally leave the plastic bib in a restaurant or run out of throwaways, bring along a clothespin or a diaper pin with which to fasten a restaurant napkin over baby's clothes.
■ Some reclosable plastic bags to hold leaky bottles, dirty bibs or clothing, and soiled diapers when a trash can isn't immediately available.
■ Sunscreen, if your destination will be sunny or snowy and your baby is six months or older.
■ A light blanket or quilt for baby to nap on or play on en route, in restaurants, and in homes that you visit. Or take along a shawl you can wear on your shoulders and use for baby when necesssary.
■ A small waterproof lap pad or changing pad to protect hotel beds and other surfaces when baby needs a change.
■ A square yard of clear, heavy-duty plastic to protect hotel furniture and rugs during feedings, and to serve as inobtrusive protection under baby's high chair in restaurants.
■ A comfort object, if your baby has one.
■ A pair of socks or booties for a barefoot baby, in case you run into some heavy air-conditioning.
■ Plastic outlet covers if your baby is a crawler or walker, to babyproof hotel rooms or homes you're visiting. You may also want to take a toilet lock if your baby is into water play.
■ A generous supply of snacks and bev-

erages. Don't rely on being able to find appropriate food for your baby on the road, in the air, or on the rails. Bring along enough food and drink for one or two more meals than you anticipate feeding, just in case. Depending on baby's culinary repertoire, take along baby food (dehydrated, if you must travel light); whole-grain crackers; small containers of bite-size dry cereal for nibbling; a small container of 'wheat germ for enriching white breads, cereals, pastas, and rices; ready-to-use formula for the bottle baby in disposable bottles (preferably of in light and unbreakable plastic); juice in a small bottle or thermos with a cup with a lid or small paper cups for cup-drinkers. Carry the three-ounce baby food jars to provide variety and avoid waste.

- A dozen plastic spoons in a plastic bag, for feeding baby en route. If there are no facilities for washing them, they can be dumped.
- Paper towels, unrolled, which are more practical, stronger, and more absorbent than napkins.
- Something old and something new to entertain your baby—the old for comfort and reliability; the new for excitement and challenge. A small activity board and a brightly illustrated board book are good choices for an older baby; a mirror, rattle, and a musical stuffed animal for a younger one. Leave home toys with a lot of pieces that can get lost or which are too bulky for easy packing and use in tight spaces. For a teether, be sure to take a couple of items to gnaw on.
- A small purse. Since you have a limited number of hands, carrying a separate handbag will be virtually impossible as well as a little risky (you'll most likely look distracted and disorganized enough to qualify as easy prey for a pickpocket). Instead, keep personal items, plane, train, or bus tickets, and your wallet, with money, credit cards, and copies of medication prescriptions, as well as baby's doctor's phone number and the names of recommended doctors at your destination, in a small, easy-to-identify-by-feel purse in the diaper bag. Or, as an alternative, keep your wallet handy in your pocket (if all of your travel outfits have safely deep pockets, you'll find life much easier).

A bag for baby's clothing. Ideal for baby's travel wardrobe is a small, lightweight, soft-sided carry-on with a shoulder or backpack strap. Since it can be kept handy in car, plane, or train, you'll be able to get at a fresh outfit without any fuss and without rummaging through your own suitcase in public. If you choose to pack baby's clothes in your suitcase, however, and that bag won't be available while you're traveling (because it's going to be either checked through on the plane, train, or bus, or buried in the car trunk), make sure you keep an extra outfit or two for baby in the diaper bag.

A medical and toiletry bag. This bag should be inaccessible to a curious baby at all times (in overhead compartments on trains and planes, for example), and should preferably have a lock or be difficult to open. Ideally, it should also be waterproof and easy to clean, and again, a shoulder strap is a plus. Keep this bag with you as you go so that medications will be available, if needed, and to protect liquids from damage by freezing in the cargo compartment of planes. It can contain:

- Any prescription medicines and vitamins to last your trip; baby acetaminophen; an antiemetic for vomiting; an antiperistaltic for diarrhea (Lomotil is not recommended for children under two); a decongestant, if recommended by the doctor.
- All medical insurance information.
- For outdoor trips, insect repellent, yellow soap for poison ivy, calamine lotion, bug-bite medicine, and a bee-sting kit if baby is allergic.
- A first-aid kit containing syrup of ipecac for accidental poisoning (but do not administer it without medical advice); bandaids and self-adhesive gauze pads; antibacterial cream (such as Neosporin); elastic bandages for sprains; thermometer; tweezers; baby nail clipper.
- Liquid baby soap, which serves as a cleanser for both hair and skin. The soaps found in hotel rooms aren't usually gentle

enough for babies.
- Baby's toothbrush, or gauze pads for tooth wiping if teeth are in.
- Multi-purpose pocketknife, with can opener and scissors.
- A night light, if your baby likes to sleep with one.

GETTING THERE IS HALF THE FUN

Whether you will be going by land, air, or rail, there are several ways of making your trip easier.

If you're flying. Planes have the advantage for family travel of usually being the fastest commercial way of getting from one point to another. You can make a flying trip pleasant (at least relatively so) as well as comfortable, if you:

- Arrive early enough to take care of pre-boarding details like luggage and seats, but not so early that you have an uncomfortably long wait in the air terminal.
- Request bulkhead seats, if you didn't reserve them. If they aren't available, try to arrange a switch after boarding.
- Preboarding is an advantage offered to those traveling with children, allowing them to settle in and stow luggage in overhead compartments before the rush. However, if you have a baby who you expect will be fidgety in close quarters (remember, you won't be able to walk the aisles while they're being used for boarding), you may want to wait and board last. If you're traveling with another adult, ask if one of you can preboard with the luggage while the other spends some extra time with baby in the open spaces of the waiting area.
- Coordinate feedings with takeoff and landing. Children (especially babies) are even more prone than adults to the ear pressure, and sometimes pain, caused by cabin air pressure changes during ascent and descent. Nursing or bottle feeding at these times (or giving finger foods or a pacifier) encourages frequent swallowing, which

helps prevent the painful pressure buildup and the fussing and crying that usually accompany it.
- If your baby does do a lot of loud complaining, accept a kind hand from friendly fellow passengers if offered, and disregard those who are ignorant and uncompassionate enough to give you dirty looks.
- Give your baby a lot to drink during the flight; air travel is dehydrating. If you're nursing, be sure you, too, take extra fluids—but remember, beverages with caffeine or alcohol don't count.
- If your baby demands warmed feedings, ask flight attendants to warm bottles and baby food for you (without their tops). But remember to shake or stir thoroughly and to carefully double-check the temperature before serving to prevent scalding accidents, since microwaves can heat unevenly.
- If you're traveling alone, feel free to ask an attendant to hold baby while you use the lavatory.
- Deplane last, to avoid the squeeze and to be sure you have time to gather up all your belongings. (Let anyone who is meeting you know that you will be last off the plane.)

If you're going by train. Traveling by train, though slower than by plane, allows children a little more mobility. Your family train trip will be easier if you remember to:

- Ask a conductor to direct you to a non-smoking car.
- Board as early as possible to find a plum seat. If a wheelchair-bound passenger (who has first call) is not positioned in front of the first seat in a car, that's a good one for a family to take because of the open space in front of it where baby can nap or play. Also a good choice is the four-seater unit at either end of most cars, which allows families to spread out comfortably. If the train is crowded and your trip is long, it may make sense to take a seat for your baby and pay for it when the conductor comes around (a check or credit card will usually be accepted). If you have only one seat, it's a toss-up whether to favor the window seat (so baby can watch the scenery go by) or the aisle (so you can get up

HIGH ALTITUDES

If you're heading to an area high above sea level, there are certain precautions that need to be taken. Because the sun's rays are more intense at higher altitudes, you need to be particularly conscientious about using sunscreens and limiting sun exposure. And because fluid requirements are increased, your baby will need several additional ounces of fruit juice or water daily while you remain at the higher altitude. In a baby who is anemic, the reduced level of oxygen in the air may increase heart and respiratory rates and cause fatigue. This is nothing to be concerned about unless your baby has an infection or other medical condition, such as a heart ailment—in which case you should consult the doctor before making the trip. But do schedule frequent rest stops.

frequently for walks if baby is fidgety).

■ Be sure to have a baby carrier if you're traveling alone and baby can still ride in one; without it you may find it impossible to go to the bathroom. (Don't park your baby even briefly with anyone, no matter how friendly, particularly as the train nears a stop.)

■ Accept help with the baggage when you board or detrain, if anyone offers, but don't let someone you don't know carry baby.

■ If your train ride will be a long one, have a varied collection of toys so you can pull out a new one when your baby tires of the old. Or do some sightseeing. Looking out the window, pointing out cars, horses, cows, dogs, people, houses, sky, clouds, is an onboard activity that has saved many a mom at the bottom of her bag of tricks.

■ Be sure to have plenty of snacks on hand. Lines for food on trains are often long and it would not be unusual to finally reach the counter only to find that the tuna sandwich you were counting on was sold out.

If you're driving. Driving is slower than other forms of transportation, more taxing on you if you're the driver, and most confining to baby. But it does give you the luxury of going at your own pace, stopping when and where you'd like, and having ready transportation at your destination. Make family auto travel safer, more pleasant, and more comfortable in these ways:

■ Be sure that there are seat belts for all adults and older children, car seats for younger ones, and that the car never moves until all are safely secured and all doors locked. In hot weather, cover vinyl-seated car seats with soft cloths, towels, or mock lamb's wool. A rolled-up towel or a store-bought headrest will keep a young baby's head from slipping down in the car seat; a blanket folded under the thighs will increase comfort and endurance.

■ Take frequent breaks (every two hours or so is ideal), since babies become restless sitting in car seats for very long stretches. When you do stop, take baby out for some fresh air, and if he or she's mobile, a crawl or walk. Use rest stops for nursing, too.

■ Alternate roles. For a change of pace and companionship for everyone, alternate driving with sitting in the back entertaining baby.

■ Attach playthings to baby's car seat with plastic links (or strings no longer than 5 inches) so that you won't have to unbelt repeatedly to retrieve tossed toys.

■ If you're driving in cold weather, especially if a storm is predicted, bring along extra clothing and blankets in case you get stranded. A car can quickly turn into a deadly icebox in subfreezing temperatures.

■ Never leave a baby in a parked car in hot or very warm weather. Even with the windows open, the car can rapidly become a deadly oven.

AT HOTELS AND MOTELS—OR OTHER HOMES AWAY FROM HOME

The first overnighter away from home with your baby can be a little unnerving. But you can survive it if you take the following precautions:

- Upon arrival at your destination, do a safety check of the room you'll be staying in – especially if your baby is mobile. Check the crib to be sure slats are no more than 2⅜ inches apart. If they are, take baby to bed with you. Be sure open windows, electrical cords, glasses, and so on aren't accessible. Cap exposed outlets.
- If you put baby on the bed for a diaper change or play, use a waterproof pad—to protect the bed from baby and baby from a possibly unsanitary bedspread.
- When you're feeding baby in the room, spread newspaper or a plastic square on the floor to protect carpeting—for courtesy's sake, and so you won't be stuck for damages.
- Don't confine an active baby. Crawling under your supervision is okay unless the carpet is visibly dirty; exploratory toddling is fine, too, but again under a watchful adult eye.
- Arrange for baby-sitters through the hotel. Meet them at the bell captain's or concierge's desk, so you'll be sure you've got the right person.

RESTAURANT SURVIVAL

At one time babies were rarely seen in public eating places. Today, many babies spend as much time in restaurants as at the playground. If yours hasn't yet had the pleasure, however, the following tips should make restaurant hopping easier on your trip or anytime:

- Plan on eating early and quickly. When you're eating out with baby, you'll have to dine on baby's schedule. not yours—even if that means being the earliest bird to catch the Early Bird Special. Choose fairly fast-paced eateries, too, so that baby will spend more time eating than waiting. And when your baby is finished eating, it's probably time to leave. Lingering over dessert and coffee is a pleasure of the past for most parents of young children.
- Call ahead to make sure the restaurant is equipped with high chairs or baby dining seats (a booster seat won't do until after baby's a year old), unless you plan to bring a portable one. The reception you get when you call, as well as whether or not such seating is available, will give you some indication as to how welcome your baby will be.
- Request a table in the back or in a quiet corner of the restaurant, where your group is least likely to offend other diners or get in the way of restaurant personnel. It will also give you more privacy if you have to spend part of the dinner hour nursing. (Be discreet.)
- Bring along a bib and, in case the restaurant is carpeted, that square of clear plastic to spread on the carpet under baby's chair.
- Bring along some toys and books for diversion between courses or when baby's finished eating. Don't take them out, however, until they're needed, and then one at a time so they won't lose their novelty before the first course arrives. Baby will probably be content to play with a spoon, flirt with a waiter, and point at the light fixtures for the first few minutes.
- Bring along some snacks (particularly finger foods that keep baby occupied) in case the food's a long time in coming or there's nothing that baby can or will eat. Again, keep these in reserve until they're needed. If your baby isn't on table foods yet, bring a jar or two of baby food and serve it up while the adults are waiting for their meal.
- Never let a child walk or crawl around a

restaurant. Such exploration could result in serious injury and damage should a waiter bearing a heavy tray of food or drink, hot or cold, be tripped up.

■ Order promptly, and ask that baby's food be brought as soon as possible. If you're with your spouse or another adult, one of you can order while the other keeps baby busy out of doors or in the lobby until some food arrives.

■ If you don't see it on the menu, ask for it. Most restaurants have a full supply of staples in the kitchen from which you can choose a meal for baby. Good choices include: cottage cheese, whole-wheat bread, cheese, hamburger (not ordered rare, because of the danger of bacteria in undercooked meat), roast or broiled chicken, soft fish (check carefully for bones), mashed or boiled potato, peas (mash them), well-cooked carrots and string beans, pasta, melon.

■ In areas where the safety of the water is questionable and sanitation a problem, avoid tap water (use carbonated bottled water and bottled juice for baby), raw vegetables, ice, dairy products that are not pasteurized and/or refrigerated, and restaurants where flies flit about and glasses look grimy.

■ Be sensitive to other diners. If your baby is crying loudly or otherwise disturbing people around you, it's time for a stroll.

■ You may find that occasionally you and your traveling companion (if you're lucky enough to have one) have to alternate shifts, eating and walking.

HAVING FUN

■ Be realistic about the itinerary. You just won't be able to keep up the same pace with a baby in tow as you would on a trip for adults only. Overschedule, and you'll end up underenjoying.

■ Be flexible about the itinerary. If you'd planned to drive straight through from Savannah to Lauderdale, but baby's had it with the car seat by Daytona, consider adding an overnight stop. If you've scheduled two days of sightseeing in Athens, but baby's crankiness is ruining the ruins for all of you by the first morning, postpone the Parthenon until another day or, perhaps, another trip.

■ Stick to sites where baby won't be confined or required to be silent for long periods of time. Outdoor ruins, parks, zoos, and even some museums can be interesting to babies and young children—even if they spend most of their time just looking at other people. Hire a baby-sitter, if possible, when you want to go to the opera, a concert or the theater.

■ Remember whose needs must come first—if anyone's going to have a good time. If baby doesn't nap or eat on time, or is repeatedly subjected to uncustomarily late bedtimes, everyone will suffer the consequences. Do what the Romans do, by all means, but only if your baby can adjust easily.

CHAPTER SEVENTEEN

When Baby Is Sick

There's nothing quite as pathetic, vulnerable, and helpless-looking as a sick baby. With the exception of a sick baby's parents.

An infant's illness, even a mild one, usually hits mommy and daddy harder than baby, especially when it's a first illness in a first child. There's the anxiety when the initial symptoms appear, the alarm when they seem to worsen or others develop, the indecision over whether or not to call the doctor and when (children almost invariably get sick in the middle of the night or on weekends, outside of the usual office hours), the pacing while waiting for the doctor's call back (interminable, even if it's only fifteen minutes), the ordeal of administering medicine, and the worry, worry, worry.

Believe it or not, things do get better. With experience, parents learn to handle a feverish infant or a vomiting toddler with less panic and more self-assurance. To reach that point more quickly, it will help to learn how to evaluate symptoms, how to take and interpret a baby's temperature, what to feed a sick child, what the most common childhood illnesses are, and how to recognize and handle a real emergency.

BEFORE CALLING THE DOCTOR

Most pediatricians want to hear from you—no matter what the time of day or night—if you think your baby is really sick. But before you dial that probably already familiar number, be sure you're armed with a written list of all the information your baby's doctor might need to know in order to accurately assess the situation. To be an effective partner in your baby's health care, you should be ready and able to provide any or all of the following information should it prove pertinent. In most simple illnesses, only two or three symptoms will be present, but running down the list will ensure you haven't missed anything. Be prepared to tell the doctor when symptoms first appeared; what, if anything, triggered them; what exacerbates or alleviates them (sitting up reduces the coughing, for example, or eating increases vomiting); and which home remedies or over-the-counter medications you've tried treating them with. It will also be helpful to let the doctor know if your baby has been exposed to a cousin with chicken pox, a sibling with diarrhea, or anyone else with a communicable illness, or if he or she has recently been injured, as in a fall. And remind the doctor of baby's age and any chronic medical problems.

Have handy the name and phone number of an open pharmacy in case the doctor needs to phone in a prescription, and a pad and pencil for jotting down any instructions you receive.

Temperature. First test for temperature with your lips on your baby's forehead. If it feels warm to the touch, get a more accurate reading with a thermometer (see page 428). Remember that in addition to illness, readings can be affected by such factors as room or air temperature (a baby's temperature is likely to be higher after playing in an overheated apartment than after coming in on a snowy day); level of activity (exercise, energetic play, and vigorous crying can all raise temperature); and time of day (temperatures tend to be higher later in the day). If baby's forehead is cool, assume there's no significant fever.

Heart rate. In some cases, knowing what your baby's heart rate is may be useful to the doctor. If your baby seems very lethargic or has a fever, take the upper arm (or brachial) pulse as shown above. The normal range in infants is between 100 and 130 beats per minute during sleep, 140 to 160 when awake, and 160 to 200 while

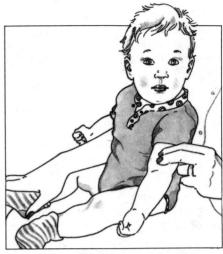

Practice taking the brachial pulse when your baby is healthy and calm.

crying. The heart rate gets progressively slower as a child gets older, and by age two is usually between 100 and 140.

Respiration. If your baby has difficulty breathing, is coughing, or seems to be breathing rapidly or irregularly, check respirations by counting how many times in a minute his or her chest rises and falls. Breathing is more rapid during activity (including crying) than during sleep, and may be speeded up or slowed down by illness. Newborns normally take about 40 to 60 breaths per minute; one-year-olds only 25 to 35. If your baby's chest doesn't seem to rise and fall with each breath, or if breathing appears labored or raspy (unrelated to a stuffy nose), report that information to the doctor, too.

Respiratory symptoms. Is your baby's nose runny? Stuffy? Is the discharge watery or thick? Clear, white, yellow, or green? Is there a cough? Does it seem dry, hacking, heavy, crowing? Does the cough bring up any mucus? (Sometimes mucus will be vomited up with a forceful cough.)

Behavior. Is there any change from the norm in your baby's behavior? Would you describe your child as tired and lethargic, cranky and irritable, inconsolable or unresponsive? Can you elicit a smile?

Sleeping. Is baby sleeping much more than usual, or seeming to be unusually drowsy? Or is he or she having trouble sleeping?

Crying. Is baby crying more than usual? Does the cry have a different sound or intensity—is it high pitched, for instance?

Appetite. Is baby eating as usual? Refusing the bottle or breast and/or turning down solids? Or eating everything in sight?

Skin. Does baby's skin appear different in any way? Is it red and flushed? White and pale? Bluish or gray? Is it moist and warm (sweaty) or moist and cool (clammy)? Or unusually dry? Are lips, nostrils, or cheeks excessively dry or cracking? Are there spots or lesions anywhere on baby's skin—under the arms, behind the ears, on limbs or trunk, or elsewhere? How would you describe their color, shape, size, texture? Does baby seem to be trying to scratch them?

Mouth. Is there swelling on the gums where teeth might be trying to break through? Any red or white spots or patches visible on the gums, inside the cheeks, or on the palate or tongue?

Throat. Is the arch framing the throat reddened? Are there white or red spots or patches?

Fontanel. If the soft spot on top of your baby's head is still open, is it either sunken or bulging?

Eyes. Do baby's eyes look different than usual? Are they glassy, vacant, sunken, dull, watery, or reddened? Do they have dark circles under them, or seem partially closed? If there is a discharge, how would you describe color, consistency, and quantity?

Ears. Is baby pulling or poking at one or both ears? Is there a discharge from either ear?

Lymph glands. Do the lymph glands in the neck appear swollen?

Digestive system. Has baby been vomiting? How often? Is there a lot of material being vomited, or are baby's heaves mostly dry? How would you describe the vomitus (like curdled milk, mucus-streaked, pinkish, bloody?) Is the vomiting forcible? Does it seem to project a long distance? Does anything seem to trigger the vomiting—eating, for example? Has there been any change in baby's bowel movements? Is there diarrhea, with loose, watery mucus, or bloody stools? Are movements more frequent, sudden, and forceful? Or does baby seem constipated? Is there an increase or decrease in saliva? Or any apparent difficulty swallowing?

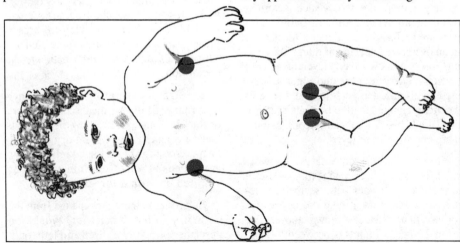

Lymph glands (locations are circled) are part of the immune system. Enlargement anywhere in the body may signal infection and should be reported to the doctor.

MOTHER'S INTUITION

Sometimes you can't put your finger on any specific symptom, but your baby just doesn't seem "right" to you. Put a call in to the doctor. Most likely you'll be reassured, but it's also possible that you will have picked up something subtle that needs treatment.

Urinary system. Are baby's diapers less wet than usual? Or do they seem wetter? Is there any noticeable change in odor or color (dark yellow, for example, or pink)?

Abdomen. Does your baby's tummy seem different in any way—flatter, rounder, more bulging? When you press it gently, or when you bend either knee to the abdomen, does baby seem to be in pain? Where does the pain seem to be—right side or left, upper or lower abdomen?

Motor symptoms. Has your baby had, or is he or she having, chills, trembling, stiffness, or convulsions? Does the neck seem to be stiff or difficult to move—can the chin be bent to the chest? Does there seem to be any difficulty in moving any other part of the body?

HOW MUCH REST FOR A SICK BABY?

In spite of well-meant advice you may get to the contrary from grandmothers, great-aunts, and neighbors, a sick baby needn't be confined to the crib or "kept quiet." You can trust your baby to listen to his or her own body and to comply with its commands. A very sick infant will relinquish the usual daily pursuits in favor of needed rest, whereas one who is just mildly ill or on the way to recovery will be active and playful. In either case, there's no need to impose restrictions of your own. Just follow baby's lead. (If anyone does need a rest when a baby's sick, it's mother.)

FEEDING A SICK BABY

Loss of appetite often accompanies illness. Sometimes, as in the case of digestive upsets, this is good since not eating gives the stomach and intestines a needed rest while they recover. Sometimes, as when there's a fever, it's not so good since the additional calories needed to fuel the fever that fights the infection may be lacking.

For most minor illnesses that don't affect the digestive system, no special diet is necessary except as noted under specific illnesses. But several general rules apply when feeding any sick baby:

Stress fluids. If your baby has a fever, a respiratory infection (such as a cold, influenza, or bronchitis), or a gastrointestinal illness with diarrhea, clear fluids and foods with high water contents (juices, juicy fruits, soups, Best-Odds gels, and frozen-juice desserts) or rehydration fluids (if necessary) will help prevent dehydration and should take precedence over solids. Offer them frequently throughout the day, even if baby takes no more than a sip at a time. Babies on formula or breast milk should suckle as often as they like, unless the doctor recommends otherwise.

Emphasize quality. Though the temptation may be to let your baby eat anything he or she will take—even if it isn't very nutritious and is loaded with sugar or salt—don't. Foods that offer little but calories are likely to sabotage your child's appetite for anything worthwhile. Since a child (like an adult) needs a lot of vitamins and minerals to help the immune system fight back, you should be sure that the little your baby is eating goes a long way nutritionally.

(When digestive disorders limit dietary intake, see page 422). And continue baby's vitamin supplement, too, unless the doctor tells you otherwise.

Play favorites. Although you don't want a sick baby to subsist on a diet of junk foods, it's okay—if baby's appetite is ailing and diet isn't restricted—to allow carte blanche with healthful favorite foods. If that means nothing but formula or breast milk and bananas for four days (or cereal three times a day, or Pumpkin Muffins, orange juice, and milk exclusively), that's okay. Try, also, to stimulate an interest in eating in an older baby with "fun" foods that look as good as they taste, such as Pancake Faces or Cottage Cheese Sundaes (all these recipes can be found in the Ready Reference).

Don't force. Even if your baby hasn't taken a bite in 24 hours, don't force. Forcing could set up a feeding problem baby might not recover from as spontaneously as he or she will from the illness. And don't worry if a few days of semi-starvation have your baby looking gaunt; babies tend to make up for lost meals after an illness, eating ravenously until lost weight is regained. Do let the doctor know about this loss of appetite.

WHEN MEDICATION IS NEEDED

Sometime during the first year, it is very likely that medication will be recommended or prescribed for your baby. Starting with the very first time, make it a habit to ask the right questions about the medication and then to use it correctly.

What You Should Know About the Medication

Either the doctor or the pharmacist will be able to answer the following questions. Be sure to jot down the responses in a notebook (or better still, in a permanent "health history") so you will have a record for ready reference now and in the future. Don't rely on your memory.

- What is the generic name of the drug? the brand name, if any?
- What is it supposed to do?
- What is the appropriate dose for your baby? (Be ready with your baby's approximate weight so that, if necessary, the doctor can calculate the dose accordingly.)
- How often should the medication be given; should baby be awakened in the middle of the night for it?
- Should it be taken before, with, or after meals?
- Should it be washed down only with certain liquids and not with others?
- What common side effects may be expected?
- What possible adverse reactions could occur? Which should be reported to the doctor? (Remind the doctor of previous reactions.)
- If your child has a chronic medical condition, might the drug have an undesirable effect on it? (Be sure to remind the prescribing doctor of the condition, since he or she may not have your baby's chart in hand.)
- If your child is taking any other medication, could there be any adverse interaction?
- How soon can you expect to see an improvement?
- When should you contact the doctor if there is no improvement?
- When can the medication be discontinued?

Giving Medication Correctly

Medicines are meant to cure, but when used improperly, they often do more harm than good. Always observe these rules when giving medication:

- Don't give a baby under three months of age any medication not prescribed for him or her by a doctor, not even an over-the-counter one. Since infants tend to keep drugs in their systems longer than older children or adults, they can quickly build up to an overdose level.
- Always make sure the medicine you're giving your child is fresh. Don't use a drug if its expiration date has passed, or if it has

changed in texture, color, or odor. Pour expired medicines down the toilet.

■ Measure medications meticulously according to the directions the baby's doctor has given you, or according to label directions on over-the-counter products. Use a calibrated spoon, dropper, or cup (all are usually available from your pharmacy) to get precise measurements (kitchen spoons are variable). To prevent spillage when using a calibrated spoon, pour the measured amount into a larger spoon before administering.

■ Keep a record of the time each dose is given (tape a sheet of paper on the refrigerator or over the changing table, or use your baby record book) so you will always know when you gave the last dose. This will minimize the risk of missing a dose or doubling up accidentally. But don't worry about being a little late with a dose; get back on schedule with the next dose.

■ Check the bottle label for care and storage directions, and follow them. Some medicines need to be stored in the refrigerator or at cool temperatures, and some must be shaken before use.

■ If directions on the label conflict with the doctor's instructions and/or those received from the pharmacist, call the pharmacist or doctor to resolve the conflict *before* giving the medication.

■ Always read the label before giving a medication, even when you're sure you have the right bottle. When administering medicine in the dark, check the label in the light first.

■ Don't give medicines prescribed for someone else (even a sibling) to your baby without the doctor's approval. Don't even use a medicine previously prescribed for your baby without the doctor's okay.

■ Don't administer medication to a baby who is lying down; this could cause choking.

■ Always give antibiotics for the prescribed length of time, unless the doctor advises otherwise, even if your baby seems completely recovered.

■ If your baby is having an adverse reaction to a medication, stop it temporarily and check with the doctor before resuming use.

■ Don't continue giving a medicine beyond the time specified by the doctor; don't start giving one again after discontinuing it without checking with the doctor first.

■ Record any medication you give your baby, the illness it was given for, the length of time it was taken, and any side or adverse effects in your baby's health history for future reference (see page 424).

Helping the Medicine Go Down

Learning how to give medication correctly is only the first step for parents, and usually the easiest. As far as many children are concerned, the cure is almost always worse than the disease; getting the medicine to go down often seems a hopeless task. And even when it does go down, it often comes right back up—all over baby, parent, furniture, and floor.

If you're lucky, your baby will be one of those who actually delights in the medicine-giving ritual and even in the taste of strange liquids—whether they are vitamins, antibiotics, or pain relievers—and who opens up like a little sparrow at the first sight of a medicine dropper. If you're not so lucky, you've got an infant who is staunchly resistant, either from the start or after becoming wiser in the ways of resistance with advancing age. There is probably nothing that will make administering medicine to such a baby a pleasure, but these tips will help get more medicine down with less trouble:

■ Chill the medication if this won't affect its potency (ask your pharmacist); the taste may be less pronounced when it's cold.

■ Use a spoon that is gently rounded rather than deep, so it can more easily be wiped clean by baby. (If it doesn't come clean during the first pass, turn it over and pull it back over baby's tongue to clean off the dregs.) If your baby doesn't take kindly to a spoon, and a dropper isn't large enough for

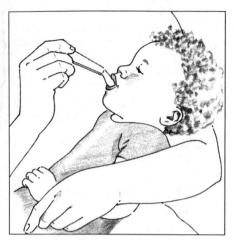

Use a medicine spoon or dropper to ease medications into baby's mouth.

the prescribed dose, ask the pharmacist for a medicine spoon or plastic syringe, which will allow you to squirt the medicine deep into baby's mouth; but don't squirt more than a baby can swallow at one time. If your baby rejects medication from a dropper, spoon, or syringe and likes a nipple instead, try putting the dose in a hand-held nursing-bottle nipple so baby can suck it out. Follow this with water from the same nipple so any medication remaining in the nipple can be taken.

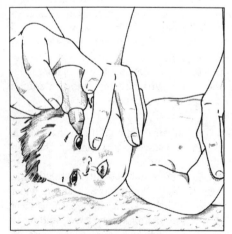

Keeping baby's head steady when using eye drops will help ensure that at least some of the medicine will hit its mark.

- Aim a spoon toward the back of the mouth, a dropper or syringe between molars or rear gum and cheek, since the taste buds are concentrated front and center on the tongue. But avoid letting the dropper or spoon touch the back of the tongue, where it could set off a gagging reflex.
- Unless you're instructed to give the medication with or after meals, plan on serving it up just before feeding. First because baby is more likely to accept it when hungry, and second because if baby does vomit it right back up, less food will be lost.
- Enlist help when you can. Holding a wriggly, uncooperative baby while trying to bring a spoon filled to the brim with medicine to an unwilling mouth without spilling would be a challenge even for a mother octopus, and can sometimes be next to impossible for the two-armed mom. If dad (or another assistant) isn't around to hold baby, try using an infant seat or a high chair as your extra pair of hands; but be sure to strap your baby in before you begin. If you have to go it alone with no seat to hold baby, try this procedure with a young medicine resister: First, premeasure the medicine and have it ready to use on a table within reach in a dropper, syringe, medicine cup, or spoon (which shouldn't be filled to the brim). Sit in a straight chair and position baby on your lap, facing forward. Put your left arm across baby's body, holding his or her arms securely. Take hold of his or her jaw with your left hand, your thumb on one cheek, your index finger on the other. Tilt baby's head backward slightly and depress cheeks gently to open the mouth. With your right hand (reverse hands if you're left-handed), administer the medicine. Keep baby's cheeks slightly depressed until the medicine is swallowed. This entire procedure should take only a few seconds; longer and your baby will begin to fight being held down.
- Approach your baby confidently with medicine—even if past experience has taught you to expect the worst. If baby knows you're anticipating a battle, you're sure to get one. You may get one anyway, of course, but a confident approach could

THE CHICKEN SOUP CURE

It turns out that old wives (and old grandmothers) weren't telling tales when they claimed their chicken soup was as curative as anything their sons the doctors could prescribe. Medical research backs up what the apron set has told us all along: a bowl of hot chicken soup, besides making us feel loved, can help combat the symptoms of colds, coughs, and flus. But when dosing your baby with this penicillin-in-a-pot, don't use commercial bouillons and broths from cubes or cans, which are astronomically high in salt and could cause serious chemical imbalances and an overload on the kidneys. Instead, don an apron and put up a pot from scratch, using chicken parts or a chicken or turkey carcass and plenty of parsley, parsnips, carrots, celery, leeks, onions, and a couple of garlic cloves. Simmer the brew until the skin falls from the bones, skimming the foam and fat as they appear on top. Strain, and feed to baby at a comfortably warm temperature in a spoon, from a cup, or in a bottle. (Don't purée the carrots for baby food, unless you're planning to serve them along with the soup they were cooked in, since most of the vitamins have cooked out into the stock.)

swing the odds in your favor.

■ As a last resort, mix the medication with a small amount (1 or 2 teaspoons) of strained fruit or fruit juice—but only if the doctor hasn't ruled out such a mix. But don't dilute the medicine in a larger quantity of food or juice since then your baby may not finish it all. Unless your baby is generally tentative about new foods, use an unfamiliar fruit or juice for mixing since the medicine may impart an unpleasant taste to a familiar one, causing baby to reject it in the future.

■ Acetaminophen that comes in "sprinkle caps," is tasteless, and can be emptied into a spoonful of juice or fruit can make giving this medicine much easier.

THE MOST COMMON INFANT HEALTH PROBLEMS

Infants in their first year of life are generally healthy, and most of the illnesses to which they are susceptible are one-time affairs (see the chart starting on page 630 for details on these). But there are some illnesses that are so common, or that tend to recur so frequently in some babies, that parents need to know as much as possible about them. They include allergies, the common cold, constipation, ear infections, and gastrointestinal illnesses with diarrhea and vomiting.

ALLERGIES

Symptoms: Depend on the organ or system inflamed by the hypersensitivity. The following are common body systems affected, and the related symptoms:

■ The upper respiratory tract: runny nose (allergic rhinitis), sinusitis (though not in infants), earache (otitis media), sore throat (as much the result of mouth-breathing of dry air as from allergy), postnasal discharge (a dripping of mucus at the back of the nose into the throat that can trigger a

TREATING BABY'S SYMPTOMS

SYMPTOM	APPROPRIATE TREATMENT
Cough	Humidified air* Increased fluids* Reduction of dairy products, for babies over six months in whom milk seems to increase mucus production Cough medication, only if prescribed Postural drainage, if recommended and taught to you by the doctor
Croupy cough	Abundant steam* A trip out of doors
Diarrhea	Increased fluids, oral rehydration (see page 422) Possible dietary changes (see page 422) Antidiarrheal medicine, only if prescribed Upright position*
Ear pain	Pain reliever, such as acetaminophen or ibuprofen*** Local dry heat to ear (hot water bottle) Decongestant, only if prescribed Antibiotics, only if prescribed for this infection Ear drops, only if prescribed
Fever	Increased fluids (see page 431) Adequate calorie intake Anti-fever medication, such as acetaminophen or ibuprofen,*** as recommended by doctor Tepid bath or sponging, if medication is inappropriate or ineffective (see page 432) Light clothing and cool room temperature (see page 431)
Itching	Calamine lotion (*not* Caladryl or other antihistaminic preparation) Comfortably hot bath (test with your elbow or wrist; not for babies under six months) Soothing tepid bath*

SYMPTOM	APPROPRIATE TREATMENT
Itching (con't)	Colloidal oatmeal bath Prevention of scratching and infection (keep fingernails short and wash with antibacterial soap; cover hands with socks or mittens during sleep) Pain reliever, such as acetaminophen (but *not* aspirin if chicken pox is a possibility)** Oral antihistamine, only if prescribed (but *not* topical antihistamines or anesthetics)
Nasal congestion	Humidified air* Salt-water irrigation* Nasal aspiration* Head elevation* Increased fluids* Decongestant, only if prescribed Nose drops, only if prescribed
Pain or discomfort from minor injury	Comfort (cuddling) Distraction (see page 441) Pain reliever, such as acetaminophen or ibuprofen*** Local heat or cold, as appropriate
Sore throat	Soothing, non-acid foods and beverages Pain reliever, such as acetaminophen or ibuprofen*** Fever treatment, if needed (see facing page) Saltwater gargle, for older children
Teething pain	Comfort (cuddling) Local cold, applied to gums (see page 224) Pressure on gums (see page 225) Pain reliever, such as acetaminophen or ibuprofen,*** only if recommended by the doctor
Vomiting	Increased fluids, in small sips (see page 422) Restricted diet (see page 422)

*See Ready Reference for tips on carrying out this treatment.
**See page 432 for precautions on giving aspirin to children.
***Available only by prescription for children under two.

chronic cough), spasmodic croup.
- The lower respiratory tract: allergic bronchitis, asthma.
- The digestive tract: watery, sometimes bloody, diarrhea; vomiting; gassiness.
- The skin: atopic dermatitis, including such itchy rashes as eczema (see page 227), hives (blotchy, itchy, raised red rash, also called urticaria), and angioneurotic edema (facial swelling, particularly around eyes and mouth, which is not as itchy as urticaria). When swelling occurs in the throat, breathing can be hampered.
- The eyes: itching, redness, watering, and other signs of conjunctivitis.

Season: Any time of year for most allergies; spring, summer, or fall for those related to pollens.

Cause: The release of histamine and other substances by the immune system in response to exposure to an allergen in persons who are hypersensitive to the allergen or a similar one (the sensitization occurs at an earlier exposure). The tendency toward allergy runs in families. The way allergy is manifested is often different in different members of the family—one has hay fever, another asthma, and a third breaks out in hives upon eating strawberries.

Method of transmission: Inhalation (of pollen or animal dander, for example), ingestion (of milk or egg whites), or injection (penicillin shot or insect sting) of the allergen.

Duration: Variable. The duration of a single allergic episode may vary from a few minutes to several hours or several days. Some allergies, such as an allergy to cow's milk, are outgrown; others change, as children get older, from one kind of allergy to another. Many allergic people have allergies of one kind or another all their lives.

RESPIRATORY SOUNDS YOU DON'T HAVE TO WORRY ABOUT

Somewhere between four and eight weeks of age, many babies develop what might best be described as a "snurgle." These are sounds produced as the infant inhales through loose mucus in the nose and throat, which probably is a product of an increased functioning by the mucus-producing glands located in the normal lining of the respiratory tract. Often these sounds are accompanied by a rattling in baby's chest that can be felt with the hand. The snurgle doesn't interfere with breathing and the infants have no problem inhaling with their mouths closed—something they can't do when they have a cold. The condition is more noticeable in babies who have high arched palates or narrower-than-usual nasal passages. This noisy breathing is not a cause for concern and usually disappears within a few weeks as baby matures.

Some babies have a "gurgle" that is noticeable when they feed and breathe in. The gurgle originates in or below the larynx, or voice box. It is often associated with tracheomalacia, a condition that is the result of an unusually soft and flexible trachea, common in many infants. There is usually no associated cough, although there may be a liquidy sounding stridor, or vibrating sound. These gurgles may continue well into the second year, but should not interfere with growth and development and require no remedial treatmeat. The condition resolves as the rings of cartilage in the airway become more rigid.

If you note a snurgle or gurgle in your newborn or very young infant, ask the doctor about it. Most likely it is completely normal. If, on the other hand, an older baby suddenly develops strange breathing sounds, call the doctor at once. A raspy noise on breathing out—usually called a wheeze—should also be reported to the doctor.

Treatment: The most successful treatment for allergy, though also often the most difficult, is to remove the offending allergen from the sufferer's life. Here are some ways in which you can remove allergens from your child's environment, whether your child is definitely allergic (difficult to determine since skin tests are not very accurate in children under eighteen months) or only possibly so:

- Food allergens. See *Dietary changes.*
- Pollens. If you suspect pollen allergy (the clue is the persistence of symptoms as long as pollen is in the air, and their disappearance when it is gone), keep your child indoors most of the time when the pollen count is high or when it is particularly windy during pollen season (spring, late summer, or fall, depending on the type of pollen), give daily baths and shampoos (to remove pollen), and use an air-conditioner in warm weather rather than opening the windows and admitting the pollen. If you have a pet, the animal can also pick up pollen when out of doors, so you should bathe him or her frequently, too. Such allergy is rare in infants.
- Pet dander. Sometimes pets themselves cause an allergy. If this is the case, or might be, try to keep your animal and your baby in different rooms, or keep the animal in the basement, garage, or backyard. (In severe cases, the only solution may be to find the pet another home.) Since horsehair can also trigger allergy, don't buy a horsehair mattress for your baby's crib.
- Household dust. These particles fill the air in your home and are breathed in, unseen, by everyone in your family. That's no problem for most people, but for someone with a hypersensitivity to these substances, it can mean misery. Limit your baby's exposure, even if you just suspect this allergy, by keeping the rooms he or she lives in as dust-free as possible. Dust daily with a damp cloth or furniture spray when baby is not in the room; vacuum rugs and upholstered furniture and damp-mop floors often; avoid chenille bedspreads, carpeting, draperies, and other dust catchers where baby sleeps and plays; wash stuffed toys frequently; keep clothing in plastic garment bags; sheathe mattresses and pillows in airtight coverings (infant mattresses usually have airtight covers); put filters over hot-air vents; install an air filter. Any curtains, throw rugs, or other such items you do have should be washed at least twice a month, or packed away. Keep humidity low.
- Molds. Control moisture in your home by using a well-maintained dehumidifier, providing adequate ventilation, and by exhausting steam in kitchen, laundry, and baths. Areas where molds are likely to grow (garbage cans, refrigerators, shower curtains, bathroom tiles, damp corners) should be cleaned meticulously with an anti-mold agent. Houseplants should be limited and firewood should not be stored in the house. Out of doors, be sure drainage around your home is good, that leaves and other plant debris are not allowed to pile up, and that plenty of sun hits the yard and house to prevent damp areas from spawning mold. Keep baby's sandbox covered in the rain.
- Bee venom. Anyone allergic to bee venom should avoid outdoor areas known to have bee or wasp populations. Carrying a bee-sting kit is mandatory for such individuals.
- Miscellaneous allergens. Many other potential allergens can also be removed from your child's world: wool blankets (cover them or use cotton or synthetic blankets); down or feather pillows (use foam or hypoallergenic polyester-filled ones) when baby's old enough to use one; tobacco smoke (no smoking in the house at all, or near baby in other locations); perfumes (use unscented wipes, sprays, and so on); soaps (use only hypoallergenic types); detergents (you may have to switch detergents or use Ivory Snow for the laundry).

Since an allergy is a hypersensitive (or oversensitive) reaction of the immune system to a foreign substance, desensitizing (usually via gradually increased injected doses of the offending allergen) is sometimes successful in eliminating allergies—particularly pollen, dust, and animal dander. Except in severe cases, however, desensitization is not usually started until a child is four years old. Antihistamines and steroids may be used to counteract the allergic response and bring down the swelling of mucous membranes in both infants and children.

Dietary changes:
- Elimination of possible dietary allergens, always using nutritionally equivalent substitutes (see The Infant Daily Dozen on page 221). Remove a suspected food allergen (cow's milk, wheat, egg whites, and citrus are among the possibilities) from your baby's diet under medical supervision; if symptoms disappear within a few weeks, you probably have discovered the culprit. You get further confirmation if the symptoms recur when the food is returned to the diet. Substitute oat, rice, and barley flours for wheat; soy or hydrolysate formula[1] for cow's milk formula; egg yolks for whole eggs; and mangoes, cantaloupe, broccoli, cauliflower, and sweet red peppers for orange juice to ensure vitamin C intake.
- Adequate fluid intake with respiratory allergies. Most nursing and bottle-fed infants get enough fluids, but many weaned babies do not.

Prevention:
- Breastfeeding, particularly when there is a family history of allergies, for at least six months, preferably for a year may help.
- Late introduction of solids, usually not until six months, and then with caution (see page 216). Even later introduction of the most serious offenders (cow's milk, egg whites, wheat, chocolate, citrus). Careful observation for reactions when food is introduced.

---

1. About 40% of babies allergic to cow's milk are also allergic to soy, so hydrolysate formula is usually a safer bet. *Do not* use so-called soy milks, since they do not provide adequate nutrition for infants. If you switch to goat's milk, vitamin supplementation will be needed because goat's milk is deficient in certain nutrients.

Complications:
- Asthma
- Anaphylactic shock, which can be fatal without treatment (but is rare).

When to call the doctor: Soon after you suspect an allergy. Call again whenever your child has new symptoms. Call immediately if there are any signs of asthma (wheezing), difficulty breathing, or signs of shock (disorientation, panting, rapid pulse rate, pale, cold, moist skin, drowsiness, or loss of consciousness).

Chance of recurrence: Some allergies disappear in adulthood never to return; others return under different guises.

Diseases with similar symptoms:
- Bronchitis (but a child who seems to have repeated bouts of this disease probably has bronchial asthma)
- The common cold (like allergic rhinitis)
- Gastrointestinal illnesses (similar to digestive tract symptoms)

THE COMMON COLD OR UPPER RESPIRATORY INFECTION (URI)

Colds are very common among babies and young children because they have not had the chance to build up immunities against the many different cold viruses.

Symptoms:
- Runny nose (discharge is watery at first, then thicker and yellowish)
- Sneezing
- Nasal congestion

Sometimes:
- Dry cough, which may be worse when baby is lying down
- Fever
- Itchy throat
- Fatigue
- Loss of appetite

Season: All year round.

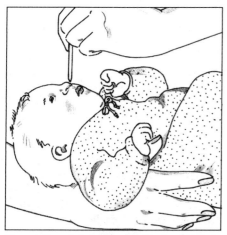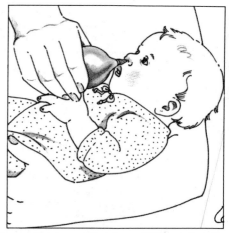

For a baby who's having trouble breathing through a stuffy nose, saline drops (left) to soften the mucus and aspiration (right) to suction it out will bring welcome relief.

Cause: More than 100 different viruses are known to cause colds.

Method of transmission: Usually spread from hand to hand.

Incubation period: One to four days.

Duration: Usually three to ten days, but in small children colds can linger longer.

Treatment: No known cure, but symptoms can be treated, as necessary:

■ Suctioning of mucus with a suction bulb (see above). If mucus is hardened, before suctioning soften with over-the-counter saline nose drops. This may be necessary to help baby to feed as well as to sleep.
■ Humidification (see page 628) to help moisten the air, reduce congestion, and make breathing easier for baby.
■ Letting baby sleep on belly rather than back, with head elevated (by raising the head of the crib or carriage mattress with a couple of pillows or other supports *under* the mattress) to ease breathing.
■ Decongestants, if needed to make it easier for baby to eat and sleep, but *only* with doctor's okay.
■ Commercial nose drops, if recommended by the physician, to ease congestion. But follow directions carefully; use

for more than a few days can cause a rebound reaction and make baby feel worse.
■ Petroleum jelly (Vaseline) or similar ointment applied lightly to outside of, and under, nose to help prevent chapping and reddening of skin. But be careful to not let it get into the nostrils, where it could be inhaled or block breathing.
■ Cough medicine, but only to ease a dry cough that interferes with sleep, and only if it is prescribed by the doctor. A cough suppressant is not usually prescribed for a baby otherwise. *Antibiotics will not help* and should not be used unless there is bacterial secondary infection.
■ Isolation, keeping the baby in the house and away from others for the first three days—which won't hasten recovery but will minimize spreading the cold to others.

Dietary changes: Baby can continue a normal diet (though many have a loss of appetite), with the following exceptions:

■ Reduce intake of milk and other dairy products, since it is possible they may thicken secretions; infants exclusively on breast milk or formula can continue on them, unless the doctor advises otherwise.
■ Increased intake of fluids to help replace those lost through fever or runny nose. If baby is old enough, drinking from a cup

THE SUDDEN COUGH

If your baby or young child suddenly begins coughing uncontrollably and does not seem to have a cold or other illness, consider the possibility that an inhaled object could be the cause. See page 454.

may be more comfortable than trying to nurse or bottle feed with a stuffy nose.
- Adequate intake of vitamin C foods. Whether or not vitamin C will prevent a cold is controversial, but some studies do show it can reduce the severity of symptoms. So including extra citrus or other juices high in vitamin C in your baby's fluid intake is a good idea.

Prevention: Careful hand washing for all the family, especially when someone has a cold, and particularly before handling baby or baby's things. Coughs and sneezes should be covered; disposable tissues rather than handkerchiefs should be used; eating utensils and towels should not be shared. If possible, no one with a cold should handle baby's toys or feeding utensils.

Complications: Colds sometimes progress to ear infections or bronchitis, and less often to pneumonia or sinusitis.

When to call the doctor: If this is a first cold; if your baby is under three months old, or under four months and has a fever over 101°F; if the temperature goes up suddenly or a fever continues for more than two days; if a dry cough lasts more than two weeks, is interfering with baby's sleep, causes choking or vomiting, becomes thick and productive or wheezy, or if breathing difficulties develop; if a thick greenish yellow nasal discharge develops and lasts more than a day, or if the discharge is streaked with blood; if there is an unusual amount of crying (with or without tugging at the ears) or a complete loss of appetite; or if baby seems really out of sorts. A cough that lasts more than three weeks in an infant or six in an older baby may require consultation with a specialist.

Chance of recurrence: Since having a cold caused by one virus doesn't make baby immune to a cold caused by another, babies, who haven't had the chance to build up immunities to many viruses, can have one cold right after another.

Diseases with similar symptoms:
- Rubella, chicken pox, and German measles begin with cold-like symptoms; check those diseases (see table starting on page 630) for additional symptoms
- Respiratory allergies
- Influenza

CONSTIPATION

This problem is rare in breastfed babies (even if they move their bowels rarely and their movements seem difficult to expel) because their movements are never hard. Constipation does, however, occur in formula-fed infants.

Symptoms:
- Infrequent bowel movements with stools that are hard (often small pellets) and hard to pass; infrequency alone, however, is not a sign of constipation and may be your baby's normal pattern
- Stool streaked with blood, if there are anal fissures (cracks in the anus caused by the passage of hard stool)
- Gastric distress and abdominal pain
- Irritability

Season: Any time, but may be more frequent in winter when less fruit is consumed.

Cause: A sluggish digestive tract, illness, insufficient fiber in diet, insufficient activity, or an anal fissure that makes defecation painful; occasionally, a serious medical condition.

Duration: May be chronic or occur just occasionally.

Treatment: Though constipation is not unusual in bottle-fed infants, symptoms should always be reported to the doctor, who can, when necessary, check for any abnormalities that might be causing it. Occasional constipation or mild chronic constipation is usually treated with dietary changes (see below); an increase in exercise may help (in infants, try moving the legs in a bicycle fashion when you see your baby having difficulty with a movement). Do not give laxatives, enemas, or any medication without the doctor's instructions.

Dietary changes: Make these only after consultation with baby's doctor:
■ Give an ounce or two of prune or apple juice by bottle, cup, or spoon.
■ For a baby on solids, add a teaspoonful of bran to morning cereal; increase intake of fruits (other than banana) and vegetables.
■ In older babies, cut back on milk if daily intake exceeds three cups.

Prevention: When solids are added to baby's diet, be sure to include only whole grains plus plenty of fruits and vegetables. Move to chunkier textures as soon as baby seems ready for them, rather than sticking to strained foods for the entire first year. Also be sure baby's fluid intake is adequate and that baby has plenty of opportunity for physical activity.

Complications:
■ Fissures
■ Difficulty with toilet training
■ Impacted stool (stool that is not passed naturally and may be painful to remove manually)

When to call the doctor: If your baby seems to be constipated often or regularly; if the problem suddenly arises when it has not been noted before; or if there is blood in the stool.

Chance of recurrence: The problem can become a "habit" if it isn't dealt with when it first occurs.

Diseases with similar symptoms:
■ Intestinal obstructions or abnormalities

DIARRHEA

This problem, too, is unusual in breastfed babies because there appear to be certain substances in breast milk that destroy many of the microorganisms that cause diarrhea.

Symptoms:
■ Liquidy, runny stools
Sometimes:
■ Increased frequency
■ Increased volume
■ Mucus
■ Vomiting

Season: Any time, but may be more common in summer, when more fruit is consumed and food spoilage is common. Rotovirus infection is more common in winter.

Cause: Very varied:
■ Illness
■ Teething
■ Sensitivity to a food in the diet
■ Too much fruit, juice (particularly apple or grape), or other laxative-type foods
■ Gastrointestinal infection (viral, bacterial, or parasitic)
■ Antibiotic medication (feeding yogurt with live cultures to a baby on antibiotics may prevent this type of diarrhea)

Method of transmission: Infectious cases can be transmitted via the feces-to-hand-to-mouth route. Also transmitted by contaminated foods.

Incubation period: Depends on the causative organism.

Duration: Usually anywhere from a few hours to several days, but some cases can become chronic if the cause is not discovered and corrected.

Treatment: Depends on the cause, but most common approaches are dietary. Sometimes medication may be prescribed. Do not give anti-diarrheal medication to an infant without the doctor's approval— some can be harmful to young children. Protect baby's bottom from irritation by changing diapers as soon as possible after they're soiled and by spreading on a thick ointment after each change. If diaper rash develops, see page 178.

A very sick baby may need hospitalization to stabilize body fluids.

Dietary changes:
- Continuing formula or breast feedings in most cases is best. Since a baby with diarrhea may develop a temporary lactose intolerance, a switch to a soy-based, lactose-free formula may be recommended if the diarrhea doesn't improve on baby's regular formula.

- High fluid intake (at least 2 ounces an hour) to replace fluids lost through diarrhea. To augment breast milk or formula, a rehydration mixture (such as Pedialyte, Resol, or Lytren), available over-the-counter at any pharmacy, is usually recommended. Offer a few sips by spoon, cup, or bottle every two or three minutes, working up to 8 ounces between loose bowel movements. Do not give sweetened drinks (such as colas), undiluted fruit juices, athletic drinks, glucose water, or homemade salt-and-sugar mixtures.

- Continuation of solids, if baby takes them regularly. The theory that it is beneficial to "rest the bowel" by withholding food in cases of diarrhea is no longer widely accepted. The sooner a baby is fed, the less severe the diarrhea will be. Starchy foods such as mashed banana, white rice or rice cereal, potatoes, pasta, or dry white toast can, depending on baby's usual diet, all be good choices. Small amounts of protein foods (chicken, cottage cheese) are also appropriate.

- If there is vomiting, solid feeding is usually not resumed until vomiting has stopped. But do offer sips of clear fluids (diluted juices or oral rehydration fluid, if prescribed), or for an older baby, ice pops made with diluted fruit juice. Offering small amounts (no more than a tablespoon or two at a time, less for a very young infant) will greatly increase the chance that it will be held down. Once vomiting has ceased, foods can be added as above.

- When stool begins to return to normal, usually after two or three days, the doctor will recommend that you begin to return your baby to a regular diet but continue limiting milk and other dairy products (other than breast milk and formula) for another day or two.

- In diarrhea that lasts for two weeks or more in a bottle-fed infant, the doctor may recommend a change in formula.

Prevention: Diarrhea can't always be prevented, but risks can be reduced:
- Attention to sanitary preparation of foods (see page 230).
- Careful hand washing by baby's caretakers after handling diapers and going to the bathroom.
- The dilution of fruit juices taken by babies; limiting total intake. (Babies and young children have been known to have chronic diarrhea as a result of drinking a quart or less of apple or grape juice a day.)

Complications:
- Diaper rash
- Dehydration, which if severe, could lead to coma and even death

When to call the doctor: One or two loose stools is not a cause for concern. But the following indicate diarrhea that may need medical attention:
- You suspect baby may have consumed spoiled food or formula.
- Baby has had loose, watery stools for 24 hours.
- Baby is vomiting (more than the usual spitup) repeatedly, or has been vomiting for 24 hours.

- There is blood in baby's stools.

- Baby is running a fever or seems ill.

Call *immediately* if baby shows signs of dehydration: decreased urine output (diapers aren't as wet as usual and/or urine is yellow); tearless and sunken eyes; a sunken fontanel; dry skin; scanty saliva.

Chance of recurrence: Likely if cause has not been eliminated; some babies are more prone to diarrhea.

Diseases with similar symptoms:
- Food allergies
- Food poisoning
- Enzyme deficiencies.

MIDDLE-EAR INFLAMMATION (OTITIS MEDIA)

Babies are very susceptible to ear infections because their eustachian tubes are short and narrow. Most eventually outgrow this susceptibility.

Symptoms: In acute otitis media

Usually:
- Ear pain, often worse at night (babies sometimes pull or rub or hold their ears, but often give no indication of pain except for crying, and sometimes not even that; crying when sucking on breast or bottle may indicate ear pain that has radiated to the jaw)
- Fever, which may be slight or very high
- Fatigue and irritability

Sometimes:
- Nausea and/or vomiting
- Loss of appetite

Occasionally:
- No obvious symptoms at all
On examination the eardrum appears pink at first, then red and bulging (though an eardrum may also appear red if baby's been crying or because of the light being used); without treatment pressure can burst the drum, releasing pus into the ear canal and relieving the pain; the eardrum heals eventually, but treatment helps to prevent further damage.

In serous otitis media (or fluid in the middle ear)

Usually:
- Hearing loss (which is temporary but can become permanent if condition persists for many months untreated).

Sometimes:
- Clicking or popping sounds on swallowing or sucking.

- No symptoms at all, other than the fluid in the ear.

Season: All year round, but much more common in winter.

Cause: Usually bacteria or viruses, though allergy can also cause middle-ear inflammation. Babies and young children may be most susceptible because of the shape of their eustachian tubes; because they are more likely to get respiratory infections, which usually precede ear infections; because they have immature immune response; or because they are often fed while lying on their backs. The eustachian tubes, which drain fluids and mucus from the ears down the back of the nose and the throat, are shorter in a baby than in an adult, so germs can easily travel through them into the middle ear. And because the tubes are horizontal rather than vertical (as in adults), drainage is poor, especially in infants who spend a lot of time on their backs. The short length also makes the tubes more subject to blockage (by swelling from allergy or from an infection, such as a cold, by a malformation, or by large adenoids). When the fluid can't drain normally, it builds up in the middle ear, causing serous otitis media. Fluid can also build up when the tube collapses because of pressure changes when traveling by plane. This fluid makes an excellent breeding place for infection-causing bacteria (usually streptococci or hemophilus influenzae).

YOUR BABY'S HEALTH HISTORY

If there isn't adequate space in your new arrival's baby book, buy a notebook to use as a permanent health history. Record all your baby's birth statistics, as well as information about each illness, medications given, immunizations, doctors, and so on. What follows is a sampling of the kinds of things to include.

AT BIRTH

Weight:	Length:	Head circumference:
Condition at birth:		
APGAR at one and five minutes:		
Results of Brazelton or other tests:		
Any problems or abnormalities:		

INFANT ILLNESSES

Date:	Recovered:
Symptoms:	
Doctor called:	
Diagnosis:	
Instructions:	
Medications given:	How long:
Side effects:	

IMMUNIZATIONS

	Date:	Reactions:
DTP:		
Boosters:		
Polio:		
MMR:		
Other:		

Method of transmission: Not direct, but children in day care may be more vulnerable. There may be a family disposition to ear infections.

Incubation period: Often follows a cold or the flu.

Duration: Varies, but treatment for acute otitis media is usually given for ten days. Serous otitis media can become chronic.

Treatment: Ear infections require medical treatment; do not try to treat on your own. Treatment usually includes:

- Antibiotics for acute otitis media, to knock out the bacterial infection. Sometimes an anti-inflammatory agent (corticosteroid) is given along with the antibiotic.
- Ear drops, only if prescribed
- Baby acetaminophen or aspirin, sometimes with codeine, for pain and/or fever.
- Heat applied to the ear in the form of a heating pad set on low, a hot-water bag filled with warm water, or warm compresses (see page 629)—any of which can be used while you are trying to reach the doctor.
- A decongestant, in the form of nose drops or spray, to help open a blocked eustachian tube, but only if prescribed. Recent studies show this medication does not speed recovery.
- Myringotomy (minor surgery to drain infected fluid from the ear through a tiny incision in the eardrum) if the eardrum appears about to burst; the incision will heal in about ten days, but may require special care until then.
- Insertion of a tiny tube to drain remaining fluids when a chronic infection doesn't respond to antibiotic therapy. This is done under general anesthesia and is a last resort for cases that don't respond to other treatments. Usually a tube is tried if fluid has remained in one ear for six months—or in both ears for four months—with no improvement. The tube falls out after nine to twelve months, sometimes sooner, and is usually successful in preventing further infections.
- Periodic ear exams until the ear (or ears) is back to normal to be sure the condition has not become chronic.
- Elimination or treatment of allergies related to repeated ear infections.

Dietary changes: Extra fluids for fever.

Prevention: A sure way to prevent otitis media is not yet known. Recent research, however, suggests that the following may reduce the risk of a baby's falling victim:

- Overall good health through adequate nutrition, plenty of rest, and regular medical care.
- Breastfeeding for at least three months.
- An upright feeding position, especially when a baby has a respiratory infection.
- An elevated sleeping position when a baby has a cold (put a few pillows *under* the head of the mattress, not under baby's head.)
- Decongestants for children with colds or allergies, particularly before an air flight, and having baby suck on breast or bottle during takeoffs and especially landings, when most ear problems occur.
- Low-dose antibiotics for children with frequent ear infections during the height of the otitis media season, or just when the child comes down with a cold (the antibiotics don't cure the cold, but they can prevent a secondary infection such as otitis media).
- Smoke-free living space.
- Home child care rather than group day-care situations, where children are more likely to come down with otitis media.

Complications:
Among others:
- Chronic otitis media with hearing loss
- Mastoid infection
- Meningitis, bacteremia, pneumonia
- Brain abscess
- Facial paralysis

When to call the doctor: Initially, as soon as you suspect your baby may have an earache. Again if symptoms do not seem to begin clearing within two days, or if baby seems worse. Even if no ear infection is suspected, call if baby suddenly doesn't seem to be hearing as well as usual.

Chance of recurrence: Some babies never have an ear infection, others have one or two in infancy and then no repeats, and still others have them repeatedly on into toddlerhood and the preschool years.

Diseases with similar symptoms: A foreign object in the ear, swimmer's ear, and referred pain from respiratory infection can mimic an earache.

WHAT IT'S IMPORTANT TO KNOW: All About Fever

Though you may remember your mother standing over you, thermometer in hand, concern in her voice, announcing, "You've got a fever—I'd better call the doctor," fever hasn't always been cause for alarm. The ancients welcomed fevers because they believed they burned out bad "humors." In the Middle Ages, fever was actually induced on occasion to fight syphilis and certain other infections. And in fact, fever was considered so beneficial that it wasn't even treated until about 100 years ago, when aspirin, with its fever-reducing capabilities, came on the scene. By the time your generation was growing up, even the slightest rise in temperature was a cause for worry, and a high fever for all-out panic.

Oddly enough, as it turns out, Hippocrates had a better notion of what fever is all about than did the modern medical community of a generation ago. Recent research has confirmed that, as Hippocrates speculated, most fevers actually do more good than harm—that they do in a sense burn out, if not the bad humors, at least the bad germs that invade and threaten the body. Instead of being a symptom to be feared and fought, fever is now recognized to be an important part of the body's immune response to infection.

Here's how scientists now believe fever plays its role. In response to such invaders as viruses, bacteria, and fungi, white blood cells in the body produce a hormone now called interleukin, which then travels to the brain to instruct the hypothalamus to turn up the body thermostat. It appears that at higher body temperatures, the rest of the immune system is better able to fight infection. Fever may also lower iron levels while increasing the invaders' need for that mineral—in effect starving them. And when it's a virus that has launched the attack, fever helps enhance the production of interferon and other antiviral substances in the body.

When an individual's body temperature suddenly rises a couple of degrees above normal (98.6°F)[2] he or she often feels, paradoxically, chilled. The chilling serves to encourage a further rise in temperature in several ways. The involuntary shivering that usually occurs signals the body to turn its thermostat up still another notch and prompts the fever sufferer to take other measures that raise the body temperature: drink hot drinks, throw on another blanket, put on a sweater. At the same time, outlying blood vessels constrict to reduce heat loss, and body tissues—such as stored fat—are broken down to produce heat (which is why it is important to take extra calories during a fever).

A very high fever occasionally causes convulsions in infants and young children, usually at the very onset of the fever. Though they are frightening for parents. doctors now believe febrile convulsions are

2. All temperature readings referred to in this chapter are oral, the standard for temperature readings, unless otherwise noted.

not dangerous. (See page 431 for safe handling of convulsions.) Studies have shown that children who have febrile convulsions show no neurological or mental impairment later on, though they are very slightly more apt to have an increased risk of epilepsy in the future (but the convulsions, it is suspected, are more likely to be a result of the tendency toward the disorder than the cause of it). Babies who have had convulsions with a fever once have a 30 to 40% greater chance of a repeat episode, and medical treatment doesn't affect that risk. Nor does treatment of a fever during the illness seem to reduce the incidence of seizures in these predisposed children, probably because the convulsions almost always occur just as the fever rises at the outset of an illness, before treatment can be given.

An estimated 80 to 90% of all fevers in babies are related to self-limiting viral infections (they get better without treatment). Most doctors today don't recommend trying to reduce such fever in babies over six months unless it is 102° or more, and some wait for significantly higher temperatures before they advise parents to get out the medicine dropper. They may, however, suggest the use of baby acetaminophen even with lower temperatures to relieve aches and pains, make a baby more comfortable, improve sleep, and sometimes, to make a nervous mother feel better. On the other hand, illnesses caused by bacteria must be treated. Antibiotics lower temperatures indirectly by wiping out the infection. Depending on the illness, the antibiotic selected, the child's level of comfort, and the height of the fever, antibiotics and fever reducers may or may not be prescribed simultaneously.

Unlike most other infection-related fever, fever related to shock from a generalized bacterial invasion of the body, as in septicemia (blood poisoning), requires immediate medical treatment to lower the body temperature.

Normally, body temperature is at its lowest (as low as 96.5° taken orally) between 2:00 and 4:00 in the morning, is still relatively low (as low as 97°) when we get up, then slowly rises over the day until it peaks between 6:00 and 10:00 in the evening at about 99°. It tends to be slightly higher in hot weather, lower in cold, higher during exercise than at rest. It's more volatile and subject to greater variation in babies and young children than in adults.

Fevers behave differently in different illnesses. In some, a fever may remain persistently elevated until a baby is well; in others it will be consistently lower in the morning and higher in the evening, spike (shoot up) periodically, or come and go with no obvious pattern. The pattern sometimes helps the doctor to make a diagnosis.

When fever is part of the body's response to illness, temperatures above 106° are rare, and those beyond 108° unheard of. But when fever is the result of the failure of the body's heat-regulation mechanism, as in heat illness, temperatures can soar as high as 114°. Such temperatures can occur when the body produces too much heat or can't cool itself effectively, either through an internal abnormality or, more commonly, through overheating caused by an external heat source, such as a sauna or a hot tub, for example, or the inside of a parked car in warm weather (air temperatures inside the car can quickly shoot up to 113° even with the windows open 2 inches and the temperature outside a moderate 85°). Overheating can also result from strenuous physical activity in hot or humid weather, or from being overdressed in warm weather. Infants and the elderly are most susceptible to heat illnesses because their temperature-regulation mechanisms are less dependable. Fever due to the failure of heat regulation is an illness in itself; and not only is it apparently not beneficial, it is dangerous and requires immediate treatment. Extremely high temperatures (over 106°) that are illness related also require immediate treatment. It's believed that when a fever is that high it ceases to be beneficial, and its positive effects on the immune response may be reversed.

TAKING BABY'S TEMPERATURE

Because the touch of lips (or back of hand) against the side of the forehead can accurately detect a fever 9 out of 10 times (except when overdressing raises skin but not rectal temperature), and because temperature taking often provokes a battle, a few doctors recommend abandoning temperature taking after a baby is six months old. Most, however, prefer a more accurate indicator of a baby's condition than a parent's kiss. Taking the temperature during the course of an illness can answer such questions as "Has the treatment effectively lowered the temperature?" or "Has the fever risen, meaning a turn for the worse?" But though temperature readings can be useful, they needn't be taken every hour on the hour, as an anxious and inexperienced parent is often wont to do. In most cases, once in the morning and once in the evening is adequate. Take it in between only if baby suddenly seems sicker. If baby seems better, and your lips testify that the fever is down, you don't really need a second opinion from the thermometer.

Core body temperatures are most often taken through the mouth, the rectum, the axilla (armpit), or the ear. Since putting a thermometer in a baby's mouth is dangerous (most doctors do not recommend taking oral temperatures until a child is four or five), you'll go one of the other routes for now.

Before you start. Try to keep your baby calm for half an hour before temperature taking, since crying or screaming could turn a slightly elevated temperature into a high one. (Though it's necessary to withhold hot or cold drinks or foods before taking an oral temperature, as they too could affect temperature readings, this precaution isn't necessary when taking rectal or axillary temperatures.)

Preparing the standard thermometer. Wash the thermometer with cold soapy water (warm or hot water can cause the mercury to expand and burst or crack the glass), rinse, then swab it with absorbent cotton dipped in rubbing alcohol. Check the mercury reading, and if it's above 96°, shake it down carefully by holding the end of the thermometer opposite the bulb firmly between your thumb and forefinger and shaking with repeated downward snaps of the wrist. If possible, do the shaking over a bed or sofa and away from hard surfaces, such as the bathroom sink, in case you lose your grip and the instrument slips from your hand. Give yourself enough room so that the thermometer won't accidentally hit something and break. Lubricate the bulb end of a rectal thermometer with petroleum jelly (Vaseline) before inserting it. Rinse an oral thermometer thoroughly in cool water to remove the taste of alcohol.

Taking the temperature. *Rectal:* Prepare the thermometer and bare baby's bottom, speaking reassuringly as you do. Then turn baby onto his or her tummy on your lap (which gives you more control and allows the legs to hang at a 90° angle, making insertion easier) or on a bed or changing table (where a small pillow or folded towel under the hips will raise the baby's bottom slightly for easier insertion). To distract baby, try singing a couple of favorite songs, or putting a favorite book or toy in baby's line of vision. Spread the buttocks with one hand, exposing the anus (the rectal opening). With the other, slip about an inch of the bulb end of the thermometer into the rectum, being careful not to force it. Hold the thermometer in place for two minutes between your index and middle fingers, using your other fingers to press the buttocks together to keep the thermometer from sliding out and to keep baby from wriggling. Remove the thermometer immediately, however, if baby begins to show very active resistance. Even if the thermometer has been in for only half a minute or so, it will have registered to within a degree of the actual temperature and you will have a rough figure to report to the doctor. Wipe the thermometer with a piece of tissue before reading. (If you're a novice, you may want to put the thermometer down—the temperature won't change—while you rediaper and safely deposit baby, then pick it up again for reading.)

Rarely, a thermometer breaks while inserted. If this happens and you can't find all the pieces, call the doctor. But don't worry; the risk of more than a scratch is slight and since the mercury is in a non-toxic form, it should do no harm to your baby (though it can damage precious metals).

Tympanic: This thermometer reads the temperature in the ear, but using it takes some skill. If you buy one (prices are coming down), have your baby's doctor show you how to use it.

Axillary, or underarm: Use this somewhat less accurate method of temperature taking when your baby has diarrhea or won't lie still for a rectal, or if only an oral thermometer is available (*never* use an oral thermometer rectally). Remove baby's shirt so that no clothing will come between thermometer and skin, and be sure the armpit is dry. Place the bulb end of the thermometer (oral or rectal) well up into the armpit, holding the arm down snugly over it and pressing the elbow against baby's

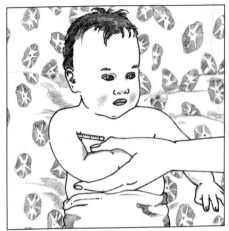
The underarm method.

side. Hold this position for at least four or five minutes, if possible—it may take as long as eight minutes to get an accurate reading. Sing songs, play a tape, put on the television—choose any activity calculated to keep your baby still for the duration.

Oral: You can begin taking oral temperatures when your child can hold the thermometer securely under the tongue with lips closed and can understand directions not to bite down on it, usually at about age four or five, occasionally earlier. For a good oral reading, the thermometer should be tucked all the way into the pocket under the tongue and held there for two to four minutes (if there is mouth breathing, it will take longer to get the temperature).

Reading the thermometer. A rectal temperature is the most accurate since it picks up temperatures from the body's core, but the oral reading is considered the standard. Temperatures obtained rectally, as they are most frequently in infants, are usually one-half to a full degree higher than those determined orally; axillary readings are about one degree lower. On an oral thermometer, 98.6°F is normal; 99.6° is the norm rectally; and 97.6° is normal for an axillary reading. A fever of 102.2° taken rectally is the equivalent of 101.2° taken orally and 100.2° by an armpit reading.

To read a mercury thermometer, hold it

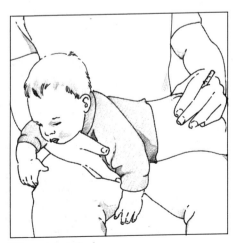
The rectal method.

in a good light and rotate it until you see the silver column of mercury. Line up the mercury between the column calibrations and the numbers, which are marked in full degrees as well as every two-tenths degree. The point where the mercury ends indicates the temperature. Write it down, along with the time it was taken. When you report the temperature to the doctor, be sure to include whether it's a rectal, axillary, or oral reading.

Storing the thermometer. After use, wash the thermometer once again with cold soapy water, rinse, and swab with alcohol. Then store it, in the case, away from such sources of heat as a sunny window, a radiator, a fireplace mantel, a clothes dryer, and the kitchen stove (heat could cause expansion of the mercury and cracking of the glass).

EVALUATING A FEVER

Behavior is a better gauge of how sick an infant is than body temperature. A baby can be seriously ill, with pneumonia or meningitis for example, and have no fever at all, or have a high fever with a mild cold.

Under the following conditions a baby with a fever requires immediate medical attention (call the doctor even in the middle of the night or go to the emergency room if the doctor can't be reached):

■ The baby is under two months old.
■ The fever is over 105°F rectally.
■ The baby has a convulsion for the first time (the body stiffens, eyes roll, limbs flail).
■ The baby is crying inconsolably (and it clearly isn't colic), cries as if in pain when touched or moved, or is whimpering, nonresponsive, or limp.
■ The baby has purple spots anywhere on the skin.
■ The baby is having difficulty breathing once you've cleared the nasal passages.
■ The baby's neck seems stiff; baby resists

having the head pulled forward toward the chest.
■ The onset of fever follows a period of exposure to an external heat source, such as the sun on a hot day or the closed interior of an auto in hot weather. Heatstroke is a possibility (see page 386), and immediate emergency medical attention is indicated.
■ A sudden increase in temperature occurs in a baby with a moderate fever who has been overdressed or bundled in blankets. This should be treated as heat illness.
■ The doctor has instructed you to call immediately should your baby run a fever.
■ You feel something's very wrong, but you just don't know what.

Under the following conditions a baby with fever needs medical attention as soon as practical:

■ The baby is two to six months old (younger babies need *immediate* attention).
■ The baby has a chronic illness, such as heart, kidney, or neurological disease, or sickle-cell or other chronic anemia.
■ The baby has had convulsions with a fever in the past.
■ The baby exhibits signs of dehydration: infrequent urination, dark yellow urine, scant saliva and tears, dry lips and skin, sunken eyes and fontanel.
■ The baby's behavior seems uncharacteristic: he or she is excessively cranky; lethargic or excessively sleepy; unable to sleep; sensitive to light; crying more than usual; refusing to eat; pulling at ears.
■ A fever that has been low grade for a couple of days spikes suddenly; or a baby who has been sick with a cold for several days suddenly begins to run a fever (this may indicate a secondary infection, such as otitis media or strep throat).
■ The fever is over 102° rectally (or whatever temperature your baby's doctor recommends you call at). Though such a temperature is not in itself an indicator of a baby's being very sick (babies can run fevers of 105° or 106° with minor illness), check with the doctor, just in case.
■ A fever isn't brought down by medication.

■ A low-grade fever (under 102° rectally) with mild cold or flu symptoms lasts for more than three days.

■ A fever lasts more than 24 hours when there are no other detectable signs of illness.

TREATING A FEVER

If your baby has a fever, take these measures as needed, unless the doctor has recommended a different course of action.

Keep baby cool. Contrary to popular belief, keeping a feverish baby warm with blankets, heavy clothing, or an overheated room is not a safe practice. These measures can actually lead to heatstroke by raising body temperature to dangerous levels. Dress your baby lightly to allow body heat to escape (no more than a diaper is needed in hot weather) and maintain room temperature at 68° to 70° (when necessary, use an air conditioner or fan if you have one, to keep the air cool, but keep baby out of the path of the air flow).

Increase fluid intake. Because fever increases the loss of water through the skin, it's important to be sure a feverish baby gets an adequate intake of fluids. For older babies, offer good sources of fluids often. These include diluted juices and juicy fruits (such as citrus and melons); water; clear soups; gelatin desserts (see page 625); and ice pops made from fruit juice. Give young infants frequent feedings of breast milk or formula. Encourage frequent sipping but don't force. If baby refuses to take any fluids for several hours during the day, inform the doctor.

Give fever-reducing medication, if necessary. If your baby is under six months old, wait until you've reached the doctor before administering any medication. If fever is over 103° rectally and/or your baby seems very uncomfortable, and you can't reach your doctor immediately, try to lower fever with a tepid sponging (see below). With older babies, the decision to give medication should be based on the doctor's prior recommendations. Ask the doctor in advance what you should do if your baby wakes up feverish in the middle of the night. At what temperature would he or she like you to administer a fever-reducing medication, give a sponging, or call? If you don't have this information in advance and if your baby is over six months old and has a middle of the night fever of over 102° with no other indications of needing immediate medical attention (see Evaluating a

---

HANDLING FEBRILE CONVULSIONS

Convulsions due to fever usually last only a minute or two. Should your baby have one, keep calm (remember such convulsions are not dangerous) and take the following steps. Keep baby unrestrained in your arms or on a bed or another soft surface, lying on one side, with head lower than body if possible. Don't try to feed or put anything into baby's mouth, and remove anything (like a pacifier) that might be in it. Babies often lose consciousness during a seizure, but they usually revive quickly without help. Any seizure that lasts five minutes or more requires immediate emergency help—dial 911 or your local emergency number.

When a seizure has ended, the baby often wants to sleep. If yours does, prop him or her in a side-sleeping position with blankets or a pillow. Then call the doctor. If you don't reach help immediately, you can give baby a sponge bath and, if he or she is more than six months old, acetaminophen to try to lower the temperature while you're waiting. But don't put baby in the tub to try to reduce the fever since another seizure could occur and water could be inhaled.

ASPIRIN OR NON-ASPIRIN?

Both aspirin and acetaminophen (Tylenol, Tempra, Panadol, Liquiprin) are antipyretics (fever reducers) and lower fever equally well, but aspirin is more effective in reducing inflammation (the heat, swelling, redness, and pain of localized infection), and possibly, in relieving pain. Given together, aspirin and acetaminophen are statistically more effective at reducing fever longer (usually about six hours). It's not clear whether or not there are any benefits if they are given alternately.

Aspirin, though a powerful and valuable drug, is associated with a wide range of common side effects. It can diminish the immune response, cause inflammation and bleeding in the gastrointestinal tract, impair platelet function (increasing the risk of all types of bleeding), and induce an attack of asthma in susceptible people. Giving aspirin to children with such viral diseases as chicken pox and influenza (flu) has been linked to the development of Reye's syndrome, and it is therefore never recommended for a baby or child who has, or is suspected of having, such an illness.

In comparison, acetaminophen, although it has been known to cause liver damage in rare cases and may occasionally trigger an allergic reaction, is remarkably free of side effects. For this reason, doctors are much more likely to recommend acetaminophen rather than aspirin for fever reduction in children. Acetaminophen comes in liquid form for infants as well as rectal suppositories for babies who can't or won't keep the liquid down.

Ibuprofen, which also lowers fever and relieves pain, is presently available for infants only by prescription.

Since all these medications can be dangerous in large doses, never give more than the doctor recommends; and when you're not using them, keep them (like all medications) safely locked away, out of the reach of babies and children.

Fever), give the appropriate dosage of baby acetaminophen (see page 628). If the temperature does not go 'down, or if it goes up, or if baby seems very uncomfortable, call the doctor. Until you are able to reach the doctor, try a tepid sponge or tub bath.

Sponging. Once a routine treatment for fever, sponging is now recommended only under certain circumstances, such as when fever-reducing medication isn't working (the temperature isn't down an hour after it is given); when trying to lower the body temperature of a baby under six months old without medication; or when trying to make a very feverish baby more comfortable.

Only tepid or lukewarm water (body temperature, neither warm nor cool to the touch) should be used for sponging. Using cool or cold water, or alcohol (once a popular fever-reducing rub), can raise rather than lower temperatures by inducing shivering, which prompts the confused body to turn up its thermostat. In addition, the alcohol fumes can be harmful if inhaled. Using hot water will also raise body temperatures and could, like overdressing, lead to heatstroke. You can sponge a feverish baby in the tub or out, but in either case the room should be comfortably warm and draft free.

■ Sponging out of the tub. Have three washcloths in a tub or basin of tepid water ready before you begin. Spread a waterproof sheet or pad, or a plastic tablecloth, on the bed or on your lap; place a thick towel over it and place baby, face up, on top of the towel. Undress baby and cover with a light receiving blanket or towel. Wring out one washcloth so it won't drip, fold it, and place it on baby's forehead (remoisten if it begins to dry at any point during the sponging). Take another cloth and begin lightly rubbing baby's skin, exposing one area of the body at a time and keeping the rest lightly covered. Concentrate on the neck, face, stomach, inside of the elbows and knees, but also include the area under the arms and around the groin. The blood brought to the surface by rubbing will be cooled as the tepid water evaporates on the skin. When the rubbing cloth begins to dry out, switch it with the third cloth. Continue rubbing and sponging your baby, alternating cloths as needed, for at least twenty minutes to half an hour (it takes this long to lower body temperature). If at any time the water in the basin cools to below body temperature, add enough warm water to raise it again.

■ Sponging in the tub. For many babies, baths are soothing and comforting, especially when they are sick. If yours is one of these, do the sponging in the tub. Again, the water should be body temperature, and you should sponge and rub for at least twenty minutes to half an hour to bring the temperature down. Do not put a baby who

has had a febrile convulsion in a tub for sponging.

What not to do. As important as knowing what to do when your baby has a fever is knowing what not to do:

■ Do not force rest. A really sick baby will want to rest, in or out of the crib. If yours wants out, moderate activity is okay, but discourage strenuous activity as this could raise body temperature further.

■ Do not give an enema, except under a doctor's directions.

■ Do not overdress or bundle a baby warmly.

■ Do not cover baby with a wet towel or wet sheet, since this could prevent heat from escaping through the skin.

■ Do not "starve a fever." Fever raises the caloric requirement and sick babies, in fact, need more calories, not fewer.

■ Do not give aspirin or acetaminophen when heatstroke is suspected.

KNOW YOUR BABY

Babies, like other people, vary in their response to pain. Some can tolerate a great deal of it (the curious crawler who falls off the sofa, get up without a whimper, and climbs right back on) and some very little (the fledgling toddler who screeches with every tumble, even when it's on a plush carpet). It's a good idea to take such differences into account when deciding how sick a baby is. For example, if your feverish baby, who is ordinarily a stoic, is pulling at one or both ears but doesn't seem to be uncomfortable, consider an ear infection and call the doctor. On the other hand,

if you've got a pain-sensitive baby, you might be wise not to fly to the phone every time he whimpers in discomfort.

Fever as a signal. Fever in a young infant, especially when there are no other symptoms of illness, suggests the possibility of a urinary tract infection (UTI). The diagnosis can be confirmed through a urinalysis. If a UTI is found, further tests may be done to determine if there is a urinary tract abnormality at the root of the infection. If there is, simple surgery can usually remedy it.

CHAPTER EIGHTEEN

First Aid Do's And Don'ts

Accidents will happen. Even the most conscientious parents and caretakers can't avert them all. What they can do, however, is prevent serious damage by knowing what to do when an accident occurs. This section can help you do that. It will be even more helpful if reinforced with a live first-aid course. But don't wait until baby tumbles down the stairs or chews on a rhododendron leaf to look up what to do in an emergency. Now—before calamity strikes—become as familiar with the procedures for treating common injuries as you are with those for bathing baby or changing a diaper, and review less common ones when appropriate (snake bites, for example, when you are going on a camping trip). See that anyone else who cares for your baby does, too.

Below are the most common injuries, what you should know about them, how to treat (and not treat) them, and when to seek medical care for them. Types of injuries are listed alphabetically (abdominal injuries, bites, broken bones, etc.), with individual injuries numbered for easy cross-reference.

A gray bar has been added to the top of these pages, making the chapter easy to locate in an emergency.

Abdominal Injuries

1. Internal bleeding. A blow to your baby's abdomen could result in internal damage. The signs of such injury would include: bruising or other discoloration of the abdomen; vomited or coughed-up blood that is dark or bright red and has the consistency of coffee grounds (this could also be a sign of baby's having swallowed a caustic substance); blood (it may be dark or bright red) in the stool or urine; shock (cold, clammy, pale skin; weak, rapid pulse; chills; confusion; and possibly, nausea, vomiting, and/or shallow breathing). Seek emergency medical assistance. If baby appears to be in shock (#44), treat immediately. Do not give food or drink.

2. Cuts or lacerations of the abdomen. Treat as for other cuts (#47, #48). With a major laceration, intestines may protrude. Don't try to put them back into the abdomen. Instead, cover them with a clean moistened washcloth or diaper and get emergency medical assistance immediately.

Bites

3. Animal bites. Try to avoid moving the affected part. Call doctor immediately. Wash wound gently with soap and water for 15 minutes. Do not apply antiseptic or anything else. Control bleeding (#47, #48, #49), and apply a sterile bandage. Try to restrain animal for testing, but avoid getting bitten. Dogs, cats, bats, skunks, and raccoons may be rabid, especially if they attacked unprovoked. Infection (redness, tenderness, swelling) is common with cat bites and may require antibiotics.

4. Insect bites. Treat insect stings or bites as follows:
- Scrape off the honeybee's stinger with the blunt edge of a knife or with your fingernail. Don't try to grasp the stinger with your nails or a tweezer—this could force more of the remaining venom into the skin.
- Remove ticks *promptly,* using blunt tweezers or your fingertips protected by a tissue, paper towel, or rubber glove. Grasp the bug as close to baby's skin as possible and pull upward, steadily and evenly. Don't twist, jerk, squeeze, crush, or puncture the tick. *Don't* use such folk remedies as vaseline, gasoline, or a hot match—they can make matters worse. Save the tick for medical examination. If you suspect Lyme disease (page 638), call the doctor.
- Wash the site of a minor bee, wasp, ant, spider, or tick bite with soap and water. Then apply ice or cold compresses (page 627) if

there appears to be swelling or pain. Follow with an application of bug-bite medication.
- Apply calamine lotion to itchy bites, such as those caused by mosquitoes.
- If there seems to be extreme pain after a spider bite, apply ice or cold compresses and call for emergency help. Try to find the spider and take it to the hospital with you, or at least be able to describe it; it might be poisonous. If you know the spider was poisonous—a black widow, brown recluse spider, tarantula, or scorpion, for example—get emergency treatment immediately, even before symptoms appear.
- Watch for signs of hypersensitivity, such as severe pain or swelling or any degree of shortness of breath, following any bee, wasp, or hornet sting. Individuals who exhibit such symptoms with a first sting usually develop hypersensitivities, or allergies, to the venom, in which case a subsequent sting could be fatal if immediate emergency treatment is not administered. Should your baby's reaction to a sting be anything more than slight pain or a bit of swelling, report this to the doctor, who is likely to recommend allergy testing. If allergy is diagnosed, it will probably be necessary for you to carry a bee-sting emergency kit with you on outings during bee season.
- It's possible, of course, for sensitization to bee venom to occur without a previously noticed reaction, especially in a baby. So should a sting victim break out in hives all over the body, experience difficulty breathing, hoarseness, coughing, wheezing, severe headache, nausea, vomiting, thickened tongue, facial swelling, weakness, dizziness, or fainting, get immediate emergency medical attention.

5. Snake bites. It's rare that a baby is bitten by a poisonous snake (the four major types in the U.S. are rattlesnakes, copperheads, coral snakes, and cottonmouths or water moccasins—and all have fangs, which usually leave identifying marks when they bite), but such a bite is very dangerous. Because of an infant's small size, even a tiny amount of venom can be fatal. Following such a bite, it is important to keep baby and the affected part as still as possible. If the bite is on a limb, immobilize it with a splint if necessary, and keep it below the level of the heart. Use a cool compress if available to relieve pain, but *do not* apply ice or give any medication without medical advice. Sucking out the venom by mouth (and spitting it out) may be helpful if done immediately, but *do not* make an incision of any kind, unless you are 4 or 5 hours from help and severe symptoms occur. If baby is not breathing, give CPR (page 448). Treat for shock (#44), if necessary. *Get prompt medical help;* and be ready to identify the variety of snake if possible. If you won't be able to get medical help within an hour, apply a loose constricting band (a belt, tie, or hair ribbon loose enough for you to slip a finger under) 2 inches above the bite to slow circulation. (Do not tie such a tourniquet around a finger or toe, or around the neck, head, or trunk.) Check pulse (see page 407) beneath the tourniquet frequently to be sure circulation is not cut off, and loosen it if the limb begins to swell. Make a note of the time it was tied.

Treat nonpoisonous snake bites as puncture wounds (#50), and notify baby's doctor.

6. Marine stings. Such stings are usually not serious, but an occasional baby or child will have a severe reaction. Medical treatment should be sought immediately as a precaution. First-aid treatment varies with the type of marine animal involved, but in general, any clinging fragments of the stinger should be gingerly brushed away with a diaper or piece of clothing (to protect your own fingers). Treatment for heavy bleeding (#49), shock (#44), or cessation of breathing (see page 448), if needed, should be begun immediately. (Don't worry about light bleeding; it may help purge toxins). The sting of a stingray, lionfish, catfish, stonefish, or sea urchin should be soaked in hot water, if available, for 30 minutes, or until medical help arrives. The toxins from the sting of a jellyfish or Portuguese man-of-war can be counteracted by applying alcohol or diluted ammonia. (Pack a couple of alcohol pads in your beach bag, just in case.)

Bleeding
see #47, #48, #49

Bleeding, Internal
see #1

Broken Bones or Fractures

7. Possible broken arms, legs, collarbones, or fingers. Signs of a break include: a snapping sound at the time of the accident; deformity (although this could also indicate a dislocation, #16); inability to move or bear weight on the part; severe pain (persistent crying could be a clue); numbness and/or tingling (neither of which a baby would be able to tell you about); swelling and discoloration. If a fractured limb is suspected, don't move the child without checking with the doctor first—unless necessary for safety. If you must move baby immediately, first try to immobilize the injured part (limb, head, neck) by splinting it in the position it's in with a ruler, a magazine, a book, or other firm object, padded with a soft cloth to protect the skin. Or use a small, firm pillow as a splint. Fasten the splint securely at the break and above and below it with bandages, strips of cloth, scarves, or neckties, but not so tightly that circulation is hampered. If no potential splint is handy, try to splint the injured limb with your arm. Check regularly to be sure the splint doesn't cut off circulation. Apply an ice pack to reduce swelling until medical attention is given. Though fractures in small children usually mend quickly, medical treatment is necessary to ensure proper healing. Take your child to the doctor or ER even if you only suspect a break.

8. Compound fractures. If bone protrudes through the skin, don't touch the bone. Cover the injury, if possible, with sterile gauze or with a clean cloth diaper; control bleeding, if necessary, with pressure (#49); and get emergency medical assistance.

9. Possible neck or back injury. If neck or back injury is suspected, don't move baby *at all*. Call for emergency medical assistance. Cover and keep child comfortable while waiting for help, and if possible, put some heavy objects (such as books) around the head to help immobilize it. Don't give food or drink. If there is severe bleeding (#49), shock (#44), or absence of breathing (see page 448), treat these immediately.

Bruises, Skin
see #45

Burns and Scalds

Important: If a child's clothing is on fire, use a coat, blanket, rug, bedspread, or your own body (you won't be burned) to smother the flames.

10. Limited thermal (heat) burns. Immerse the burned extremity in cool water or apply cool (50° to 60°) compresses to burns of the trunk or face. Continue until baby doesn't seem to be in pain anymore, usually about half an hour. Don't apply ice, which could compound the skin damage, and don't break any blisters that form. After soaking, gently pat burned area dry and cover with nonadhesive material (such as a non stick bandage, or in an emergency, aluminum foil). Burns on the face, hands, feet, or genitals should be seen by a doctor immediately. Any burn, even a minor one, on a child under a year old warrants a call to the doctor.

11. Extensive thermal (heat) burns. Keep baby lying flat. Remove any clothing from the burn area that does not adhere to the wound. Apply cool wet compresses to the injured area (but not to more than 25% of the body at one time). Keep the baby comfortably warm, with legs higher than heart if they are burned. Do not apply pressure, ointments, butter or other fats, powder, or boric acid soaks to the burn. If baby is conscious and doesn't have severe mouth burns, nurse or give water or another fluid. Transport the child to the doctor's office or ER at once or call for emergency medical assistance.

12. Chemical burns. Caustic substances (such as lye and acids) can cause serious burns. Gently brush off dry chemical matter from the skin and remove any contaminated clothing. Immediately wash the skin with large amounts of water, using the antidote, if any, recommended on the chemical container or using soap if available. Call a physician, the Poison Control Center, or the ER for further advice. Get immediate medical assistance if there is difficult or painful breathing, which could indicate lung injury from inhalation of caustic fumes. (If a chemical has been swallowed, see #41.)

13. Electrical burns. Immediately disconnect the power source, if possible. Or pull victim away from the source using a dry nonmetallic object such as a broom, wooden ladder, rope, cushion, chair, or even a large book—but not your bare hands. Initiate CPR (page 448) if baby is not breathing. All electrical burns should be evaluated by a physician, so call your baby's doctor or go to the ER at once.

14. Sunburn. If your baby (or anyone else in the family) gets a sunburn, treat it by applying cool tap-water compresses (see page 627) for 10 to 15 minutes, three or four times a day, until the redness subsides; the evaporating water helps to cool the skin. In between these treatments, apply Nutraderm, Lubriderm, or a similar bland moisturizing cream, or calamine liniment, which has the added benefit of drying out blisters. Don't use petroleum jelly (Vaseline) on a burn because it seals out air, which is needed for healing. And don't give antihistamines unless they are prescribed by the doctor. For severe burns, steroid ointments or creams may be prescribed, and large blisters may be drained and dressed. Though there have been some claims to the contrary, aspirin won't prevent damage to the skin; but a baby pain reliever, such as acetaminophen, may reduce the discomfort.

BE PREPARED

■ Discuss with your baby's doctor what the best plan of action would be in case of injury—calling the office, going to the emergency room (ER), or following some other protocol. Recommendations may vary, depending upon the seriousness of the injury, the day of the week, and the time of day.

■ Keep your first aid supplies (see page 39) in a childproof, easily manageable kit or box so it can be moved as a whole to an accident site. And, if possible, make the next phone you buy a portable, so that it can be taken to the site of any accident in or around your home.

■ Near each telephone in your home, post the numbers of the doctors your family uses, the Poison Control Center, the nearest hospital emergency room (or the one you plan on using), your pharmacy, the Emergency Medical Service (911 in many areas), as well as the number of a close friend or neighbor you can call on in an emergency. Keep a card with the same listings in your diaper bag.

■ Know the quickest route to the ER or other emergency medical facility.

■ Take a course in baby CPR, and keep your skills current and ready to use with periodic refresher courses and regular home practice on a doll. Also become familiar with first-aid procedures for common injuries.

■ Keep some cash reserved in a safe place in case you need cab fare to get to the ER or a doctor's office in an emergency.

■ Learn to handle minor accidents calmly, which will help you keep your cool should a serious one ever occur. Your manner and tone of voice (or those of another caretaker) will affect how your baby responds to an injury. Panic or worry on your part could upset your baby. And a baby who is upset is less likely to cooperate in an emergency and will be harder to treat.

■ Remember that TLC (tender loving care) is often the best treatment for minor injuries. But tailor your comfort to the degree of seriousness of the hurt. A smile, a kiss, and a little reassurance ("You're all right") are all a little bump on the knee may need. But a painful pinched finger will probably warrant a heavy dose of kisses and probably some distraction. In most cases, you will need to calm a baby before giving first aid. Only in life-threatening situations (which are fortunately rare, and in which babies are not usually up to being obstreperous) will taking some time to quiet baby interfere with the outcome of treatment.

Chemical Burns
see #12

Convulsions

15. Symptoms of a seizure or convulsion include: collapse, eyes rolling upward, foaming at the mouth, stiffening of the body followed by uncontrolled jerking movements, and in the most serious cases, breathing difficulty. Brief convulsions are not uncommon with high fevers (see page 427). Deal with a seizure this way: clear the area around baby, but don't restrain except if necessary to prevent injury. Loosen clothing around the neck and middle, and lay baby on one side with head lower than hips. Don't put anything in the mouth, including food or drink, breast or bottle. Call the doctor. When the convulsion has passed, sponge with cool water if fever is present, but don't put baby into a bath or throw water in his or her face. If baby isn't breathing, begin CPR (see page 448) immediately.

Cuts
see #47, #48

Dislocations

16. Shoulder and elbow dislocations are

common among toddlers—mostly because they are often tugged along by the arm by adults in a hurry. A deformity of the arm or the inability of the child to move it, usually combined with persistent crying because of pain, are typical indications. A quick trip to the doctor's office or the ER, where an experienced professional will reposition the dislocated part, will provide virtually instant relief. Apply an ice pack and splint before leaving, if pain seems severe.

Dog Bites

see #3

Drowning

17. Even a child who quickly revives after being taken from the water unconscious should get medical evaluation. For the child who remains unconscious, have someone else call for emergency medical assistance, if possible, while you begin CPR (see page 448). Even if no one is available to phone for help, begin CPR immediately and call later. Don't stop CPR until the child revives or help arrives, no matter how long that takes. If there is vomiting, turn baby to one side to avoid choking. If you suspect a blow to the head or a neck injury, immobilize these parts.

Ear Injuries

18. Foreign object in the ear. Try to shake the object out by turning the baby so the ear faces down and shaking the head very gently. If that doesn't work, try these techniques.
■ For an insect, use a flashlight to try to lure it out.
■ For a metal object, try a magnet to draw it out.
■ For a plastic or wood object, dab a drop of quick-drying glue (don't use one that might bond to the skin) on a straightened paper clip and touch it to the object if it is visible. Do not probe into the inner ear. Wait for the glue to dry, then pull the clip out, hopefully with the object attached. Don't attempt this if there's no one around

to help hold baby still.
If the above techniques fail, don't try to dig the object out with your fingers or an instrument. Instead, take baby to the doctor's office or the ER.

19. Damage to the ear. If a pointed object has been pushed into the ear or if your baby shows signs of ear injury (bleeding from the ear canal, sudden difficulty hearing, swollen earlobe), call the doctor.

Electric Shock

20. Break contact with the electrical source by turning off the power, if possible, or separate the child from the current by using a dry nonmetallic object such as a broom, wooden ladder, robe, cushion, chair, or even a large book. Call for emergency medical assistance, and if baby isn't breathing, begin CPR (see page 448).

Eye Injury

Important: Don't apply pressure to an injured eye, touch the eye with your fingers, or instill medications without a physician's advice. Keep baby from rubbing the eye by holding a small cup or glass (or an eyecup) over it or by restraining both hands, if necessary.

21. Foreign object in the eye. If you can see the object (lash or grain of sand, for example), wash your hands and use a moist cotton swab to gently attempt to remove it from baby's eye. You can also try to wash the object out by pouring a stream of tepid (body temperature) water into the eye while someone holds baby still, if necessary. If this is unsuccessful, try pulling the upper lid down over the lower for a few seconds.
If after these attempts you can still see the object in the eye or if baby still seems uncomfortable, proceed to the doctor's office or the ER since the object may become embedded or may have scratched the eye. Don't try to remove an embedded object yourself. Cover the eye with a sterile gauze pad taped loosely in place, or with a few clean tissues or a clean handkerchief to

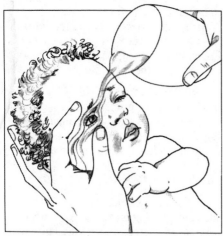

Baby won't enjoy an eye bath, but it's crucial for washing away a corrosive substance.

alleviate some of the discomfort en route.

22. Corrosive substance in the eye. Flush the eye immediately and thoroughly with plain lukewarm water (poured from a pitcher, cup, or bottle) for 15 minutes, holding the eye open with your fingers. If just one eye is involved, keep baby's head turned so that the unaffected eye is higher than the affected one and the chemical run-off doesn't drip into it. Don't use drops or ointments, and don't permit baby to rub the eye or eyes. Call the doctor or the Poison Control Center for further instructions.

23. Injury to the eye with a pointed or sharp object. Keep baby in a semi-reclining position while you seek help. If the object is still in the eye, do not try to remove it. If it isn't, cover the eye lightly with a gauze pad, clean washcloth, or facial tissue; do not apply pressure. In either case, get emergency medical assistance immediately. Though such injuries often look worse than they are, it's wise to consult an ophthalmologist any time the eye is scratched or punctured, even slightly.

24. Injury to the eye with a blunt object. Keep baby lying face up. Cover the injured eye with an ice pack or cold compress (page 627). If the eye blackens, if baby seems to be having difficulty seeing or keeps rubbing the eye a lot, or if an object hit the eye at high speed, consult the doctor.

Fainting

25. Check for breathing, and if it is absent begin CPR *immediately* (see page 448). If you detect breathing, keep baby lying flat, lightly covered for warmth if necessary. Loosen clothing around the neck. Turn baby's head to one side and clear the mouth of any food or objects. Don't give anything to eat or drink. Call the doctor immediately.

Finger and Toe Injuries

26. Bruises. Babies, ever curious, are particularly prone to painful bruises from catching fingers in drawers and doors. For such a bruise, soak the finger in ice water. As much as an hour of soaking is recommended, with a break every 15 minutes (long enough for the finger to rewarm) to avoid frostbite. Unfortunately, few babies will sit still for this long, though you may be able to treat for a few minutes by using distraction or force. A stubbed toe will also benefit from soaking, but again it often isn't practical with an infant who won't cooperate. The bruised fingers and toes will swell less if kept elevated.

If the injured finger or toe becomes very swollen very quickly, is misshapen, or can't be straightened, suspect a break (#7). Call the doctor immediately if the bruise is from a wringer-type injury or from catching a hand or foot in the spokes of a moving wheel.

27. Bleeding under the nail. When a finger or toe is badly bruised, a blood clot may form under the nail, causing painful pressure. If blood oozes out from under the nail, press on it to encourage the flow, which will help to relieve the pressure. Soak the injury in ice water if baby will tolerate it. If the pain continues, a hole may have to be made in the nail to relieve the pressure. Your doctor can do the job or may tell you how to do it yourself.

TREATING A YOUNG PATIENT

Babies are rarely cooperative patients. No matter how uncomfortable the symptoms of their illness or how painful their injuries, they're likely to consider the cure worse. It won't help to tell them that the calamine lotion will make chicken pox itch less or that the ice pack will keep a bruised finger from swelling. Even older children, who are capable of understanding such reasoning, are almost certain to resist it. But it may help to use distraction while trying to treat a baby or young child's illness or injury. Entertainment (begun before the treatment, and hopefully, before the tears have started) in the form of a favorite music box, video, or audio tape; a toy dog that yaps and wags its tail; a choo-choo train that can travel across the coffee table; or a parent or sibling who can dance, jump up and down, or sing silly songs can help make the difference between a successful treatment session and a disastrous one. Or try sailing some boats in the soaking water; taking a teddy's temperature; giving a doll a dose of medicine; putting an ice pack on doggie's "boo-boo."

How forceful you are about treatment will depend on the severity of the illness or injury. With a mild stuffy nose, aspirating the mucus may not be worth the battle. But if the stuffy nose is interfering with baby's sleep or eating, then the battle may be necessary. A slight bruise may not warrant upsetting yourself and a baby who's rejecting the ice pack. A severe burn, however, will certainly merit the cold soaks, even if baby screams during the entire treatment. In most cases, try to treat at least briefly—even a few minutes of ice on a bruise will reduce the bleeding under the skin and even thirty seconds of temperature taking will give a fairly good idea of baby's condition. And when baby's upset outweighs the benefits of the treatment, abandon it.

28. Torn nail. For a small tear, secure with a piece of adhesive tape or a band-aid until the torn nail grows to a point where it can be trimmed. For a tear that is almost complete, trim away along the tear line and cover with a band-aid until the nail is long enough to protect the fingertip once again.

29. Detached nail. Completely remove the nail if it is still partly attached. Soak the finger or toe for 20 minutes in cold water, if possible, then apply antibiotic ointment and cover with a nonstick band-aid. For the next three days, soak once a day in warm salt water (½ teaspoon salt to 1 pint water) for about 15 minutes. Apply antibiotic ointment and cover with a fresh band-aid after each soaking. By the fourth day dispense with the ointment as long as healing continues, but continue the daily soakings for the rest of the week. Keep the nail bed covered with a band-aid until the nail is completely grown in. If the redness, heat, and swelling of infection occur at any point, call the doctor.

Frostbite

30. Babies are extremely susceptible to frostbite, particularly on fingers and toes, ears, nose, and cheeks. In frostbite, the affected part becomes very cold and turns white or yellowish gray. Should you note such signs in your baby, immediately try to warm the frosty parts against your body—open your coat and shirt and tuck baby inside next to your skin. As soon as possible, get to a doctor or an emergency room. If that isn't feasible immediately, get baby indoors and begin a gradual rewarming process. Don't put a baby with frostbite right next to a radiator, stove, open fire, or heat lamp, because the damaged skin may burn; don't try to quick-thaw in hot water, which can also add to the damage. Instead, soak affected fingers and toes directly in water that is about 102°—just a little warmer than normal body temperature and just slightly warm to the touch. For unsoakable parts, such as nose, ears, and cheeks, use compresses (wet washcloths or towels) of the same temperature, but don't apply pressure. Continue the soaks until color returns to the skin, usually in 30 to 60 minutes (add warm water as needed), nursing baby or giving warm (not hot) fluids by bottle or cup as you do. As frostbitten skin rewarms it becomes red and slightly swollen, and it may blister. If baby's injury hasn't been seen by a doctor up to this point, it is important to get medical attention now.

If, once the injured parts have been warmed, you have to go out again to take baby to the doctor (or anywhere else), be especially careful to keep the affected areas warm en route, as refreezing of thawed tissues can cause additional damage.

After prolonged exposure to cold, a baby's body temperature may drop to below normal levels. This is a medical emergency known as hypothermia—no time should be wasted in getting a baby who seems unusually cold to the touch to the nearest emergency room. Keep baby warm next to your body en route.

Head Injuries

31. Cuts and bruises to the scalp.
Because of the profusion of blood vessels in

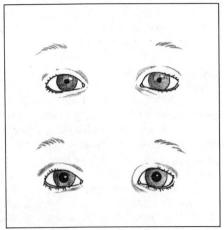

Pupils should become smaller in response to light (above) and larger once the light is removed (below).

the scalp, heavy bleeding is common with cuts to the head, even tiny ones, and bruises there tend to swell to egg size very quickly. Treat as you would any cut (#47, #48) or bruise (#45). Check with the doctor for all but very minor scalp wounds.

32. Possibly serious head trauma.
Most babies experience several minor bumps on the head during the first year. Usually these require no more than a few make-it-better kisses from mommy, but it's wise to observe a baby carefully for 6 hours following a severe blow to the head. Call the doctor or summon emergency medical assistance immediately if your baby shows any of these signs after a head injury:

- Loss of consciousness (a brief period of drowsiness—no more than two or three hours—is common and nothing to worry about)
- Convulsions
- Difficulty being roused (check every hour or two during daytime naps, two or three times during the night for the first 6 hours following the injury to be sure baby is responsive; if you can't rouse a sleeping baby, check for breathing; see page 448)
- More than one or two episodes of vomiting
- A depression or indentation in the skull
- Inability to move an arm or leg
- Oozing of blood or watery fluid from the ears or nose
- Black-and-blue areas appearing around the eyes or behind the ears
- Apparent pain for more than an hour that interferes with normal activity and/or sleep
- Dizziness that persists beyond one hour after the injury (baby's balance seems off)
- Unequal pupil size, or pupils that don't respond to the light of a penlight by shrinking (see illustration) or the removal of the light by growing larger
- Unusual paleness that persists for more than a short time

While waiting for help, keep your baby lying quietly with head turned to one side. Treat for shock (#44), if necessary. Begin CPR (page 448) if baby stops breathing.

Don't offer any food or drink until you talk to the doctor.

Heat Injuries

33. Heatstroke typically comes on suddenly. Signs to watch for include hot and dry (or occasionally, moist) skin, very high fever, diarrhea, agitation or lethargy, confusion, convulsions, and loss of consciousness. If you suspect heatstroke, wrap your baby in a large towel that has been soaked in ice water (dump ice cubes in the sink while it's filling with cold tap water, than add the towel) and summon immediate emergency medical help, or rush baby to the nearest emergency room. If the towel becomes warm, repeat with a freshly chilled one.

Hypothermia
see #30

Insect Bites
see #4

Lip, Split or Cut
see #34, #35

Mouth Injuries

34. Split lip. Few babies escape the first year without at least one cut on the lip. Fortunately, these cuts usually heal very quickly. To ease pain and control bleeding, apply an ice pack. Or let an older baby suck on an ice pop or a large ice cube under adult supervision (switch to a fresh ice cube when the first has become small enough to choke on). If the cut gapes open, or if bleeding doesn't stop in 10 or 15 minutes, call the doctor. Occasionally a lip injury is caused by baby chewing on an electrical cord. If this is suspected, call the doctor.

35. Cuts inside the lip or mouth. Such injuries, too, are common in young children. An ice pack for young infants, or an ice pop or a large ice cube for older children to suck on under adult supervision (switch to a fresh ice cube when the first has become small enough to choke on),

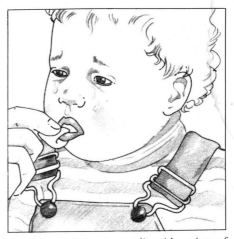

Applying pressure to a cut lip with a piece of gauze held between thumb and forefinger will stop the bleeding.

will relieve pain and control bleeding inside the lip or cheek. To stop bleeding of the tongue if it doesn't stop spontaneously, squeeze the sides of the cut together with a piece of gauze or clean cloth. If the injury is in the back of the throat or on the soft palate (the rear of the upper mouth), if there is a puncture wound from a sharp object (such as a pencil or a stick), or if bleeding doesn't stop within 10 to 15 minutes, call the doctor.

36. Knocked-out tooth. If a permanent tooth is dislodged, it should be rinsed gently under running water while being held by the crown (not the root). It can then be reinserted into the gum, if possible, or held in the mouth or in tap water or milk en route to the dentist, who may be able to reimplant it if no more than 30 to 45 minutes have elapsed since the accident. But there is little chance that the dentist will try to reimplant a dislodged baby tooth (such implantations often abscess and rarely hold), so precautions to preserve the tooth aren't necessary. But the dentist will want to see the tooth to be sure it's whole. Fragments left in the gum could be expelled and then inhaled or choked on by the baby. So take the tooth along to the dentist or to the ER if you are unable to reach a dentist.

37. Broken tooth. Clean dirt or debris carefully from the mouth with warm water and gauze or a clean cloth. Be sure the broken parts of the tooth are not still in baby's mouth—they could cause choking. Place cold compresses (see page 627) on the face in the area of the injured tooth to minimize swelling. Call the dentist immediately for further instructions.

Nose Injuries

38. Nosebleeds. Keeping baby in an upright position or leaning slightly forward, pinch both nostrils gently between your thumb and index finger for 5 to 10 minutes. (Baby will automatically switch to mouth breathing.) Try to calm baby, because crying will increase the blood flow. If bleeding persists, try packing the bleeding nostril with a wad of absorbent cotton and pinch for 10 minutes more and/or apply cold compresses. If this doesn't work and bleeding continues, call the doctor—keeping baby upright while you do. Frequent nosebleeds, even if easily stopped, should be reported to baby's doctor.

39. Foreign object in the nose. Difficulty breathing through the nose and/or a foul-smelling, sometimes bloody, nasal discharge may be a sign that something has

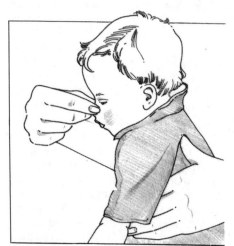

Pinching the nostrils stems the flow of a bloody nose.

been pushed up the nose. Keep baby calm and encourage mouth breathing. Remove the object with your fingers if you can reach it easily, but don't probe or use tweezers or anything else that could injure the nose if baby moves unexpectedly or that could push the object farther into the nasal canal. If you can't remove the object, blow through your nose and try to get baby to imitate your action. If this fails, take baby to the doctor or emergency room.

40. Blows to the nose. If there is bleeding, keep baby upright and leaning forward to reduce the swallowing of blood and the risk of choking on it (#38). Use an ice pack or cold compresses (page 627) to reduce swelling. Check with the doctor to be sure there is no break.

Poisoning

41. Swallowed poisons. Any nonfood substance is a potential poison. If your baby becomes unconscious, and you know of or suspect the ingestion of a dangerous substance, begin emergency treatment immediately. Place baby face up on a table and check for respiration (see page 448). If there is no sign of breathing, begin CPR promptly. Call for emergency medical assistance after 2 minutes, then continue CPR until baby revives or until help arrives.

The more common symptoms of poisoning include: lethargy, agitation, or other behavior that deviates from the norm; racing, irregular pulse and/or rapid breathing; diarrhea or vomiting (baby should be turned on one side to avoid choking on vomitus); excessive watering of the eyes, sweating, drooling; hot, dry skin and mouth; dilated (wide open) or constricted (pinpoint) pupils; flickering, sideways eye movements; tremors or convulsions.

If your baby has several of these symptoms (and they cannot be explained in any other way), or if you have evidence that your baby has definitely or possibly ingested a questionable substance, do not try to treat it on your own. Do not give your baby anything by mouth (including food or drink; the activated charcoal blend known as universal antidote; or anything to induce vomiting, such as syrup of ipecac, salt water, or egg whites). Instead, call the doctor, the local Poison Control Center, or the hospital emergency room *immediately* for instructions. Call even if there are no symptoms—they may not appear for hours. Take with you to the phone the container the suspected substance came in, label intact, as well as any of the remaining contents. Report the name of the substance (or of the plant if your baby ingested greenery) and how much of it you know or believe baby took, if it's possible to determine that. Also be prepared to supply your baby's age, size, weight, and symptoms.

With many poisons, you will be advised to induce vomiting with syrup of ipecac in order to empty the stomach of as much of the poison as possible.[1] Give the dose recommended by the Poison Control Center or the doctor. (If you have no ipecac available, ask medical personnel about using liquid dish—*not* dishwasher—detergent to induce vomiting.) If vomiting does not occur within 20 minutes, repeat the dose—but only once. If you succeed in inducing vomiting, collect the vomited material in a deep pan or bowl. If you are instructed to go to the emergency room or doctor's office, take the vomitus along for analysis. (It may be easier to carry it in a jar with a lid or a heavy zip-lock-type plastic bag, but bring along a clean bowl or pail in case baby heaves again.) Also be sure to take the suspect substance (bottle of pills, container of cleaning fluid, branch of philodendron).

Vomiting is not usually induced in babies under six months of age because of the greater risk of choking in young infants. In babies six months to one year of age, it should be induced only under medical supervision. Vomiting should not be induced at any age when a corrosive substance (such as bleach, ammonia, or drain cleaner) or anything with a kerosene, benzene, or gasoline base (furniture polishes, cleaning fluid, turpentine) has been ingested. Nor when the victim is unconscious, drowsy, or having convulsions or tremors. In some cases, liquid charcoal, which absorbs the poison, is the preferred treatment.

42. Noxious fumes or gases. Fumes from gasoline, auto exhaust, and some poisonous chemicals and dense smoke from fires can all be toxic. Get a baby who has been exposed to any such hazards to fresh air (open windows or take the child outside) promptly. If baby is not breathing, begin CPR (see page 448) *immediately* and continue until breathing is well established or help arrives. If possible, have someone else call the Poison Control Center or an emergency medical service while you continue CPR. If no one else is around, take a moment to call for help yourself after 2 minutes of resuscitation efforts—and then return immediately to CPR. Unless an emergency vehicle is on its way, transport baby to a medical facility promptly, but not if doing so means discontinuing CPR or if you were also exposed and your judgment is impaired. Have someone else drive. Even if you should succeed in establishing breathing, immediate medical attention will be necessary.

Puncture Wounds
see # 50

Scrapes
see #46

Severed Limb or Digit

43. Such serious accidents are rare, but knowing what to do when one occurs can mean the difference between saving and losing a limb or digit. Take these steps as needed immediately:

■ Try to control bleeding. With several sterile gauze pads, a clean diaper, a sanitary napkin, or a clean washcloth apply heavy pressure to the wound. If bleeding continues, increase pressure. Don't worry about doing damage by pressing too hard. Do not

---

1. If you use up your ipecac, be sure to replace it.

apply a tourniquet without medical advice.
■ Treat shock if present. If baby's skin seems pale, cold, and clammy, pulse is weak and rapid, and respiration is shallow, treat for shock by loosening clothing, covering baby lightly to prevent loss of body heat, and elevating legs on a pillow (or folded garment) to force blood to the brain. If breathing seems labored, raise baby's head and shoulders slightly.
■ Re-establish breathing, if necessary. Begin CPR immediately if baby isn't breathing (see page 448).
■ Preserve the severed limb or digit. As soon as possible, wrap it in a wet clean cloth or sponge, and place in a plastic bag. Pack the bag with ice and tie it shut. Do not place part directly on ice, don't use dry ice, and don't immerse it in water or antiseptics.
■ Get help. Call or have someone else call for immediate emergency medical assistance or rush to the ER, calling ahead so they can prepare for your arrival. Be sure to take along the ice-packed limb; surgeons may be able to reattach it. During transport, keep pressure on the wound and continue other lifesaving procedures, if necessary.

Shock

44. Shock can develop in severe injuries or illnesses. Signs include cold, clammy, pale skin; rapid, weak pulse; chills; convulsions; and frequently, nausea or vomiting, excessive thirst, and/or shallow breathing. To treat, position baby on back. Loosen restrictive clothing, elevate legs on a pillow or folded garment to force blood to the brain, and cover baby lightly to prevent chilling or loss of body heat. If breathing seems labored, raise baby's head and shoulders very slightly. Get emergency medical assistance.

Skin Wounds

Important: Exposure to tetanus is a possibility whenever the skin is broken. Should your child incur an open skin wound, check to be sure tetanus immunization is up-to-date. Also be alert for signs of possible infection (swelling, warmth, tenderness, reddening of surrounding area, oozing of pus from the wound), and call the doctor if they develop.

45. Bruises or black-and-blue marks. Encourage quiet play to rest the injured part, if possible. Apply cold compresses, an ice pack, or cloth-wrapped ice for half an hour. (Do not apply ice directly to the skin.) If the skin is broken, treat the bruise as you would a cut (#47, #48). Call the doctor immediately if the bruise is from a wringer-type injury or if it resulted from catching a hand or foot in the spokes of a moving wheel. Bruises that seem to appear out of nowhere or that coincide with a fever should also be seen by a doctor.

46. Scrapes or abrasions. In such injuries (most common on knees and elbows) the top layer (or layers) of skin is abraded, or scraped off, leaving the area raw and tender. There is usually slight bleeding from the more deeply abraded areas. Using sterile gauze or cotton or a clean wash cloth, gently sponge off the wound with soap and water to remove dirt and other foreign matter. If baby strenuously objects to this, try soaking the scrape in the bathtub. Apply pressure if the bleeding doesn't stop on its own. Cover with a sterile nonstick bandage. Most scrapes heal quickly.

47. Small cuts. Wash the area with clean water and soap, then hold the cut under running water to flush out dirt and foreign matter. Apply a sterile nonstick band-aid. A butterfly bandage (see illustration) will keep a small cut closed while it heals. Check with the doctor about any cuts on a baby's face.

48. Large cuts. With a sterile gauze pad, a fresh diaper, a sanitary napkin, a clean washcloth, or if necessary, your bare finger, apply pressure to try to stop the bleeding, elevating the injured part above the level of the heart, if possible, at the same time. If bleeding persists after 15 minutes of

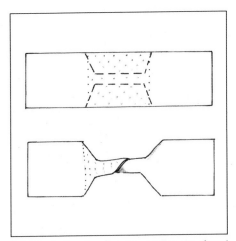

A butterfly bandage keeps a gaping cut closed so it can heal. Trim down a regular band-aid and make one complete twist to form a strong butterfly.

pressure, add more gauze pads or cloth and increase the pressure. (Don't worry about doing damage with too much pressure.) If necessary, keep the pressure on until help arrives or you get baby to the doctor or ER. If there are other injuries, try to tie or bandage the pressure pack in place so that your hands can be free to attend to them. Apply a sterile nonstick bandage to the wound when the bleeding stops, loose enough so that it doesn't interfere with circulation. Do not use iodine, Burrows solution, or other antiseptic without medical advice. Take baby to the doctor's office (call first) or the ER for wounds that gape, appear deep, or don't stop bleeding within half an hour.

49. Massive bleeding. Get emergency medical attention by calling your local Emergency Medical Service (EMS) or rushing to the nearest ER if a limb is severed and/or blood is gushing or pumping out. In the meantime, apply pressure on the wound with gauze pads, a fresh diaper, a sanitary napkin, or a clean washcloth or towel. Increase the packing and pressure if bleeding doesn't stop. Do not resort to a tourniquet without medical advice as it can sometimes do more harm than good. Maintain pressure until help arrives.

50. Puncture wounds. Soak the injury in comfortably hot, soapy water for 15 minutes. Consult the baby's doctor or go to the ER. Do not remove any object (such as a knife or stick) that protrudes from the wound, as this could lead to increased bleeding. Pad it, if necessary, to keep it from moving around. Keep baby as calm and still as possible to avoid thrashing and making the injury worse.

51. Splinters or slivers. Wash the area with clean water and soap, then numb it with an ice pack (see page 629). If the sliver is completely embedded, try to work it loose with a sewing needle that has been sterilized with alcohol or the flame of a match. If one end of the sliver is clearly visible, try to remove it with tweezers (also sterilized by flame or alcohol). Don't try to remove it with your fingernails, which might be dirty. Wash the site again after you have removed the splinter. If the splinter is not easily removed, try soaking in warm, soapy water for 15 minutes, three times a day for a couple of days, which may help it work its way out. If it doesn't, or if the area becomes infected (indicated by redness, heat, swelling), consult the doctor. Also call the doctor if the splinter was deep and your baby's tetanus shots are not up to date.

Splinters or Slivers
see #51

Sunburn
see #14

Teeth, Injury to
see #36, #37

Toe Injuries
see #26, #27, #28, #29

Tongue, Injury to
see #35

LABEL YOUR IPECAC

Though it's a good idea to keep a bottle of syrup of ipecac among your first-aid supplies, this emetic (vomiting inducer) should never be administered without medical advice. To be certain that it isn't, tape a wide piece of adhesive with the warning "DO NOT USE WITHOUT INSTRUCTIONS FROM THE DOCTOR OR THE POISON CONTROL CENTER" across the face of the bottle. Add the telephone number of the Poison Control Center and the baby's doctor, both of which should also be posted next to all the phones in your home. And don't be afraid to use ipecac that is outdated. It is known to be 100% effective and safe up to four years after its expiration date. Keep a spare bottle, similarly labeled, in your diaper bag for visiting and travel.

Some recent studies indicate that liquid charcoal may be a preferable treatment in some cases of poisoning. Check with your local Poison Control Center to see if they recommend stocking liquid charcoal in your medicine chest.

RESUSCITATION TECHNIQUES FOR BABIES

The instructions that follow should be used only as reinforcement. You must, for your child's sake, take a course in baby CPR (check with baby's doctor, a local hospital or Y, or the Red Cross for the location of a class in your community) in order to be sure you can carry out these life support procedures correctly. Periodically, reread these guidelines or those you receive at the course and run through them step by step on a doll (*never* on your baby or any other person, or even on a pet) at least once a month so you will be able to perform them automatically should an emergency occur. Take a refresher course now and then—both to brush up on your skills and to learn the latest techniques.

The protocol below should be begun only on a baby who has stopped breathing, or on one who is struggling to breathe and turning blue (check around the lips and fingertips).

If a baby is struggling to breathe but hasn't turned blue, call for emergency medical assistance immediately or rush to the nearest emergency room. Meanwhile, keep baby warm and as quiet as possible, and in the position he or she seems most comfortable in.

If resuscitation seems necessary, survey baby's condition with Steps 1-2-3:[1]

1. Check for Unresponsiveness

Try to rouse a baby who appears to be unconscious by calling by name loudly, "Annie, Annie, are you okay?" several times. If that doesn't work, try tapping the soles of baby's feet. As a last resort, try gently shaking or tapping baby's shoulder—do not shake vigorously and don't shake at all if there is any possibility of broken bones, or of head, neck, or back injury.

---

1. This protocol is based on the latest rescue procedures of the American Red Cross and the American Heart Association, and was prepared with the assistance of Barbara Hogan of the Emergency Care Institute of Bellevue Hospital in New York. The training you receive may be somewhat different, and should be the basis for your action.

2. Seek Help

If you get no response, have anyone else present call for emergency medical assistance while you continue to Step 3. If you are alone with baby and feel sure of your CPR skills, proceed without delay, periodically calling loudly to attract help from neighbors or passersby. If, however, you are unfamiliar with CPR and/or feel paralyzed by panic, go the nearest phone immediately with the baby (assuming there are no signs of head, neck, or back injuries) or better still bring a portable phone to baby's side, and call your local EMS (emergency medical service). The dispatcher will be able to guide you as to the best course of action.

> *Important:* The person calling for emergency medical assistance should be certain to stay on the phone as long as necessary to give complete information and until the EMS dispatcher has concluded questioning. The following should be included: name and age of baby; present location (address, cross streets, apartment number, best route if there is more than one route); condition (is baby conscious? breathing? bleeding? in shock? is there a heartbeat?); cause of condition (poison, drowning, fall, etc.), if known; phone number, if there is a phone at the site. Tell the person calling for help to report back to you after calling.

3. Position Baby

Move baby as a unit, carefully supporting head, neck, and back as you do, to a firm, flat surface (a table is good because you won't have to kneel, but the floor will do). Quickly position baby face up, head level with heart, and use A-B-C[2] to survey his or her condition.

A: Clear the Airway

Use the following head-tilt/chin-lift technique to try to open the airway, unless there is a possibility of a head, neck, or back injury. If such an injury is suspected, use

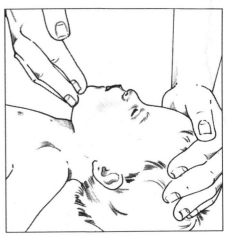

Head tilt/chin lift.

the jaw-thrust technique (below) instead.

> *Important:* The airway of an unconscious baby may be blocked by a relaxed tongue or epiglottis or by a foreign object. It must be cleared before baby can resume breathing.

Head tilt/chin lift. Place the hand nearest baby's head on the forehead and one or two fingers (not the thumb) of the other hand under the bony part of the lower jaw at the chin. Gently tilt baby's head back slightly by applying pressure on the forehead and lifting the chin. Do not press on the soft tissues of the underchin or let the mouth close completely (keep your thumb in it if necessary to keep the lips apart). Baby's head should be facing the ceiling in what is called the neutral position, with the chin neither down on the chest nor pointing up in the air. The head tilt necessary to open the airway in a child over one year may be somewhat greater (the neutral-plus

---

2. If you suspect a head, neck, or back injury, go to step B to look, listen, and feel for breathing before moving baby. If breathing is present, don't move baby unless there is immediate danger (as from fire or explosion) at the present site. If breathing is absent, and rescue breathing cannot be accomplished in the position baby is in, roll baby to a face up position as a unit so that head, neck, and body move as one without twisting.

position). If the airway does not open in a neutral position, move on to check for breathing (B).

Jaw thrust, for use when neck or back injury is suspected: With your elbows resting on the surface where baby is lying, place two or three fingers under each side of the lower jaw, at the angle where the upper and lower jaw meet, and gently lift the jaw upward to a neutral position (see head tilt, above).

>*Important:* Even if baby resumes breathing immediately, get medical help. Any baby who has been unconscious, stopped breathing, or nearly drowned requires medical evaluation.

B: *Check for Breathing*

1. After performing either the head tilt or the jaw thrust, look, listen, and feel for 3 to 5 seconds to see if baby is breathing: Can you hear or feel the passage of air when you place your ear near baby's nose and mouth? Does a mirror placed in front of baby's face cloud up? Can you see baby's chest and abdomen rising and falling (this alone isn't proof of breathing, since it could mean baby is trying to breathe but isn't succeeding)?

If normal breathing has resumed, maintain an open airway with head tilt or jaw thrust. If baby regains consciousness as well (and has no injuries that make moving inadvisable), turn him or her to one side. Call for emergency medical assistance now if someone else hasn't already called. If baby starts to breathe independently, and also starts to cough forcefully, this may be the body's attempt to expel an obstruction. *Don't interfere with the coughing.*

If breathing is absent, *or* if baby is struggling to breathe and has bluish lips and/or a weak, muffled cry, you must get air into the lungs immediately. Continue below. If emergency medical assistance has not been summoned and you are alone, continue trying to attract neighbors or passersby.

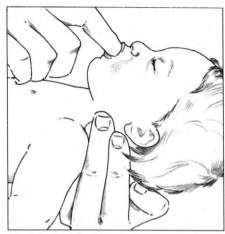

Clearing the baby's mouth of vomitus or foreign matter.

2. Maintain an open airway by keeping baby's head in a neutral position (or neutral-plus position, if needed, with a baby over a year) with your hand on the forehead. With a finger of the other hand, clear baby's mouth of any *visible* vomitus, dirt, or other foreign matter. Do not attempt a sweep if nothing is visible.

>*Important:* If vomiting should occur at any point, immediately turn baby to one side, clear mouth of vomitus with a finger, reposition baby on back, and quickly resume rescue procedures.

3. Take a breath through your mouth and place your mouth over baby's mouth and nose, forming a tight seal (see illustration). With a baby over a year old, cover just the mouth, and pinch the nostrils closed with the fingers of the hand that is keeping the head tilted back.

4. Blow two *light, slow* breaths of 1 to 1½ seconds each into baby's mouth, pausing between them to turn your head slightly and take a breath. Observe baby's chest with each breath. Stop blowing when the chest rises, and wait for the chest to fall before beginning another breath. In addition listen and feel for air being exhaled.

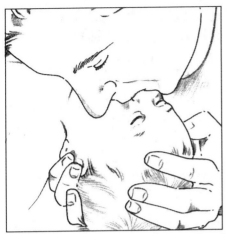

In rescue breathing for infants, both mouth and nose must be covered.

Important: Remember, a small baby needs only a small amount of air to fill the lungs. Though blowing too lightly may not expand the lungs fully, blowing too hard or too fast can force air into the stomach, causing distension. If at any point during rescue breathing baby's abdomen becomes distended, don't try to push it down—this might cause vomiting, which could present the risk of vomitus being aspirated, or inhaled, into the lungs. If the distension seems to be interfering with chest expansion, turn baby to one side, head down if possible, and apply gentle pressure to the abdomen for a second or two.

5. If the chest does not rise and fall with each breath, readjust the head-tilt/chin-lift (or jaw-thrust) position and try two more breaths. Blow a bit harder if necessary. If the chest still does not rise, it is possible that the airway is obstructed by food or a foreign object—in which case move quickly to dislodge it, using the procedure in "When Baby Is Choking" on page 454.

For a baby over a year, and sometimes for a large younger baby, it may be necessary to tilt the jaw a bit more to the neutral-plus position in order to open the airway

and ventilate (get air into) baby; retilt and try two more breaths. If that doesn't work, extend the chin further and try again; repeat until the chin is pointing straight up. If the chest still does not rise, proceed to "When Baby Is Choking."

C: Check Circulation

1. As soon as you've determined with two successful breaths that the airway is clear, check for a pulse. With an infant under a year, try to find the brachial pulse in the arm closest to you: keeping one hand on baby's head to maintain an open airway, use the other to pull baby's arm away from the body and turn it palm up. Use your index and middle fingers to try to locate the pulse between the two muscles on the inside of the middle arm, between the shoulder and elbow; see page 407. (With an older baby, take the carotid pulse in the neck). Since it's dangerous to give CPR to a baby whose heart is beating, do a thorough search; be sure to give yourself a full 5 to 10 seconds to locate the pulse. (Parents should practice finding their baby's pulse under non-emergency conditions so they can find it in a hurry under stress.)

2. If you find no pulse, begin CPR (see page 452) immediately. If you find a pulse, baby's heart is beating. Begin rescue breathing immediately (page 452) if breathing has not resumed spontaneously.

Activate Emergency Medical System

If the EMS has not yet been called and there is someone available to make the call, have them do so now. If a call was made before baby's condition was assessed, have the caller contact the dispatcher again to give further information on baby's condition: whether or not baby is conscious, is breathing, and has a pulse. Do not take time to call yourself if baby requires rescue breathing or CPR. Proceed without delay, periodically calling loudly to attract help from neighbors or passersby.

RESUSCITATION: RESCUE BREATHING

1. Blow into baby's mouth as described above at a rate of roughly one breath every 3 seconds (20 breaths per minute) for a baby under a year old (breathe, one and two and three and breathe), and once every 4 seconds (15 breaths per minute) for a baby older than a year. Watch to be sure baby's chest rises and falls with each breath.

2. Check for baby's pulse after a minute of rescue breathing to be sure the heart has not stopped. If it has, go to CPR. If it hasn't, look, listen, and feel for spontaneous breathing (see page 450) for 3 to 5 seconds. If baby has begun breathing independently, continue to maintain an open airway and check breathing and pulse frequently while waiting for help to arrive; keep baby warm and as quiet as possible. If there is no spontaneous breathing, continue rescue breathing, checking for the pulse and breathing once every minute.

Important: The airway must be kept open for rescue breathing to be effective. Be sure to maintain baby's head in the neutral position during rescue breathing.

3. If you're alone and emergency medical help has not yet been summoned, call as soon as independent breathing has been established. If within a few minutes baby hasn't starting breathing independently, carry the child in the football hold to a phone, continuing rescue breathing as you go. On the phone, simply report, "My baby isn't breathing," and quickly but clearly give all pertinent information (see above). Don't hang up until the dispatcher does; if possible, continue rescue breathing while the dispatcher is speaking; then get back to rescue breathing immediately.

Important: Do not discontinue rescue breathing until the baby is breathing independently or until medical professionals arrive to take over.

CARDIOPULMONARY RESUSCITATION (CPR): Babies Under One Year[3]

Important: In CPR, rescue breaths, which force oxygen into the lungs where it is picked up by the bloodstream, must be alternated with chest compressions, which artificially pump the oxygen-laden blood to the vital organs and the rest of the body.

1. Continue with baby face up on a firm, flat surface. Baby's head should be level with the heart.

2. Continue to maintain baby's head in a neutral position with one hand on the forehand. Place a small rolled towel, diaper, or other support under baby's shoulders and lift them just a bit, which will also help maintain an open airway. Do not cause the head to dip back more than slightly (see illustration page 449).

3. Position the three middle fingers of your free hand on baby's chest: imagine a horizontal line from nipple to nipple; place the pad of the index finger just under the intersection of this line with the breastbone, or sternum (the flat bone running midline down baby's chest between the ribs); the area to compress is one finger's width below this point of intersection.

4. Using two or three fingers, compress the sternum straight down to a depth of ½ to 1 inch (your elbow should be bent). At the end of each compression, release the pressure without removing your fingers from the sternum and allow it to return to its normal position. Develop a smooth compression-relaxation rhythm that allots equal

3. One year is the arbitrary cutoff chosen by the American Heart Association, the American Red Cross, and the American Academy of Pediatrics for switching from infant to child resuscitation procedures. The child's size may be a factor in some cases, but experts say that a slight error either way is not critical.

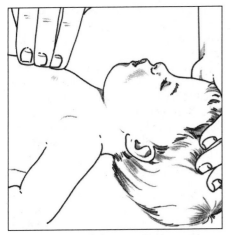

Compressions on infants can be done with two or three fingers.

time to each phase and avoids jerky movements.

5. After every fifth compression, pause with your fingers still in position on the sternum and deliver one slow rescue breath of 1 to 1½ seconds. Watch for the chest to rise. (If it doesn't, remove your fingers from the breastbone and lift the chin and blow again.) Aim for a rate of 100 compressions per minute, with a rescue breath after every five compressions. Count at a more rapid rate than you would if counting seconds: one, two, three, four, five—breathe.

6. After about a minute, take 5 seconds to check for the brachial pulse. If there is no pulse, give one slow rescue breath, then continue the compression/ventilation cycles of CPR, checking every few minutes for a pulse. If a pulse if found, discontinue chest compressions. Look, listen, and feel for 3 to 5 seconds for spontaneous respiration. If breathing is present, keep airway open and baby warm and quiet, and continue to monitor baby's breathing. If baby is still not breathing, continue with rescue breathing alone as described above.

7. After one minute of CPR, if you are alone and have not been able to attract anyone who could call for emergency medical assistance up until now, go quickly to a phone (carrying baby with you, if possible, or bringing the phone to where baby is) and summon help; then immediately return to rescue procedures as needed.

Important: Do not discontinue CPR until breathing and heartbeat are re-established or until medical relief arrives.

CARDIOPULMONARY RESUSCITATION (CPR): Babies Over One Year

1. Continue with the child face up on a firm, flat surface. There should be no pillow under the child's head; the head should be level with the heart. The child's head should be in the neutral-plus position (pages 449 to 450) to keep the airway clear.

2. Position your hands: with your middle and index fingers, locate the lower margin of the rib cage on the side nearest you; follow the margin of the rib cage down to the notch where the ribs and the breastbone, or sternum (the flat bone running down baby's chest between the ribs), meet; place the middle finger of the hand nearest baby's feet on this notch and the index finger down next to it; place the heel of your other hand just above the index finger with the long axis of the heel lengthwise, so that the two fingers and your hand line up along the sternum.

Important: Do not apply pressure to the tip of the sternum (called the xiphoid process). Doing so could cause severe internal damage.

3. Compress the chest with the heel of your hand to a depth of 1 to 1½ inches. The only contact should be between the heel of your hand and the flat lower half of the sternum—do not press on the ribs during compressions. Allow the chest to return to its resting position after each compression without lifting your hand from the chest.

Develop a compression-relaxation rhythm that allots equal time to each phase and avoids jerky movements.

4. At the end of every fifth compression, pause, and with baby's nostrils pinched closed, deliver a slow breath of 1 to 1½ seconds. Chest compressions must always be accompanied by rescue breathing to ensure a steady supply of oxygen to the brain (a child without a heartbeat is not breathing and is not getting oxygen). Aim for a rate of 80 to 100 compressions a minute, with a breath after every five compressions. Count at a more rapid rate than you would if counting seconds: one, two, three, four, five—breathe.

5. After about a minute, take 5 seconds to check for a pulse. If there is no pulse, give one slow breath with the nostrils pinched closed, then continue compression/ventilation cycles of CPR, checking periodically for a pulse. If a pulse is found, discontinue chest compressions. But if baby is still not breathing, continue with rescue breathing alone.

6. If you have not been able to attract help by calling, and emergency medical assistance has not been summoned, take a moment to go to a phone and call now; then immediately return to rescue procedures as needed. If possible, carry baby with you to the phone in a football hold and continue rescue breathing as you go.

Important: Do not discontinue CPR until breathing and heartbeat are re-established or until medical relief arrives.

WHEN BABY IS CHOKING

Coughing is nature's way of trying to dislodge an obstruction in the airway. A baby (or anyone else) who is choking on food or some foreign object and who can breathe, cry, and cough forcefully should not be interefered with. But if after two or three minutes baby continues to cough, call for emergency medical assistance. And when the choking victim is struggling for breath, can't cough effectively, is making high-pitched crowing sounds, and/or is turning blue (usually starting around the lips), the following rescue procedures should be pursued. They should also be pursued *immediately* if the baby is unconscious and not breathing, *and* if attempts to open the airway and breathe air into the lungs (see Steps A and B, pages 449 to 450) are unsuccessful.

Important: An airway obstruction may also occur because of such infections as croup or epiglottitis. A choking baby who seems ill needs immediate attention at an emergency care facility. *Do not* waste time in a dangerous and futile attempt to try to relieve the problem.

For Babies Under One Year (Conscious or Unconscious)

1. **Get help.** If someone else is present, ask them to phone for emergency medical assistance. If you're alone and unfamiliar with rescue procedures, or if you panic and forget them, take the baby to a phone or take a portable phone to where the child is and call for emergency medical assistance *immediately.* It's also usually recommended that even if you're familiar with rescue procedures, you take the time to call yourself before the situation worsens.

2. **Position baby.** Straddle baby face-down along your forearm, head lower than trunk (at about a 60° angle; see illustration). Cradle baby's chin in the curve between your thumb and forefinger. If you are seated, rest your forearm on your thigh for support. If baby is too big for you to comfortably support on your forearm, sit in a chair or on your knees on the floor and place baby face down across your lap in the same head-lower-than-body position.

3. **Administer back blows.** Give five

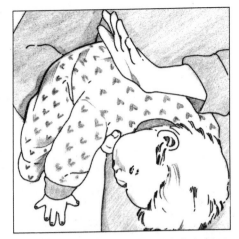

Back blows can often expell an inhaled object.

consecutive forceful blows between baby's shoulder blades with the heel of your free hand.

4. Administer chest thrusts. If there is no indication that the obstruction has been dislodged or loosened (forceful coughing, normal breathing, the object shooting out), place the flat of your free hand on the back, and supporting the head, neck, and chest with the other hand turn the child over, again with the head lower than the trunk. Support the head and neck with your hand, and rest your forearm on your thigh for support. (A baby who is too large to hold in this position can be placed face up on your lap.) To position your hand, imagine a horizontal line from nipple to nipple. Place the pad of your index finger just under the intersection of this line with the sternum (the flat breastbone running midline down baby's chest between the ribs). The area to compress is one finger's width below this point of intersection. Position two fingers (three, if you aren't achieving effective compression with two—but be careful to stay within the area from one finger's width below the nipple line to above the end of the sternum) along the sternum on baby's chest. Deliver five chest thrusts, compressing the sternum to a depth of ½ to 1 inch with each, and allowing the sternum to

return to its normal position in between compressions without removing your fingers. These are similiar to chest compressions but are performed at a slower rate—about 1 to 1½ seconds apart (one and, two and, three and, four and, five).

If baby is conscious, keep repeating the back blows and chest thrusts until the airway is cleared or the baby becomes unconscious. If baby is unconscious, continue below.

5. Do a foreign body check. If there is no indication that the obstruction has been dislodged or loosened (forceful coughing, normal breathing, the object shooting out), check for a visible obstruction. Open the mouth, by placing your thumb in baby's mouth, and grasp the tongue and lower jaw between your thumb and forefinger. Depress the tongue with your thumb as you lift the jaw up and away from the back of the throat. If you see a foreign object, attempt to remove it with a sweep of a finger. Do not sweep the mouth if you do not see an obstruction, and do not try to remove a visible obstruction with a pincer grasp, as you might force the object farther into the airway.

6. Do an airway check. If baby is still not breathing normally, open the airway with a head-tilt/chin-lift maneuver and attempt to administer two slow breaths with your mouth sealed over baby's nose and mouth, as on page 451. If the chest rises and falls with each breath, the airway is clear. Check for spontaneous breathing, Step B, and continue procedure as necessary.

7. Repeat sequence. If the airway remains blocked, keep repeating the sequence above until the airway is cleared and baby is conscious and breathing normally, or until emergency help has arrived. Don't give up, since the longer the baby goes without oxygen, the more the muscles of the throat will relax, and the more likely the obstruction can be dislodged.

THE UNSUSPECTED INHALED OBJECT

If your baby seems to choke on something and then with or without emergency treatment seems better, watch carefully for any signs of continued problems such as an unusual tone when crying or talking; decreased breathing sounds; wheezing; unexplained coughing; or blueness around the lips or fingernails, or of the skin generally. If any of these signs is apparent, take baby immediately to the emergency room. It's possible an object has lodged in the lower respiratory tract.

For Children Over One Year (Unconscious)

1. Position baby. Place child face up on a firm, flat surface (floor or table). Stand or kneel at the child's feet (don't sit astride a small child) and place the heel of one hand on the abdomen in the midline between the navel and the rib cage, fingers facing toward the child's face. Place the second hand on top of the first.

2. Administer abdominal thrusts. With the upper hand pressing against the lower, use a series of 6 to 10 rapid, inward-and-upward abdominal thrusts to dislodge the foreign object. These thrusts should be gentler than they would be for an adult or older child. And be careful not to apply pressure to the tip of the sternum or to the ribs.

3. Do an airway check. If the child is still not breathing spontaneously, tilt the head and administer two slow mouth-to-mouth breaths, while pinching the nostrils closed. If the chest rises and falls with each breath, the airway is clear. Check for spontaneous breathing, Step B (see page 450), and continue the procedure as necessary.

4. Repeat sequence. If the airway remains blocked, continue repeating the sequence above until the airway is cleared and baby is conscious and breathing normally, or until emergency help has arrived. Don't give up, since the longer the child goes without oxygen, the more the muscles of the throat will relax, and the more likely the obstruction can be dislodged.

> *Important:* Even if your baby recovers quickly from a choking episode, medical attention will be required. Call baby's doctor or the emergency room.

For Children Over One Year (Conscious)

1. Position yourself. Stand behind the child and wrap your arms around his or her waist.

2. Position your hands. The thumb side of one fist should rest against the child's abdomen in the midline, slightly above the naval and well below the tip of the breastbone.

3. Administer abdominal thrusts. Grasp the positioned fist with your other hand and press it into the child's abdomen with a quick upward thrust (the pressure should be less than you would use on an adult). Repeat until you see the object ejected or the baby begins breathing normally.

CHAPTER NINETEEN

The Low-Birth-Weight Baby

Most parents-to-be expect their babies to arrive right around the due date, give or take a couple of days or weeks. And indeed, the majority of babies do arrive on schedule—allowing them sufficient time to prepare for life outside the uterus, and their parents sufficient time to prepare for life with a baby.

But about 300,000 times a year in the United States, that vital preparatory time is cut unexpectedly— and sometimes perilously—short when baby is born prematurely and/ or too small. Some of these babies weigh in just a few ounces under the 2,500 gram (5-pound 8-ounce) low-

birthweight cutoff, and are able to quickly and easily catch up with their full-term peers. But others, robbed of many weeks of uterine development, arrive so small that they can fit in the palm of a hand; and it can take months of intensive medical care to help them do the growing they were supposed to have done in the womb.

Many parents, too, are far from ready when birth comes too early. For them, the first postpartum days, sometimes weeks or months, are filled not with writing thank you notes, learning to diaper, and getting adjusted to having a baby in the house, but with reading hospital charts, learning to insert nasogastric tubes, and getting adjusted to *not* having a baby in the house.

Though the low-birthweight baby (whether born early or not) is still at higher risk than larger babies, rapid advances in medical care for tiny infants have made it possible for the great majority of them to grow into normal, healthy children. But before they are carried proudly home from the hospital, their parents often experience many agonizing days and sleepless nights.

FEEDING BABY: Nutrition for the Preterm or Low-Birthweight Infant

The feeding of the preterm infant is a science that itself hasn't reached term; there is still much to be learned about the nutritional needs of babies who arrive before their expected due date. But what is known, or suspected, grows each year, as neonatologists and neonatal intensive care nurses try to devise and perfect the best methods for nourishing babies who must be fed outside the uterus at a time when they should still be getting fed inside it.

One of the still unclear areas of knowledge—and one critical to the rest of the picture—is how much weight a preterm baby should gain each week. There are many variables that affect weight gain, including birth size, hereditary factors (babies of Asian women may be smaller and grow more slowly than those with a Nordic heritage, for example), atmospheric conditions (growth is slower at high altitudes than at sea level), and overall health. Some experts now believe that the growth potential of premature infants has been underestimated in the past, possibly because inadequate feeding led to inadequate weight gain, and inadequate weight gain became the accepted norm. As nutritional understanding has increased, and along with it average weight gains, the expectations have been upped. The 2½- to 5-ounce (70- to 140-gram) weekly gain once considered an appropriate goal for premies is rapidly being replaced by a suggested 3¼ to 7½-plus ounces (90 to 210 grams). Whatever the projected weight gain, it's unlikely to begin until the premature infant's condition has stabilized. You can expect your premature infant, like the full-term baby, to lose some weight before beginning to gain.

It's also now recognized that the nutritional requirements of a preterm infant differ considerably from those of a baby born at term. Neither full-term breast milk nor ordinary baby formula—both of which term babies thrive on—are adequate for premies. These tiny babies need a diet closer to what they would have received if they were still in the uterus, including more protein, calcium, phosphorus, zinc, sodium, and possibly other nutrients. And they need to obtain these nutrients in as concentrated a form as possible because they are able to take only very small amounts of food at a time—partly because their stomachs are small, and partly because their immature digestive systems are sluggish, making the passage of food a very slow process.

When a very small neonate (newborn) is rushed to the intensive care nursery, an intravenous solution of water, sugar, and certain electrolytes is usually given to prevent dehydration and electrolyte depletion. After that initial feeding, very premature babies (those who arrived earlier than 30 to 33 weeks of gestation) will be fed by a method not dependent on sucking (such as

PORTRAIT OF A PREMIE

The parents of full-term newborns may be surprised when they first see their babies. The parents of preterm infants are often shocked. The typical premie weighs between 1,600 grams (about 3½ pounds) and 1,900 grams (about 4 pounds 3 ounces) at birth, and some weigh considerably less. The smallest can fit in the palm of an adult hand and have such tiny wrists and hands that a wedding band could be slipped over them. The premie's skin is translucent, leaving veins and arteries visible. It seems to fit loosely because it lacks a fat layer beneath it, and often it is covered with a fine layer of body hair, or lanugo. Skin coloring changes when the infant is handled or fed. Because brown fat (the fat layer that keeps us warm) is absent, the baby is unable to keep itself warm. The premie's ears may be flat, folded, or floppy because the cartilage that will give them shape is lacking.

Sexual characteristics are usually not fully developed—testicles may be undescended, the foreskin in boys and the inner folds of the labia in girls may be immature, and there may be no areola around the nipples. Because neither muscular nor nerve development is complete, many reflexes (such as grasping, sucking, startle, rooting) may be absent. And because of lack of strength and wind, the baby may cry little or not at all. He or she may also be subject to periods of breathing cessation, known as apnea of prematurity.

But being a premie is only a temporary condition. Once preterm newborns reach forty weeks of gestation, the time when, according to the calendar, they should have been born, they very much resemble the typical newborn in size and development.

via a nasogastric tube going through the nose and into the stomach) since such babies usually have not yet developed this reflex. Larger premies (at least 1,300 grams, or 2 pounds 14 ounces) who arrive at 30 weeks of gestation or later may be able to skip such gavage feedings and can often be put right to the breast, though they usually have to wait longer if they are to go to bottle feeding.

Since small premies can't self-regulate yet, feeding is very carefully monitored: How much fluid, protein, calcium, and so on is the baby taking? How much is being excreted in urine and stool? How much is left in the stomach? How are blood gases (oxygen, for example) affected by feedings? The calculations, once done exclusively by hand, are now often turned over to a computer for very rapid and accurate processing so that the diet of each infant can be individually programmed. The baby's condition can provide clues to nutritional deficiencies: white streaks or white hair is a sign of protein malnutrition; poor skin integrity and cracking of the lips are signs of zinc deficiency; loss of pigmentation and chronic anemia are signs of inadequate copper.

Many experts favor breast milk over formula for the premature baby, just as they do for the full-term infant. One reason is the presence of many important substances not found in cow's milk, including maternal antibodies, hormones, and enzymes, particularly lipase, which dramatically improves a baby's ability to absorb much-needed fat. But not just any breast milk will do. It's been found that the milk produced by mothers who've just delivered premature babies has, thanks to the body's infinite wisdom, more of the things these babies need (protein, nitrogen, sodium, lactose, and chloride) than does the breast milk of a woman who's delivered at term. So while

EXPRESSING MILK FOR A PREMATURE BABY

The decision to breastfeed a preterm baby is not always an easy one, even for women who planned on nursing at term. A major attraction of breastfeeding, close mother-child contact, is usually absent, at least at first, and is replaced by a mother-machine-child affair that is difficult as well as lacking in satisfaction. But though almost all women find pumping their breasts exhausting and time-consuming, most hang in there knowing that this is the one way in which they can contribute to the well-being of the baby from whose care they otherwise feel excluded.

The following tips can make the effort to feed a preterm baby in the best possible way more efficient and less tedious:

■ Keep in mind that if you were given magnesium sulfate for toxemia, you may not have milk for as long as two weeks.

■ See page 91 for tips on expressing breast milk. Ask about in-hospital facilities for expressing breast milk. If your hospital does not have a special room (with comfortable chairs, a breast pump, and disposable sterilization units) set aside for mothers to use, ask if one can be set up, or for information on borrowing or renting a breast pump. Your local La Leche League should be able to help you if the hospital can't.

■ Begin expressing milk as soon after delivery as possible, even if your baby isn't ready to take it. Express every two to three hours (about as often as a newborn nurses) if your baby is going to use the milk immediately; every four hours or so if the milk is going to be frozen for late use. You may find getting

up to pump once in the middle of the night helps build up your milk supply; or you may value a full night's sleep more. Empty your breasts each time to get all the higher-fat hind milk.

■ It's likely you will eventually be able to express more milk than your tiny baby can use. Don't cut back, however, figuring you're wasting too much. Regular pumping now will help to establish a plentiful milk supply for the time when your baby takes over where the machine leaves off. In the meantime, the excess milk can be dated and frozen—in the hospital or at home—for later use.

■ Don't be discouraged by day-to-day or hour-to-hour variations in supply. Such variations are normal, although you wouldn't be aware of them if you were nursing directly. Also normal when milk is expressed mechanically are an apparently inadequate milk supply and/or a drop in production after several weeks. Your baby will be a much more efficient stimulator of your milk supply than even the most efficient pump. When actual suckling begins, your supply is almost certain to increase quickly.

■ When baby is ready for feeding by mouth (usually not until at least 1,300 grams, or 2 pounds 14 ounces, and 30 weeks are reached), ask if you can try to breastfeed rather than have baby put to the bottle, since new studies show that low-birthweight babies take to the former more easily than to the latter. But don't worry if yours does better on the bottle—use it while your baby gets the hang of breastfeeding.

your own milk (or that of another mother of a premature infant) will be good for your baby, term milk won't be. And if it comes from a milk bank, where milk is routinely heat-sterilized, it will have the added disadvantage of having had the critically important lipase destroyed. Thus, if it's at all possible, nursing should be considered even if you weren't planning to breastfeed.

Sometimes, however, even the milk of a premie's mother isn't adequate for the baby. Since some of them, particularly very tiny ones, need even more concentrated nutrition—including more calories, protein, calcium, and phosphorus, and possibly more of such other nutrients as zinc, magnesium, copper, and vitamin B_6—the breast milk being fed through a tube or a bottle may be fortified as needed. If a baby is nursing directly, fortification may be given via intravenous or gavage feeding, or by a supplemental nutrition system, which allows simultaneous nursing and supplementation (see page 101). When possible, it's preferable not to give it to nursing infants via a bottle since this could lead to nipple confusion.

When a mother can't or doesn't wish to nurse, the highly concentrated formulas designed especially for premature babies (but not regular formulas) are a very good substitute. The intake of formula must, however, be very carefully monitored. Too much formula would be hard for the immature system to handle; too little would not support adequate growth. Soy formulas (because their calcium and phosphorus are not as well absorbed) are not ordinarily used for premature babies.

WHAT YOU MAY BE CONCERNED ABOUT

GETTING OPTIMUM CARE

"How do I know that our premature baby—she's only a little more than 2½ pounds—is getting the best possible care?"

In order to avoid duplication of services and expenses and to be sure that enough specialized medical care is available, the hospital system in this country is arranged in three levels. Small community hospitals make up level one—they provide care for noncomplicated cases of all types, including low-risk deliveries and normal newborns, but do not have neonatal intensive care units for very premature, low-birthweight, or sick newborns. Second-level hospitals have somewhat more sophisticated facilities, can care for more complicated cases including many high-risk deliveries, and do have neonatal intensive care units that can care for most babies in trouble. Third-level, or tertiary, hospitals are the major medical centers, boasting the most highly trained specialists, the most sophisticated facilities, and state-of-the-art neonatal intensive care units (NICUs) ready to care for the tiniest and sickest of newborns.[1]

Though healthy babies, including premies who weigh in at more than 2,250 grams (close to five pounds), do equally well at first-, second-, and third-level hospitals, very small babies (those who are at the highest risk) do best at major medical centers. Having your baby at such a facility is the best guarantee you can get of good care. If your baby is not in a tertiary hospital, discuss the possibility of having her transferred to one with her pediatrician, the present NICU staff, and the staff at the medical center you are considering.

Wherever your baby is, your input will be important in ensuring optimum care. Become knowledgeable about low-birthweight babies in general, and about any special problems your baby has, by reading books and by asking questions. Whenever you're uncomfortable or unhappy about the course your baby's treatment is taking, raise your concerns with her pediatrician and/or the hospital nurses or neonatologists. You may be satisfied with their explanation, or perhaps things can be done differently. If you aren't satisfied, ask for a consultation with another neonatologist. If you feel uncomfortable challenging doctors, find a friend or relative to act as advocate.

1. In some hospitals, this unit is called an intensive care nursery (ICN).

THE NEONATAL INTENSIVE CARE UNIT OR INTENSIVE CARE NURSERY

A first look at a neonatal intensive care unit can be frightening, especially if your baby is one of the tiny, helpless patients in it. (That's why it's a good idea for all expectant parents to routinely take that look during their prenatal tour of the hospital.) Knowing what you're looking at, however, can keep your fears from overwhelming you. Here's what you're likely to see in a typical neonatal intensive care unit or intensive care nursery:

- Babies naked or clad in diapers; in many hospitals they will be wearing little knit stocking caps to prevent heat loss through the head.
- Babies on "warming beds," adjustable mattresses set under warming lights. Very sick babies are often cared for on these to allow easy access for carrying out procedures, such as insertion of feeding tubes.
- Babies in isolettes (what used to be called incubators), see-through bassinets that are totally closed except for four portholes, two on either side. In some hospitals, isolettes will be fitted with water mattresses, which simulate floating in the amniotic fluid in the

uterus and may improve breathing, or even with miniature hammocks.
- Tubes and wires and lines—from babies to monitors, to IV bottles, or to other apparatus that supply nourishment, clear respiratory secretions, monitor temperatures, breathing, heart rate, and oxygen consumption, draw blood samples at regular intervals, and carry out many other important functions.
- Monitors to record vital signs and to warn, by setting off an alarm, of any ominous changes. These monitors pick up information via leads that are either stuck on the skin with gel or inserted by needle just under the skin.
- Plastic hoods or ventilators for the administration of oxygen and to assist breathing.
- Suction setups at each cribside for periodically removing excess respiratory secretions.
- Lights for phototherapy (bili lights) for babies with jaundice. The babies undergoing this treatment will be naked except for eye patches to protect their eyes from the light.

LACK OF BONDING

"We'd expected to bond with our baby right after birth. But since she arrived six weeks early and weighed only 3½ pounds, she was whisked away before we had a chance to even touch her. We're worried about the effect this will have on her—and on our relationship with her."

During this stressful time, the last thing you need is another worry. And the last thing you need to worry about is bonding at birth. Love and attachment between parent and child develops over many months, even years, blossoming over a lifetime rather than bursting miraculously into full bloom

during the first few moments of life. So instead of regretting the past and those first few moments (or even days) you've lost, start making the most of the present and of the months of parenthood that lie ahead. Though it isn't necessary to begin bonding at birth, you may be able to initiate the process while your baby is still in the hospital. Here's how:

Ask for a picture, along with a thousand words. If your baby has been moved from the hospital you delivered in to another hospital for upgraded intensive care (possibly essential to her survival), and you are not yet able to be discharged, ask that pictures of her be brought to you. Your husband or the hospital staff can take them, and you can enjoy looking at them until you're able to look at the real thing. Even if more tubing and gadgetry is visible than baby, what you see will likely be less frightening and more reassuring than what you might have imagined. As helpful as a picture may be, you'll still want those thousand words—from your husband, and later the medical staff—describing every detail of what your baby is like and how she's getting along.

Relinquish daddy. While you're unable to visit your baby, your husband can spend extra time with her rather than visiting exclusively with you. You'll be more lonely, but at least you'll know that someone who loves your child will be with her. As soon as you're out of the hospital, you should each spend as much time as possible with the baby. But be certain not to neglect any older children at home since they will need you more than ever — neglect housework, business, and everything else first.

Feast with your eyes. Just watching her in her isolette or warming mattress may help bring you closer.

Lay on the hands. Though it may seem that such a tiny and vulnerable infant is better off not being touched, studies have shown that premature infants who are stroked and lightly massaged while they are in intensive care grow better and are more alert, active, and behaviorally mature than babies who are handled very little. The nurses in the NICU will show you how to scrub (washing hands and arms up to the elbows) and don a hospital gown before reaching through the isolette portholes to get acquainted with your baby. Start with her arms and legs, since they are less sensitive at first than the trunk. Try to work up to at least twenty minutes of gentle stroking a day.

Carry on a conversation. To be sure, it will be a one-way conversation at first— your baby won't be doing much talking, or even crying, while she's in the NICU. She

may not even appear to be listening. But she will recognize your voice—and her daddy's. They will be the only familiar voices in the ICN at first (she's heard them for months from the uterus), and hearing them will be comforting to her.

See eye to eye. If your baby's eyes are shielded because she's getting phototherapy for the treatment of jaundice, ask to have the bili lights turned off and her eyes uncovered for at least a few minutes during your visit so that you can make eye-to-eye contact, an important part of parent-child bonding.

Take over for the nurses. As soon as your baby's out of immediate danger, the NICU nurse will probably be happy to show you how to diaper, feed, and bathe her, and even do some simple medical procedures for her. Caring for her during your visits will help make you more comfortable with the role of mother, while giving you some valuable experience for the months ahead.

Don't hold back. Many parents remain detached from their premature babies for fear of loving and losing. But that's a mistake. First, because the odds are very much with your preterm baby; the great majority survive to be healthy and normal. And second, because if you do hold back and the unthinkable happens, you'll always regret the moments you lost. The loss would be harder, not easier, to take.

INTRAUTERINE GROWTH RETARDATION

"My baby wasn't premature, but she was just under five pounds. The doctor said it was because of intrauterine growth retardation. Does this means she will be mentally retarded?"

As ominous as it may sound, intrauterine growth retardation, often shortened to IUGR, has nothing to do with any kind of mental or physical retardation after birth, only with growth retardation while in the uterus. The vast majority of infants with IUGR end up having normal IQs and neurological function. IUGR appears to be nature's way of ensuring a fetus's survival in a uterus where, for some reason, she is not getting an adequate supply of nutrients through the placenta. The reduction in size allows a baby to get along well on the reduced intake of nutrients. Doctors surmise that this protective mechanism is called into action when the placenta isn't functioning at optimal efficiency, limiting the passage of nutrients to the fetus, or when the mother's nutrition is inadequate, because of poor diet, smoking, illness, or other, unknown factors.

The baby's brain also appears to be protected by this survival mechanism, usually continuing to grow normally by taking more than its share of nourishment from what is available. That's why most babies with IUGR have heads that are even larger in relation to their bodies than are those of full-size newborns.

Though a low-birthweight baby is at high risk for many complications during the early days of life, most will do well with proper neonatal care. With good nutrition, preferably beginning with breast milk, you can expect your baby to start thriving; and by the end of her first year she'll probably have caught up on many, or even on all, fronts with her peers. But should you decide to become pregnant again, try to determine first, with the aid of your doctor, what might have been responsible for the poor growing environment in your uterus so that your next baby won't have to struggle with the same problems prenatally.

LONG HOSPITALIZATION

"The first time I saw our baby in the intensive care nursery I was devastated. It's horrible to think that our baby will spend the first weeks—maybe months— of his life in a sterile hospital room."

Walking into an intensive care nursery may be an upsetting experience, but it's likely you'd be much more upset if there were no such facility available for your baby.

Someday we may have a better way of dealing with premature infants who experience no medical problems. In Bogota, Colombia, for example, a system of kangaroo-style newborn care has evolved, which eliminates sterile hospital nurseries and allows a mother to go home shortly after delivery. But instead of transferring her new baby to a crib or cradle, she carries him in a sling at her breast, where he can nurse on demand around the clock for the next few weeks of life. Even small preterm infants with no complications seem to thrive in this warm, cozy, nourishing environment. But unless and until such a system or a similar one is deemed safe and approved for use here, parents of premies will have to wait until their babies reach four or five pounds and a gestational age of 37 to 40 weeks before taking them home— or about as long as they would have had to wait if the babies had been carried to term.

Feeling anxious in such a situation is not only normal but healthy. Mothers who are anxious after the birth of a premature baby go on to be better at mothering than those who aren't. But the anxiety needs to be channeled into productive activities:

Hit the shops. Since your baby arrived ahead of time, you may not have had time to order baby furniture, layette items, a diaper service, and the like. If so, now's the time to get that shopping done. If you feel superstitious about filling your home with baby things before baby is discharged from the hospital, put in your orders pending his homecoming. You'll not only have taken care of some necessary chores, you'll also have filled some of the interminable hours of baby's hospitalization and made a statement (at least to yourself) that you are confident of bringing him home.

Strike up a partnership. Parents of a premie often begin to feel that their baby belongs to the doctors and nurses, who seem so competent and do so much for him, rather than to them. Instead of trying to compete with the staff, try working together with them. Get to know the nurses (which will be easier if your baby has a "primary" nurse in charge of his care at each shift), the neonatologist, the residents. Let them know you'll be happy to do little chores or errands for your baby—which can save them time and help you feel useful.

Get a medical education. Learn the jargon and terminology used in the NICU. Ask a staff member (when he or she has a free moment) to show you how to read your baby's chart; ask the neonatologist for details about your baby's condition—and for clarification when you don't understand. Parents of premies often become experts in neonatal medicine, throwing around terms like "RDS" and "intubation" with the aplomb of a neonatologist.

Be a fixture at your baby's side. Some hospitals may let you move in, but even if you can't, you should spend as much time as possible with your baby, alternating shifts with your husband. This way you will not only get to know your baby's medical problems, but your baby as well. (If you have other children at home, however, they'll also need you now. Be certain that they get a substantial piece of mom and dad's time, too.)

Make your baby feel at home. Even though the isolette's only a temporary stop for your baby, try to make it as much like home as possible. Ask permission to put friendly looking stuffed animals around your baby and tape pictures (perhaps including stimulating black-and-white enlargements of snapshots of mommy and daddy) to the sides of the isolette for his viewing pleasure. And tuck in a baby music box for a little night and day music. Remember, however, that anything you put in the baby's isolette will have to be sterilized and should not interfere with life-sustaining equipment. Also be sure to keep noise levels low.

Ready your milk supply. Your milk is the perfect food for your premature baby (see page 459). Until he's able to nurse, pump your breasts for indirect feedings and in order to keep up your milk supply. Pumping will also give you a welcome feeling of usefulness.

SIBLINGS

"We have a three-year-old daughter, and we don't know what to tell her about her new premature sister."

Children, even children as young as yours, are able to understand and handle a lot more than we adults usually give them credit for. Trying to protect your daughter by keeping her in the dark about the condition of her new sibling will only make her anxious and insecure—particularly when you and your husband suddenly, and to her, inexplicably, start spending so much of your time away from home. Instead, enlighten her fully. Explain that the baby came out of mommy too soon, before she had grown enough, and has to stay in a special crib in the hospital until she's big enough to come home. With the hospital's okay, take your older daughter for an initial visit, and if it goes well and she seems eager, take her regularly. Children are just as likely to be fascinated by the wires and tubes as they are to be scared, particularly if their parents set the right tone—confident and cheerful rather than nervous and somber. Have her bring a present for the baby, to be placed in the isolette, which will help her feel that she's a part of the team caring for her new sibling. If she would like to, and if you have the staff's permission, let her scrub and then touch the baby through the portholes. Like you, she will feel closer to the baby when she finally comes home if she has some contact now. (Read about sibling relationships in Chapter 26.)

BREASTFEEDING

"I've always been determined to breast-feed my baby, and since she was born prematurely, I've been pumping milk to be fed to her through a tube. Will she have trouble switching to nursing later?"

So far, so good. From birth your baby has been provided with the best possible food for a premature newborn—her mommy's milk—in the only way such a tiny baby is able to take nourishment, through a tube. Naturally, you're concerned that she be able to continue to get this perfect food once she graduates to suckling.

A recent study, however, indicates you have little to worry about. It showed that premature infants weighing as little as 1,300 grams, or nearly 3 pounds, were not only able to suckle at the breast, but were more successful at it than they were with the bottle. It took these infants between one and four weeks longer to become proficient at sucking from the bottle than at suckling from the breast. In addition, their bodies responded better to breastfeeding. When they nursed their oxygen levels fluctuated little, while during bottle feeding they showed significant drops in oxygen levels, with these levels staying down for varying periods after feeding. And they were comfortably warmer when being breastfed than when getting the bottle, which is important because premies, whose thermostats aren't operative, have trouble keeping themselves warm. This study and others like it show that the small preterm infant has the sucking reflex at 30 weeks, rather than at the 33- to 36-week point previously believed, and suggest that the prevalent practice of waiting until a preterm infant nurses well on a bottle before putting her to breast should be reconsidered.[2]

---

2. If the neonatal intensive care staff at your baby's hospital is not familiar with the study, refer them to the *Journal of Maternal Child Nursing*, April 1987. The study was done by Paula Meier, D.N.Sc., RN, at Michael Reese Hospital in Chicago.

Once you do put your baby to the breast, you'll want to make conditions as conducive to success as possible:

- Read all about breastfeeding, beginning on page 49, before getting started.
- Be patient if the neonatologist or nurse wants your baby monitored for temperature and/or $TCPO_2$ (oxygen) changes during breastfeeding. This won't interfere with the breastfeeding itself and it will protect your baby by sounding an alarm in case she is not responding well to the feeding.
- Be sure you're relaxed, and that your baby is awake and alert but not crying frantically with hunger. A nurse will probably see to it that she is dressed warmly for this momentous event.
- Ask the staff if there is a special nursing area for premie moms, or at least a private corner with an armchair for you and your baby.
- Get comfortable, propping your baby on pillows, supporting her head. Many women find a football hold comfortable (see page 52) as well as easy on the nipples.
- If your baby doesn't yet have a rooting reflex (she probably doesn't), help her get started by placing your nipple, with the areola, into her mouth. Compress it with your fingers to make it easier for her to latch onto, and keep trying until she succeeds.
- Use your finger to press the breast away from her nose so your baby can breathe.
- Watch to be sure your baby is getting milk. The first few minutes of sucking may be very rapid, a non-nutritive sucking aimed at stimulating let-down. Your breasts are used to mechanical pumping and will take a while to adjust to the different motions of your baby's mouth, but soon you will notice that the suckling has slowed and that your baby is swallowing. This lets you know that let-down has occurred.
- If your baby doesn't seem interested in your breast, try expressing a few drops of milk into her mouth to give her a taste of what's in store.

- If it's okay with the hospital staff, nurse your baby for as long a period as she's willing to stay at the breast. Experts who've studied breastfeeding of premature babies recommend letting them remain at the breast until they've stopped active sucking for at least two minutes. Small premies have been known to nurse for close to an hour before being satisfied.
- Don't be discouraged if the first session, or even the first several sessions, seem unproductive. Many full-term babies take a while to catch on, and pretermers deserve the same chance.
- Ask that any feedings at which you cannot nurse be given by gavage rather than by bottle. If your baby is given bottle feedings while you're trying to establish breastfeeding, nipple confusion could interfere with your efforts. If human milk fortifier or other fortification is given to your baby to supplement the breast milk, ask that it, too, be given by gavage or by the supplementary nutrition system (see page 101).

You'll be able to tell how well your baby is doing on the breast by following her daily weigh-in. If she continues gaining about 1 to 2% of her body weight (about 15 to 30 grams for a 1,500-gram, or 3⅓-pound, baby) daily, or about 3½ to 7½ ounces a week, she'll be doing fine. By the time she reaches her original due date, she should be approaching the weight of a full-termer—somewhere around 6 to 8 pounds.

CATCHING UP

"Our son, who was born nearly two months early, seems very far behind compared with other three-month-olds. Will he ever catch up?"

He's probably not "behind" at all. In fact, he's probably just where a baby conceived when he was should be. Traditionally, in our culture, a baby's age is calculated from the day he was born. But this system is misleading when assessing the growth and development of premature infants since it fails to take into account that at birth they have not yet reached term. Your baby, for example, was just a little more than *minus* two months old at birth. At two months of age he was, in terms of gestational age (calculated according to his *original* due date), equivalent to a newborn; and now, at three months, he's more like a one-month-old. Keep this in mind when you compare him to other children his age or to averages on development charts. For example, though the average baby may sit well at seven months, your child may not do so until he's nine months old, when he reaches his seventh month corrected age. If he was very small or very ill in the neonatal period, he's likely to sit even later. In general, you can expect motor development to lag more than the development of the senses (vision and hearing, for example).

Experts use the gestational age, usually called "corrected age," in evaluating a premature child's developmental progress up until he's two or two and a half. After that point, the two months or so differential tends to lose its significance—there isn't, after all, much developmental difference between a child who is four years old and one who is two months shy of four. And as your baby gets older, the behavior gap between his corrected age and his birth age will diminish and finally disappear, as will any developmental differences between him and his peers (though occasionally, extra nurturing may be needed to bring a premie to that point). In the meantime, if you feel more comfortable using his corrected age with strangers, do so. Certainly do so when assessing your baby's developmental progress.

Instead of looking for specific behaviors from your baby at specific times, relax and enjoy his progress as it comes, providing support as needed. If he's smiling and cooing, smile and coo back at him. If he's starting to reach for things, give him the opportunity to practice that skill, too. When he can sit propped up, prop him in different surroundings for a while each day.

But always keep his corrected age in mind, and don't rush him. Pushing too hard too soon could have negative repercussions. For one, your baby could begin to feel inadequate if he can't do what you expect of him when you expect it. For another, you may use up so much enthusiasm pushing him when he isn't ready that when he is ready, you may have run out of baby-stimulating steam.

Use the infant stimulation tips in this book (pages 163, 263, 380), gearing them to your baby's behavior rather than his age, and be careful to stop when he signals that he's had enough. You can, additionally, encourage motor development by placing your baby on his abdomen, facing outward toward the room rather than toward the wall, as often and for as long as he'll tolerate it. Since premies and low-birthweight babies spend most of their early weeks, sometimes months, on their backs in isolettes, they often resist this position, but it's a necessary one for building arm and neck strength.

If, of course, your baby is far behind developmentally even after making allowances for his prematurity, and if he seems to stay that way, read page 317 and check with his doctor.

HANDLING BABY

"So far I've only handled our baby through the portholes of her isolette. But I'm worried about how well I'll be able to handle her when she finally comes home. She's so tiny and fragile."

When your baby finally makes that long-anticipated trip home, she may actually seem pudgy and sturdy to you, rather than tiny and fragile. Like many premies, she'll probably have doubled her birthweight before hitting the requisite four or five pounds necessary for discharge. And chances are you won't have any more trouble caring for her than most new mothers have caring for their full-term babies. In fact, if you have a

chance to do some baby care at the hospital (something you should insist on) in the weeks before your baby's homecoming, you'll actually be ahead of the game. Which is not to say it will be easy—rare is the new mother who finds it so.

If you're wondering how well you and your baby will do without a nurse or neonatologist looking over your shoulder, ready to step in if anything goes wrong, be assured that hospitals don't send home babies who are still in need of full-time professional care. Still, some mothers, particularly those who come home with such extra paraphernalia as breathing monitors or oxygen hoods, find it comforting to hire a baby nurse who has had experience with premies and their medical care to help them through the first week or two. Consider this option if you're anxious about going it alone.

GUILT

"I know that I wasn't as careful during my pregnancy as I should have been and I feel it was my fault that our son came so early."

There's probably not one mother of a premature baby who doesn't look back and regret something she did during pregnancy that she might have done better—something that might have contributed to her baby's early arrival. Such feelings of remorse are normal, but not productive. It's almost impossible to be sure just what factor or factors are responsible for your baby's early arrival, and even if you are sure, assigning blame is not going to help your baby. What your baby needs now is a mother who is strong, loving, and supportive, not one who is floundering in guilt. Read Chapter 20, which concerns newborns with medical problems, for some suggestions on how to deal with your feelings of guilt, anger, and frustration. It may also help to talk to other parents of premies; you will find they share many of your feelings. Some hospitals have parent support groups; others feel parents do better consulting with the staff than with other parents. Do what seems to help you most.

Of course, next to taking the best possible care of your baby who's already been born, the most productive thing you can do is to make sure you take the best possible care of your next baby (if you decide to have one) before birth. Though not all cases of prematurity can be prevented, a great many can be. Consult with your obstetrician before becoming pregnant again to discuss your medical history, and follow a prepregnancy plan for getting your body and your eating and lifestyle habits into optimum shape (see *What to Expect When You're Expecting* and *What to Eat When You're Expecting*).

PERMANENT PROBLEMS

"Though the doctor says our baby is doing well, I'm still afraid that he'll come through this with some kind of permanent damage."

One of the greatest miracles of modern medicine is the rapidly increasing survival rate for premature infants. At one time, a baby weighing in a 1,000 grams (about 2 pounds 3 ounces) had no chance of making it. Now, thanks to the advances in neonatology, many babies who are born even smaller than that can be expected to survive.

Of course, along with this increased survival rate has come an increase in the number of babies with moderate to severe handicaps. Still, the odds of your baby's coming home from his hospital stay both alive *and* well are very much in his favor. Only an estimated 10% of all premies and 20% of those between 1½ and 3½ pounds end up with major handicaps. The risks of permanent disability are much greater for those who are born at 23 to 25 weeks and/or weigh less than 750 grams (25 ounces); still, of the 40% of these infants who survive, more than half do well.

Overall, better than 2 out of 3 babies born prematurely will turn out to be perfectly normal, and most of the others will have only mild to moderate handicaps. IQ will most often be normal, though preterm infants do have an increased risk of learning problems.

For a couple of years, even if your baby is absolutely normal, you can expect him to lag behind others of the same birth age. His progress is likely to follow more closely that of children of his corrected age. And if he was very small, or had serious complications during the neonatal period, he is very likely to lag behind his corrected age-mates too, particularly in motor development.

Premature infants may also display one or more neuromuscular abnormalities. They may not lose such newborn reflexes as the Moro, tonic neck, or grasp reflexes as early as term infants, even taking corrected age into account. Or their muscle tone may be abnormal, in some cases causing the head to droop excessively, in other cases causing the legs to be stiff and the toes to point. Though such signs my be worrisome in full-term babies, they usually aren't in pretermers. (Still, they should be evaluated by the physician, and physical therapy should be begun if necessary).

Slow developmental progress in a premie is not only *not* cause for alarm, it is to be expected. If, however, your baby seems not to be making *any* progress week to week, month to month, or if he seems unresponsive (when he's not ill), speak to his doctor. If the doctor doesn't share your concerns, but doesn't allay them either, ask for a second opinion. Occasionally a mother, who sees her baby day in and day out, catches something the doctor misses. If there turns out to be no problem, which will most often be the case, the second opinion will help to erase your fears. And if a problem is discovered, the early diagnosis could lead to treatment as well as ongoing training and care, which may make a tremendous difference in the ultimate quality of your baby's life.

CAR SEATS

"My baby seems lost in the car seat we borrowed. Wouldn't she be safer in my arms?"

It's not only unsafe but illegal for a baby (premature or full term) to ride in mommy's (or anyone else's) arms rather than in a car seat. This presents a serious problem, however, to parents of low-birth-weight babies. Not only are their small bodies often lost in a regular car seat, but they may also have trouble breathing in the semi-propped position the seat requires. One study has shown that some preterm infants show a decreased oxygen supply while riding in a car seat, and that this deficit may last for as long as thirty minutes or more afterward. Some may also experience short periods of apnea (breathing cessation) in car seats. Much better for such infants is a new crash-tested infant car bed, in which the infant is prone rather than propped and which protects her in case of accident without compromising breathing.[3] Check with your local juvenile furnishings store to see if one is available locally. If for any reason you can't obtain such a bed or a seat designed for a premie, you may want to limit the amount of auto travel you do with your baby for the first month or two at home, especially if she has had spells of apnea previously. Or ask her doctor about monitoring her breathing when she's in an ordinary car seat, at least for a while, to see if she is experiencing any problems.

To help your baby ride more comfortably in a car seat, roll a towel or small blanket and arrange it so that it cradles her head, or buy a ready-to-use head roll designed for infant car seats. If there's a big space between your baby's body and the harness (or anywhere else in the seat), use another folded towel or blanket to fill it in.

The same breathing problems may occur in young premature babies in infant seats and baby swings, so don't use either without the doctor's approval.

A REPEAT WITH THE NEXT BABY

"Will the fact that our first son was premature make it more likely that our second baby will be?"

Whether or not you're at high risk for a repeat premature delivery depends primarily on just what the cause of the first one was. If the suspected cause was something that is within your control—if such risk factors as smoking, heavy drinking, drug use, poor nutrition, inadequate weight gain, and/or physical stress (a job requiring constant standing or heavy physical labor, for example) were part of your pregnancy profile—then you simply (or maybe not so simply) have to change your lifestyle to protect any future babies. If your doctor believes you are one of the small percentage of women in whom sexual intercourse seems to trigger labor prematurely, your lovemaking may have to be restricted during part or all of your pregnancy. If diagnostic tests point to hormonal imbalance as the reason for your premature labor, hormone replacement therapy may help you carry to term.

Other risk factors linked to prematurity are less easily controlled or eliminated, but they can often be modified. These include:

Infection. If an acute infection led to your first preterm delivery, you aren't likely to experience a repeat; but be sure you're clear of venereal disease (including chlamydia) and urinary tract and vaginal infections, and are immune to rubella, before conceiving again. If you do contract an infection during pregnancy, have it treated medically as soon as possible. (But be sure the treating doctor knows you are expecting.)

Incompetent cervix. If your cervix

---

3. The Swinger Infant Car Bed from Evenflo and the Cosco Dream Ride meet the needs of premies.

dilated prematurely under the weight of the growing fetus (probably because of muscular weakness), stitching it closed early on in a new pregnancy should prevent a recurrence.

Structural abnormalities of the uterus. Once diagnosed, these abnormalities can often be surgically corrected.

Placenta previa. If your placenta was too low in the uterus, close to, partially covering, or fully covering the cervix, and is again next time (though it won't necessarily be), complete bed rest may ward off early labor.

Chronic maternal illness. If you have diabetes, heart disease, hypertension, or

SPECIAL CARE TIPS
FOR PRETERM BABIES

■ Read the month-by-month chapters in this book; they apply to your preterm baby as well as to full-termers. But remember to adjust for your baby's corrected age.

■ Keep your home warmer than usual, about 72° or so, for the first few weeks that your baby is at home. The temperature regulating mechanism is usually functioning in premature infants by the time they go home, but because of their small size and greater skin surface in relation to fat, they may have difficulty keeping comfortable without a little help. In addition, having to expend a great many calories to keep warm could interfere with weight gain. If your baby seems unusually fussy, check the room temperature to see if it's warm enough, and feel baby's arms, legs, or the nape of the neck to be sure it isn't too cool. (Don't, however, overheat the room.)

■ Buy diapers made for premies, if necessary. You can also buy baby clothes in premie sizes, but don't buy too many—before you know it, your baby will have outgrown them.

■ Sterilize bottles, if you're giving them. Though it may be an unnecessary precaution for a term baby, it's a good one to take for premies, who are more susceptible to infection. Continue for a few months, or until baby's doctor gives you the okay to pack away the sterilizer.

■ Feed your baby frequently, even though this may mean spending most of your time nursing or bottle feeding. Premies have very small stomachs, and may need to eat as often as every two or three hours. They also may not be able to suckle as efficiently or effectively as full-termers, and so they may take longer—as long as an hour—to drink their fill. Don't rush feedings.

■ Unless your baby is getting formula containing all the required nutrients, give a baby multivitamin supplement as prescribed by the doctor. Preterm babies are at greater risk of becoming vitamin deficient than full-termers and need this extra insurance.

■ Don't start solids until your doctor gives the go-ahead. Generally, solids are introduced to a preterm infant when weight reaches 13 to 15 pounds, when more than 32 ounces of formula is consumed daily for at least a week, and/or when the corrected age is six months. Occasionally, when a baby is not satisfied with just formula or breast milk, solids may be started as early as three months, corrected age, or five or six months, chronological age.

■ Treat your baby just as you would a full-term infant. Parents of babies who were born prematurely tend to think of their children as particularly fragile. They are often overly cautious (they worry that baby's too warm or too cold, or isn't eating enough or sleeping enough); overly indulgent (baby always gets his or her way); and overly attached (mothers often have difficulty separating from their premies). No limits are set and the baby, rather than the parents, is usually in charge. Such an atmosphere can interfere with normal development and turn out a dependent, demanding, unhappy child.

some other chronic illness, good medical care, sometimes including bed rest, can often prevent premature delivery; consult your doctor.

Stress. If physical or emotional stress contributed to your baby's early arrival, try to reduce it next time around. Get professional help if necessary.

Age. This is a prematurity risk factor you can't change—if you were over 35 the first time, you will be even older the next time. But you can improve your chances of carrying to term by being sure you get optimum medical care not only from your doctor, but from yourself as well. Eliminating or modifying every alterable risk factor above can reduce your excess risk almost to

that of a younger woman.

Whether or not the reason for your previous premature delivery is known, see your doctor before becoming pregnant again. Discuss what you can do to reduce the risk of your delivering prematurely again. Follow doctor's orders religiously— even if that means cutting back on your lovemaking, work, and other activities. Also discuss the possibility of monitoring contractions at home with a device that can be hooked up by phone to the physician's office or hospital. Since the monitor can usually spot contractions before you can, it often allows medical action—in the form of tocolytic drugs that stop contractions, bed rest, or other steps—to be taken early enough to forestall labor.

WHAT IT'S IMPORTANT TO KNOW: Health Problems Common in Low-Birthweight Babies

Prematurity is risky business. Tiny bodies are not fully mature, many systems (heat regulatory, respiratory, and digestive, for example) aren't yet fully operative, and not surprisingly, the risk of neonatal illness is greatly increased. As the technology for keeping such babies alive improves, more attention is being given to these conditions, most of which are rare or unknown among full-term babies, and successful treatment is becoming more and more the norm for many of them. New treatments are being developed almost daily and so may not be detailed here—but do ask your neonatologist or pediatrician about recent advances. The medical problems that most frequently complicate the lives of preterm infants include:

Respiratory distress syndrome (RDS). Because of immaturity, the premature lung often lacks pulmonary surfactant, a de-

tergent-like substance that gives the lung surfaces their elastic properties. Without surfactant the tiny alveoli, or air sacs, of the lungs collapse like deflating balloons with each expiration, forcing the tiny baby to work harder and harder to breathe. Babies who have undergone severe stress in the uterus, usually during labor and delivery, are less likely to lack surfactant as the stress appears to speed lung maturation.

RDS was once frequently fatal, but nearly 80% of babies who develop RDS today survive, thanks to an increased understanding of the syndrome and new ways of treatment such as continuous positive airway pressure (CPAP), which is administered through tubes in the nose or mouth, or via a plastic oxygen hood. The continuous pressure keeps the lungs from collapsing until the body begins producing sufficient surfactant, usually in three to five days. Sometimes, when lung immaturity is detected before delivery and delivery can safely be delayed, RDS can be prevented entirely by the administration, prior to birth, of a hormone to speed lung maturation and production of surfactant. Also promising as a way of preventing or reducing the severity of RDS is the instillation of artificial or human surfactant into a premature infant's lungs before the first breath is taken. For children in respiratory distress, extracorporeal membrane oxygenation (ECMO), which employs a type of heart-lung machine, gives temporary support to the failing heart and lungs and provides a healing rest. (ECMO is used for many types of respiratory failure, not just that associated with RDS.)

Bronchopulmonary dysplasia (BPD). In some babies, particularly those with low birthweight, long-term oxygen administration and mechanical ventilation appear to combine with lung immaturity to cause BPD, or chronic lung disease. The condition is usually diagnosed when a newborn requires increased oxygen after the twenty-eighth day of life. Specific lung changes are generally seen on X-ray, and these babies frequently gain weight slowly and are subject to apnea. A few continue to require oxygen when they go home, others have fluids restricted or are put on diuretics or bronchodilators to prevent complications, and all require a high caloric intake to improve growth. Often the condition is outgrown as the lungs mature.

Hypoglycemia. Low blood sugar can make an adult feel dizzy, jittery, or irritable, but in a newborn it can be much more serious, causing brain damage and retardation if left untreated. It's most commonly a problem in babies born of multiple births in which the smaller or smallest weighs less than 4½ pounds and in babies of diabetic moms (who usually have high, rather than low, birthweights). Hypoglycemia is routinely screened for during the first 24 to 48 hours, and if it's found, treatment to normalize sugar levels is begun immediately.

Patent ductus arteriosus. In the fetal circulatory system there is a duct connecting the aorta (the artery through which blood from the heart is sent to the rest of the body) and the left pulmonary artery (the one leading to the lungs) called the ductus arteriosus. This duct shunts blood away from the nonfunctioning lungs and is kept open during gestation by high levels of prostaglandin E (one of a group of fatty acids produced by the body) in the blood. Normally, levels of prostaglandin E fall at delivery and the ductus begins to close within a few hours. But in about half of very small premature babies (those weighing under 1,500 grams, or 3 pounds 5 ounces), and in some larger babies, levels of prostaglandin E don't drop and the ductus remains open, or "patent." In many cases there are no symptoms, except perhaps a little shortness of breath on exertion and/or blueness of the lips, and the duct closes by itself in the neonatal period. Occasionally, however, severe complications occur. Treatment with an antiprostaglandin drug (indomethacin) is often successful in closing the duct; when it isn't, simple surgery generally does the job.

Retinopathy of prematurity (ROP). This condition, also called retrolental fibroplasia, can lead to significant scarring and distortion of the retina of the eye, increased risk of myopia (nearsightedness), amblyopia (wandering eye), nystagmus (involuntary rhythmic movements of the eye), and even blindness. ROP is extremely common among very small babies—it afflicts 4 out of 5 babies who weigh under 750 grams (about 1 pound 10 ounces) as compared to only 3 in 100 of those who weigh 1,500 to 1,750 grams (3 pounds 5 ounces to 3 pounds 14 ounces). It was once thought to be caused by excessive oxygen administration, but it is now believed that the problem in many cases is an imbalance of oxygen in the baby's blood and that a variety of other factors (possibly including bright light in the nursery, maternal diabetes, or maternal antihistamine use during the last two weeks of pregnancy) probably also contribute to the condition. A newborn with ROP should be seen by a pediatric ophthalmologist. Close monitoring of blood gases in the infant when oxygen therapy is given is now routine and does seem to help minimize damage. Vitamin E given orally or intramuscularly also seems to help,[4] but blood levels need to be monitored regularly so the dosage can be changed as the baby grows. Aggressive therapy with cryosurgery (freezing to destroy the excess growth of blood vessels in the eye and to prevent further detachment of the retina) may be effective in preventing blindness. (Iron supplements are not usually given to infants with ROP who do not have iron deficiency anemia until the retinas are mature or the condition has resolved, so don't give a supplement without the doctor's approval.)

Intraventricular hemorrhage. The immature brain of a fetus contains the germinal matrix, a gelatinous structure filled with veins, arteries, and capillaries, which disappears at about 38 weeks. Infants born before it disappears are at high risk of hemorrhage because of the fragility of these vessels and the great amount of blood flow through them. Intraventricular hemorrhage is extremely common among preterm infants, striking 30 to 40%, most often within the first 72 hours of life. Hemorrhages are graded on a four-step scale, with grade I the least severe and grade IV the most severe. Grade IV requires close observation to correct any further problems that develop—for example, hydrocephalus. Regular follow-up cranial ultrasounds are usually ordered for grades III and IV until the hemorrhage is resolved. Babies with the more severe-grade hemorrhages are also at greater risk for seizures immediately, and handicaps later on. Treatments are being developed to prevent and/or treat the condition, including one in which temporary muscle paralysis is in-duced to reduce the fluctuation of blood flow in the brain.

Necrotizing enterocolitis. The symptoms of this bowel disease, in which tissue in the intestine becomes damaged and dies, usually appear between the second and twentieth day, almost always in low-birth-weight babies. They include abdominal distention, bilious vomiting, apnea, and blood in the stool. A great many theories have been advanced in an attempt to pinpoint the cause, none totally satisfactory. It seems most likely that a combination of factors, possibly including the use of formula (breastfed babies are less likely to be stricken), are involved. A baby with necrotizing enterocolitis is usually put on intravenous feedings, and treatment will depend on symptoms. If there is serious deterioration of the intestine, surgery is usually performed to remove the damaged portion.

Apnea of prematurity. Though apnea, periods of breathing cessation, can occur in any newborn, this problem is much more common among premature infants. Apnea of prematurity is diagnosed when a baby has such periods that last more than fifteen seconds or that are shorter but are associated with bradycardia, a slowing of the heart rate. When apnea is observed, testing is often done to determine if the infant needs monitoring (see page 183). Monitoring for apnea of prematurity is usually unnecessary past six months, but during that time the monitor has to be adjusted as the baby's heart rate goes through the normal slowing down that comes with growth (if it isn't, there may be a lot of false alarms for slow heart rate). This type of apnea, if it doesn't recur after a baby has reached his or her original due date, is not related to SIDS (sudden infant death syndrome).

Jaundice. Premature babies are much more likely to develop jaundice than are full-term infants. Read about the condition and its treatment on page 70.

---

4. Vitamin E is no longer given intravenously to newborns because it causes serious complications.

CHAPTER TWENTY

The Baby With Problems

After nine months of hoping for a healthy, perfect baby, it is devastating to give birth to a child who is anything less than that. And no one who hasn't been dealt such a blow can possibly understand the pain involved. Still, the vast majority of parents do recover from their initial feelings of helplessness, hopelessness, and despair. As they learn to cope with the complexities of having a baby with birth defects, they begin to see past the problems to the child underneath, a child who, above all, needs what all children need: love, attention, and discipline.

Some find that the problem, which at first seemed so frightening, is easily corrected or at least alleviated with surgery, medication, or other treatment. Others learn that there is little or nothing that can be done to make their baby perfect. But even these families often find that raising a handicapped baby adds another dimension to their lives, that they achieve a sense of fulfillment they might never have experienced otherwise. They find that though they often must work long and hard to stimulate their child physically and intellectually, the rewards are all the more gratifying, and well worth the extra effort involved. And as time passes they often discover that their child, in addition to teaching them something about pain, has taught them a lot about love.

While much of the general information in this book is useful to parents of a child born with birth defects, this chapter deals with some of the adjustments and decisions that are unique to their situation. It may also be helpful to read Chapter 19 for other concerns, such as long-term hospitalization.

FEEDING BABY: Can Diet Make a Difference?

All parents want their offspring, disabled or not, to be the best they can be. And ensuring optimum nutrition—from birth on—is one way to help children develop to their greatest potential, whatever that potential might be. While a good diet can't change the fact that a child has a birth defect, or may not even improve his or her condition, it can have an impact on general health and can affect behavior, learning ability, and development. There's no evidence, however, that dietary manipulation (feeding a special diet, for example, or giving vitamin megadoses) can significantly improve the medical condition of a child born with a birth defect, except in cases where the defect is diet related.

For the child with no such unusual dietary needs, the best in nutrition begins with breast milk, when possible, or commercial infant formula, and then the Best-Odds Diet, page 221.

WHAT YOU MAY BE CONCERNED ABOUT

FEELING RESPONSIBLE

"Our doctor just told us that our baby isn't completely normal. I can't help feeling that I'm somehow responsible—that I could have done something to prevent his problem."

Parents often feel responsible for the bad things that happen to their children; even a tumble precipitated by a toddler's own clumsiness can elicit a parental "What did I do wrong?" When a child is born with a birth defect, the guilt can be overwhelming and debilitating. Parents may feel that it was something they did that was responsible for the child's condition, even though most often the cause was out of their control. Guilt can be particularly strong when one or both parents felt ambivalent about having a baby, as most parents-to-be do at some point. They may conclude that their unspoken thoughts were to blame for the child's condition—that it must be their punishment for not really wanting the baby.

And as untrue as this may be, such parents often need repeated reassurance to convince them that they are not to blame.

Occasionally, as in the case of fetal alcohol syndrome, the development of a birth defect can be traced to a mother's actions, making the guilt all the more difficult to handle. It's important to remember, however, that alcoholism is as much a disease as is diabetes—that an alcoholic mother didn't drink because she was immoral or wanted to hurt her baby, but because the disease was controlling her. Though she can't undo what's been done, she can seek professional help now to deal with her problem and to prevent any further negative impact on this baby and babies she may have in the future.

Whether it's founded or unfounded, guilt won't do you, your husband, or your baby any good—and it could do all of you a great deal of harm. Instead of wasting emotional energy on self-flagellation, concentrate on the positive steps that can be taken to make your baby's future, and your family's, the best it can be.

FEELING ANGRY

"Ever since I gave birth to my daughter, who has Down syndrome, I've been angry at everyone—the doctors, my husband, my parents, other mothers with normal babies, even the baby."

Why wouldn't you be angry? Your dreams of nine months, or maybe longer, have been shattered. You look around at friends, neighbors, relatives, strangers at the supermarket with their normal babies, and you think bitterly, "Why not me?" The fact that asking this question yields no satisfying answers further fuels your frustration. You may be angry at the doctor who delivered your baby (even if he or she wasn't at fault), at your spouse (even without logical reason), at your normal children (even though you know it's not their fault they're healthy and the new baby isn't).

Accept your anger as normal, but also recognize that, like guilt, it isn't a particularly productive emotion. Being angry takes a lot of energy—energy which really should be focused on your baby and her needs. You can't change the past, but you can make a difference in your child's future.

NOT LOVING THE BABY

"It's been almost a month since our daughter was born with a birth defect, and I still don't feel close to her. I wonder if I ever will."

Your feelings aren't at all unusual. Even parents with normal babies often take months to feel really close to their newborns. Initial rejection turns to ambivalence, then acceptance, and finally to love. For parents with handicapped infants, the process is, understandably, more gradual, with the first two reactions usually more exaggerated. Moving on to acceptance usually requires that a mother give up the idealized baby she carried in her mind's eye and open her heart to the child she does have. Interacting lovingly with your baby, singing lullabies, cuddling, stroking, and kissing will help make the love grow and will help you to discover and focus on your baby's endearing qualities (all children have them).

If you don't feel closer to your baby as time passes, then seek counseling from someone experienced in working with parents of children with birth defects, or join a self-help group of such parents in your community. Your doctor or hospital should be able to direct you.

"Doctors tell us our little boy may not make it, so we're afraid to get too attached to him."

Parents of babies whose lives are in jeopardy often share this fear of loving and losing, and consciously avoid bonding with their newborns. But in general, studies show, parents who allow themselves to get to know their critically ill babies (even if only through the portholes of an incubator) end up having an easier time coping if the child doesn't survive than do those who try to stay aloof. Perhaps this is because they are able to say, "At least we loved him while we had him," and because they can truly grieve (you can't mourn for something you never had), a process necessary for them to resolve their feelings about their terrible loss. Showering love on your critically ill infant, in a sense providing him with a reason for living, can also have a significant impact on his will to survive, and might actually help to pull him through.

WHAT TO TELL OTHERS

"Our son's birth defect is very obvious. People don't know what to say to me when they see him, and I don't know what to say to them."

When people meet a child with a birth defect, their loss for words is often as obvious as the defect. They want to say the right thing, but they don't know what that is. They want to be kind and supportive, but they don't know how. They want to congratulate you on the birth of your baby, but feel almost as though condolences would be more appropriate. You can help them, and yourself, by acknowledging their discomfort, opening the way for them to express their feelings. If you're feeling able to, let them know you understand if they're uneasy, that most people are at first, and that it's perfectly natural. Beyond this, all that a casual friend need be told is that though your newborn is not the child you expected, he's yours, you love him, and you intend to treat him as normally as possible—and hope that they will do the same.

Of course, this is a rational approach to the question, and you may not feel rational at first. You may want to ignore strangers, and sometimes even friends and family, or to lash out if they are thoughtless or un-kind. Don't feel bad if you're too upset to be able to put others at ease. With time and, if necessary, sensitive individual counseling or group therapy, you'll become better able to cope.

Friends and relatives who will be in closer, more frequent contact with your baby will need to know more. In addition to being encouraged to be open about their feelings, they will have to be educated about your child's problems and special needs. Provide them with reading material about your child's medical problems, ask the baby's doctor to speak with them, en-courage them to talk informally to other family members of children with birth de-fects, or refer them to a support group. Include them in your baby's care—give them the opportunity to hold, diaper, bathe, and play with him. In time they, too, will come to see him as the lovable baby he is. Sometimes close relatives, particularly grandparents, feel guilty ("Did I contribute a faulty gene?"), or angry ("Why couldn't you give us a healthy grandchild?"), or think they have all the answers ("Feed him

this food," "Go to that doctor"). If your efforts to involve them in your baby's life and educate them about his problems don't help to overcome such attitudes, and if their negative input continues to threaten the del-icate equilibrium of your nuclear family, keep lines of communication open, but don't let their problem become yours.

In spite of your best efforts, there will always be people who—probably because of their own insecurities—will make cruel and thoughtless comments, undervalue your child because he is different, and feel uncomfortable around him. There will be times when both you and he will be hurt by their intolerance. As much as you might like to educate the world, it isn't possible. You'll just have to learn to hold your head high and ignore the narrow-minded people you can't reach.

HANDLING IT ALL

"We love our new baby, even with all her problems and the special care she re-quires, but with another small child to care for and care about, I feel totally overwhelmed and unable to cope."

Raising a child with a birth defect can be both physically and emotionally drain-ing—particularly for the mother, on whom most of the responsibility usually falls, even if she's also employed outside the home. The pointers in Chapters 23 and 24, which can help any new mother, can also help you. But you'll need more:

More breaks. If you are a full-time mother (and many mothers of handicapped children are, choosing to postpone return-ing to their jobs), then you've got to find ways of getting out of the house, away from the stress of caring for your child day in and day out. Take off at least a few hours a week, leaving the baby with a relative, friend, trusted sitter, or baby nurse. Have dinner with your husband, lunch with a friend, play a few sets of tennis, see a movie or a concert, or just browse through a mall—whatever will relax you most. Escaping for an hour or two every day—to go for a jog, get a facial or haircut (looking your best will give you a psychic boost), pick up a couple of books at the library—is even better if you can arrange it. If you have another child, then try to take some of your breaks with him or her; both of you will benefit.

More release. Don't bottle up your worries, fears, complaints—air them with your spouse, your mother or sister, your best friend, your doctor, other women in your situation, or a professional counselor if necessary. You may not feel ready to face a self-help group for parents of children with similar problems at first, but you may find this helpful later on. Keeping a journal is another way to express your feelings and work out your anxieties. Record problems and progress, what you've done and what needs to be done. Seeing your life on paper may help make it seem more manageable.

More help. You can't do it alone. If you can't pay for help with household and child-care chores, you will need to rely on

---

BE A FRIEND IN DEED

Few people know what to do or say when they hear that a friend, relative, neighbor, or casual acquaintance has given birth to a child with a birth defect, a child who is seriously ill, or one who dies at or shortly after delivery. There are no pat answers; every individual and every situation is unique. But in general, these approaches are the ones likely to help the most:

■ *Lend an ear.* Don't say "I know how you feel." You don't, and hopefully never will. Don't say "You've got to be brave," or offer any other advice. The new parents in crisis will get plenty of advice from the professionals. What they need from you is love, support, and a willing ear. Listen to what's on their minds and in their hearts without being judgmental or offering your viewpoints. Let them vent their feelings, whatever those feelings may be (you can expect them to be angry at times, despondent at others) and empathize with them—this will be the best therapy.

■ *Become informed.* If the parents seem to want to talk about their baby's problems, listen. But if they've told the terrible tale too many times already, get your information second- or third-hand from a relative or friend so they needn't relive it again. To be better able to understand what they are going through, read this chapter (and if relevant, the previous one) and get further

information, if you feel you need it, from the March of Dimes or from an organization that deals with the baby's specific condition.

■ *Use body language.* Often when words fail, the squeeze of a hand, a loving hug, a sympathetic look will get the message that you care across.

■ *Keep in touch.* Because we don't know what to say or do, we often take the coward's way out and avoid the friend who is going through a crisis. Those who have been on the receiving end of such behavior almost always say, "I'd rather hear the wrong words than none at all." Those phone calls, visits, and invitations are more important now than at any other time and shouldn't be neglected. And though you shouldn't force your company on someone who would rather suffer their pain alone, don't give up after one "We're not up to it yet." Try again soon.

■ *Help out.* There are innumerable tasks friends and family can take over when new parents are mourning the loss of an infant or are faced with one who is hospitalized or needs a great deal of attention. Cook a meal, baby-sit for older children, do the laundry, offer to vacuum, wield the dust cloth, or take over with the baby for an hour or two if possible. Any way in which you can lighten the burden will doubtless be appreciated.

friends and family more than most. You needn't feel guilty about it, as long as you don't take the time and energy given by others for granted. Though you may feel like the sole beneficiary of their kindness, they also benefit—perhaps even more—by helping.

GETTING THE RIGHT DIAGNOSIS

"According to our family doctor, our son has a very serious congenital disorder. I just can't believe it—everyone in our family is so healthy."

Serious illness, especially in our children, is difficult to accept. The first reaction is almost always denial: we cling to the hope that someone's made a mistake. The best way to resolve your nagging doubts is to double-check the diagnosis—no one, after all, is infallible. So if you haven't already, do have your child thoroughly examined by an experienced neonatologist, one familiar with the condition that's been diagnosed, and be sure that all appropriate tests are carried out, both to verify the diagnosis and to uncover any other problems that may exist. You can help ensure an accurate diagnosis by giving examining physicians as much information as possible about your family's medical history (including any familial genetic discorders) and your pregnancy history and behavior (including tobacco use, alcohol or drug consumption, medications taken, illnesses, especially with accompanying fevers, use of hot tubs, and so on). Your *candid* answers may, in fact, help a doctor to pinpoint an elusive diagnosis.

If the consulting doctor concurs with the first, you can be pretty sure their diagnosis is correct—and taking your child from doctor to doctor won't change the facts. Though there's always that one-in-a-million chance that even several doctors are wrong, the odds are much better that a problem does exist and that you, like most other parents of children with birth defects, are trying hard to deny it.

Be certain that you're completely clear about what the diagnosis is. The first time parents are told their newborn child has a birth defect, it's not unusual for most of the details to be washed away in a tide of overwhelming shock. What they hear is "Your child isn't normal"; beyond that, everything's a blur. So request a second meeting with the doctor when your head is a little clearer (don't expect your thinking to be very focused for a while). In addition to the information you get from the doctors and/or nurses caring for your baby, seek out information in books, from parents in similar situations, and from organizations concerned with handicapped children and/or your baby's particular problem, or from the local or national March of Dimes office.[1] Don't rely, however, on advice from well-meaning but uninformed neighbors or family friends—it's likely to be based more on mythology than on medicine.

Before you take your baby home, ask his doctor exactly what you can expect (in terms of behavior, development, medical problems) and what warning signs you need to be on the lookout for, as well as what you and the rest of your family can do to help your baby reach his potential. Take notes so that you'll have them to refer to when you go home.

---

1. The following organizations may be able to help: The Clearing House on the Handicapped, Switzer Building, Room 3132, 330 C Street SW, Washington, DC 20202, (202) 732-1241; The Coordinating Councils for Handicapped Children, 20 East Jackson Boulevard, Room 900, Chicago, IL 60604, (312) 939-3513; The Association of Birth Defect Children, 3526 Emorywood Lane, Orlando, FL 32812, (407) 859-2821; The National Information Center for Children and Youth with Handicaps, PO Box 1492, Washington, DC 20013, (703) 522-3322. For the names of organizations involved with specific disorders, contact The National Health Information Center (NHIC), PO Box 1133, Washington, DC 20013-1133, (800) 336-4797 (toll free).

WHETHER OR NOT TO ACCEPT TREATMENT

"Our baby boy was born without part of his brain. The doctors say he has no chance of living, but they want to operate on him to keep him alive a little longer. We don't know what to do."

While the issue of whether or not babies who have no hope of long-term survival should be treated and kept on life-support systems has become a major ethical one for society, it is now a painfully personal one for you. Your decision is one that, if at all possible, probably shouldn't be made without first talking it over with your family, a religious counselor, the baby's doctors, and the hospital ethicist, if there is one. In many cases there will be time for such reasoned decision making. Even when there isn't, and time is of the essence, there is usually a chance to talk with your baby's doctors and, possibly, a hospital chaplain. The doctors can usually tell you the quality of life you can expect your child to have if kept alive, and whether treatment will improve the quality of his life or only prolong his dying. The chaplain can explain the religious issues involved, and the ethicist, your legal rights and responsibilities as well as the ethical issues. When you make your decision, consider all the information and counsel you've received, but do what you believe in your heart to be right—because no matter what it is, that's the decision you will be able to live with best.

In some cases, parents of children for whom there is no hope have found some solace in being able to donate some of their baby's organs to save the life of another sick infant. This isn't always feasible—sometimes for medical reasons, sometimes for legal ones—but do ask your doctor and hospital authorities about the possibility of organ donation if it interests you.

GETTING THE BEST CARE AND TREATMENT

"We're determined to give our baby, in spite of his handicaps, the best possible chance in life. But we're not sure how to do it."

Your determination to help your child greatly increases his chances of enjoying a productive and satisfying life. But there's much more you can do, and the earlier you begin the better. Most babies with serious birth defects get the best start in a major medical center, but occasionally a community hospital is equipped with an excellent neonatal intensive care unit (NICU). A hospital near your home has the benefit of allowing you to visit regularly, which sometimes will compensate for a lack of scientific sophistication. To minimize the effects of a lengthy hospitalization, if that will be necessary, see pages 461 and 464.

Wherever your child is treated, you'll want to have him cared for by a physician who specializes in dealing with his particular birth defect—though often day-to-day care can be provided by a local pediatrician or family doctor under the supervision of the specialist. With many birth defects, a team approach to treatment is best. The team may include physicians from various specialties, psychologists, physiotherapists, nutritionists, social workers, as well as a neonatologist and, usually, the baby's own doctor. If you aren't sure how to locate the appropriate specialist or specialists, and the hospital staff can't help you, you can contact the March of Dimes (914-428-7100), the National Institute of Child Health and Human Development (301-496-5133), or the National Health Information Center (800-336-4797).

Though excellent medical care and, often, early educational intervention will be crucial to your child's development, in most cases the home environment you create will be even more significant in determining how well he is prepared for life and whether or not he reaches his maximum potential. The primary need of most children born with birth defects is to be treated like other children—to be loved and nurtured, but also to be disciplined and expected to meet standards (which should, of course, take into account their individual limitations). And like other children, they need to feel good about themselves—to know that each step forward, no matter how small, is appreciated and applauded, and that they won't be expected to live up to the baby next door, only to their own possibilities.

A wide range of therapies, as well as high-tech aids—everything from adapted playground equipment and toys to special education software, laser canes (for sight-impaired children), cochlear implants (to aid hearing), and robotic devices—are now available to help you help your handicapped child grow, develop, and enjoy. Ask a member of your child's care team about them, or check with the appropriate organization for information.

It should be reassuring to know that the majority of children with handicaps grow up psychologically sound, are well accepted by their peers and others, and have a risk of adjustment problems only slightly higher than that faced by children without handicaps.

EFFECT OF BABY ON SIBLINGS

"We're planning to raise our Down syndrome baby ourselves, but we're worried about how well our normal three-year-old daughter will handle the changes that she'll bring to her life."

More and more parents are choosing to raise their handicapped child at home—a decision that often turns out to be good not only for the child and the parents, but for the rest of the family as well. Having a handicapped sibling at home can have a profound positive impact on the other siblings, making them, on average, more patient and understanding than other children and more adept at getting along with different kinds of people.

Your other child will need to have some special times with both parents (as impossible as this may sometimes seem, it's absolutely crucial). Children who feel neglected in such a situation often act up, manifest psychosomatic illnesses, and even play dumb in school to gain back parental attention. Most don't need counseling or therapy—just a little extra understanding. They need to be reassured that they aren't selfish or bad if they want their needs attended to, or if they sometimes feel resentful or ashamed of their sibling. They may also need reassurance that what has happened to her isn't going to happen to them, and may need extra support when they bring friends home.

An older sibling may also need special attention if the handicapped sibling is institutionalized. ("Why isn't my baby sister home with us?" "Was she bad?" "If I'm bad, will I be sent away, too?") Again, understanding and a reassuring explanation will be necessary. If a child continues to seem anxious about the situation, counseling is probably a good idea.

Many older siblings of handicapped children benefit from talking to others in their position. Many hospitals and organizations sponsor programs for siblings; check into this possibility in your area. Such a program gives children a chance to talk about their worries in a safe and supportive environment, and to learn that they're not alone. For a newsletter and more information, ideas, and the latest research on the problems of siblings of handicapped children, write the Sibling Information Network, c/o Connecticut University Affiliated Program on Developmental Disabilities, 991 Main Street, Suite 3A, East Hartford, CT 06108, or call them at (203) 282-7050.

EFFECTS ON YOUR MARRIAGE

"My husband and I have cried a lot together since our son was born with a birth defect, but that's been the extent of our relationship. I'm afraid we'll never have emotional energy to spend on each other again."

All new parents find that having a baby in the house restricts the amount of time they spend as a couple. Parents of babies born with a handicap discover the restrictions on romance and intimacy to be even greater, since caring for the baby zaps not just physical strength, but emotional reserves as well. But the baby you came together to create is not inevitably going to tear you apart. Though it might seem that the cumulative effects of months and years of living with a handicapped child might weaken even the sturdiest marital relationships, they rarely do. Most marriages, it appears, not only hold up under the strain, they are strengthened by it. (Though there is a slightly increased risk of divorce when a child is chronically ill over a long period of time.) To help improve the chances that your marriage will become one of the happy statistics, make sure that:

The work is shared. No one can single-handedly care for a handicapped child and still have the energy left to be a loving partner to a spouse. If your husband works all day while you stay at home, let him take over some of the baby care responsibilities in the evening so you can have a break. If he's considering taking on a second job to ease the financial strain of your not working, it might be better for you to take a part-time job and to transfer more of the child-care load to him. Hired or volunteer relief child care, for at least a few hours a week, and/or household help can also ease the burden and free up some time and energy for each other.

Each partner gets enough support from the other. Both of you have hurts that need healing; both of you need to make adjustments in your lives. (Many people fail to realize that the father of a handicapped child may be as much in need of emotional support as the mother.) Facing the future as a team will be infinitely more productive and satisfying than facing it as individuals. Share your problems and concerns, and protect each other from outside assault (from overly critical grandparents, for example).

You make time for each other. All new parents need to make a concerted effort to make time alone for each other—or the time just doesn't happen. And as particularly difficult as it may be for you and your husband, you need to do the same. See page 582 for tips.

You give yourselves time. Romance may be the furthest thing from your minds right now, and it may take a few months before any desire returns. This is the rule among most newly delivered couples, and is even more likely in your situation. So instead of pressuring yourselves to perform sexually when you're not emotionally ready, wait until you are. And remember, you don't have to make love to show love. Hugging and hand holding—sometimes even a good cry together—may be, more than anything, what both of you need right now.

A REPEAT WITH THE NEXT BABY

"We would like to have another baby within a year or so, but we're afraid that our daughter's birth defect might repeat in our next child."

As common as this fear is among parents of children born with birth defects, it is in most cases unfounded; their chances of having a normal baby are often as good as those of other parents. But in order to predict the risk in your particular case, the cause of your baby's problem needs to be determined. There is a wide range of possibilities:

Genetic. If your baby's defect is determined to be genetic (passed on by genetic material from you and/or your husband), a genetic counselor or, often, the baby's doctor will probably be able to give you precise odds on the likelihood of a repeat. In some instances, you will also be able to test future fetuses for the defect early in pregnancy, giving you the option to terminate should it turn up.

Environmental. If the birth defect was the result of a one-time event—such as an exposure during pregnancy to infection, chemicals, X-rays, medications, or other factors that interfered with normal fetal development—it is not likely to repeat unless the exact set of circumstances recur at the same critical point in pregnancy.

Lifestyle. If the defect can be traced to your smoking, alcohol consumption, drug abuse, or poor nutrition, for example, it is not likely to repeat in subsequent pregnancies unless the lifestyle mistakes are repeated.

Maternal factors. If your baby's problems seem related to your age, the shape or size of your uterus, or other unchangeable factors, they might repeat, though the risk can sometimes be reduced. For example, if you are past 35 and have a Down syndrome baby, prenatal testing can diagnose the disorder in future pregnancies. Or if your uterus is misshapen, surgery may be able to reshape it.

Multifactorial. When a variety of factors are involved, predicting future outcomes may be more complicated, but the doctor or a genetic counselor can still be helpful in such cases.

Unknown. Sometimes there is no apparent reason for a baby's birth defect. Usually such cases do not repeat. But if no one can say why your baby was not born completely normal, it would be a good idea to discuss the situation with a doctor familiar with genetic counseling before becoming pregnant again.

Before making a decision to become pregnant, be sure you are doing so for the right reasons. To deliver a healthy baby in order to compensate for one that wasn't healthy is not fair to the new child. Speak to your baby's doctor or to a family therapist if you feel in conflict.

If you do decide to become pregnant again, your obstetrician should be completely familiar with your previous history so that you can be monitored throughout pregnancy for any possible problems. But with good medical care and good self-care (you are your doctor's best partner), your odds of delivering a normal and healthy baby will be very good.

A DIFFERENT BIRTH DEFECT NEXT TIME

"I'm not so worried about having another child with the same birth defect— I can be tested for that. What I'm worried about is having one with a different defect."

Even if the chances of a repeat of your first child's defect in your next baby may be somewhat higher than average (and this isn't always the case), the same would not be true of other unrelated defects. In fact, you and your husband have just as good a chance of producing a child free of other birth defects as any other set of parents.

As reassuring as these odds should be, it's normal to still harbor some nagging fears after what you've already gone through. To help ease them, talk to your doctor, consult a genetic counselor, and follow the precautions listed above.

WHAT IT'S IMPORTANT TO KNOW: The Most Common Birth Disorders

If your child hasn't been diagnosed as having a birth disorder but you've noticed symptoms associated with any of the following problems, don't panic—what you notice may indicate something far less serious than you're imagining. But do check with your baby's doctor. It may take more than a phone call to allay your fears; an examination or special testing may be necessary. If a problem does turn up, early recognition and prompt medical attention and therapy can often be beneficial, even correct the problem completely.

COMMON BIRTH DISORDERS

AIDS/HIV-Perinatal

What is it? HIV infection usually has no symptoms, but it often eventually causes AIDS, a serious immune disorder.

How common is it? Becoming more common as more women are infected.

What causes it? The human immunodeficiency virus (HIV), most often passed on from mother to child during pregnancy, childbirth, or breastfeeding.

Treatment. Antiviral drugs for HIV positive mother during pregnancy, for child after birth.

Prognosis. Now improving; many children have survived for several years.

Anencephaly

What is it? A neural tube defect in which the failure of the neural groove to close normally early in pregnancy leads to lack of brain development, and all or a major part of the brain is absent.

How common is it? Very rare in full-term babies, since 99% of fetuses with the defect are miscarried.

Who is susceptible? Not known.

What causes it? Not known at present. Heredity is probably involved in some way, along with adverse prenatal environment.

Related problems. All body systems are affected negatively.

Treatment. None, and most doctors agree that no medical intervention is best, though the baby should be kept as comfortable as possible.

Prognosis. The condition is incompatible with life. Organ donations to help others are difficult because of present laws.

Autism

What is it? An inability, that dates from birth or develops within the first two and a half years of life, to develop normal human relationships, even with parents. Babies don't smile or respond to parents or anyone else in any way, and dislike being picked up or touched. There are usually extreme problems in speaking (including bizarre speech patterns such as echolalia, in which the child echoes the words just heard rather than replying), strange positions and mannerisms, erratic and inappropriate behavior (compulsiveness and ritualism, screaming fits and arm flapping), and, sometimes, self-destructiveness. The child may have normal intelligence but appear to be retarded or deaf because of lack of responsiveness. Autism may sometimes be confused with childhood schizophrenia, and occasionally may precede it.

How common is it? There are an estimated 2 to 7 cases per 10,000 babies.[2]

Who is susceptible? Male children are three to four times more likely to be autistic than females.

What causes it? Probably, according to a recent study, autosomal recessive inheritance: both parents must pass on recessive genes for the baby to be affected. There seem to be some differences in brain wave patterns in autistic children, which may be related to their condition. It is not related to parenting.

Related problems. Behavior and developmental problems.

Treatment. At present there is no cure, but some children can be helped with behavior modification therapy, stimulation, special training, and, sometimes, drugs. When possible, the child remains at home, but sometimes the stress is more than a family can tolerate, and institutionalization becomes necessary. Day-care programs can sometimes help alleviate the stress while allowing the child to remain at home. Counseling is often helpful for the rest of the family.

Prognosis. At present, about a third of children recover sufficiently to function fairly normally, but most remain autistic and need special institutional care. Outlook is best when a child can be taught to use meaningful speech before age five.

Cancer

Rare in early infancy. Many infant cancers are highly curable today.

Celiac Disease

What is it? Also called celiac sprue or gluten-sensitive enteropathy (GSE), this is a condition in which there is sensitivity (not allergy) to gliadin, which is found in gluten

(a component of wheat and other grains), characterized by faulty food absorption and loss of appetite, poor growth, pot belly, consistently foul-smelling, fatty diarrhea, and sometimes anemia, beginning at about six to twelve months. May be mistaken for cystic fibrosis.

How common is it? An estimated 1 in 3,000 in the general population; females are affected twice as often as males and whites from northwestern Europe most often (it is rare in blacks, Asians, Jews, and others of Mediterranean descent).

Who is susceptible? Children of parents who both carry the gene for the condition.

What causes it? Unclear, but most likely some combination of environmental factors and genetic disposition. Possibly linked to a defect in a gene that causes antigliadin antibodies to be produced; it is suspected that antibodies combine with gliadin to attack and flatten villi in the intestines, causing malabsorption and other symptoms.

Related problems. Symptoms of malnutrition such as developmental delay, fluid retention, late teething, and rickets.

Treatment. Gluten-free diet, which usually begins to work in three to six weeks and which must be adhered to for life. Nutritional supplementation and, sometimes, steroids may also be prescribed.

Prognosis. Usually, a normal life on a gluten-free diet.

Cerebral Palsy

What is it? A neuromuscular disorder caused by damage to the brain. Motor impairment may be mild to disabling. The infant may have difficulty sucking or retaining the nipple; drool constantly; seldom move voluntarily; have arm or leg tremors with voluntary movements; have legs that are hard to separate; have delayed motor development; and use only one hand or, later, use hands but not feet, crawl in a strange fash-

---

2. Occasionally a child who seems to be autistic is helped by the elimination of foods to which he is allergic. See page 413.

ion, and walk on tiptoes. Muscle tone may be excessively stiff or floppy, but this may not be apparent until three months or so. Exact symptoms differ in each of the three different types of CP: spastic, athetoid, and ataxic.

How common is it? Decreasing in frequency because of safer childbirth (except in the tiniest newborns) and better treatment of jaundice. About 15,000 cases a year.

Who is susceptible? Premature and low-birthweight babies, boys slightly more often than girls, white infants more often than blacks.

What causes it? Estimated 50% of cases are related to prenatal causes (including maternal infection or other illness, radiation, malnutrition); 33% related to the birth (including unusually prolonged or rapid labor, prolapsed cord, depressed maternal vital signs); 10% postnatal trauma (such as falls or other accidents), infection (of the brain), pathological jaundice, and lack of oxygen (as when breathing is interrupted); 7% mixed causation.

Related problems. Sometimes, seizures; speech, vision, and hearing disorders; dental defects; mental retardation.

Treatment. No cure, but early treatment can help a child live up to potential. May include: physical therapy, braces, splints, or other orthopedic appliances; special furniture and utensils; exercise; surgery, when needed; medication for seizures or to relax muscles if needed.

Prognosis. Varies with case. Child with a mild form, given proper treatment, may live a nearly normal life. Child with a severe form may be completely disabled. Disease does not get progressively worse.

Cleft Lip and/or Palate

What is it? A split, sometimes extensive, sometimes slight, occurs where parts of upper lip or palate (the roof of the mouth) fail to grow together. Some babies have only

cleft lip, more have only cleft palate. About 40% of affected babies have both.

How common is it? About 5,000 children a year, or approximately 1 in 700 births.

Who is susceptible? More common among Asians and Native Americans, less common among black Americans. Also more common among premature babies and those with other defects.

What causes it? Heredity plays a role in about 1 in 4 cases; after having a baby with a cleft, the odds of having another one increase slightly. But illness, certain medications, lack of essential nutrients (particularly folic acid), and other factors that adversely affect the prenatal environment may also interfere with normal development of lip and palate, possibly in combination with each other and/or heredity.

Related problems. Because sucking is usually difficult, feeding may be a serious problem, so special procedures are necessary (usually an upright position, small amounts, a nipple with large holes or a special syringe). Ear infections are also common and need to be controlled.

Treatment. Usually a combination of surgery (sometimes in the first few months of life), speech therapy, dental adjustments (often including braces later in life), and psychological counseling.

Prognosis. Usually excellent with treatment.

Clubfoot

What is it? An ankle or foot deformity that occurs in three forms. In the most severe and least common, equinovarus, the foot twists inward and downward. If both feet are "clubbed," the toes point toward each other. The most common type of club foot, calcaneal valgus, is milder. The foot is sharply angled at the heel and points upward and outward. In the mildest form of clubfoot, metatarsus varus, the front part of the foot is turned inward. This type may not be diagnosed until the baby is a few months old, though it is present at birth. Clubfoot is not painful and doesn't bother the baby until it's time to stand or walk.

How common is it? Affects 1 in 400 babies.

Who is susceptible? Boys are twice as likely to have clubfoot as girls.

What causes it? Not the position in the uterus, as was once believed (cases of this sort correct themselves after birth). Probably a combination of heredity and environmental factors, such as infection, drugs, and disease, in most cases; but some cases are related to spina bifida, nerve diseases, or muscle diseases.

Related problems. The foot can't move up and down as it normally would in walking; the child walks as though on a peg leg. When both feet are affected, the child may walk on the sides or even tops of feet, leading to damage to this tissue and to abnormal leg development. Psychological problems may arise because of the abnormality. Occasionally there may be other defects as well.

Treatment. Mild cases may be treated by exercise alone. Plaster casts or surgery are used in more severe cases to force the twisted foot gradually and gently into place so that it can move up and down normally. Shoes connected with bars may also be used at night.

Prognosis. With expert early treatment, most grow up to wear regular shoes, take part in sports, lead active lives.

Congenital Heart Defect

What is it? Any heart defect, minor or major, that is present at birth. Though the defects can usually be diagnosed with a stethoscope, further tests such as X-rays, ultrasound, and ECGs will be needed to verify abnormalities. Depending on the type of defect, one or more functions of the heart may be adversely affected. Symptoms may show up at birth, or not become apparent until adulthood. Cyanosis, or bluing of the skin, particularly around fingers, toes and lips, is the most common symptom.

How common is it? About 1 out of 175 babies in the U.S. is born with a heart defect.

Who is susceptible? Children of mothers who had rubella during pregnancy, Down syndrome children, and those with affected siblings (though their increased risk is slight).

What causes it? In most cases, scientists just don't know. Certain infections (such as rubella, or German measles) and some chemicals (thalidomide, amphetamines, or alcohol, for example) are capable of causing heart abnormalities prenatally, but such abnormalities may sometimes be the result of a random genetic error.

Related problems. Sometimes, poor weight gain and growth, fatigue, weakness, difficulty breathing or sucking (because of weakness from heart failure).

Treatment. Surgery (either immediately or later in childhood), which varies according to the defect present, and sometimes drugs or a heart transplant can remedy heart defects. (Even a defect that causes no symptoms may require treatment to prevent problems later in life.) Sometimes a heart defect can be diagnosed before birth and medication given to correct it.

Prognosis. Most congenital heart defects are treatable, but some very serious ones may be disabling or even fatal. Most children with murmurs can lead normal lives with no restrictions on activities.

Cystic Fibrosis (CF)

What is it? A condition in which there is a generalized dysfunction of the exocrine glands, the glands that discharge their secretions through an epithelial surface (such as the skin, the mucous membranes, the linings of the hollow organs). When sweat glands are affected, perspiration is salty and profuse, and excessive perspiration can lead to dehydration and shock. When the respiratory system is affected, thick secretions may fill the lungs, causing chronic coughing and increased risk of infection. With digestive system involvement, mucus secretions may make first bowel movements after birth difficult to pass, causing intestinal obstruction. The pancreatic ducts may also be obstructed, resulting in deficiencies of the pancreatic enzymes and inability to digest protein and fat. The stools, containing the undigested materials, are usually frequent, bulky, foul-smelling, pale, and greasy. Weight gain is poor, appetite ravenous, abdomen distended, arms and legs thin, and skin sallow. Sweat-test screening is available to pick out possible cases, but lack of meconium bowel movement after birth, salty skin, and poor weight gain along with good appetite can be early indications.

How common is it? Relatively rare.

Who is susceptible? More common in those with central European ancestry (1 in 2,000 births) than in American blacks, native Americans, or those of Asian ancestry (1 in 17,000).

What causes it? Autosomal recessive inheritance: both parents must pass on recessive genes for a child to be affected.

Related problems. Pneumonia, because of respiratory secretions, is common. Also pancreatic insufficiency, insufficient insulin production, abnormal glucose tolerance, cirrhosis of the liver, and hypertension, among others.

Treatment. The earlier the better, to prevent development of symptoms when possible. No cure exists, but treatment helps a child lead a more normal life. For sweat gland malfunction, generous salting of foods and salt supplements during hot weather. For digestive problems, pancreatic enzymes given by mouth with meals and snacks, limitation of fat, supplementation with fat-soluble vitamins (A, D, E, and K). For various types of intestinal blockages (meconium ileus, rectal prolapse, and so on) associated with CF, both surgical and nonsurgical treatment is available and usually successful. For respiratory problems, copious fluid intake to thin secretions, usually daily respiratory physical therapy (including postural drainage, to help loosen and remove secretions), and oxygen therapy as needed. Room air is best kept cool and dry. Infections are treated with large doses of antibiotics. Initial studies indicate that treatment with anti-inflammatory agents (such as prednisone) may help reduce bouts of illness. If researchers find the gene (they have already located a genetic marker, a gene that seems to be inherited with CF), a cure may be possible.

Prognosis. Most cystic fibrosis babies once died in childhood, usually because of respiratory failure; today with early diagnosis, aggressive treatment (particularly at one of the major CF centers), and strong family support, more than half live to the age of 21, and many are now reaching their 30s, 40s, and 50s, and have busy, active lives. Some have married, and though males with CF are sterile, several women have successfully borne children. The outlook for those born now is even better.

Deformation

What is it? An abnormality in one or more organs or parts of the body.

How common is it? About 2 in every 100 babies has some deformity of this type.

Who is susceptible? An extra large fetus in a crowded uterus, or any fetus in a malformed or small uterus, or in a uterus with fibroids, an inadequate supply of amniotic fluid, or an unusual placental site; a fetus who shares the uterus with one or more siblings. Deformations are most common in babies of small and first-time mothers, and when there is an abnormal presentation such as a breech.

What causes it? Conditions in the uterus, such as those just mentioned, that put undue pressure on one or more developing parts of the fetus.

Related problems. Depends on abnormality.

Treatment. In most cases, none is necessary since the deformed part will gradually resume normal shape. Some conditions, however, such as scoliosis, clubfoot, and hip dislocations do require treatment.

Prognosis. Good, for most conditions.

Down Syndrome

What is it? A set of signs and symptoms that usually include mild to severe mental retardation, specific facial features (more obvious in some than in others), an oversized tongue, and a short neck; they may also include a flat back of the head, small ears (sometimes folded at the tops), and a flat wide nose. Hearing and vision may be poor, and various internal defects (particularly of heart or GI tract) may also exist. Down syndrome children are often short and have loose muscle tone (responsible for some of the delayed development). They are also usually very sweet and lovable.

How common is it? Down syndrome affects about 2,800 babies a year, or approximately 1 in 1,300.

Who is susceptible? Babies of parents who have already had a baby with the birth defect, or of a mother or father with a chromosome rearrangement, or of a mother over 35 (the risk increases with age). All ethnic groups and economic levels are affected.

What causes it? In 95% of the cases, an extra chromosome contributed by either the mother or the father, so that baby has 47 instead of 46 chromosomes. This cause of Down syndrome is called Trisomy 21, because three number-21 chromosomes are present (normally there are two). About 4% of the time, certain other accidents affecting chromosome number 21 are responsible. For example, sometimes a piece of a normal chromosome 21 breaks off and attaches to

another chromosome in the parent (this is called a translocation). The parent remains normal because he or she still has the right amount of genetic material. But if this augmented chromosome is passed on to a child, the child can have an excess of chromosome 21 material, resulting in Down syndrome. Very rarely, an accident during cell division in the fertilized egg results in an extra chromosome in some but not all cells. This is called mosaicism, and affected children may have only some Down syndrome characteristics because only some of their cells carry the excess chromosome.

Related problems. Dental problems, poor eyesight and hearing, heart disease, gastrointestinal defects, thyroid dysfunction, early aging (including Alzheimer's disease), higher risk for respiratory illnesses, as well as leukemia and other cancers.

Treatment. Prenatal tests can diagnose Down syndrome in the fetus. Surgery, after birth, can correct heart and other serious medical abnormalities; in some countries, surgery is performed to make appearance more normal, but benefits are unclear. Early specialized education programs improve the IQs of Down syndrome children who are mildly or moderately retarded.

Prognosis. Most children with Down syndrome have greater capabilities than previously believed, and early intervention can bring these abilities out, leaving fewer than 10% severely retarded. Many can be mainstreamed to a certain age in school, some even go to college. Most later find places in sheltered homes and workshops; some live and work independently; and some even marry. The average life span, once the hurdles of the first two to ten years are surmounted, is 55, more than twice what it was in the past.

Fetal Alcohol Syndrome (FAS)

What is it? A group of signs and symptoms that develop during gestation in a child whose mother drinks heavily during pregnancy. The most common are low birthweight, mental deficiency, deformities of the head and face, limbs, and central nervous system; the neonatal mortality rate is high. Less obvious effects may occur in children of moderate drinkers.

How common is it? About 1 in 750 live births.

Who is susceptible? Babies of women who drink heavily. (It is estimated that 30 to 40% of women who drink heavily during pregnancy have babies with FAS.)

What causes it? Ingestion of alcohol—usually five or six drinks of beer, wine, or distilled spirits a day—during pregnancy.

Related problems. Developmental problems.

Treatment. Therapy for individual handicaps.

Prognosis. Depends on extent of problems.

Heart Defect—see Congenital Heart Defect

Hydrocephalus (Water on the Brain)

What is it? Absorption of the fluid that normally bathes the brain is blocked, and the fluid collects. The pressure spreads apart the loosely connected parts of the skull, causing the head to become enlarged. This enlargement is often the first clue to the problem. Often occurs along with spina bifida, or following surgery to close an open spine. The scalp skin may be shiny and thin, neck muscles may be underdeveloped, eyes may look strange, cry may be high pitched, and baby may suffer from irritability, lack of appetite, and vomiting.

How common is it? Relatively rare.

Who is susceptible? Not clear, though

infants with spina bifida are at increased risk.

What causes it? At birth, a defect in the membrane that is supposed to absorb cerebrospinal fluid; later, injury (sometimes from surgery to correct spina bifida) or a tumor.

Related problems. Retardation if fluid is not drained away regularly; complications with shunts, including infection and shunt malfunctions.

Treatment. Under anesthesia, a special tube is inserted through a hole drilled in the skull into the brain to drain the excess fluid into either the abdominal cavity, the pleural cavity (surrounding the lung), or directly into a major blood vessel. The head gradually returns to normal size, but frequent checkups are necessary to be sure all is going well and the tube has not become blocked. Doctors are now trying to develop a treatment that doesn't require surgery.

Prognosis. Poor if the problem is well advanced by the time the baby is born. Good if treatment is begun early enough; this can usually prevent retardation. Complications can worsen the prognosis. Treatment before birth has not been successful.

Malformation

What is it? An organ or part of the body appears abnormal. Sometimes several organs or body parts are affected, and grouped together, they form a syndrome that indicates a particular disease (such as Down syndrome). Sometimes there is just one isolated malformation—such as a stunted limb.

How common is it? Probably fewer than 1 in 100 newborns is born with a noticeable malformation, usually a mild one.

Who is susceptible? Those with similar malformations in other family members; those whose parents, most often mothers, are exposed to certain dangerous environmental hazards before or after conception.

What causes it? Abnormal differentiation or organization during the development of the embryo, because of either a genetic or chromosomal abnormality or an environmental factor (such as X-ray or infection).

Related problems. Depends on the syndrome.

Treatment. Varies with the defect.

Prognosis. Depends on the malformation. (See individual conditions, such as spina bifida, Down syndrome, etc.)

Open Spine—see Spina Bifida

PKU— (Phenylketonuria)

What is it? A metabolic disorder in which the individual is unable to metabolize a protein called phenylalanine. The buildup of phenylalanine in the bloodstream can interfere with brain development and cause serious retardation.

How common is it? 1 in 14,000 births in the U.S.

Who is susceptible? When both parents carry the trait, they have a 1 in 4 chance with each pregnancy of having a child with PKU. Low incidence among Finns, Ashkenazi Jews, and blacks.

What causes it? Autosomal recessive inheritance: both parents must pass on recessive genes for a child to be affected.

How is it diagnosed? Because damage can occur during the first few months when babies appear normal, a blood test for PKU is routinely required within a few days of birth.

Related problems. Without treatment, children become irritable, restless, and destructive; they may have a musty odor, dry skin or rashes, and some have convulsions. They are usually physically well developed, and frequently blonder than others in their families.

Treatment. A diet low in phenylalanine (which means low in such high-protein foods as breast milk, cow's milk, or regular cow's milk formula, and meat) begun immediately and continued for at least eight years to prevent retardation.[3] Though the sooner treatment begins the better, hope for a normal life is not entirely lost for children whose treatment may be delayed somewhat. Blood levels of phenylalanine are routinely monitored during treatment. Someday, medication to help with phenylalanine metabolism may be available.

Prognosis. Usually a normal life with special diet.

Pyloric Stenosis

What is it? A probably congenital condition in which thickening or overgrowth of the muscle at the exit of the stomach causes a blockage, leading to increasingly more severe and more forceful projectile vomiting (spewing a foot or more) usually starting at two or three weeks of age, and accompanied by constipation. The thickening can usually be felt as a lump by the doctor; spasms of the muscle are often visible.

How common is it? 1 boy in 200; 1 girl in 1,000.

Who is susceptible? Males more often than females; sometimes tends to run in families.

What causes it? It isn't known what triggers development.

Related problems. Dehydration.

Treatment. Surgery, after baby's fluid levels have been normalized, is safe and almost always completely effective.

Prognosis. Excellent.

---

3. Some studies suggest it may be wise to maintain these dietary measures through the reproductive years, at least in women, and as long as feasible in males; it is certainly suggested for women who are pregnant or planning to be.

Sickle-Cell Anemia

What is it? An anemia in which red blood cells (usually round) are abnormal (sickle shaped) and do a poor job of carrying oxygen to body cells, often getting stuck in and blocking blood vessels. Symptoms (such as fatigue, shortness of breath, joint swelling, especially in fingers and toes, and severe bone pain) don't usually appear until six months of age, but testing should diagnose immediately after birth.

How common is it? 1 in 400 to 600 black children; lower incidence in others.

Who is susceptible? Primarily blacks of African descent, but also whites of Mediterranean/Middle Eastern heritage. Risk is 1 in 4 if both parents are carriers, 4 in 4 if both have the disease.

What causes it? Autosomal recessive inheritance: both parents must pass on recessive genes for child to be affected. Periodic crises can be triggered by infection, stress, dehydration, and inadequate oxygen.

Related problems. Poor growth, delayed puberty, narrow body, curved spine and barrel chest; infection, particularly pneumococcal. Premature death common.

Treatment. Penicillin daily beginning at two months, at least through age five. Also symptomatic relief: pain relievers, blood transfusions, oxygen, fluids. Full series of immunizations, including pneumococcal vaccine. Parent education and genetic counseling also important.

Prognosis. Fair. Still, most live past young adulthood, and some reach middle age and beyond.

HOW DEFECTS ARE INHERITED

All the good and beautiful things a baby is are a result of the genes he or she inherited from both parents, as well as the environment in the uterus during the nine months of gestation. But the not-so-good things a baby is born with—a birth defect, for instance—are also a result of genes and/or environment. Usually the genes a parent passes on to a child are inherited from his or her own parents, but occasionally a gene changes (because of an environmental insult or some unknown factor) and this mutation is passed on.

There are several kinds of inherited disorders:

■ Polygenic disorders (such as clubfoot and cleft lip) are believed to be inherited through the interaction of a number of different genes in much the same way that eye color and height are determined.

■ Multifactorial disorders (such as some forms of diabetes) involve the interaction of different genes and environmental conditions (either prior to birth or after it).

■ Single-gene disorders can be passed on through either recessive or dominant inheritance. In recessive inheritance, two genes (one from each parent) must be passed on for the offspring to be affected. In dominant inheritance, just one gene is needed, and it is passed on by a parent who also has the disorder (by virtue of having the gene). Single-gene disorders can also be sex linked (hemophilia, for example). These disorders, carried in genes on the sex-determining chromosomes (females have two X-chromosomes and males one X and one Y), are most often passed from carrier mother to affected son. The male child, having only one X chromosome, has no opposite gene to counteract the one carrying the defect and is affected with the disorder. A female child receiving the gene on an X chromosome from her mother has also received a normal X chromosome from her father, which makes her a carrier but leaves her unaffected by the disorder.

WHEN A BABY DIES

You've waited for this baby for nearly nine months. You've dreamed about it, felt it kick and hiccup, heard its heartbeat. You've picked out a crib, ordered a tiny layette, prepared your friends, family, and life for the new arrival—and now you're going home empty-handed.

There's probably no greater pain than that inflicted by the loss of a child. And though nothing can banish the hurt you're feeling, there are steps you can take now to make the future more bearable, and to lessen the inevitable depression that follows such a tragedy.

- If death is near, consider organ donation.
- See your baby, hold your baby, name your baby. Grieving is a vital step in recovering from your loss. But you can't grieve for a nameless child you've never seen. Even if your child is malformed, experts advise that it is better to see him or her than not because what is imagined is usually worse than the reality. Holding and naming your baby will make the death more real to you, and ultimately, easier to deal with. So will arranging for a funeral and burial, which will also give you another opportunity to say goodbye. And the grave will provide a permanent site where you can visit your baby in future years.
- Discuss autopsy findings and other details with the doctor to harden the reality of what happened and to aid you in the grieving process. You may have been given a lot of details in the delivery room, but medications, your hormonal status, and your sense of shock probably prevented you from fully understanding them.
- If possible, ask not to be sedated in the hours after you hear the news. Though it will ease your pain momentarily, it will tend to blur your recollections and the reality of what happened. Again, this makes it harder to get on with your grieving, as well as depriving you and your spouse of the chance to support one another.
- Save a photo (many hospitals take them) or other mementos, so that you'll have some tangible objects to cherish when you think about your lost baby in the future. As morbid as this may sound, experts say it helps. Try to focus on positive attributes—big eyes and long lashes, beautiful hands and delicate fingers, a headful of hair.
- Ask friends or relatives not to remove all vestiges of the preparations you made for baby at home. Tell them you will do it yourself. As well-meaning as their gestures might be, coming home to a house that looks as though a baby was never expected will only add to your sense of unreality.
- Cry·—for as long and as often as you feel you need to. Crying is part of the mourning process. If you don't cry now, it will remain unfinished business that you may find you have to attend to later.
- Expect a difficult time. For a while you may feel depressed; you'll probably have trouble sleeping, fight with your husband, neglect your other children. You will probably feel the need to be a child yourself, to be the one who is loved, coddled, and cared for. All this is normal.
- Recognize that fathers grieve, too, but that their grief may in some cases be or appear to be shorter-lived and/or less intense, partly

Rh Disease

What is it? A condition in which a child inherits a blood type from the father that is incompatible with the mother's. If the mother has antibodies to the father's blood (from a previous pregnancy, an abortion, miscarriage, or blood transfusion), these antibodies attack the baby's blood.

How common is it? Much less common since the development of preventive techniques; still, about 7,000 infants a year are affected in the U.S.

Who is susceptible? A baby who inherits Rh-positive blood from his or her father and has a mother with Rh-negative blood.

What causes it? Antibodies in mother's blood attack baby's blood cells, recognizing them as foreign.

because, unlike mothers, they haven't carried their baby inside them for so many months. And they often have different ways of dealing with their distress. They may, for example try to bottle it up, to be strong for their wives. But then the pain often comes out in other ways: bad temper, irresponsibility, loss of interest in life—or they may use alcohol in an attempt to feel better. Unfortunately, a grieving father may not be much help to his wife, nor she to him, and both may need to seek support elsewhere.

■ Don't face the world alone. If you're putting off getting back into circulation because you dread the friendly faces asking, "Oh, what did you have?" take a friend who can field the questions for you on the first several trips to the supermarket, playground, bank, and so on. Be sure that those at work, at church or synagogue, at other organizations in which you're active, are informed before you return so you don't have to do any difficult explaining.

■ Expect your pain to lessen over time, but be prepared for the possibility that it will never go away entirely. The grieving process, with nightmares and intrusive recollections, is often not fully completed for as long as two years, but the worst is usually over in three to six months after the loss. If after six to nine months your grief remains the center of your universe, if you lose interest in everything else and can't seem to function, seek help. Seek help, too, if from the beginning you haven't been able to grieve at all.

■ See support. Like many other parents, you may derive strength from joining a self-help group for parents who have lost infants. But beware of letting such a group become a way of sustaining your rage or grief. If after a

year (sooner, if you're having trouble functioning) you're still having problems coming to terms with your loss, you should seek individual therapy.

■ Turn to religion, if you find it comforting. Some bereaved parents feel too angry with God to do this, but for many faith is a source of great solace.

■ Don't expect that having another baby will resolve any unresolved grief. Do become pregnant again, if that's what you both want—first observing whatever waiting period the doctor recommends. But don't try to conceive in order to feel better, assuage guilt or anger, or gain peace of mind. It won't work, and it could put an unfair burden on any new arrival. Any decision about your future fertility—either to have another baby or to undergo sterilization—should be postponed until the period of deepest sorrow has passed.

■ Recognize that guilt can compound grief and make adjusting to a loss more difficult. If you felt ambivalent about having a baby (as many women do) and now feel your baby's death is your punishment, if your mother wasn't nurturing and you fear you aren't either and that's why you lost your baby, if you feel insecure about your womanhood and now believe your doubts have been confirmed (you couldn't produce a live baby), or if you feel you have failed your family and friends, seek professional support to help you understand that such feelings are in no way responsible for your loss. If you feel guilty even thinking about getting your life back to normal because you sense it is somehow disloyal to your dead baby, it may help to ask your baby, in spirit, for forgiveness or permission to enjoy life once again.

Related problems. Blood disease, brain damage, or death before or shortly after birth.

Treatment. Often a complete blood transfusion of the baby with a blood incompatibility. Some babies may not need a transfusion immediately but do require one at 4 to 6 weeks because of severe anemia. Prevention, with the injection of a vaccine called Rh immune globulin for Rh-negative mothers within 72 hours of the birth (or miscarriage or abortion) of a baby or fetus that is Rh-positive is the best treatment. This vaccine almost always prohibits the development of antibodies and protects future children. A dose of the vaccine may also be given about midway during pregnancy. Doctors are trying to develop a treatment for women who already have developed antibodies.

Prognosis. Usually good, with treatment.

Spina Bifida (Open Spine)

What is it? The bony spine, or backbone, that helps protect the spinal cord is normally open for the first few days of prenatal development but then closes. In spina bifida, the closing is incomplete. The resultant opening can be so slight that it causes no problems and is not noticed except through an X-ray taken later for other reasons, though a small dimple or tufts of hair may be visible on the covering skin. Or it can be large enough that part of the covering of the spinal cord (the meninges) protrudes through, covered by a purplish red cyst or lump (a meningocele), which can range in size from an inch or two in diameter to the size of a grapefruit. If this meningocele is low on the spinal column, it can cause weakness in the legs. In the most severe form of spina bifida, the spinal cord itself protrudes through the opening (a myelomeningocele). It often has little or no skin protecting it, allowing spinal fluid to leak out. The area is often covered with sores, the legs are paralyzed, and bladder and bowel control become a problem later, though some children do attain this control.

How common it it? Affects 1 in 2,000 babies born in the U.S., though it has been estimated that 1 in 4 may have hidden spina bifida. The more severe form of the condition is fortunately the least common.

Who is susceptible? Children of mothers who already have an affected child have a 1 in 40 risk; with two affected children in the family, the risk rises to 1 in 5. Cousins of affected children have a two-fold increase in risk. It is three or four times more common among the poor than among the wealthy, is more frequent in Ireland and Wales, and is less common in Israel and among Jewish people in general.

What causes it? Not known at present.

Heredity is probably involved in some way along with adverse prenatal environment. Nutrition may be involved—recurrences have been reduced by the administration of vitamin supplements containing folic acid to mothers before conception and through the first two months of pregnancy.

Related problems. Infection when spine is visibly open. Also hydrocephalus (water on the brain) in about 70 to 90% of cases (see page 491). Impaired bladder and bowel control.

Treatment. None is needed for a slight defect. Cysts can be removed surgically and water on the brain drained. But though surgery can remove the most severe cysts, covering the opening with muscle and skin, the paralysis in the legs can't be cured. Physical therapy, and later leg braces and crutches or a wheelchair, will probably be needed. Casts may be applied to prevent or minimize deformity. Prior to surgery, it is important not to put pressure (even in the form of clothing) on the cyst. Team approach to treatment, with a range of specialists, is usually best.

Prognosis. Depends on severity of the condition. Most children with less severe conditions can have active and productive lives; most females will be able to bear children, but their pregnancies will be in the high-risk category. Quick treatment of hydrocephalus can generally prevent retardation.

Tay-Sachs Disease

What is it? Children with this lipid-storage disease, in which there is a congenital deficiency of an enzyme needed for breaking down fatty deposits in the brain and nerve cells, appear normal at birth. But about six months later, when the fatty deposits begin to clog cells, the nervous system stops working and children begin to regress—they stop smiling, crawling, and turning over, lose the ability to grasp, gradually become blind, paralyzed, and unaware of their surroundings. Most die by age three or four.

How common is it? Rare (fewer than 100 cases each year in the U.S.).

Who is susceptible? Mostly descendants of Central and Eastern European (Ashkenazi) Jews. Nearly 1 in 25 American Jews are carriers of the Tay-Sachs gene, and 1 in 3,600 Ashkenazi babies is affected.

What causes it? Autosomal recessive inheritance—one gene from each parent is necessary for child to be affected.

Related problems. Concern about future children; there is a 1 in 4 chance of an affected child with each pregnancy.

Treatment. None, though researchers are trying to find a way of replacing the missing enzyme. Those with Ashkenazi backgrounds should be tested for the gene before conception or during early pregnancy. If both parents have the gene, then amniocentesis can be performed to see if the fetus has inherited the disease. An option: therapeutic abortion.

Prognosis. Disease is invariably fatal.

Thalassemia

What is it? An inherited form of anemia in which there is a defect in the process necessary for the production of hemoglobin (the oxygen-carrying red blood cells). The most common form, thalassemia B, can range from the very serious form, called Cooley's anemia, to thalassemia minima, which has no effect but shows up in blood or genetic testing. Even in serious cases, infants appear normal at birth, but gradually become listless, fussy, and pale, lose their appetites, and become very susceptible to infection. Growth and development are slow.

How common is it? One of the more common inherited diseases in the U.S. About 2,500 people are hospitalized annually for treatment.

Who is susceptible? Most frequently, those of Greek or Italian descent; also those from Middle Eastern backgrounds, southern Asians, and Africans.

What causes it? Autosomal recessive inheritance: an affected gene must be inherited from each parent for the child to have the most serious form of the disease.

Related problems. Without treatment, the heart, spleen, and liver all become enlarged, and the risk of death from heart failure or infection multiplies. Eventually bones become brittle, distorting appearance.

Treatment. Frequent blood transfusions of young blood cells, and sometimes bone marrow transplants for children with the most severe form of the disease. Buildup of iron, which can lead to heart failure, can be treated with medication. Prenatal diagnosis is available to determine if a fetus is affected.

Prognosis. Excellent for those with minor forms of the disease; those with moderate disease also become normal adults, though puberty may be delayed. Of those with severe disease, more children are now living into their teens and twenties, though the threat of heart failure and infection are still great.

Tracheal-Esophageal Fistula

What is it? A congenital condition in which the upper part of the esophagus (the tube through which foods move from throat to stomach) ends in a blind pouch and the lower part, instead of connecting to the upper, runs from the trachea (windpipe) to the stomach. Since this makes taking food by mouth impossible, vomiting, choking, and respiratory distress occur on feeding. Excessive drooling occurs since saliva can't be swallowed. Food getting into lungs can cause pneumonia, and even death.[4]

---

4. There are several other, much less common, deformities of the trachea and esophagus.

How common is it? 1 in 4,000 live births.

Who is susceptible? Sometimes babies of women who had excessive amniotic fluid in pregnancy; one-third of victims are born prematurely.

What causes it? A defect in development, possibly due to hereditary or environmental causes.

Related problems. In a small percentage, heart, spine, kidney, and limb abnormalities also occur.

Treatment. Immediate surgery can usually correct condition.

Prognosis. If no other abnormalities, and surgery corrects the problem, outlook is very good.

Water on the Brain, see Hydrocephalus

CHAPTER TWENTY-ONE

CHAPTER TWENTY-ONE

The Adopted Baby

This is it. You're about to become, or have just become, adoptive parents. You've been waiting for months—or, more likely, years—for this moment. But now that it's upon you, you're filled with trepidation. Along with joy, you feel uncertainty and a sense of inadequacy. Just like birth parents.

As an adopting parent, this chapter is for you. But so is most of the rest of this book. Your baby is like other babies, and you are like other mothers (except that you don't experience the physical symptoms of postpartum) and other fathers.

WHAT YOU MAY BE CONCERNED ABOUT

GETTING READY

"My friends who are pregnant are involved in all kinds of preparations—childbirth classes, looking over hospitals, choosing pediatricians. But I don't know where to start in preparing for our adopted baby's arrival."

Instead of surprising mothers with their babies without benefit of notice, Mother Nature wisely designed "gestation." This waiting period before birth (or hatching)

was meant to give parents a chance to prepare for the arrival of their offspring. A chance for the mother bird to feather her nest, the expectant lioness to prepare her lair, and nowadays anyway, for the mother and father human to decorate a nursery, take classes, make key decisions about breastfeeding, child care, and pediatricians, and generally prepare themselves emotionally, intellectually, and physically for becoming a family.

For the couple about to adopt a baby, the waiting period is not usually a predictable and manageable nine months, as it is for other expectant parents. For some, usually those who go the agency route, the entire process may drag on for years, but the big day itself arrives unexpectedly, not leaving enough time for reality to set in, much less for preparations to be made. It's much like the shock of being told you're pregnant one day and being delivered of a baby the next. For others, usually those who adopt privately, definite arrangements may be made to adopt a particular baby far in advance of the infant's due date, giving the adoptive parents-to-be the opportunity to go through pre-baby preparations that are not dissimilar in many ways to those of biological expectant parents. But no matter how much or how little time you have between learning you are going to become a parent and the actual arrival of your baby, there are some steps you can take to make the transition smoother:

Shop ahead. Read Chapter 2 of this book; most of the preparations for the arrival of a baby are the same whether you're adopting or birthing. If you are uncertain as to the date, scout around for the crib, carriage, layette, and so on in advance. Have everything picked out (brand names, style numbers, sizes) and listed along with the store names and telephone numbers so that you can call for delivery the moment you hear from the adoption agency or lawyer. (Check in advance with the stores to be sure that your choices will be in stock.) If you are going the private adoption route and have an approximate arrival date, many stores will allow you to put your order in and then will hold delivery until you call. Should the adoption fall through, they will return your money. Such advance purchasing is a lot better than trying to do the shopping after the baby arrives, when you're busy trying to get acquainted and adjusted. But don't overbuy. Adoptive parents often wait so long for their babies that they end up with a drawerful of six-month sizes that go unworn.

Find out how adoptive parents feel. Talk to other couples who have adopted infants about their concerns, their problems, and their solutions; and read some books on the subject. Find an adoptive parent support group and attend a few sessions—your clergyman, pediatrician, lawyer, or adoption agency may be able to direct you in locating individuals or groups.

Find out how newborns feel. Read up on childbirth so that you have some idea of what your baby has gone through when he or she finally does arrive. You'll learn that after a long, hard struggle to be born, babies may be tired—something that birth parents understand because they are tired, too. Adoptive parents, usually exhilarated and excited rather than exhausted by their baby's arrival, tend to overstimulate the newborn rather than allowing for needed rest.

Learn the tricks of the trade. Take a parenting class that gives instruction in such basics as bathing, diapering, feeding, and carrying baby. Or plan on hiring a baby nurse who is as good at teaching baby care as she is at practicing it, for a day or two, or longer if you prefer, to help out with the basics (see page 14). But be sure to hire a nurse who helps rather than intimidates.

Take a good look at babies. Visit friends or acquaintances with young babies, or stop in at a hospital nursery at visiting time, so that a newborn won't seem such a foreign creature to you. Read about newborn characteristics in Chapter 3.

Pick your pediatrician. It's as important for you to have your pediatrician selected in advance as it is for the expectant couple (see page 25). You'll want someone who will be able to check your baby out on the very first day he or she is with you. A pre-baby interview will give you a chance to ask questions and voice concerns about becoming adoptive parents. And because the newborn's health is a special concern—unlike birth parents, adoptive parents can decide not to take a handicapped infant—you will want the pediatrician to be available almost at a moment's notice to consult with doctors when the baby is born and to give you advice on the prognosis if there is a problem.

Consider breastfeeding. Some adoptive mothers are able to breastfeed their babies, at least partially. Check with your gynecologist to discuss the possibility, and see page 503.

NOT FEELING LIKE A PARENT

"Not having gone through pregnancy and childbirth, holding a child born to someone else, I don't feel much like a mother to our adopted son and I'm afraid I never will."

You don't have to be an adoptive mother to have trouble adapting to the role of mother. Most first-time birth mothers experience the very same self-doubts as they hold their newborns. Becoming a mother doesn't begin with conception and culminate in the moments directly after birth; motherhood evolves over the course of days, weeks, months, and years of loving and caring. Though many women don't feel like mothers during those first challenging days, virtually all do eventually.

Still, while you are struggling to reach that point you may, like many adoptive parents, wish that you could somehow erase the fact of the adoption—that then presto! you would feel like a parent. But biological closeness doesn't guarantee emotional closeness, and though as an adoptive parent you may have a hard time accepting yourself as a mother, your baby will have no such difficulty. You—who love, shelter, and provide for all his needs—are the real

thing to him. And you'll know that long before you hear his first "mama."

Do keep in mind, however, that all babies are not created equally affectionate. Some tend not to be cuddly and don't enjoy being touched a lot (see page 156), but this has nothing to do with what their parents do or don't do. If you have such a baby, don't blame yourself or the fact that he's adopted.

FEELING INADEQUATE

"There must be some biological reason why I feel so inept as a mother. Ever since we got our little girl four days ago, I can't seem to do anything right—from changing a diaper to giving her a bath."

Join the club—which, by the way, is by no means exclusive to adoptive mothers. How well a new mother or father handles the first few weeks on the parenting job has nothing to do with levels of hormones; more likely, it has to do with levels of experience and anxiety. If you've never held a tiny infant before your own, much less changed or bathed one, it's not surprising you're feeling all thumbs. Even for those who've confidently handled newborns as baby-sitters or big sisters (or even nurses or doctors), being suddenly charged with absolute, 24-hour-a-day responsibility for your own small and helpless human being can bring out strong feelings of inadequacy and ineptitude.

For any new mother, hiring a baby nurse for a couple of days for a little on-the-job training (but make sure she's the kind who wants to teach rather than take over) can help instill confidence and speed transition from bumbling novice to self-assured pro. So will parenting classes and reading the first chapters of this book, particularly the Baby-Care Primer on page 73. And, of course, time.

LOVING THE BABY

"I've heard that birth mothers fall in love with their babies right in the delivery room. I'm afraid that because I didn't carry and deliver this baby, I'm never going to be able to love her in the same way."

That all mother-baby love affairs begin in the delivery room is yet another motherhood myth. Your fears are shared by a large proportion of birth mothers who are surprised and disappointed to find they are not overcome by a great tide of love when they first hold their babies—and neither you nor they have anything to be concerned about. The seed of mother-baby (or father-baby) love doesn't sprout miraculously at first meeting, but takes time and nurturing to grow.

And it grows for adopting parents just as it does for birth parents. Studies show that adoptive families form good strong bonds, particularly when the child is adopted before the age of two. That the relationships are solid and loving is reflected in the fact that on psychological tests, adopted children often are shown to be more confident than non-adopted children, tend to view the world more positively, feel more in control of their lives, and see their parents as more nurturing than non-adopted children do.

BABY'S CRYING A LOT

"Our newly adopted baby girl seems to cry a lot. Are we doing something wrong?"

There aren't any healthy new babies who don't cry, and many of them happen to cry a lot—it is, after all, their only way of communicating. But sometimes, crying is increased by overstimulation. Many adoptive parents are so excited about the arrival of their new babies and so eager to show them off that they expose them to a steady stream of visitors. Just because you aren't exhausted from delivery doesn't mean your baby's not. Give her a chance to rest. Slow down, handle her gently, speak to her quietly. After a couple of weeks in a calm atmosphere, you may find she's crying less. If not, she may have colic, which is no reflection on you or your care, just a very common pattern of behavior in the first three months of life.

POSTADOPTION BLUES

"If postpartum blues are supposed to be hormonal, how come I've been feeling depressed since we brought our adopted son home?"

If the baby blues were strictly hormonal, adoptive parents and birth fathers wouldn't suffer from it. But many do. Actually, a wide range of factors contribute to what is commonly called postpartum depression, or the baby blues. And many of them have nothing to do with hormones or the stresses of delivery. Whether you adopt or deliver, your life as a new mother is suddenly very different, much less orderly, much more out of your control. Perhaps you miss the stimulation of work, feel you have no time for yourself or your spouse, and are concerned about managing on one income, at least for a while. Or maybe you feel unsure of yourself as a mother. As an adoptive mother you may be worried about bonding with this new baby (can you love him as you would a biological child?), wonder if he'll turn out to be healthy, if he'll grow up to be like you and your husband or like his biological parents. Or you may feel a tinge of disappointment that this baby, much as you're thrilled to have him, isn't biologically yours (this feeling will pass as the baby comes more and more to feel like your very own, and as you realize that, to him, you are the only parents he has).

You may also be worried that your baby's birth mother might change her mind during the waiting period, which is as long as sixty days in some states. This can also lead to sleepless nights, anxious days, and a heavy case of baby blues.[1]

But since it is likely that at least some of the causes of your depression are the same as for traditional postpartum depression, many of the cures may help you, too. See page 545 for tips to help you shake the blues and let you enjoy your new role more.

NOT BEING ABLE TO BREASTFEED

"After years of trying to conceive, we've given up and are adopting. I've accepted that, but I am very disappointed that I won't be able to nurse when our baby arrives."

Once a baby's born, there's just about nothing that a biological mother can do that an adoptive mother can't. And in this age of medical miracles, that even goes, to a certain extent, for breastfeeding. Though some mothers of adopted infants never succeed in inducing lactation at all, and most will never lactate enough to feed their babies exclusively from the breast, a few dedicated souls do manage to breastfeed their babies at least partially. And those adoptive mothers who attempt to induce lactation, even those who fail to produce milk, reap the benefits of the special intimacy nursing affords.

Breastfeeding will be possible only if the baby you are adopting is a newborn, not yet habituated to sucking on an artificial nipple, and if you have no medical condition (such as a history of breast surgery) that might prevent your producing milk.

Should you decide to try to breastfeed your baby, the following steps will increase your chances of success:

1. When the waiting period is over, be sure to finalize the adoption in court. Some parents forget to do this and thus do not have legal custody of their children, which could lead to serious complications later.

■ Ask yourself why you're eager to breastfeed. If you're trying to prove your worth as a woman or to deny to yourself or to others, consciously or subconsciously, that your baby is adopted, you should reconsider. It's important for you to come to terms with the fact that you were unable to conceive and that your baby is adopted; if you don't, you and baby may run into problems later. If you simply want to give your baby the best nutritional start possible and to share the emotional pleasures of nursing with your new arrival, go ahead and give it a try.

■ Ask yourself whether or not you are willing to put everything else in your life on hold while you try to establish lactation. You may have to nurse almost constantly and face weeks, even months, of trial, tribulation, and frustration, with nothing to show for them but disappointment. Are you ready to accept the idea that you may not succeed? And that if you do, you may be able to supply only part of your baby's nourishment?

■ Will your spouse and other family members be understanding and supportive? Without such support, your chances of success are practically nil.

■ See your obstetrician to discuss your hopes of trying to breastfeed your adopted baby, and to be sure that no condition exists that will make breastfeeding impossible or inadvisable in your case. If he or she doesn't seem to know anything about the subject (this wouldn't be unusual) or is not supportive, ask for a referral to a doctor who is familiar with lactation induction—possibly a pediatrician. If your doctor can't supply a referral, call the La Leche League in your community or in the nearest large city for the name of a physician who can help you; they may also be able to recommend a lactation consultant.

■ If you know in advance approximately when you will get your baby (as when you have arranged to adopt the child of a particular expectant mother), you should begin to try to stimulate lactation a month or so before the due date. To do this you will need a breast pump, preferably an electric one since a manually operated pump will take so much energy that you will almost certainly give up before you succeed.[2] (Some women enjoy enlisting their husbands in the effort to stimulate lactation.) See page 91 for information on expressing milk; if you successfully produce milk before your baby arrives, bottle and freeze it for future use or donate it to a milk bank.

Once you have your baby in your arms, try putting him to breast and see if he is satisfied with what you have to offer. Look for a sensation of let-down in your breasts and signs of adequate intake (such as contentment after feeding, wet diapers, frequent bowel movements). If he doesn't appear satisfied, hook up a supplemental nutrition system (see page 101), its bottle filled with formula recommended by baby's doctor, and let him take as much as he likes. (See page 99 for more tips on determining whether or not a baby is getting enough breast milk and on how to increase your milk supply.)

■ If you won't know when you will be getting your baby until virtually the last minute, order a supplemental nutrition system (SNS) to be delivered when you get the word—or purchase one and keep it on hand. That way, when your baby arrives you will be able to try to stimulate milk production together via suckling while he is nourished by formula. Divide baby's quota of formula (as recommended by his doctor) into at least eight (and preferably ten) feedings, so you can nurse every two or three hours. When baby is hungry, put the formula into the supplementary feeding bottle and put him to your breast. Let him suckle as long as he wishes to (assuming your nipples aren't too sore), even after he's emptied the bottle. Once your milk comes in, if it does, try to start each meal with breastfeeding, augmenting the breast milk with formula through the SNS if your baby still seems hungry.

■ If you're having trouble with milk let-down, ask your doctor about prescribing an oxytocin nasal spray and/or a medication such as chlorpromazine or theophylline. One of these may stimulate the pituitary to produce prolactin (a hormone essential in milk production), but neither should be used for longer than a week or so.

■ Get plenty of rest, relaxation, and sleep; even a woman who has just given birth can't produce adequate milk if she's tense and overtired.

■ Follow the Best-Odds Breastfeeding Diet (page 534), being particularly careful to get enough calories and fluids and to take a vitamin-mineral supplement.

■ Don't give up too soon. A pregnant woman's body usually has nine months to prepare for lactation; give yours at least two or three months to get it going. If your baby was bottle fed at first, getting the hang of nursing may take even longer. Be persistent. If he doesn't feed at the breast a lot at first, supplement his stimulation of your nipples by expressing milk by hand or with a pump.

If in spite of all your hard work you don't succeed at producing milk, or don't produce enough to make you the sole supplier of your baby's nourishment (some biological mothers don't either), you should feel comfortable abandoning your efforts, knowing you and your baby have already shared some of the important benefits of breastfeeding. Or you can continue nursing, supplementing your baby's intake of breast milk, if any, with formula, either through the supplemental nutrition system or with a bottle.

GRANDPARENTS' ATTITUDES

"My folks already have three grandchildren they dote on. And I'm very upset that they don't seem to be excited about the baby boy we've just adopted."

---

2. Call a local hospital, your family doctor, an obstetrician, or the pediatrician you intend to use for your baby for information on the location of rental stations for electric pumps.

It's easy for your parents to become attached to their biological grandchildren. They've borne their own children and slip easily into loving the children their children have borne. But they may be a little unsure whether they will be able to love an adopted grandchild as easily or as well—even as many adoptive parents are unsure—and may stay aloof for fear they will fail. Perhaps, too, they haven't yet resolved any feelings of disappointment (or guilt) they may have had about your not being able to conceive—they may even believe deep in their hearts that you still can—or anger if you're adopting by choice.

It's understandable that you feel hurt by your parents' seeming lack of interest in your baby, but don't be tempted to retaliate by excluding them from his life. The more you include them, the sooner they will grow to accept and love him.

Ideally, it's best to involve grandparents in preparing for the arrival of an adopted grandchild just as they would be, or have been, involved in preparing for a biological one. Enlist them in shopping for furniture and a layette, in picking out teddies and musical mobiles; consult with them on possible colors for the baby's room, and on possible names for the baby. Choosing a family name for your child may make him feel more like "real" family to them.

After you bring the baby home, seek your parents' advice on feeding and burping, bathing and diapering, even if you don't really need it. If they live nearby, ask them to baby-sit when it's convenient. If you're planning a ritual circumcision, baby naming, or christening, invite them to play a major role in the planning and in the celebration themselves. If you're not having a religious ceremony, consider having a "welcome baby" party for relatives and friends. Being able to show the baby off will make them feel more like grandparents.

If you feel comfortable doing so, talk to them about your perception of their feelings. Tell them that with this kind of new experience, uncertainties are natural—you've had some yourself. If they get a chance to vent their feelings, they may begin to feel more comfortable with them—and with you and the baby. If you can't raise the subject, perhaps a clergyman, doctor, respected relative, or family friend can do it for you.

Most of all, give your parents plenty of time to get to know your baby; to know a baby is usually to love him. Be sure that you're not being oversensitive or defensive, and just imagining that your baby is being treated differently. If in the end they still seem not to accept him fully, try to cover your hurt and keep family ties tied, with the hope that closeness will come gradually over the years.

UNKNOWN HEALTH PROBLEMS

"We've just adopted a beautiful little girl. She seems perfect, but I keep worrying that some unknown hereditary problem will surface."

Adopted or not, the genetic makeup of every child is uncertain. And every parent worries occasionally about possible unknown defects. Fortunately, really serious genetic defects are rare, and most parental worry unnecessary. It would be helpful to you, however, to get as complete a health history on both the baby's biological parents as possible, to provide to the baby's doctor and in case of future illness. Also try to arrange, when drawing up adoption papers, for some way to trace the adoptive mother (possibly by being supplied with her social security number) so that should an unlikely crisis arise and your baby need help from the birth mother (a bone marrow transplant, for instance), you would be able to find her.

But while an adopted baby is not any more likely to have an inherited disorder than is one who isn't adopted, she is more

subject to infection. Because she doesn't
come equipped with the same germs as her
adoptive mother and father, she is less
likely than a biological child to have antibodies to infectious organisms in her new
environment. Take some extra precautions
for the first few weeks:
- Be sure feeding equipment is carefully
sterilized (see page 56).
- Wash your hands before handling your
baby, her bottle, or anything that may go
into her mouth or come in contact with her
hands.
- Limit visitors. Though the temptation to
show her off is great, wait a few weeks
before exposing her to large numbers of
people. (She can use the rest, too.)

If your baby has come from abroad,
particularly from Southeast Asia, she may
also be harboring an infection or parasites
that would be rare here. Her pediatrician
should know her country of origin and
should check her for diseases indigenous to
that area of the world upon her arrival here.
Immediate treatment of any problems uncovered will not only assure your baby of a
good start in life, unhampered by disease,
but it will also protect the rest of your
family and other contacts.

DEALING WITH FRIENDS AND FAMILY

*"A few close friends knew we were going
to adopt a baby. But now that she's here
we have to tell everyone we know. I'm not
sure how to go about this."*

Whether they've adopted or delivered, the
traditional way for new parents to spread
their happy word is to send announcements
to friends and family, and sometimes, to
local papers. In your case, the announcement should make it clear that the baby is
adopted ("We're delighted to announce the
adoption of . . ."). Enclosing a picture of the
baby will help make her seem more real to
friends and family.

When talking to anyone about your
baby, start right off saying "our baby" or
"my baby." In referring to the parents who
conceived her, use the words "birth" or
"biological" parents, rather than "real" or
"natural." *You* are baby's real parents, and
the more you hear yourself say it, the more
you—and everyone else—will come to accept it. If you have other biological children, don't call them "my own" children or
permit other people refer to them in that
way.

TELLING BABY

*"Even though our son is still an infant, I
can't help worrying about how and when
we're going to tell him that he's adopted."*

It's no longer a question, as it once was, of
whether or not to tell a child that he's
adopted. Today, experts agree that children
need to know and have the right to know
about their adoption, and should find out
about it from their parents—not through
inadvertent slips by relatives or taunts from
neighborhood kids. There's less agreement
about when to tell, though support seems to
be growing for the idea of gradually introducing a child to the fact that he's adopted
from infancy on, so that the news doesn't
come as a shock later.

You can start right now, while your baby
is tiny and still doesn't really understand
what you are saying. Just as a birth mother
talks about the day her baby was born, you
can talk about the day you brought your
baby home: "That was the best day of our
lives!" And when you're gurgling and
cooing at him, you can say, "We're so
happy we adopted you!" and "We were so
lucky to be able to adopt a baby as wonderful as you." Though your baby won't be
able to understand, even in the simplest
terms, what "adoption" means until he's
three or four years old, early exposure to
the concept will make it seem natural, and
the eventual explanation of it less threatening and easier to cope with.

CHAPTER TWENTY-TWO

The First Postpartum Days

WHAT YOU MAY BE FEELING

You may experience all of these phys-ical and emotional aftereffects of childbirth at one time or another during the first postpartum week, or you may note only a few of them. You may also have some less common symptoms. Report any unusual or severe symptoms to a hospital nurse or your practitioner.

Physically:

- Chills, hunger, and thirst in immediate minutes after delivery
- Bloody vaginal discharge (lochia) turn-ing pink then brownish toward end of first week
- Cramping (afterpains) in abdomen even after first 24 hours
- Perineal discomfort and/or pain and

numbness, if you had a vaginal delivery (especially if you had stitches)
- Exhaustion, particularly if labor was diffi-cult or lengthy
- Incisional pain and, later, numbness in the area, if you had a cesarean delivery (especially if it was your first)
- Discomfort when sitting or walking if you had stitches
- General body soreness if you pushed for a long time
- Broken capillaries (in eyes, on face) if pushing was lengthy or difficult
- Difficulty urinating for a day or two
- Difficulty and discomfort with bowel move-ments for the first few days; constipation
- Hemorrhoids
- A slight fever just after delivery, perhaps

because of dehydration
- Excessive sweating for the first few days; night sweats
- Hot flashes
- Chills for the first few days
- Breast discomfort and engorgement between the second and fifth (sometimes later) postpartum day
- Sore or cracked nipples if you are breastfeeding, after several days of nursing
- Fluid retention and swelling for the first few days of breastfeeding

Emotionally:

- Elation, depression, or both alternately
- Feelings of inadequacy and trepidation about mothering, about breastfeeding if you're nursing
- Frustration, if you're still in the hospital but would like to leave
- Little interest in sex, or less commonly, increased desire (but intercourse won't be okayed by your doctor until at least three weeks postpartum, more often six)

WHAT TO EXPECT AT YOUR IN-HOSPITAL CHECKUPS

The exact procedures will vary from hospital to hospital and practitioner to practitioner, but in general you can expect the following to be checked immediately after delivery:

- The placenta and amniotic membranes, to be certain they are intact
- The location and firmness of the fundus (the top of your uterus)
- Your level of anxiety, excitement, and restlessness
- Your pulse and blood pressure (your pulse will initially be accelerated and your blood pressure elevated because of excitement and exertion, but should be back to normal within a few hours)

In the hours that follow delivery, and then less often during the rest of your hospital stay, the following will probably be checked periodically:

- Your pulse, blood pressure, and respirations
- Your temperature (it may be elevated slightly during the first 24 postpartum hours, often due to dehydration)
- The location of the fundus (it rises above the level of your navel for a couple of days,

then begins to descend; it should be in the center of your abdomen—if it's to the right of center, the bladder will be checked for distension)
- The firmness of the fundus (if it's soft, it may be massaged to help expel clots)
- Your perineum, for color and condition of stitches, if any
- The lochia, for amount and rate of flow (if it's initially heavy it will be checked very frequently to be sure the rate slows; if it seems to spurt, the doctor will check for lacerations) and for color
- Your bladder, for distension
- Your breasts, to determine if your milk has come in and to check the condition of the nipples
- Your legs, for signs of thrombosis (blood clots in the veins)
- Your incision, if you had a cesarean section
- The aftereffects of medication, if any

You will also be asked:
- Whether you have urinated, and then if you are urinating regularly, and whether or not you have any burning or discomfort on urination
- Whether you have had a bowel movement if you're in the hospital more than a

day or two, and whether regular bowel habits have been reestablished
■ About discomfort or pain you may be experiencing

You will probably be instructed about:
■ Care of the perineum
■ Post-surgical care, including care of the incision if you had a cesarean

■ Simple postpartum exercises
■ Breastfeeding and breast care, if you are nursing
■ Breast care, if you are not nursing
■ Basic baby care

If necessary, medication may be prescribed for constipation, pain, or infection, or to dry up your milk if you're not nursing.

WHAT YOU SHOULD BE EATING:
Surviving Hospital Food

There have been reports in medical journals about seriously ill patients, particularly those recovering from major surgery, starving to death on hospital food. Starvation isn't likely to be your problem in the postpartum ward, but in most hospitals it will be a challenge to put together a nutritious meal from the choices offered—a challenge that will require careful scrutiny of menus.

Depending on the time of day you deliver and on hospital policy, you may or may not be able to order your first hospital meals. If they are preselected for you, keep in mind that this may have been done without considering the fact that you are a newly delivered mother with special dietary needs, particularly if you are nursing. So prepare for the worst, and pack a few nutritious postpartum snacks in your hospital bag. Good take-alongs include: whole-grain, juice-sweetened cakes or cookies to appease your sweet tooth and provide some bulk to get you started on the road to regularity; some citrus or other fresh fruit, or raisins or other dried fruit, again for fiber, as well as for vitamins and minerals; a flask of wheat germ to sprinkle on pasta or pancakes or any other refined-grain food you find on your meal tray; a packet or two of nonfat dry milk to add to breakfast cereal or coffee to supplement your liquid milk

intake; a small container of unprocessed bran in case your bowels need extra encouragement. Check with the hospital staff to see if there is a patients' refrigerator in which you can store items brought from home—and be sure to label them with your name and room number.

Of course, your special dietary requirements shouldn't stand between you and the after-delivery celebration you've been looking forward to. Whatever that treat you've been craving—a hot fudge sundae, cream cheese and smoked salmon on a bagel, an ice cream cake, imported chocolate truffles—you'll have earned it. Special-request it from a family member or friend.

When you do get your meal order cards, spend some thoughtful time going over them and consider these points before you check off your selections:

You need milk (or another calcium source) to make milk. If you don't get five servings daily while you're nursing, the calcium needed for milk production is likely to be drawn from your own bones, making you a good candidate for osteoporosis years from now. Getting it while in the hospital shouldn't be too difficult. Order at least one container of milk with each meal (all hospitals will be able to provide you with skim or low-fat milk if you specify). Round out your requirement with more milk at snack time or with the equivalent in other calcium foods, such as cheese (1¼ ounces of Swiss, 1½ ounces of Cheddar, or 2 ounces of mozzarella equal a cup of milk), yogurt (1 cup), dark green leafy vegetables (2 cups of broccoli or 1½ of kale), tofu coagulated with calcium (8 ounces). If you don't like drinking a lot of milk straight, fortify cereal (hot or cold), soups, or coffee with nonfat dry milk from home. Each ⅓ cup you sprinkle is one less cup of liquid milk you have to drink. If you don't use dairy products for any reason, use nondairy sources of calcium and take a calcium supplement for insurance. If you use goat's milk, be sure it's pasteurized and that you are taking a lactation vitamin formula.

You need plenty of fiber to activate your bowels. Not to mention plenty of vitamins and trace minerals to speed your general recovery. To make sure you get all of the above, pass your pencil by the white bread, rolls, and bagels on the menu cards and place your x's beside the "whole wheat" at all meals (or, if whole wheat isn't listed, write it in as a special request). Select whole-grain cereals (such as oatmeal or shredded wheat) for breakfast, opt for a bran muffin over the blueberry, dried prunes over prune Danish, a fresh apple over applesauce. If the hospital's "whole-wheat" bread is clearly a commercial "wheat" bread made partly or primarily with white flour, ask a visiting well-wisher to bring in a loaf of the real thing (for re-sandwiching tuna or accompanying scrambled eggs). If whole-grain cereals aren't on the menu, fortify what is with wheat germ and/or bran from your own private stash.[1] If dried prunes are stewed with sugar and fresh fruit isn't available, have some brought from home.

You need protein to regain and maintain your strength and to make milk. Getting enough should be easy. Even if you're nursing, a single serving of 3 ounces of meat, poultry, or fish, 3 eggs, ¾ cup cottage cheese, or a complete vegetable-protein combination (grains and legumes, for example) at lunch and another at dinner—plus your milk—should easily cover your protein requirement, which will be down to three servings from the four you needed during pregnancy. If you're not nursing, you will need only two servings. Forgo dishes that are fried or heavily sauced if you want to get a head start taking off pregnancy pounds and to have an easier time digesting your food.

You need vitamins and minerals, especially vitamin C, for healing. Order a salad and at least one cooked vegetable (preferably including a green leafy or yellow), plus fresh fruit and fruit juice every day. Be wary of syrupy compotes and canned fruits that are heavy with sugar but light on nutrients. For vitamin C, look for citrus, strawberries, melon, red or green peppers, and cauliflower or broccoli that hasn't been boiled beyond nutritional recognition. If you can't find what you're looking for on hospital menus, request "care packages" from home or the nearest fruit market.

You need iron to replace what was lost with blood during and following delivery. Take your prenatal iron supplement or one that your doctor has just prescribed, but try to eat some iron-rich foods as well. Even if you normally eat red meat infrequently, order some beef or even liver for at least one meal and nibble on dried fruit between meals. If you prefer meatless sources of iron, scan the menu for chick peas or other beans or peas, spinach, or sardines. And continue taking your prenatal iron supplement.

You need fluids. An adequate fluid intake will help you to urinate and move your bowels sooner and more easily, will aid in the production of milk, and will replace

---

1. If you do use bran, remember that it decreases the absorption of calcium taken with it and that it can't do its work without plenty of fluid to wash it down and out.

body fluids lost through postpartum perspiration. In addition to milk (which is only two-thirds liquid), drink fruit and vegetable juices (if the ones the hospital offers don't excite you, request one that does—a bottle of sparkling cider, for instance, or strawberry-apple juice—from outside sources), order soups, and ask for a pitcher of water to keep next to your bed.

You don't need empty calories. Much as you may be tempted to try every dessert on the hospital menu, keep in mind that every empty calorie now does one of two things: it replaces a nutrition-packed calorie that you need for recuperation (and milk production, if you're nursing) or, added to all the nutrient-dense calories you need, it gives you more calories than you should be taking if you intend to start dropping pregnancy pounds. Treat yourself to no more than one nutrition-empty dessert a day during your hospital stay, choosing those you feel you really can't live happily without. Opt, when given the choice, for ice cream, custards, or puddings (which at least contain some calcium and protein) over cakes, cookies, and pastries. (You'll probably be disappointed with the desserts, anyway; these aren't the desserts you get at your favorite restaurant or bake yourself.) In between splurges, especially if your stay is long, satisfy that ache in your sweet tooth with some juice-sweetened cookies from the health-food store.

WHAT YOU MAY BE CONCERNED ABOUT

FEELINGS OF FAILURE

"For nine months I had an image of what my delivery would be like: natural, loving, peaceful. But it turned out to be none of these. My disappointment and sense of failure is so great that I've been crying on and off since my son was born two days ago."

A century ago, when all deliveries were "natural," women were grateful just to survive childbirth. Today, safe deliveries are so routine that they're almost taken for granted. And many women have come to expect, even demand, in addition to a good physical outcome, certain emotional rewards. When they don't end up getting them, they experience a sense of letdown and failure.

Part of the problem lies with those books and classes that prepare couples unrealistically for childbirth, emphasizing the "experience" itself rather than the outcome. Though childbirth education can do a lot to help expectant couples participate in and cope with labor and delivery, it can sometimes give them the notion that childbirth is a test that one passes or fails. And then, if the big event doesn't turn out to be the glorious climax-to-pregnancy they've witnessed on film and read about in books—if they agreed to a pitocin drip to encourage contractions after twenty hours of fruitless labor, if they screamed obscenities instead of panting with Madonna-like serenity, if their wills as well as their bodies were violated by a scalpel in an episiotomy or a cesarean—these women (and often their husbands) feel they've failed.

Yet they haven't. Because the ultimate criteria by which you can judge successful delivery are a healthy mother and a healthy baby. A woman's performance through the nine months of pregnancy—how she eats, drinks, cares for her body—is far more significant than what she does during the fourteen or so hours of labor and delivery. And passing precious moments of new motherhood crying over what might have been is wasteful.

A labor that fulfills your greatest expectations is ideal, and perhaps you'll have it if there's a next time. But its importance is negligible when weighed against those 7 or 8 pounds of healthy baby filling the bassinet beside your bed. Any delivery— or set of parents—that produced your very special newborn can't (and shouldn't) be called a failure.

BROKEN TAILBONE

"I was really shocked when my doctor told me that my tailbone was broken during delivery. I've never heard of such an injury."

You've probably never heard of a broken tailbone, or coccyx, because such an occurence is very rare. But as you now know, it does happen. More common is injury to the muscles of the pelvic floor, which can result in muscular spasm and tenderness in the area. Either can cause what is medically termed coccygodynia, or pain in the region of the coccyx at the base of the spine. Most women find the pain is most severe when they are sitting on a hard surface or straining (not just sitting) at the toilet. Lying down or sitting on a cushion or a rubber ring, or "donut," usually offers relief.

Treatment may include heat applications and massage of the buttocks to relax the area, and, possibly, intrapelvic massage. With treatment, pain gradually lessens and is usually gone in a month or two.

BLACK AND BLOODSHOT EYES

"My eyes were bloodshot after delivery, and now I look like I'm getting two black eyes."

Childbirth can not only leave a woman looking as though she's been through the wringer, it can leave her looking as though she's been in the ring. The pushing during a long, hard second stage of labor can break small blood vessels in and around the eyes, causing bloodshot and even black eyes. This is especially likely to occur when a woman holds her breath at the peak of a push and pressure builds up in her head. If your appearance makes you cringe every time you pass a mirror, or if you're concerned that visitors may be shocked when they see your shiners, go "incognito" for a while with slightly tinted glasses.

Do, of course, discuss the condition and any treatment with your practitioner. In most cases, cold compresses for ten minutes several times a day will be soothing and may even hasten healing; in extreme cases, a consultation with an ophthalmologist may be in order.

You should be able to pack the dark glasses away in a few days to a few weeks. Until then, don't feel self-conscious—all eyes will be on your baby, not on your eyes.

ABDOMINAL CRAMPING

"I've been having cramplike pains in my abdomen, especially when I'm nursing."

The last thing you want to feel after hours of labor is more contractions, but that's very likely what you're experiencing. These "afterpains" are apparently caused by the normal postpartum contractions of the uterus as it goes about the important work of pinching off blood vessels torn by the separation of the placenta and of returning to prepregnancy size and location. Afterpains are more likely to be felt by, and are more intense in, women whose uterine musculature is lacking in tone because of previous births or excessive stretching (as with twins); many first-time mothers aren't even aware of them. This cramping is likely to be more pronounced during nursing because suckling releases the contraction-stimulating hormone oxytocin.

If the pain is severe enough to interfere with your sleep or if the tension it causes interferes with your nursing, a mild anal-

WHEN TO CALL YOUR PRACTITIONER

During the first six postpartum weeks, there remains the possibility of a post-childbirth complication. It could be signaled by one or more of the following, all of which require *immediate* consultation with your practitioner:

■ Bleeding that saturates more than one pad an hour for more than a few hours. Have someone take you to the emergency room or call 911 if you can't reach your doctor immediately. En route or while waiting for emergency help to arrive, lie down and keep an ice bag (or a securely tied plastic bag filled with ice cubes and a couple of paper towels to absorb the melting ice) on your lower abdomen (directly over your uterus, if you can locate it, or at the focus of the pain), if possible.

■ Bright red bleeding any time after the fourth postpartum day. But don't worry about an occasional bloody tinge to your discharge, a brief episode of painless bleeding at about three weeks postpartum, or an increased flow that slows down when you do.

■ Lochia that has a foul odor. It should smell like a normal menstrual flow.

■ Large blood clots in the lochia. Occasional small clots in the first few days, however, are normal.

■ An absence of lochia during the first two weeks postpartum.

■ Pain or discomfort, with or without swelling, in the lower abdominal area beyond the first few days after delivery.

■ After the first 24 hours, a temperature of over 100° for more than a day. Many women run temperatures as high as 100.4°

right after delivery due to dehydration, and some run a low-grade fever when their milk comes in, but these fevers are of no concern.

■ Sharp chest pain, which could indicate a blood clot. Call 911 or have someone take you to the emergency room if you can't reach your doctor immediately.

■ Localized pain, tenderness, and warmth in your calf or thigh, with or without redness and pain when you flex your foot—which could be signs of a blood clot in a leg vein. Rest, with your leg elevated, while you try to reach your doctor.

■ A lump or hardened area in a breast once engorgement has subsided, which could indicate a clogged milk duct. Begin home treatment (see page 557) while waiting to reach the doctor.

■ Localized pain, swelling, redness, heat, and tenderness in a breast once engorgement has subsided, which could be signs of mastitis, or breast infection. Begin home treatment on page 556 while waiting to reach the doctor.

■ Localized swelling and/or redness, heat, and oozing at the site of a cesarian incision.

■ Difficult urination; pain or burning when urinating; a frequent urge to urinate that yields little result; scanty and/or dark urine. Drink plenty of water while trying to reach the doctor.

■ Depression that affects your ability to cope, or that doesn't subside after a few days; feelings of anger toward your baby, particularly if those feelings are accompanied by violent urges.

gesic may be ordered for you. Don't hesitate to take it; such medication won't affect your baby because it doesn't pass into the colostrum in any significant amounts, and it may help you. The pain should subside naturally within two to seven days. If it doesn't, or if the analgesics don't relieve it, check with your practitioner.

CHEST PAIN

"I delivered yesterday—after three hours of pushing—and today my chest hurts when I breathe. Is something wrong?"

You wouldn't expect to do three hours of pushups and not feel sore. And you can't expect to do three hours of baby pushing without feeling the effects of your workout. Which muscles will be sorest will depend on which you tensed and released most as you pushed; the aches and pains might be in the area of the rib cage, in the back, the legs, even in the shoulders.

Of course, such pain can occasionally indicate a more serious problem—such as a blood clot or internal bleeding—so it should be reported to the nurse on duty promptly and to your practitioner at the first opportunity. If the pain is indeed muscular, it should gradually diminish over the next several days. Heat (in the form of hot baths or showers or a heating pad) may be suggested to relieve the discomfort, or a pain medication may be prescribed.

BLEEDING

"I knew I could expect a bloody discharge after delivery, but when I got out of bed the first time and saw the blood running down my legs, I was really frightened."

Don't be alarmed. This discharge of leftover blood, mucus, and tissue from your uterus, known as lochia (from the Greek for "of childbirth"), is normally as heavy as (sometimes a little heavier than) a menstrual period for the first three postpartum days. It may total up to two cups before it begins to taper off, but it often seems more copious than it really is. And a sudden gush upon getting out of bed in the first few days is common, and no cause for concern. Since blood, primarily from torn vessels at the placental site, is the predominant ingredient of lochia during the immediate postpartum period, the discharge is quite red at first. Then as healing progresses and the bleeding slows, the discharge gradually turns to a watery pink, then to brown, and finally to a yellowish white over the next week or two.

Sanitary napkins, *not* tampons (which could cause infection), should be used to absorb the flow, which may continue on and off for as little as two weeks or as long as six, and may occasionally be tinged with a bit of blood. Sometimes it seems to stop for a day or so, and then resumes. Women who do too much too soon sometimes note a recurrence of actual bleeding after the first week—a clear sign to slow down because physical exertion is interfering with the healing process. Some women experience what seems to be a "small period" about three weeks postpartum. This episode of painless bleeding is normal as long as it doesn't become profuse or prolonged, or repeat—in which case your doctor should be consulted.

Anything more than a slightly bloody discharge after the first week should be reported to your practitioner since it could indicate that a small fragment of placenta may still be clinging to the wall of the uterus, or that the site at which the placenta was attached to the uterus hasn't healed completely. In either case a D and C (dilatation and curettage), in which the doctor dilates the cervix and scrapes away any remaining pieces of placenta from the uterine wall or dead tissue from a poorly healed placental site, usually stops the bleeding. Also inform your practitioner if brownish or yellowish lochia persists longer than six weeks, since this could indicate infection, especially when associated with fever and/ or abdominal pain or tenderness.

Breastfeeding and intramuscular or intravenous oxytocin (routinely ordered by some doctors following delivery) may both reduce the flow of lochia by stimulating uterine contractions and help to shrink the uterus back to normal size more quickly. Some practitioners will massage the fundus (the top of the uterus) gently for a while after delivery to encourage uterine contractions. The shrinking of the uterus is vital because it pinches off exposed blood vessels at the site where the placenta separates from the uterus, preventing hemorrhage.

If the uterus is too relaxed and contractions weak, excessive bleeding may occur. This is most likely when the uterus has been overworked during a long or traumatic delivery or was overdistended because of multiple births, a large baby, or excess amniotic fluid; when the placenta was oddly placed or separated prematurely (abrupted); when fibroids prevented symmetrical contraction of the uterus; or when the mother was in a generally weakened condition at the time of delivery (due to anemia, preeclampsia, or extreme fatigue, for example).

More uncommon is postpartum hemorrhage that occurs because of lacerations to the genital tract. Rarely, hemorrhage is due to a previously undetected bleeding disorder. Infection can also cause postpartum hemorrhage right after delivery or weeks later.

Most postpartum hemorrhages occur without any warning about seven to fourteen days after delivery. Since this relatively rare complication of childbirth can be life threatening, prompt diagnosis and treatment are vital. Any of the first six symptoms on the When to Call Your Practitioner list on page 513 can be a sign of impending hemorrhage (or, in some cases, of postpartum infection) and should be reported immediately.

THROMBOPHLEBITIS

"I had a c-section and the doctor instructed me to put on elastic stockings first thing in the morning. Why?"

An ounce of prevention, even if it comes in the form of uncomfortable elastic stockings, is worth at least a pound of cure. Once in a great while, following a surgical delivery, a traumatic vaginal one, or a period of protracted bed rest (which makes circulation sluggish), a blood clot develops in a leg vein and the vein becomes inflamed. Women with varicose veins are more susceptible to the problem, and

sometimes pressure from the stirrups during delivery seems to precipitate it. Called thrombophlebitis, this condition is a much less common postpartum problem today than it was forty years ago when women weren't even allowed to dangle their feet over the side of the bed until a week or more after delivery, and when traumatic deliveries were more common.

Elastic stockings plus early ambulation (walking around as soon after delivery as is safe and practical) can usually prevent the problem. If for any reason (you were given a spinal anesthetic, for instance) you are confined to bed after delivery for more than eight hours, doing simple leg exercises such as those on page 524 will help to improve the circulation of blood in your legs. If you feel a sharp pain on doing any exercise, particularly one in which you flex the foot (turning your toes up toward your body), stop exercising and notify the nurse.

There are basically two kinds of thrombophlebitis. When a clot forms in a superficial vein near the surface of the skin, the symptoms are tenderness and warmth right over the affected area and possibly a red line visible through the skin. Keeping the legs elevated and applying moist heat will usually resolve the problem quickly. When a deeper vein is involved, the area along the path of the vessel becomes painful, slightly swollen, and exquisitely tender. Flexing the foot may cause pain in the calf, apparently because this movement stretches the inflamed vein. Occasionally, swelling of the leg may be extreme. Deep-vein thrombophlebitis is very serious, since the blood clot can break away and move to the lungs, and requires prompt treatment to dissolve the clot. Therapy usually includes: absolute bed rest with the affected leg elevated, warm heat, elastic stocking or bandage, and anticoagulant medication to reduce the clotting ability of the blood. If such treatment is unsuccessful, which is rare, the vein may have to be tied off surgically.

PAIN IN THE PERINEAL AREA

"I didn't have an episiotomy, and I didn't tear. Why am I so sore?"

You can't expect some seven or eight pounds of baby to pass by the perineum without having some impact. Even if your perineum was left intact during the baby's arrival, the area has still been stretched, bruised, and generally traumatized. Discomfort, ranging from mild to not-so-mild, is the very normal result. Time will be the best healer, but if discomfort is great, try some of the remedies below.

"I'm afraid my episiotomy may be infected. It's very sore and really hurts when I laugh."

The perineal soreness experienced by a vaginal deliverer is likely to be compounded if the perineum was torn or surgically cut in an episiotomy and then sutured. And though it won't hurt only when you laugh, it's likely to hurt more when you do—and when you cough or

PERINEAL CARE

Scrupulous attention to perineal care is necessary to prevent infection not only of the repair site when there's been an episiotomy or a laceration, but of the reproductive and urinary tracts in the woman who's recently delivered. The following steps are usually recommended:

■ Wash your hands before *and* after going to the bathroom or changing a sanitary pad.

■ Change sanitary pads at least every four to six hours. Secure them snugly so that they don't slide back and forth.

■ Place and remove pads front to back to avoid dragging germs from the rectum to the vagina.

■ Pour or squirt warm water (or an antiseptic solution, if one was recommended by your practitioner) over the area after going to the bathroom. Pat dry with gauze pads, paper wipes, or medicated pads (which the hospital may supply), always from front to back.

■ Keep your hands—and anyone else's—off the area until healing is complete.

Though discomfort is likely to be greater with a repair (with itchiness around the stitches possibly accompanying soreness), these suggestions are usually welcomed by all recently delivered mothers:

■ Warm sitz baths, hot compresses, or heat lamp exposure. If you use the tub for a sitz bath, ring for the nurse immediately should you feel faint while in the bath. To avoid burns when using a heat lamp, use one in the hospital only under supervision; at home use only with instructions from your practitioner.

■ Chilled witch hazel on a sterile gauze pad or a rubber glove filled with crushed ice applied to the site of discomfort. Or line your sanitary napkin with medicated pads at each change.

■ Anesthetic sprays, creams, or pads; mild pain medications, if prescribed by your physician.

■ No pressure positions. Lying on your side and avoiding long periods of standing or sitting can decrease strain on the area. Sitting on a pillow or a rubber ring (called a "donut") may help, as may tightening your buttocks before sitting.

■ Kegel exercises (see page 528). Do these as frequently as possible after delivery and right through the postpartum period to stimulate circulation to the area, which will promote healing. Don't be alarmed if you can't feel yourself doing them at first; the perineum will be numb right after delivery. Feeling will return to the area gradually over the next few weeks.

sneeze, as well. (Laughing, coughing, and sneezing can't, however, cause your stitches to open up, nor can going to the bathroom.) Like any freshly repaired wound, the site of an episiotomy or laceration will take time to heal—usually seven to ten days. Pain alone during this time, unless it is severe, is not an indication that infection has developed.

While you're in the hospital, a nurse will check your stitches periodically for inflammation or other indications of infection. But infection is very unlikely if good perineal hygiene has been practiced.

GETTING OUT OF BED

"I feel ready to be up and about, but the nurse said I can't get out of bed until eight hours after delivery."

The six- to eight-hour bed rest rule is routine in many hospitals—partly because a woman's body has taken a beating and needs a rest, and partly because dizziness and even fainting, which can result in falls and serious injury, are common in those early postpartum hours.[2] So that you don't hurt yourself (or your baby, if you're carrying him or her), as well as for the hospital's protection, most hospitals insist on eight hours of bed rest postpartum. You may not even be allowed to go to the bathroom and may have to use a bedpan, instead. If you do get the okay for trips to the toilet, you will probably not be allowed to go alone.

It's easy for women who deliver at night or in the wee hours to obey this rule—by sleeping away the eight or so postpartum hours (not uninterrupted, of course, since they will be awakened for baby feedings). But to those who deliver by day, being confined to bed when they're raring to go can be trying. Still, doctor probably knows best: you will feel stronger when you do get

2. This is due to a sudden drop in blood pressure, the kind you may have experienced during pregnancy when you got up too suddenly.

up if you treat yourself to some well-deserved rest first. Your episiotomy or laceration repair, if any, will have begun to heal by the end of that eight-hour period, any soreness will interfere less with walking, and your vaginal discharge will have diminished somewhat.

And consider this: it may be a long time before you'll be enjoying the luxury of spending an entire eight-hour stretch in bed again. Savor the experience while you can.

DIFFICULTY WITH URINATION

"It's been several hours since I gave birth, and I haven't been able to urinate yet."

During the first 24 postpartum hours, many women experience difficulty in passing urine. Some feel no urge at all; others feel the urge but are unable to fulfill it. Still others do urinate, but with accompanying pain and burning. There are a host of factors that may interfere with the return of normal bladder function after delivery:

■ The holding capacity of the bladder increases because, with the enlarged uterus out of the way, it suddenly has more room in which to expand—thus the need for urination may be less frequent.
■ The bladder, bruised or otherwise traumatized during delivery due to pressures during childbirth, may have become temporarily paralyzed. Even when full, it may not send the usual voiding signals.
■ Drugs or anesthesia may decrease the sensitivity of the bladder or the alertness of the mother to its signals.
■ Low fluid intake and fluid loss through perspiration during labor and delivery can combine with inadequate fluid consumption following childbirth to cause dehydration. The result—little urine to excrete.
■ Pain in the perineal area may cause reflex spasms in the urethra (the tube that carries the urine from the bladder), making urination difficult. Swelling of the perineum

may also interfere with urination.
■ Urine may burn or sting the sensitive site of a fresh episiotomy or laceration repair, making a woman hesitant to urinate. This can be alleviated somewhat by standing astride the toilet while urinating so that the flow comes straight down, without touching sensitive tissue.
■ Any number of psychological factors may also inhibit the ability to urinate—lack of privacy, fear that voiding may cause pain, embarrassment or discomfort over using a bedpan or needing assistance in the bathroom.

In spite of these impediments it's essential that the bladder be emptied within six to eight hours—to avoid urinary tract infection, loss of muscle tone in the bladder from overdistension, and bleeding due to a distended bladder's interfering with the normal postpartum descent of the uterus. You can expect, therefore, that a nurse will ask you at least once a shift if you've urinated. You may be asked to void for the first time into a container, so that your output can be measured. And your bladder may be checked to be sure it's not distended with unpassed urine.

If you haven't urinated within eight hours or so of delivery, you may be catheterized (your bladder emptied of urine via a slim tube inserted into the urethra). But you can probably get the waterworks going more quickly and avoid catheterization (or if you have been catheterized following a cesarean, resume urinary function when the catheter has been removed) by trying the following:

Take a walk. Getting out of bed and going for a stroll as soon after delivery as you're allowed will help activate your bladder (*and* your bowels).

Take a drink. An adequate fluid intake will also help activate your bladder.

Go it alone. If you're self-conscious with an audience and feel you can manage on your own, ask the nurse to wait outside your room the first time you try to urinate. She

can rejoin you when you've finished to give you a demonstration of perineal care and to help you back to bed if necessary.

Bed down with the bedpan. Dismiss your inhibitions and psych yourself into using the bedpan if you're too weak to walk to the bathroom, if hospital policy requires maternity patients to stay in bed for the first eight postpartum hours, or if your bladder seems intent on emptying drip-by-drip. Sitting on a bedpan (if it's metal, ask to have it warmed) can facilitate urination because it allows you to go the moment you feel the urge. It may help to arrange for privacy (have the curtain around your bed drawn if you're sharing a room), to pour a little warm water over the perineal area, to have a faucet in your room turned on, and to sit rather than lie on the bedpan.

Go hot or cold. Warm the area up in a sitz bath or cool it down with ice packs, whichever seems to induce urgency for you.

Try that trickle trick. Running the water in the sink really does help encourage your own faucet to flow. So does running warm water over the perineal area.

HAVING A BOWEL MOVEMENT

"I delivered almost a week ago and I haven't had a bowel movement yet. I think fear of opening my episiotomy stitches is making me constipated."

The passage of the first bowel movement after childbirth is a milestone of the postpartum period, one that doesn't come as soon as many women would like.

Several factors, both physical and psychological, may postpone the immediate return of normal bowel function after delivery. For one thing, the abdominal muscles that assist in elimination have been stretched during childbirth, making them less effective at this task. For another, like the bladder, the bowel itself may have been traumatized during labor and delivery, leaving it sluggish. In addition, it may be relatively empty thanks to increased activity (perhaps with diarrhea) in early labor, possibly an enema before delivery and some evacuation during it, decreased food intake through delivery, and perhaps little appetite in the immediate postpartum period because of excitement or exhaustion.

Perhaps the most potent inhibitors of postpartum bowel activity are psychological: the fear of splitting open the stitches; the embarrassment over lack of privacy in the hospital; and the pressure to perform.

Although reregulating your system is rarely either effortless or instantaneous, there are several steps you can take to make it easier and speedier:

Don't worry. Nothing will keep you from moving your bowels more effectively than worrying about moving your bowels. Don't worry about your stitches popping—they won't (though it may sometimes feel as though they will). And don't worry if it takes a few days to get your plumbing back into smooth working order—it just takes longer for some women than others.

Request roughage. Select whole grains, fresh fruits and vegetables, and stewed prunes from the hospital menu, if possible. Supplement these with bowel-stimulating food brought in from outside. Apples, raisins, prunes and other dried fruit, nuts, bran muffins, and wheat bran cereal or unprocessed wheat bran will help. Beware of chocolate, however. This classic gift for hospital patients tends to constipate.

Keep the liquids coming. To compensate for fluids lost during labor and delivery, and to help soften stool if you're constipated, you must increase your intake of fluids—especially water and fruit juices. But turn to prune juice only if all else fails since a glass of prune juice can be a very strong laxative.

Get off your bottom. You won't be running marathons the day after delivery, but you should be able to take short strolls through the corridors. An active body encourages active bowels. Kegel exercises, which can be done very soon after delivery, will help tone up the rectum.

Follow your urges. Try to answer immediately whenever nature calls, even if it's in mid-feeding (return baby to the bassinet) or if you have a roomful of company (ask them to leave for a few minutes if you'd like more privacy, or use the bathroom in the hall).

Don't strain. Straining on the toilet won't open your episiotomy or laceration repair, but it can lead to, or aggravate, hemorrhoids. Place your feet on a low stool or box to simulate the squatting position (the natural one for moving your bowels) and avoid straining.

The doctor may also recommend a stool softener to get things moving.

Once the first bowel movement has passed, you will probably breathe a great sigh of relief. But keep in mind that constipation may return if you become lax once you're back home and ignore these preventive measures. The first few bowel movements may pass with unaccustomed discomfort. But as stools soften and you become more regular, the discomfort will ease.

HEMORRHOIDS

"For nine months I escaped hemorrhoids. Now, postpartum, I suddenly have them."

Hemorrhoids, also called piles (they resemble a pile of marbles or grapes), are actually varicose veins of the rectum or anus. They may be painful, itchy, and/or burning, and they sometimes bleed. Internal hemorrhoids are found far up in the rectum, external ones right on the skin just beyond the anal sphincter.

Hemorrhoids often develop during pregnancy, particularly during the last trimester. Childbirth, because of the extreme pressure exerted on the rectum and anus during pushing, may make them worse or can even make them a problem for the first time. In new mothers who didn't have hemorrhoids before pregnancy, the bothersome symptoms usually lessen or disappear after the immediate postpartum period. In the meantime, taking the following steps can help minimize discomfort and may hasten that departure:

■ Maintain regularity. Constipation aggravates hemorrhoids, so be sure to follow the tips on page 519 for avoiding it. In some cases your practitioner may recommend a stool softener. (Do *not* take mineral oil, which can deplete your body of nutrients.)
■ Apply heat or cold, whichever offers more relief. Warm sitz baths of about twenty minutes' duration are usually recommended, but some women find ice packs or chilled witch hazel soaks more soothing. Or you might try alternating hot and cold treatments.
■ Keep the perineal area scrupulously clean. At first, rinse the area with water after each bowel movement, using a peri-bottle (a plastic squirt bottle, usually provided by the hospital, for keeping the perineal area clean) as directed. When you can begin wiping, use moistened, unscented white toilet tissue (which is less irritating than colored) and wipe from front to back.
■ Sleep or rest on your side, not on your back, and avoid long periods of standing (not a good idea right now, anyway) or sitting (when you do sit, use a rubber ring, or donut, if that makes you more comfortable).
■ Do Kegel exercises (page 528) to improve circulation to the area.
■ Use medicated suppositories or topical anesthetics as recommended by your practitioner.
■ If hemorrhoids protrude, ask the nurse to show you how to tuck them back in.

If bleeding and/or discomfort continues in spite of your best efforts, check with your physician to rule out any more serious condition and to see if more radical therapy might be needed to deal with your hemorrhoids.

EXCESSIVE PERSPIRATION

"I've been waking up at night soaked with perspiration. Is this normal?"

What your doctor may sometimes refer to as diaphoresis, but is more commonly and less politely referred to as sweating, is one of the ways in which your body rids itself of pregnancy-accumulated fluids during the days following delivery (frequent urination is another). Sometimes perspiration continues to be a problem for several weeks—occasionally accompanied by hot flashes and/or chills—because of postpartum hormonal adjustments. Though you needn't worry about these symptoms, do make sure essential fluids lost through the skin are replaced, particularly if you're breastfeeding, by increasing your intake of liquids. An absorbent towel placed over your pillow may help make you more comfortable if you do most of your perspiring in bed.

Once you're back at home, it's a good idea to take your temperature if you're sweating excessively, and as a precaution, to report it to your doctor if it's over 100° orally.

ENGORGED BREASTS

"My milk finally came in, and my breasts are swollen to three times their normal size—and so hard, engorged, and painful that I can't bear to put on a bra. Is this what I have to look forward to until I wean my baby?"

If painfully tender, granite-hard breasts the size of an exotic dancer's were what mothers had to look forward to for the duration of the breastfeeding experience, most babies would be weaned before they entered their second week of life. The engorgement that arrives with a mother's milk can temporarily make nursing agonizing for her and, because the nipples are flattened by the swelling, frustrating for baby. The condition may be more severe when a baby isn't put to breast until 24 to 36 hours after birth.

Engorgement occurs rather suddenly, usually over a few hours, most often on the third or fourth postpartum day, but it can occur as early as the second day or as late as the seventh. It's more uncomfortable for some women than for others, is more severe with first babies, and also occurs later with first babies than with subsequent ones. Some lucky women get their milk without experiencing any discomfort or noticeable engorgement at all, especially if they are nursing regularly from the start.

Happily, engorgement and its distressing effects disappear within a matter of days. Until then, you can use cold packs, warm showers, alternate warm and cold showers, or a mild analgesic recommended by the doctor to reduce discomfort. (If you take a pain reliever, take it just before feeding.) Expressing a bit of milk by hand or with a breast pump can help to get the flow started and ease engorgement enough to allow your baby to grasp the nipple for suckling. Using an oxytocin nasal spray prescribed by your doctor or applying warm soaks just before nursing to encourage milk let-down may also bring some relief.

Don't be tempted, however, to skip or skimp on feedings because of pain; the less your baby sucks, the more engorged you will become. The more you nurse your newborn, on the other hand, the more quickly engorgement will subside. If your baby doesn't nurse vigorously enough to relieve the engorgment in both breasts at each feeding, use a breast pump to do this yourself.

"I just had my second baby. My breasts are much less engorged than with my first. Does this mean I'm going to have less milk?"

It's common for the breasts to engorge less with second and subsequent pregnancies. Perhaps the breasts, having gone through all this before, have less difficulty adjusting to the influx of milk, or perhaps the experienced mother can get her baby started nursing more easily and more quickly, re-

sulting in more efficient emptying of the engorged breast.

Very rarely, a lack of engorgement and of a sensation of milk let-down does indicate inadequate milk production, but only in first-time mothers. Many women, even first-timers, who don't experience engorgement turn out to have copious milk supplies nevertheless. There's no reason to worry that a milk supply might be inadequate unless a baby isn't gaining well (see page 99).

DRYING UP YOUR MILK

"I'm not nursing. I understand that drying up the milk can be painful."

Whether or not you're nursing, your breasts will become engorged (overfilled) with milk sometime between your second and seventh postpartum day, most often on the third or fourth. This can be an uncomfortable, even painful, experience—but it is blessedly temporary.

Medications to suppress lactation are no longer on the market. Such medications didn't always relieve engorgement, and if they did, the engorgement often returned a week or two after they were discontinued. They also occasionally caused serious side effects. So it is now recommended that nonnursing mothers take nature's course, letting the body take care of suppressing milk production. The breasts are designed to produce milk only as needed—if you don't nurse, production eventually ceases. Though sporadic leaking may occur for several days or even weeks, the worst of the engorgement shouldn't last more than 12 to 48 hours. During this time, ice packs, mild pain relievers, and possibly squeezing a few drops of milk from the breasts may be helpful. Hot showers and soaks, however, though soothing, may stimulate milk production and aren't a good idea. Wear a well-fitting, supportive bra until your breasts return to prepregnancy size, which may not be until six weeks postpartum.

HOSPITAL CONFUSION

"My doctor told me to stay in bed until noon today. At nine in the morning, an aide came in and said I should get up and she would take me for a walk. Who do I listen to?"

In a hospital, as in any other institution, mistakes can be made. That's why it's important for you to take some responsibility for your own care. If something doesn't make sense—you're getting conflicting messages, a treatment is painful or uncomfortable, someone wants to give you a medication you think you already took or said you didn't want—speak up. If your nurse can't clear up the problem, ask to see the head nurse. If you're still not satisfied, call your doctor or midwife, or ask for a consultation. For non-medical issues, find out if the hospital has a patient advocate on staff—most do—and turn there for help.

GOING HOME

"I had a relatively easy labor, my son is doing fine, and I feel terrific. I'd like to go home early, but everyone tells me I should stay in the hospital and rest."

This is one case in which listening to "everyone" might be a good idea. Childbirth takes its toll no matter how effortless and rapid the labor and delivery. And though in your present state of euphoria you may not feel that you need to rest, you'll find out otherwise very quickly if you do too much too soon. Your attitude is likely to change from "Why should I rest?" to "What's rest?" before the month is out.

So the question isn't whether or not you need rest—you do—but where you'll be most likely to get it. For the woman who's coming home to relatives, friends, and/or hired help who will make it possible for her to take it easy, early discharge can bring welcome relief from the regimentation and relatively impersonal atmosphere of hospi-

tal life. On the other hand, for a woman who's returning with babe in arms to a home full of other children and devoid of help, the hospital stay, though brief and imperfect, often represents an idyllic, peaceful calm before the storm.

Also relevant to your decision is how much your personality will allow you to rest if you do go home, even if you're going home to lots of help. If you're not the kind of person who can lie idly by for a couple of days watching other people do your laundry, cook your meals, and tidy your home, you're better off with the enforced vacation from household responsibilities that a postpartum hospital stay brings.

Of course, while a hospital stay sometimes isn't medically necessary for you, it may be for your baby. And unless you don't mind being separated, you'll have to remain in the hospital for as long as your baby's doctor requires him to, unless that stay is prolonged.

"I was surprised to be told by my doctor that I was expected to go home only 24 hours after my baby was born. What's the big rush?"

With health-care costs spiraling, medical economists are looking in every hospital nook and cranny for ways to cut them. Thus: the 24-hour discharge. It can also be argued that after an uncomplicated vaginal delivery, the very best place for a mother and her baby is at home. There are familiar surroundings and favorite foods (at least for mom), loving family, and no exposure to hospital germs.

Of course, something could go wrong at home. So if you are discharged early, faithfully follow the medical instructions you are given for you and your infant (ask that they be put in writing). If you note any warning signs that a problem might be developing in you (see page 513) or in your baby (see page 70), contact the appropriate practitioner *immediately*. To help you over some of the early hurdles, ask for a home visit from a nurse or lactation consultant (many women have trouble getting started breastfeeding on their own) or an early office visit to the doctor (most doctors schedule them). It's also a good idea to ask to have your infant's PKU test done between the third and fifth days of life (earlier tests may not be valid). And remember, getting the okay to go home doesn't give you carte blanche to start going out on the town, scrubbing floors, or even dusting the living room. If you don't take it easy, you might end up back in the hospital—and there go those cost savings.

RECOVERY FROM A CESAREAN SECTION

"I had a c-section. How different will my recuperation be from that of a woman with a vaginal delivery?"

Recovery from a cesarean section is similar to recovery from any major abdominal surgery—with a delightful difference: Instead of losing an old gall bladder or appendix, you gain a brand new baby.

Of course, there's another difference slightly less delightful. In addition to recovering from the surgery itself, you'll also be recovering from childbirth. Except for a neatly intact perineum, you'll experience all the same postpartum discomforts you would have if you'd delivered—vaginally—afterpains, lochia, breast engorgement, fatigue, hair loss, excessive perspiration, the baby blues, and, if you had a longish period of labor, the exhaustion and other aftereffects of that as well.

As for your surgical recovery, you can expect the following in the recovery room.

Careful monitoring until anesthesia wears off. If you had general anesthesia, your memory of the time in the recovery room may be fuzzy or totally absent. Since everyone responds differently to drugs and each drug is different, whether you are clear-headed and alert in a few hours or not for a day or two will depend upon your body and upon the medications you were given. If you feel disoriented or if you have

hallucinations or bad dreams, your husband or an understanding nurse can help you return to reality quickly.

It takes longer to shake the effects of a spinal or an epidural block than those of general anesthesia. Numbness will wear off from the toes up, and you will be encouraged to wiggle your toes and move your feet as soon as you can. If you had a spinal block, you will have to remain flat on your back for eight to twelve hours. You may be allowed to have both your husband and your baby visit you in the recovery room.

In some cases your doctor may elect to continue your epidural for several hours or more postpartum, extending the effects of the anesthesia but easing your pain.

Incisional pain. Once the anesthesia wears off, your incision is going to hurt—though just how much depends on many factors, including your personal pain threshold and whether or not you've had a previous cesarean (subsequent recoveries are less uncomfortable than the first one). You will probably be given pain medication as needed, which may leave you with a woozy or drugged feeling. It will also allow you to get some needed sleep. You needn't be concerned if you're nursing: the medication won't pass into your colostrum in any meaningful amount, and by the time your milk comes in you probably won't need any more pain relief medication.

Possibly, nausea. If you do experience nausea, you may be given an antiemetic preparation to try to prevent vomiting. If you vomit easily, you might want to talk to your doctor about giving you such a medication before you even begin to feel queasy.

Encouragement to do breathing and coughing exercises. These help rid your system of any leftover general anesthetic, and help to expand your lungs and keep them clear to prevent the complication of pneumonia. Done correctly, they may cause discomfort, but you may be able to minimize it by holding a pillow against your incision while performing them.

Regular evaluations of your condition. A nurse will check your vital signs (temperature, blood pressure, pulse, respiration), your urinary output and vaginal discharge, the dressing over your incision, and the firmness and location of your uterus. She will also check your IV and urinary catheter.

Once you have been moved to your hospital room, you can expect:

Continued evaluation of your condition. Your vital signs, dressing, urinary output and vaginal discharge, and your uterus, as well as your IV and catheter (while they remain in place), will be checked regularly.

Removal of the catheter after 24 hours. Urinating on your own may be difficult at this point, so try the tips on page 517. If you can't urinate on your own, the catheter may be reinserted until you can.

Afterpains. Like the woman who's gone through a vaginal delivery, you can expect to begin feeling afterpains about 12 to 24 hours after delivery. See page 515 for more about these contractions, which help bring your uterus back to prepregnancy shape.

A gradual return to a normal diet. About 24 hours after surgery, or soon after your bowels begin to show signs of activity (by moving or passing gas), your IV will be discontinued and you will be allowed fluids by mouth. Over the next few days, you will gradually return to your usual diet. Even if you're famished, don't try to circumvent doctor's orders by having someone sneak in a Big Mac. Take it slow getting back to your usual fare, or you may find yourself with unnecessary digestive discomfort. If you are breastfeeding, be sure to get plenty of fluids.

Referred shoulder pain. Irritation of the diaphragm from air in the abdomen following surgery can cause a few hours of sharp pain referred to the shoulder. An analgesic may help, and it won't get into your colostrum.

Possible constipation. Like the mom who went through a vaginal delivery, you may have difficulty having a bowel movement for a few days. That's not a reason for concern, especially since you haven't eaten very much that can come out, anyway. Once you are eating, a stool softener and/or a laxative may be prescribed to help move things along. You could also try the tips on page 518, but don't introduce the roughage until you get the doctor's okay. If you haven't had a movement by the fourth or fifth or sixth postpartum day, you may be given a suppository or an enema.

Encouragement to get physical. Even before you are out of bed, you will probably be urged to start wiggling your toes, flexing your feet and pressing them against the end of the bed, and turning from side to side. You can also try these simple exercises: (1) Lie flat on your back, one leg bent at the knee, the other extended, while tightening your abdomen slightly. Slide the bent leg slowly down on the bed; repeat, reversing legs. (2) Lie flat on your back, both knees pulled up, feet flat on the bed, and raise your head a few inches for about 30 seconds. (3) On your back, knees bent, tighten your abdomen, and reach with one arm across your body to the other side of the bed, at about waist level; reverse. These exercises will improve circulation, especially in your legs, reducing the chance of developing a blood clot. But be prepared to find some quite painful, at least for the first 24 hours or so.

To get out of bed between 8 and 24 hours after surgery. You will first be helped to a sitting position, supported by the raised head of the bed. When you're ready to stand up, the process will be gradual, probably like this: using your hands for support, you will slide your legs over the side of the bed and dangle them for a few minutes. Then, slowly, you'll be helped to step down onto the floor. If you feel dizzy, which is normal, sit back down. Steady yourself for a few more minutes before trying again. Once standing, take a couple of steps. These may be extremely painful (though not everyone finds them so). Stand as straight as you can, and fight any temptation to hunch over to ease the discomfort. This difficulty in getting around is only temporary. In fact, you may soon find yourself more mobile than the vaginal deliverer next door—and you will certainly have the edge in sitting.

To wear elastic stockings. These improve circulation and are intended to prevent blood clots in the legs.

Gas pain. As your digestive tract (temporarily put out of business by surgery) begins to function again, trapped gas can cause considerable pain, especially if it presses against your incision line. Discomfort may be worse when you laugh, cough, or sneeze. Tell your nurse or doctor about your problem. You may be advised to walk up and down the corridor, or to try lying on your left side or on your back, with your knees drawn up and taking deep breaths while holding a pillow against your incision. If these tactics don't work, you may be given an enema or a suppository to help evacuate the gas. Narcotics are not usually recommended for gas pain because they can prolong the difficulties, which ordinarily last just a day or two. If pain remains severe, however, a tube inserted in your rectum to help the gas escape may spell relief.

Time with your baby. You can't lift your baby yet, but you can cuddle and feed him or her. (Place the baby on a pillow over your incision for feeding.) Depending on how you feel, and on hospital regulations, you may be able to have modified rooming-in. Some hospitals even allow full rooming-in following c-sections, which will be easier if your husband or mother or a friend can be with you a good deal of the time.

Sponge baths. Until your stitches or clips are removed (or absorbed), you probably won't be allowed a tub bath or shower. So enjoy the spongings.

Removal of stitches or clips. If your stitches aren't absorbable or if you have clips, they will be removed four to six days after delivery. And although the procedure isn't very painful, you may find it uncomfortable. When the dressing is removed, look at the incision with the nurse or doctor (even if you're squeamish) so you'll know what it looks like. Ask how soon you can expect the area to heal completely, what changes in appearance to expect with healing, and what kinds of changes might indicate a need for medical attention.

You can expect to go home about four to seven days after delivery.

WHAT IT'S IMPORTANT TO KNOW: Getting Back Into Shape

Back when you were pregnant, looking the part was part of the fun. Remember the thrill of buying your first pair of maternity jeans? The elation of watching your belly swell from a scarcely noticeable bulge to a larger-than-life watermelon? And the momentous day when you could finally walk down the street confident that everyone you passed could see that you were pregnant, and not just unpleasingly plump?

Once delivery day has come and gone, however, looking pregnant quickly loses its appeal. No woman wants to look as though she's still toting a baby in her belly once she's started toting a newborn in her arms.

For many women it's not pregnancy pounds that keep them looking pregnant; most are shed without much effort in the first six weeks postpartum. Rather, it's stretched-out abdominal muscles that stand between those new mothers and their old prepregnancy silhouettes.

Unfortunately, simply waiting it out won't work. Pregnancy-stretched muscles regain some of their tone as time goes by, but won't ever return to their prepregnancy condition without a concerted exercise effort. Leave your tummy muscles to their own devices, and you'll find that their sagging increases as the years pass, and with each baby you deliver.

And exercise postpartum will do more than help you pull your tummy in. Abdominal routines will improve general circulation and reduce the risk of back problems, varicose veins, leg cramps, swelling of ankles and feet, and the formation of clots in blood vessels. Perineal exercises will help you avoid stress incontinence (leaking of urine), which sometimes occurs after childbirth; dropping, or prolapse, of the pelvic organs; and will tighten your perineum so that making love, once you resume it, will be as good or better than ever. Regular exercise will also promote healing of your battered uterine, abdominal, and pelvic muscles, hastening their return to normal and preventing further weakening from inactivity, as well as help your pregnancy-and-delivery-loosened joints return to normal (or nearly so). If excess pounds are a problem, exercise will help you shed them (you can burn the 100 calories of a baked potato in just twenty minutes of brisk walking). And finally, exercise can provide psychological benefits, improving your ability to handle stress and to relax, while minimizing the possibility of postpartum depression.

If you have the time, opportunity, and inclination, sign up for a postpartum exercise class, or buy a postpartum exercise book or video (the American College of Obstetricians and Gynecology has produced a good one[3]) and fit an at-home program into your schedule. If the idea of an intense exercise program seems unappealing, regularly doing just a few simple exercises aimed a your particular problem areas (such as tummy, thighs, buttocks) can also get you back into shape. Add a daily brisk walk or other aerobic activity to your agenda and you will have put together an adequate exercise program. Before you begin any exercise program, of course, be sure you have your doctor's okay.

GUIDELINES FOR SAFE AND SANE POSTPARTUM EXERCISE

■ If you've had an uncomplicated delivery and are in good health, you can follow the simple exercise program beginning on page 528. If you had a surgical or difficult delivery, or if you have medical problems, consult your doctor about when you can start exercising and which exercises would be appropriate.

■ Stick to a schedule. Exercise done only sporadically is useless and thus a waste of your precious time. Muscle-toning exercises (leg lifts, sit-ups, and pelvic tilts, for example) are best done daily in short takes; two or three 5-minute sessions a day will tone you up better than one 20-minute workout. Once you begin doing aerobic exercises (brisk walking, jogging, bicycling, and swimming, for example), aim for at least three 20-minute sessions of sustained activity a week—though 40 minutes

3. For information on ordering this and other videos from the American College of Obstetricians and Gynecologists, call ACOR Programs, (800) 332-3373.

four or five times weekly may be a better goal for strengthening bones and preventing osteoporosis later in life.[4]

■ Don't rush. Muscle-toning exercises are most effective when done slowly and deliberately, with adequate recovery time between repetitions. It's during the recovery periods that muscle buildup occurs.

■ Start slowly if you haven't exercised recently or are doing unfamiliar exercises. Do only a few repetitions the first day, and increase the number gradually over the next week or two. Don't do more than the recommended amount, even if you feel great. Stop your workout as soon as you begin to tire.

■ Avoid competitive sports until you get your doctor's okay to participate.

■ Because your joints are still unstable and your connective tissue lax, avoid jumping; rapid changes of direction; jerky, bouncy, or jarring motions; and deep flexion or extension of joints. Also avoid knee-chest exercises, full sit-ups, and double leg lifts during the first six weeks postpartum.

■ Do muscle-toning exercises on a wood floor or tightly carpeted surface to reduce shock and provide sure footing.

■ Do five minutes of warm-ups (very light stretching exercises, slow walking, or stationary biking against low resistance) before you begin exercising. Cool down at the end of each session with some gentle stretching exercises, but to avoid damaging loose joints, don't stretch to the maximum for the first six weeks.

■ Get up slowly to avoid dizziness from a sudden drop in blood pressure, and to equal-ize circulation, keep your legs moving for a few moments (by walking, for example) when you stand up.

■ Once you begin doing aerobic exercises, be careful not to exceed your target heart rate. Ask your doctor what that is or find it in the table on page 528.

■ Avoid vigorous exercise in hot weather or when you have a fever. Once the six-week postpartum period is over, you can begin exercising in warm weather by dropping back to less than half your usual level of activity and working back up gradually. Try to exercise early in the morning or in the evening—when the heat is generally less intense. Wear light-colored, lightweight clothing and an open mesh hat or cap when exercising in the sun.

■ Drink plenty of fluids before and after exercising, and if the weather is very hot or you are perspiring a great deal, have something to drink as you go, as well. Water is best; avoid sugar-sweetened drinks, including those marketed especially for athletes.

■ Stop exercising immediately and notify your doctor if you experience any of the following symptoms: pain, faintness, dizziness, blurred vision, shortness of breath, palpitations (your heart seems to tremble, flutter, or race), back pain, pubic pain, nausea, difficulty walking, or a sudden increase in vaginal bleeding (if brown or pink lochia turns red after exercise, you are overdoing).

■ Don't use your baby as an excuse for not exercising. Most babies love lying on mommy's chest during a calisthenics session; snuggling in a baby carrier while she pedals a stationary bike, works a rowing machine, skiing machine, or treadmill; and being pushed in the stroller or carriage while mommy walks or jogs. But don't bounce an infant around in a baby carrier while you jog or prop up on your bike a baby who can't sit independently.

---

4. It's generally agreed that an exercise that is extremely strenuous, such as jogging, is best not done daily. The body needs a day of recovery in between to help prevent injury.

HEART RATE GUIDELINES FOR POSTPARTUM EXERCISE

Your Age	Limit Yourself to This Heart Rate* (beats per minute)	Maximum Heart Rate for Your Age (beats per minute)
20	150	200
25	146	195
30	142	190
35	138	185
40	135	180
45	131	175

*Figures represent 75% of the maximum heart rate for each age group. Under proper medical supervision, more strenuous activity yielding heart rates that exceed these limits may be okay.

Source: ACOG Home Exercise Programs, 1985

A POSTPARTUM EXERCISE PROGRAM

All the following exercises are done in the basic position—lying on your back with your knees bent—though Kegels can be done in any position at all. Phase One exercises can be done while you're in your bed—in the hospital or at home; the others are best done on a hard surface, such as the floor. (If you invest in an exercise mat, it can do double duty as a play mat for baby.) Remember, this exercise program is appropriate only for women who've had uncomplicated vaginal deliveries and are in good health. Others need to consult their physicians.

Phase One: Twenty-four Hours After Delivery

Kegel exercises. You may have been doing these all during pregnancy, and you can resume them almost immediately after delivery. (If you've never done them, see below for directions.) At first, with your perineum still numb from the beating it took during delivery, you won't be able to feel yourself doing the Kegels. You can Kegel in bed, while reading or nursing or in the tub. Though you can try doing Kegels while you are urinating—contract to stop, relax to release the flow of urine—as a way of learning how to do these exercises, it is-

KEGEL EXERCISE

Firmly tense the muscles around your vagina and anus. Hold for as long as you can, up to eight or ten seconds, then slowly release the muscles and relax for several seconds.

Repeat. Do at least 25 repetitions at various times during the day, while sitting, standing, lying on your back or taking a bath.

NOTE TO ADOPTIVE MOTHERS

Being a new mother is exhausting and stressful, whether you personally went through childbirth or not. Exercise is a wonderful way to reduce tension, keep your figure, improve your health, and have fun with your baby. And it sets a good example for your child. So an exercise program such as this one is important for you, too, though you needn't worry about the caveats for the mother going through postpartum. If you don't already exercise regularly, consider beginning now.

n't recommended that you routinely do them during urination. As muscle tone improves, you'll be able to restrict the flow to just a few drops between each Kegel repetition. Both you and your sex life can benefit from your continuing to perform Kegels even beyond the postpartum period; and doing them during sexual intercourse is one of the best ways to combine your body's business with its pleasure.

Deep diaphragmatic breathing. Start in the basic position (see page 530). Place your hands on your abdomen so you can feel it rise as you inhale slowly through your nose; tighten the abdominal muscles as you exhale slowly through your mouth. Repeat just a couple of times at first to avoid hyperventilation. (If you feel dizzy, faint, experience tingling or numbness of fingers and toes, or blurred vision, breathe in and out into a paper bag or into your cupped hands.) Increase the number of breaths by two each day until you're up to ten. The exercise can be repeated several times during the day.

Phase Two: Three Days After Delivery

Now that your body is beginning to re-

cover from some of the more immediate effects of childbirth, you can begin doing some more serious exercising. Before you begin, however, be certain that the recti abdominis (the pair of vertical muscles that run down the center of your abdominal wall) didn't separate during pregnancy. This separation, called "diastasis," is fairly common, especially in women who have had several children, and it will get worse if you do even mildly strenuous exercise before it closes up. Ask your practitioner about the condition of your recti abdominis muscles, or perform this self-examination: as you lie in the basic position, raise your head slightly with your arms extended; then feel for a soft lump below your navel. Such a lump would probably indicate recti abdominis separation. You can help correct it with this routine: assume the basic position; inhale, cross your hands over your abdomen, then use your fingers to draw the separated halves of your rectus muscles together as you breathe out, raising your head slowly. Repeat three or four times, twice daily. Once the separation has closed, or if you didn't have one to start with, you can progress to the exercises that follow.

PHASE TWO: THE EXERCISES

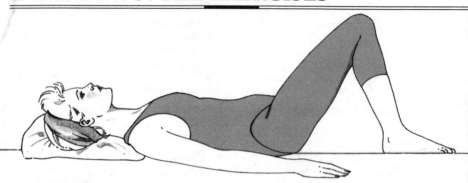

The basic position. *Lie on your back with your arms at your sides, palms down. Your knees should be bent, feet placed about 12 inches apart, and flat on the floor.*

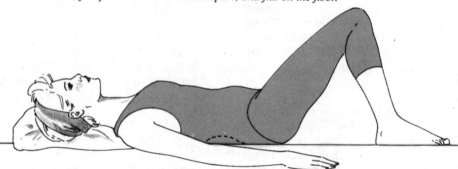

The pelvic tilt. *Assume the basic position. Inhale as you press the small of your back against the floor. Then exhale and relax, allowing your back to arch normally. Repeat three or four times to start, gradually increasing to 24.*

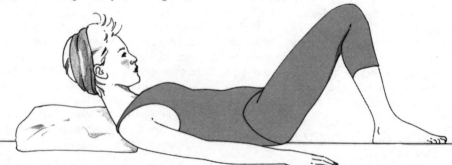

Head lifts. *Assume the basic position. Inhale deeply. Raise your head very slightly, exhaling as you do. Lower your head slowly, while inhaling. Raise your head a little higher each day, gradually working up to lifting your shoulders slightly off the floor. Don't do full sit-ups for three or four weeks, and then only if you have very good abdominal muscle tone.*

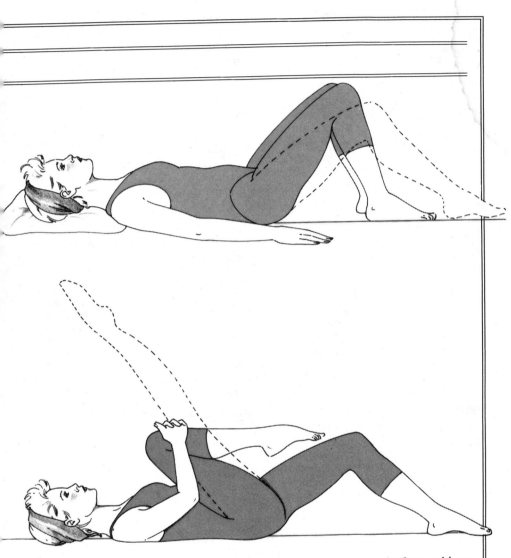

Leg slides. *Assume the basic position. Slide your right foot, sole flat on the floor and knee bending as you go, back toward your buttocks while pressing the small of your back against the floor. Slide your leg back down. Repeat with your left leg. Start with three or four slides per side, and increase gradually until you can do twelve or more comfortably. After three weeks, try modified leg lifts: keeping the opposite leg bent, slowly lift one leg at a time slightly off the floor, then slowly lower it. If you can do these comfortably, start with three or four lifts per leg, gradually increasing the number to twelve each. Once you have this down, bring the lifted leg into your chest, straighten it up as far as it will go, then lower it slowly back to the ground. Repeat this twelve times with each leg.*

Phase Three: Four to Six Weeks Postpartum— Exercise for Life

Starting yourself on an aerobic exercise program after the first four to six weeks— and staying with it as your baby grows—is important not only for your good health and longevity, but for your baby's; a mother who exercises regularly is likely to have children who will follow in her sneakersteps. But get your doctor's okay to proceed, especially if you had a difficult

delivery. You can choose to exercise to a videotape or in an aerobics class, or you may decide to embark on a running, bicycling, rowing, skiing, or swimming program of your own.[5]

---

5. Though swimming provides excellent aerobic exercise, improving cardiorespiratory fitness as well as jogging or walking does, it does not provide weight-bearing exercise, which research is beginning to show can help strengthen bones and ward off osteoporosis later in life. It may also be less useful in weight reduction.

EXERCISE AND BREASTFEEDING

Life is never simple. Exercise is good for you. Breastfeeding is good for your baby. But recent studies show that many babies turn their noses up at breast milk after their moms have exercised vigorously. Apparently, the exercise increases levels of lactic acid, which makes the milk taste sour. Levels remain elevated for at least 90 min-

utes. So by all means exercise, but try to do so immediately following feedings so that your baby's next meal won't be scheduled until those levels come down. If that isn't possible, try to pump and store your milk before your workout, then feed the pre-exercise milk in a bottle when you're ready.

CHAPTER TWENTY-THREE

Surviving The First Six Weeks

WHAT YOU MAY BE FEELING

During the first six weeks postpartum, you will be recovering from childbirth and delivery. You will probably experience many of the following to some degree at one time or another.

Physically:

- Continuing vaginal discharge (lochia), turning pink, then brownish, then yellowish white
- Fatigue, sometimes bordering on exhaustion
- Some pain, discomfort, and numbness in the perineum, if you had a vaginal delivery (especially if you had stitches)
- Diminishing incisional pain, continuing numbness, if you had a cesarean section (especially if it was your first)

- Continuing bouts of constipation (although it should be easing up)
- Gradual flattening of your abdomen as your uterus returns to prepregnancy location in the pelvis (but only exercise will bring you completely back to prepregnancy shape)
- Gradual loss of weight (you may lose all your pregnancy gain by the end of two months, or not until the end of the first year)
- Breast discomfort and nipple soreness, if you're nursing, until breastfeeding is well established
- Achiness in arms and neck; backache (from carrying and feeding baby)
- Noticeable hair loss
- Swollen neck glands; throat dryness and constriction

Emotionally:

- Elation, depression, or both alternately
- Either a sense of being overwhelmed or a growing feeling of confidence, or both alternately

- Decreased sexual desire (even if your practitioner has given you the okay to resume) or increased desire (more rare)

WHAT YOU CAN EXPECT AT YOUR SIX-WEEK CHECKUP

Your practitioner will probably schedule you for a checkup four to six weeks after delivery; if you had a cesarean, you may also see the doctor at one to three weeks postpartum for a check of your incision. At six weeks you can expect the following to be checked, though the exact content of the visit will vary depending upon your particular needs and your practitioner's philosophy:

- Blood pressure

- Weight, which will probably be down by 17 to 20 pounds or more from predelivery weight

- Shape, size, and location of your uterus, to see if it has returned to its prepregnancy state

- Cervix, which will be on its way back to its prepregnancy condition, but will still be somewhat engorged; the surface may possibly be eroded

- Vagina, which will have contracted and regained much of its muscle tone

- Episiotomy or laceration repair site, if any; or, if you had a surgical delivery, the site of your incision

- Breasts, for any abnormalities

- Hemorrhoids or varicose veins, if you have had either during pregnancy or postpartum

- Your plans for birth control; if appropriate, a diaphragm will be fitted or birth control pills prescribed (see page 569)

Have any questions about your recovery or general health ready (bring a list, so you won't forget anything).

WHAT YOU SHOULD BE EATING: The Best-Odds Postpartum Diet

If you worked hard to revamp your eating habits during pregnancy, now isn't the time to abandon them, temporarily or permanently. And if you didn't eat right during pregnancy, you couldn't pick a better time to start good habits than now. Though a nutritious diet plan can include a few more perks postpartum than it did during pregnancy, careful eating will be essential if you're going to keep up your energy level, gradually take off those extra pounds put on during the nine months of pregnancy, and, if you're nursing, produce enough milk.

NINE BASIC DIET PRINCIPLES FOR NEW MOTHERS

Good nutrition is vital for a speedy recovery from childbirth and for the maintenance of the abundant energy, optimum health, and vibrant spirits necessary for top-notch mothering. It is also crucial to successful nursing. While neglecting nutrition essentials when you're breastfeeding won't necessarily reduce your milk supply, at least not for a couple of months (even women who are severely undernourished can often produce milk for a while), it may affect the nutritive value of your milk and shortchange your own body nutritionally. Whether you decide to nurse or not, these nine basic principles can serve as a guide to eating well during the postpartum period:

Make most bites count. Though each bite isn't as vital now as it was when you were sharing every one with your gestating baby, it's still important to make as many of them as possible count toward nutrition. Careful food selection will help ensure a plentiful supply of quality breast milk, enough energy to survive sleepless nights and endless days, and a speedier return to prepregnancy shape. And don't waste bites when you're cheating, either; splurge only on those empty-calorie foods that provide optimum gastronomic pleasure.

All calories are not created equal. No matter who in the family you're feeding, the 1,500 calories (derived mostly from nutritionless, even dangerous, saturated fats and sugar) in *one* typical fast-food meal aren't nutritionally equal to the 1,500 calories (from protein and complex carbohydrates, laden with vitamins and minerals) in *three* well-balanced meals. Also compare: the 235 calories in a slice of frosted devil's food cake with the 235 calories in half a cantaloupe mounded with ½ cup of ice milk or the 160 calories in ten french fries with the 160 calories in a baked potato

topped with 2 tablespoons of yogurt and chives and ⅔ cup of broccoli flowerets.

Starve yourself, cheat your baby. Missing meals now is not as hazardous as missing them when you're pregnant, but a consistently irregular eating schedule can cut into your own reserves, giving you less energy for mothering. If you're nursing, severely inadequate nutrition—such as might develop on certain fad diets—could in time seriously reduce your milk supply.

Stay an efficiency expert. To keep your postpartum weight going down and your nutrition up, it's still important to select foods dense in nutrition in relation to their calorie content—tuna fish over bologna for lunch, pasta primavera over fettuccine Alfredo for dinner. If your problem is losing too much weight, look for foods high in both nutrition and calories but low in bulk, such as avocado and nuts, but stay away from foods like popcorn that fill you up without filling you, or your nutritional requirements, out.

Carbohydrates are a complex issue. And complex carbohydrates, unrefined, are just the kind you want to concentrate on postpartum (actually forever—for a lifetime of good nutrition for yourself and your family). Whole-grain breads, cereals, and cakes, brown rice, dried beans, peas, and other legumes provide fiber (as important now as during pregnancy to ensure regularity) and plenty of vitamins and minerals—most of which are absent from refined grains even when they're enriched.

Sweet nothings—nothing but trouble. The average American consumes a whopping 150 pounds of sugar in its various disguises a year. Some of this comes right from the sugar bowl, and is sprinkled on cereals and fruits or stirred into coffee or tea. A fair amount is taken, not unexpectedly, in cakes, cookies, candies, pastries, and pies. But a surprising proportion comes from such unlikely sources as soups, salad dressings, breakfast cereals, breads, hot dogs, luncheon meats, and processed, canned, or frozen main courses and side dishes (hidden in the form of sucrose, dextrose, honey, fructose, corn syrup, and so on).

If your sugar intake is just average, you're consuming over 800 nutritionless or empty calories a day. For a new mother who wants to make sure she gets her Daily Dozen without gaining a dozen (or more) pounds in the process, an occasional sugary treat won't create nutritional havoc, but consuming a great many empty calories a day will.

Eat foods that remember where they came from. Foods that are highly processed lose a lot of their nutrition in the process, and people who consume them frequently, in turn, become nutritional losers. Often processed foods also contain unhealthy excesses of saturated fat, sodium, and sugar, as well as artificial colors and other chemical additives, none of which enhance the diet, and the last of which can occasionally contaminate breast milk (see page 553). The closer the food you eat is to its natural state, the better for your baby— and for you.

Make good eating a family affair. Include the whole household in your Best-Odds eating, and your baby will grow up in a home where good nutrition is natural. You will extend not only your child's (or children's) lifespan, but those of your husband and yourself as well.

Don't sabotage your diet. Though you can go back to a morning cup of caffeinated coffee and an occasional alcoholic beverage even if you're nursing, much more caffeine or alcohol can definitely affect you and your baby adversely, as can any amount of tobacco or illicit drug use (see page 539).

THE BEST-ODDS DAILY DOZEN FOR POSTPARTUM AND BREASTFEEDING

If you're familiar with the Best-Odds Diet, you already know that you needn't sit down with a ledger, a calculator, and volumes of nutritive value tables before each meal in order to be sure you're getting the nutrients you need (to produce milk and stay healthy yourself if you're breastfeeding, or just to stay healthy if you're not). All you have to do is get your Daily Dozen.[1]

Calories. You'll need enough of these to keep up your energy levels (as a new mother, you will need more energy than ever before) and, if you're nursing, your milk supply. But not so many that you won't continue to gradually lose those pregnancy pounds. If you're breastfeeding, you'll need about 400 to 500 extra calories a day above what you would need to maintain your pre-pregnancy weight (double that if you're nursing twins, triple for triplets). You can reduce that number a little after the first six postpartum weeks if you don't seem to be losing weight, but you shouldn't cut calories drastically because your body could start producing ketones, metabolic byproducts that (by passing into your milk) could be harmful to your nursing baby.[2] In addition, melting body fat quickly releases any toxic chemicals stored in the fat into your bloodstream and then into your breast milk.

---

1. Note that some foods can provide more than one Daily Dozen serving. Broccoli, for example, can provide a green leafy, a vitamin C, and in somewhat greater quantity, a calcium serving. Many dairy products provide both protein and calcium servings, and some fruits and vegetables supply both yellow or green leafy and vitamin C servings.

2. Some recent research indicates that nursing mothers, especially in later months, may need fewer than the usually quoted 400 to 500 extra calories daily. Your weight should be your guide.

If you're not nursing, you should be able to lose those unwanted pregnancy pounds and fuel your recovery by eating the approximate number of calories you would need to maintain your prepregnancy weight.[3] After the first six weeks postpartum, when recovery is complete and dieting is safer, you can reduce that number by 200 to 500 calories a day, but don't go on a stringent diet without medical supervision.

Nursing or not, weighing yourself regularly is the best way of determining whether your calorie intake is high, low, or just right. As long as you are losing pregnancy pounds gradually and stop losing once your desired weight is reached, you're on target. Adjust your calories up or down if you're not. Keep in mind, too, that it's always wiser to increase exercise than to dramatically decrease calories. If you can't brake a too rapid weight loss, see your doctor.

Protein—three servings daily if you're nursing, two if you're not. One serving equals any of the following: 2½ to 3 glasses skim or low-fat milk; 1¼ cups evaporated skim milk; 1¾ cups low-fat yogurt; ¾ cup low-fat cottage cheese; 3 ounces Swiss cheese; 2 large eggs plus two whites; 5 egg whites; 3 to 3½ ounces fish, meat, or poultry; 5 to 6 ounces tofu; 5 to 6 tablespoons peanut butter; 1 protein combination of legumes and grains (see page 361).[4] Nursing mothers of twins or triplets need an extra serving for each additional baby. Vegans, those vegetarians who eat no animal protein, should add an extra protein serving daily since the quality of vegetable protein is not as high as that of animal protein.

---

3. To find out how many calories it takes to sustain your prepregnancy weight, multiply your prepregnancy weight by 12 if you're sedentary, 15 if you're moderately active, and up to 22 if you're very active.

4. The portion sizes of these combinations are for toddlers. An adult serving would be about four times as large.

Vitamin C foods—two servings daily if you're nursing, at least one if you're not. One serving equals any of the following: ½ cup strawberries; ¼ small cantaloupe; ½ grapefruit; 1 small orange; ½ to ¾ cup citrus juice; ½ large kiwi, mango, or guava; ⅔ cup broccoli or cauliflower; 1 cup cabbage or kale; ½ medium green bell pepper or ⅓ medium red bell pepper; 2 small tomatoes or 1 cup tomato juice.

Calcium—five servings daily if you're nursing, three plus if you're not. One serving equals any of the following: ¼ cup Parmesan cheese; 1¼ to 1½ ounces most other hard cheeses (such as Swiss or Cheddar); 1 cup skim or low-fat milk; ½ cup evaporated skim milk; ⅓ cup nonfat dry milk; 1¾ cups low-fat cottage cheese; 1½ to 1¾ cups broccoli, collards, or kale; 3 tablespoons blackstrap molasses; 4 ounces canned salmon or 3 ounces sardines, with bones; 9 ounces tofu prepared with calcium. Mothers nursing twins, triplets, or more will need an extra calcium serving for each additional baby, and may want to use calcium-enriched dairy products or calcium supplements to get their quota. Vegetarians who don't use dairy products may find it difficult to meet the requirement from purely vegetable sources unless they are fortified with calcium (orange juice, for example) and may need calcium supplements. Though lack of calcium when nursing isn't likely to affect breast milk composition, the calcium drawn from a mother's bones to produce breast milk may make her more susceptible to osteoporosis later in life.

Green leafy and yellow vegetables and yellow fruits—at least three servings daily if you're nursing, two or more if you're not. One serving equals any of the following: 4 apricot halves; ⅛ cantaloupe; ¼ large mango; 1 large yellow (not white) peach; ¾ cup broccoli; ½ small carrot; ¼ to ½ cup cooked greens; ¼ cup winter squash, or ⅛ cup sweet potato, or 1 tablespoon unsweetened canned pumpkin; 1 large tomato; ½ red bell or chili pepper.

Other fruits and vegetables—two or more servings daily. One serving equals any of the following: 1 apple, pear, banana, or white peach; ⅔ cup cherries or grapes; 1 cup cranberries; 1 slice pineapple; 2 cups watermelon; 5 dates; 3 figs; ¼ cup raisins; 5 or 6 asparagus spears; 1 cup bean sprouts, eggplant, or onions; ⅔ cup parsnip, snow peas or green peas; 1 small potato; ¼ head iceberg lettuce; ½ cup mushrooms or summer squash.

Whole grain and other concentrated complex carbohydrates—six or more servings daily whether you're nursing or not. One serving equals any of the following: ½ cup cooked brown rice, wild rice, millet, kasha (buckwheat groats), unpearled barley, bulgar, or triticale; ¼ cup whole cornmeal (before cooking); 1 serving cooked or ready-to-eat whole-grain cereal; 2 tablespoons wheat germ; ¼ cup unprocessed bran; 1 slice whole-grain bread; ½ whole-wheat bagel or English muffin; 1 small or ½ large whole-wheat pita; 2 to 6 whole-grain crackers; 2 brown rice cakes; ½ cup lentils, beans, or split peas; ⅔ cup lima beans or black-eyed peas; 1 ounce whole-wheat or high-protein pasta; 2 cups air-popped popcorn. Vegetarians should not count a carbohydrate serving as filling both a protein and carbohydrate requirement. Keep in mind, especially if you have trouble keeping weight on, that federal guidelines now recommend up to 11 servings a day of grain foods.

Iron-rich foods—one or more daily. Iron is found in varying amounts in beef, blackstrap molasses, carob, chick-peas and other dried legumes, dried fruit, Jerusalem artichokes, oysters (but don't eat them raw), sardines, soybeans and soy products, spinach, and liver.[5] It is also found in wheat germ, whole grains, and cereals that are iron-fortified.

High-fat foods—small amounts daily. While an adequate fat intake was essential during pregnancy, and your body was able to handle even those foods high in cholesterol with impunity, it is now once again necessary for you to consider limiting fat in your diet and carefully selecting the type of fat you do consume. It is generally agreed that the average adult should get no more than 30% of his or her total calories from fat; those at high risk for heart disease should limit their intake even more rigidly. This means that if your ideal weight is 125 pounds, you need 1,875 calories daily, no more than 30% of those, or 62 grams, from fat. That's the equivalent of 4½ fat servings (at 14 grams per) a day. If you're lighter, you will need fewer servings; if you're heavier, more. You can expect that you will get roughly one serving from drips and drabs in low-fat foods. The rest can come from fatty foods. One half fat serving equals: 1 ounce of hard cheese (Swiss, Cheddar, etc.); 1½ ounces mozzarella, provolone; 2 tablespoons grated Parmesan; 1½ tablespoons light cream, pecans, peanuts, or walnuts; 2 tablespoons whipped cream; 1 tablespoon cream cheese; 1 cup whole milk or whole-milk yogurt; ½ cup regular ice cream; 6 ounces tofu; ¼ small avocado; 1 tablespoon peanut butter; 3½ ounces dark meat or 7 ounces light meat turkey or chicken (no skin); 4 ounces fatty fish (such as salmon); 9 french fries; 1 egg yolk; 2 small biscuits or 1 average muffin; 1 slice of cake or 3 cookies (these vary with recipes). Full servings equal: 1 tablespoon olive, safflower, corn, canola, or other vegetable oils, butter, margarine, or regular mayonnaise; 2 tablespoons regular salad dressing; 3 to 6 ounces lean meat or 1 to 1½ ounces fattier cuts; ¾ cup tuna salad.

Salty foods—limited quantities. While salt was necessary in pregnancy, you need to begin limiting it now. As a rule, avoid highly salted foods such as salted pea-

5. Eat liver only rarely in spite of its great nutritive value because of its very high cholesterol content and because it is a storehouse for the chemicals, including questionable ones, to which an animal is exposed.

nuts, potato chips, and pickles. Look for un-salted cheeses and snack foods, reduced- or low-sodium prepared foods. Unless some-one in your family is on a sodium-restricted diet, salting lightly to taste when cooking is okay. But remember that any family food you're planning to also feed to your baby or young child should go unsalted to the table—because infants can't handle a great deal of sodium and because exposing them to salt will help give them a taste for it.

Fluids—at least 8 cups daily if you're nursing, 6 to 8 if you're not. You will need to add 4 more cups if you're nursing twins. Water (preferably fluoridated), fruit and vegetable juices, milk, soups, and seltzer are all good fluid choices. But beware of too much of a good thing: excessive fluids (more than 12 cups a day if you're nursing one child) can inhibit breast milk production.

Vitamin supplements. Take a preg-nancy/lactation formula daily if you're breastfeeding—not as a replacement for a good diet, but as insurance because no-body's diet is perfect. If you eat no animal products (not even milk and eggs), you should be certain your supplement contains at least 4 micrograms of vitamin B_{12} (which is found naturally only in animal foods), 0.5 milligrams of folic acid, and if you don't get at least half an hour's dose of sunshine daily, 400 milligrams of vitamin D (the amount fortifying a quart of milk).

Even if you're not breastfeeding, you should continue taking your pregnancy vi-tamins for at least the first six weeks post-partum. After that, a standard multiple vitamin/mineral supplement will fill in the nutritional gaps if you find you don't al-ways have the time or opportunity to eat as well as you'd like. A supplement designed for women in the child-bearing years will provide the extra iron needed to replace iron that might have been depleted with preg-nancy and/or postpartum bleeding and will again be lost when menstruation resumes. While you're nursing, your supplement should contain zinc.

IF YOU'RE NOT BREASTFEEDING

Though good nutrition is important for all mothers postpartum, there are some basic differences in dietary needs between bot-tle-feeding and breastfeeding moms that you should be aware of. For one, if you're not breastfeeding, you can't continue eating for two. (If you did, you would soon end up looking like two.) For another, because what you eat and drink will no longer have a direct effect on your baby (unless it tam-pers with your temperament or energy level), you'll be able to be somewhat less rigid when it comes to sugar, caffeine, diet soft drinks, and alcohol. Be aware, how-ever, that caution and moderation are still necessary. Consider the following:

■ Excess sugar in the diet can cause tooth decay, obesity and/or malnourishment, and once a "sugar high" has ended, deep lows in energy and spirit often follow.

■ Excess caffeine can lead to jitteriness, emotional instability, and at doses of 10 cups of coffee or more, ringing in the ears, delirium, irregular heartbeat, muscle ten-sion, and trembling.

■ Saccharin is suspected of being a weak carcinogen, and though moderate intakes of aspartame (Equal, Nutrasweet) have not been shown to be hazardous, the effects of excessive amounts over long periods are as yet unknown.

■ Excesses of alcohol can impair your abil-ity to cope sanely and safely with the tasks of mothering and can aggravate postpartum depression—not to mention the potential physical and emotional damage to the entire family over the long haul. A mother who drinks more than lightly (one to two drinks daily) puts her child at risk.

■ Excesses of any or all nutritionally empty foods (such as sugar) or beverages (such as wine, beer, hard liquor, or soft drinks) can interfere with your intake of necessary nutrients.

■ Any amount of tobacco use by you can in-

crease your child's risk of a variety of illnesses as well as deprive him or her of a parent prematurely.
■ The use of any illegal drug (cocaine, marijuana, heroin, crack, and so on) or the abuse of legal drugs (uppers, downers) can be damaging to your relationship with your child, threaten your child's health and safety (as well as your own), and be catastrophic to any future pregnancies.

WHAT YOU MAY BE CONCERNED ABOUT

GETTING EVERYTHING DONE

"I've been home with my new daughter for only two days and I'm already falling behind on everything: cleaning, laundry, dishes, literally everything. My once immaculate house is now a mess. I've always considered myself a competent person—till now."

Take the responsibility of caring for a newborn baby for the first time. Days and nights that seem like one endless feeding. Add a few too many visitors. A generous helping of postpartum hormonal upheaval. Possibly, a fair amount of clutter accumulated during your stay in the hospital. And the inevitable mountain of gifts, boxes, wrapping paper, and cards to keep track of. It's only natural to feel that as your new life with your baby is beginning, your old life—with its order and cleanliness—is crumbling around you.

Don't despair. Your inability to keep up with both baby and house during the first days at home in no way predicts your future success at mothering. (You can't, after all, judge an inexperienced employee's future performance on the basis of her first two days at a demanding new job.) Things are bound to get better as you regain your strength, become familiar with the basic baby-care tasks, and learn to be a little less rigid. It will also help to:

Get hold of yourself. Dwelling anxiously on what you have to do makes facing it twice as difficult. Relax. Focus on what's really important: getting to know and enjoy your newborn. Banish thoughts of household chores while you're with her (relaxation techniques learned in childbirth class may help you to do this). When you look around you later on, the clutter and chaos will still be there, but you'll be better able to deal with it.

Get rest. Paradoxically, the best way to start getting things done is to start getting more rest. Give yourself a chance to recuperate fully from childbirth and you will be better able to tackle your new responsibilities.

Get help. If you haven't already arranged for household help—paid or unpaid—and taken steps to streamline housekeeping and cooking chores, now's the time to do so (see page 16). If necessary, remind your spouse that yours is a two-parent home (but gently, especially if he's not yet used to the idea; see page 544). Think of ways that he (or someone else you can rely on) can help ease your load—by calling you before leaving work in the evening for a list of last-minute items to pick up at the store, or dropping off the drycleaning on the way to work, or vacuuming and/or picking up where needed while you give the baby the last feeding of the evening (waking in the morning to at least a semblance of neatness can give your spirits a real boost).

Get your priorities straight. What's

most important? The condition of your house or your new baby? Is it more important to get the vacuuming done while baby's napping or to put your feet up and relax so you can be refreshed when she awakens? Is it really essential to touch up those wash-and-wear shirts, or would taking the baby out for a walk in the stroller be a better use of your time? Keep in mind that doing too much too soon can rob you of the energy to accomplish anything well, and that while your house will someday be clean again, your baby will never be two days (or two weeks, or two months) old again.

Get organized. Lists are a new mother's best friend. First thing every morning, while you're nursing (if you can manage it) or while your husband is giving baby her bottle or playing with her, jot down a list of what needs to be done. Divide your priorities into three categories: chores that must be taken care of as soon as possible, those that can wait until later in the day, and those that can be put off until tomorrow—or next week, or indefinitely. Assign approximate times to each activity, taking into account your personal biological clock (are you useless first thing in the morning, or do you do your best work at the crack of dawn?) as well as your baby's (as best as you can determine it at this point).

Though organizing your day on paper doesn't always mean that everything will get done on schedule (in fact, for new mothers it rarely does), it will give you a sense of control over what may now seem like a largely uncontrollable situation; plans on paper are always more manageable than plans whirling frenetically through your head. You may even find, once you've made your list, that you actually have less to do than you'd thought. Don't forget to cross off completed tasks for a satisfying feeling of accomplishment. And don't worry about what's not crossed off—just move those items to the next day's list.

Another good organizational trick of the new mother trade: keep a running list of baby gifts and their givers as they're re-ceived. You think you'll remember that Cousin Doris sent that darling blue-and-yellow sweater set, but after the seventeenth sweater set has arrived, that memory may be dimmed. And check off each as the thank-you is sent so you don't have to ponder, "Did I or didn't I thank Aunt Jane?"

Get simplified. Use a one-step product on the kitchen floor, paper plates at the dinner table, frozen vegetables instead of fresh; order in pizza one night, pick up a selection from the local salad bar the next; take whatever steps are practical to cut down the time it takes to do necessary chores. Keep supplies and equipment close to where you will be using them to reduce the number of trips you have to make from room to room. Pack away for now knickknacks and other items that take special care (they'll have to go once baby begins to crawl, anyway).

Get a jump on tomorrow tonight. Once you've bedded baby down each night, and before you collapse onto the sofa for that well-deserved rest, summon up the strength to take care of a few chores so that you'll have a head start on the next morning. Restock the diaper bag. Prepare formula and fill the bottles. Measure out the coffee for the coffee pot. Sort the laundry. Lay out clothes for yourself and the baby. In ten minutes or so, you'll accomplish what would take you three times as long—at least—with baby awake. And you'll be able to sleep better (when she lets you) knowing that you'll have less to do in the morning.

Get good at doubling up. Learn to do two things at once. Wash the dishes or grate carrots for the meat loaf while you're on the phone. Balance your checkbook or fold the laundry while you catch the news on TV. Read a book or tell an older child a story while you nurse a sleepy baby (an alert one needs more attention). There still won't be enough hours in the day, but this way you may only crave 36 instead of 48.

Get out. Unless the weather's inclement,

plan an outing every day. This won't help you get the dusting done or the floors washed, but it will make these tasks seem less urgent.

Get to expect the unexpected. The best laid plans of mothers often (actually *very* often) go astray. Baby's all bundled up for an outing, the diaper bag is ready, your coat is on, and suddenly the distinct gurglings of a bowel movement can be heard from under all baby's gear. Off comes coat, bunting, diaper—ten minutes lost and a tight schedule is knocked totally out of kilter. To allow for such unexpected turns of events, build extra time into your daily schedules.

Get the joke. If you can laugh at your predicament, you're less likely to cry. So keep your sense of humor—even in the face of total disorder and utter clutter. Not only will this help you to keep your sanity, it will save your child from being one of those adults who looks back on a childhood where nobody smiled—because everyone was too busy maintaining order.

Get used to it. Living with a baby means living with a certain amount of mayhem most of the time. And as baby grows, so will the difficulty of keeping the mayhem in check. No sooner will you scoop the blocks back into their canister than she will dump them back out again. As fast as you can wipe mashed peas off the wall behind her high chair, she can redecorate with strained peaches. You'll put safety latches on the kitchen cabinets, and she'll figure out how to open them, covering the linoleum with your pots and pans.

And remember, when you finally pack your last child off to college, your house will be immaculate once again—and so lonely that you'll be ready to welcome the pandemonium they bring home on school vacations.

NOT BEING IN CONTROL

"For the last ten years I've run my business, my household, and every other aspect of my life quite effectively. But ever since I came home with my little boy, I can't seem to get control of anything."

There's been a coup in your home—as there is in the homes of all new parents. And the man who would be king in your castle isn't a man at all, but a newborn baby boy. As powerless as he may seem, he is quite capable of disrupting your life and usurping the control you once had over it. He won't care if you customarily take your shower at 7:15 and your coffee at 8:05, if you favor a leisurely cocktail at 6:30 and dinner promptly at 7:00, if you enjoy dancing into the wee hours on Saturday night and sleeping luxuriously late the morning after. He'll demand feedings and attention when he wants them, without first checking your schedule to see if it's convenient. Which means your routine and many of your old, comfortable ways may have to be abandoned for several months, if not several years. The only schedule that will matter, particularly in these early weeks, is his. And that schedule, at first, may have no discernible pattern you can latch onto. Days, and especially nights, may pass as a blur. You may often feel more like an automaton (and if you're nursing, a milk cow) than a person, more servant than master, wielding not the slightest measure of power over your life.

What to do? Hand the scepter over graciously—at least for now. With the passage of time, as you grow more competent, confident, and comfortable in your new role, and as your baby becomes more capable and less dependent, you will regain some of the control you've lost. Don't, however, expect to regain absolute power.

You might as well accept the fact that your life will never be quite the same, but then, would you really want it to be?

REGAINING YOUR FIGURE

"I knew I wouldn't be ready for a bikini right after delivery, but I still look six months pregnant a week later."

Though childbirth produces more rapid initial weight loss than the Scarsdale, Stillman, and Mayo Clinic diets combined (an average of 12 pounds at delivery), few women are satisfied with the results. Particularly after they catch a glimpse of their postpartum silhouettes in a mirror and see that they still look distressingly pregnant. The good news is that most are able to pack away their pregnancy jeans within the month. The bad news: the old jeans may not fit the way they used to for a while longer.

How quickly you return to your prepregnant shape and weight will depend on how many pounds and inches you put on during pregnancy—and where they settled. Women who gained between 20 and 30 pounds on a good diet and at a gradual and steady pace may be able to shed it all, without dieting, by the end of the second month or so. On the other hand, those who overindulged and gained more than was necessary to produce a healthy, good-size baby—particularly if the weight was gained in uneven spurts on junk food—may find the return to postpartum shape more challenging.

No matter what your weight gain, sticking to the Best-Odds Postpartum and Breastfeeding Diet now should lead to slow, steady weight loss—with no loss of energy. Non-nursers can, once the six-week postpartum recovery period has passed, go on a sensible, well-balanced reducing diet with exercise to drop whatever pounds remain. Nursing mothers who aren't losing weight can reduce calorie intake by a couple of hundred a day and increase activity to encourage weight loss without cutting into milk production. They will usually take off any remaining excess poundage when they wean their babies.[6]

But there are several reasons for that postpartum pregnant look that have nothing to do with weight gain. One is 5 pounds or so leftover fluids, which will bloat your belly for the first few days after delivery but will flush out naturally, on their own, within the week. Another is the still-enlarged uterus, which continues to give the abdomen a pregnant appearance until it is finally reduced to prepregnancy size and has slipped back into the pelvis, usually by the end of the sixth postpartum week. But the major and most persistent reason most women continue to look a little pregnant well after delivery is stretched out abdominal muscles and skin. For most women, even after weight loss is accomplished, returning the abdomen to prepregnancy tone will require more than waiting for time and nature to take their course. In fact, it will sag for a lifetime unless a concerted exercise effort is made (see Getting Back into Shape on page 525).

There are, alas, some body changes that will stay with you no matter how many sit-ups and leg lifts you do and how carefully you monitor your diet—though you may not even be aware of them. Most common is a change in body configuration due to the loosening of the joints during pregnancy (to facilitate delivery) and their tightening up again postpartum. The changes may be either imperceptible or significant enough to increase a shoe or dress size. Women who have had c-sections may also note a slight alteration in the shape of the abdomen that won't yield to exercise.

---

6. A nursing mother should never reduce her caloric intake drastically, however, since excessive burning of her own body fat could result in the release of ketones (byproducts of fat metabolism) and of toxic chemicals or drugs stored in the fat into her milk, which could be harmful to her baby.

SHARING BABY CARE

"I feel guilty asking my husband for help with our new baby, especially at night—after all, he works all day and has to get up early in the morning. Yet I'm exhausted handling her all by myself."

There's no more demanding job than the one you now hold; you'll need and deserve all the help you can get from your partner-in-parenthood. Having a job outside the home—even a particularly grueling one—doesn't automatically exempt a man from taking on work inside the home, especially when that work is created by the arrival of a new baby that's half his doing. And when you're tempted to feel guilty about asking for help, remind yourself that you've been working all day, too, at a job that is almost undoubtedly more tiring and stressful (as much because of the newness as the nature of the work) than your mate's. And unless he's a professional baby nurse, helping you out with baby care will be a refreshing and satisfying break from the demands of his day, rather than an exhausting and tedious extension of them. And even if he is a professional baby nurse—or a pediatrician, or a school teacher, or if he works with little ones in some other capacity—taking care of his own child will still be uniquely rewarding.

Of course, you may have to do some persuading to gain his full cooperation, and some initial labor negotiations may have to take place to work out a baby-and-house-care program that is mutually acceptable. Ideally it is one that takes some of the burden off you without placing too much on him. (The initial deal can be renegotiated should you return to work.) Begin with these steps:

Speak up. Perhaps your husband isn't even aware that you need his help—maybe you're working too hard at making it look effortless. Or that you want his help—maybe he's gotten the impression you'd rather do it yourself, or that you think he's not competent to care for a baby. Sit down with him at a quiet time, when the baby's asleep and you're both fairly relaxed, and explain your needs calmly and rationally. You might find that your doing all the baby care is bothering him as much as it is you.

Teach him a thing or two. If lack of confidence and experience are keeping your husband from trying his hand at baby care, he will benefit from a few lessons. First demonstrate, then talk him through, several diaper changes. Have him observe and assist at bath time and in dressing the baby. Teach him a basic lullaby and share your most successful rocking technique with him (but remember, daddies generally hold babies differently than mommies do, and his own method may be even more successful than yours). Be a patient instructor, and don't give up (or let him give up) if he takes ten minutes to change his first dirty diaper, if baby comes out of the first bath still soapy, or if he puts her dress on backwards. Keep in mind (and remind him) that fathers (like mothers) are made, not born, and that he has the innate capacity for mastering the fine art of baby care. At first, it may seem easier to change a diaper yourself than to watch him struggle through it. But eventually your efforts will pay off—as your husband becomes a thoroughly capable parenting partner.

Leave him alone. That is, with the baby. Occasionally devise (deviously, if need be) reasons why daddy and baby must be left alone together. Start with short periods of time—say fifteen or twenty minutes—and build up from there. Forced to perform in a sink-or-swim situation, most new fathers surprise themselves and their mates by staying afloat. This will build his self-confidence and give him a chance to get to know the baby, which will in turn make him feel better disposed toward helping out.

Overlook his mistakes. Unless something he's doing might endanger the baby (throwing her up in the air, for instance), don't be quick to comment on your husband's flubs. He's more likely to learn from his own mistakes (or your good example) than from your criticism. When you do need to show him the error of his ways, do so gently, to avoid undermining his self-confidence and creating hostility. And be ready to learn from him.

Set up a standard operating policy. For some people, drawing up and keeping to a schedule (Monday, Wednesday, and Friday nights you change the diapers and he gives the bath, Tuesday and Thursday nights you bathe, he diapers, and so on) is the only way to ensure all the jobs will get done and the work will be divided fairly. For others, particularly those who see no need to keep score, divvying up responsibilities as they come along ("Could you change her diaper while I finish the dishes?") is a workable system. For still others, assigning duties according to personal strengths works best. If your husband's a four-star chef but you burn water, let him take over the kitchen. If baby seems to think dad's got more rhythm than you, let him do the rocking. But if he's hopelessly inept at holding a squirming, wet baby—even after repeated practice—you take over the bath chore.

Share the nights. Even if you're nursing, there's no reason why your husband should sleep through every night when you and baby don't. There's more to the middle-of-the-night routine than feeding. Dad can pick baby up, diaper her if that's necessary, then bring her to bed for you to breastfeed. Depending on who's got more strength, either of you can return the little darling to her crib or cradle when feeding is done. But baby will probably be less likely to waken if the deed is done by dad, since the closeness of your breasts might prompt her to ask for seconds. If you're bottle feeding, either partially or totally, nighttime feedings can be divided between the two of you according to a mutually agreeable schedule. Maybe he takes all the feedings before 2 A.M. and you take all that follow. Or you alternate nights.

In spite of the best of intentions and the greatest goodwill, you may still end up doing the lioness' share of the child-rearing work. Many men, even if they believe intellectually in equality of the sexes (and especially if they don't) and were eager to participate in labor and delivery (and especially if they weren't), are just not ready to accept a full share of child-care tasks. Some may equate being a good father with being a good provider and feel that they are more than pulling their weight in the family by working longer hours. Others, because they have no role models on which to build (they were fatherless, or their own fathers steered clear of child-rearing duties), are uncomfortable and uncertain when confronted with parenting responsibilities. Old attitudes die hard.

If your husband, for whatever reason, fails to share the load with you, try to understand why this is so and to communicate clearly where you stand. Don't expect him to change overnight, and don't let your resentment when he doesn't trigger arguments and stress. Instead explain, educate, entice; in time, he'll meet you—partway, if not all the way.

DEPRESSION

"I have everything I've always wanted: a wonderful husband, a beautiful new baby girl—why do I feel so miserable?"

Roughly one-half (some estimates go as high as 90%) of all new mothers ask the same question, complaining of weepiness, unhappiness, anxiety, and mood swings during the first week or so after delivery. This bout of "baby blues" is probably related to the precipitous drop in estrogen and progesterone after childbirth, and usually clears up within a few days, though some women find it comes and goes over the first six weeks.

Less common (it probably affects 25% of first-time mothers and 20% in subsequent pregnancies) and longer lasting (it often begins during the first six weeks and can persist for months) is true postpartum depression. Hormone variations offer one explanation for this depression. The fact that sensitivity to hormonal fluctuations varies from woman to woman is believed to explain, at least partially, why it is that although all women experience the same shift in hormonal levels after delivery, not all suffer mood changes. Depression can also be triggered by the hormonal changes related to weaning.

But there are a host of other factors that are believed to contribute to postpartum depression. Some of these non-hormonal factors may explain why fathers and adoptive mothers, who have no postpartum hormone changes to blame, are also subject to such depression:

The end of the pregnancy. For women who passed the nine months in relative misery—with morning sickness, varicose veins, backaches, and indigestion—the end of pregnancy is something to celebrate. But if you thoroughly enjoyed pregnancy, its conclusion may be something to mourn, particularly if more children are not on your agenda. You may feel a sense of loss and emptiness, and miss the uniquely intimate sensation of carrying your baby inside you. You may even regret the disappearance of your bulging belly, to which you'd grown fondly accustomed.

A feeling of anticlimax. Childbirth—the big event you'd trained for and anticipated for so long—is over.

The shift from center stage to backstage. Your baby is now the star of the show. Visitors flock to stand at the nursery window rather than sit at your bedside inquiring after your health. Your husband, who may have kept you on a pedestal for nine months, may now be so busy doting on his newborn child that, however unintentionally, he ends up ignoring you when you need his adoration most. With a wave of the obstetrician's wand, you've done a reverse Cinderella—the pregnant princess has become the postpartum peasant. This change in status will accompany you home. When you go out with the baby now, people may be less quick to offer assistance—as you struggle to fold a stroller, juggle a baby and a diaper bag, and hail a cab—than when you were pregnant and were carrying the baby almost effortlessly inside of you. Strangers won't glance at your tummy and beam anymore, friends won't comment on your radiance; all eyes will be on the baby and all compliments and smiles directed at her.

Hospitalization. Eager to get home and begin mothering, you may be frustrated by the lack of control you have over your life and your baby's in the hospital, and a prolonged stay may compound your frustration. If this is not your first baby, you may miss your older child or children, feel guilty about being away from them, and worry about how they're doing—particularly if this is the first time you've been separated.

Going home. It's not unusual to feel overwhelmed and overworked by the responsibilities that greet you ("What do I do first?"), especially if you have no help and if dishes, dust, and dirty clothes have been allowed to pile up while you've been away. Returning to a house that's now crowded with baby things (your home has been taken over by this tiny invader) may also be unsettling.

Disappointment. In your newborn: she is so small, so red, so puffy, so unresponsive—not the cuddly, all-smiles Ivory Snow baby you pictured. About the birth and/or in yourself: if unrealistic expectations of an idealized childbirth experience weren't realized, you may feel (unnecessarily) that you're a failure. About motherhood: it isn't at all what you expected, and the letdown is depressing.

Exhaustion. Fatigue following childbirth, compounded by the rigors of caring for a newborn, can make you feel unable to meet the multiple challenges you face.

Lack of sleep. People deprived of sleep, whether they are airline pilots, prisoners of war, or doctors in training, can experience severe mood changes. New mothers are no exception.

Physical discomfort or pain. Your episiotomy or cesarean incision burns, your breasts are uncomfortably engorged, your hemorrhoids are excruciating, and those afterpains are a pain. It's not easy to be cheerful when you hurt so much.

Feelings of inadequacy. Virtually every new mother doubts her ability to handle the role. If you're a total novice, you may wonder "Why did I have a baby if I can't take care of it?" If you're a veteran who had reached the point of handling one child with aplomb but are now overwhelmed by two, you may wonder "Why did I have another?" If you seem to get less respect in the role of mother than you did when you held a paying job, you may feel like less of a person. And it's disheartening not to feel good about yourself.

Feelings of guilt. Maybe you really didn't want this baby when you became pregnant, and even though you do now, you feel guilty. Or you feel guilty about not loving her at first sight, or not thinking she's beautiful, or not enjoying the tedium of motherhood. Or about having to go back to work in the near future, or not bringing in income if you're planning to stay home. Guilt, no matter what the cause, can be very depressing.

Mourning for the old you. Your carefree, possibly career-oriented self has passed (at least temporarily) with your baby's birth. So has your self- and/or couple-oriented way of life—time-consuming hobbies, frequent dining out, classes, or movies may realistically have to take a back burner for a while.

Unhappiness over your appearance. Before you were fat and pregnant; now, to your over-critical eyes, you're just plain fat. You can't stand wearing maternity clothes anymore, but nothing else fits.

Lack of support. If you don't have enough support—from family and friends, but especially from your spouse—facing the job of new mother may be overwhelming and depressing.

Nonbaby-related stress. Problems—family, job, financial—that aren't related to your new baby can nevertheless induce postpartum depression.

Though there's no sure cure for postpartum depression other than the passage of time, there are ways of minimizing it (some physicians are using gradually decreasing doses of hormones successfully) and of fading those baby blues:

■ If the blues arrive at the hospital, ask your husband to bring in a romantic dinner for two; limit visitors if their chattering grates on your nerves, invite more of them if they cheer you up. If it's the hospital environment that's getting you down, inquire about early discharge (see page 522).

■ Fight fatigue by accepting help from others, by being less compulsive about doing things now that can wait until later, and by trying to grab a nap or rest period when your baby is napping. Use baby feeding times as your rest periods—nurse or bottle feed in bed or in a comfortable chair with your feet up.

■ Follow the Best-Odds Nursing or Postpartum Diet (page 534) to keep your strength up. Avoid sugar (especially in combination with chocolate), which can act as a depressant in some people.

■ If you enjoy a drink, unwind with your husband over a cocktail during the baby's dinner hour or enjoy a glass of wine during your own, but be careful not to overdo—even moderate amounts of alcohol can exacerbate your depression and, if you're nursing, intoxicate your baby.

■ Treat yourselves to dinner out, if possible. If not, make believe. Order dinner in (or maybe your husband will cook), dress up, create a five-star-restaurant ambience with candlelight and soft music. And keep your sense of humor handy, in case baby decides to interrupt your romantic interlude.

■ Communicate to your husband any feelings of under-appreciation you may be experiencing. He may not realize that you need him as much as the baby does.

■ Ask for help with the house, the baby, other children—from your husband, your mother, your neighbors, your friends, or whoever's willing, able, and available. If you can't get all the help you need for free, and if you can afford it, consider hiring someone (a teenager, an elderly neighbor) to free you up for an hour or two a day—so you can freshen up, take a bath or a nap, prepare dinner, or do whatever else you need to do.

■ If your problem is coping with the new baby plus a toddler, or more—the depression usually increases geometrically with each baby—see the tips in Chapter 26.

■ Look your best so you'll feel your best. Walking around, hair unkempt, in a robe all day would depress anyone. Shower before your husband leaves in the morning (you may not get a chance later); comb your hair; put on makeup if you ordinarily wear it.

■ Get out of the house. Meet a friend for lunch, window shop, traipse through a museum—with the baby, or if you can enlist a volunteer to stay home with her, without.

■ Get active. Exercise can help chase away the baby blues and, at the same time, get rid of any postpartum flab that might be compounding your depression. (See page 525.)

■ Make some time for yourself. Set aside half an hour or so a day just for you, and pretend you're a lady of leisure. While your baby naps or someone else watches her, read the newspaper (unless current events depress you), make a dent in that novel, watch a video movie, do an exercise routine, catch up on your letter writing, pamper yourself with a facial, a manicure, or a bubble bath.

■ If you think your misery might like some company, get together with any new mothers you know and compare frustrations. If you don't know any, find some. Ask your pediatrician for names of new mothers in your neighborhood and start a new-mothers group. Contact women who were in your childbirth class and organize a weekly re-union. Take a postpartum exercise or parenting class (most welcome babies).

■ If yours is the kind of misery that wants to be alone, indulge in some solitude. Though ordinary depression generally feeds on itself, some experts believe that this is not true of the postpartum variety. If spending time with cheerful people only makes your mood worse, avoid socializing for a while. Don't, however, leave your husband out in the cold. Husbands, too, are susceptible to postpartum depression, and yours may need your support as much as you need his.

■ *Seek professional help immediately* if your depression persists for more than one week and is accompanied by sleeplessness (you can't sleep even when the baby does); lack of appetite; loss of interest in yourself and your family; a feeling of hopelessness, helplessness, and lack of control; suicidal urges; the wish that the baby were gone or had never come; thoughts of harming the baby; other weird thoughts or fears, hallucinations or delusions.

Though severe postpartum depression that requires professional therapy is relatively rare—estimated at less than 1 in 1,000—more than 3,000 women in this country suffer from it annually. On the chance that you could be one of them, get a professional diagnosis in a hurry if you have the symptoms of severe depression described here. Don't allow yourself to be put off by "Oh, it's the baby blues—you'll get over it" or "Just buck up and you'll be fine." Prolonged maternal depression can interfere with mother-child bonding and interaction, and is often detrimental to an infant.

If you are unsure of where to turn, ask your obstetrician, nurse-midwife, family doctor, cleric, or a friend who has had a good counseling experience to refer you, or call a community mental health center. Contact a postpartum depression support group if there's one in your community, or find out about starting one.[7] If you see a non-medical therapist, you should also have a medical doctor involved in your treatment, because postpartum depression has a hormonal component.

If at any time you feel a strong urge to hurt your baby, whether you think you're depressed or not, go immediately to a neighbor's house, call a doctor (yours or your baby's) or someone who can get to where you are in a hurry (a friend, your husband, your mother), or dial 911. You can be helped.

"I feel terrific, and have since the moment I delivered three weeks ago. Is all this good feeling leading up to one terrific case of the blues?"

Unfortunately, feeling good isn't nearly as newsworthy as feeling bad. You'll find no shortage of coverage in magazines, newspapers, or books of the roughly 50% of newly delivered women who are affected to some degree by postpartum depression; but you'll see little or nothing written about the other 50% who aren't, and who feel terrific after giving birth.

Baby blues are common, but they're by no means inevitable. And there's no reason to believe that if you've been feeling buoyant, you're in for an emotional dunking. Since most cases of postpartum depression occur within the first week after birth, the odds are pretty good that you've escaped them. If you'd like to improve the odds even further, see the tips for fading those baby blues (page 545). They can prevent as well as cure.

Some women have mild mood swings postpartum as they did during pregnancy—they feel overwhelmed and inadequate one day (baby didn't sleep at all, spit up all over a new blouse, and leaked a bowel movement on the couch), euphoric and competent the next (baby took three three-hour naps, got rave reviews in the supermarket, and smiled a first smile). Such mood swings are both normal and temporary.

Very occasionally a woman does develop a delayed case of postpartum blues, sometimes at the time of weaning her baby from the breast. Anyone who at any time develops the symptoms of severe depression described on page 548 should seek immediate professional help.

FEELING INADEQUATE

"I really thought I could handle it. But the moment our little boy was handed to me, all my confidence dissolved. I feel as though I'm a total flop as a mother."

Though the ultimate rewards of motherhood are greater than those of any other occupation, the stresses and challenges are greater, too—particularly at the beginning. After all, there's no other job in the world that thrusts you, without previous training or experience and without supervisory guidance, into fully responsible eighteen-to twenty-hour shifts. What's more, there's no other job that offers as little feedback during the first weeks to let you know how you're doing. The only person who could possibly give you a job evaluation is a largely unresponsive, unpredictable, and uncooperative newborn who doesn't smile when he's satisfied, doesn't hug you when he's grateful, sleeps when he should be eating, cries when he should be sleeping, hardly even looks at you for more than a couple of minutes, and doesn't seem to know you from the next-door neighbor. A sense of satisfaction in a job completed seems totally absent. Virtually every job you do—changing diapers, making formula, washing baby clothes, feeding baby—is quickly undone and/or needs redoing almost immediately. It's not surprising that you feel like a failure at your new profession.

Even for a seasoned pro the postpartum period is no picnic; for a novice, it can seem like a never-ending series of blunders, bumbles, mishaps, and misadventures. And yet there are better times in sight

7. For information on such groups, contact: Depression After, the Delivery Support Group, PO Box 1282, Morrisville, PA 19067; 215-295-3994.

(though you may have trouble envisioning them); competence at mothering is closer than you'd now imagine. In the meantime, keep these points in mind:

You're unique. And so is your baby. What works for another mother and baby may not work for you, and vice versa. Avoid making comparisons.

You're not the only one. More first-time mothers than ever before have had no previous experience with newborns. And even among those who've had some, very few manage to glide through those first weeks as though they'd been doing it all their lives. Remember, mothers are not born, they are made on the job. Hormones do not magically transform newly delivered women into able mothers; time, trial and error, and experience do. If you have the opportunity of sharing your worries with other new mothers, you will be reminded that though you are unique, your concerns as a new mother aren't.

You need to be babied. In order to be an effective mother, you've got to baby yourself a little. Tell yourself, as your own mother would, that you need to eat right and get enough rest, particularly in the postpartum period, and that moderate exercise to keep your energy level up and a bit of relaxation now and then to elevate your spirits are important, too.

You're both only human. You shouldn't expect or demand perfection from either yourself or your baby—now, or at any point in your relationship.

Your instincts can be trusted. Give them a chance instead of self-doubting them away. In many cases, even the greenest mother knows more about what's right for her baby than more experienced friends and relatives or baby books.

You needn't go it alone. While you should trust your own instincts and shouldn't make comparisons, there's a lot of good advice and comforting support out there you can benefit from. Seeking it from grandmas, sisters, or friends, or in books or magazines doesn't brand you as incompetent, but as open-minded and willing to learn. Judiciously sift through information acquired from others, test out what seems right for you and your baby, discard what doesn't.

Your mistakes can help you grow, and they won't count against you. Nobody's going to fire you (though on a particularly bad day you may wish that you could quit) if you make mistakes. Mistakes are an important part of learning to be a mother. You can expect to continue making them at least until your children are off to college. And if at first you don't succeed, just try, try something else (the baby only screams louder when you rock him in your arms side to side, so try holding him over your shoulder and swaying back and forth).

Your love won't always come easy. It's sometimes difficult to relate lovingly to a newborn—a basically unresponsive creature who takes greedily but doesn't offer much in return (except dirty diapers). And it may be some time before you stop feeling like a fool, babbling in baby talk and crooning off-key lullabies, and before you can hug and kiss this tiny bundle naturally and unselfconsciously. (See page 264 for tips on talking to baby.)

Your baby is forgiving. Forget to change his diaper before a feeding. Let soap drip into his eye during his shampoo. Get a turtleneck stuck halfway over his head. Your baby will forgive and forget these and a multitude of other minor sins—as long as he gets the message that you love him loud and clear. If he does, he will even forgive you when you're too frazzled to smile at him or when you let him cry for an extra few minutes because you're in the bathroom or a pot is boiling over on the stove.

The ultimate rewards are fantastic. Think of motherhood as a long-term project, with results that will be unfolding in the months and years ahead. When you see your baby's first smile, watch him reach for a toy, laugh out loud, pull himself up, say "Mommy, I love you," you will know that you've done a good job, that you have indeed accomplished something very special.

VISITORS

"I feel like a real heel, but I'm tired of the steady stream of visitors at our door since our son was born."

Short of hanging a "quarantine" or "gone fishin'" sign on your front door, there's little you can do to keep your baby's admirers away entirely. There's no more powerful magnet to friends, family, and neighbors, after all, than a newborn. But there are ways of minimizing the number of visits, and of making those that are unavoidable less burdensome:

■ Limit visitors the first week or two to immediate family and close friends. You can put the blame on "doctor's orders," since most agree that visitors should be limited during the first few postpartum weeks.

■ Buy or borrow a telephone answering machine and tape a message that gives all the pertinent baby data to callers—date of birth, weight, name—as well as the information that visitors are limited. Return the calls at your convenience, inviting close friends and family to visit at specific times.

■ Ask visitors to call ahead; don't be afraid to say that a suggested stop-in time is not convenient, but do propose an alternative when possible.

■ Be the hostess with the leastest, for now. Put a bowl of fruit on the coffee table and some paper cups next to the kitchen sink if that makes you feel any better, but don't offer more elaborate refreshments—save your energy for feeding the baby.

■ Don't be shy about letting guests know when they've overstayed their welcome. A not so subtle hint, such as "I've got to grab a nap while baby's napping," should get the point across. Of course, for those who don't take hints, there's nothing wrong with a candid request to leave.

■ Consider "showing" your baby at a single event—perhaps a baptism, a ritual circumcision, a baby naming, or a welcome-baby party—and let friends know they will have a chance to see him then. Get grandmas or other relatives or close friends to help set up the party so that you won't overwork. Keep it simple (unless you can afford a catered affair), sticking to a limited menu of cheese, crackers, and wine, or coffee and cake.

Whatever you do, don't feel guilty because you aren't eager for visitors. You are going through a very complex adjustment period, and you have a right to want—and to have—some peace, quiet, and privacy.

DOING THINGS RIGHT

"I'm so worried that I'm going to make a wrong move that I spend hours researching every little decision I make about my baby. I want to make sure I do everything right for her, but I'm driving myself and my husband crazy."

No one can do *everything* right—not even a mother. We all make mistakes—mostly little ones, occasionally bigger ones—in raising our children, and most of the time they make it to adulthood just fine. (In fact, it's through making a few mistakes and learning from them that we become more effective parents.) In addition, it's not always possible to know what's "right" in a particular situation; what's right for one mother and baby may in some cases be wrong for another.[8]

---

8. There are exceptions, however. In matters of safety, for example. It is *always* right to strap an infant in a car seat, even for short rides, and *always* right to keep poisonous substances locked out of a baby's reach. And in matters of health, no medical decision should be made without consultation with your baby's doctor.

Even reading all the literature and consulting experts won't always give you all the answers. Getting to know your baby and yourself, and learning to trust your instincts and good sense, is often a better route to making decisions you both can live with. It's true, for example, that some babies love to be snugly swaddled, but if yours cries whenever she's wrapped up tightly in a receiving blanket, consider that she would rather be free to kick up her heels. And the experts may tell you young babies like to listen to high-pitched sounds, but if yours clearly responds more positively to a deep voice, come down an octave. Trust yourself and your baby—you may not always be right, but you won't go too far wrong.

POSTPARTUM TUB BATHS

"I seem to be getting a lot of contradictory advice about whether or not tub baths are safe in the postpartum period. Are they?"

At one time new mothers weren't permitted to set foot in a tub until at least one month after delivery because it was believed that bacteria from the bath water would cause postpartum infection. Today, it's known that still bath water does not enter the vagina, and infection from bathing is no longer considered a threat. Some physicians, in fact, recommend tub baths in the hospital (when available) on the theory that bathing removes lochia from the perineum and from between the folds of the labia more efficiently than showering. In addition, the warm water is comforting to the sore episiotomy site, relieves swelling in the area, and soothes hemorrhoids.

Still, your doctor may prefer that you hold off on bathing at least until you go home, sometimes even later. If you're eager to bathe (which may be especially true if you have no shower at home), discuss the question with him or her; you may be able to get a dispensation. If you do bathe dur-

ing the first week or two following delivery, be sure the tub is well scrubbed before it's filled. (But be sure you're not the one who does the scrubbing.) And get help getting into and out of the tub during the first few postpartum days, when you still may be shaky. Whether you are using the shower or tub, be certain to always use a clean washcloth and towel, washing your breasts and nipples first (with water only), and then the perineum (with mild soap and water), before going on to the rest of you. Don't be afraid of opening any stitches as you wash; you won't.

TIME SPENT BREASTFEEDING

"Why didn't somebody tell me I'd be nursing my baby 24 hours a day?"

Maybe because you wouldn't have believed it. Or because nobody wanted to discourage you. Either way, now you know. Nursing is, for many mothers, a nearly round-the-clock job in the early weeks. But take heart; as time passes, you'll spend less of it as a captive of your baby's eager sucking. As breastfeeding becomes solidly established, the number of feedings will begin to tail off. By the time your baby's sleeping through the night, you'll probably be down to five or six feedings, taking a total of only three or four hours out of your day.

In the meantime, put everything else that's clamoring to be done out of your mind; relax and savor these special moments that only you can share with your baby. Make double use of them by keeping a baby journal, reading a book, or scheduling your day on paper. Chances are that once your baby is weaned, you'll look back and think how much you miss nursing.

CONTAMINATION OF BREAST MILK

"Does everything I eat or drink get into my breast milk? Could any of it harm my daughter?"

Feeding your baby outside the womb doesn't require quite the degree of careful monitoring of your own diet that feeding her inside the womb did. But for as long as you're breastfeeding, a certain amount of restraint is needed in what goes into you in order to ensure that everything that goes into your baby is safe.

The basic fat-protein-carbohydrate composition of human milk isn't dependent on what a mother eats. If a mother doesn't consume enough calories and protein to produce milk, her body will tap its own stores for milk production until the stores are depleted. Certain vitamin deficiencies in a mother's diet, however, can alter the vitamin content of her breast milk. So can excesses of certain vitamins. A wide variety of substances, from seasonings to medications, can also show up in breast milk, with varying implications for the newborn.

To keep breast milk safe and healthful, and up to your baby's taste specifications:

■ Follow the Best-Odds Nursing Diet (page 534).
■ Avoid foods to which your baby seems sensitive. Garlic, onions, cabbage, and chocolate are common offenders, provoking bothersome gas in some, though by no means all, babies. Some, particularly those with very discriminating palates, will simply reject the breast after you've eaten a food that imparts a strong or unfamiliar flavor to their accustomed beverage.
■ Take a vitamin supplement especially formulated for pregnant and/or lactating mothers. With the exception of vitamin C, which appears to enter the breast milk in only tiny amounts, *do not* take any other vitamins without the advice of your physician.
■ Do not smoke. Many of the toxic substances in tobacco enter the bloodstream, and eventually your milk. Though the long-term effects of these poisons on your baby aren't known for sure, one can safely speculate that they aren't positive. On top of that, it is known that second-hand smoke from parental smoking can cause a variety of health problems in their offspring.

■ Do not use any recreational drugs (other than an occasional single alcoholic beverage). Take medicines only with medical approval. Most drugs pass into breast milk to some extent — some appearing to have no effect on a nursing baby at all, others a mild transient effect, and still others a significant detrimental effect. But not enough is known about the long-term effects of medications on the nursing infant to recommend that a mother take any drug without first weighing the risks against benefits.

All medications which pose even a theoretical risk to the nursing baby carry a warning—on either the label, the package, or both. When the benefits outweigh the possible risks, your physician will probably okay the occasional use of certain of these (cold medications or mild pain relievers, for example) without medical consultation and prescribe others when your health requires it. Like an expectant mother, a nursing mother does neither herself nor her baby a favor by refusing prescribed medication under such circumstances. Do be sure, of course, that any doctor who prescribes a medication for you is aware that you are breastfeeding.

For the most up-to-date information on which drugs are believed safe and which aren't, check with your child's pediatrician or your local chapter of the March of Dimes Birth Defects Foundation. The most recent research indicates that most medicines (including acetaminophen, ibuprofen, most sedatives, antihistamines, decongestants, antihypertensives, antibiotics, and antithyroid drugs) are compatible with nursing. Some, however, including anticancer drugs, lithium, and ergots are clearly harmful. Others, including aspirin, many tranquilizers, antidepressants, and antipsychotics are suspect.

In some cases, a medication can safely be discontinued for the duration of nursing; in others, it is possible to find a safer substitute. When medication is needed short term, nursing can be interrupted temporarily (with breasts pumped and milk discarded). Or dosing can be timed for just after nursing or before baby's longest sleep period. Often non-drug treatments (see page 578) can be used.

■ Drink alcoholic beverages only rarely. Until recently, it was believed that one or two drinks a day would be harmless to the nursing infant, but a recent study suggests that as little as one glass of wine a day could slow both large and small motor development in the baby. More study needs to be done, but to be safe rather than sorry, limit alcohol intake. Alcohol has other drawbacks as well. It dehydrates, causing the loss of fluids needed for milk production. In large doses, it can make baby sleepy, sluggish, unresponsive, and unable to suck well. In very large doses, it can interfere with breathing. Alcohol can also impair your own functioning (whether you're nursing or not), making you more susceptible to depression, fatigue, and lapses in judgment, weakening your let-down reflex, and making you less able to care for, protect, and nourish your baby. And like any nutritionally vacant food or beverage, too much alcohol can add excess calories (and thus pounds) or divert your appetite from necessary nutrients. So drink only rarely. And then limit your intake to one or two drinks (one drink equals 12 ounces of beer, 5 ounces of wine, or 1½-ounces of distilled liquor). If you can't limit your drinking, or stop at two, you have a problem. Seek help from a physician or Alcoholics Anonymous.

■ Restrict your intake of caffeine. One or two cups of caffeinated coffee, tea, or cola a day won't affect your baby or you. More probably will, making one or both of you jittery, irritable, and sleepless. The caffeine also acts as a diuretic, drawing valuable fluids out of your body. And too many nutritionless beverages, caffeinated or not, can spoil your appetite for nutritious beverages and foods.

■ Don't take laxatives; some will have a laxative effect on your baby. To combat constipation, step up your fiber and fluid intake, and exercise more.

■ Take aspirin or acetaminophen only with your doctor's approval, and never exceed the prescribed dose or frequency. Since ibuprofen is excreted into the breast milk in only tiny amounts, ibuprofen medications may be considered a safer choice for the nursing mother.

■ Avoid excessive quantities of chemicals in the foods you eat. An occasional diet soda won't hurt, but frequent consumption of those containing saccharin isn't a good idea. Aspartame-sweetened soft drinks appear to be a better choice since aspartame is secreted into the breast milk in only tiny amounts. Whether you're nursing or not, however, heavy use of aspartame isn't wise because all of its long-term effects are not yet known. Do not use it at all if either you or your baby has PKU. And though no food additive currently in general use has been proven toxic to a baby who gets it via mother's milk, several are suspect. So it is prudent to limit your total intake of foods containing long lists of additives, including preservatives, artificial colors and flavors, and stabilizers.

■ Don't drink herbal teas. Some of the herbs found in true herbal teas (unlike those in flavored decaffeinated teas) are powerful drugs, possibly harmful to a nursing infant. So stay away from any unprescribed herbs or herbal teas that contain any ingredient not ordinarily found in your diet (orange rind and dried apples, for instance, should be okay).

■ Minimize the incidental pesticides in your diet. A certain amount of pesticide residue in your diet (from produce, for example), and thus in your milk, is virtually unavoidable and not likely to be harmful. But it's wise to try to keep such residues to a minimum by purchasing, when possible, produce that is certified organically grown; peeling or scrubbing other vegetable and fruit skins with dish detergent and water and rinsing well; choosing low-fat milk products, lean meats, white-meat poultry with the skin removed; and eating organ meats rarely (the pesticides and other chemicals ingested by animals are stored in fat, fatty skin, and such organs as the liver and brain).

■ Avoid eating freshwater fish (such as trout, perch, whitefish, salmon, and striped bass) that might have been contaminated by industrial wastes in lakes and rivers. Exceptions can be made if you know that they've come from safe waters (farm-raised trout or catfish, for instance, should be okay). Most deep-water ocean fish are considered safe to eat, but swordfish and tuna, which can contain high levels of methylmercury, should be eaten infrequently. Periodically, fish from certain off-shore areas are found to be unsafe. If you're unsure about a particular fish, contact your local Environmental Protection Agency (EPA) or health department.[9]

SORE NIPPLES

"Breastfeeding is something I always wanted to do. But my nipples have become so excruciatingly sore that I'm not sure I can continue nursing my son."

At first you wonder if your newborn will ever catch on; then before you know it, he's suckling so vigorously your nipples become sore, even painful. The problem is not uncommon, and in fact most women suffer at least a little nipple soreness before breastfeeding becomes well established. But in the vast majority of these women, soreness peaks at about the twentieth feeding, nipples start to toughen up, and nursing becomes more

9. If you believe you have had extensive exposure to PCBs (through your work, eating a lot of contaminated fish, or some other source), have your breast milk tested before you decide to breastfeed your baby. If you have high levels of PCBs in your breast milk, you may be advised not to nurse.

comfortable. For some women, however, particularly those with delicate or fair skin or whose babies are very vigorous nursers, the nipples get worse before they get better, cracking, becoming exquisitely tender, and sometimes bleeding. Nursing sessions can become torture.

Fortunately, there is relief at the end of the tunnel even for these women, though sometimes no for a month or six weeks. In the meantime, these precautions will help alleviate the discomfort:

■ Be certain your baby has the entire areola (the dark area around the nipple) in his mouth when nursing, and not just the nipple. Not only will his sucking on the nipple alone make you sore, but he won't get much milk. If engorgement makes it difficult for him to grasp the full areola, express a little milk manually or with a breast pump before nursing to reduce the engorgement and make it easier for him to get a good grip.

■ Expose nipples to air whenever possible, but especially after nursing. Just lower the blinds and leave the flaps of your nursing bra down as you go about your business at home.

■ Remove any waterproof lining from your bra (again, to encourage air circulation), and don't insert waterproof pads.

■ If only one nipple is sore, don't favor it by nursing more on the other one. But do nurse first on the less sore one, since your baby's sucking will be most vigorous at the beginning of a feeding session. If both nipples are sore, alternate the breast you start with at each feeding. If possible, reduce nursing periods to five minutes on each side, and nurse more often.

■ Let nature—not cosmetic companies—take care of your nipples. Nipples are naturally protected and lubricated by skin oils; commercial preparations should be used only when nipple cracking is severe, and then should be as pure as possible. Ultra-purified, medical-grade lanolin, and A & D ointments are effective; petroleum-based ointments and petroleum jelly itself (Vaseline) are not. Clean the nipples only with water—never with soap, alcohol, tincture of benzoin, or pre-moistened towelettes—whether they are sore or not. Your baby is protected from your germs by antibodies in your milk, and the milk itself is clean.

■ Rotate nursing positions so a different part of the nipple will be compressed at each feeding; but always keep baby facing your breasts.

■ Relax for fifteen minutes or so before feedings—listen to music, watch TV, cat-nap, do relaxation exercises—to banish the tension that could inhibit milk let-down. Or try a glass of wine or beer occasionally to enhance let-down. Or encourage it with an oxytocin nasal spray prescribed by your doctor, or with warm breast soaks or a warm shower prior to nursing sessions. If let-down doesn't occur, your baby will have to suckle desperately to get milk, adding to soreness.

LEAKING AND SPRAYING

"My breasts leak a lot. Sometimes I even spray milk across the room. It's messy and embarrassing."

The good news is that leaky breasts are full of milk; the bad news is there isn't a great deal you can do to stem the flow, though it will probably ease up sometime in the second month, once your baby's demands and your supply equalize. In the meantime, there are a few tricks you can try:

■ Wear breast pads in your bra to absorb any leaking milk; but be sure to change them frequently to avoid setting up conditions of warmth and moisture in which bacteria can breed.

■ Wear clothes that camouflage the milk stains—dark prints do this best—and that are washable.

■ Try crossing your arms tightly across your breasts when you feel let-down occurring in public; the pressure may curb let-down.

■ Try not to go very long between feedings, but if you must, express some milk when your breasts become too full.

MASTITIS

"My little boy is an enthusiastic nurser, and though my nipples were a little cracked and sore, I thought everything was going pretty well. Now, all of a sudden, one breast is very tender and hard—worse than when my milk first came in."

For most women the course of breastfeeding, after a shaky initial startup, is relatively smooth. But for about 1 in 20—and it sounds like you're one of them—mastitis (an inflammation of the breast) comes along to complicate matters. This infection can occur anytime during lactation, but is most common between the tenth and twenty-eighth postpartum days.

Mastitis is usually caused by the entry of germs, often from the baby's mouth, into a milk duct through a crack or fissure in the skin of the nipple. Since cracked nipples are more common among first-time breastfeeders, whose nipples are not used to the rigors of infant sucking, mastitis strikes these women more often. The symptoms of mastitis include severe soreness, hardness, redness, heat, and swelling over the affected duct, with generalized chills and usually fever of about 101° to 102°—though occasionally the only symptoms are fever and fatigue. Prompt medical treatment is important, so report any such symptoms to your doctor immediately. Prescribed therapy may include bed rest, antibiotics, pain relievers, and ice or heat applications.

Though nursing from the affected breast will be painful, you should not avoid it. In fact, you should let your baby nurse frequently to keep the milk flowing and avoid clogging. Empty the breast thoroughly by hand or with a pump after each feeding if your baby doesn't do a thorough job himself. Don't worry about transmitting the infection to your baby; the germs that caused the infection probably came from his mouth in the first place.

Delay in treating mastitis could lead to the development of a breast abscess, the symptoms of which are excruciating, throbbing pain; swelling, tenderness, and heat in the area of the abscess; and temperature swings between 100° and 103°. Treatment generally includes antibiotics and, frequently, surgical drainage under local anesthesia. If you develop an abscess, breastfeeding on the affected breast must be halted temporarily, though you should continue to empty it with a pump until healing is complete and nursing can resume. In the meantime, your baby can continue nursing on the healthy breast.

LUMP IN BREAST

"I've suddenly discovered a lump in my breast. It's tender and a little red. Could it be related to nursing—or something worse?"

Finding a lump in a breast strikes fear in any woman. But fortunately, what you describe is almost certainly related to nursing—a milk duct has probably become clogged, causing milk to back up. The clogged area usually appears as a lump that is red and tender. Though not serious in itself, a clogged duct can lead to breast infection, so it shouldn't be neglected. The basis of treatment is to keep milk flowing:

■ Empty the affected breast thoroughly at each feeding. Offer it first and encourage baby to take as much milk as possible. If there still seems to be a significant amount of milk left after nursing (if you can express a stream, rather than just a few drops), express the remaining milk by hand or with a breast pump.

■ Keep pressure off the clogged duct. Be sure your bra isn't too tight or your clothes too constricting. Rotate your nursing positions to put pressure on different ducts at each nursing.

■ Be sure that dried milk isn't blocking the nipple. Clean any away with sterile cotton dipped in cooled boiled water.

■ Don't stop nursing, if at all possible. Now is not the time to wean your baby, or to cut back on nursing. This would compound the problem.

Occasionally, in spite of your best efforts, infection develops. If the tender area becomes increasingly painful, hard, and red, and/or if you develop a fever, call your doctor (see page 556).

HAIR LOSS

"My hair, which was really luxuriant during pregnancy, now seems to be falling out in handfuls."

Don't panic, and don't order a hairpiece. This fallout is normal and can be quite heavy, but it will stop well in advance of baldness—though an occasional new mom may begin to wonder if it will. Ordinarily, the average person sheds 100 head hairs a day, each of which is replaced by new growth. When a woman is pregnant (or taking oral contraceptives), hormonal changes slow normal hair loss considerably, making the hair thicker and more luxuriant than ever before. But this reprieve from normal hair loss lasts only as long as the pregnancy. During the first three to six months after delivery (or after one stops taking the pill), all the hairs that were scheduled to have fallen out during pregnancy are shed. Regrowth can't keep up with the loss at first, and so hair looks much thinner than usual.

By the end of your baby's first year, your hair should be back to prepregnancy thickness. In the meantime, a good haircut may minimize the problem.

RENEWED BLEEDING

"My discharge turned to pink toward the end of my first postpartum week and got even lighter the next. Now, after fourteen days, all of a sudden it's red again, and heavier."

If you find your discharge is either reddish or a little heavier than it has been recently, it may mean nothing more than that you are more active than you should be. In which case a slower pace, with self-enforced, feet-up rest periods, should return your lochia to normal. On the other hand, if menstrual-like bleeding either continues beyond the first week or suddenly recurs later in the postpartum period, you should imme-diately call the practitioner who attended your delivery. If you can't reach him or her right away and bleeding is heavy, saturating a sanitary pad in one hour or less for a few hours, go to the nearest emergency room. If it's not that heavy, be certain to make contact with the practitioner within a few hours (or, if it's the middle of the night, first thing in the morning) so that you can be examined—either vaginally or via a sonogram—to determine the source of your bleeding.[10]

Abnormal vaginal bleeding after the first week postpartum suggests the possibil-ity that the placental site is not healing (involuting) properly or that a fragment of placenta remains in your uterus (this can happen even if the placenta seemed whole when checked at the time of delivery). Ei-ther condition could result in life-threaten-ing hemorrhage if not treated promptly. Lack of involution usually responds to a treatment including rest, antibiotics, and sometimes medication to help the uterus contract. Retained placental fragments often requires hospitalization, with surgery, careful curettage (scraping) of the lining of

the uterus, antibiotic therapy, and possible blood transfusions. Recovery is usually rapid and hospital discharge is frequently permitted as soon as 24 hours after admis-sion. In most instances, arrangements can be made for a nursing baby to be brought to the mother for feedings during hospitaliza-tion. If this isn't possible, a temporary alter-native feeding plan can be implemented (see page 91).

POSTPARTUM INFECTION/FEVER

"I've just returned home from the hospi-tal and I'm running a fever of about 101°. Could it be related to childbirth?"

Thanks to Dr. Ignaz Semmelweis, the chances of a new mother's developing childbirth (or puerperal) fever today are extremely slight. It was in Vienna in 1847 that this young Hungarian physician dis-covered that if birth attendants washed their hands before delivering a baby, the risk of childbirth-related infection was greatly reduced. (At the time, his theory was considered so outlandish that he was driven from his post, ostracized, and later died a broken man.) And thanks to Sir Alexander Fleming, the British scientist who developed the first infection-fighting antibiotics, the occasional case that does occur is easily cured.

The most severe cases of postpartum infection usually begin within 24 hours of delivery. While a fever on the third or fourth day could indicate postpartum infec-tion, it could also be caused by a cold or flu virus or some other minor problem. Occa-sionally a low-grade fever of about 100° accompanies engorgement when your milk first comes in.

There are several types of postpartum infection, and the symptoms vary accord-ing to the site at which the infection took hold. A slight fever, vague lower-abdominal pain, and sometimes a foul-smelling vag-inal discharge characterize endometritis, an

---

10. Some women experience a mini-period about three weeks postpartum, but it is brief and not as heavy as that described above. Even if you suspect that this is the reason for your bleeding, report it to your doctor.

infection of the lining of the uterus (the endometrium), which is particularly vulnerable after childbirth until the site where the placenta detached has healed. Endometritis is most likely to occur if a fragment of the placenta remains in the uterus; it can spread from the endometrium to the uterus and even into the bloodstream. When a laceration to the cervix, vagina, or vulva becomes infected, there will usually be pain and tenderness in the area and sometimes a foul-smelling thick discharge, abdominal or flank pain, or difficult urination. With certain types of postpartum infection, fever spikes as high as 105° and is accompanied by chills, headache, and malaise. Sometimes there is no obvious symptom but fever.

Treatment with antibiotics is very effective, but it should begin promptly. You should therefore report any fever during the first three postpartum weeks to the doctor—even if you also have cold or flu symptoms—so that its cause can be determined and treatment started, if necessary.

LONG-TERM CESAREAN RECOVERY

"I am just now going home, a week after a cesarean. What next?"

The process of recovery is a bit more extended if you've had a surgical delivery rather than a vaginal one. Over the next several weeks, you can expect:

To need plenty of help. Reliable paid help—a baby nurse and/or a housekeeper—is ideal for at least the first week, when your strength and energy levels will be at low tide. If hiring is not financially possible, you'll need extra help from your husband, supplemented when he's not home by rotating shifts of relatives and friends. It's best not to do any lifting (including the baby) or any housework for at least the first week back home. If you must lift the baby, have the crib mattress set at waist level and lift so as to put the strain on your arms

rather than your abdomen. If you have to bend, bend at the knees, not at the waist.

To have little or no pain. But if you do hurt, a mild pain reliever should help. Don't take any medication, however, if you are breastfeeding, unless you've got an okay from your baby's doctor.

To note progressive improvement at the incision site. Your incision will be sore and sensitive for a few weeks, but this will gradually lessen as it heals. A light bandage and loose clothing will help protect it from irritation. Occasional pulling and twitching sensations, other transient pains, and eventually itching can be expected with healing. All will subside over the course of the next few weeks. Numbness of the abdomen around the scar can last longer, possibly several months. Lumpiness of the scar tissue will diminish (unless you are prone to keloids, or thick scar tissue), and the scar may turn pink or purplish before it finally fades. If pain returns or worsens, if the area around the incision turns an angry red or becomes swollen, or if you notice a brown, gray, green, or yellow discharge coming from the wound, the incision may have become infected. Report such symptoms to your doctor promptly. A clear fluid discharge should also be reported, though it may be perfectly normal.

To wait at least four weeks before resuming sexual intercourse. Your doctor may recommend that you wait anywhere from four to six weeks before engaging in intercourse (though other kinds of lovemaking are certainly permissible). When you get the green light will depend on how your incision is healing and when your cervix returns to normal. (See page 560 for tips on making postpartum lovemaking more successful. Also see Postpartum Contraception, page 569.) You are, incidentally, much more likely to find early postpartum intercourse comfortable than are women who delivered vaginally.

To be allowed to start exercising once you are free of pain. Since the muscle tone of your perineum probably hasn't been compromised much, you may not need to do Kegel exercises (though they're a good pelvic toner for anyone). When your doctor gives the go-ahead, concentrate instead on those abdominal muscles (see page 528). Make "slow and steady" your motto; get into an exercise program gradually and continue it daily. Expect it to take several months before you're back to your previous level of fitness.

RESUMING SEXUAL RELATIONS

"My doctor says I have to wait six weeks before having sex again. A friend tells me this isn't necessary."

It's fairly safe to assume that your doctor is more familiar with your medical condition than your friend is. Though a doctor may in some instances okay intercourse as early as two weeks postpartum, your physician's restriction is probably based on what he or she believes is best for you, taking into consideration the kind of labor and delivery you had, whether or not you had an episiotomy or a laceration repair, and the speed of your healing and recovery. Some practitioners, however, apply the six-week prohibition routinely to all their postpartum patients, regardless of individual circumstances. If you think this may be the case with your doctor, and you're feeling up to making love, ask if he or she will consider bending the rules for you. This will be possible only if your cervix has healed and the lochia has stopped completely. If you do get the go-ahead, you may still decide to postpone intercourse if it causes severe pain in your perineal area.

Should your request be denied, however, it's wise to follow doctor's orders. Waiting the full six weeks couldn't hurt (at least not physically), while not waiting might.

WHAT IT'S IMPORTANT TO KNOW: Making Love Again

Is the honeymoon over? Has the romance faded now that there's a little fledgling sharing your love nest? Will you ever feel that heady rush of abandon in bed again? For that matter, will you ever stop feeling tired long enough to feel anything else at all?

For most women, even those who lived highly memorable love lives before delivery, doubts that any kind of sexual relationship with their husband will ever resume, at least on a regular basis, are nagging and numerous. Though a very few women do find themselves amorous in the immediate postpartum period (alas, even before they have been given the okay to consummate their desires and sometimes before their mates feel ready) because of genital engorgement, most women find the postpartum period (and sometimes a several-month stretch following it) a sexual wasteland.

WHY THE LACK OF INTEREST?

There's no shortage of reasons why you may not feel like making love now, among them:

■ Readjusting hormones can zap sexual desire during the postpartum period, and later if you're breastfeeding.
■ Temporary physiologic changes can cause a reduction in both the rapidity and

the intensity of sexual response.

■ Your libidos (yours and your spouse's) usually lose when they compete with sleepless nights, exhausting days, dirty diapers, and the endless needs of a demanding newborn.

■ Fear of pain, of doing some internal damage, of your vagina being stretched out, or of becoming pregnant again too soon may nip any romantic buds before they blossom.

■ A painful first intercourse postpartum can make the thought of further attempts unappealing. Pain on subsequent tries can make lovemaking extremely awkard and uncomfortable. Such pain may continue for a while even after the perineum is healed.

■ Discomfort because of decreased vaginal lubrication, a result of hormonal changes during the postpartum period and during lactation in women who are breastfeeding, can also dull desire. The problem usually lasts longer in nursing mothers, but can continue for as long as six months even in those who aren't breastfeeding.

■ Uneasiness because of lack of privacy, particularly if baby's in the room with you, can quench desire. Your head believes what you've heard—that your baby will be oblivious to and unaffected by your lovemaking—but your body balks at the idea.

■ Mothering may be taking all the loving and nurturing you have to give right now and you may sometimes be unable to summon any up for anyone else, even your husband.

■ Breastfeeding may be satisfying your sexual needs (without your realizing it), making you less receptive to your husband's overtures. Though nursing mothers may sometimes be interested in sex earlier, at least one study shows a decrease in sexual feelings and activity while breastfeeding.

■ Leaking of breast milk, stimulated by sexual foreplay, may make either you or your husband uncomfortable, physically as well as psychologically. Or you may not want to have your breasts touched by your mate at all, seeing them as nurturing rather than sexual right now and finding such foreplay annoying.

■ There are so many other things that you feel you need or want to do that sex may seem less important now—if you have a spare half hour, lovemaking may not be at the top of the list.

EASING BACK INTO SEX

To help you overcome some of the most common postpartum sexual difficulties:

Lubricate. Altered hormone levels during the postpartum period (which may not normalize in the nursing mother until her baby is partially or totally weaned) can make the vagina uncomfortably dry. Use a lubricating product (like K-Y Jelly) or lubricating vaginal suppositories until your own natural secretions return.

Medicate. If necessary, ask your practitioner to prescribe a topical estrogen cream to lessen pain and tenderness.

Take a nip. Don't get drunk, of course (since overindulgence, as Shakespeare pointed out, "provokes the desire, but it takes away the performance"), but if you drink, do indulge in a glass of wine with your husband before making love, to help both of you relax physically and emotionally. The alcohol will also numb some of your pain, lessen your fear of it, and lessen his fear of causing it. If you don't drink, try relaxation or meditation techniques instead.

Exercise. Kegel exercises (see page 528) will help to tone the pelvic muscles, which are associated with vaginal sensation and response during intercourse.

Vary positions. Side-to-side or woman-on-top positions allow more control of depth of penetration and put less pressure on a sore perineum. Experiment to find what works best for you.

WHAT CAN YOU DO ABOUT IT?

In spite of the bleak outlook for lovemaking at present, there's promise for the future. You will surely live to love again, with as much pleasure and passion as ever—and maybe, because you have been brought closer by sharing parenthood, even more. In the meantime, there are many steps you can take to improve both interest and performance right now:

Don't rush it. It takes at least six weeks for your body to recover completely, and sometimes much longer—especially if you had a difficult vaginal delivery or a cesarean section. Your hormonal balance may not return to normal until you resume menstruating, which, if you are breastfeeding, may not be for several months or more. Don't feel obligated to jump into bed the minute your practitioner gives you permission. If you don't feel up to it—mentally, emotionally, or physically—wait a while.

Express love in other ways. Intercourse isn't the only way for a couple to love. If you're not ready to go all the way, try cuddling and caressing in front of the TV, backrubs in bed, and hand holding while strolling in the park with baby. As for any couple getting acquainted (and you, after all, are becoming reacquainted physically), romance en route to the bed is an important first step. If you're not too pooped to pop, you can even try mutual masterbation. But some evenings, there may be nothing more satisfying than the intimacy that is shared lying in each other's arms.

Expect some discomfort. Many women are surprised and disheartened to find that postpartum intercourse can really hurt. If you've had an episiotomy or a laceration that required stitching, you may indeed experience some degree of pain or discomfort (ranging from mild to severe) for weeks, even months, after the tissues have outwardly healed. You may have pain with intercourse, though probably less of it, if you delivered vaginally, perineum intact—and even if you had a cesarean. To minimize pain, try the tips in Easing Back into Sex, page 561.

Don't expect perfection. Don't count on perfectly orchestrated orgasms at your very first return engagement. Many women don't have orgasms for several weeks or even longer when they start making love again. But with time, caring, and patience, the thrill does return and sex becomes as satisfying as ever.

If you can't beat baby's schedule, work around it. Falling into each other's arms when and where the spirit moves may no longer be possible. Instead, you may have to make time by that spirited little alarm clock in the crib. Baby is napping at 3 o'clock on Saturday afternoon; drop everything and head for the bedroom. Or if the little angel has been predictably sleeping from 7 to 10 every evening, plan ahead for a romantic interlude. If he or she wakes up crying just as your evening is reaching a climax, try to see the humor in your plight. You can, incidentally, if you can concentrate, keep your baby waiting for a couple of minutes if need be. Should sexual encounters with your spouse continue to be less frequent for a while (sometimes for a long while), strive for quality rather than quantity.

Keep your priorities straight. If making love is important to you, reserve for it by cutting corners elsewhere (in areas that won't affect your family's physical or emotional well-being). Go an extra day before running the vacuum, use frozen vegetables instead of fresh, keep the family in easy-care clothes. If you spend your entire day at full throttle, trying to be super mom, homemaker, and perhaps career woman as well, you won't have the strength left to do anything in bed but close your eyes.

Talk about it. A good sexual relationship is built on trust, understanding, and communication. If, for instance, you're too exhausted one night from 24-hour baby care to feel sexy, don't beg off with a headache. Instead, 'fess up. If your husband has been sharing baby-care responsibilities from the beginning, he's very likely to understand (he may, in fact, be too fathered-out some nights himself). If he hasn't, and he doesn't understand your exhaustion, this may be the time to explain that your handling all the baby and house care yourself is wearing you out, and that if he would help out, even a little, you might be left with more energy at night.

Communicate, too, about problems like a dry vagina or pain during intercourse. Tell your spouse what hurts, what feels good, what you'd rather put off until next time.

Don't worry about it. The more you worry about a lack of libido, the less libido you're likely to have. So face the facts of postpartum life, relax, and take your sexual relationship one night at a time, confident that the romance will return to your life.

SLIGHT SPOTTING ALERT

Occasionally, a couple of months postpartum, a new mother notes very slight spotting after intercourse or just anytime. This may be due to the growth of skin flaps at the site of the incision or tear. These skin flaps are easily repaired. Report such spotting, or any degree of bleeding postpartum, to your practitioner.

CHAPTER TWENTY-FOUR

Enjoying The First Year

WHAT YOU MAY BE FEELING

By the end of the first six weeks postpartum, your body should have recovered from the traumas of pregnancy, labor, and delivery. You may, however, expect to experience one or more of the following during the first year.

Physically:

- Further loss of weight, until you reach your prepregnancy weight or another goal
- Further flattening of your abdomen, particularly if you exercise
- Extreme fatigue, at least until your baby sleeps through the night

- A return of menstruation if you are not breastfeeding, or if you have reduced the number of nursings or weaned your baby
- Backache and other aches and pains from toting baby

Emotionally:

- Reduced sexual desire, at least at first
- Exhilaration, frustration, boredom
- A gradual increase in confidence and a lessening of the feeling of being overwhelmed

WHAT YOU SHOULD BE EATING: The Best-Odds for a Healthy Future

Eating regularly during your baby's first year is difficult enough, but eating well often seems impossible. Yet good diet is imperative if you are to keep up your energy, maintain good health, and if you're nursing, produce quality breast milk. So it's important to continue to get your Postpartum Daily Dozen (see page 534) and to follow the Nine Basic Principles of a Healthy Diet.

If you're nursing, your diet will have to change as your baby's does. As baby takes more and more nourishment from other sources—formula, cow's milk, solid foods—and less and less breast milk, you will have to reduce your caloric intake. But this doesn't require counting calories, just keeping a close eye on the scale. If it shows your weight going up when it should go down or stay level, then you are taking in too many calories. If you are losing when you shouldn't be, or losing very rapidly, then you're not eating enough. Adjust accordingly.

Once you've weaned your baby from the breast, or if you've never nursed at all, the Best-Odds Postpartum Diet can continue to be a blueprint for healthy eating in the years to come. Follow it, not only to feel better and live longer, but to set a good example for that new little baby of yours.

WHAT YOU MAY BE CONCERNED ABOUT

FINDING OUTSIDE INTERESTS

"As much as I'm committed to being a full-time mother, I'm starting to feel suffocated by staying home with my new daughter. There's got to be more to life than changing diapers."

In the first few months of a baby's life, when the demands of feeding and caring for her are round-the-clock and seemingly endless, about all a new mother has the time or inclination to crave is sleep. But once baby has settled into a routine and mother into a manageable rhythm, the dreary doldrums may settle over the frenetic fog of earlier weeks. Instead of finding yourself with too much to do and not enough time in which to do it, you may find yourself with too much time and not enough to do with it. The challenge gone from getting through a day's baby-care chores, you may well begin to feel like a wind-up mother going mechanically through the motions, and to crave the stimulations and satisfactions of life beyond the four walls of home. And particularly if you were involved in many activities before—a career, hobbies, school, athletics, community work—you may start to feel those four walls closing in, and start doubting your self-worth as well as your decision to stay home with your baby.

Yet a rich, full, satisfying lifestyle and life with baby are not, as they may seem now, mutually exclusive. The important first step toward achieving such a lifestyle is to recognize that woman (or man) cannot live by baby alone—though your mother, or others of her generation, may have taken twenty years to find that out. Even if you adore every moment with your baby, you still need intellectual stimulation and the chance to communicate with someone who can say more than ah-goo, ah-goo (cute as that may be). There are a variety of ways of achieving these goals, and of reclaiming the sense of self you feel you've lost:

Through Your Baby

You can look upon your baby as an obstacle to entry into the grownup world—or as a ticket to it. The following will give you a shot at finding adult interaction through your baby:

Play groups. Locate an existing group

or seek out mothers interested in joining you to set up a new one up by putting up a notice at the baby's doctor's office, at your church or synagogue, on your building complex, supermarket, or community bulletin board. Try for a group with mothers whose interests match yours.

Baby classes. Classes designed for babies are often more valuable for their mothers. By signing up for such a class (first making sure it's appropriate and safe for your baby; see page 330), you'll have the weekly opportunity to meet and talk with other women, many of whom have chosen to stay home with their babies.

Mothers' discussion groups. Join an established one, or become involved in setting up a new one. Invite guest speakers (a local pediatrician, a nurse, a librarian, an author, and others who can address your needs as mothers and/or as women); jointly hire a baby-sitter or sitters for the children. Meet in homes, a church, synagogue, school—or wherever there's space available—weekly, every other week, or monthly.

The local playground or play area. Where babies play, mothers can't be far behind. The playground is not only a great place for infants (even when too young to be mobile, they find watching the children and the activity fascinating) and older babies (when they can sit well, they usually love the swings, and many can tackle the slide and climbing areas before they are a year old), it is also an ideal place for mothers to meet other mothers and set up "play dates." These dates, too, are more for the benefit of the mothers at this point than they are for their babies, who aren't yet capable of "playing together."

Through Personal Enrichment Activities

Being a full-time mother doesn't mean you can't be anything else. Continue to pursue old interests, or find new ones, through any of the following:

A course at a local college. Take it for credit, or just for fun or intellectual enrichment.

An adult education class. They are proliferating all over the country and offer everything from aerobics to Zen.

A study group or class at your church or synagogue. While you were working you might not have found time to take a course in biblical criticism or comparative religion. Now's your chance.

An exercise class. Challenging the body activates the mind. In addition, an exercise program, particularly one that offers child care or combines mother exercise with baby exercise, is a good place to meet other women with similar interests.

Active sports. Playing tennis or golf or another favorite sport regularly will help keep both body and mind well toned, as well as provide companionship.

A museum or art gallery. Become a member of a local museum and you can visit regularly, studying one exhibit each time. (It will be even more fun if you go with another parent.) Added benefits for baby: early exposure to art and artifacts is visually and intellectually stimulating (infants are often fascinated by paintings and sculpture) and will help keep young minds open to them later.

Educational video or audio tapes. Watch videos while doing household chores or nursing, listen to audios while driving; keep up with an old interest or explore a new one (learn a foreign language via Walkman, for instance). Educational tapes are often available at no charge at the public library.

Books. They can take you anywhere, anytime. They can teach, challenge, and entertain. Take a book you're reading everywhere you go—read while you nurse, on a stationary bike, while baby naps, before bed.

Through Good Works

The crisis in volunteerism grows as more

and more women work at paying jobs full-time, and as society continues to further downgrade work that isn't paid. If you're not in the paid work force, then your local charities and community service organizations need you. Choose an organization you already belong to (Junior League, Hadassah, your church sisterhood) or join a new one, and offer your services. If you don't know where to start, you can contact a central clearinghouse for volunteers if there is one in your city, or you can ask at your local school, hospital, house of worship, or poverty center where volunteers are needed. The possibilities are endless: tutoring a child or adult in English or other subjects; visiting the elderly (they'll doubly appreciate your visit if you bring your baby along) or shut-ins; cheering patients at hospitals; serving meals at a soup kitchen; and so on.

Or use volunteer work to keep your professional skills from becoming rusty. Teach a course in your area of expertise at your local church, synagogue, or adult learning center; write a newsletter; design a direct-mail campaign; or provide medical care or legal counsel pro bono.

Through Paid Work

Being a full-time mother doesn't mean you can't be a part-time worker. A few hours a week at work related to your present field or a field you'd like to break into can keep you in touch, provide adult contacts, and offer escape from your daily routine. See page 587 for suggestions on how to find or create such work options, particularly those you can pursue from your home.

Making Baby Fit In

Though baby may be the cause of the lack of stimulation in your life, she doesn't have to stand in the way of a cure. In virtually every situation, her needs can be attended to at the same time yours are.

Take her along. In a baby carrier or stroller, she will enjoy (or sleep through) short visits to museums or galleries. She'll also, in some cases, be able to accompany you on your volunteer assignments (such positions are often far more flexible than paid ones) and to less formal courses, such as those given at community centers (try to time baby's feeding and/or nap to coordinate with the lecture to reduce the risk of her distracting you or others; bring quiet toys for an older baby).

Leave her with someone. Accept offers of assistance from relatives and friends. Or consider the possibility of co-op baby-sitting with another mother of a young child (you sit for both babies on Mondays while the other mother goes out, then she reciprocates on Thursdays).

Hire a baby-sitter. If you can afford it, this is usually the most reliable source of relief.

Depend on dad. Schedule your outside activities when your husband will be at home (play tennis or go to an aerobics class on the weekend, take French literature in the evening). Though this will cut down on the amount of time you spend together as a family, it will give daddy more time alone with baby, something he might not ordinarily have if he works full-time—and a wonderful plus for their relationship.

Use child care. Some colleges offer nursery facilities for children of students, some exercise programs offer baby-sitting, a very few workplaces offer day care for children of employees. If there are other mothers of infants or young children in a class or course you're taking, ask if they'd like to chip in for a communal sitter. The advantage of having on-site care is greatest if you're breastfeeding exclusively.

LEAVING BABY WITH A SITTER

"I don't work outside the home, but I do occasionally leave my nine-month-old son with a sitter—and always feel guilty when I do."

As every employer knows, no worker can stay on the job round the clock and round the calendar, and still be effective. And as a self-employed mother, you'll have to recognize this fact, too. No matter how much you enjoy your child and how much he enjoys you, you'll both benefit from some time apart. Take it—and don't feel guilty.

STRETCHED VAGINA

"Now that our son is sleeping through the night, my husband and I have finally resumed a fairly active sex life. The problem is that I seem roomier than before I delivered, and making love is less satisfying for both of us."

Most women come out of vaginal deliveries more roomy than when they went in. Often, the change isn't significant enough to be noticed by either partner. Sometimes, as when conditions were previously too cramped for comfort, it's welcomed. Occasionally, however, a vaginal delivery—particularly when no episiotomy was performed—can leave a woman who was "just right" before stretched out enough to markedly decrease the pleasure she and her husband experience during intercourse.

The passing of time may help tighten things up a bit, and so can keeping up with your Kegels. (If you haven't been doing Kegel exercises throughout pregnancy and postpartum, it's not too late to start now; see page 528.) Repeat these muscle toners as many times as you can during the day; get into the habit of doing them while you're cooking, watching TV, nursing, or reading—even during intercourse.

Very rarely, the muscles don't tighten up. If six months have passed since delivery and you still feel that you're too slack, it may be useful to discuss with your practitioner the possibility of surgical repair to snug things up. The procedure is a minor one, but it can make a major difference in your love life.

RETURN OF MENSTRUATION

"I weaned my daughter two months ago and I still haven't gotten a period. Could something be wrong?"

The resumption of the menstrual cycle in women who've been nursing can vary widely. Some women, especially those with substantial fat reserves, produce enough estrogen while they're nursing to start menstruating again before weaning, sometimes as early as six weeks to three months postpartum. But others, particularly those who have nursed for a long time, nursed exclusively, or had irregular menstrual periods before pregnancy, may not menstruate until several months after they've weaned their babies. Be sure, however, that you're eating enough and haven't been losing weight too quickly; strenuous dieting, especially when combined with strenuous exercise, can temporarily stall the return of the menstrual cycle. And mention the situation to your practitioner at your next checkup, which will probably be scheduled some time after the sixth month postpartum.

In women who aren't nursing their babies, the cycle can resume anywhere between four weeks and three months postpartum. Again, a delay in the start of menstruation could be the result of undernutrition due to overzealous dieting.

If you haven't yet had a period, don't count on this to prevent your becoming pregnant. See below for information on more reliable means of contraception.

GETTING PREGNANT AGAIN

"I want to wait at least two years before having another baby. A friend of mine said not to worry about birth control because she heard you can't get pregnant if you're nursing."

Your friend is only a little bit right, which means that if you depend on nursing as a contraceptive, you could end up a little bit pregnant. Some women who breastfeed find their menstrual periods don't return at all while they are nursing, and sometimes not for months past weaning; this usually means they aren't ovulating and can't conceive. The factors that seem to boost the ovulation-suppressing effects of breastfeeding include: low levels of body fat (hormones produced by body fat can stimulate menstruation); frequent nursings (more than three times a day may keep menstruation away); late weaning (often, the longer weaning is postponed, the longer ovulation is delayed); and delayed introduction of supplementation to breastfeeding (formula, solids, even water can all reduce breast milk intake, signaling the body that it's time to resume menstruating).

Many nursing mothers, however, particularly those who have excess fat stores or whose babies are only partially breastfed, do resume menstruating and can become pregnant. The catch: it's impossible to predict who will or won't menstruate while nursing. That wouldn't be a problem if everyone had a "sterile" menstrual period before ovulating again for the first time. Then the arrival of menstruation would warn that it's time to resume using contraception. But this is just not the case. Some women ovulate and conceive again before their periods return, and they can go from pregnancy to pregnancy without ever menstruating in between.

If you would be devastated by another pregnancy now (your body might be, even if your mind could accept it), you should use a more reliable form of contraception

than nursing. The following all have advantages and disadvantages, and the choice is a personal and individual one that should be based on your physical condition, your lifestyle, your doctor's recommendation, and your own feelings and circumstances. All are effective when used correctly and consistently, but only sterilization is 100% certain to prevent conception.

Oral contraceptives. Today's low-dose oral contraceptives work basically by suppressing ovulation and are very effective at preventing conception. But many women are confused about their safety. And it's no wonder. Scientific evidence seems to careen crazily back and forth. The following is what is known as this book goes to press. Check with your doctor to learn the latest.

The risk of heart attack, stroke, and blood clots is increased in OC users, so they aren't recommended for women at high risk for these cardiovascular problems (see below). The risks increase with extended use—longer than five years.

Though OCs appear to protect against certain forms of cancer (ovarian and endometrial, for example), some recent studies point to a connection between the Pill and breast cancer in some women (those who went on the Pill early, before a pregnancy, and took it for more than three years). On the plus side, OCs appear to protect against nonmalignant breast disease, ectopic pregnancy, ovarian cysts, and iron-deficiency anemia (due to less bleeding with the menses), and reduce the risk of arthritis and the incidence of menstrual cramping. Other benefits, for some women, are diminished premenstrual tension and very regular periods.

If you're breastfeeding, the Pill is probably not the birth control method for you since the hormones in it can suppress lactation. (Your doctor may, however, okay the use of a progestin-only pill after breastfeeding is well established.) It's also not usually recommended for women over 45, women over 35 who smoke (some say 35 should be the cutoff even for women who don't smoke), those who have a history of blood clots (thromboses), heart attack, stroke, angina, known or suspected breast or endometrial cancer, liver tumors, undiagnosed vaginal bleeding (which could indicate a malignancy), or jaundice during pregnancy. The Pill may also be unsuitable for women with a history of fibroids in the uterus, diabetes, high blood-cholesterol levels, high blood pressure (or a history of it during pregnancy), obesity, depression, gall bladder disease, or exposure to DES prenatally. Women with a history of migraines, asthma, epilepsy, or kidney or heart disease may find the Pill worsens their condition; if they elect to take it, very close medical monitoring is needed.

Oral contraceptives provide the most effective nonpermanent method of birth control (most failure is due to a user's missing a day or taking pills in the wrong order) and they allow for spontaneity in lovemaking. But some women report side effects, most commonly fluid retention; weight changes; nausea and vomiting; breast tenderness; abdominal cramps; skin discoloration; an increase in bladder and vaginal infections; an increase or decrease in sex drive; hair loss; intolerance to contact lenses (because of fluid retention); and menstrual irregularities (spotting, breakthrough bleeding, or rarely, amenorrhea, or total cessation of menstruation). Less common are reports of depression, listlessness, or tenseness. Many of these side effects are less severe or less common with the new low-dose combination pills and the progestin-only minipills, though menstrual irregularities are more common with these. Side effects often diminish or disappear completely after the first few cycles of pill use.

If you're planning to have another baby, fertility may take longer to return if you're using OCs than if you're using a barrier contraceptive. Ideally, you should switch to a condom or diaphragm about three months prior to the time you plan to try to conceive. About 80% of women ovulate within the first three months after stopping the Pill, 95% within a year—though you should check with your doctor after six months if you still aren't pregnant.

If you decide to try the Pill, your doctor will help you determine which type is best for you based on your menstrual cycle, weight, age, and medical history, and will select the lowest possible dose compatible with your needs (most women do best on less than 50 micrograms of estrogen). Then it's up to you to use this birth control method intelligently. Take it regularly; if you miss even one pill, or if you have diarrhea or vomiting (which can interfere with absorption of the pill by your body), use backup protection (such as a condom and foam) until your next period. See your doctor every six months to one year for monitoring of your health; report any problems or signs of complications that show up

ORAL CONTRACEPTIVE WARNING SIGNS

If you are taking an oral contraceptive and experience any of the following symptoms, call your physician *immediately*. If your doctor can't be reached, go to the nearest emergency room.

- Sharp pains in the chest
- Coughing up of blood
- Sudden shortness of breath
- Pain or tenderness in the calf or thigh

- Severe headache
- Dizziness or faintness
- Muscle weakness or numbness
- Disturbed speech
- Sudden partial or complete loss of vision, blurred vision, flashing lights
- Severe depression
- Yellowing of the skin
- Severe abdominal pain

IUD WARNING SIGNS

A woman wearing an IUD should call her doctor immediately if she experiences any of the following:

- A missed or delayed period, followed by spotty, scanty, or irregular bleeding
- Cramping, tenderness, sharp pain in the pelvis or lower abdomen (after the discomfort of the initial insertion has passed)
- Fainting or an urge to have a bowel movement associated with such pain

- Such pain that radiates down the legs, or pain in the shoulder
- Unusual or abnormal vaginal bleeding, with or without pain (other than the not abnormal spotting or staining following the initial insertion)
- Unexplained chills and fever
- Painful intercourse
- Genital sores or vaginal discharge

---

between visits, and be sure to inform anyone prescribing medication of any kind that you are on oral contraceptives (some drugs interact adversely with the Pill). Limit caffeine intake, *do not smoke,* and because oral contraceptives increase the need for certain nutrients (though they decrease the need for others), take a daily vitamin supplement that contains the RDA of vitamins B_6, B_{12}, C, riboflavin, zinc, and folic acid.

If you have trouble remembering to take pills, ask your doctor about the new 5-year hormonal implant that suppresses ovulation and builds up cervical mucus to block sperm. Implanted in the arm, it's effective and can be removed anytime you want to conceive.

IUD, or intrauterine device. This type of birth control (it is not strictly speaking a contraceptive, since it interferes with implantation rather than conception) was out of favor for several years because of suspected risks and legal battles.

Today, however, the IUD is making a comeback. At least two companies in the U.S. are producing devices approved by the FDA and more are expected to follow suit. But to protect users and themselves, they are marketing exclusively to doctors and clinics who agree to supply IUDs only to women who are 25 years of age or older, who have at least one child, and who are in a mutually monogamous relationship. Doctors are also

required to fully inform patients of the risks of IUD use.

For many women, particularly those who don't plan to have more children, these risks are outweighed by the benefits. The major one: once it is inserted, it can be forgotten about for at least a year (often up to four, depending upon the device), except to check regularly (monthly is a good idea) for the string attached to it. This allows for a spontaneous sex life with no pausing to find and insert a diaphragm or put on a condom, and no need to remember to take a daily pill. In addition, the IUD does not interfere with breastfeeding nor does it affect the nursing infant.

The IUD should not be used by a woman who is exposed to multiple partners, or has a partner who is. Nor should it be used by a woman with a history of PID (pelvic inflammatory disease) or ectopic pregnancy; known or suspected uterine or cervical malignancy or premalignancy (or even an unexplained abnormal Pap smear); abnormalities of the uterus or an unusually small uterus; menstrual or other bleeding irregularities (the IUD can increase menstrual flow and cramping); postpartum or postabortion infection within the past three months; or by a woman who recently delivered a baby, or experienced a miscarriage or abortion. Allergy or suspected allergy to copper rules out the use of a copper IUD.

Possible complications include cramping

(which can be severe) during insertion and, rarely, for a few hours or even days following; uterine perforation; accidental expulsion (it might go unnoticed and leave you unprotected); and tubal or pelvic infections. The intrauterine device is extremely effective in preventing pregnancy, although when pregnancy does occur while one is still in place, it can cause complications.

Diaphragm. The diaphragm is a dome-shaped rubber cap that is placed over the cervix, the mouth of the uterus, to block the entry of sperm. It is an effective birth control method when used properly with a spermicidal gel to inactivate any sperm that might get past the barrier. Aside from possible increases in the risk of toxic shock syndrome (TSS) from leaving the diaphragm in for prolonged periods (contrary to directions) or of urinary tract infections and an occasional allergic reaction triggered by either the spermicide or the rubber, the diaphragm is safe. In fact, used with a spermicide, it appears to reduce the risk of pelvic infections that can lead to infertility. And it in no way interferes with lactation or affects a nursing baby.

The diaphragm must be prescribed and fitted by a medical professional. *Refitting is essential after childbirth,* as the size and shape of the vagina may have changed. The diaphragm has the disadvantage of having to be inserted before each intercourse, left in for six to eight hours, and removed within 24 hours. (Some experts suggest it's prudent to remove it within twelve to eighteen hours, and some recommend women insert their diaphragms nightly when they brush their teeth to avoid neglecting to use it in a moment of passion). And since the diaphragm is inserted through the vagina, this method is unappealing to some women.

The cervical cap. Approved by the FDA in the late 1980s for use in the U.S., the cervical cap is similar to the diaphragm in many ways. It must be fitted by a physician, must be used with a spermicide, and

does its job by preventing the entry of sperm into the uterus. Its success at preventing pregnancy is about the same as the diaphragm, though theoretically the diaphragm's figures are better. The cap offers a couple of additional advantages. Shaped like a large thimble, the pliable rubber cap, whose firm rim fits snugly around the cervix, is only about half the size of the diaphragm; and it can be left in place for 48 hours rather than the 24-hour outside limit recommended for the diaphragm. Odor and difficulty inserting the cap may, however, present problems for some women.

The vaginal sponge. A more recent addition to the birth control arsenal, the sponge, like the diaphragm, the cervical cap, and the condom, is considered a barrier method of contraception, one that blocks the entrance to the uterus, keeping sperm from swimming up to meet an ovum. But its major contraceptive effect is probably through the spermicide it releases. It seems somewhat less effective than the diaphragm, but when it contains nonoxynol-9, it appears to reduce the risk of contracting such sexually transmitted diseases as gonorrhea and chlamydia. It can, however, increase the risk of the less serious vaginal infection candida. Fears that use of the sponge might cause birth defects, cancer, or TSS haven't proved out, and in fact, there is some evidence that the sponge may inhibit the development of TSS. But some people are allergic to the spermicide used. And some women are uncomfortable inserting the sponge into the vagina.

The sponge is growing in popularity because it requires neither a visit to the doctor nor a prescription, it is relatively easy to use (you insert it yourself, like a diaphragm), it allows for greater spontaneity than other barrier methods (providing continuous protection for a full 24 hours after insertion), and it is believed to have no effect on the nursing infant. It should not be left in longer than recommended, and great care should be taken to remove the entire sponge (a piece left in could cause odor and infection). And it should not be used during the six-week postpartum period or shortly after a miscarriage, abortion, or D and C, without a physician's approval.

Condom. A sheath for the penis made of latex or natural skin (from the intestines of a sheep) and often called a rubber, the condom is a very effective if used conscientiously, though it is somewhat less foolproof than the Pill. Its effectiveness, as well as its ability to combat pelvic infection, is enhanced if it is used with a spermicidal agent or jelly, and if care is taken to see that it is undamaged before use. The condom is totally harmless, though the latex or any spermicide used with it may spark an allergic reaction in some people. It has the advantage of not requiring a doctor's visit or prescription, of being easily available and easy to carry, and of reducing the risk of transmitting infections, such as gonorrhea, chlamydia, and AIDS (the latex variety is better at preventing passage of the AIDs virus). Because it in no way interferes with breastfeeding or affects the nursing infant, and because it doesn't require postpartum refitting (as does the diaphragm), it is an ideal "transitional" method for many women. Some find, however, that because it must be put on before intercourse (and not until erection), it interferes with spontaneity. Others find that putting on the condom can be part of the lovemaking. Care should be taken when sheathing the penis to leave a small reservoir at the tip of the condom (some have one built in) to hold the semen. The penis should be withdrawn before the erection is totally lost and while the condom is held on. The use of a lubricating cream (or a lubricated condom) will help make insertion more comfortable when the vagina is dry after pregnancy and during lactation.

Spermicide foams, creams, jellies, suppositories, and contraceptive films. Used alone, these antisperm agents are fairly effective at preventing pregnancies.

They are easy to obtain without a prescription and don't interfere appreciably with lovemaking, but they can be messy.

Calendar-rhythm method. This approach, which depends on keeping careful records of when one menstruates and avoiding intercourse during the middle of the cycle when ovulation usually takes place, is impossible to use before periods have resumed. Because of the irregularity of the menstrual cycle in many women, it has been the least effective of the various popular birth control methods. For this reason, and because of the much greater effectiveness of Natural Family Planning (NFP; see below), women who wish to use a form of contraceptive that is natural and doesn't contradict religious teachings, prefer NFP.

Natural family planning. A refinement of the calendar-rhythm method, NFP depends on using one or more body signs or symptoms to determine the time of ovulation. The more factors a couple takes into consideration, the better the success rate. These factors include mucus changes in the vagina (the mucus is clear and can be pulled into strings at ovulation); basal body temperature changes (the baseline temperature, measured first thing in the morning, drops slightly just before ovulation, reaches its lowest point at ovulation, and then immediately rises to a high point before returning to the baseline for the rest of the cycle; see diagram); and cervical changes (the normally pink cervix becomes bluish). Intercourse is avoided from the first sign that ovulation is about to occur until three days after.

Though it's possible to use natural family planning without the help of a physician, learning the latest techniques from an informed professional can increase the effectiveness of this (or any) type of birth control.

Because NFP is much more effective at preventing pregnancy than the calendar-rhythm method, and because it, too, is

CALCULATING
THE CALENDAR RHYTHM METHOD

The calendar method   A woman keeps a record of her monthly menstrual cycles for three to six months. She then calculates:
- Day A = the number of days in her shortest cycle minus 18
- Day Z = the number of days in her longest cycle minus 11

Thus if her longest cycle is 30 days and her shortest 28, she figures:
- Day $A = 28–18 = 10$
- Day $Z = 30–11 = 19$

Her fertile period (unsafe for intercourse if she does not want to become pregnant) runs from A to Z, days 10 to 19 of her menstrual cycle, counting the first day of her menstrual period as 1.

sanctioned by religious groups that find other forms of birth control objectionable, NFP has largely replaced the older method.

Surgical sterilization. Tubal ligation (the tying of the fallopian tubes) for women and vasectomy (the tying or cutting of the *vasa deferentia,* the tubes that transport sperm from testicles to penis) for men must be considered permanent, though occasionally it is possible to reverse them (newer techniques may be easier to reverse). Sterilization is also increasingly safe, with no known long-term health effects, and virtually foolproof. The occasional failure one hears of generally is due not to a failure of the method, but rather to

a slipup in the surgery or carelessness on the part of a man who fails to use other birth control methods until all viable sperm have been ejaculated.

Sterilization is frequently the choice of couples who feel their family units are complete, and is the most widely used form of birth control in the United States. Some women opt to have their tubes tied immediately after delivering their last child.

DIAGNOSING A NEW PREGNANCY

"I had a baby about ten weeks ago, and I

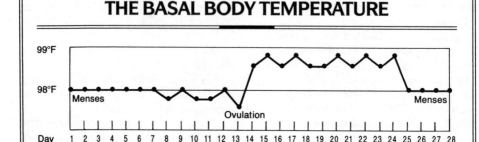

THE BASAL BODY TEMPERATURE

The basal body temperature   The BBT can help to pinpoint more accurately the unsafe period of ovulation. To get the BBT, the woman takes her temperature every morning *immediately* on awakening, before

speaking, sitting up, etc. In most women the temperature will drop and then rise abruptly at the time of ovulation as seen above. Three full days after ovulation, intercourse can be resumed.

started feeling a little queasy yesterday. How soon can you get pregnant again, and if you're nursing, how can you tell?

A new pregnancy at ten weeks postpartum is unusual, particularly in a nursing mother (who isn't likely to ovulate until breastfeedings begin to be supplemented), but it's not unheard of. Unless you or your partner have been sterilized, you run the risk of conceiving any time you have intercourse, even if you use birth control and especially if you don't. A postpartum pregnancy, however, may be difficult to recognize. This is particularly true if you haven't resumed menstruating, since the first tip-off most women get that they might be pregnant is a missed period. If you're nursing, another pregnancy clue many women rely on —tender and enlarged breasts with increased vascularization—may be obscured. However, you may begin to notice other clues that you may have conceived once a new pregnancy is established: a diminished milk supply because different sets of hormones operate in pregnancy and lactation (but such a drop in production may also be due to exhaustion, not nursing enough, or other factors); morning sickness or queasiness (which could also result from something you ate or a gastrointestinal virus); or frequent urination (this could instead be due to a urinary tract infection).

If you have any reason to suspect you are pregnant, or even if you're just unreasonably nervous about the possibility, use a home pregnancy test or go to your doctor or a clinic for a blood test. In the unlikely event that you turn out to be pregnant, see an obstetrician, midwife, or your family doctor as soon as possible. A new pregnancy within a year of childbirth puts a tremendous strain on the body, and you'll need close medical supervision, extra rest, and plenty of good nutrition. As long as you feel up to it, you can continue breastfeeding your baby. If you feel utterly exhausted, you may want to supplement with formula or even wean completely. Discuss the options with your doctor. If you do breastfeed while pregnant it will be extremely important to consume enough extra calories (about 300 for the fetus and another 200 to 500 for milk production), protein (five servings a day), and calcium for both baby making and milk making (the equivalent of six servings a day), as well as to get plenty of rest.

EXHAUSTION

"I expected to feel run-down during the postpartum period, but it's been three months since I had my baby and I'm still exhausted. Could something be wrong?"

Many a new mother has dragged herself to her doctor's office complaining of overwhelming chronic fatigue—convinced she's fallen victim to some fatal malady. The nearly invariable diagnosis? A classic case of new motherhood.

Rare is the woman (or man, if he's a full-time parent) who escapes this parental fatigue syndrome, characterized by physical exhaustion that never seems to ease up and an almost total lack of energy. And it's not surprising. There's no other job as emotionally and physically taxing as mothering in the first year. The strain and pressure are not limited to eight hours a day or five days a week, and there are no lunch hours or coffee breaks to spell relief. For the first-time mother, there is also the stress inherent in any new job: mistakes to be made, problems to solve, a lot to learn. If all this isn't enough to produce exhaustion, the new mother may also have her strength sapped by breastfeeding, by toting around the load of rapidly growing infant and accompanying paraphernalia, and by night after night of broken sleep.

The new mother who goes back to an outside job may also suffer from fatigue and exhaustion—from trying to do two jobs well. She gets up early to attend to several mommying jobs, often including nursing, before she even leaves for her job away from home. That job may or may not be a respite, depending on how stressful it is, but when she returns home, unless she has a full-time housekeeper or a particularly helpful and competent spouse, she will still have cooking, cleaning, laundry, and baby care to contend with. To top it all off, she can be up with the baby half the night and still be expected to be alert and cheerful in the morning. Exhaustion would be inevitable for Supermom herself.

Of course, it's a good idea see your doctor to be sure there is no medical cause for your exhaustion. If you get a clean bill of health, be assured that in time, as you gain experience, as your routine becomes routine, and as your baby begins sleeping through the night, the unrelenting fatigue will gradually disappear (though you may not feel totally "caught up" on your rest until your children are all in school). And your energy level should pick up a bit, too, once your body adjusts to the new demands. In the meantime, be sure to eat well, get some exercise, and try the tips for relieving postpartum depression, many of which may also help reduce fatigue.

ACHES AND PAINS

"I've been having backaches and a nagging pain in my neck, arm, and shoulder ever since our son was born."

Nothing quite compares to carrying a baby and an overstuffed diaper bag around all day. And this weighty burden almost always explains those aches and pains in the neck, arms, wrists, fingers, shoulders, and backs of new moms – and increasingly, as they share more of the load, of new dads.

Recognizing the cause of your afflictions is the first step toward relieving them. (Often, mothers and the doctors they consult fail to make this connection, with batteries of unnecessary tests the common result.) The next step is to try to alleviate the problem with a combination of preventive and curative measures:

■ If you haven't yet taken off all of your pregnancy weight, gradually do so now. Excess weight puts unnecessary strain on your back.

■ Exercise regularly, concentrating on those exercises that strengthen the abdominal muscles, since they support the back, and those that strengthen the arms (see page 525 for a basic postpartum exercise program).

■ Assume a comfortable position for feeding baby. Don't slouch, and be sure your back is supported—if you can't slide all the way to the back of the chair, tuck a pillow behind you. Use pillows or armrests, as needed, to support your arms as you hold baby and direct breast or bottle. And don't cross your knees.

■ Learn to bend and lift correctly. Place feet shoulder-width apart and bend at the knees, not at the waist. When lifting baby or anything else, put the weight on your arms and legs rather than on your back.

■ Don't stretch to reach high places; stand on a footstool instead.

■ Be conscious of your posture. Walk, sit, and lie with your buttocks tucked under and abdomen tilted inward (this is called a "pelvic tilt").

■ Sleep on a firm mattress, or put a board under an overly soft one. A mattress that sags in the middle will have you sagging, too. Lie on your back or side (but not your stomach) with your knees bent.

■ If you push a carriage or stroller, be sure the handles are at a comfortable height for you. If they aren't, see if you can have them adjusted, or if they're too short, buy extenders.

■ If shoulder pain is a problem, carry the diaper bag in the crook of your arm rather than on your shoulder, or use a backpack.

■ Use a heating pad or warm bath to temporarily relieve muscle discomfort and spasm.

■ Try not to stand for long periods of time; if you must, keep one foot on a low stool with

your knee bent. If you're on a hard-surfaced floor, use a small rug as a cushion underfoot.
■ Instead of walking the floor night after night with a colicky infant in your arms, try using a swing (once he's six weeks old) or a rocker to comfort him.

URINARY INCONTINENCE

"Ever since my second child was born, I find that I leak a bit of urine when I cough or laugh or strain to lift something.".

Your problem is probably stress incontinence, which is fairly common in women after childbirth, particularly in those who've had several children. The usual cause is weak muscle tone in the vaginal wall that supports the urethra and bladder. The bladder may push through the weakened musculature, causing a cystocele, or bulge, which is actually a hernia. A small cystocele may not even be noticed, but a large one may droop down to or even through the vaginal opening and can cause some discomfort in addition to the incontinence. Doing two or three hundred Kegel exercises spread out over the course of a day every day for a couple of months (see page 528) may help to strengthen the muscles in the vaginal wall and eliminate the problem. In severe cases, surgery may be recommended to remedy the condition. Unfortunately, unless the uterus is also removed, the cystocele may recur because of the weight of the uterus, especially a pregnant one, pressing down on the bladder and pushing it once again into the vaginal wall.

FRIENDSHIPS

"I feel uncomfortable with my friends who don't have children, but I don't know any women with young babies and feel very lonely."

Major changes in one's life—a new school, a new job, a new marriage, a move to a new community, a divorce, children leaving the nest, retirement, widowhood—almost always have some effect on relationships. The arrival of a baby is no different. Yet somehow, many women seem more uncertain about how to deal with the changing balance of friendships when they become mothers than at almost any other time. Perhaps that's because nothing quite changes the way you see yourself and the way others see you as much (though for some women, a divorce or widowhood also has the effect of redefining them as people).

Many factors can contribute to changes in your social life post-baby. For one, you undoubtedly have a lot less time and energy for socializing. For another, until you go back to paid employment—whether that's six weeks or six years after your baby is born—you'll feel somewhat removed emotionally as well as physically from the circle of friends that revolved around your job or career. For still another, your interests, if they haven't already, will begin to change. As much as you still might enjoy a conversation centered around foreign policy, films, literature, or gossip, you've probably recently developed an interest in discussing the merits of baby exercise classes or the efficacy of various diaper rash preparations, sharing thoughts on how to quiet a crying baby or how to get more sleep, bragging about baby's first successful attempt at turning over or cutting a first tooth. Yet another factor upsetting your social life: some single friends seem less comfortable with you. This may be partly because you share less in common and partly because some of them, consciously or unconsciously, are envious of your new family. And finally, friendships that are only job-deep (or partying- or tennis-deep) often don't have what it takes to survive change.

What most women are searching for is a way to integrate the women they were with the mothers they've become—without diminishing either. That isn't easy. Trying to stay completely within the old circle denies that you're a mother now. Abandoning old friends and spending time only with other new mothers denies the old you. Making new friends while keeping some of the old will probably be the happiest and most fulfilling of compromises, one which satisfies all the women you are.

See your old friends socially on occasion—for lunch, the ballet, a seminar. They'll want to hear about your baby and your new lifestyle (but not exclusively) and you'll want to hear what's new and what's the same, at work and with their relationships. Try to stick to subjects you have in common, whatever brought you together in the first place. You may find yourself feeling a little uncomfortable at first, but pretty soon you'll know which friendships are going to continue and which it makes sense to put on hold, except perhaps for birthdays and holidays. You may be surprised to find that one or more old friends become very involved in your new life and offer a great source of support. And those old friends you lose touch with may suddenly seek you out again when they begin to have families of their own.

Making new friends among the new mothers in your community is relatively easy. It only requires your turning up at places where mothers of babies congregate (at playgrounds, exercise classes, mothers' groups, play groups, your church or synagogue). Seek out those who share not only your interest in babies but also some of your other interests, so that these friendships can be multi-dimensional and so that you'll have more to talk about than diapers and day care—though you'll find babies will often be the subject of choice.

DIFFERENT MOTHERING STYLES

"My closest friend is relaxed and disorganized, doesn't worry if her seven-month-old doesn't get his lunch until dinnertime, drags him to parties until all hours—and is in no hurry to return to work. I'm compulsive about everything—

bedtimes, meals, clean laundry—and I went back to work part-time when my son was three months old. Who's doing something wrong?"

Nobody. Each mother has to mother in the way that's most comfortable for her. You would probably have a nervous breakdown trying your friend's laissez-faire mothering style, and she would do likewise trying yours. The only time you need fear you're doing something wrong is when your baby tells you—by fussing or crying a lot, by seeming depressed and unresponsive, or by not thriving physically—that he's not satisfied with your approach to mothering. If that happens you've got to make some adjustments—because babies, like mothers, are individuals, with different styles.

A baby who is happy and healthy is saying to his mother, no matter what her style, "You're doing a great job!"

BREASTFEEDING DURING ILLNESS

"I've just come down with the flu. Can I still breastfeed my baby without her getting sick?"

Breastfeeding your baby is the best way to strengthen her resistance to your germs (and other germs around her) and to keep her healthy. She can't catch cold or flu germs through your breast milk, though she can become infected through other contact with you. To minimize the spread of infection, always wash your hands before handling your baby or her belongings and also before feedings; if she ends up getting sick in spite of your precautions, see the treatment tips on page 414. To speed your own recovery as well as keep up your milk supply and your strength while you have a cold or flu, drink extra fluids (a cup of water, juice, soup, or decaffeinated tea every hour while you're awake), be sure to take your vitamin supplement, try to get your Daily Dozen (being particularly certain to meet your vitamin C requirements), and rest when you can. If you have a lot of congestion, drinking juices instead of milk for a couple of days may help reduce it (though this theory is controversial). Check with your doctor if you need medication—*don't* take any without medical approval.

If you come down with a "stomach virus," or gastroenteritis, you should again take precautions against infecting your baby—though the risk is small, since breastfed babies appear to be protected against most such infections. Wash your hands, especially after you've gone to the bathroom, before touching your baby or anything that she might put into her mouth. Take plenty of fluids (particularly diluted fruit juices or decaffeinated teas[1]) to replace those lost through diarrhea or vomiting, but limit solids to such bland items as white toast, converted rice, boiled or baked potatoes without the skin, cream of wheat or cream of rice, bananas, applesauce, and Best-Odds gelatin desserts (see page 625).

Though common colds and flus can't be transmitted through breast milk, some forms of hepatitis can. If you come down with this disease, discuss with your baby's doctor the advisability of discontinuing nursing. AIDS may also be transmitted through breast milk; an infected mother should discuss the advisability of nursing with a pediatrician familiar with AIDS.

"I have a cold sore; can my baby boy catch it?"

The cold sore, or fever blister, which usually develops on the lip or around the mouth, is caused by a herpes virus, but a different strain from the one that causes genital herpes. Most people are first infected as children, with the initial episode often including fever as well as sores in the mouth. After the acute phase passes, the virus usually lies dormant in the body for months or even years. During times of physical or emotional stress, it may be reactivated. The most obvious symptom of

the flare-up is a blister that oozes and later scabs over. It's only during the blister phase that the virus is transmissible, but it appears that not everyone is susceptible.

To avoid passing the infection on to your baby, wash your hands very thoroughly before handling him or anything that goes into his mouth (including his hands, bottle, or pacifier, and your nipples)—and no kissing or drinking from the same cup! Lactobacillus (the bacterial culture used to make yogurt), available in tablet form at your pharmacy and taken as directed, often helps to ward off a threatening cold sore at the first tingle or at least to stop one from becoming full blown. Try that treatment or ask your doctor to suggest another.

If you have an active genital herpes infection, you should be careful to wash your hands thoroughly after using the bathroom and before you feed your baby; use condoms to protect your spouse unless he's already infected. To keep baby away from the sores and from any clothing that touches them, slip into a clean robe or cover your lap with a fresh towel before feeding or handling him. Since herpes can be very risky for a newborn, be especially careful if the infection flares shortly after you deliver.

PERSISTENT DEPRESSION

"I can't seem to shake my postpartum depression. My son's already four months old, but I have no energy. I don't feel like doing anything or seeing anybody or even leaving the house. My husband says I need help, but I keep hoping I'll come out of it on my own."

Maybe you will come out of it on your own, and maybe you won't. In about one in a thousand cases, postpartum depression is so severe and so persistent that expert treatment is needed to bring the new mother to emotional equilibrium. Your prolonged depression suggests that you may be that one

---

1. The once popular diarrhea cure of cola, ginger ale, or other carbonated beverages is no longer recommended because sugar appears to increase diarrhea.

in a thousand. There's no point in suffering (or making your family suffer) any longer on the chance that you may beat the blues yourself—get help now. Talk to your obstetrician or family doctor first. He or she may be able to help you; if not, you will be referred to a specialist. Because your problem is more likely to be physical (caused by a hormone imbalance) than emotional, a medical doctor is likely to be able to help more quickly and more satisfactorily than a nonmedical therapist. Hormone therapy may be helpful in some cases.

Whomever you turn to for help, do it quickly. The sooner you shed the baby blues, the sooner you can start enjoying your baby and your new life as a mother.

FINDING TIME FOR YOURSELF

"I'm so busy seeing to my new daughter's needs that I never have time to see to my own. Sometimes I don't even have a chance to take a shower."

Little things can mean a lot to the mother of a young baby. And often these little things that others take for granted—going to the bathroom when you feel the urge, having a cup of coffee while it's still hot, sitting down for lunch—become luxuries she can no longer afford.

Still, it's important to *make* time you can call your own. Not only so that you (and your husband) will remember that your needs count, but so that your baby, as she grows in awareness, will recognize this, too. "Mother" needn't be synonymous with "martyr." You don't have to suffer frequent urinary tract infections from infrequent trips to the bathroom, or indigestion from eating on the go, or chronically and depressingly greasy hair from postponing showers. Though it will, indeed, take a lot of judicious juggling to meet your own needs without neglecting your baby's, it will be well worth it for both of you. After all, a happier mother is a better mother.

How to best make time for yourself will depend on such factors as your schedule, your priorities, and just what it is you want to find time for. But the following tips can help put a little more personal time in your life:

Let baby cry. Not for half an hour, but certainly it won't hurt if you put her safely in her crib and let her fuss while you brush your teeth or put on some mascara and lipstick.

Include baby. Sit down to lunch with your baby. If she's not yet on solids, put her in a baby seat on the table and chat with her as you eat. Or take your lunch to the park if she's more content in her stroller and if weather permits. Place her in her baby seat on the bathroom floor while you attend to personal needs—she'll be getting early potty training while you get relief. Or play peekaboo with her from behind the curtain while you shower.

Depend on daddy. Shower while he breakfasts with her in the morning, or give yourself a facial while he takes her for a walk on Saturday afternoon. Don't feel guilty about turning baby over to him in his spare time; a mother's work (whether full- or part-time) is more consuming and demanding than any paid job.

Exchange favors. Trade baby-sitting services with other mothers who also need to free up some time. Sit for a friend's baby and your own one afternoon or morning a week while she does whatever it is she needs to get done; she reciprocates another day.

Hire help. You may not be able to afford even a part-time baby-sitter, but you probably can afford a young teenager to entertain your baby while you prepare dinner or attend to other chores at home.

BABY FORGETTING YOU

"I'm going to be starting back to work in a

couple of weeks. What worries me most is that my baby won't know me when I get home at night."

This concern is at the top of the worry list of virtually every mother who has to leave her baby—even briefly—for any reason. But it's a worry that can quickly be crossed off the list. Babies know their mothers very early, recognize their voices almost at birth, and don't forget them even if they are away for the day.

QUALITY TIME

"I hear a lot about the importance of spending quality time with your children. Well, even though I spend virtually all my time with my son, I'm so busy that I'm not sure there's any quality to it."

Along with the proliferation of the working mother (a misnomer, since *all* mothers work) came the popularization of the concept of "quality time": if a mother couldn't spend a lot of time with her child, the least she could do was make the best of the time she did spend with him. The theory seemed to imply that quantity was no longer important. But there's quality in quantity, too. You don't have to drop everything, sit down on the floor, and play with your baby all day long to provide him with quality care. You give quality time every time you change his diaper and smile at him, every time you feed him and talk to him, every time you bathe him and splash around with bath toys. You do it even when you chat with him from the kitchen as he races around in his walker, sing to him while you're driving in the car, lean over to tickle him in his playpen as you vacuum by, or sit him down with some blocks while you sit down with the bills.

Quality parenting time is time spent relating to your child in passive as well as active ways, and something that a loving and responsive mother who spends a lot of time with her child can hardly avoid providing. You'll know if you're succeeding just by watching your baby—does he smile, laugh, respond, seem basically content? If the answers are yes, he's getting quality time.

"As a mother who works outside the house full-time, I worry that I don't spend enough quality time with my daughter."

An employed mother is under enough pressure without having the added pressure of worrying about whether the time she spends with her child or children is of the proper quality (which, incidentally, isn't the kind of pressure that enhances performance). If you do have limited time with your baby, the impulse is to make every minute count. Accepting the impossibility of this (there will be moments when you'll need to do things other than child care, moments when she'll want to turn her interests elsewhere; days when you'll be in a lousy mood, days when she'll be) will, ironically, be the first step in ensuring your time with her is well spent. The following are other steps you can take:

Act natural. No need to don your Supermom cape before you walk through the door. All your daughter wants is *you*. And no need to fill every minute you have with her with stimulating activities. Instead, be spontaneous, and take your cues from your baby (she may be too pooped at day's end for active play). Quality time is time spent together, whether it's eating together, cuddling together, or just being together in the same room (even if you're not doing the same thing).

Involve your baby. Take her with you into the bedroom while you change from your work clothes, and otherwise include her in your routine when you get home from work. She can play with the empty envelopes while you open the mail, empty the market bags while you put away groceries, or bang on pots and pans while you prepare dinner.

Tell her about your day. This will serve

two purposes. One, it will ensure that you're communicating with her (she loves to listen to you talk, even if she doesn't understand what you're saying). Two, unloading your day's experiences will help you unwind and make a faster transition from your job to your homelife.

Give your house short shrift. With time at a premium, devote less of it to matters that matter less (cleaning, cooking, and clothes care for instance). Take shortcuts in dinner preparation wherever possible (cook double quantities, freeze half to reheat another night; use frozen vegetables; get your green leafies from the local salad bar). Let the dust accumulate all week, and wait until the weekend to tackle it all at once with your husband. Or if you can afford it, hire someone to clean once a week. Use no-iron clothes, skipping the touch-ups, and send out your shirts if they have to be perfect.

Keep your dinner on the back burner. Or don't put it on at all until your baby's gone to bed. Late meals may not be best for digestion, but they'll give you more time to spend with your baby while she's awake (give her your undivided attention while she dines) and more time to spend with your husband when she's asleep (when he can be the center of attention). Though family dinnertimes are important later on, they're not really necessary now. At this age, in fact, meals with baby can be so stressful that instead of enhancing togetherness, they can give it a bad name.

Tune out distractions. You can't give your baby quality time while you're catching the six o'clock news. Save television watching, radio listening, and phone-call making for after your baby's gone to bed. Turn on the answering machine to postpone talking to incoming callers until after her bedtime, too.

Don't shut out your husband. In your quest for quality time with your baby, don't forget time spent as a family. Include your husband in whatever you're doing with the baby, from bathing to tickling. Also keep in mind that time he spends with her alone is important, too, for several reasons. It allows him to enjoy the pleasures of participatory parenting, something many fathers of generations past missed. It gives your baby the benefits of closeness with two unique individuals. And it doubles her quality time.

FINDING TIME FOR ROMANCE

"My husband and I are both so busy—with our jobs, our new son, the house—that we rarely find any time for each other. And when we do, we're too tired to make the most of it."

The three that baby makes isn't necessarily a crowd, but he can crowd your days and nights so much that you have no time left for the company of two. The period of new parenthood is actually one during which it is very easy for couples to grow apart instead of closer. Yet your relationship with your husband is the most significant in your life—more important even than the relationship with your child (children grow up and leave the nest, but hopefully your mate will be yours into old age). It was your love for each other that created your family in the first place, and it's that love that can best nurture and sustain it.

Nevertheless, the husband-wife relationship is the most easily taken for granted. If either of you neglected your jobs or your baby, the consequences would be clear and swift. Even the results of neglecting such home chores as cleaning and cooking would quickly become evident. But the results of neglecting a marriage often are not apparent at first; still; they can erode a relationship before the partners even realize it.

So give your relationship its due now and make a conscious effort to keep the love-lights glowing or, if they seem to have flickered out, to rekindle them. Rethink your priorities and reorganize your time in any way you have to, but free some up to spend alone together. One way is to put your baby on a reasonably early-to-bed schedule (see page 173 for tips on how) and settle back for some quality time with each other. Share a leisurely late dinner (no TV, no phone calls, no reading the daily paper, and hopefully, no crying baby allowed). A glass of wine may help you unwind (unless it leads to three or four, which may unravel you completely); candlelight and soft background music will help set the romantic mood.

Every such evening need not culminate in coitus. Indeed, intercourse may turn out to be a relatively rare treat in the exhausting early months—it may even be a treat you won't be very interested in for a while. Right now, verbal intercourse can be even more beneficial to your relationship than the sexual variety. But resist the temptation to talk exclusively about the baby; that would defeat the purpose of your interlude.

Try to wangle a romantic night out on the town at least once a month; more often would be even better. Have dinner, see a movie, visit with friends, or do whatever it is you enjoy doing together most. Also try to arrange for a baby-free hour or two on weekends to pursue a shared interest. Hire a sitter, swap sitting time with a neighbor, or enlist a grandparent (this is a great deal for everyone concerned).

If you can't seem to squeeze a regular rendezvous into your current schedule, a reevaluation of that schedule is in order. Perhaps you're trying to do too much. One or both of you may have to cut back working hours, drop a class, miss a ballgame or bowling night, or reduce TV watching.

JEALOUSY OF DADDY'S ATTENTION TO BABY

"As terrible as this sounds, I'm finding that I'm jealous of the time my husband spends with our daughter. I sometimes *wish he'd devote half as much attention to me."*

As harmless—even as heartwarming—as a budding romance between father and infant may seem to an outsider, it can be genuinely threatening to a woman who's not used to sharing her husband's affection, particularly if she's enjoyed his solicitous attention during nine months of pregnancy.

Although your feelings of jealousy will probably subside on their own once the family dynamics have had some time to work themselves out, there are several steps you can take to deal with them in the meantime:

Be assured. The first thing you need to do to overcome the feelings you're experiencing is to recognize that they're normal and common—not petty, evil, selfish, immoral, or otherwise shameful. Dump that guilt.

Be grateful. Consider how lucky you are to be married to the kind of man who's eager to spend time with his baby. Though active participation from the male partner in parenting is increasingly common, it's by no means standard. Take advantage of the time they spend together to catch up on chores or personal needs. Watch with appreciation the love that's blossoming between the two of them, and try to support it; the bonds they're building now will last a lifetime, through the terrible twos and even the turbulent teens, and will make your daughter a better woman (or make your son a better man).

Be a part of it. Father and baby should certainly share some time alone together, but sometimes a third player will be welcome. Join that tickle fest (he gets the ribcage, you get the toes), flop down on the bed beside them as they read a book, sit down and make their two-way game of "catch" on the rug three-way.

Be honest and open. Don't just sulk from the sidelines when daddy and baby leave you out of the loving action. In the excitement of discovering a new best buddy, your husband may not realize that he's been shutting out his (relatively) old one; he may even believe he's helping you out. Tell him, without being offensive or putting him on the defensive, how you feel and exactly what he can do about it (for example, tell *both* of you how pretty you look, give *both* of you a kiss and hug when he comes and goes, snuggle spontaneously with *both* of you). He can't fulfill your needs unless he knows what they are.

Be there for him. Remember, a relationship that works, works two ways. You can't ask your husband to devote more attention to you without your reciprocating. Make sure you, too, haven't been spending all your time, energy, and affection on the baby, unwittingly leaving none of the above for him. Dote on him, and you're bound to find him doting back.

Be there for baby, too. Maybe your husband is consciously or subconsciously trying to compensate for attention he feels your baby isn't getting from you. Perhaps you're so busy with other responsibilities (a job, housework, volunteer work, sports, or whatever) that you have little time left for your child. If that's the case, be grateful she's getting parental attention somewhere, and consider reassessing your priorities to make certain that she gets more of it from you.

JEALOUSY OF DADDY'S PARENTING SKILLS

"I thought that mothers were supposed to be naturally better at parenting than fathers. But my husband has a way with our son—making him laugh, calming him down, rocking him to sleep—that I don't. And that makes me feel inadequate and insecure."

Every parent enters parenthood with something to offer his or her baby, with no one contribution more valuable or desirable than another, at least not as far as the little beneficiary is concerned. Some parents are better at the fun-and-games aspects of baby raising (roughhousing, getting a good giggle going, playing peekaboo), some at the nuts-and-bolts tasks (feeding, bathing, getting baby dressed without a struggle). Some, like your husband, display a knack for building rapport with baby.

Still, it isn't surprising for one parent to be a little envious of the other's talents. But it's possible to shake such feelings:

Consider yourself lucky. The father who's able and willing to participate so fully and successfully in baby care is a precious commodity and can take a lot of the pressure off mom. Let him practice his baby magic whenever possible. For any partnership to be productive (and parenting should be a partnership), each partner should contribute what he or she knows and can do best.

Don't be a female chauvinist. Sexual stereotypes that depict women as naturally better at parenting than men are inaccurate and, ultimately, destructive to all concerned. There is no child-care responsibility other than breastfeeding that all mothers are more naturally suited to than all fathers, or vice versa. Some parents (no matter what gender) have a natural knack for parenting skills, some have to work hard at mastering infant care. Given the opportunity, any parent of either sex can overcome a lack of natural aptitude in time.

Give yourself more credit. You may not realize how much you do for your baby and how well you do it—though your baby almost certainly does, and he couldn't do without you.

And give yourself a chance. Just because certain parenting skills don't come as easily to you as they do to your husband doesn't mean they'll always be elusive. If you're breastfeeding, you may find that once you've weaned your baby and the distraction of breast milk is past, you'll be able to calm him on your chest as well as your husband does. With practice and a lessening of self-consciousness, you will also learn to sing the lullabies and silly songs your baby loves, to play finger games and make funny faces, and to rock him with a comforting rhythm.

Instead of mimicking what seems to work for your husband, start doing what comes naturally to you. Your odds for success will be better if you don't start out with a defeatist attitude, which your smarter-than-you-think baby is sure to sense. Also make sure you get the chance to give yourself a chance. If your baby-care assignments all seem to be the more tedious, less rewarding ones (changing diapers or giving the dreaded shampoo, for instance), negotiate some changes in the duty roster with your husband. When he takes over some of the less glamorous tasks, you will be freed up for some of the fun ones.

And remember, no matter how good a relationship dad and baby develop, there will always be times when no one else will do for your child but you, and you'll hear those soon to be familiar words: "I want my mommy."

FEELING UNAPPRECIATED AS A WOMAN

"Ever since our son was born, I've felt that my husband sees me only as the mother of his child, not as the woman he loves."

A man doesn't usually grow up thinking of his own mother as a sexual being, or if he does, he quickly learns to sublimate such thoughts. When the woman he loves, and who is the sexual being in his life, becomes a mother, his feelings about her often become confused. She frequently adds to his dilemma by acting more like a mother than a mate as she busily tries to master the new and challenging role of mother.

Though this is a common problem in new families, it isn't an insolvable one and resolving it is one of the most significant steps you can take to ensure your baby will grow up in a happy, intact home. You *can* be both mother to your child and wife and lover to your spouse; it only takes a little extra effort.

Make yourself feel like a woman. Caring for your looks is a good place to begin. Clean and well-groomed hair (an easy-care haircut will help), simple makeup (if you customarily wear it, or if you feel you need it now that you're getting less sleep), and fresh clothes (a shirt baby has spit up on isn't going to inspire romance) will not only make you feel more attractive, they will help your husband to see you as a desirable woman. Hoping to start the day that way every day would, for most new mothers, be unrealistic; but attaining that state before a husband's key turns in the door in the evening may not be. Even on the worst of days, when a shampoo is impossible, when you feel lucky to find a sweatshirt that doesn't clash with your jogging pants, you can take five minutes for a quick face wash and mini-makeover: put on some mascara and blush, run a brush through your hair, dab on some of your favorite scent. You'll feel better and your efforts won't be lost on your spouse.

Make him feel like a man. Most new mothers transfer their focus from their husband to their baby, at least initially. That's good for the perpetuation of the species, but not so good for the perpetuation of the marriage. Make it a point to romance your husband as you would like to be romanced. Hug him unexpectedly from behind while he's washing the dishes, squeeze his hand when he passes the baby shampoo, lavish him with compliments when he comes home with a new haircut, kiss him anytime (and anywhere) at all. Cook his favorite meal, give him an unbirthday present, ask him how his day went instead of just complaining about yours.

Share the baby. Making your husband

feel more comfortable as a father may help him feel more like a man, reduce any resentment about sharing you with the baby, and make him more a part of your new life, which in turn may help rekindle the romantic flame for both of you. Encourage him to participate in baby care without nagging him to do so, making it seem more like a privilege and a pleasure than a chore. And be sure to praise, not criticize, his efforts—even if they're clumsy at first.

THINKING ABOUT THE NEXT BABY

"I'm nearly forty and had my first baby nearly a year ago. I know it's early to be thinking about another, but I don't have many fertile years left."

Today, decisions about spacing offspring often have less to do with the latest psychological literature on what's best for baby than on the exigencies of time. Many women are trying to squeeze in a second or third baby before they reach forty, or soon thereafter.

It's best to wait at least a year after the birth of one child before becoming pregnant with the next. Many moms and babies have, it's true, come through closer spacings with no problems, but a year's hiatus gives a mother's body adequate time to heal and recover strength (particularly important if the first baby was delivered by cesarean section). It also allows for nursing the first child for a full year if desired. What it doesn't allow for, unfortunately, is optimum time for that child to be the baby of the family. It's probably not ideal to be displaced by a younger sibling when you're barely out of diapers yourself; and today, most babies still aren't even at 21 months. The experts are divided on what is ideal, though most suggest a two- to four-year wait, which some (but not all) studies indicate gives children a slight edge. But gener-

alities don't work for every family, and the best time for you to have another baby is when you and your spouse feel your family is ready.

Since waiting longer than a year is not always an acceptable option, you should also know that close spacing of children can work well. It offers some pluses that two- to four-year spacing doesn't, particularly once the first few years of chaos, sleepless nights, and endless diapers are over: the siblings may be closer chums; and the same toys, movies, activities, and vacations may interest both. With plenty of love, attention, and preparation your oldest can make the transition from baby to older sibling with a minimum of trauma (see page 601).

If you are seriously thinking about becoming pregnant again soon, see your doctor for a complete checkup now; take care of any dental problems, too. Then, in the two or three months before you start trying to conceive, start preparing your body:[2]

■ Wean your baby, if you haven't already. Or in the competition for nutrients, someone's bound to lose—and it's most likely to be the unborn baby. Setting up such a sibling rivalry isn't healthy or recommended. You too may suffer if your stores are drained of calcium and other essential nutrients.

■ Follow the Best-Odds Prepregnancy Diet (see footnote number 2), and encourage your husband to improve his diet, too. Continue taking a pregnancy vitamin supplement.

■ Get or stay in shape with exercise and try to bring or keep your weight as close to ideal as possible. Do not diet strenuously, however, in the few months before conception, and *don't* try to lose weight once you've become pregnant.

■ Discontinue using birth control pills or spermicides at least two months (or better still, three) before the time you plan to begin trying to conceive. Switch to condoms until you're ready to begin trying.

---

2. For a more detailed prepregnancy plan, see our book *What to Expect When You're Expecting.*

- Avoid excesses in alcohol during the pre-pregnancy stage; stop drinking altogether once you start trying to conceive. If you smoke or use other "recreational" drugs, quit before you try to conceive. Your husband, too, should abstain from alcohol and drugs while you are trying to conceive. If either of you can't quit, get help.
- Once you've begun trying to conceive, limit prescription and over-the-counter drugs to those your doctor approves for use during pregnancy.
- Also once you begin trying, avoid exposure to X-rays or potentially hazardous chemicals.
- Relax. Excess stress in your life can prevent your conceiving, and too much tension during pregnancy isn't good for your fetus, your older baby, or you.

WHAT IT'S IMPORTANT TO KNOW: To Work or Not to Work

Many women, because of a variety of pressures—societal, career, financial—don't have the option of staying at home after their babies are born. However, for those who have a choice, the process of decision making is often agonizing. Childcare experts—because they are in disagreement—offer these mothers little guidance. Some believe there is no harm and possibly some benefit when a mother takes a job and leaves her baby in a child-care situation. Others believe just as strongly that there is the potential for more than a little damage to the infant in a two-paycheck family, and urge that one parent (for practical reasons it's usually the mother) stay at home, at least part-time, until the baby is three years old.

Research is no more helpful. Study results are contradictory. Primarily this is because such research is both difficult to do and difficult to evaluate. (How do you judge the effects on her offspring when a mother holds a paying job? Or doesn't hold one? Which effects are important to evaluate? Which are difficult to quantify? Are there some we can't even predict? Will problems show up early or not until adulthood?) In addition, the research is often colored by the bias of the researcher.

A recent study demonstrates the difficulties. It found that children in day care from as early as seven months can have enhanced language skills and thinking ability—but only if the day care program is a good one, where children are talked to a lot. On the other hand, the study also showed a link between the amount of time spent in day care and the attitude of mother toward infant and toddler toward mother. The more time spent in day care, the less sensitive mothers seemed toward infants at six months, 15 months, and 36 months. In addition, children with a lot of time in day care were less affectionate toward their mothers at ages 24 and 36 months. Does this mean that putting your child in day care will scuttle your efforts at bonding with your child? Not necessarily. It just may be that parents who put their children in day care early and for longer periods start out with less of an attachment—and the results would not have been any different if those parents stayed at home. They might even have been worse.

With no clear-cut evidence on the longterm risks or benefits of a mother's working outside the home to go on, the full weight of making this decision falls entirely on the parents. If you're pondering the question, asking yourself the following questions may help you sort out the best way to go.

What are your priorities? Consider carefully what is most important in your life. List your priorities in order on paper. They may include your baby, your family, your career, financial security, the luxuries of life, vacations, study—and may be vastly different from those of the woman next door or the woman at the next desk. After charting your priorities, consider whether returning to employment or staying at home will best meet the most important of them.

Which full-time role suits your personality best? Are you at your best at home with the baby? Or does staying home make you impatient and tense? Will you be able to leave worries about your baby at home when you go to your job, and worries about your job at the office when you're home with the baby? Or will an inability to compartmentalize your life keep you from doing your best at either job?

Would you feel comfortable having someone else take care of your baby? Do you feel no one else can do the job as well as you can? Or do you feel secure that you can find (or have found) a person (or group situation) that can substitute well for you during your hours away from home?

How do you feel about missing the major milestones? The first time your baby laughs, sits alone, gets up on all fours and crawls, or takes a step—will you mind hearing about it secondhand? Will you feel saddened and slighted if the sitter is the one your baby runs to when hurt? Do you feel you can learn to tune in to your baby's unspoken needs and feelings by just spending evenings and weekends together?

How much energy do you have? You'll need plenty of emotional and physical stamina to rise with a baby, get yourself ready for work, put in a full day on the job, then return to the demands of your baby, home, and husband once again. Often, what suffers most when energy is lacking in the two-paycheck family with young children is the relationship between husband and wife.

How stressful are your job and your baby? If your job is low stress and your baby's a piece of cake to care for, the duo may be relatively easy to handle. If your job is high pressure and your baby is, too, will you find yourself unable to cope with both, day in and day out?

If you do return to employment, will you get adequate support from your spouse or from some other source? Even a mother from the planet Krypton couldn't do it all alone. Will your husband be willing to do his share of baby care, shopping, cooking, cleaning, and laundry? Or are you able to afford outside help to take up the slack?

What is your financial situation? Will your not working threaten your family's economic survival, or just necessitate cutting down on the extras you've been enjoying? Are there ways of cutting back so that the loss of your income won't hurt so much? If you go back to work, how much of a dent will job-related costs (clothes, commutation, child care) make in your income?

How flexible is your job? Will you be able to take time off if your baby or your baby-sitter is sick? Or come in late or leave early if there's an emergency at home? does your job require long hours, weekends, and/or travel? Are you willing to spend extended time away from the baby?

How will not returning to your job affect your career? Putting a career on hold can sometimes set you back when you return to the working world. If you suspect this will happen to you (though many women discover, when they return, that their fears haven't materialized), are you willing to make this sacrifice? Are there ways to keep yourself in touch professionally during your at-home years without making a full-time commitment?

Is there a compromise position? Maybe you can't have it all and remain sane, but you may be able to have the best of both worlds by looking for a creative compromise. The possibilities are endless and depend on your skills and work experience. If your skills are valuable to someone full-time, then you should be able to sell them part-time. It's possible a current or previous employer, or somebody new, will hire you on a flexible, reduced, or job-sharing schedule. Or maybe you can be a free-lance consultant rather than a full-time employee. Perhaps you can do some or all of your work at home, or bring your baby to the office part-time (some women have done this successfully full-time). Or take your baby with you to see clients and on assignments (again, something a few determined women have managed to pull off). When you have the choice, it's usually better to work four or five half-days than two or three full ones—that way you won't be apart from your baby for long stretches.

If you sell real estate, show houses twice a week; tutor two or three afternoons for pay if you're a teacher; see clients a couple of nights a week if you're a therapist; teach some self-help health classes if you're a nurse; take in typing if you're a secretary; or work part-time for a group or in a clinic if you're a doctor. If you enjoy teaching, start a class in your area of expertise (anything from cooking to creative writing, from aerobic exercise to exercising rights in housing court, from how to fix a car to how to prepare tax returns) at a local Y, your church or synagogue, or an adult learning center.

Or run a part-time business out of your home. If you're an accountant or an advertising copywriter, find a few clients whose accounts you can handle from your den; if you're a writer, editor, or graphic designer, look for free-lance assignments. If you've a knack for knitting, design sweaters to sell to baby boutiques; if you make an incomparable carrot cake, package your creations for a local gourmet shop.

If you decide to work out of your home, for yourself or someone else, you may still need a sitter for at least part of your working hours. But you can also plan to work while baby naps and after he or she's in bed for the night, and to do pickups and deliveries with baby in tow. Getting help with the household chores is important so that you won't have to give up too much of your time with the baby.

Whatever choice you make, it's likely to require some measure of sacrifice. As committed as you might be to staying home, you may nevertheless feel a pang or two (or more) of regret when you talk to friends who are still pursuing their careers. Or as committed as you might be to returning to your job, you may experience regret when you pass mothers and their babies on their way to the park while you're on your way to the office.

Such misgivings are normal, and since few perfect situations exist in our imperfect world, they're something you'll have to learn to live with. If, however, they begin to multiply and you find dissatisfaction out-weighing satisfaction, it's time to reassess the choice you've made. A decision that seemed right in theory when you made it may seem all wrong in practice now—in which case you shouldn't hesitate to reverse or alter it, if at all possible.

And when everything isn't as idyllic as you'd like, remember that children who get plenty of love are very resilient. Even the wrong decision, if there is such a thing, isn't likely to leave permanent scars.

WHEN TO RETURN TO YOUR JOB

There's no predictably perfect point at which someone can say, "Okay, now you can go back to your job. Your baby will be fine and so will you." If you decide to go back to work during the first year, when you pick up that briefcase or lunchbox will depend in part on your job and the amount of maternity leave you were able to wangle and in part on when you and your baby are ready. And that's highly personal and highly individual.

If you have the choice, experts suggest you wait at least until you've "attached" or "bonded" with your baby and feel competent as a mother. Bonding can take three months (though if your baby has had colic, you will probably just be starting to become friends at this point), or it can take five or six. Unfortunately many women with difficult babies hurry back to their jobs, assuming someone else can do a better job with the baby than they can. With the task of bonding incomplete, some of these women never do reach the point of feeling competent at mothering—which could be detrimental to the mother-child relationship.

Support is growing nationally for longer maternity leave with some job guarantees. As a nation we're far behind much of the rest of the world. While more than 100 other countries guarantee some sort of parental leave, only about 40% of working women in the U.S. get any leave at all, and for most of these six weeks without pay is it. Canadian workers are guaranteed up to 41 weeks of leave with job security and 60% pay, Italians get up to five months with 80% pay, and West Germans 18 weeks at full pay. We should not only be able to do as well—we should be able to do better.

CHAPTER TWENTY-FIVE

Becoming A Father

For the nine months of your wife's pregnancy, the direct care of your baby was pretty much out of your hands—not by choice, but thanks to the quirks of reproductive biology. You could stand by, offering love and support, but you couldn't take over the responsibility of nurturing your baby even for a moment.

Now that the cord's been cut, the rules of the game have changed. No longer do you need special biological equipment for the job of child care. You don't even need experience. All you need is the will to chip in and parent. Not as your wife's chief assistant and bottle washer, but as her partner in the wonderful, unpredictable, exhausting, exhilarating, enlightening, ever-challenging business of parenting.

WHAT YOU MAY BE CONCERNED ABOUT

YOUR DIET AND YOUR BABY

"I gave up a lot of my favorite foods when my wife was pregnant so I could support her efforts to eat right for our baby. But enough's enough. Now that our son's here, shouldn't I be able to eat what I like?"

Your baby's nutritional dependence doesn't end with the cutting of the umbilical cord. Until he's grown and has moved out of your home, your child will likely be what you (and the rest of the family) eat. Elect to breakfast on donuts or Danish, snack between meals on potato chips or cookies, wash down your lunchtime sandwich with Coke, leave over your carrots and zucchini at dinner, and you're setting a dietary example that he's sure to follow.

Another significant reason to take your diet seriously, even while your child is a young infant, is to increase the odds that you'll be around when he's older, and that you'll be a healthy, productive father to him as he grows. The diseases that are most likely to take your life, or the lives of other American males, prematurely—cancer, heart disease, stroke, diabetes—can all be prevented to some degree by eating right.

Continue to eat a diet high in fiber-rich complex carbohydrates (such as whole-grain cereals and breads, high-protein or whole-grain pastas, dried peas and beans, fruits and vegetables), low in sugar, salt, fat (especially hardened or saturated fats), and cholesterol, and moderate in protein—for baby's sake as well as your own.

And don't sabotage the benefits you give your baby through good diet by smoking. Children of smoking parents have considerably more illness than children of non-smokers, and they are more likely to smoke themselves. They are also more likely to be colicky. If you're a smoker and have had difficulty quitting, seek help from your doctor or join a smoking cessation program or group.

A DISAPPOINTING DELIVERY

"My wife and I had our hearts set on a natural childbirth. But delivery didn't go as we'd hoped and she ended up needing medication. I was upset then, and I still feel a sense of disappointment."

Like many women experiencing childbirth today, many husbands have come to believe that the labor and delivery experience is a test to be passed or failed. If medication, an episiotomy, or even a cesarean proves nec-

essary, these husbands consider the birth a failure and often end up feeling not only disappointed but angry. These attitudes are usually born in childbirth education classes and in pregnancy books that emphasize the joy of the birth experience over a safe outcome, and that pressure couples to "go natural" under almost any circumstance. The implication is that when a woman asks for medication it's because she's inexcusably weak, not because the pain is unbearably strong. Descriptions of the birthing process can be more idealistic than realistic, often calling the pain of childbirth "discomfort" in spite of the fact that research has shown it to be the most severe pain experienced by humans.

That's not to say that the birth experience never turns out to be a perfect and perfectly natural one, just that more often it doesn't. And in the long run, it really doesn't matter whether it does or not. As long as both mother and child come out of the birthing or delivery room healthy, childbirth was a success and both parents have every reason to be happy. By making your wife feel that you're dissatisfied with her "performance" (even indirectly) if medical intervention proved necessary, you may heighten her own feelings of inadequacy and intensify her disappointment—both of which can put her at increased risk for postpartum depression. Instead, let her know how proud you are of her, how you admire her courage, how happy you are that both she and the baby came through the ordeal in good shape, and how much both of them mean to you.

BONDING

"I expected to be overwhelmed with affection for my baby the first time I held her in the birthing room, but I wasn't. She's so unresponsive, so red and puffy, so unlike what I'd imagined she'd be."

To a first-time parent who's never even seen a minutes-old newborn before, disappointment and dismay are as likely to be first reactions to the just-delivered offspring as love and affection. As with any romance, your love affair with your baby will require plenty of time and nurturing to develop and deepen. Even those new parents who seem to fall in love with their babies "at first sight" find their relationships growing richer as the months pass.

Relax. As your baby becomes more responsive, so will you. And what you'll feel once you've had a chance to get to know her will have far more impact on your future than what you feel at your first meeting.

If, however, you don't begin to feel any love toward your baby in the weeks ahead, and especially if you feel anger, hostility, or violent urges, seek immediate psychological counseling from your family physician, a family therapist, a psychiatrist, or another mental health professional.

"My wife had an emergency cesarean and I wasn't allowed to be with her. I didn't hold our son until 24 hours later, and I'm afraid bonding will suffer."

Until the 1970s, fathers rarely witnessed the birth of their children, and none had even heard of the concept of "bonding." Nevertheless, most developed loving relationships with their sons and daughters. And though in recent years, witnessing the birth of their offspring has enriched the lives of many men, it hasn't guaranteed a lifetime of father-child closeness.

Being able to share the moment of delivery with your wife is certainly ideal, and being deprived of that opportunity is reason for disappointment—particularly if you spent months training together for childbirth. But it's no reason for a less than loving relationship with your baby. What really bonds you with your baby is day-to-day contact—diapering, bathing, feeding, cuddling, lullabying, playing. He will never care that you didn't share in the moment of birth or the first hours after it, but he will surely miss you if you aren't there when he needs you from then on.

WIFE'S POSTPARTUM DEPRESSION

"We have a beautiful and healthy baby girl, just what my wife has always wanted. Still, she's been weepy and unhappy ever since she came home from the hospital."

A number of factors—from a sense of letdown over not being pregnant anymore to frustration over still looking as if she is—combine with hormonal upheaval to trigger postpartum depression in about half (some estimates go as high as 90%) of all newly or recently delivered women. Fortunately for the vast majority (about 999 in 1,000), the depression is neither severe nor long lasting, and usually resolves within the first couple of weeks postpartum.

Though hormonal changes may contribute to postpartum depression, you don't have to be an endocrinologist—only a loving and attentive husband—to help banish it. Try to:

Lighten her load. Fatigue, a major contributor to depression, is an inevitable component of the postpartum period. Be sure that your wife has all the help she needs—from you when you're around, and from others when you're not.

Brighten her day—and night. When the new arrival becomes the center of everyone's attention, the new mother often feels neglected. She may also feel inadequate (having much to learn about the care and feeding of an infant) as well as unattractive (having several pregnancy pounds still to shed). Here, too, you can make a difference. Compliment her at unexpected moments on how good she is with the baby, how radiant she looks, how slim she's getting, how motherhood becomes her. Cheer her up with little gifts—flowers, a new book, a pretty nightgown—but not chocolates, which will only feed the depression and the pounds.

Take her away from it all. Time alone together is critical not only for her sake but also for the sake of your relationship. Make some time daily for the two of you (see page 582 for help).

If your wife's depression lasts more than two weeks, is accompanied by sleeplessness, lack of appetite, expressions of hopelessness and helplessness, or suicidal or violent urges, don't wait any longer for it to pass. Insist that she seek help—from either her obstetrician, the family doctor, or a skilled therapist. A very occasional new mother needs psychiatric care to clear the hurdles of the first few months of motherhood.

Once in a while, the depression holds off until the new mother weans her breastfed baby. As with any depression, it should be treated if it persists.

YOUR DEPRESSION

"How come my wife feels terrific since our son was born, and I'm the one with postpartum depression?"

Today's fathers are becoming more involved in pregnancy, childbirth, and child care than ever before. Short of carrying the fetus and nursing the baby, there's virtually nothing they're not getting into—including postpartum depression. In fact, a full 62% of dads in one study were found to be suffering from the "baby blues." Though there's been some speculation that hormones are somehow the cause, there's been no evidence to support the theory. It's much more likely that any number of the following contributing factors are combining to bring you down at what you may have expected would be one of the highest points of your life:

Financial stress. Rare is the father who is exempt from financial concerns once there's another mouth to feed, body to clothe, mind to educate, and future to plan for. The stress can be compounded when one paycheck in a two-paycheck family

suddenly disappears, even temporarily.

Feeling like a third wheel. A father who's become accustomed to being the center of his wife's life may be chagrined to suddenly discover himself on the sidelines, watching her attention being lavished on a noisy newcomer.

A love life lost. Many men find their sex lives are curtailed, at least temporarily, which is depressing enough. But on top of that they fear that the romantic relationship they once enjoyed with their wives will never be completely revived.

Changed relationships. A husband who had been dependent on his wife for the fulfillment of a variety of needs may be upset to find she's suddenly unavailable because she's busy filling someone else's needs. Conversely, a husband used to having his wife depend on him may be unnerved to find that she, having found a dependent of her own, no longer is. Until he adjusts to the changing family dynamics, a new father can feel emotionally out of kilter.

Altered life style. You needn't have had a full social calendar before baby's arrival to be depressed about not having any social life at all now that he's here. At least for a while, even a movie or a dinner with friends may be elusive, and staying home night after night can certainly spark a dark mood in anyone but the most naturally reclusive new father.

Sleep deprivation. Though the father who routinely answers his baby's calls is likely to be most worn out by middle-of-the-night wakings, even the father who doesn't is bound to feel the effects of night after night of disturbed sleep. The physical exhaustion soon takes an emotional toll, often in the form of depression.

Being aware of the possible causes of your "baby blues" may help you to escape, or at least manage, them—particularly if you take steps to modify their effects (see tips throughout this chapter). Then again, it's possible that your depression will linger for a few weeks no matter what you do and then disappear as unexpectedly as it arrived. If it doesn't, and if it starts to interfere with your functioning and/or with your relationship with your wife and/or your child, speak to your family doctor or contact a therapist.

FEELING UNSEXY

"The delivery of our new daughter was miraculous to watch. But seeing her emerge from my wife's vagina seems to have turned me off to sex."

Human sexual response, compared to that of other animals, is an extremely delicate mechanism. It's at the mercy not only of the body, but of the mind as well. And the mind can, at times, play merciless havoc with it. One of those times, as you probably already know, is pregnancy. Another, as you are now discovering, is the postpartum period.

It's very possible that your sudden disinterest in sex has nothing to do with having seen your baby born. Most brand-new fathers, whether they've viewed delivery or not, find both the spirit and the flesh somewhat less than willing for a while—although there's certainly nothing abnormal about those who don't. There are many very understandable reasons: fatigue, especially if the baby is waking frequently at night; uneasiness over loss of privacy, especially if your baby is sharing your room; fear that she will awake crying at the most inopportune moment; concern that intercourse may hurt your wife, even though the doctor has given you a green light; and finally, general physical and mental preoccupation with your newborn, to whom your energies are sensibly directed at this stage in her life.

In other words, it's probably just as well that you aren't feeling sexually motivated, particularly if your wife, like many women in the early months of motherhood, isn't either. Just how long it will take for your interest (and hers) to return is impossible to predict. As with all matters sexual, there's a wide range of normal. For some couples, the urge will precede even the doctor's go-ahead. For others, six months or more may pass before l'amour and le bébé begin to coexist harmoniously. (Some women find desire lacking until they stop breastfeeding, although on the average, breastfeeding mothers find passion rekindled earlier than non-breastfeeders.)

Some fathers, however, even if they've been prepared for the experience in class, do emerge from childbirth feeling that their "territory" has been "violated," that the special place that had been reserved for loving has suddenly taken on an all-too-functional purpose. If that's actually the case with you, you will need to—first intellectually and then emotionally—begin to accept the idea that the vagina's sexual and reproductive functions are equally important and equally miraculous. Neither excludes the other, and in fact, they are very much interconnected. Most importantly, the vagina is a vehicle for childbirth only briefly, but it is a source of pleasure for you and your wife for a lifetime.

"Fondling my wife's breasts used to be an important part of our sexual foreplay. Now that she's breastfeeding, that's becoming a big problem."

Like the vagina, breasts were designed for both fun and function. And although these purposes are not only not mutually exclusive, but are actually interdependent in the grand scheme of things (if sex weren't fun, there wouldn't be as many babies to nurse), they can conflict temporarily during lactation.

Many couples, either for aesthetic reasons (leaking milk, for instance) or because they feel uncomfortable using their baby's source of nourishment for their own sexual pleasure, find breastfeeding a very definite turnoff. Others, however, find it a sexual turn-on, possibly because of its inherently sensual nature. Either reaction is perfectly normal.

If you feel that your wife's breasts are too functional to be sexy now, if leaking occurs on stimulation and you find that to be unpleasant, or if your touching them dampens your wife's ardor, simply leave them out of sexual foreplay until baby is weaned. And don't worry—all uneasiness will pass once breastfeeding ceases.

Be sure, however, to be open and honest with your wife now; taking a sudden, unexplained, hands-off approach to her breasts could leave her feeling that motherhood has somehow made her unappealing. Be sure, too, that you're not harboring resentment against the baby for using "your" breasts; as strange as it may seem, many men do.

"The first time we had sex after the baby was born my wife had a lot of pain. Now I'm so afraid of hurting her again that I've been avoiding sex."

You may hurt your wife more by avoiding sex than by initiating it. More than ever before, your wife needs to feel attractive, desirable, and wanted—even if she herself is hesitant to engage in intercourse because of fear of pain or lack of desire. Although your intentions are certainly noble, your steering away from lovemaking may lead to the development of beneath-the-surface anger and resentment in either or both of you, which could jeopardize your relationship.

But before you approach her again sexually, approach her verbally. Tell her your concerns, and find out what hers are. Decide together whether you want to wait a little longer before trying again, or whether you want to make love despite the discomfort. Keep in mind that you needn't worry about causing physical harm if your wife's practitioner has examined her and given the go-ahead. Whatever you decide, the tips on page 560 will help minimize the pain and maximize the pleasure when lovemaking resumes. And remember, too, that postponing intercourse doesn't mean banishing romance from your lives. Intercourse is by no means the only way two people can enjoy each other and show their love. Right now,

you may find just as much fulfillment lying in each other's arms.

EXCLUSION FROM BREASTFEEDING

"My wife is breastfeeding our son. There's a closeness between them I can't seem to share, and I feel left out."

There are certain immutable biological aspects of parenting that undeniably exclude you, the father: you can't be pregnant, you can't labor and deliver (which many would consider a definite plus), and you can't breastfeed. But as millions of new fathers discover each year, your natural anatomical limitations don't have to relegate you to spectator status. You can share in nearly all the joy, anticipation, trials, and tribulations of your wife's pregnancy, labor, and delivery—from the first kick to the last push—as an active, supportive partner. And though you'll never be able to put your baby to breast (at least not with the kind of results your baby's looking for), you *can* share in the feeding process:

Be your baby's supplementary feeder. There's more than one way to feed a baby. And though you can't nurse, you can be the one to give any supplementary bottles. It will not only give your wife a break (whether in the middle of the night or in the middle of dinner), it will give you extra time for closeness with your baby. Don't waste an opportunity by propping the bottle in the baby's mouth. Strike a nursing pose, with your baby snuggled close to your chest.

Don't sleep through the night. Sharing the joys of feeding also entitles you to share the sleepless nights. Even if your baby's not getting supplementary bottles, you can be a part of nighttime feeding rituals by rising to get baby out of the crib, doing any necessary diaper changing, and bringing him to his mommy for nursing. Should he still be awake after the feeding, you can rock and soothe him to sleep before putting him back to bed. Here, your not being the nursing parent works in your favor; since your baby doesn't feel or smell breasts filled with milk, he is much more likely to be calmed by you than by his mother.

Watch in wonder, and appreciate. Enormous satisfaction can be had in simply observing the wondrous miracle that is breastfeeding. Next time you feel left out, take a few minutes to sit with your wife and baby and witness the love that passes between them as they nurse—it's bound to make you feel closer to both of them.

Participate in all the other daily rituals. Nursing is the *only* daily child-care activity limited to mothers. And chances are if you make at least one, or better still several, of these chores (such as bathing, dressing, feeding solids, changing diapers) your responsibility, you'll be too busy building your own relationship with your baby to be envious of your wife's.

JEALOUSY OF MOTHER'S ATTENTION TO BABY

"I love my new daughter, but I also love my wife—and as much as I hate to admit it, I'm jealous of all the time she spends with her. She doesn't seem to have any energy left for me."

There may be a companionable new twosome in your family, but it shouldn't leave you feeling as though three's a crowd. Though it's natural that your wife should be somewhat preoccupied with the baby, it shouldn't be at the expense of your relationship as a couple—a relationship that is vital to your future as a family, and that needs nurturing to survive the assaults of parenthood, now and in the future. To help deal with your feelings (which, though normal and common, can become destructive

if allowed to fester) and to preserve and improve your own twosome, take these steps:

Make your feelings known. Perhaps your wife isn't aware that as she's getting to know your baby she's losing touch with you. Tell her how you feel, but in a constructive discussion, rather than a destructive tirade. Let her know you appreciate the terrific job she's doing as a mother, but remind her that full-grown men, too, need regular doses of tender loving care—though they may not always be as vocal as babies in demonstrating that need.

Make a threesome. Since you can't (and wouldn't want to) beat them, join them. As time alone with each other becomes a more and more precious and elusive commodity, concentrate on spending more time together as a family—stretching that mother-baby twosome into a cozy threesome—which you may find will strengthen the bonds between you as a couple. Pitching in with baby care will give your wife more time to devote to you, while giving you less inclination (and energy) to feel jealous.

Make a deal. Negotiate for some private time with your wife. Try to arrange to set aside an hour each night (after the baby's asleep and before the television goes on) for the two of you to spend together eating dinner (if it isn't too late), sipping wine or tea, unwinding, chatting (hopefully not just about the baby), getting to know each other again. And bargain to reserve at least one night a month (more, if possible) for a special and romantic evening out. But be understanding when she falls asleep at a movie or while you're trying to have an adult conversation—her exhaustion can't be willed away by either of you.

Make a little whoopee. Romance is a two-way street. And it's possible that your wife is feeling as neglected by you since the baby's been born as you are by her. So go out of your way to cast that romantic spell: be spontaneous (flowers for no reason), flirtatious (hug her from behind as she bends over to pick up that diaper), lavish her with compliments (especially when she needs them most). Play a determined Romeo, and it won't be long before she's your Juliet again.

In spite of all your efforts, and even your wife's good intentions, you may find that she still seems distant. That's not unusual in women for anywhere between six weeks to six months after the birth of a baby. This attitude may be part of a built-in protective mechanism that keeps a new mother from cohabiting too soon after delivery, prevents her from conceiving too quickly, and ensures that her attention and energies are focused on the newborn. It isn't a reflection on her husband or a barometer of her love for him. Be patient, and it will pass. If, however, the estrangement lasts well into the second half of the year, and talking about it doesn't help, professional counseling may be needed.

FEELING INADEQUATE AS A FATHER

"I want to be involved with caring for the baby, and I want to help my wife out. But I've never had any experience with an infant, and I'm feeling completely useless."

You're a pioneer, treading where the vast majority of past generations of fathers either dared not or cared not to tread. Like any pioneer, you probably have neither hands-on nor passed-on (if your own father didn't participate in baby care) experience to count on. Little wonder, then, that you're feeling a little insecure at the outset.

It's a feeling, however, that's bound to be short-lived. The willingness to try and a lot of love to offer are the only qualifications needed to succeed at parenting. Though those with some baby care under their belts may get off to a faster start, even a novice

like you will be running (and rocking, and bathing, and changing) neck-and-neck with them within a couple of months. In the meantime, you needn't worry about your baby's suffering because of your inexperience. First of all, he can tolerate a lot more manhandling than you'd think—and he won't "break" if your touch is tentative or awkward. Second, he'll be a good sport as you learn. He has no frame of reference, no "perfect" father to measure you against. As long as his immediate needs are attended to, even in a bumbling way, and he senses your good intentions, he's bound to accept you—imperfections, inexperience, and all.

Studies show that fathers exhibit the same physiological responses to a baby's crying as mothers, and they can be just as sensitive to a baby's cues (although because they're less likely to spend as much time around baby as a mother, they're less likely to sharpen this sensitivity and respond accordingly). Some fathers, in fact, once the initial trepidation has worn off, demonstrate even greater natural ability for parenting than their female partners. And babies aren't blind to this: by their first birthdays, babies are as likely to object to being separated from father as from mother, and a full 25% are more likely to go to their dads than their moms when given the choice.

If your wife has had previous experience caring for babies, or is taking to the job more readily than you, have her show you the ropes. If she's as green as you, learn as you go, together (the tips in the Baby-Care Primer will help). You'll both be pros the next time around.

HANDLING BABY

"I'm afraid I'm not gentle enough when I handle my new daughter."

One of the benefits of a baby's having two parents is that she has the opportunity to experience the love and attention of two different people. Often the mother is more gentle and slower paced, sings to her baby in a high, soft voice, and has a soft body to snuggle up against; she's usually the one that a baby comes crying to for comfort. The father is often a little rougher, more lively, and fast paced in his handling; his voice is deeper and his body harder; he's the one baby most frequently turns to for fun and games. A baby quickly comes not only to accept the differences between parents, but to enjoy them. (The degrees of gentleness and roughness vary from person to person, of course. Working mothers are more likely to resemble fathers in the way they relate to their children, and in an occasional family the ways mother and father treat their baby may even be totally reversed.)

While it's all right to handle your baby a little more energetically, real roughhousing is dangerous; see page 187.

BABY'S CRYING

"Our little boy is colicky and it's so bad that sometimes I just don't want to come home."

The sound of a screaming baby isn't a pleasure to come home to—even for the most loving father. And it isn't a pleasure to stay home with, either—even for the most dedicated mother. Your wife undoubtedly harbors some secret fantasies of sneaking out of the house when your baby starts his daily wailing marathon, and not returning until he's screamed himself to sleep. Unless you've got regular help, however, it isn't likely that either of you will be able to escape. But you can reduce the agony somewhat and retain your sanity by following the tips on surviving colic on page 122. And happily, as bad as things are, you can be pretty sure they will soon get better. Most colic disappears miraculously when baby reaches three months.

If, in the meantime, the crying makes you angry, try some strenuous exercise or a punching bag to release your hostilities. If at any time it makes you feel angry enough that you fear you might hurt the baby, speak to a doctor, cleric, or therapist immediately, or telephone the local Child-Abuse Hotline.

UNFAIR BURDEN

"I work a long day at the office while my wife stays home with our daughter. I don't mind helping out a little on the weekend, but I resent her pressuring me to give her a hand on weeknights—particularly in the middle of the night."

Caring for your baby when you come home from work, a time when you used to relax and unwind from the pressures of the day, may seen an unfair burden; it does to many husbands of women who don't work outside the home. But it's actually an incomparable opportunity in disguise. In previous generations, few fathers were given a chance to spend significant amounts of time with their babies, which was a shame. As a member of a more enlightened generation, you're getting the chance to get to know your daughter as you couldn't otherwise. You may miss the evening news or a before-dinner nap in the recliner, but you'll find that an even better way to relax and unwind is with your baby. Nothing can make you forget a personnel problem, a botched job, or a lost deal faster than conversing in coos with your baby as you change her diapers, watching her splash and giggle in the tub, or rocking her gently to sleep. And while you're forgetting your workaday cares, you'll also be building a collection of moments to remember.

Which is not to say that every moment you spend with your little one, particularly in the middle of the night, will be one you'll want to remember (some will pass in such a thick, sleepy fog that you wouldn't be able to remember them even if you wanted to). Like any job, baby care has its quota of anxiety and drudgery.

And this job—with its pluses and minuses—is the one your wife does all day while you're at work. Her workday is at least as physically and emotionally demanding as yours (more so if she's nursing). She needs relief in the evening more than you need the rest you'll be giving up by helping her. Sure, you'll have to rise in the early light of morning to start another day at work, but so will she—and unlike you, she won't be able to take lunch hours, coffee breaks, and often, not even bathroom breaks.

And next time you walk the floor with your colicky baby while your wife prepares dinner, remember that soon the rewards of your involvement in baby care will begin to outweigh the stresses. At first, it will be the smiles and gurgles meant just for you, then a breathless "da-da" when you come through the door, then a finger raised for your kiss to make a boo-boo better. Later, and for years to come, compensation will come in the form of a closer relationship with your child that will not only bring joy, but will also make the more difficult times a little easier.

Of course, sometimes both your wife *and* you will need a break from child care, so be sure that once in a while there's a night out for just the two of you.

NOT ENOUGH TIME TO SPEND WITH BABY

"I work long hours, often staying late at the office. I want to spend more time with my new son, but I don't seem to have any."

If there was ever something worth making time for, that little baby of yours is it. As terrific a job of parenting as one parent can do, two can do it twice as well. Baby boys who get lots of attention from their fathers are brighter and happier by the time their half-year birthday rolls around than boys who don't. So it's not just you who stands to lose if you don't spend time with your son. (Little girls, too, grow up more confident when they are close to their dads.)

Make more time for your baby, even if it means taking time from other important activities in your life. Organization may help. Try to dovetail your working hours and your baby's waking ones. If you don't have to be in the office until ten, spend the early morning with him; if you don't get home until eight, see if your wife can arrange his schedule so that he naps early in the evening, then is up for a visit with you before bedtime (of course, this will cut into time alone with her). If a lot of extracurricular activities (whether nighttime meetings or weekend sports) keep you from your baby's side, cut back on them. The organizations and teams will still be there when your baby is a little older—at which point his schedule will be more regular and easier to work around.

Especially if you're not able to make a great deal of time for your baby, it's important to make the most of the time you do have. Don't read the paper at the breakfast table, sit glued to the six o'clock news before dinner, or sleep until noon on Saturday. Instead, wield the baby spoon at breakfast, give the bath at six o'clock, take the baby to the playground on Saturday morning.

You can also make time for your baby by including him, when feasible, in your other activities. If you've got a few errands to run, strap him in a baby carrier and take him along. If jogging is on your schedule, tuck him in a carriage or stroller and increase your aerobic effort by pushing as you go (but *don't* jog with him in a baby carrier). And if you've got some chores to do, prop him securely in a baby seat and let him watch as you provide a blow-by-blow description of what you're doing.

CHAPTER TWENTY-SIX

From Only Child To Older Child

When you brought your first child home from the hospital, you and your husband were novices at parenting, with lessons to be learned, adjustments to be made, and the challenge of forming an attachment to a new member of the family waiting to be faced. When you bring a second child home, you'll already be seasoned pros when it comes to parenting; instead of you, it will be your older child who will need to do most of the learning, make most of the adjustments, and work the hardest at forming an attachment to the newborn. It won't be any easier for your older child than it was for you, and considering age and level of maturity, it may be considerably more difficult. Following the suggestions and tips in this chapter won't make the transition from only child to older child effortless for your firstborn (or for you), but it can help to make it smoother.

The best tip of all? Relax. Children take their cues from the adults around them. If you're anxious about how your child is going to react to having a new sibling, your child will be anxious, too.

WHAT YOU MAY BE CONCERNED ABOUT

PREPARING AN OLDER CHILD

"We have a two-and-a-half-year-old and we're expecting another baby. How can we best prepare our first child so she won't feel threatened?"

Pregnancy and childbirth have become a family affair. Like fathers in the 70s, siblings in the 80s are no longer excluded from the nine months of preparation and excitement that will culminate in the arrival of a new brother or sister. Instead of trying to piece together what is about to happen from hushed whispers among adults and mysterious talk about cabbage patches and storks, today's firstborns are often involved in the pregnancy from the early months on.

Preparation of a sibling is at least as complicated as the preparation of the expectant parents. The first step, of course, is to tell the older child that her mother is pregnant. Just when this should be done has generated some controversy among child-care experts. For a long while, the prevailing belief was that young children should not be told very early in a pregnancy because an early announcement would leave too much "waiting" time—and waiting is something that children are usually not very good at. More recently, however, it's been suggested that children begin to sense something is "going on" very early. Perhaps they overhear serious or excited grownup conversations, see their mother not feeling well or being distracted, note other changes around the house—and they wonder "What are they keeping from me? What is going to happen?" And often the fears born of ignorance are far worse than the reality—and worse, too, than a long and sometimes boring wait. Letting a child know early also gives you more time to help her adjust to the idea of a sibling and to work out her feelings ahead of time. It may make sense to wait until test results

are obtained if you're having amniocentesis, or until the danger period is over if you have a history of miscarriages—although your child may be more upset if you're confined to bed and she hasn't been told why.

Once the kitten's out of the bag, there are a number of steps that parents can take to make the expected arrival less threatening to the child already in residence—and perhaps even eagerly anticipated:

■ Make any planned major changes in your child's life early in the pregnancy if you haven't had a chance to make them before conception. For example, get her enrolled and settled in a preschool or play group so that she'll have an out-of-home experience to escape to once the baby's arrived, and won't feel she's being put out because of the baby. Begin toilet training her or weaning her from the bottle now, rather than just after your new baby's birth. Any significant changes not made within a month or two of the baby's due date should probably be postponed until a couple of months after the birth, if possible.

■ Get your child used to spending a little less time alone with you. If you never have before and will need to after the baby arrives, start leaving her with a baby-sitter for short periods during the day. If daddy hasn't been very involved in caring for her up till now, ease him into the feeding, bathing, and bedding down routines so that he will make a skillful stand-in for you when you're in the hospital and when you're busy with the new baby. Initiate some regular father-firstborn fun activities (Sunday morning breakfast out, Saturday afternoon at the playground, an after-dinner story hour), rituals that can continue to be enjoyed far into your new addition's first year. Be careful, though, not to withdraw too far from your firstborn; she needs to be reassured (through loving actions, not in so many words) that the arrival of a baby won't mean the loss of her mommy.

■ Be honest and open about the physical changes you're undergoing. Explain that you're tired or grumpy because "making a baby" is hard work, not because you're tired of her or sick. But don't use the pregnancy as an excuse for not picking her up as much as you used to; picking up a child is not in any way threatening to your pregnancy unless your doctor has for some reason, such as premature dilatation of your cervix, forbidden it. If you can't pick her up because your back is killing you, blame your back, not the baby—and give her extra hugs from a sitting position. If you need to lie down more often, suggest she lie down with you and nap, read her a story, or watch TV together.

■ Introduce your child to the new baby while it's still in the uterus. Show her month-by-month pictures of fetal development that seem appropriate for her age, explaining that as the baby grows so will mommy's tummy, and that when the baby is big enough it will be ready to come out. As soon as kicks are easily seen and felt by outsiders, let her experience the baby's movements herself. Encourage her (but don't push her if she resists) to kiss, hug, and talk to the baby. When referring to the baby, call it "our baby" or "your baby" to give her a sense that it belongs to her as well as to you. Explain that there's no way to tell whether it's a brother or a sister (unless, of course, you've learned the sex in advance through amniocentesis), and make a game out of guessing.

■ Take your child to at least one or two prenatal visits (and if she seems interested and isn't disruptive, take her to all of them) so she will feel like more than a player in the unfolding pregnancy drama. Hearing the heartbeat will help make the baby more of a reality for her. If a sonogram photograph has been taken, show her that, too. But be sure to bring a snack and a book or favorite toy to the practitioner's office in case of a long wait or a waning attention span. And if she decides she doesn't care for a return visit, abide by her wishes without pressuring her to change her mind.

■ Involve your child in any baby preparations she shows interest in. Let her "help" you pick out furnishings, a layette, toys—and even let her select an inexpensive monstrosity or two herself. Go through her old baby clothes and toys together to select items which might be recyclable—but don't push her to hand down anything until she wants to. Let her open any baby gifts that arrive before the baby.

■ Familiarize your child with babies in general. Show her photos of herself as a baby, and tell her what she was like (be sure to include some stories that will show her how much she's grown up since then). If possible, take her to a hospital nursery to look at the newborns (so she will know they aren't as "pretty" as older babies). If you have friends with small babies, arrange for the two of you to spend some time with them. Point out babies everywhere—in supermarkets, in the park, in picture books. So that she'll be prepared for reality, explain that babies do very little besides eat, sleep, and cry (which they do a lot of), and that they don't make good playmates for quite a while. If you're planning to nurse, explain that baby will drink milk from mommy's breasts (just as she did, if she did), and if you have a friend who is nursing, arrange a casual visit at feeding time.

■ In trying to prepare your child, don't raise issues that may never materialize. For instance, don't tell her "Don't worry, we'll love you just as much as the new baby," or "We'll still have plenty of time for you." Such statements, although well intentioned, can set your child up for worries about how well she'll be able to compete with her new sibling for your love and attention.

■ If you're planning to have your older child vacate a crib for her expected sibling, do it several months in advance of your due date. If she's not ready for a bed, buy her another crib—preferably one that can convert to a junior bed. If you'll be moving her to a different room, do this, too, well in advance, and have her help with the decor and furnishings. Put the emphasis on her graduating to a new bed or new room because she is growing up, rather than on her being displaced from the old by the baby.

■ If you have a car and your older child has been sitting in the middle back seat, move her car seat to a side back seat now; if she's big enough (see page 42), put her in a belt-positioning booster. Put a doll in an infant seat in the middle seat for a few weeks before baby's due to accustom her to a travel companion.

■ Try out names you're considering on your child, involving her in the selection process. "Naming" the baby will help make her feel closer to him or her. (Of course, it would be courting disaster to give your preschooler complete creative control over the process; you'll have to make the final determination, unless you want your second child named Big Bird.)

■ If there's a sibling class available in your neighborhood—some hospitals offer them—enroll your child. It's important for her to know that there are other children in the same spot she's in—about to have a new sibling. Even if she's taking a class, and especially if she isn't, prepare her further by reading her books on the subject—there are many "new baby" books geared to her age group on the market.

■ As your due date draws near, prepare your child for your spending some time at the hospital when the baby arrives. Have her help you pack your suitcase and encourage her to add something of hers that she would like you to take along to keep you company—a teddy bear, a picture of her, or a picture she's drawn, for instance. Be sure that whoever is going to be caring for her is fully familiar with her routines, so there won't be any break from them at this sensitive time. Tell her in advance who the caretaker will be (best mommy substitutes are daddy, grandma, grandpa, another familiar relative, a regular sitter, or a close family friend), and assure her you will come home in a few days. If the hospital permits sibling visits (many do), tell her when she will be able to visit you and the baby. Whether she will be able to

visit or not, a prebirth tour of the hospital, if one can be arranged, will make her feel more comfortable about your being away.

■ Don't suddenly shower her with gifts or special outings in the weeks before delivery. Instead of placating her, such unaccustomed overindulgence may well give your child the sense that something terrible is about to happen, and that you're trying to soften the blow. It may also give her the idea that baby's impending arrival is bestowing her with valuable bartering power and lead her to attempt to trade good behavior for presents and favors in the future. Buy just a couple of small but thoughtful gifts to give her after the baby arrives—perhaps one to give at the hospital and one for when you get home, for her being such a big help while mommy was away. For a fairly young child, a batheable baby doll that's just the right size for her arms is often a good gift; later she can bathe, "nurse," or diaper her baby doll while mommy takes care of the real thing. Shop with her for (and let her wrap) a small gift for the baby "from her" that she can bring to the hospital on the occasion of their first meeting.

■ In your efforts to prepare your first child for the birth of your second, don't overdo it. Don't let your pregnancy and the expected family addition become the primary focus of your household, or the dominant topic of conversation. Remember that there are, and should be, other concerns and interests in your preschooler's life—and that they deserve your attention, too.

SIBLINGS AT THE BIRTH

"We're delivering our second baby at a maternity center, and we have the option of having our three-year-old son attend the birth. But we're not sure how healthy it would be for him."

When your generation was being delivered, childbirth was for mothers only. Fathers paced the floors of hospital waiting rooms, and siblings never made it to the hospital at all, passing their mothers' labors at grandmother's house watching Captain Kangaroo and being indulged with chocolate chip cookies, only vaguely aware, if at all, of what was going on. Today, fathers are usually present at the big event (they sometimes even "deliver" their babies and cut the cords themselves), and children have moved into the waiting rooms. The next logical step, according to some, is to allow the children to join the rest of the family in the delivery room. And indeed, a few hospitals and some maternity centers have opened their birthing room doors to brothers and sisters of all ages.

While virtually everyone agrees that the father's move into the delivery room has been a positive one, there has been a great deal of controversy over the wisdom of letting siblings follow in their father's footsteps. Though theoretical benefits are suggested (less rivalry or better attachment between siblings; less trauma for the child, who doesn't feel deserted when the mother goes off to pick up his "replacement"), the major reason children attend sibling births seems to be that their parents want them there. And the possible negative results appear to outweigh any positive ones. For one thing, childbirth can be an unsettling and difficult experience for a child to understand—with the blood, grunts, groans, and sometimes screams from mother and the unbaby-like look of the emerging newborn. (At least one study shows, however, that not all children are distressed by viewing a birth; some are merely bored, especially during a long labor, and some actually become actively involved.) For another, though complications are uncommon in the typical low-risk labor and delivery, there is no way of predicting whether all will go smoothly. Should an emergency cesarean become necessary or should something be seriously wrong with the newborn, the resultant flurry of activity and change in atmosphere—probably necessitating the child's unceremonious eviction—could be truly frightening, possibly with long-term impact. In addition, having a child in the

room during active labor or pushing can be distracting and inhibiting to the mother (she may want to cry out, but feel hesitant in front of him). And as mother and dad focus on the work of delivering the new child and then express wonder and excitement at its arrival, the older child may feel left out.

On the other hand, most experts concur that under normal circumstances, having an older sibling greet his new brother or sister immediately *after* the actual birth offers all of the benefits of attending the birth but presents none of the risks. And if your hospital allows this option, it's a good one to pick up. If it doesn't, speak to your doctor about trying to effect a change in policy or at least wangling an exception. If that fails, remember that a delay in meeting will not doom sibling harmony—there are plenty of other ways to build a loving relationship between your children.

If you do decide to have your child present at the birth, be certain he is very well prepared (he should see films and pictures of births, watch you practice your breathing exercises, and if possible, attend a sibling class on childbirth), and that you have food, books, toys, and other diversions to keep him occupied when your contractions don't. If at any point he wants to leave, let him—without showing any disappointment. Be sure another familiar adult is waiting outside to stay with him or to take him home or to grandma's in case of such a change of heart.

SEPARATION AND HOSPITAL VISITS

"Will visiting me in the hospital make my older child miss me more than if she doesn't see me at all?"

Quite the contrary. Being out of your child's sight doesn't mean you'll be out of her mind. Seeing you at the hospital will assure her that you're all right, that you haven't gone off and left her for another child, and that she's still important in your life. And studies show that children who don't visit their mothers are more likely to show hostility to them upon homecoming. ("I don't like you, mommy—you left me all alone!") In most hospitals, she will also be allowed to see, sometimes even touch and "hold," her new baby brother or sister, which will give her a sense of reality about this new sibling and make her feel an important part of the new baby excitement.

You can make the hospital visits—and the separation—go more smoothly if you do the following:

■ Be sure your child is prepared in advance for the visit. She should know how long she's going to stay, and that she's going to have to go home without you and the baby. And tell her if regulations will limit her to seeing the baby through the nursery window.

■ Be sure you're prepared for your child's visit. If you're expecting her to rush headlong into your arms and fall in love at first sight with her new sibling, you may be disappointed. It's very possible that she'll give either you or the baby or both of you the cold shoulder, that she'll seem tentative or out of sorts, that she'll burst into angry or sorrowful tears upon leaving. Such negative or neutral reactions are common, are not a cause for concern, and are better than no visit at all. Keep your expectations realistic and you'll be pleasantly surprised if all goes smoothly—and you won't be unduly upset if they don't.

■ If you leave for the hospital in the middle of the night, or when your older child is in nursery school or otherwise away from home, leave her a note that can be read to her when she wakes up or returns. Tell her that "our" baby is ready to come out, that you love her, and that you'll see her or speak to her soon. If it's practical (grandma or someone else can come along to stay with her) and possible (the hospital allows it), take her along to the hospital to await baby's arrival. Have a bag for her, as you do

for yourself. It should include a change of clothing, diapers (if she wears them), playthings, and snacks you know she will enjoy. If labor is lengthy (it is less likely to be the second time around) and you are confined to the labor room, have daddy come out and deliver regular bulletins, possibly even have lunch with her in the cafeteria. Of course, if her bedtime comes up before the baby comes out, you will probably want to have her taken home so she can sleep in her own bed; if she is still around when the baby arrives, try to arrange for her to visit—at least with you, and possibly with her new sibling.

■ Make sure to place a picture of your older child on your bedstand, so she'll know that you've been thinking of her when she comes to visit.

■ If it's possible, have whoever is bringing your child to visit you stop at a store on the way so that she can buy you and her new sibling small presents. Exchanging gifts (this is the time to give her that little something you picked up for her before delivery) will help break the ice and make her feel important. The practice of giving a gift "from the baby" is common, but most kids see right through the ploy, and it's not a good idea to start this relationship with a deception, however innocent.

■ Hold a little "birth-day" party for the new enlarged family in your hospital room. Have a cake (the older child will probably be pleased that she can have a piece and her new sibling can't), candles (she can blow them out), and a few decorations (let her choose them).

■ Have the same person who brings your child to visit take her home. If daddy takes her and then stays on for an extended visit while she's sent home with a grandparent or friend, she may feel doubly deserted.

■ Between visits, or if she can't visit, keep in touch by phone (avoiding sensitive times such as right before bed, if you feel that the sound of your voice may upset her) and by writing notes that daddy can read to her. She may feel good, too, about making a drawing or two for you to display in your hospital room. Have daddy or a favorite relative take her out to dinner or on some other special outing so that it will be clear that the new baby isn't the only thing everyone is interested in these days—and make sure that conversation during the outing doesn't center around the baby unless she wants it to.

■ Arrange to go home early, if you want to and can, so that your older child can begin sharing in the new baby experience sooner, and so that the separation time is reduced.

EASING THE HOMECOMING

"How can I make coming home with the baby less traumatic for my older son?"

An older sibling usually has mixed feelings when it comes to the homecoming. He knows that he wants his mother to come home, but he's not quite as sure about the baby she's planning to bring with her. In a way he likes the idea—having a new baby in the house is exciting and different, and if he's old enough, it's something to boast to his friends about. But he's probably at least a little nervous when he ponders how his life is going to change once that baby's carried through his front door and deposited in what used to be his crib.

How you handle the homecoming will influence, at least initially, whether your child's greatest expectations or worst fears about the new baby are realized. Here's how to accentuate the positive and minimize the negative:

■ Consider giving your child an active role in the homecoming, having him come to the hospital with his daddy to take you and the new baby home. This will work only if grandma or another familiar adult is along (so that daddy can be free to take care of the paperwork and such) and if hospital policy permits.

■ Or have him help with preparations for the baby at home (he can lay out diapers and cotton balls and so on for the baby, for example) while daddy goes to pick you up. Try to come into the house first (perhaps daddy can wait in the car with the baby) so that you can greet your older child privately for just a few minutes.

■ Start right off using the baby's name, rather than always referring to the new sibling as "the baby." This will give your older child a sense that this baby is really a person, not just an object.

■ Limit visitors for the first few days at home—for your own health and sanity, and for your older child's sake. Even the most well-meaning of visitors tend to go on endlessly about a new baby, all but ignoring the older child. Those visitors you can't deny immediate access to (such as grandparents, aunts and uncles, and close friends) should be briefed in advance not to be overly and obviously effusive toward the baby, and to give plenty of attention to the older sibling. You can also suggest that visitors come when he's in school or after he's gone to bed. Limiting visitors for the first week or so has other benefits—more time for you to regain your strength and more opportunity for the bonding of your expanding family.

■ Focus much of your attention on your older child, particularly in the early days, when the baby will probably be sleeping a good deal of the time. Hang his drawings on the refrigerator, applaud toileting if he's newly trained, tell him how proud you are about his being such a good big brother, be quick with praise and slow with anger. Avoid the mistake of parents who worship at the new baby's crib ("Oh, look at those tiny fingers!" or "Isn't she beautiful!" or "See, she's smiling!"), leaving the older child feeling very much an unnecessary and unappreciated appendage. But don't go to the extreme of never kissing, hugging, or showing affection for the baby in front of the sibling, either. If you do, the child will be confused ("I thought we were supposed to love this baby. Is it possible my parents will soon stop loving me, too?") or see right through your plan or beyond it ("They're pretending not to like the baby so I won't know that they really like her more than me"). Instead, bring the older child into the talk about the baby: "Look at those tiny fingers; do you believe yours were once so small?" or "Isn't she beautiful? I think she looks just like you" or "See, she's smiling at you; I think she loves you already." Your child will feel more comfortable if you freely display natural affection for the new baby (without overdoing it), as well as for him.

▪ Allow your older child to open all the baby gifts and (assuming they aren't breakable or dangerous) to play with them for a bit if he wishes, even if they're clearly "baby" toys, pointing out that they're the baby's presents but that he can play with them until she's old enough to appreciate them. Some wise visitors remember to bring a small gift for the older child; but should several days pass and truckloads of baby gifts come in with nothing for the older sibling, have grandma or daddy bring home something special just for him. You can also show him some of the gifts he received as a newborn, explaining that now it's his new baby's turn to get gifts. And if the influx of gifts really seems excessive, put away those that don't come to his attention. Eventually, those cards and gifts will stop coming.

▪ If your older child decides he wants to stay home from nursery school for a few days, let him. This will assure him that you aren't pushing him out of the house so you can enjoy the baby, and it will give him some opportunity to bond with the baby. (But decide in advance, with his consultation, just how long his vacation will be so that he doesn't get the idea that he can stay home permanently.) Don't, however, force your child to stay home if he would rather go to school. He may feel the need to be in a place where there is no baby, and where there are other centers of interest.

OPEN RESENTMENT

"My toddler is openly resentful of the new baby. He tells me he wants him to go back to the hospital."

You obviously can't carry out your child's wishes, but you can—and should—let him express them. Though his feelings may seem very negative, the fact that he is able to vent them is very positive. Every older sibling feels a certain measure of resentment toward the new intruder (or to his mother for bringing the intruder in); some just express it more overtly than others. Instead of implying to your older child that he's bad to feel that way ("Oh, that's a terrible thing to say about the baby!"), tell him that you understand that it isn't always fun to have a new baby in the house—for him or you. Let him talk out his resentment if he wants to, but don't dwell on the subject. Move on quickly to something upbeat ("How about if we bundle the baby up and go to the playground together?").

Some children don't feel free to express negative feelings toward a new baby, and it's a good idea to encourage them to talk about how they feel. One way to do that is to confide your own mixed feelings: "I love the baby, but sometimes I hate having to get up in the middle of the night to feed him" or "Boy, with our new baby I hardly ever have a free moment for myself." Another is to tell and/or read stories about older siblings with mixed feelings about new arrivals. If you are an older sibling yourself, you can talk about how you felt when a new baby came along.

"My daughter shows no hostility toward her new brother. But she's been acting very moody and disagreeable with me."

Some older siblings don't see any point in confronting a newborn (after all, you can't get a rise out of him no matter what you do) or feel too inhibited to show their hostilities toward him (they've been told too often that they're supposed to be loving and affectionate). The next best target, one they feel they can torment with less guilt and more satisfying results, is mommy. It is, after all, mother who is spending hours feeding the baby, diapering the baby, rocking and cuddling the baby, and spending much less time than she used to with her. A firstborn may vent her feelings toward her mother by throwing tantrums, exhibiting regressive behavior, refusing to eat, or rejecting her mother entirely and turning to her father or someone else (a baby-sitter, for instance) as a "favorite." This type of behavior is a common and normal part of the period of adjustment to the new baby.

As at any developmental stage, it's important to deal with disagreeableness calmly and to not take it personally. Try to respond with patience, understanding, reassurance, and extra attention. And remember, this too will pass—usually within a few months.

YOUR OWN RESENTMENT

"Since our second child arrived, I've felt pulled in all directions and often find myself resenting the demands for time and attention from my older son, which makes me feel very guilty."

You're overtired and overpressured—it's not surprising that you have hostile feelings that need venting. And it's also not surprising that you're tempted to vent them on your older child (though some women choose their husbands as the would-be targets) rather than your newborn. Like an older sibling who redirects his anger at his mother, you probably recognize that an infant isn't an acceptable object of disaffection. You probably also believe, at least unconsciously, that now that your firstborn is an older child he should be more mature—if only he would "act his age," you probably reason, everything else would be so much easier. An unrealistic and unjust, but common, belief. (Besides, your child probably is acting his age.)

Though such feelings aren't unusual among second-time mothers, they often do come as a surprise to those mothers who spent their second pregnancies worrying that they wouldn't be able to love their new child as much as their first. They're shocked to see how easily and quickly the new baby creeps into their hearts, and feel fickle and guilt-ridden when they find themselves begrudging their older child his requests for time and attention.

Recognizing your negative feelings and accepting the reasons for them is an important step in overcoming them. This may be the first time in your life that you feel anger or resentment toward your children, but it won't be the last. Such feelings occur even in the best of human relationships. But as you settle into a comfortable rhythm as a mother of two, more adroit at sharing yourself with both your children, you'll find the feelings will dissipate. (If they don't, or if they become more severe, talk to your doctor or see a counselor who can help you work them out.)

EXPLAINING GENITAL DIFFERENCES

"My three-year-old daughter is obsessed with her new brother's penis. She wants to know what it is and why she doesn't have one. I don't know what to tell her."

Try the truth. As young as your daughter is, if she's old enough to ask questions about her body and her brother's, she's old enough to get some honest answers. It can be quite a shock for a little girl to see something on her baby brother that she doesn't have (or for a little boy to note the absence of a penis on his baby sister; is it possible that he'll lose it, too? he wonders). The simple explanation that boys (and men, like daddy) have penises and girls (and women, like mommy) have vaginas is probably all that is needed, and will help your child understand one fundamental difference between males and females. Be sure to use the proper names for these body parts just as you would for the eyes, nose, or mouth, and add more information only if it's requested—though you may want to let her know that girls have vaginas so that when they grow up they can have babies and boys have penises so they can be fathers. If your child asks to know more than you can comfortably impart, look for a book for parents that can help you with the task, and/or for one written and illustrated at your child's level that you can read to her.

NURSING IN FRONT OF AN OLDER CHILD

"I'm planning to nurse my second baby, but I'm worried about doing so in front of my four-year-old son."

Though there's speculation that seeing the parent of the opposite sex fully undressed may be harmful to a child preschool-age and older, there's no reason to believe any damage can be done if a boy watches his mother nurse. In fact, it's more likely to be harmful if you go out of your way to keep your son away from you while you nurse—considering how much time is spent nursing a newborn, you'd be seeing very little of your older child. And besides baby's nap time, there'll no more undivided time you can give your son than when you're nursing. Almost any quiet activity, from reading a story to playing a game of Candyland, can be pursued during feeding sessions.

If you're uncomfortable about your son's seeing your breasts (although they're almost certain not to be stimulating to him, particularly in that context), nurse discreetly. But don't overreact if he does catch a glimpse or if he reaches a curious hand over for a squeeze. Many experts agree that both prudery, which could give a child the idea that there's something bad or unclean about the human body and its functions, and blatant exhibitionism, which dampens respect for personal privacy and could lead to unwanted stimulation, probably help to

build unhealthy attitudes toward sexuality.

THE OLDER CHILD WHO WANTS TO NURSE

"My two-and-a-half-year-old son, watching me nurse the baby, has been saying he wants some milk, too. I thought the interest would pass if I ignored it, but it hasn't."

The best way to cure an older sibling (up to three or four years old) of the desire to nurse is to let him know that he can. (A child more than four years old should understand that nursing is for babies.) Often, just your okay will be enough, and he won't feel the need to pursue the issue further. If he does, let him. You may feel uncomfortable, but he'll feel that he's being given access to this mysterious and special relationship the baby has with you. Chances are one nip is all he'll need to make him realize that babies don't have it so good after all. The warm, watery, unfamiliar, poor-excuse-for-milk fluid he extracts almost certainly won't be worth the effort involved (and he may well give up before the milk ever makes it to his mouth). His feelings of curiosity satisfied, he'll probably never ask to nurse again, and he'll likely feel more sympathy for the baby (who's stuck drinking that stuff when he's guzzling apple juice and "real" milk and gobbling raisins and peanut butter and jelly sandwiches) than jealousy.

If he continues to show an interest in nursing, or if he objects to baby's indulging, it's probably not a breast to suck on that he's after, but a breast (and a mommy) to snuggle up against and some of the attention he feels the baby's always getting when nursing. Including your older child in the nursing sessions may be all that's necessary to quell his interest in taking to the breast. There are several simple ways to do this. Before you sit down to nurse, for example, say "I'm going to give the baby some milk now. Would you like some juice?" or "Would you like your lunch now, while baby is eating?" Or take the quiet opportunity offered by nursing to read him a story, help him do a puzzle, or listen to records with him (good because you don't have to use your hands), steadfastly resisting the temptation to watch TV or catch up on phone calls instead. And be sure, too, that your firstborn gets plenty of hugging and cuddling when you're not feeding the baby.

REGRESSIVE BEHAVIOR

"Ever since her sister was born, my three-year-old daughter has started acting like a baby herself. She talks in baby jargon, wants to be picked up all the time, and even has toileting accidents."

Even fully grown adults can't help sometimes envying a newborn her undemanding existence ("Oh, that's the life!" they'll sigh as a sleeping baby is wheeled by them in a cushy carriage). It's not surprising that a youngster, barely out of the carriage herself and just beginning to master some of the myriad of responsibilities that come with growing up, would yearn for a return to babyhood when confronted with an infant sibling. Especially when she sees that acting like a baby works very well for her new sister, who is allowed to lie in the lap of luxurious leisure (not to mention the lap of her mommy), who is carried everywhere, catered to endlessly, opens her mouth to whimper and receives precisely what she wants when she wants it (instead of receiving a sharp "Stop that whining!").

Rather than pressuring your older daughter to "be a big girl" at this sensitive time, baby her when she wants to be babied—even if it means caring for two "babies" at once. Give her the attention she is craving (rock her in your arms when she's tired, carry her up the stairs once in a while, feed her when she demands it) and don't chide her when she regresses to one-word sentences (even if it grates on your

nerves), wants to take her milk from a bottle (even if she never has before), or if her toilet habits take a sudden turn for the infantile. At the same time, encourage her to act her age by being especially lavish with praise when she is particularly grown up—when she cleans up after herself, is a big help to mommy, or goes on the potty. Offering such praise in front of others will reinforce its benefits. Remind her that she was your first baby, and now she's your big girl. Point out, too, the special things that she can do that her sister can't, such as enjoying ice cream at a birthday party, zooming down the slide at the playground, or having pizza out with mommy and daddy. Bake with her while baby is napping, enlist her help when food shopping, send her on a picnic with daddy, take her to see a movie while the baby stays with a sitter. In her own time, she will figure out for herself the advantages of being the older child and will decide to leave her baby past behind.

THE OLDER SIBLING HURTING THE NEW BABY

"I left the room for a minute and was horrified when I returned to find my older son jabbing his baby sister with a toy. She wasn't hurt this time, but it seemed as though he was trying to make her cry on purpose."

Although such an assault would seem, on the surface, nothing more than a sadistic attempt to harm an unwanted newcomer, this isn't usually the case. Though there may be an element of hostility involved (and this is only natural, considering the upheaval a newborn causes in an older sibling's life), these seemingly malicious attacks are often merely innocent investigations. Your son may have been trying to make his sister cry not out of malevolence, but out of curiosity to find out how this strange little creature you've brought home works (just as he is constantly examining and probing everything else in his environment). The trick is to react to such a situation without overreacting. Impress upon your older child, by example and by involving him in baby care when you're around, the importance of being gentle with the baby. When he gets rough, react calmly and rationally, avoiding angry, guilt-provoking recriminations for him (if he's into tormenting you, he will enjoy having triggered your outburst) and hysterical protectiveness for her (which can reinforce any feelings of jealousy). Avoiding the explosive response is even more vital if the baby has actually been hurt; making an older child feel guilty about what he has done, whether it was intentional or not, can leave permanent emotional scars and serves little positive purpose.

When it comes to older sibling hurting younger, prevention is preferable to punishment. No matter how well you believe your older child has gotten the message, don't leave the two of them alone together again until your older child is of an age—probably around five years old—to understand what damage he can do. Younger children do not really have a sense of the extent of injury they can inflict with their actions, and they can inflict serious harm unintentionally.

AVOIDING JEALOUSY

"I'm wondering how I can divide myself fairly so that both my four-year-old son and his new baby brother get the attention they need, and so the older child won't be jealous."

As much as a second you (or at least a second pair of arms) would prove helpful at this time in your life, that isn't possible. There will be only one of you to go around, and that fact leaves you divided at least two ways for many years to come. The question is how to make the division in a way that will be best for your preschooler as well as for his new brother.

Later on in your child-rearing years, the split will have to be pretty much equal; the amount of time you spend with one child will have to be matched fairly evenly by the amount of time you spend with the other (just as every apple or slab of cake will have to be divided precisely to satisfy both children). Now, however, a little lopsidedness in favor of your older child is not only acceptable, it's best. Consider, first, that your older child is used to being an only child, and to not sharing your attention (save with your husband), and that your baby, happily unaware of who's getting more of you, will be basically content as long as his fundamental needs are being met. In addition, for a while, the baby will be getting a considerable amount of attention from significant and nonsignificant others, while your older child, looking on from the sidelines, will be largely ignored. Consider, too, that unlike your firstborn, who came home from the hospital to a relatively quiet home, your new baby has been born into a very active household, with plenty of parent-children interaction to keep his senses occupied and stimulated. If he sits on your lap while you're building a block city or fitting together puzzle pieces with your older son, or nestles in a baby carrier while you push your older son's swing, he's receiving as much stimulation as if you were playing with him directly. Finally, remember that there's another "caretaker" in your home now—your older son—who will be giving lively attention to your baby.

And though doing "double duty" will no doubt prove tricky, increasingly so as your baby nears demanding toddlerhood, you will soon become very adept at it. You'll learn to share your attention with your older child without cutting into your time with the younger not only by taking care of the needs of both at once (nursing or bottle feeding the one while reading a story to or doing a puzzle with the other, for instance), but also by appointing your firstborn as your chief assistant. He can fetch diapers for the baby when he's wet, sing and dance for the baby when he's cranky, and help you fold and put away the baby's laundry—matching those little socks is a chore for you, but a challenge and a learning experience for a child. Feeling useful will help keep him from feeling neglected.

But the older sibling needs more than shared time—he needs an unbroken span of time alone with you every day. If you don't have household help, finding such time may be difficult, but it's nevertheless essential. Baby's nap time (assuming your baby naps well during the day) is ideal if you can resist the urge to do the laundry, tidy up the house, or read the daily paper (these may have to wait until both children are in bed). So is early evening when daddy is home and can entertain the baby for a while. (Don't forget your older child will appreciate time alone with his father, too.)

In addition to seeing that your older child gets his fair share of attention, there are other steps you can take to modify the jealousy factor. For one, you should always refer to the infant either by his name or as "ours" or "yours"—never "mine." For another, try to avoid making the older child's life revolve around the younger's: "Keep quiet—baby's sleeping" or "You can't sit on my lap—baby's nursing" or "Stop poking the baby—you'll hurt him!" You can get the same (or even a better) result by keeping "don't" directives to a minimum and rephrasing them more positively: "Baby's sleeping. Let's see if we can whisper so he won't wake up." Or "How about sitting on this chair right next to me so we can be close together while I'm nursing?" Or "Baby really loves it when you stroke him gently like this."

Though you should limit the times you say you can't play with him or get something for him because you're busy with the baby, it's unrealistic to attempt to never use the baby as an excuse; that's a part of life with a sibling that your older child will just have to learn to accept. It will be easier for him if you continue to remind him of the benefits of being the older child, and if

sometimes you turn the tables. Say to the baby (even if your child may have doubts about baby's comprehension), "You're going to have to wait a minute for your diaper change because I have to give your brother his snack," or "I can't pick you up now because I have to tuck your big brother in."

Since you can spread yourself only so thin, you'll probably have to engage in some benign neglect of home and hearth in order to avoid neglecting your children. It will be more important to sit down and watch"Sesame Street"with your preschooler than to run the vacuum over the living room rug, more important to take the family to the park than to spend the day slicing and chopping foods for dinner. Limit housekeeping chores to the very essential (and/or, if you can't live with the lived-in look and if you can afford it, get someone else to help with them), keep the baby in disposable diapers (or use a diaper service) and the rest of the family in no-iron clothes, use frozen vegetables (they're at least as nutritious as fresh) when necessary, and keep meals simple (including those for baby; see page 247 for the merits of commercial baby food). Enlist your older child to help with such chores as dusting, opening vegetable packages, or setting the table; at first his help may seem more a hindrance, but with a little practice, you'll be surprised to find that he'll become more of a help.

LACK OF JEALOUSY

"I was all prepared for sibling rivalry when we decided to have another baby. But throughout the pregnancy and in the four months since her brother's arrival, my daughter hasn't shown any jealousy. Is that healthy?"

As you already know, your daughter has a personality all her own. Her reactions to the arrival of a new sibling may be completely different from those of a peer, and yet be just as normal and healthy. Though many children do show hostility toward a new baby in the family, such feelings aren't inevitable, or necessary for the development of a strong sibling relationship. A child who seems delighted with a new sibling isn't necessarily hiding feelings of jealousy; she may just be secure enough to feel unthreatened by the new arrival. She may, however, once the helpless little newcomer takes to the floors as a crawler, find some solid ground for resentment as he tears up her books, scatters her blocks on the floor, and chews the fingers off her favorite doll.

Still, in the meantime, you should be sure that she gets as much time and attention as her new sibling, even if she isn't demanding it. If you unintentionally begin to take her for granted because she's being such a good sport about the new baby, she may start to feel neglected and eventually become resentful.

And because almost every child feels some negative feelings toward a sibling somewhere along the way, make sure she knows it's okay to have such feelings, and give her ample opportunity to express them.

SIBLING ATTACHMENT

"I wonder how I can help my older child to feel more connected to his new baby brother."

Mothers and fathers bond with their new babies by interacting with them while taking care of them. And there's no good reason why siblings can't do the same. With close adult supervision, even the youngest of older siblings can share in baby's care and begin to feel a sense of attachment to the baby—and an easing of postpartum jealousy. Depending on the age of the older child, he can participate in a variety of ways, including the following:

Diapering. A school-age child can actually change a wet diaper with mom standing nearby; a toddler can help by fetching a clean one, handing mom a diaper wipe, patting down the adhesive tape on a disposable, or entertaining the wriggling baby during the process.

Feeding. If your baby is bottle fed, or takes a relief bottle occasionally, even a fairly young child can hold it for him. If your baby is on the breast exclusively, your older child can't actually do the feeding, but he can snuggle next to you with a book while you nurse his sibling.

Burping. Even a toddler can pat baby's back to bring on an after-meal burp—and they usually delight in the results.

Bathing. Bath time can be a fun time for the whole family. An older sibling can pass the soap, wash cloth, or towel, pour rinse water (temperature-tested by an adult) over baby's body, and entertain baby with his own bath toys or with singing. But don't let a sibling under twelve be baby's only chaperone at bath time—not even for a moment.

Baby-sitting. While an older sibling can't take total responsibility for a younger one until he's a teen (never allow a preschooler to mind a baby alone for even a minute), he can be dubbed "baby-sitter" when you're close by. Babies find no one quite as amusing as their older siblings, and finding that they have the ability to entertain baby is ego-boosting to senior sibs.

ESCALATING WARFARE

"My daughter was very loving towards her little brother from the time he was born. But now that he's crawling and able to get into her toys, she's suddenly turned on him."

For many older siblings, a newborn doesn't pose much of a threat. He's helpless, basically immobile, incapable of grabbing away books or breaking up dolly tea parties. Give him several months to develop reaching, crawling, cruising, and other motor skills, and the picture takes a turn from the idyllic. Even older children who have been loving (at least most of the time) to a younger sibling up to this point may suddenly begin to display hostility. And you can hardly blame them—a miniature barbarian has just invaded their turf. Their crayon boxes have been looted, their books violated, their dolls plundered.

To defend her turf, an older sibling (tension is usually greatest if the age difference between the two siblings is three years or less) often begins screaming at, hitting, pushing, and knocking down the baby. Sometimes there is a mix of affection and aggression in the actions: what begins as a hug ends up with baby on the floor crying. The action often accurately reflects the child's conflicting inner feelings. As the parent, you have to walk a narrow tightrope in such a situation—protecting the younger sibling without punishing the older. Though you should make it clear to your older child that it's not permissible to hurt her younger brother intentionally, you should also make it clear that you understand and sympathize with her plight and

her frustrations. Try to give her the chance to play without him around part of the time (while he naps, is in the playpen, or is otherwise occupied). Particularly when she has guests over, respect her privacy and property and be sure that her younger sibling does, too. Spend some extra time with her, and intervene on her behalf whenever the baby takes away or tries to destroy her belongings, instead of always urging her to "let him—he's only a baby." But do give her plenty of praise on occasions when she comes to this mature realization on her own.

Fairly soon, the tables will turn. Little brother, tired of being pushed around and strong enough to do some intentional pushing (and hair pulling and biting) of his own, will start fighting back. This usually occurs near the end of the first year, and is followed by a couple of years or more of mixed feelings between siblings—a confusing combination of love and hate. And you can expect these years, when you'll often feel more like a referee than a parent, to be a constant challenge to your patience and your ingenuity—as well as a joy.

PART THREE

Ready Reference

Best-Odds Recipes

FOR THE FIRST YEAR AND BEYOND

They don't know a bisque from a brioche or a pâté from a pot-au-feu, but babies and toddlers are some of the most discriminating eaters on the gastronomic scene. And discriminate they do—against vegetables, protein foods, and just about everything their parents would like them to eat. At mealtimes, pleasing them is a long shot, displeasing them a cinch, and getting them to take in their quota of the Daily Dozen a near impos-

sibility—or so it too often seems.

But there is hope—and help—on the next few pages. Though the recipe hasn't been created that will make every baby "open wide for the choo choo," those that follow stand a good chance of making it through a majority of young tunnels. All will go a long way in nourishing your little food critic and in satisfying, in most cases, several nutritional requirements at once.

SUPER CEREAL

One bowl of this powerhouse cereal, and your toddler will be leaping tall block buildings in a single bound.

Makes 1 toddler portion

⅓ cup oat circles or other unsweetened whole-grain dry cereal
1 tablespoon wheat germ

2 tablespoons instant nonfat dry milk
2 dried apricots, finely chopped
½ cup whole milk

Mound the first four ingredients in a small cereal bowl in the order given, pour the milk over all, and serve immediately.

Best-Odds Toddler Servings per portion: 1 Protein; 1½ Whole Grain; 1 Calcium; 1 Yellow Fruit; some Iron

FRUITED CHEESE BREAD

Even a baby determined to live on bread alone can't help but thrive when the bread is packed with protein, calcium, and minerals. Bake ahead, slice, and freeze for fussy mornings or afternoon snacks.

Makes 2 loaves, 9½ × 5½ × 3 inches

4 to 4½ cups whole-wheat flour
¾ cup wheat germ
1 teaspoon salt
2 packages active dry yeast
1 cup water
½ cup apple juice concentrate
¼ cup vegetable oil
1 cup unsalted low-fat cottage cheese
1 whole egg
2 egg whites
¾ cup rolled oats
1½ cups shredded low-sodium Swiss cheese (about 6 ounces)
1 cup chopped dried currants, raisins, or dates

1. Combine 3½ cups of the flour, the wheat germ, and the salt in the bowl of an electric mixer. Remove 1½ cups of the mixture and combine with the yeast. Make a well in center of remaining flour and return yeast mixture to the well.

2. Combine the water, juice concentrate, oil, and cottage cheese in a saucepan and heat over medium heat until very warm. Gradually add this mixture to the yeast mixture in the well, stirring as you do. Beat together at medium speed, scraping the sides of the bowl as needed, for 2 minutes.

3. Add the egg, egg whites, and another ½ cup flour to the dough; beat the dough again, scraping sides of bowl as needed, for 2 minutes. Blend in the rolled oats.

4. Turn out the dough onto a lightly floured board. Knead until smooth and elastic, about 8 to 10 minutes (or knead in mixer or processor, following appliance directions). If the dough remains too sticky, add the remaining flour, 2 tablespoons at a time, as needed. Place in a large bowl oiled with a little more vegetable oil, turning to grease on all sides. Cover tightly with foil. Set bowl in a warm place until dough has doubled in bulk, about 1 hour.

5. Punch down the dough. Turn it out onto a lightly floured board. Knead in the Swiss cheese and the fruit. Divide the dough in half. Shape each half into a loaf and place each loaf in a 9½ × 5½ × 3-inch loaf pan that has been well greased with additional vegetable oil. Brush the top of each loaf lightly with oil, cover with a towel, and let rise in a warm place until doubled, about 1 hour.

6. Fifteen minutes before baking the loaves, preheat the oven to 375°F.

7. Bake until the loaves are nicely browned and the bottoms sound hollow when tapped, about 35 to 40 minutes.

Best-Odds Toddler Servings in 1 slice or ¹⁄₁₀ loaf: 2 Grain; 1½ Protein; ½ Other Fruit; ½ Calcium; some Iron

LOW-SODIUM BAKING POWDER

Ordinary double-acting baking powder is very high in sodium and is a major source of sodium in the American diet. Since excess sodium is not good for babies (or anyone else), we suggest using low-sodium baking powder, available in health food stores, for baking these Best-Odds recipes. If you use ordinary baking powder, use ⅔ as much (2 teaspoons for every 3 called for).

PUMPKIN MUFFINS

Yellow-vegetable nutrition in a delectable disguise. Keep frozen for days when baby won't take vegetables straight.

Makes about 24 muffins

Vegetable cooking spray
1½ cups apple juice concentrate
¼ cup vegetable oil
2 whole eggs
4 egg whites
1½ cups canned, unsweetened, solid-pack
  pumpkin
1¼ cups raisins
1½ cups whole-wheat flour
½ cup wheat germ
4½ teaspoons low-sodium baking powder
2 teaspoons ground cinnamon

1. Preheat the oven to 400°F. Coat 24 muffin tin cups with vegetable cooking spray or line each with a cupcake paper. Set aside.

2. Combine the juice concentrate, oil, eggs, egg whites, pumpkin, and raisins in a blender jar. Purée until the raisins are chopped.

3. Mix together the flour, wheat germ, baking powder, and cinnamon in a large mixing bowl. Gradually add the pumpkin mixture, blending with an electric mixer set on low, or mix slowly by hand, just until well combined.

4. Pour the batter into the prepared muffin tins, filling each cup two-thirds full. Bake for 15 to 20 minutes. The muffins are done when a toothpick inserted into the center of one comes out clean (or with just a crumb or two attached).

Best-Odds Toddler Servings in 1 muffin: 2 Yellow; 1+ Whole Grain; 1 Other Fruit; ½ Protein

PANCAKE FACES

Smiles on the pancakes are bound to bring smiles to the high chair. Serve them plain or with fruit-only preserves, yogurt blended with fruit-only preserves, sliced bananas, sautéed apples or pears, or unsweetened applesauce. Freeze leftover pancakes for easy and nutritious finger food anytime.

Makes about 24 small pancakes

1 cup whole milk
¼ cup nonfat dry milk
2 tablespoons apple juice concentrate
1 tablespoon butter or margarine, melted
1 whole egg
2 egg whites
¾ cup whole-wheat flour
⅓ cup wheat germ
1½ teaspoons low-sodium baking powder
Vegetable cooking spray
Chopped raisins
Dried apricots cut into thin strips

1. Combine the ingredients through the baking powder in a blender, and process just until smooth. Let the mixture stand for 15 minutes.

2. Spray a nonstick skillet or griddle with vegetable cooking spray. Heat over medium-high heat until very hot. Reduce the heat to medium, stir the batter, and spoon it onto the griddle to make 3-inch pancakes.

3. Using bits of raisin and strips of apricot, add facial features to the pancakes. When the surface of the pancakes begins to bubble and the bottoms are nicely browned, about 2 minutes, turn and brown the other side, about 1 minute more.

4. Serve the pancakes face side up with any of the suggested accompaniments.

Best-Odds Toddler Servings in three 3-inch pancakes: 1 Protein; 1 Whole Grain; ¼ Calcium; some Iron

GOLDEN-NUGGET OATMEAL FLAPJACKS

The whole family will flip for these fruity pancakes. Serve them with yogurt, unsweetened applesauce, fresh berries, juice-sweetened apricot preserves, or Dried Apricot Purée (see page 624).

Makes about 48 silver-dollar-size pancakes

1 cup whole milk
¼ cup apple juice concentrate
2 tablespoons butter or margarine, melted
1 whole egg
2 egg whites
1 cup whole-wheat flour
½ cup rolled oats
½ cup wheat germ
2½ teaspoons low-sodium baking powder
¼ cup nonfat dry milk
1½ teaspoons vanilla extract
1 teaspoon ground cinnamon (optional)
½ cup dried apricots, finely chopped
Vegetable cooking spray

1. Beat the whole milk, juice concentrate, butter, egg, and egg whites together in a large bowl. Add in the remaining ingredients through the vanilla (or cinnamon, if using) and beat just until smooth. Fold in the chopped apricots.

2. Spray a skillet or griddle with vegetable cooking spray. Heat over medium-high heat until very hot. Reduce the heat to medium and spoon batter to make 2-inch pancakes. When the surface of the pancakes begins to bubble and the bottoms are nicely browned, about 2 minutes, turn and brown the other side, about 1 minute more.

Best-Odds Toddler Servings in four 2-inch pancakes: ⅔ Whole Grain; ½ Protein; some Calcium; ⅙ Fat

CROQUE BEBE

Your baby doesn't have to speak a word of French (or English, for that matter) to enjoy the intriguing taste and bountiful nutrition of these French toast-style grilled cheese sandwiches.

Makes 1 sandwich

1 egg
¼ cup milk
2 slices (about 2 ounces) low-sodium Swiss or Cheddar cheese
2 slices low-sodium whole-grain bread
Vegetable cooking spray

1. Beat the egg and milk together lightly in a bowl large enough to hold the bread.

2. Layer the cheese between the bread slices. Soak the sandwich in the egg mixture, turning it until the liquid is absorbed.

3. Spray a nonstick skillet with vegetable cooking spray. Heat over medium-high heat until hot. Reduce the heat to medium and brown the sandwich on both sides.

Best-Odds Toddler Servings in ½ sandwich: 2 Whole Grain; 1 Calcium; 1 Protein

BANANA FRENCH TOAST

One of baby's favorite flavors—banana—enhances the appeal of this French toast; nonfat dry milk adds a jolt of protein and calcium. It makes a nutritious breakfast, lunch, or supper as well.

Makes 4 slices

1 egg
2 tablespoons banana-orange juice concentrate
2 tablespoons apple juice concentrate
½ small banana
¼ cup nonfat dry milk
4 slices low-sodium whole-grain bread
Vegetable cooking spray

1. Combine the ingredients through the milk in a blender and process until smooth. Transfer the mixture to a bowl large enough to hold the bread.

2. Soak the bread in the concentrate mixture, turning the slices until all the liquid is absorbed.

3. Spray a nonstick skillet with vegetable cooking spray. Heat over medium-high heat until hot. Reduce the heat to medium-low. Add the bread and cook until the bottoms are nicely browned, about 3 minutes. Turn and cook the second side, about 2 minutes. Serve warm.

Best-Odds Toddler Servings in 1 slice: 2 Whole Grain; ¾ Protein; ½ Other Fruit; ¼ Calcium

Variation: Omit banana and banana-orange juice concentrate and use 4 tablespoons apple juice concentrate.

COTTAGE CHEESE SUNDAE

Hold the hot fudge and the ice cream. A baby with unspoiled taste buds will be just as happy with this naturally sweet, naturally nutritious version. Serve any time of the day, and vary according to seasonal availability of fruit.

Makes 1 toddler portion

¼ cup sliced fresh fruit (bananas, cantaloupe, peaches, strawberries)
¼ cup unsalted low-fat cottage cheese
1 tablespoon dairy sour cream (omit for children older than two)
2 tablespoons juice-sweetened preserves
1 tablespoon wheat germ

Arrange fruit in a ring on a small plate. Fill the center of the ring with cottage cheese. Top with the remaining ingredients.

Best-Odds Toddler Servings per portion: 1½ Protein; 1 Whole Grain; 1 Other Fruit (if bananas or white peaches are used); 1 Vitamin C (if strawberries or cantaloupe is used); 1 Yellow Fruit (if cantaloupe or yellow peaches are used); ½ Fat

FUNNY FINGERS

The protein of your choice will become baby's choice under this crispy coating. Serve Funny Fingers as finger food, of course.

Makes 1 toddler portion

1 ounce fresh fish fillet, such as sole, flounder, or haddock, or boneless chicken breast; or 1½ ounces tofu
¼ cup fine whole-wheat bread crumbs (see Note)
1 tablespoon grated Parmesan cheese (optional)
Dash garlic powder
½ teaspoon mayonnaise
Vegetable cooking spray

1. Preheat the oven to 350°F.

2. Cut the fish (checking carefully for bones), chicken, or tofu into ½-inch strips.

3. Combine the bread crumbs, grated cheese, if using, and the garlic powder in a small bowl, stirring until well blended.

4. Spread the mayonnaise on the fish, chicken, or tofu strips, then roll them in the crumb mixture. Arrange the strips in a shallow pan sprayed with vegetable cooking spray. Bake for 5 minutes; turn, and bake 5 minutes more.

Best-Odds Toddler Servings per portion: 1½ Protein; 1 Whole Grain; ⅓ Calcium

Note: You can make your own bread crumbs in a blender or food processor, using cubes of your favorite bread that has gone slightly stale. Store unused crumbs in the freezer until needed.

BABY'S FIRST CAKE

Even if the doctor's red light on eggs hasn't been lifted yet, you can let 'em eat cake—if it's this fruit-studded but eggless wonder.

Makes 1 single-layer 8-inch-square cake

Vegetable cooking spray
1 cup plus 2 tablespoons apple juice concentrate
½ cup whole raisins
½ cup chopped raisins
½ cup chopped dates
¼ cup (4 tablespoons) butter or margarine
1½ teaspoons ground cinnamon
¾ cup whole-wheat flour
½ cup wheat germ
4½ teaspoons low-sodium baking powder

1. Preheat the oven to 325°F. Coat an 8-inch square nonstick baking pan with vegetable cooking spray. Set aside.

2. Combine the juice concentrate, dried fruits, butter, and cinnamon in a small saucepan. Simmer over low heat until the butter is melted. Remove from the stove and let cool.

3. Combine the flour, wheat germ, and baking powder in a mixing bowl. Gradually blend in the fruit mixture, stirring just until mixed. Do not overmix.

4. Pour the batter into the prepared baking pan. Bake about 30 minutes. The cake is done when a toothpick inserted into the center comes out dry. Cover loosely with foil during baking if the cake starts to brown.

5. To keep the cake from becoming dry and too hard for baby to gum, cover with aluminum foil or store in a plastic bag as soon as it has cooled slightly.

Best-Odds Toddler Servings in ¹⁄₁₆ cake: 1½ Other Fruit; 1 + Whole Grain; ⅓ Protein

GOLDEN CAKE

Vitamin A finds its way into another unexpectedly delicious place; this time, a light but homey cake, scented with cinnamon. Freeze in squares for convenient serving.

Makes 1 single-layer 9-inch-square cake

1 cup dried apricots, finely chopped
1½ cups apple juice concentrate, or more if needed
1 cup whole-wheat flour
½ cup wheat germ
3 teaspoons low-sodium baking powder
1½ teaspoons ground cinnamon
2 egg whites, lightly beaten
¼ cup vegetable oil
Vegetable cooking spray
½ cup juice-sweetened apricot preserves or Dried Apricot Purée (recipe follows)

1. Preheat the oven to 350°F.

2. Combine the apricots with 1 cup of the juice concentrate in a small saucepan. Bring to a boil, then lower the heat and simmer, uncovered, until the apricots are soft, 5 to 15 minutes. Drain, reserving juice in a liquid measuring cup and setting apricots aside.

3. Blend the flour, wheat germ, baking soda, and cinnamon together in a large mixing bowl. Add the egg whites and the remaining ½ cup juice concentrate; stir to blend.

4. If necessary, add enough juice concentrate to the reserved juice to make ½ cup liquid. Stir in the oil and heat just until hot. Add the liquid and the reserved apricots to the flour mixture. Stir just until smooth.

5. Pour the batter into a nonstick 9-inch square pan coated with vegetable cooking spray. Bake until the top springs back when lightly touched and the sides have begun to pull away from the pan, about 35 minutes. While still warm, spread with apricot preserves or purée. Cool, and serve.

Best-Odds Toddler Servings in one 2-inch square: 1 Whole Grain; ½ Protein; ½ Yellow Fruit; Iron

DRIED APRICOT PURÉE

A quick and easy homemade fruit spread, rich in vitamin A and iron.

Makes about 1½ cups purée

1 cup dried apricots
1 cup apple juice concentrate

Combine the ingredients in a saucepan, and simmer, uncovered, until the fruit is soft, 5 to 15 minutes. Purée in a blender or food processor until smooth. Use as a spread on cake or bread, or as a topping for yogurt or cottage cheese.

Best-Odds Toddler Servings in 2 tablespoons: 1½ Yellow Fruit; 1 Other Fruit; some Iron

FIRST BIRTHDAY CAKE

Carrots disappear magically from a toddler's plate when they come in a cake. Frost for birthdays and other special occasions, but also keep a supply of plain squares in the freezer for snacking and daily desserts.

Makes 1 double-layer 9-inch-square cake

2½ cups thinly sliced carrots
2½ cups apple juice concentrate (you will use slightly less than this)
1½ cups raisins
Vegetable cooking spray
2 cups whole-wheat flour
½ cup wheat germ
2 tablespoons low-sodium baking powder
1 tablespoon ground cinnamon
¼ cup vegetable oil
2 whole eggs
4 egg whites
1 tablespoon vanilla extract
¾ cup unsweetened applesauce
Cream Cheese Frosting (recipe follows)

1. Combine the carrots with 1 cup plus 2 tablespoons of the juice concentrate in a medium-size saucepan. Bring to a boil, then lower the heat and simmer, covered, until carrots are tender, 15 to 20 minutes. Purée in a blender or food processor until smooth. Add the raisins and process until finely chopped. Let mixture cool.

2. Preheat the oven to 350°F. Line two 9-inch-square cake pans with waxed paper and spray the paper with vegetable cooking spray.

3. Combine the flour, wheat germ, baking powder, and cinnamon in a large mixing bowl. Add 1¼ cups juice concentrate, the oil, eggs, egg whites, and vanilla; beat just until well mixed. Fold in the carrot purée and applesauce. Pour the batter into the prepared cake pans.

4. Bake until a knife inserted in the center comes out clean, 35 to 40 minutes. Cool briefly in the pans, then turn out onto wire racks to cool completely. When cool, frost with Cream Cheese Frosting.

Best-Odds Toddler Servings in one 2-inch frosted square: 3 Yellow Vegetable; 2 + Other Fruits; 1½ Whole Grain; 1 + Protein; some Iron; 1 Fat

CREAM CHEESE FROSTING

The traditional foil for carrot cake—but without the sugar.

Frosts one 2-layer cake

½ cup apple juice concentrate
1 pound light cream cheese
2 teaspoons vanilla extract
½ cup finely chopped raisins
1½ teaspoons unflavored gelatin

1. Set aside 2 tablespoons of the juice concentrate.

2. Process the remaining juice concentrate, the cream cheese, vanilla, and raisins in

a blender or food processor until smooth. Transfer to a mixing bowl.

3. Stir the gelatin into the 2 tablespoons juice concentrate in a small saucepan; let stand 1 minute to soften. Heat to boiling and stir to dissolve gelatin.

4. Beat the gelatin mixture into the cream cheese mixture until well blended. Refrigerate just until the frosting begins to set, about 30 to 60 minutes. Frost the cake.

OATMEAL RAISIN COOKIES

Even the baby who hasn't yet sprouted a sweet tooth can gum these cakey treats.

Makes 3 to 4 dozen cookies

Vegetable cooking spray
1 cup whole-wheat flour
¾ cup wheat germ
½ cup rolled oats
1 tablespoon low-sodium baking powder
2 teaspoons ground cinnamon
1 cup apple juice concentrate
¼ cup vegetable oil
2 egg whites or 1 whole egg
¾ cup raisins

1. Preheat the oven to 375°F. Coat 2 cookie sheets with vegetable cooking spray. Set aside.

2. Mix the flour, wheat germ, oats, baking powder, and cinnamon in a large mixing bowl.

3. Combine the juice concentrate, oil, egg, and raisins in a blender. Blend at medium speed until the raisins are chopped. Pour the mixture into the dry ingredients, and stir together.

4. Drop the batter by heaping teaspoons onto the prepared sheets, about 1 inch apart. Flatten each mound with the back of a fork. Bake, being careful not to let the cookies brown and become crispy, about 8 to 10 minutes. Let the cookies

cool slightly on the sheets before removing to a plastic bag. (This will prevent the cookies from becoming hard.) Wait until cookies are completely cool before closing the plastic bag. Continue baking cookies until the batter is finished. Cookies can be frozen.

Best-Odds Toddler Servings in 2 to 3 cookies: 1+ Whole Grain; ¾ Other Fruit; ½ Protein; some Iron

APPLE-CRANBERRY CUBES

They wiggle, they jiggle, they shake, and they shiver—and these cubes of fruit gel haven't a drop of sugar in them to spoil the fun. The perfect answer, too, when a sick baby won't, or shouldn't, eat anything solid and refuses liquids.

Makes 4 toddler portions

1 tablespoon unflavored gelatin
¼ cup water
1½ cups unsweetened apple-cranberry juice
¼ cup apple juice concentrate

1. Mix together the gelatin and the water in a medium-size bowl; let stand to soften, 1 minute.

2. Meanwhile, in a small saucepan, bring the apple-cranberry juice to a boil. Add the juice to the gelatin mixture and stir until the gelatin is thoroughly dissolved. Add the juice concentrate. Pour the mixture into an 8-inch-square baking tin, and chill until firm. Cut into cubes and mound in a pretty dessert dish.

Best-Odds Toddler Servings in ¼ recipe: 1 Other Fruit

Variation: Use apple juice instead of apple-cranberry for babies or children with gastrointestinal viruses.

BANANA-ORANGE GEL

Same wiggle, with a little more kick.

Makes 4 toddler portions

1 tablespoon unflavored gelatin
½ cup water
1 cup fresh orange juice
½ cup banana-orange juice concentrate
1 small banana, sliced

1. In a small saucepan, stir the gelatin into the water; let stand to soften, 1 minute. Heat over medium-high heat just to boiling.

2. Stir in the juice and juice concentrate until the gelatin is thoroughly dissolved.

3. Pour half the mixture into an 8-inch-square baking tin and freeze until thickened, about 10 minutes. Add a layer of sliced banana and cover with the remaining gel mixture. Refrigerate until firm.

4. To serve, cut into four squares.

Best-Odds Toddler Servings in one portion: 1 Other Fruit

PEACHY YOGURT

Commercial frozen yogurts have as much sugar in them as ice cream—some even more. This one only tastes as though it does.

Makes 4 toddler portions

2 cups whole-milk plain yogurt
1 cup peeled, sliced fresh yellow peaches
¼ cup apple juice concentrate

1. Combine all ingredients in a blender and process until smooth.

2. Prepare according to the directions for your ice-cream maker. Or, pour into an 8-inch-square baking tin and freeze until mushy. Scrape mixture into a large mixing bowl and beat until fluffy. Repeat the freezing-beating process once or twice more. Then freeze until desired texture is reached. If the dessert freezes too hard, let it defrost until spoonable.

Best-Odds Toddler Servings in ¼ recipe: 1+ Yellow Fruit; 1 Protein; 1 Calcium

Common Home Remedies

The doctor recommends suctioning baby's nose to ease the congestion of a cold. Cold compresses, you hear, are the best way to treat a burn. And steam is ideal for treating a baby with the croup. But just how do you suction a baby's nose? What is a cold compress? And how do you build up enough steam to ease the croup? This guide to home remedies will give you the answers.

COLD COMPRESSES

Fill a basin (a styrofoam bucket or cooler is best) with cold tap water and a tray or two of ice cubes. Dip a clean washcloth into the water, wring it out, and place it over the affected part. Re-chill the cloth when the cold dissipates.

COLD SOAKS

Fill a basin (a styrofoam bucket or cooler is best) with cold water and a tray or two of ice cubes. Immerse the injured part for 30 minutes, if possible. Repeat in 30 minutes, if necessary. Do not apply ice directly to baby's skin.

COOL COMPRESSES

Fill a basin with cool water from the tap. Dip a washcloth or towel into the water, squeeze it out, and apply to injured part. Re-dip when the cloth no longer seems wet and cool.

EYE SOAKS

For eyes, dip a clean washcloth in warm,

DOSAGE CHART FOR COMMON INFANT-FEVER MEDICATION*

Tempra	Drops	Syrup
Under 3 months		
13 pounds**	½ dropper	¼ teaspoon
3 to 9 months		
13 to 20 pounds**	1 dropper	½ teaspoon
10 to 24 months		
21 to 26 pounds	1½ droppers	¾ teaspoon
2 to 3 years		
27 to 35 pounds	2 droppers	1 teaspoon

Tylenol or Panadol	Drops	Elixir
Under 3 months		
6 to 11 pounds**	½ dropper	
4 to 11 months		
12 to 17 pounds**	1 dropper	½ teaspoon
12 to 23 months		
18 to 23 pounds	1½ droppers	¾ teaspoon
2 to 3 years		
23 to 35 pounds	2 droppers	1 teaspoon

*These are acetaminophen preparations; aspirin should not be given without a doctor's recommendation.

**Do not give medication to babies under six months old without the doctor's recommendation. Give medication every four hours as needed, but no more than 5 times daily. If weight range and age don't correlate, use the dosage appropriate for baby's weight.

not hot, water (test it for comfort on your inner wrist or forearm), and apply to baby's eye for 5 to 10 minutes every 3 hours.

HEATING PAD

A hot-water bottle, which has no cords or heating element, is usually safer to use with an infant. If you use a heating pad, re-read directions before each use, be sure the pad and cord are in good condition, and cover entirely with a cloth diaper if the pad doesn't have a cloth covering. Keep the temperature low, do not leave baby, and use no more than 15 minutes at a time.

HOT COMPRESSES

See "Warm compresses." Never use hot compresses on a baby.

HOT SOAKS

Fill a basin with water that feels comfortably hot on your inner wrist or arm (not to your fingers). Never use water you haven't tested first. Immerse injured part in basin.

HOT-WATER BOTTLE

Fill a hot-water bottle with water that is just

warm to the touch. Wrap the bottle in a towel or cloth diaper before applying to baby's skin.

HUMIDIFIER

See "Steam."

ICE PACK

Use a commercial ice pack you keep in the freezer or a plastic bag filled with ice cubes (and a couple of paper towels to absorb the melting ice) and closed with a twist tie or rubber band. Also usable: an unopened can of frozen juice concentrate; an unopened package of frozen food. Do not apply ice directly to a baby's skin.

INCREASED FLUIDS

Frequently nurse the baby who is solely breastfed. Give formula to a bottle baby, unless the doctor says not to. Give water between feedings, and when baby is taking juice dilute half-and-half with water. But do not force fluids unless the doctor tells you to. When baby is vomiting, tiny sips of fluids spaced out stay down better than larger quantities. (See specific illnesses for preferred fluids.)

NASAL ASPIRATION

With baby held upright, squeeze bulb of aspirator (see illustration, page 419) and place tip carefully in one nostril. Slowly release bulb to draw mucus into it. Repeat with second nostril. If mucus is dried and caked, irrigate with salt water (see below) and aspirate again.

SALT-WATER IRRIGATION

Though it's possible to use a homemade salt solution (add ⅛ teaspoon salt to ½ cup cooled boiled water), commercial saline so-

lutions are safer. Put two drops in each nostril with clean small dropper to soften crusts and clear congestion. Wait 5 to 10 minutes and suction with a nasal aspirator. Do not use irrigation or commercial nose drops for more than three days, because such use can worsen congestion.

STEAM

Use a cold-mist humidifier or a steam vaporizer placed out of baby's reach to moisten the air; or place a bowl of hot water on a hot radiator (out of baby's reach) or a kettle or pot of hot water on the stove in the same room as baby.[1] For quick and abundant steam for a baby with croup (see page 634), close the bathroom door, turn on the hot water in the shower full blast, and fill the room with steam. Remain with baby in the bathroom until the croupy cough stops. If cough has not improved in ten minutes, check with the doctor.

WARM COMPRESSES

Fill a basin (a styrofoam bucket or cooler is best) with warm (it should not feel uncomfortable on your upper arm), not hot, water. Dip a clean washcloth in the water, wring it out, and place it over affected part as directed by baby's doctor.

1. Since germs and molds can multiply in a cold-mist humidifier, wash yours daily according to manufacturer's instructions when it's in use. It's generally recommended that the tank be cleaned with dish detergent and water, then rinsed with a mild solution of chlorine bleach and water. At each use it should be refilled with fresh water. Cold mist vaporizers are most likely to send germs and mold into the air; steam vaporizers are less likely to, but present a burn hazard. Best are ultrasonic units, which eject no live molds and very few bacteria into the air. But because the ultrasonic units pulverize not only bacteria and mold but minerals in the water, straight tap water, with its normal mineral content, should not be used in them. The mineral particles emitted by the humidifier are fine enough to be breathed into the deepest parts of the lungs and could increase risk of colds and flu, and aggravate chronic respiratory illnesses. Use distilled water or filter tap water to remove the minerals.

Common Childhood Illnesses

Though the physician will usually be the one to diagnose your baby's ill- nesses, you may find the basic information in this chart helpful as you try to sort out

DISEASE/SEASON/ SUSCEPTIBILITY	SYMPTOMS		
	NON-RASH	(numbers indicate order of appearance)	RASH
BRONCHIOLITIS (inflammation of the smaller branches of the bronchial tree) **Season:** Respiratory synctial viruses (RSV), winter and spring; parainfluenza viruses (PIV), summer and fall. **Susceptibility:** Greatest in those under 2 years, especially under 6 months, or with a family history of allergy.	1. Cold symptoms. 2. *A few days later:* Rapid, shallow breathing; wheezing on breathing out; low-grade fever for about 3 days. *Sometimes:* Chest does not seem to expand with breathing in; pale or bluish color.		

the possibilities and prepare to seek medical help. Keep in mind that not every child has a textbook case of every illness. Your child's symptoms, duration of disease, and so on may vary from those listed here.

The details of how to treat specific symptoms (such as a cough, diarrhea, or an itch, for example) or of how to handle a fever are omitted from the chart to avoid repetition. For information on treating symptoms, see page 414; for treating a fever, see page 431.

To aid in diagnosis, symptoms are numbered if they can be expected to appear at different times in the course of the illness. Rashes are listed separately for quick and easy comparison.

Scientists aren't always certain how disease is transmitted. But most frequently germs seem to be passed to a healthy person through droplets from the sneezes or coughs of an infected individual; on bits of dust in the air (airborne); via direct contact (touching the infected individual, most often hand-to-hand); via indirect contact (touching an object contaminated by the infected person); via respiratory secretions (mucus, phlegm) either directly or indirectly; via feces, directly or indirectly; via body fluids (tears, saliva, blood, pus, urine) by direct or indirect contact; via sexual activity or contact with sexual fluids; through contaminated food; or through animal or insect vectors, or carriers. Depending on the infectious organism, a person may be more susceptible to infection when general health is poor, when there is an open wound, sore, or other break in the skin, or when there has been no immunity developed.

The risk of contracting most diseases can be reduced by keeping your baby in general good health (immunizations, regular medical checkups, good nutrition, adequate rest), practicing good hygiene (washing hands after using the toilet or changing diapers and before handling baby or food, disposing of soiled diapers and tissues in a sanitary fashion), and isolating anyone with an infectious disease in your home as best you can (separate linens, dishes, utensils).

Even if this chart tells you everything you want to know about a particular childhood illness, it is no substitute for medical advice. Consult your baby's doctor as recommended.

CAUSE/TRANSMISSION/ INCUBATION/DURATION	CALL THE DOCTOR/ TREATMENT/DIET	PREVENTION/RECURRENCE/ COMPLICATIONS
Cause: Various viruses, most often RSV or PIV; rarely, bacteria. **Transmission:** Usually via respiratory secretions by direct contact or on household objects. **Incubation:** Varies with causative organism; usually 2 to 8 days. **Duration:** Acute phase may last only 3 days; cough from 1 to 3 weeks or more.	**Call the doctor immediately or go to the ER** if doctor can't be reached. **Treatment:** Hospitalization; possibly, antiviral drug. **Diet:** If food can be taken by mouth, frequent small meals.	**Prevention:** No vaccine available; avoid exposure of infants with a family history of respiratory allergy **Recurrence:** Can recur, but symptoms may be milder. **Complications:** Heart failure; bronchial asthma.

DISEASE/SEASON/ SUSCEPTIBILITY	SYMPTOMS	
	NON-RASH (numbers indicate order of appearance) RASH	
BRONCHITIS (inflammation of the bronchial tree and often the windpipe, or trachea) **Season:** Varies with causative microorganism. **Susceptibility:** Greatest in children under 4 years.	1. *Usually:* Cold symptoms. 2. *Abrupt onset of:* Fever, about 102°; harsh cough, worse at night, sometimes paroxysmal, with vomiting; greenish or yellow sputum; wheezing or whistling on breathing out, especially with a family history of respiratory allergy; lips and fingernails tinged blue.	
CHICKEN POX **(Varicella)** **Season:** Late winter and spring in temperate zones. **Susceptibility:** Most people are infected as children.	Slight fever; malaise; loss of appetite; severe itching.	Flat red spots turn into pimples, then blister, crust and scab; new crops continue to develop for 3 to 4 days, mostly on the body.
CONJUNCTIVITIS **(Pinkeye;** inflammation of the conjunctiva, or lining of the eye)	*Depending on cause, may include:* Bloodshot eyes; tearing; discharge; burning; itching; light sensitivity. Usually begins in one eye, but may spread to the other.	

CAUSE/TRANSMISSION/ INCUBATION/DURATION	CALL THE DOCTOR/ TREATMENT/DIET	PREVENTION/RECURRENCE/ COMPLICATIONS
Cause: Usually a virus; less often, bacteria, but secondary bacterial infection is common. Cough made worse by tobacco smoke. **Transmission:** Usually via respiratory secretions. **Incubation:** Varies with causative organism. **Duration:** Fever lasts 2 or 3 days; cough 1 or 2 weeks or more.	**Call the doctor** if cough is severe, or lasts more than 3 days. **Treatment:** Symptomatic, for cough, if needed; in some cases, antiobiotics. **Diet:** Increase in clear fluids.	**Prevention:** Proper care of a baby with a common cold (page 418). **Recurrence:** Some children are particularly susceptible, and get bronchitis with every cold. **Complications:** Otitis media (ear infection).
Cause: Varicella-zoster virus. **Transmission:** Person-to-person via droplets, and airborne; very contagious from 1 to 2 days before onset until all lesions are scabbed. **Incubation:** Usually 14 to 16 days, but can be as short as 11 or as long as 20. **Duration:** First vesicles crust in 6 to 8 hours, scab in 24 to 48; scabs last 5 to 20 days.	**Call the doctor** to confirm diagnosis; **call immediately** for high-risk children; **call again** if symptoms of encephalitis appear. **Treatment:** for itching (page 414) and fever (page 431). DO NOT GIVE ASPIRIN.	**Prevention:** Avoidance of exposure in infants; VZV immunization of those over 12 months. **Recurrence:** Extremely rare; but dormant virus may flare up as shingles later in life. **Complications:** Rarely, encephalitis; anyone on steroids or those who are immunocompromised can become seriously ill. **In expectant mothers,** possible risk to fetus; contact physician if exposure occurs.
Cause: Many, including viruses, bacteria, chlamydia, allergens, parasites, fungi, environmental irritants, blocked tear duct (see page 108), and silver nitrate drops at birth. **Transmission:** For infective organisms, eye-hand-eye. **Incubation:** Usually brief. **Duration:** Varies: silver nitrate, 3 to 5 days; virus, 2 days to 3 weeks (can become chronic); bacteria, about 2 weeks; others, until allergen, irritant, or duct blockage is removed.	**Call the doctor** to confirm diagnosis; **call again** if condition worsens or does not start to improve. **Treatment:** Eye soaks; separate bed linens and towels to prevent spread of infection; elimination of irritants, such as tobacco smoke, when possible; drops or ointment prescribed for bacterial and herpes infections, possibly for viral conjunctivitis (to prevent secondary infection), and to relieve discomfort of allergic reaction.	**Prevention:** Good hygiene (separate towels when family member is infected); avoidance of allergens and other irritants. **Recurrence:** Some people are more susceptible and more likely to have recurrences. **Complications:** Blindness (rare, except with gonorrheal infection); chronic eye inflammation; eye damage from repeated attacks.

DISEASE/SEASON/ SUSCEPTIBILITY	SYMPTOMS	
	NON-RASH (numbers indicate order of appearance)	RASH
CROUP (Acute Laryngotracheitis) **Season:** Varies; usually occurs at night. **Susceptibility:** Young children.	Hoarseness; sharp, barking cough; crowing, wheezing, or grunting sound on breathing in. *Sometimes:* Difficulty breathing.	
EAR INFECTION (Otitis media)	See page 423.	
ENCEPHALITIS (inflammation of the brain) **Season:** Depends on cause. **Susceptibility:** Varies with cause.	Fever; drowsiness; headache. *Sometimes:* Neurological impairment; coma at a late stage.	
EPIGLOTTITIS (inflammation of the epiglottis) **Season:** Winter months in temperate climates. **Susceptibility:** Not common in children under 2.	Low-pitched cough; muffled voice; difficulty breathing and swallowing; drooling. *Sometimes:* Protruding tongue; fever. Child seems ill.	
FIFTH DISEASE (Erythema Infectiosum) **Season:** Early spring. **Susceptibility:** Greatest in children 2 to 12 years old.	*Rarely:* Joint pain.	1. Intense flush on face (slapped-cheek look). 2. *Next day:* Lacy rash on arms and legs. 3. *3 days later:* Rash on inner surfaces, fingers, toes, trunk, and/or buttocks. 4. Rash may reappear on and off with exposure to heat (bath water, sun) for 2 or 3 weeks.

CAUSE/TRANSMISSION/ INCUBATION/DURATION	CALL THE DOCTOR/ TREATMENT/DIET	PREVENTION/RECURRENCE/ COMPLICATIONS
Cause: Usually, virus (most often parainfluenza or adenovirus; occasionally, bacteria or inhaled object. **Transmission:** Probably, person-to-person; contaminated objects; droplet spray. **Incubation:** 2 days (usually follows cold or flu). **Duration:** ½ hour; may recur over several days.	**Call the doctor immediately** if steam doesn't bring relief; if baby looks blue, has blue lips, or is drooling excessively; or if you suspect an inhaled object. **Initial treatment:** Steam (see page 629). **Follow-up:** Humidifier. **Diet:** Reduce intake of dairy products, especially if mucus is heavy. Sleep in same room as baby to reassure and to be handy for treating another attack.	**Prevention:** Supply humidified air to baby with cold or flu. **Recurrence:** Tends to repeat in some children. **Complications:** Breathing problems; pneumonia; ear infection about 5 days after recovery.
Cause: Bacteria or viruses (often a complication of another disease). **Transmission:** Depends on cause; some viruses transmitted via insects. **Incubation:** Depends on cause. **Duration:** Varies.	**Call the doctor immediately or go the ER** if you suspect encephalitis. **Treatment:** Hospitalization is required.	**Prevention:** Immunization against diseases for which this is a complication, for example measles. **Recurrence:** Unlikely. **Complications:** Neurological damage; can be fatal.
Cause: Bacteria, most often hemophilus influenzae (Hib). **Transmission:** Probably, person-to-person, or inhalation of droplets. **Incubation:** Less than 10 days. **Duration:** 4 to 7 days or longer.	**Call 911 immediately or go to the ER.** While waiting for help, keep baby upright, leaning forward, with mouth open and tongue out. **Treatment:** Hospitalization; establishment of airway; antibiotics.	**Prevention:** Hib immunization. **Recurrence:** Slight possibility. **Complications:** Can be fatal without prompt medical attention.
Cause: Possibly, human parvovirus. **Transmission:** Probably person-to-person. **Incubation:** 4 to 14 days; usually 12 to 14. **Duration:** 3 to 10 days, but rash may reappear on and off for up to 3 weeks.	**Call the doctor** only if you need confirmation of diagnosis or if other symptoms occur. **Treatment:** None. **Diet:** No changes.	**Prevention:** None. **Recurrence:** Possible. **Complications:** Only in those who are immune deficient or pregnant (can cause miscarriage, though most women are immune by the time they conceive).

DISEASE/SEASON/ SUSCEPTIBILITY	SYMPTOMS	
	NON-RASH (numbers indicate order of appearance)	RASH
GASTROINTESTINAL UPSET	See Diarrhea, page 421.	
GERMAN MEASLES (Rubella) **Season:** Late winter and early spring. **Susceptibility:** Any unimmunized person.	None in 25% to 50% of cases. 1. *Sometimes:* Slight fever; swollen neck glands.	2. Small (1/10-inch), flat, reddish pink spots on face. 3. Rash spreads to body, and sometimes, to roof of mouth.
HAND-FOOT-MOUTH DISEASE (Vesicular Stomatitis) **Season:** Summer and fall in temperate climates. **Susceptibility:** Greatest in babies and young children.	1. Fever; loss of appetite. *Often:* Sore throat and mouth (discomfort nursing); difficulty swallowing.	2. *In 2 or 3 days:* Lesions in mouth; then fingers, maybe feet, buttocks, sometimes arms, legs, and less often face. Mouth lesions usually blister.
HERPANGINA **Season:** Mostly, summer and fall in temperate climates. **Susceptibility:** Greatest in babies and young children. Occurs alone or with other diseases.	1. Fever (100° to 104°, even 106°); sore throat. 1. or 3. Painful swallowing. *Sometimes:* Vomiting; loss of appetite; diarrhea; abdominal pain; lethargy.	2. Distinct grayish white papules in back of mouth or throat that blister and ulcerate (5 to 20 in number).
HERPES SIMPLEX (Cold Sores, Fever Blisters) **Season:** Any, but sunshine can precipitate flare-up of virus. **Susceptibility:** Most primary infections occur in childhood.	*Primary infection:* Fever (can be 106°); sore throat; swollen glands; drooling; bad breath; loss of appetite. *Often:* No symptoms. *Subsequent flare-ups: Possibly:* headache. Infection can also occur in the eye.	*Primary infection:* Sores in mucous membranes of mouth. *Subsequent flare-ups:* Welt forms on or near lip, tingles and itches, then blisters and oozes (painful stage), finally crusts and scabs (may itch).
HYDROPHOBIA	See **Rabies.**	

CAUSE/TRANSMISSION/ INCUBATION/DURATION	CALL THE DOCTOR/ TREATMENT/DIET	PREVENTION/RECURRENCE/ COMPLICATIONS
Cause: Rubella virus. **Transmission:** 7 to 10 days before rash appears until possibly 7 days after rash appears; via direct or droplet contact. **Incubation:** 14 to 21 days; usually 16 to 18. **Duration:** A few hours to 4 or 5 days.	**Call the doctor** if a non-immune pregnant woman is exposed. **Treatment:** None. **Diet:** No changes.	**Prevention:** Immunization (MMR). **Recurrence:** None; one case confers immunity. **Complications:** Very rarely, thrombocytopenia or encephalitis.
Cause: Coxsackie virus. **Transmission:** Mouth-to-mouth; feces-to-hand-to-mouth. **Incubation:** 3 to 6 days. **Duration:** About 1 week.	**Call the doctor** to confirm diagnosis. **Treatment:** Symptomatic (page 414). **Diet:** Soft foods will be more comfortable.	**Prevention:** None. **Recurrence:** Possible. **Complications:** None.
Cause: Coxsackie virus. **Transmission:** Mouth-to-mouth; feces-to-hand-to-mouth. **Incubation:** 3 to 6 days. **Duration:** 4 to 7 days, but healing can take 2 to 3 weeks.	**Call the doctor** to confirm diagnosis; **Call immediately** if convulsions or other symptoms occur. **Treatment:** Symptomatic. **Diet:** Soft foods will be more comfortable.	**Prevention:** None. **Recurrence:** Possible. **Complications:** None.
Cause: Herpes simplex virus (HSV) remains in body and can be reactivated by sun, stress, teething, a cold, fever. **Transmission:** Direct contact with lesion, saliva, stool, urine, or eye discharge; or with household articles within hours of contamination. **Incubation:** Possibly, 2 to 12 days. **Duration:** Scab falls off within 3 weeks.	**Call the doctor** only if baby seems ill. **Treatment:** Over-the-counter ointment may help; antiviral drugs in high-risk children. **Diet:** For primary infection, soft, non-acid foods; during subsequent flare-up, plain yogurt with live cultures may help. (A crushed lactobacillus tablet added to the yogurt will increase effectiveness.)	**Prevention:** Avoid triggering factors when possible. **Recurrence:** Latent infection can flare up anytime. **Complications:** Eye involvement.

DISEASE/SEASON/ SUSCEPTIBILITY	SYMPTOMS	
	NON-RASH (numbers indicate order of appearance)	RASH
INFLUENZA (Flu; upper respiratory infection, or URI) **Season:** More often in cold months; often in epidemics. **Susceptibility:** Anyone, but very old and very young can become sicker.	*Sometimes:* None noted. 1. *Usually, abrupt onset of:* Fever (100.4° to 104°); shivering; malaise; dry, unproductive cough; diarrhea/vomiting; achiness (adults). 2. *Often, 3 or 4 days after onset:* Cold symptoms. 3. *Sometimes, for next 1 or 2 weeks:* Productive cough; fatigue.	1. or 2. *Often:* Intermittent or variable, fever, malaise, headache, mild neck stiffness, and achiness. *Sometimes,* as disease spreads: headache, fatigue, aches and pains, nervous system involvement. 3. *Late disease, if untreated:* chronic arthritis, especially in knees; further central nervous system involvement; *rarely,* heart damage.
LYME DISEASE **Season:** May 1 to Nov. 30, with most cases in June and July. **Susceptibility:** Everyone; heaviest concentration of cases in Northeast, but disease is spreading.	1. or 2. *Often:* Fatigue; headache; fever and chills; generalized achiness; swollen glands near site of bite. *Sometimes:* Conjunctivitis; swelling around the eyes; intermittent behavioral changes due to involvement of the nervous system; swelling of the testicles; sore throat; non-productive cough. 3. *Weeks to years later:* Joint pain (arthritis); heart abnormalities.	1. *Usually:* An often bull's-eye-shaped red rash (*erythema migrans*) at site of tick bite, which usually expands over days to weeks to form larger red rash. 2. *Sometimes:* If disease spreads, multiple rashes develop, similar to, but often smaller than the primary lesion.
MEASLES (Rubeola) **Season:** Winter and spring. **Susceptibility:** Anyone not already immune.	1. *For 1 or 2 days:* Fever; runny nose; red, watery eyes; dry cough. *Sometimes:* Diarrhea; swollen glands.	2. Tiny white spots like grains of sand appear inside of cheeks (Koplik spots); may bleed. 3. Dull, red, slightly raised rash begins on forehead, behind ears, then spreads downward giving a red-allover look.

CAUSE/TRANSMISSION/ INCUBATION/DURATION	CALL THE DOCTOR/ TREATMENT/DIET	PREVENTION/RECURRENCE/ COMPLICATIONS
Cause: A variety of influenza viruses. **Transmission:** Inhalation of respiratory droplets; use of contaminated articles. Communicable from 5 days before symptoms appear. **Incubation:** 1 to 2 days. **Duration:** Acute phase, a few days; convalescent phase, 1 to 2 weeks.	**Call the doctor** if baby is under 6 months, if symptoms are severe or continue 3 days, or if fever is over 102°. **Treatment:** Symptomatic; in severe cases antiviral drugs may be prescribed. DO NOT GIVE ASPIRIN. **Diet:** Extra fluids.	**Prevention:** Annual immunization for certain high-risk infants; antivirals for others (ask the doctor and see page 153); avoiding crowds in flu season. **Recurrence:** Common. **Complications:** Secondary bacterial infections: otitis media, bronchitis, croup, pneumonia. Also Reye's syndrome.
Cause: A spirochete. **Transmission:** Spread by bite of the pinhead-size deer tick (which is carried by deer, mice, and other animals, and can jump from them to humans) and, possibly, other ticks. Since ticks take a long time to inject bacteria, prompt removal may prevent infection. **Incubation:** 3 to 32 days. **Duration:** Without treatment, possibly years.	**Call the doctor** if you suspect anyone in your family may have been bitten by a tick. **Treatment:** Antibiotics appear essential to defeat disease; effective even at late stages. **Diet:** No changes.	**Prevention:** Protective coverup clothing when out of doors in infested areas; removal of ticks; alertness to possible tick bites; *prompt removal of ticks.* **Recurrence:** Possible; there is no lasting immunity. **Complications:** Neurological, cardiac, motor abnormalities. *For latest information, call Lyme Disease Hotline: 800-886-LYME.*
Cause: Measles virus. **Transmission:** Direct contact with droplets from 2 days before to 4 days after rash appears. **Incubation:** 8 to 12 days. **Duration:** About a week.	**Call the doctor** for diagnosis; **recall immediately** if cough becomes severe, if convulsions or symptoms of pneumonia, encephalitis, or otitis media occur, or if fever goes up after going down. **Treatment:** Symptomatic; warm soaks, dim lights if eyes are sensitive (but bright light not harmful). **Diet:** Extra fluids for fever.	**Prevention:** Immunization (MMR); strict isolation of infected persons. **Recurrence:** None. **Complications:** Otitis media, pneumonia, encephalitis; can be fatal.

DISEASE/SEASON/ SUSCEPTIBILITY	SYMPTOMS		
	NON-RASH	(numbers indicate order of appearance)	RASH
MENINGITIS (inflammation of the membranes around the brain and/ or the spinal cord). **Season:** Varies with causative organism; for Hib, winter. **Susceptibility:** Depends on causative organism; for Hib, greatest for infants and young children.	Fever; high-pitched cry; drowsiness; irritability; loss of appetite; vomiting; bulging fontanel. *In older children, also:* stiff neck; sensitivity to light; blurred vision and other signs of neurological ills.		
MENINGOENCEPHALITIS (a combination of meningitis and encephalitis)	See **Meningitis** and **Encephalitis.**		
MUMPS **Season:** Late winter and spring. **Susceptibility:** Anyone not immune.	1. *Sometimes:* Vague pain; fever; loss of appetite. 2. *Usually:* Swelling of salivary (parotid) glands on one or both sides of jaw, below and in front of ear; ear pain; pain on chewing, or on taking acid or sour food or drink; swelling of other salivary glands. No symptoms at all in about 30% of cases.		
NONSPECIFIC VIRAL ILLNESSES **Season:** Mostly summer. **Susceptibility:** Mostly young children.	*Vary, but may include:* Fever; loss of appetite; diarrhea.		Various types of rashes are seen with NSV.

CAUSE/TRANSMISSION/ INCUBATION/DURATION	CALL THE DOCTOR/ TREATMENT/DIET	PREVENTION/RECURRENCE/ COMPLICATIONS
Cause: Most often, bacteria, such as Hib; also viruses, which cause less serious disease. **Transmission:** Depends on organism. **Incubation:** Varies with organism; for Hib, probably less than 10 days. **Duration:** Varies.	**Call the doctor immediately** if you suspect meningitis, **or go to the ER** if doctor can't be reached. **Treatment:** For viral meningitis, symptomatic; for bacterial, hospitalization required; antibiotics plus other drugs, possibly glycerol. **Diet:** Extra fluids for fever.	**Prevention:** Hib immunization for Hib infections; stringent health-care rules in day-care centers. **Recurrence:** None with Hib; one attack confers immunity. **Complications:** Hib and other bacterial forms can do lasting neurological damage, and can be fatal; viral forms usually do no long-term damage.
Cause: Mumps virus. **Transmission:** Usually 1 or 2 days (but could be as long as 7 days) prior to onset until 9 days after onset via direct contact with respiratory secretions. **Incubation:** Usually 16 to 18 days, but can be 12 to 25. **Duration:** 5 to 7 days.	**Call the doctor** for diagnosis; **call back immediately** if there is vomiting, drowsi-ness, possible headache, back or neck stiffness, or other signs of meningo-encephalitis either along with or following the mumps. **Treatment:** Symptomatic for fever and pain; cool compresses applied to cheeks. **Diet:** Non-acid, non-sour soft diet.	**Prevention:** Immunization. **Recurrence:** Very slight chance of recurrence if only one side was affected. **Complications:** Meningoencephalitis; other complications rare in infants, but can be serious in adult males.
Cause: Various enteroviruses. **Transmission:** Feces-to-hand-to-mouth; possibly mouth-to-mouth. **Incubation:** 3 to 6 days. **Duration:** Usually a few days.	**Call the doctor** to confirm diagnosis; **call again** if baby seems worse or if new symptoms appear. **Treatment:** Symptomatic. **Diet:** Extra fluids for diarrhea, fever (see pages 421, 431).	**Prevention:** None. **Recurrence:** Common. **Complications:** Very rare.

DISEASE/SEASON/ SUSCEPTIBILITY	SYMPTOMS NON-RASH (numbers indicate order of appearance) RASH	
OTITIS MEDIA	See page 423.	
PERTUSSIS (Whooping Cough) Season: Late winter/early spring. **Susceptibility:** Half of all cases occur in babies under 1 year.	1. *Catarrhal stage:* Cold symptoms with dry cough; low-grade fever; irritability. 2. *Paroxysmal stage, 1 or 2 weeks later:* Coughing in explosive bursts with no breaths between; thick mucus expelled. *Often:* Bulging eyes and protruding tongue; pale or red skin; vomiting; profuse sweating; exhaustion. *Sometimes:* Apnea, in infants; hernia, from cough. 3. *Convalescent stage:* Cessation of whooping and vomiting; reduced coughing; improved appetite and mood. Mild in immunized children.	
PHARYNGITIS	See **Sore Throat**	
PNEUMONIA (Inflammation of the lung) Season: Varies with causative factor. **Susceptibility:** Anyone, but especially the very young, very old, and those with chronic illnesses.	*Commonly, after cold or other illness, baby seems suddenly worse, with:* Increased fever; productive cough; rapid breathing; blueness; wheezy, raspy, and/or difficult breathing; abdominal bloating and pain.	

CAUSE/TRANSMISSION/ INCUBATION/DURATION	CALL THE DOCTOR/ TREATMENT/DIET	PREVENTION/RECURRENCE/ COMPLICATIONS
Cause: Bordetella pertussis bacteria. **Transmission:** Direct contact via droplets; most communicable during catarrhal stage, less so later; antibiotics reduce period of communicability. **Incubation:** 7 to 10 days; rarely more than 2 weeks. **Duration:** Usually 6 weeks, but can last much longer.	**Call the doctor promptly** for persistent coughing. **Treatment:** Hospitalization for infants; antibiotics (may help reduce symptoms in first stage, communicability later); oxygen; mucus suctioning; humidification. **Diet:** Frequent small feedings; fluid replacement; intravenous feeding if necessary.	**Prevention:** Immunization (DTP) **Recurrence:** None; one attack confers immunity. **Complications:** Many, including: otitis media; pneumonia; convulsions. Can be fatal, especially in infants.
Cause: Various organisms, including bacteria, myco-plasma, fungi, viruses, and protozoa, as well as insult by chemical or other irritant or inhaled object. **Transmission:** Varies with cause. **Incubation:** Varies with cause. **Duration:** Varies with cause.	**Call the doctor** for productive or persistent cough; or if a slightly sick baby seems worse or has increased fever or cough; **call immediately or go to ER** if baby has difficulty breathing, turns a bluish color, or seems very sick. **Treatment:** Symptomatic. Most cases can be treated at home. Antibiotics, if needed. **Diet:** Fluids; adequate nutrition.	**Prevention:** Hib immunization for Hib infections; protection of susceptible infants against illness. **Recurrence:** Many types can recur. **Complications:** Riskiest for those infants weakened by other illnesses or low birthweight.

DISEASE/SEASON/ SUSCEPTIBILITY	SYMPTOMS NON-RASH (numbers indicate order of appearance) RASH	
RABIES (Hydrophobia) **Season:** Anytime, but more rabid dogs in summer. **Susceptibility:** Anyone.	1. Local or radiating pain, burning, sensation of cold, itching, tingling at bite site. 2. Slight fever (101° to 102°); lethargy; headache; loss of appetite; nausea; sore throat; loose cough; irritability; sensitivity to light and noise; dilated pupils; rapid heart-beat; shallow breathing; excessive drooling, tearing, sweating. 3. *2 to 10 days later:* Increased anxiety and restlessness; vision problems; facial weakness; fever up to 103°. *Often:* Fear of water, with liquids expelled; frothy drooling. 4. *About 3 days later:* Paralysis.	
RESPIRATORY SYNCYTIAL VIRUS (RSV) **Season:** Winter and early spring in temperate climates; rainy season in tropics. **Susceptibility:** Anyone, at any age, but about 66% contract by age 1, most by age 3.	Range from mild cold-like symptoms to bronchiolitis and bronchopneumonia, with: Cough, wheezing; sore throat; painful breathing; malaise; inflamed mucous membranes of nose and throat. *Sometimes:* Apnea (especially in premies).	
REYE'S SYNDROME **Season:** Anytime. **Susceptibility:** Mostly children who are given aspirin during a viral illness such as chicken pox or influenza.	*1 to 7 days following a viral infection:* Persistent vomiting; lethargy; rapidly deteriorating mental state (irritability, confusion, delirium); rapid heartbeat and respiration. *May progress to:* Coma.	

CAUSE/TRANSMISSION/ INCUBATION/DURATION	CALL THE DOCTOR/ TREATMENT/DIET	PREVENTION/RECURRENCE/ COMPLICATIONS
Cause: Rabies virus. **Transmission:** From an infected animal, via a bite; rarely, licking of an open wound; scratches or abrasions; possibly, close exposure to a rabid bat or other animal. **Incubation:** 5 days to 1 year or more; 2 months is average. **Duration:** About 2 weeks from start of symptoms to point of paralysis.	**Call the doctor** following a bite by any animal you do not know for certain has been vaccinated against rabies. **Treatment:** Restrain animal; see first aid instructions for animal bites (page 435); Postexposure prophylaxis (PEP) with human rabies immune globulin (HRIG) and human diploid cell vaccine (HDCV) will be given if animal can't be found or turns out to be rabid; tetanus booster will be given as needed. Hospitalization if disease is not headed off. **Diet:** No dietary changes.	**Prevention:** Immunization of pets and individuals at high risk; teaching babies caution with strange animals; community effort to keep strays off street and wild animal population rabies-free. **Recurrence:** None. **Complications:** Disease if left to natural course, untreated, is fatal. Once symptoms occur, mortality rate high, even with treatment.
Cause: Respiratory syncytial virus (RSV). **Transmission:** Via eyes or nose through contact with infected person or contaminated articles from 3 days to 4 weeks from onset. **Incubation:** Usually 5 to 8 days. **Duration:** Varies with illness caused.	**Call the doctor** if baby with cold symptoms has difficulty breathing (nostrils flare), is wheezing, has a raspy cough, or has very rapid respiration (see page 407). **Treatment:** Symptomatic; may also include antiviral drug and hospitalization, if needed. **Diet:** For symptoms only.	**Prevention:** Isolation, careful handwashing, avoidance of exposure to smoke; RSV immune globulin in high-risk infants; no vaccine as yet. **Recurrence:** Possible, but usually as upper respiratory infection after age 3. **Complications:** Lower respiratory disease in 33% infants (2.5% require hospitalization); otitis media.
Cause: Unknown, but appears to be related to such viral illnesses as chicken pox and influenza, and to aspirin use during them. **Transmission:** Unknown. **Incubation:** Unknown, but seems to occur within days of onset of viral infection. **Duration:** Varies.	**Call the doctor immediately** if you suspect Reye's Syndrome, **or go to the ER.** **Treatment:** Hospital treatment is vital.	**Prevention:** Avoid giving aspirin with viral diseases such as chicken pox or influenza. **Recurrence:** None. **Complications:** Can be fatal, but survivors usually have no lasting problems.

DISEASE/SEASON/ SUSCEPTIBILITY	SYMPTOMS	
	NON-RASH (numbers indicate order of appearance)	RASH
ROSEOLA INFANTUM **Season:** Year-round, but more common in spring and fall. **Susceptibility:** Greatest in babies and young children.	1. Irritability; loss of appetite; fever (102° to 105°). *Sometimes:* Runny nose; swollen glands; convulsions. 2. *On 3rd or 4th day:* Fever drops and baby seems better.	3. Faint pink spots that turn white upon pressure on body, neck, upper arms, and sometimes, face and legs. In some cases, there may be no rash.
SCARLET FEVER **(Scarlatina)** **Season:** Year-round, but more common in cold months. **Susceptibility:** Greatest among school-age children; less common in those under 3 and in adults.	Similar to strep throat, but often heralded by vomiting and characterized by rash.	Bright red rash on face, groin, and under arms; spreads to rest of body and limbs; leaves skin rough, peeling.
SORE THROAT, VIRAL **(Tonsillitis; Pharyngitis)** **Season:** Fall, winter, and spring. **Susceptibility:** More often, older children.	Moderate fever (101° to 103°); fatigue; throat pain or discomfort; some difficulty swallowing; irritability and fussiness. Throat appears red and tonsils may be swollen. *Sometimes:* Hoarseness; coughing.	

CAUSE/TRANSMISSION/ INCUBATION/DURATION	CALL THE DOCTOR/ TREATMENT/DIET	PREVENTION/RECURRENCE/ COMPLICATIONS
Cause: Probably virus. **Transmission:** Unknown; not highly contagious. **Incubation:** 5 to 15 days. **Duration:** 3 to 6 days.	**Call the doctor** to confirm diagnosis; **call back** if fever persists for 4 or 5 days, if baby develops convulsions or seems ill. **Treatment:** Symptomatic. **Diet:** Increased fluids for fever.	**Prevention:** None known. **Recurrence:** Apparently, none. **Complications:** Very rare.
Cause: Streptococcus bacteria. **Transmission:** Direct contact with infected person. **Incubation:** 2 to 5 days. **Duration:** About 1 week in infants under 6 months, but runny nose and general crankiness can last 6 weeks; about 1 to 2 weeks in older babies.	See **Strep Throat.**	**Prevention:** Isolation of infected persons, and good preventive hygiene. **Recurrence:** Can occur. **Complications:** See **Strep Throat.**
Cause: Various viruses, most often adenovirus; also enterovirus. (Chronic sore throat may be due to allergy; tobacco smoke; hot, dry air, or other factors.) **Transmission:** Depends on causative virus; probably respiratory route with adenovirus. **Incubation:** Depends on causative virus; 2 to 14 days with adenovirus. **Duration:** 1 to 10 days.	**Call the doctor** if you suspect baby has a sore throat, so throat culture can be taken to rule out strep. **Treatment:** Symptomatic. Acetaminophen for pain. (Babies are too young for gargling or sucking on lozenges.) DO NOT GIVE ASPIRIN. **Diet:** Soft cold foods may be easier for a baby on solids to tolerate. Fluids.	**Prevention:** Isolation of infected person, and good hygiene. In chronic sore throat, the removal of the cause. **Recurrence:** Possible. **Complications:** Unlikely, except in children with suppressed immunity.

DISEASE/SEASON/ SUSCEPTIBILITY	SYMPTOMS		
	NON-RASH	(numbers indicate order of appearance)	RASH
STREP THROAT (**Streptococcal Pharyngitis**) **Season:** October through April. **Susceptibility:** Most common in school-age children.	*In infants under 6 months:* Fever; moderate inflammation of the throat. *In older babies:* Low-grade fever; mild sore throat. *Sometimes:* No symptoms noted. *In chronic strep:* Runny nose; fluctuating temperature; crankiness; loss of appetite; pallor. *In older children:* High fever; red pussy throat; trouble swallowing; swollen tonsils and glands; abdominal pain.		
TETANUS (Lockjaw) **Season:** When more time is spent out of doors. **Susceptibility:** Anyone not immunized.	*Localized:* Spasm and increased muscle tone near the wound. *Generalized:* Involuntary muscle contractions that can arch back, lock jaw, twist neck; convulsions; rapid heartbeat; profuse sweating; low-grade fever; difficult sucking, in infants.		
TONSILLITIS	See **Sore Throat.**		
UPPER RESPIRATORY INFECTION (URI)	See **Common Cold** (page 418) and **Influenza.**		
WHOOPING COUGH	See **Pertussis**		

CAUSE/TRANSMISSION/ INCUBATION/DURATION	CALL THE DOCTOR/ TREATMENT/DIET	PREVENTION/RECURRENCE/ COMPLICATIONS
Cause: Streptococcus pyogenes, a group of Group A streptococcus bacteria. **Transmission:** By direct contact with infected individual from 1 day before onset to 6 days after, but antibiotics reduce communicability to 24 hours. Highly contagious. **Incubation:** 2 to 5 days. **Duration:** About 1 week in infants under 6 months, but runny nose and general crankiness can last 6 weeks. About 1 to 2 weeks in older babies.	**Call the doctor** initially for diagnosis (throat culture will confirm); **call again** if fever doesn't drop in 2 days, or if new symptoms appear. **Treatment:** Symptomatic. Antibiotics to prevent complications. **Diet:** Soft cold foods may be easier for a baby on solids to tolerate. Fluids.	**Prevention:** Isolation of infected persons, and good hygiene. **Recurrence:** Possible. **Complications:** Infection can spread to ears, mastoids, sinuses, lungs, brain, kidneys, skin (impetigo). Rheumatic fever less common but does occur in infants; also joint pain and rashes.
Cause: Toxin produced by bacteria called Clostridium tetani, which spreads through the body. **Transmission:** Transmitted via contamination by the bacteria of a puncture wound, a burn, a deep scrape, or an unhealed umbilical cord. **Incubation:** 3 days to 3 weeks, but an average of 8 days. **Duration:** Several weeks.	**Call the doctor immediately or go to the ER** if unvaccinated baby incurs susceptible wound. **Treatment:** Medical treatment essential: Tetanus toxoid to prevent development of disease; tetanus antitoxins; muscle relaxants; antibiotics; respirator.	**Prevention:** Immunization (DTP); sanitary care of umbilicus; avoidance of outdoor injuries when possible. **Recurrence:** None. **Complications:** Many, including: Ulcers; pneumonia; abnormal heart rate; blood clot in lung. Can be fatal.

HEIGHT AND WEIGHT CHARTS

Record your baby's weight and length at birth in a permanent health record, and update his or her progress at each visit to the doctor. To chart measurements on these graphs, find baby's age along the bottom of the page and weight (in kilograms and pounds) or length (in centimeters and inches) along the side. Put a color dot at the

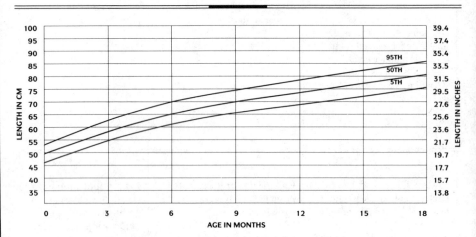

GIRLS HEIGHT CHART

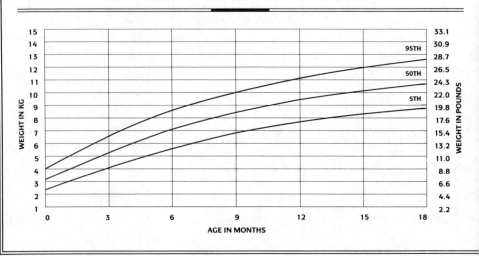

GIRLS WEIGHT CHART

point where the two come together. To see your baby's progress, connect the dots as they are added. Ninety out of every one-hundred children fall within the fifth and ninety-fifth percentiles. Though those in the top and bottom five percent may come by their size genetically and be doing well, some may be growing too slowly or gaining too quickly. If your baby falls into either of these groups, discuss your concern with the doctor. Check with the doctor, too, about any sudden variation from the typical pattern (in height or weight or both), though such a variation may be perfectly normal for your baby.

BOYS HEIGHT CHART

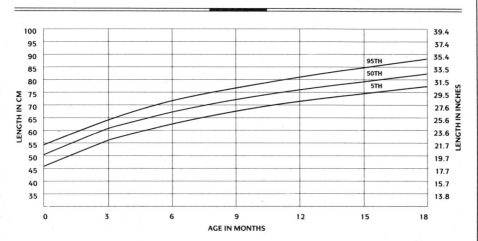

BOYS WEIGHT CHART

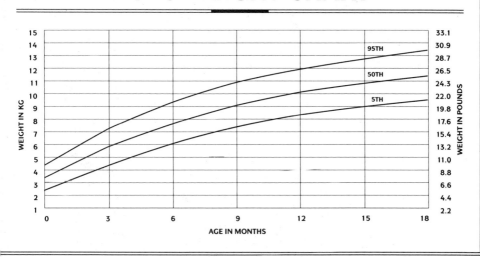

Index

A

Abscess, breast, 557
Abdomen
    cramping in, postpartum, 513
    in sick baby, 409
    injuries to, 434
    lump in, postpartum, 529
    muscles of, postpartum, 529
    pain in, postpartum, 513, 558
    shape of, postpartum, 543
Abrasions, first aid for, 446
Accidents to baby
    falls, 346
    parental reaction to, 346
    prevention of, 292
Accidents caused by baby
    handling of, 339
Acetaminophen, 432
    and breast milk, 554
    dosages for babies, 628
    side effects of, 432
Acne, infant, 96
Acquired Immune Deficiency Syndrome, 485
Active baby, 158
Adaptability, poor, 159
ADD (Attention Deficit Disorder), 379
Additives in food, 242
Advenovirus, 635
Adopted baby, 499
    and friends and family, 506
    breaking the news to, 506
    breastfeeding and, 503
    grandparents and, 504
    health problems in, 505
    hiring baby nurse for, 501
    loving, 502
    of foreign birth, 506
    picking doctor for, 500
    preparing for, 499
Adoption
    and baby blues, 502
    and breastfeeding, 9, 503
    and loving baby, 502
    and not feeling like a mother, 501
    and parental insecurity, 501
Adoptive mother and exercise, 529
Adoptive parents, 501
Advice, unasked for, 228
Afterpains, 513

Aggressiveness in older child, 611
AIDS, 485
    and breastfeeding, 9
Air, indoor
    pollution of, 238
Airway
    clearing of, in CPR, 448
    suctioning of, at birth, 45
Alar, 244
Alcohol, 359, 536
    and making love, 561
    baby sitter, use by, 193
    in breast milk, 554
    in mother's diet, 539
Allergy(ies), 413
    and breast milk, 3
    causes of, 416
    food, 220, 231, 232, 418
    prevention of, 418
    symptoms of, 413
    to cow's milk, 114, 143
    treatment of, 416
Altitudes, high, 403
Aluminum pots, 248
Anemia, 255
Anencephaly, 485
Anesthesia and breastfeeding, 51
Angel hair, 396
Anger, parental
    because of crying baby, 128
    handling of, 338, 340
    over abnormal baby, 477
    toward baby, in severe depression, 548
    toward older child, 609
Animal bites, 435
Anterior fontanel, 106
Anti-cancer foods, 244
Antiseptic cream, 39
Apgar test, 47, 48
Apnea, 183
    and car seats, 470
    of prematurity, 184, 474
Appearance of newborn, 65
Appetite
    changes in, 99, 370
    decrease in, 370
    erratic, 312
    in newborn, 64
    in sick baby, 408
    increase in, 371
    loss of, 314

    loss of, and teething, 224
    poor, 370
Apple-cranberry cubes, 625
Apples, chemicals in, 244
Apricot, purée, dried, 624
Arm pain, in new parents, 576
Artificial sweeteners, 242
Aspartame, 242
    in breast milk, 554
Aspirin, 432
    and Reye's syndrome, 432
    in breast milk, 554
    side effects of, 432
Asthma, 416
Atopic dermatitis, 179
Attachment
    fear of, to sick newborn, 477
    of siblings, 614
    to security object, 310
    see also, Bonding
Attention deficit disorder, 379
Autism, 485
Auto safety, 302

B

Babies
    comparing development of, 146
    differences in development of, 138
Babinski reflex, 48
Baby, difficult, 156
Baby blues, 545
    how to beat, 547
    in adoptive mother, 502
Baby care, 73
    bathing, 73
    burping, 76
    diapering, 77
    dressing, 80
    feeling incompetent at, 549
    feeling incompetent at, as adoptive mother, 501
    lifting and carrying, 81
    of the ears, 81
    of the nails, 83
    of the nose, 84
    on outings, 84
    sharing with spouse, 544
Baby carrier
    advantages of, 147
    choosing, 42

precautions, 147
Baby food
 appropriate texture for,
  248
 commerical, 247
 freezing of, 248
 home-prepared, 248
 ingredients to avoid in, 248
 instant or dehydrated, 248
 junior style, 267
 proper preparation of, 248
 stage 2, 267
Baby oil, 38
Baby sitter
 age of, 136
 alcohol use and, 193
 baby's separation anxiety
  with, 373
 check list for, 189
 choosing a, 190
 competition with, 27
 drug abuse and, 193
 guilt over using, 568
 health of, 193
 leaving baby with, 188
 not leaving baby with, 188
Baby supplies, 35
Baby swing, 43
Baby talk
 embarrassment over using,
  162
 getting comfortable with,
  160
Baby's first cake, 623
Baby-bottle mouth, 254
Baby-sitting services, 191
Back carrier
 readiness for, 148
 safe use of, 228
Back, baby sleeping on, 120
Backache in new parents, 576
Backyard safety, 299
Baking powder, 619
Baking soda
 and depletion of vitamins,
  248
 high sodium content of,
  619
Banana french toast, 621
Banana, as first food, 219
Banana-orange gel, 626
Barbecue, safety near, 390
Basal body temperature, 574
Basic position for exercise, 530
Bassinet, 40
 benefits of, 119
Bathroom safety, 298
Baths
 fear of, 252
 for treating fever, 432
 how to give, 73

in the big tub, 250
 postpartum, 552
Battery breast pump, 93
Bed
 switching toddler to, 377
 sharing with baby, 186
Bed rest, postpartum, 517
Bedroom, sharing with baby,
  177, 185
Bedtime
 difficulties, 315
 nursing baby to sleep at,
  175
 problems at, with weaned
  baby, 366
 routine, 315
Bee sting
 first aid for, 435
 severe reaction to, 435
Bee venom allergy, 417
Behavior
 in sick baby, 407
 indicating serious illness,
  430
 unpredictable, 372
Belly button
 care of, 88
 healing of, 106
 swelling of, 107
Belly, baby sleeping on, 120
Benzopyrenes in indoor air,
  239
Best-odds diet
 for infants, 220
 for breastfeeding mothers,
  534
 for non-breastfeeding
  mothers, 539
 for the first year, 564
 for toddlers, 357
 postpartum, 534, 564
 starting, early, 305
Bicycle breast pump, 92
Biking with baby, 318
Bilirubin, 70
Birth certificate, 88
Birth control, 569
 see also, individual
  methods
Birth control pills, 569
Birth defects
 and fetal alcohol syndrome,
  476
 causes of, 484
 explaining, to others, 477
 getting information on,
  480, 481
 getting right diagnosis for,
  480
 inheritance of, 493
 most common, 485

repeat of, with next baby,
  483
Birth defect(s), baby with a,
  475
 and diet, 476
 and siblings, 482
 anger over, 477
 attachment or bonding to,
  477
 coping with, 478
 diagnosis of, 480
 ethical decisions
  concerning, 481
 guilt over, 476
 helping parents of, 479
 optimum care for, 481
 parental love for, 477
 prognosis for, 482
Birth weight, 47
 differences in, 61
Birthday party, first, 363
Birthmarks, 67
Bite(s)
 animal, 435
 bad, 254
 insect, 435
 marine, 436
 snake, 435
Biting
 and teething, 223
 nipples, while nursing, 268
 playful, 333
Bladder, postpartum, 517
Bleeding
 first aid for, 446
 from nose, 444
 massive, 447
Bleeding, postpartum
 abnormal, 513
 normal, 514
 renewed, 558
Blinking, 327
Blisters
 from herpes, 579
 nursing, 106
 on gums, 69
Blood clots in lochia, 513
Blood in spitup, 131
Blood in stool, 420, 423
Blood pressure, postpartum,
  508, 517
Blueness of skin
 temporary, 111
 in breathing emergency,
  448
Body changes in mother,
  postpartum, 543
Bonding, 61
 of mother and baby, 61
 fear of, to sick newborn,
  477

of father and baby, 592
of siblings, 614
with hospitalized newborn, 462
Bones, broken, first aid for, 436
Books
best, for beginners, 289
expanding baby's repertoire, 354
introducing, to baby 264
Boredom with staying home, 565
Bottle
for breastfed baby, 249
propping of, 57
rejection of, 249
Bottle feeding
advantages of, 5
changing your mind about, 131
deciding about, 2
feelings about, 7
getting started, 54
safety, 54
supplies for, 39
techniques, 57
tips, 59
with love, 55
Bottles
and breastfeeding, 51, 249
and tooth decay, 254
attachment to, 366
choosing, 39
propping of, 57
rejection of, 249
sterilizing of, 56
weaning from, 366
Bouncing, risks of for infant, 148
Bowed legs, 146, 344
Bowel movement, postpartum, 518
Bowel movements
and solids, 249
black, 210
changes in, 249
color of, in newborns, 72
explosive, 113
frequency of, 112
frequent, runny, 421
less frequent, 187
straining with, 113
strange-looking, 317
texture of, 112
undigested food in, 249
Boy–girl differences, 375

Brachial pulse, 407
Brain
inflammation of, 634

inflammation of membranes, 640
injury to, 442
Brain, absence of and ethical decisions, 481
Brazelton neonatal assessment scale, 49
Bread, fruited cheese, 619
Breads for baby, 267
Breast
abscess of, 557
baby favoring one, 156
engorgement, 520
inflammation of, 556
lump in, 557
rejection of, 311
Breast massage, 94
Breast milk
adequacy of, 99, 100
after weaning, 344
alcohol in, 554
benefits of, 3
benefits of, for preterm babies, 459
caffeine in, 554
collection of, 95
components of, 3
contaminated fish and, 555
contamination of, 553
drugs in, 553
drying up of, 521
effects of tobacco in, 553
excessive vitamins in, 553
exercise and, 532
expressing, 91, 94
produced by newborns, 46
increasing supply of, 101
laxatives in, 554
medications in, 553
pain relievers in, 554
storing of, 95
strong flavors in, 553
supplementing, for premies, 460
supply of, and sleeping through night, 102
Breast milk jaundice, 71
Breast pumps, 92
Breast shells/shields, 24, 102
Breast, rejection of one, 156
Breastfeeding
advantages of, 3
and adopted baby, 503
and adoption, 9
and breast surgery, 10
and cancer, 10
and drug abuse, 10
and fathers, 8
and lack of freedom, 188

and love making 7, 561, 595
and medication, 9
and mother's health, 9
and night wakening, 261
and oral contraceptives, 569
and PKU, 10
and pregnancy, 575
and relaxation, 8
and working away from home, 170
as birth control, 5, 569
basics, 52
changing your mind about, 131
contraindications for, 9
deciding about, 2
during illness, 578
father's exclusion from, 596
feelings about, 7
getting started, 49
in front of older child, 610
jaundice and, 71
loss of interest in, 155, 311, 323
myths about, 8
problems with, 99
sore nipples from, 555
the premature baby, 466
time spent, 552
tips, 59
supplementation of, 102, 144
see also, Nursing
Breasts
and breastfeeding, 8
engorgement of, 520
enlargement of, in newborn, 46
leaking from, 556
lack of engorgement of, 100, 521
preparation of, for breastfeeding, 24
rejection of, 155, 311, 323
Breath holding, 328
Breathing
cessation, 184
checking baby's, 118
checking for in CPR, 450
cessation incident, 183
emergencies, 184
emergencies, CPR for, 448
lapses, in premies, 474
noisy, 416
problems in premies, 470
Breathing exercises, postpartum, 529
Bronchiolitis, 630
Bronchitis, 632
Bronchopulmonary dysplasia (BPD), 473

Bruises, first aid for, 446
Brushing teeth, 253
Bumpers, crib, 40
Burns,
    first aid for, 437
    prevention of, 297
Burping baby, 59, 76
Butter, 351
Butterfly bandage, 447

C

Café au lait spots, 68
Caffeine
    in breast milk, 554
    in food and drink, 241
    in mother's diet, 539
Cake
    Baby's first, 623
    carrot, 624
    eggless, 623
    First birthday, 624
    Golden, 623
Calcium
    in breast milk, 3
    in breastfeeding diet, 537
    in infant diet, 221
    in postpartum diet, 537
    in toddler diet, 360
Calcium-rich foods, 359
Calories
    in infant diet, 221
    in postpartum diet, 535, 536
    in toddler diet, 357, 359
    needed for breastfeeding,
        536
Camera flash, safety of, 132
Cancer
    and breastfeeding, 5, 10
    and rejection of breast, 156
    and sunburn, 386
    foods to prevent, 244
    in infants, 486
Candida albicans infection, 69
Candidal dermatitis, 179
Car safety, 302
Car seats
    choosing, 41
    for premature babies, 470
    safe use of, 78
    types of, 42
Carbohydrates
    complex vs. simple, 358,
        535
    dietary recommendations
        for, 350
    see also, Complex
        carbohydrates
Carbon monoxide in indoor air,
    239

Caretakers for baby, selecting,
    190
    see also, Baby sitters;
        Child care
Carotene, excess of, 361
Carriage, baby, 41
Carrier, baby, 42
Carrying baby, 81
Catheter, postpartum, 518, 524
Cats, and baby, 23
Cause and effect, teaching, 353
Cavernous hemangioma, 68
Celiac disease, 486
Center for Science in the
        Public Interest, 244
Cephalohematoma, 46
Cereal, as first food, 218
Cereal, super, 618
Cerebral palsy, 486
Cervical cap, 572
Cervix, at 6 weeks, 534
Cesarean section
    and exercise, 559
    and sexual intercourse, 559
    gas pain following, 525
    getting up after, 525
    going home after, 525
    incisional pain from, 523
    long-term recovery from,
        559
    removal of stitches
        following, 525
    short term recovery from,
        523
Chafing dermatisis, 179
Change, baby who resists, 159
Changing diapers,
    difficulty, 203
    directions for, 77
Changing table, 40
Charcoal, liquid, for poison
        treatment, 448
Checkups, baby's
    in-hospital, 45
    1st month, 90
    2nd month, 141
    4th month, 201
    6th month, 246
    9th month, 304
    12th month, 356
Checkups, mother's
    in-hospital, 508
    6 weeks postpartum, 534
Cheek rubbing, and teething,
    224
Cheeks, swollen, 392
Chemical burns, first aid for,
    437
Chemicals in breast milk, 554
Chest pain, postpartum, 512,
    513

Chicken fingers, 622
Chicken pox, 632
    immunization against, 152
Chicken soup as a cure, 413
Child care
    and your child, 199
    choosing, 190
    corporate, 199
    for mother's activities, 567
    for sick child, 199
    group day care, 195
    in-home, 191
    in-home day care, 198
Childbirth, disappointment
        with, 511, 592
Childproofing the home, 291
Chills, postpartum, 507,
    508
Chin rash, and teething, 223
Chin, quivering, 67
Choking, first aid for
    in babies over 1 year, 455
    in babies under 1 year, 454
Cholesterol
    and breastfeeding, 4
    dietary recommendations
        for, 350
    in baby's diet, 347
Christmas trees, 395
Chronic lung disease, 473
Circulation, checking for in
        CPR, 451
Circumcision
    and cancer, 17
    and infection, 17
    care of, 135
    pros and cons, 17, 18
Circumcised penis, care of, 86
"Clap hands," 319
Classes for baby, 330
Cleanliness and baby, 285
Cleft lip and/or palate, 487
    and breastfeeding, 10
Clogged milk duct, 557
Clothes for baby
    how to choose, 36
    how to put on, 80
    what to buy, 37
Club foot, 487
Coccyx, broken, 512
Cold compresses, 627
Cold soaks, 627
Cold sore, 579, 636
Cold weather concerns, 393
Cold, common, 418
    and loss of appetite, 155
    prevention of, 420
    symptoms of, 418
    treatment of, 419
    when to call the doctor for,
        420

Colic
    and parental smoking, 20
    and siblings, 124
    coping with, 126
    effects of, 124
    father's reaction to, 599
    medication for, 123
    possible causes of, 123
    prevalence of, 122
    symptoms of, 123
    tips for surviving, 125
Color changes in infant, 111
Colostrum, 64
Comfort objects, 309
Comforting a crying baby, 128
Commercial baby food, 247
Communicable diseases, 630
Comparing babies, 146
Complex carbohydrates, 358
    in infant diet, 221
    in postpartum diet, 535, 538
    in toddler diet, 362
Complexion, baby's, 68, 96
Conception, and breast-feeding, 5, 569
Concepts
    introducing to baby, 265
    teaching, 352
Condom, 573
Congenital heart defects, 488
Congenital pigmented nevi, 68
Conjunctivitis, 632
Constipation, 420
    causes of, 421
    dietary changes during, 421
    in bottle babies, 113
    in breastfed baby, 113
    in mother, postpartum, 518
    prevention of, 421
    symptoms of, 420
    treatment of, 421
    when to call the doctor for, 421
Consumer, your role as, 244
Continuous positive airway pressure (CPAP), 472
Contraception, 569
Contractions, postpartum, 513
Control
    giving baby some, 340
    lack of, as new mother, 542
    lack of, in severe depression, 548
Convulsions, first aid for, 438
Convulsions, febrile, 427
    how to handle, 431
Cooing, 145
Cookies, oatmeal raisin, 626
Cool compresses, 627
Coombs test, 47

Coping
    as new mother, 540
    with handicapped baby, 478
    with postpartum depression, 547
Copper pots, 248
Cornstarch, 38
Corporal punishment, 339
Corporate day care, 199
Cottage cheese sundae, 622
Cough medicine, 419
Coughing
    and teething, 223
    as an affectation, 225
    sudden, 420
    treatment for, 414
Cow's milk
    allergy to, 143
    and anemia, 255
    inappropriateness of, 178
    weaning to, 254
Coxsackie virus, 637
CPR, 448
    for babies over 1 year, 453
    for babies under 1 year, 452
Crackers for baby, 267
Cradle, 40
    benefits of, 119
Cradle cap, 144
Cramping, abdominal, postpartum, 513
Cranberry-apple gelatin, 625
Crawling
    age of, 282
    types of, 282
Cream cheese frosting, 624
Creativity, stimulating, 265
Crib
    choosing, 40
    portable, 43
    graduating from, 377
    transferring to new baby, 603
Crib death (SIDS), 181
Croque bébé, 621
Crossed eyes, 107
Croup, 634
    treatment for, 414
Cruising, 322
Crying, baby's
    anger at, 128
    and father, 599
    comfort for, 128
    coping with, 126
    in adopted baby, 502
    in sick baby, 408
    prevalence of, 122
    reasons for, 122
    when to call the doctor for, 129
Crying it out, 261

Cup, introducing, 229
Cuts, first aid for, 446
Cystic fibrosis, 488
Cytomegalovirus (CMV), 197

D

D and C, postpartum, 514
Daily dozen
    for new mother, 536
    for infants, 221
    for toddlers, 359
Dairy products
    cholesterol in, 349
Dairy protein combinations for toddlers, 362
Daminozide, 244
Day and night, confusing, 118
Day care
    evaluating group, 195
    evaluating home, 197
    nutrition provided in, 197
    safety rules for, 197
    health concerns in, 196
Deafness, 96
    and loud music, 132
Death of a baby
    coping with, 494
    helping parents, 479
Decongestants, 419
Deformation, in newborns, 489
Dehydration, signs of, 430
Delivery, disappointment with, 511, 592
Demand feeding, 50, 111
Dental emergencies, 443
Dental health, 253
Dentist, pediatric, 254
Denver Developmental Screening Test, 139
Depression, postpartum, 545
    and father, 593
    in adoptivive mother, 502
    in father, 594
    persistent, 580
Dermatitis, diaper, 179
Detergent for baby's laundry, 115
Development
    apparent lapses in, 369
    comparisons of infant, 146
    differences in, 138
    in premature baby, 467
    slow, 317
Developmental milestones, 45
    1st month, 89
    2nd month, 140
    3rd month, 169
    4th month, 200
    5th month, 215

6th month, 245
7th month, 266
8th month, 278
9th month, 303
10th month, 321
11th month, 341
12th month, 355
Diaper bag
    choosing, 42
    packing for travel, 400
    stocking, 84
Diaper pail, 40
Diaper pins, 38
Diaper rash, 178
    ointment for, 180
    on penis, 181
    treatment of, 179
Diaper wipes, 38
Diapering baby, difficulty, 203
Diapers
    changing, 77
    diaper-service cloth, 19
    disposable, 19
    home-laundered cloth, 20
Diaphragm, 572
Diaphragmatic breathing
    exercise, 529
Diarrhea, 112, 421
    and teething, 224
    causes of, 421
    dietary changes during,
        422
    due to food allergy, 220
    in milk allergy, 114
    prevention of, 422
    symptoms of, 421
    treatment for, 414, 422
    when to call the doctor for,
        423
Diet for baby with birth
    defect(s), 476
Diet, infant
    cholesterol in, 347
    fiber in, 349
    in sickness, 409
    see also, Best-Odds diet
Diet, mother's
    in the first year, 564
    in the hospital, 509
    postpartum, 534
Difficult baby, 156
Digestive upset
    due to food allergy, 220
    in sick baby, 408
Diphtheria
    immunization against, 149
Dirt
    eating, 286
    playing in, 287
Discipline, 335
    permissive, 336

strict, 336
Diseases, communicable, 630
Dislocations, 438
Doctor, baby's
    check list for calls to, 406
    choosing, 25
    credentials of, 29
    family doctor as, 26
    fees charged by, 31
    locating, 28
    pediatrician as, 26
    poor relationship with, 34
    prenatal interview with, 32
    type of practice of, 27
    when to call, for fever, 430
    working with, 33
    See also, Checkups;
        specific illnesses
Doctor, mother's, when to call
    postpartum, 513
Dog bites, 435
Dogs
    and baby, 23
    fear of, 335
Dominant inheritance, 493
Down syndrome, 490
Dressing baby, 80
    for out of doors, 110
    in changeable weather, 393
    in cold weather, 393
    in hot weather, 385
Dried apricot purée, 624
Drooling
    and epiglottitis, 634
    and teething, 223
Drowning, first aid for, 439
"Drownproofing" baby, 392
Drug abuse,
    and breastfeeding, 10
    in baby sitter, 193
Drugs, 359, 536, 540
    in breast milk, 553
    See also, Medication
Dry skin in winter, 394
DTP immunization, 149
    and SIDS, 184
    common reactions to, 150
    recommended schedule for,
        153
    reducing risk of, 149
    severe reactions to, 150
    when to call the doctor
        following, 150

E

Ear infection, See Otitis media
Ear pulling
    and ear infection, 423
    teething, 224

as a habit, 226
Early rising, 260
Ears
    care of, 81
    and hearing, 96
    in sick baby, 408
    inflammation of, 423
    injury to, 439
    in newborn, 66
    object in, 439
    pressure in, in flight, 402
    protruding, 66
    treatment for pain in, 414
Eating
    chokable items, 286
    dirt, 286
    motivation for, 371
    spoiled food, 286
    See also, Best-Odds Diet;
        Foods; Solids
Eating habits
    establishing good, 305
    fussy, 312
    messy, 325
    poor, 370
    irregular, 370
Eczema, 227
Egg whites
    avoiding raw, 231
    introducing, 220
Eggs
    cake with no, 623
    cholesterol in, 350
    introducing, 220
Eighth month, 278
Elbow, dislocation of, 438
Electric breast pump, 93
Electric burns, first aid for, 437
Electric shock, first aid for, 439
Eleventh month, 341
Emergencies, medical
    breathing, CPR, for, 448
    choking, first aid for, 454
    telephone numbers for, 438
    first aid for, 434
    preparation for, 438
Emergency medical service
    (EMS), calling, 449
Employment, returning to, 12,
    587
    and breastfeeding, 170
    best time for, 171, 589
    compromising on, 588
    deciding about, 587
    financial factors in, 588
    personality factors in, 588
Endometritis, 558
Enemas, 113, 433
Enterovirus, 641
Environmental hazards, 236
EPA hotline number, 238

Epiglottitis, 634
Episiotomy, healing of, 516
Epstein's pearls, 69
Erections in babies, 286
Erythema infectiosum, 634
Erythema toxicum, 69
Evaporated milk formula, 54
Exercise for baby, 210
    classes, 210, 212
Exercise for mother
    aerobic, 532
    after cesarean, 524, 559
    as example to baby, 212
    benefits of, 526
    breast milk and, 532
    breathing, postpartum, 529
    in hot weather, 527
    postpartum, 525, 530
    practical program for, 528
    safe guidelines for, 526
Exertion, postpartum, 514
Exhaustion
    in new mother, 575
    postpartum, 507
Expressing breast milk, 91
    by hand, 94
    for premature baby, 460
    pumps for, 92
    techniques for, 93
Eye soaks, 627
Eye drops
    at birth, 47
    instilling, 412
Eyes
    blinking of, 327
    color of, 66
    corrosive substance in, 440
    crossed, 107
    dilated pupils in, 442
    discharge from, 108
    discharge from, in
        newborns, 72
    drops in, at birth, 47
    foreign object in, 439
    in sick baby, 408
    inflammation of, 632
    injury to, 439, 440
    in newborn, 46, 65
    teary, 108
    and vision, 97
Eyes, mother's, postpartum
    blackened, 512
    blood-shot, 512
"Eyes, nose, mouth," 319

F

Face rash
    and teething, 223
    in eczema, 227

    See also, Rashes
Falls, 346
Falls, preventing, See Safety
Family
    and diet, 359
    and healthy eating, 536
Family bed, 186
Family physician, 26
    see also, Physician
Family planning, 569
    natural, 573
Fast foods, 350
Fasting, risks of, 535
Fat
    animal, 351
    dietary recommendations
        for, 350
    foods high in, 362
    hydrogenated, 351
    in cooking, 350
    in infant diet, 222, 347
    in postpartum/
        breastfeeding diets, 538
    in toddler diet, 347, 362
    monounsaturated, 538
    saturated, 538
    storage of chemicals in,
        243
    types of, 351
Fat baby, 206
Father
    and baby's crying, 599
    and breastfeeding, 8, 595,
        596
    and roughness with baby,
        599
    and wife's depression, 593
    as postpartum help, 12, 16
    becoming a, 591
    depression in, postpartum,
        594
    diet of, and baby, 591
    envy of, 583
    feelings of inadequacy in,
        598
    jealousy of baby in, 597
    lack of libido in, 595
    lack of time of, 600
    not feeling like a, 501
    pressures on, 599
    responses of, 598
    sharing baby care with, 544
Fatigue, 533, 564, 575
Favoring one breast, 156
Fears in baby, 334
    of strangers, 309
    of tub baths, 252
Fears, irrational in postpartum
        depression, 548
Febrile convulsions, 427
    how to handle, 431

Feeding baby
    at the table, 307
    coarser textures, 267
    coping with the mess of,
        325
    ensuring adequate nutrition
        when, 370
    establishing good habits
        when, 305, 348
    finger foods, 279
    from a cup, 229
    from the breast, 49
    in cold weather, 384
    in the beginning, 59
    in warm weather, 385
    problems with, 314
    safely, 230
    schedule for, 111
    solids, 202, 216
    the role of fat in, 348
    when sick, 409
    who wants to self feed, 314
    with a bottle, 54
    with expressed milk, 91
    with supplementary
        bottles, 142
    See also, Bottle feeding;
        Breastfeeding; Solids;
        Weaning
Feeding chair
    choosing, 43
    portable, 43
    safe use of, 235
    use of, 234
Feeding preterm or small baby,
        458
Feet
    crooked, 146
    flat, 310
    treatment for abnormalities
        of, 146
Female characteristics, 375
Fetal alcohol syndrome (FAS),
        491
    and birth defects, 476
Fever, 426
    and teething, 224
    assessing, 430
    convulsions during, 427
    in bacterial infections, 427
    in blood poisoning, 427
    in failure of heat-
        regulation, 427
    in heat illness, 427
    in viral infections, 427
    requiring emergency
        medical attention, 430
    role of, in infection, 426
    sponging for, 432
    starving a, 433
    treatment for, 414, 431

when to call the doctor for,
     430
  with dehydration, 430
  See also, specific diseases
Fever blister, 579, 636
Fever, in mother
  postpartum, 507, 508, 513,
     558
  with mastitis, 556
Fever-reducing medicines
  when to give, 431
  types of, 432
Fiber, dietary, 349
  postpartum, 509, 510
Fifth disease, 634
Fifth month, 215
Figure, mother's, 526, 543
  after 6 weeks, 533
  changes in, 543
Finger foods, 279
  to avoid, 280
Finger injuries, first aid for,
     440
  bleeding under the nail,
     440
  bruises, 440
  torn nail, 441
Finger, severed, 445
Fire prevention, 297
Fireplace safety, 395
First Aid, 434
  distracting baby during, 441
  supplies for, 39, 438
First birthday
  cake, 624
  party, 363
First month, 89
First year, mother's, 564
  emotional symptoms in,
     564
  physical symptoms in, 564
Fish
  as finger food, 280
  benefits of, in the diet, 349
  from contaminated waters,
     241
  unsafe, during lactation,
     555
  unsafe, raw, 241
Fish fingers, 622
Flash, camera, 132
Flat feet, 310
Floor, eating food from, 285
Flossing, 253
Flu, 638
  immunization against, 153
Fluids
  for diarrhea, 422
  for sick baby, 409
  in breastfeeding diet, 539
  in infant diet, 222

in postpartum diet, 539
  in toddler diet, 363
  increased, 629
  postpartum, 510
  with fever, 431
Fluoride
  adequate intake of, 134
  supplementation with, 134
Fontanels, 106, 201
  in sick baby, 408
Food
  additives in, 242
  contaminants in, 241
  eating from floor, 285
  proper preparation of, 248
  removing chemicals from,
     231
  spoiled, 286
  unsafe for babies, 241
Food allergy, 231, 418
  and starting solids, 232
  elimination diet for, 233
  most common offenders in,
     232
  reducing risk of, 232
  treatment of, 418
Food, baby, 247, 267
Food hazards, 241
  in perspective, 242
Food safety, 230, 231
  in summer, 392
Foods
  first, 218, 219
  mashed or chopped, 267
  natural, 358
Foot size, change in
  postpartum, 543
Football hold, 83
Footprints, baby's, 47
Foreign language, teaching a,
     161
Forgetting a skill, 369
Formaldehyde, 240
Formula
  heating of, 55
  on outings, 84
  safe preparation of, 55
  selection of, 54
  storage of, 55
  types of, 54
Fourth month, 200
Fractures, first aid for, 436
French toast, banana, 621
Frequent bowel movements,
     112
Friend with sick baby, helping,
     479
Friendships, changes in, 577
Frostbite
  first aid for, 441
  preventing, 394

recognizing, 394
Frosting, cream cheese, 624
Frozen yogurt, peachy, 626
Fruit
  contamination of, 242, 244
  for mother, postpartum,
     510
Fruit, other
  choices of, 361
  in infant diet, 222
  in postpartum/
     breastfeeding diets, 538
  in toddler diet, 361
Fruit, yellow, *See,* Yellow Fruit
Fruited cheese bread, 619
Fundus, massaging of,
  postpartum, 508, 514
Fungus infection
  in diaper area, 179
  in mouth, 69
Funny fingers, 622
Furniture for baby
  choosing, 40
  safety of, 40

G

Gagging
  in newborn, 66
  on medication, 412
Games babies play, 318
Garlic, in breast milk, 553
Gas, passing of, 114
Gases, noxious, 445
Gate, safety
  choosing, 43
  using, 300
Gelatin desserts
  apple-cranberry, 625
  banana-orange, 626
Gender differences, 375
Genitals
  discovering, 286
  explaining differences in,
     to child, 609
  in newborn, 46
  touching of, 287
German measles, 636
  immunization against, 151
Germs
  contact with strangers', 110
  on food from floor, 285
Gifted babies, 271
Gifts, safe, 397
Girls, as different from boys,
     375
Goat's milk, 114
Golden cake, 623
Golden-nugget oatmeal
  flapjacks, 621

Grains, *See,* Whole grains
Grandparents
  and adopted baby, 504
  and baby with birth defects,
    478
  as postpartum help, 13, 16
  disagreement with, 14, 270
  lack of, 14
  rights of, 270
  spoiling baby, 270
Grazing, 272
Green leafy vegetables
  choices of, 361
  in infant diet, 221
  in postpartum/
    breastfeeding diets, 537
  in toddler diet, 361
Grilled cheese sandwich,
  French-style, 621
Group day care, 195
  benefits/disadavantages of,
    195
  how to find, 195
  what to look for in, 195
Growth
  normal, 351
  spurts, 99
  swings in, 350
Guilt
  over baby with defects, 476
  over premature delivery,
    468
  over using baby sitters, 568
Gums
  cysts on, 69
  hematoma on, in teething,
    224
Guns, toy, 214

H

Habits
  blinking, 327
  breath holding, 328
  hair rolling, pulling of, 328
  head banging, 326
  pacifier use, 117, 177
  rhythmic, 326
  teeth grinding, 328
  thumb sucking, 204
  see also, Eating habits
Hair
  care of, 333
  newborn, 46
  rolling, pulling of, 328
  sparse, 311
Hair loss, postpartum,
  557
Hallucinations, 548

Hand-foot-mouth disease, 636
Handedness, 290
Handicapped baby, 475
  and diet, 476
  ethical decisions
    concerning, 481
  optimum treatment for,
    481
  prognosis for, 482
Hands
  bluish color of, 111
  temperature of, 109
Head
  banging, rocking, 326
  circumference of, 47
  flat spot on, 120
  injury to, 442
  in newborn, 65
  pointy, at birth, 46
  when to call the doctor for
    injury to, 442
Head lifts, 530
Health history, baby's, 424
Health maintenance
    organization (HMO),
    33
Health problems
  in mother, and
    breastfeeding, 9
  in adopted baby, 505
Hearing, 96
  and loud music, 132
  and speech, 146
  loss of, with otitis media,
    423
  stimulating in early months,
    165
  stimulating in older baby,
    265
Heart
  congenital defects of, 488
  irregularities of, 209
  murmur, 209
  raising a healthy, 349
heart rate
  measuring, 407
  target, in exercise, 528
heat illness, 427
  first aid for, 443
  see also, Hot weather
Heating pad, 628
Heatstroke
  first aid for, 443
  preventing, 386
  recognizing, 386
Height, in infants, 350
Hemangioma, cavernous,
  68
Hemophilus influenzae b (Hib),
  152
  vaccination schedule, 153

when to omit immunization
  for, 152
Hemorrhage, postpartum, 558
  signs of, 513
Hemorrhoids, postpartum, 519
Hepatitis B
  and breastfeeding, 9
  immunization against, 152
  vaccination for, 152
Herbal teas, 241
  in breast milk, 554
Hernia
  inguinal, 154
  umbilical, 107
Herpangina, 636
Herpes, 579, 636
  preventing spread of, 579
Hib (hemophilus influenzae b),
  152, 635, 641
Hiccups, 112
High chairs
  safe use of, 235
  see also, Feeding chairs
High intensity baby, 159
Hitting, 369
HIV
  and breastfeeding, 9
  in infants, 485
Hives, 416
HMOs, 33
Holiday safety, 395
Holly, 395
Home
  childproofing, 291
  dangers in the, 293
  managing, 540
  mess in the, 293
  safety in the, 292
Home day care, 198
Homecoming with baby and
  older sibling, 607
Homosexuality, 376
Honey, dangers of, 221
Hopelessness, feelings of, 548
Hormonal changes
  and depression, 546
  and breast rejection, 156
Hospital
  confusion, postpartum,
    522
  discharge from, 44, 50
  discharge from, postpartum,
    522
  early discharge from, 50
  what to take to, 43
Hospitalization, long, for
  newborn, 464
Hospitals, types of, 461
Hot compresses, 628
Hot flashes, postpartum, 508
Hot soaks, 628

Hot water bottle, 628
Hot weather
    keeping baby cool in, 385
    precautions, 385
    safety in, 385
Hotels and motels, 404
House calls, 30
Humidifier, 629
Humor, and discipline, 338
Hunger, in newborn, 64
    constant, 60
    sudden, 99
Hunger, postpartum, 507
Husband
    feeling unappreciated by,
        585
    relationship with, 582
    sharing baby care with, 544
Hydrocele, 135
Hydrocephalus, 491
Hydrolysate formula, 114
Hydrophobia, 644
Hyperactivity, 379
Hypertension and sodium, 275
Hypoglycemia
    in premature infants, 473
Hypospadias, 136
Hypothermia (low body
        temperature), 442

I

Ibuprofen, 432
    and breast milk, 554
Ice cream, fruit-juice
        sweetened, 363
Ice pack, 629
Icterus, 70
Identification precautions, 47
Illness, 406
    and breastfeeding, 4
    and parental smoking, 20
    see also, Sick baby
Illness, mother's, and
        breastfeeding, 578
Illnesses
    allergy, 413
    common cold, 418
    communicable, 630
    diarrhea, 421
    ear inflammation, 423
    in newborns, 485
    in premies, 472
    most common, 413
    symptomatic treatment of,
        414
Immunization, 148
    and SIDS, 184
    benefits of, 148
    postponement of, 152

risks of, 149
    recommendations for, 153
Impetigo, 179
Implant, birth control, 571
In-home child care, 191
    advantages/disadvantages,
        191
    getting adjusted to, 194
    interviewing for, 192
    where to find, 191
Inadequacy, feelings of
    as a mother, 549
    as an adoptive mother, 501
    as father, 598
Incisional pain, following
        cesarean, 533
Independence
    baby's struggle for, 379
    vs. insecurity, 372
Inexperience at mothering, 549
Infant development
    rates of, 138
    see also, Developmental
        milestones
Infant seat, 41
Infectious diseases, 630
Influenza, 638
    immunization against, 153
Inhaled object, choking on, 455
Initial withdrawal baby, 159
Insect bites/stings
    prevention of, 389
    treatment of, 435
Insecurity vs. independence,
    372
Intellectual development, 275
    in gifted children, 271
    stimulating, in early
        months, 168
    stimulating, in older baby,
        265
    stimulating, in toddler, 381
    see also, Language
        development
Intelligence, 138, 271
Intensive care nursery (ICN),
    461, 462
Intercom, 42
Intercourse
    and breastfeeding, 561
    best positions for, 561
    father's lack of interest in,
        596
    fear of causing injury
        during, 596
    fears about, 561
    lack of interest in, 560
    pain during, 561
    resumption of, 560
    ways ot improve, 562
    see also, Sexual relations

Interests outside the home, 565
Internal bleeding, 434
Intertrigo, 179
Intrauterine device (IUD), 571
Intrauterine Growth
        Retardation (IUGR),
        463
Intraventricular hemorrhage,
    474
Inverted nipples, 24, 155
Iodized salt, 363
Ipecac, syrup of, 448
IQ in infancy, 138
    and intelligence later, 271
Iron
    bran and absorption of, 256
    deficiency, 256
    in baby cereals, 218
    need for, postpartum, 510
    supplementation, 134, 256
Iron supplement, 134
    and black stool, 210
Iron-rich foods, 362
    in infant diet, 222
    in postpartum/
        breastfeeding diets, 538
    in toddler diet, 362
Irregular baby, 158
Irritability
    and teething, 223
Isolettes, in NICUs, 462
Itching
    treatment for, 414
IUD, 571
    warning signs, 571

J

Jaundice, 70
    and breastfeeding, 71
    in premature infants, 474
Jealousy
    sibling's, 612
    father's, 597
    mother's, 583, 584
Jellyfish, sting of, 436
Jerusalem cherry, 395
Juices, 231, 371
Jumpers, 234

K

Kegel exercises, 528
Kernicterus, 71
Ketones, 536
Kidneys
    infection of, 433
    defects of, 498
Kitchen safety, 297
Knock-knees, 344

L

La Leche League, 51
Lactase deficiency, 114
Lactation
    suppression of, 521
    see also, Breastfeeding
Lactose intolerance, 114
Language development, 139, 145
    different rates of, 146
    encouraging in toddler, 352
    first words in, 281
    nonverbal, 374
    stimulating, in early months, 160
    stimulating, in older baby, 264, 265
    unclear, 345
Language, second, 161
Lanugo, 46
Laryngotracheitis (croup), 634
Laundering baby's clothes, 115
Laxatives, 113, 519, 421
    in breast milk, 554
Lead, as environmental hazard
    in drinking water, 237
    in gasoline emissions, 237
    in newspapers/magazines, 238
    in paint, 237
    in soil, 238
Leaking breasts, 556
Left-handedness, 290
Leg pain, postpartum, 515
Leg slides, 531
Legs
    bowed, 344
    and early walking, 308
    knock-knees, 344
    shape of, 146
    treatment for abnormalities of, 146
Legumes, in protein combinations, 361
Length, 350
    at birth, 47
Let-down, milk
    factors interfering with, 102
    slow, and rejection of breast, 155
    stimulating, 94, 556
Libido, lack of, 560, 595
Lifestyle, changing, 11
Lifting baby, 81
Light-sensitive baby, 157
Limb, severed, 445
Limits, setting, 336
Linens, for baby, 38
Lip blisters, 106, 636
Lip, split, first aid for, 443

Liquiprin, 432
Lochia, 514, 533
    abnormal changes in, 558
    absence of, 513
    blood clots in, 513
    foul smelling, 513
Lockjaw (tetanus), 648
Loose bowel movements, 112
Love, parental
    for abnormal baby, 477
    for adopted baby, 502
    for new baby, 62
Low-birthweight baby
    and breast milk, 459
    best care for, 461
    feeding of, 458
    home care of, 471
    nutritional needs of, 458
    weight gain of, 458
    worries about handling, 468
Low-sensory threshold baby, 157
Low-sodium baking powder, 619
Lump in abdomen, postpartum, 529
Lump in breast, 557
Lyme disease, 389, 435, 638
Lymph glands, swollen, 408

M

Magazines, lead content of, 290
Making love, 560
Male characteristics, 375
Malformation in newborn, 491
Manipulation by baby, 274
March of Dimes, 481
Margarine, 351
Marine stings, 436
Marriage
    effects of new baby on, 582
    effects of sick baby on, 483
Massage
    baby, 210
    breast, 94
Mastitis, 556
Masturbation, 287
Maternity leave, 590
Mattress crib, 40
Meal skipping, 357
Measles, 638
    immunization against, 151
Medication for baby
    getting it down, 411
    giving correctly, 410
    questions to ask about, 410
Medication for mother
    and breastfeeding, 9

and contamination of
        breast milk, 514, 553
    when breastfeeding, 65
Medicine chest
    how to stock, 39
Medicine spoon, 412
Meningitis, 640
Meningoencephalitis, 640
Menstruation
    and breastfeeding, 5
    resumption of, 568
Messy baby, copy with, 283
Middle ear inflammation, 423
Milia, 68
Milk duct, clogged, 557
Milk, cow's, 178
    allergy to, 114
    best type of, for baby, 360
    calcium equivalents for, 360
    ensuring intake of, 360
    pasteurization of, 360
    serving straight, 306
    weaning to, 254
    whole vs. skim, 254
Mineral oil, 113
Misbehavior
    dealing with, 335
    with parent, 275
Mistletoe, 395
MMR (measles, mumps, rubella) immunization, 151
    common reactions to, 151
    recommended schedule for, 153
    when to omit, 152
Molds, allergy to, 417
Mongolian spots, 68
Monitoring baby's breathing, 183
Mood swings in mother
    at 6 weeks, 534
    postpartum, 508
Moro reflex, 47
Motels and hotels, 404
Mother
    anxiety in, 540
    not feeling like a, 501
    part-time employment for, 567
    personal enrichment for, 566
    shape of, postpartum, 526
    tension in, and rejection of breast, 156
    volunteer work for, 567
Mother love
    for abnormal baby, 477
    for adopted baby, 502
    seeming lack of, 62

variations of, at birth, 62
Mother's diet
    and rejection of breast, 155
    and breastfeeding, 534, 536
    postpartum, 534, 536
Mother's health
    and breastfeeding, 9
    and weaning, 324
Mother's intuition, 409
Mothering
    boredom with, 565
    coping with, 10, 540
    different styles of, 578
    exhaustion from, 575
    feeling inadequate at, 549
    feeling inadequate at, as adoptive mother, 501
    preparing for, 11
Motor development, large, 139
    stimulating in older baby, 263
    stimulating in toddler, 380
    stimulating in early months, 167
    through exercise, 210
Motor development, small, 139
    stimulating in early months, 167
    stimulating in older baby, 263
    stimulating in toddler, 381
Motor symptoms, in sick baby, 409
Mouth
    development of, 4
    fungus infection in, 69
    gum cysts in, 69
    in sick baby, 408
    injuries to, 443
    white patches in, 69
    yellowish white spots in, 69
Mouthing
    of chokable items, 286
    of dirt, 286
    of newspapers and magazines, 290
    of spoiled foods, 286
Muffins, pumpkin, 620
Mumps, 640
    immunization against, 151
Muscle pain, in parents, 576
Music
    and baby's hearing, 132
    for older baby, 264
    for toddlers, 378
    introducing, 166
Mycoplasma, 643
Mylicon drops, 123
Myringotomy, 425

N

Nail trimming, 83
Nails, injuries to, 440, 441
Nakedness, parental, 345
Name, choosing baby's, 21
Nanny organizations, 192
Naps
    and nighttime sleep, 119
    changing patterns in, 315
    giving up, 315
    length of, 226
    number of, 226
Nasal congestion
    nasal aspiration for, 419, 629
    treatments for, 415
National Health Information Center, 481
National Institutes of Child Health and Human Development, 481
Natural family planning, 573
Natural foods, 358, 536
Navel, swelling of, 107
Neatness, teaching, 284
Necrotizing enterocolitis, 474
Negative baby, 159
Negativism, 379
Neonatal intensive care units (NICU), 461, 462
Nevus flammeus, 68
Nevus simplex, 68
Newborn, 45
    abilities of, 45
    appearance of, 65
    characteristics of, 46
    fear of handling, 95
    tests for, 47, 48, 49
    with birth defects, 475
    with problems, 475
Newspapers, lead content of, 290
Next baby
    chance of repeat problems, 483
    planning for, 586
Night and day, confusing, 118
Night lights, 316
Night waking
    and crying it out, 261
    and hunger, 175
    and premature infants, 262
    and systematic awakening, 261
    at 3 months, 175
    at 6 months, 260
    at 7 months, 269
    at 12 months, 367
    breaking habit of, 260
    when to call doctor for, 262

in baby who used to sleep through, 367
    in early infancy, 116
    see also, Sleep problems
Nine basic diet principles
    for new mothers, 535
    for toddlers, 357
Ninth month, 303
Nipple confusion, 72
Nipples
    and breastfeeding, 8, 102
    biting of, by baby, 268
    cleaning of, 555
    cracked, 555
    inverted, 24
    inverted, in infant, 155
    sore, 555
Nipples, bottle
    types of, 40
    wrong size openings, 58
"No"
    effective use of, 337
    when baby says, 380
Noise
    fear of, 334
    when baby is sleeping, 116
Non-aspirin medication, 432
Non-sexist child rearing, 375
Nose
    bleeding from, 444
    foreign object in, 444
    injuries to, 444
    of newborn, 66
Nose care, 84
Nose drops, 419
Nose, stuffy
    treatment for, 415
Noxious fumes, 445
Nudity, parental, 345
Number concepts, 354
Nurse, baby, 14
Nurses' registries, 191
Nursing
    all day, 173
    and lack of freedom, 188
    and working, 170
    frequent, 99
    loss of interest in, 155, 311, 323
    baby to sleep, 175, 316
    see also, Breastfeeding
Nursing blisters, 106
Nursing-bottle mouth, 254
Nutrition Action Health Letter, 244

O

Oatmeal flapjacks, 621
Oatmeal raisin cookies, 625

Obesity, 206
  and breastfeeding, 4
Odor-sensitive baby, 160
Oils, dietary, 351
Ointment, diaper rash, 180
Older child, 601
  see also, Sibling, older
Omega-3 fatty acids, 349
"One, two, buckle my shoe,"
  320
Onions, in breast milk, 553
Open spine (spina bifida), 496
OPV immunization, 149
Oral contraceptives, 569
  danger signs, 570
Orange-banana gelatin, 626
Organ donation, 481, 494
Organic foods, 243
Organizing the day, 540
Osteoporosis, 509
Other fruits and vegetables, 361
Otitis media (middle ear
        inflammation), 423
  and loss of appetite, 155
  causes of, 423
  prevention of, 425
  symptoms of acute, 423
  symptoms of serous, 423
  treatment of, 425
  when to call doctor for, 426
Out-of-doors safety, 299
Outings with baby, 84, 110
Outsiders, contact with, 110
Overdressing baby, 109
Overheating
  in baby carrier, 147
  and fever, 427
  and risk of SIDS, 181
Overweight baby, 206
Ovulation
  cervical changes during,
    573
  mucus changes during, 573
Oxytocin, postpartum use of,
  514

P

Pacifier
  for crying baby, 117
  safe use of, 40
  use at 3 months, 177
  use in the hospital, 71
Pain, postpartum, 513
  in back of arms, 576
  following cesarean, 533
  following delivery, 513
  in perineal area, 516
  medication for, 514
Pain
  teething, 223

  treatment for, 415
Paint, lead in, 237
Palmar grasping reflex, 48
Panadol, 432
  dosage for, 628
Pancake faces, 620
Pancakes, golden-nugget
    oatmeal, 621
Parainfluenza virus, 635
Parents
  inadequacy as, 501
  not feeling like, 501
  of adopted baby, 501
  of sick baby, 483
  rights of, 270
Part-time work, 567,
  589
Particulate matter in indoor air,
  239
Patent ductus arteriosus, 473
Peachy yogurt, 626
Pediatric nurse-practitioner, 27
Pediatrician, 26
  see also, Doctor; Physician
"Peek-A-Boo," 319
Pelvic tilt, 530
Penis
  abnormalities of, 136
  care of, 85
  erection of, 287
  sore on, 181
  see also, Circumcision
Perfection, striving for, 551
Perianal dermatitis, 179
Perineum, postpartum
  care of, 516
  pain in, 516
Personal enrichment, 566
Perspiration, excessive,
    postpartum, 520
Pertussis, 642
  immunization against, 149
  when to omit
    immunization, 151
Pesticides
  household, 236
  in breast milk, 554
  in food, 242
  safe use of, 237
Petroleum jelly, 38
Pets
  allergy to, 417
  and baby, 22
Pharyngitis, 647
Phenylketonuria (PKU), 492
  and breastfeeding test for,
    47
Phimosis, 17
Photo flashes, 132
Physical aggressiveness, 369
Physical exam of infant, 90

Physician
  choosing, 25
  credentials, 29
  fees, 31
  locating, 28
  poor relationship with, 34
  type of practice of, 27
  visits to, see, Checkups
  when to call, see,
      individual ailments
  working with, 33
Pigeon-toes, 146
Pillow, use of, 136
Pinkeye, 632
PIV (parainfluenza virus), 631
PKU, see, Phenylketonuria
Placenta
  checking at birth, 45
  retained, 514, 558
Plants, poisonous, 301
Plastic bags, danger of, 136
Play groups, 331
Play sand, unsafe, 239
Playground safety, 302
Playing with baby, 318, 381
  see also, Stimulating baby
Playing with peers, 368
Playpen
  choosing, 43
  impatience with, 288
  overuse of, 289
Playthings, 212
  see also, Toys and
      playthings
Pneumonia, 642
Poinsettia, 395
Poison
  in the home, 294
  teaching baby about, 300
Poisoning, first aid for, 444
Poisonous plants, 301
Polio, immunization against,
  149
Pollen allergy, 417
Polygenic inheritance, 493
Pony- or pigtails, 333
Pool safety, 390
Poor adaptability baby, 159
"Pop goes the weasel," 320
Popsicle panniculitis, 392
Portwine stain, 68
Postadoption blues, 502
Posterior fontanel, 106
Postpartum
  best-odds diet for, 534
  constipation, 518
  depression, 545
  emotions at 6 weeks, 534
  feeling good during, 549
  fever, 559
  first few days of, 507

getting up, after cesarean, 525
getting up, after vaginal delivery, 517
immediate emotions, 508
immediate physical symptoms of, 507
infection, 558
lochia during, 514
pain, 513, 514, 516, 533
pain medication in, 65
perspiration, 520
physical symptoms of, at 6 weeks, 533
tub baths during, 552
urination problems of, 517
Postpartum depression, 545
absence of, 549
and father, 593
factors contributing to, 546
danger signs in, 548
in adoptive parents, 502
in father, 594
minimizing, 547
where to get help for, 548
Postpartum help
father as, 12, 16,
grandparents as, 16
other sources of, 16
Postpartum infection, 558
signs of, 513, 514
Postpartum psychosis
warning signs of, 548
Postpartum recovery
and breastfeeding, 5
Pots
aluminum, 248
copper, 248
nonstick, 238
Practitioner, when to call
postpartum, for mom, 513
see also, Doctor
Pregnancy, a new, 569
and breastfeeding, 575
and oral contraceptives, 570
diagnosing, 575
preventing, 5, 569
Premature baby, 457
and breast milk, 459
and car seat, 470
appearance of, 459
best care for, 461
breastfeeding of, 466
common health problems of, 472
expressing breast milk for, 460
fears about handling, 468
guilt concerning, 468
home care for, 471
nutritional deficiencies in, 459

risk of permanent damage in, 469
slower development in, 467, 469
Premature delivery
causes of, 470
fear of a repeat, 470
Prenatal interview, with baby doctor, 32
Preparing for baby, 2
Preteeth, 69
Preterm baby, 457
see also, Premature baby
Pronunciation, unclear, 345
Pronouns, 160, 264, 353
Propping baby to sitting, 204
Protein
dietary recommendations for, 350
in breast milk, 3
in breastfeeding diet, 537
in infant diet, 221
in postpartum diet, 537
in toddler diet, 359
postpartum, 510
Protein foods, 359
cholesterol in, 349
Pulling up, 308
delay in, 347
encouraging baby in, 347
readiness for, 308
safely, 308
Pulse, taking, 407
Pumpkin muffins, 620
Puncture wounds, 447
Punishment, 338
Pupils, dilated, 442
Pushing baby's development, 275
Pyloric stenosis, 492

R

Rabies, 435, 644
Radioactive iodine in breast milk, 554
Radon, 240
Rashes
in common childhood illnesses, 630
in eczema, 227
in hives, 416
in infants, 96
in newborns, 68, 69
see also, Skin
Reading
developing early interest in, 289
expanding, repertoire, 354
Recessive inheritance, 493

Recipes, 618
Records, health, 424
and twins, 105
Recti abdominis muscles, 529
Reflexes in newborn, 47
Regressive behavior in older child, 611
Rejection of breast
and cancer, 156
and hormonal changes, 156
and teething, 224
and weaning, 156, 311
Relactation, 131
Relaxation and breastfeeding, 8
REM sleep, 115
Remedies, home, 627
Rescue breathing, 452
Respiration, 407
Respiratory Distress Syndrome (RDS), 472
Respiratory sounds, 416
Respiratory symptoms, 407
Respiratory syncytial virus (RSV), 631, 644
Rest, for sick baby, 409
Restaurant, eating in, with baby, 404
Resuscitation techniques, 448
Retinopathy of prematurity (ROP), 473
Retrolental fibroplasia, 473
Reward and punishment, 338
Reye's syndrome, 644
Rh disease, 494
Rhythm method, calendar, 573
calculating, 574
Rickets, 345
Right, doing things, 551
Right-handedness, 290
Rights
children's, 340
parental, 340
"Ring-a-round the rosies," 319
Rocking baby, 119, 128
Rocking chair, 42
Romance, finding time for, 582
Room temperature
for premature babies, 471
in summer, 386
in winter, 394
Room, sharing with baby, 177, 185
Rooming in, 63
and breastfeeding, 50
Rooting reflex, 48
Roseola infantum, 646
Roughhousing, 187, 287
RSV (respiratory syncytial virus), 631, 644
Rubella, 636
immunization against, 151

Rubeola (measles), 638
Runny nose
in cold weather, 394
with cold, 418

S

Saccharin, 242
in mother's diet, 539
Safety
around fireplaces, 395
around water, 390
at holiday time, 395
at home, 292
equipment for, 296
fire, 297
for toddlers, 381
for young infants, 137
from poisoning, 294
in car, 78, 302
in food preparation, 230
in gift giving, 397
in summer, 389
in the bathroom, 298
in the kitchen, 297
in the playground, 302
of toys and playthings, 213
out-of-doors, 299
teaching baby about, 299
Saline
irrigation of nose, 419, 629
nose drops, 419
Salmon patch, 68
Salt and salty foods
in infant diet, 222
in postpartum/
breastfeeding diets, 538
in toddler diet, 363
intake of, 257
iodized, 363
limiting, 306
to avoid, 363
see also, Sodium
Sand, unsafe, 239
Saturated fat, 538
Scalds, first aid for, 437
Scarlet fever, 646
Schedules
baby who resists, 158
erratic, 542
establishing regular, 173
feeding, 111
irregular, 174
living without, 174
sleeping, 116
Scooting, 283
Scrapes, first aid for, 446
Scrotum, swelling of, 135
Sea urchin, sting of, 436
Seasonal concerns, 384

Seats, hook on
safety tips for, 235
Seborrheic dermatitis, 179
of the scalp, 144
Second language, 161
Second month, 140
Security objects, 309
Seizures
first aid for, 438
Self feeding, 314
refusal of, 372
Senses
overstimulation of, 157
stimulation of, 165
Separation anxiety
at night, 367
in older babies, 373
Seventh month, 266
Sex differences, 375
Sex-linked inheritance, 493
Sexual relations, resumption
of, 560
see also, Intercourse
Sexual stereotypes, 375
Sexuality in infants, 286
Shaking baby, 288
Shampoo
how to give, 86
what to use, 38
Sharing baby care, 544
Shock, first aid for, 446
Shoes
fitting, 332
for the nonwalker, 250
for walkers, 331
selecting, 331
Shots for immunization, 148
Shoulder pain,
in new parents, 576
postpartum, 524
Shoulder, disclocation of, 438
Shyness, 368
Sibling information network,
482
Sibling, older, 601
and baby's homecoming,
607
and colic, 124
and hospital visits, 465,
605
and nursing, 610
and prenatal visits, 603
and sick newborn, 482
at the delivery, 604
avoiding jealousy in, 612
bonding of, to baby, 614
classes for, 604
explaining genitals to, 609
hostility to parent in, 608
hurting baby, 611
increase in hostility of, 614

lack of jealousy in, 613
mother's resentment of, 609
open resentment in, 608
preparing, for baby, 602
regression in, 611
separation from, 605
switching, from crib, 603
when to tell, 602
Sick baby, 406
and child care, 199
evaluation of, 406
feeding of, 409
Sickle-cell anemia, 493
tests for, 47
SIDS, 181
see also, Sudden Infant
Death Synrome
Sight, in infants, 97
Silver nitrate, for eyes
at birth, 47
Sitting
late, 273
position, propping to, 204
pulling to, 201
Sitting, postpartum, 507
Six weeks postpartum, 533
emotions, 534
physical symptoms, 533
Skin flaps postpartum, 563
Sixth month, 245
Skin
birthmarks on, 68
changes in color of, 111
dryness, in winter, 394
in infant acne, 96
in sick baby, 408
mottling of, 111
of newborn, 46
red spots on, 69
whiteheads on, 68
wounds of, 446
yellowing of, 70
Sleep
and noise, 116
best positions for, 120
during meals, 60
in hours after birth, 64
moving baby during, 120
refusal to, after meals, 60
restless, 115
tips for improving, 119
Sleep patterns
changes in, 315
in infancy, 115, 116
in sick baby, 408
Sleep problems
and feeding, 224
and milk supply, 102
and premature infants, 262
and teething, 316
at bedtime, 315

at naptime, 315
checking with doctor about, 262
confusing of night and day, 118
dealing with at 6 months, 261
early waking, 260
in baby who used to sleep through, 367
night waking, 269, 367
night waking at 6 months, 260
night waking at 3 months, 175
Sleeplessness, in mother, 548
Slivers, removal of, 447
Slow development, 317
Smell, sense of, 165
Smell-sensitive baby, 160
Smile, first, 108
Smiling, 145
Smoked meats and fish, 241
Smoking
and baby's health, 20
quitting, 20
Snacking, 272
and fussy eating, 313
Snake bites, 435
Sneezing, 107
Snowburn, 394
"So big," 319
Soap
use of, 180
Soap, use of on baby, 76
Social development, 139
Social Security number, 88
Social skills
encouraging in infant, 167
encouraging in older baby, 265
encouraging in toddler, 381, 382
lack of, 368
sharing, as a, 368
Socks, 332
Sodium
content of foods, 258
in baking powder, 619
in breast milk, 3
intake in infancy, 257
recommended intake, 258
see also, Salt and salty foods
Soft spot, on head, 106
in sick baby, 408
Solids
allergic reaction to, 220
criteria for introducing, 203
first, 218, 219

introducing, 216
introducing, in premies, 471
when to start, 202
Songs and rhymes, introducing, 264
Sore throat, 646
treatment for, 415
Sound-sensitive baby, 157
Southeast Asia, baby from, 505
Soy formula, 114
Soy milk, danger as formula substitute, 54
Spanking, 339
Spastic movements, 177
Speaking to baby
at 6 months, 264
in early months, 160
Speech
development of, 281
encouraging in, early months, 160
encouraging, in older baby, 264
encouraging, in toddler, 352
unclear, 345
use of nonverbal, 374
see also, Language development
Spermicide foam, creams, jellies, 573
Spider bites, 435
Spina bifida (open spine), 496
Spitting up, 97
Spitup
blood in, 131
cleaning up, 98
Splinters, removal of, 447
Spoiling
a young baby, 130
after 6 months, 268
and grandparents, 270
Sponge bath
for fever, 432
how to give, 74
Stair safety, 300
Standing
early, 204
encouraging pulling up to, 347
pulling up to, 308
Startle reflex, 47, 66
Steam, 629
Stepping reflex, 48
Sterilization, surgical, 574
Sterilizing bottles, 56
Stimulating baby
at year's end, 380
creating environment for, 163
in the early months, 163

in the middle months, 263
Stimulation-sensitive baby, 160
Stingray, sting of, 436
Stitches, removal of, following cesarean, 525
Stomach, mother's
sleeping on, and breast-feeding, 103
Stool
black, 210
bloody, 420, 423
changes in, 249
color of, in newborns, 72
colorful, 317
frequent, 421
liquid, runny, 421
softeners, 519
specks in, 317
strange-looking, 317
texture of, 112
undigested food in, 249, 317
Stranger anxiety, 309
Strangers
explaining birth defects to, 478
baby's contact with, 110
Strawberry marks, 67
Strep throat, 646
Streptococcus bacteria, 647
Stroller, 41
Sucking satisfaction
and breastfeeding, 4, 102
and pacifier, 117
thumb sucking, 204
Suckling, ineffective, 101
Sudden infant death syndrome (SIDS), 181
explanation of, 182
fear of, 181
incidence of, 181
information on, 183
monitoring baby for, 183
risk factors for, 182
Sugar
and dental health, 253
banning of, in first year, 305
in breastfeeding diet, 535
in postpartum diet, 539
in toddler diet, 358
milk, and baby-bottle mouth, 255
types of, 358
Sugar water, 51
Summer concerns, 385
Sunburn, first aid for, 437
Sunscreens, 388
Suntan, sunburn
in winter, 394

preventing, 387
risks of, 386
signs of, 389
Super cereal, 618
Superbaby, raising a, 275
Supplemental nutrition system, 101
Supplementing breastfeeding, 142
  occasionally, 144
  reasons for, 142
  what to use for, 142
  when baby isn't thriving, 144
  when to begin, 142
  winning baby over, 143
  with backup bottles, 143
Supplements, dietary
  in breastfeeding diet, 539
  in infant diet, 222
  in postpartum diet, 539
  in toddler diet, 363
  see also, Vitamin supplements
Swaddling
  directions for, 87
  rejection of, 98
Sweets
  and dental health, 253
  in toddler diet, 358
  limiting, 305
  postpartum, 511
  see also, Sugar
Swim classes, 390
Swing, infant
  choosing, 43
  for crying baby, 128
Swollen glands, in mother, 533
Swollen lymph glands, 408
Symptomatic treatments, 414
Symptoms
  in sick baby, 406
  of common diseases, 630
  treating, 414
  see also, specific diseases
Syringe breast pump, 92
Syringe, for medication, 412
Systematic awakening, 261

T

Tail bone, broken, 512
Talk, teaching baby to, 352
Talking to baby, 160, 264
Tanning devices, 388
Tantrums, 380
Taste, sense of, 165
Tay Sachs disease, 496
TB, see, Tuberculosis

Td immunization
  for older children, 151
  recommended time for, 153
Tear duct, blocked, 108
Teeth
  and iron supplements, 273
  and nutrition, 253
  brushing of, 253
  decay in, from bottle use, 254
  grinding of, 328
  possible decay in, 273
  stains on, 273
  widely spaced, 254
Teething, 223
  and loss of interest in nursing, 155
  and sleep problems, 316
  early, 69
  late, 311
  order of, 225
  relief for, 224
  symptoms of, 223
  treatment for pain of, 415
Television watching and babies, 378
Temperature, dressing baby for, 109, 385, 393, 471
Temperature, basal body, 574
Temperature, body
  abnormally high, 427
  abnormally low, 442
  and premature babies, 471
  assessing, 407
  axillary, or armpit, 429
  estimating, with lips, 428
  in heat illness, 427
  in infection, 427
  normal, 427
  normal axillary, 430
  normal oral, 430
  normal rectal, 430
  oral, 429
  rectal, 428
  taking baby's, 428
Tempra, 432
  dosage for, 628
Tenth month, 321
Terrible twos, 380
Testicle
  swelling of, 135
  undescended, 154
Tetanus, 648
  booster, 446
  immunization against, 149
Thalassemia, 497
"The itsy bitsy spider," 319
Thermometers
  breaking of, 429
  reading of, 429
  types of, 39

Thin baby, 208
Third month, 169
Thirst, postpartum, 507
"This little piggy...," 319
Thriving, lack of, 99
Throat
  dry, postpartum, 533
  in sick baby, 408
Throat sore, 646
Thrombophlebitis, postpartum
  prevention of, 515
  signs of, 515
Thrush, 69
  and loss of appetite, 155
Thumb sucking, 204
Ticks
  removal of, 435
  treating bites of, 435
Tidemark dermatitis, 179
Time
  father's lack of, 600
  for romance, 582
  mother's lack of, 580
  quality, with baby, 581
Tobacco, 359, 536, 539
  in breast milk, 553
Toe injuries, first aid for, 440
  bleeding under the nail, 440
  bruises, 440
  severed toe, 445
  torn nail, 441
Toilet training, 329
Toiletries for baby, 38
Tonic neck reflex, 48
Tooth
  broken, 443
  knocked out, 443
Toothpaste, 253
TOPV immunization, 149
  recommended schedule for, 153
Touch-sensitive baby, 157
Touch, sense of, stimulating, 165
Toxic erythema, 69
Toy chest, 41
Toys and playthings
  and sexual stereotypes, 376
  for toddlers, 381
  philosophical objections to certain, 214
  safety of, 213
  selecting, 212
Tracheal-esophageal fistula, 497
Tracheomalacia, 416
Travel with baby, 397
  and hotels and motels, 404
  and restaurant eating, 404
  by auto, 403

by train, 403
medical precautions for, 397
medical supplies to take, 402
packing for, 400
planning ahead for, 397
Travel without baby, when breastfeeding, 173
Tremolite in play sand, 239
Trigger breast pump, 92
Tub baths, 250
fear of, 252
postpartum, 552
how to give, 75
Tub seat, 41
Tub, infant, 41
Tubal ligation, 574
Tuberculosis (TB)
and breastfeeding, 9
testing baby for, 356
testing baby sitter for, 193
Tubes, insertion for otitis media, 524
TV watching and babies, 378
Twelfth month, 355
Twins, 104
Tylenol, 432
dosage, 628
see also, Acetaminophen

U

Umbilical cord
care of, 87
cutting of, 45
healing of, 106
Umbilical hernia, 107
Underdressing baby, 109
Underweight baby, 208
Undescended testicles, 154
Unhappy baby, 159
Unpredictability, in baby, 372
Urinary incontinence (leaking), after childbirth, 577
Urinary system
in sick baby, 409
Urinary tract infection (UTI), 433
Urination, postpartum
difficulty with, 517
painful, burning, scant, 513
Uterus
at 6 weeks, 534
immediately postpartum, 508
involution of, postpartum, 514

V

Vaccination, 148
Vagina
at 6 weeks postpartum, 534
stretched by childbirth, 568
Vaginal discharge
abnormal changes in, 558
absence of, 513
blood clots in, 513
foul smelling, 558
in newborn girls, 46
postpartum, 514, 533
Vaginal dryness, 561
Vaginal lubrication, 561
Vaginal sponge, 572
Valuables, protecting from baby, 291
Vaporizer, 629
Varicella, 632
Varicella vaccine, 152
Variety, in diet, 306
Vasa deferentia, 574
Vaseline, 38
Vegetables
as first foods, 219, 221
chemical contamination of, 242
in toddler diet, 361
postpartum, 510
Vegetables, green leafy, see, Green leafy vegetables
Vegetables, other
choices of, 361
in infant diet, 222
in postpartum/ breastfeeding diets, 538
in toddler diet, 361
Vegetables, yellow, see, Yellow vegetables
Vegetarian diet
and baby vitamin supplements, 257
and breastfeeding, 256
dairy protein combinations for, 362
for baby, 256
vegetable protein combinations for, 361
Vernix caseosa, 46
Vesicular Stomatitis, 636
Violent feelings, 130, 599
Viral illnesses, nonspecific (NSV), 640
Vision, 97
Visitors, postpartum, 551
Visual perception
stimulating in early months, 165
Visually-sensitive baby, 157

Vitamin C foods
choices of, 359
in breastfeeding diet, 537
in infant diet, 221
in postpartum diet, 537
in toddler diet, 359
postpartum, 510
Vitamin D supplementation, 133
Vitamin K, 47
Vitamin supplements, 132
in breastfeeding diet, 539
in infant diet, 222
in postpartum diet, 539
in toddler diet, 363
see also, Supplements, dietary
Vitamins, excess, 241, 553
Volunteer work, 567
Vomiting, 98
in milk allergy, 114
treatment for, 415

W

Waking baby, 60
Waking early, dealing with, 260
Waking patterns
in early infancy, 116
Walker, 233
avoiding overuse of, 234
selection of, 43
safe use of, 233
Walking
and illness, 365
delayed, 365
early, 308
encouraging, 365
pushing, 308
risks in learning, 346
Walking reflex, 48
Walking, postpartum, 507
Washing baby's clothes, 115
Water
and babies, 390
safety, 390, 392
Water on the brain (hydrocephalus), 491
Water, drinking
contaminated, 238
lead in, 237
supplementary, 102, 137
unsafe, 241
Weaning from the breast
at baby's insistence, 311
best time for, 323
early, 185
from the bottle, 366
from the breast, 342
in summer, 392

keeping comfortable
  during, 344
bedtimes after, 366
readiness for, and breast
  rejection, 156
sudden, 344
Weaning from bottle at one
  year, 255
Weight
  at birth, 47
  controlling, in infant, 207
  differences in, at birth, 61
  inadequate gain of, in
    infant, 99
  loss after birth, 47, 70
  swings in, 350
Weight loss postpartum, 533
Weight problems
  efficient feeding for, 358
Weight, baby's
  below average, 208
  excessive, 206
  inadequate gain of, 99, 208
  increasing gain of, 209
Weight, postpartum, 543
  and breastfeeding, 5
  control of, 535
  loss of, 533
  too rapid loss of, 543
Weird thoughts, in depression,
  548

What to Expect When You're
  Expecting, 43
What You May Be Feeling first
  month, 89
  during first year, 564
  first few days postpartum,
    507
What You May Be Feeling
  during first six weeks,
    533
What Your Baby May Be Doing
  1st month, 89
  2nd month, 140
  3rd month, 169
  4th month, 200
  5th month, 215
  6th month, 245
  7th month, 266
  8th month, 278
  9th month, 303
  10th month, 321
  11th month, 341
  12th month, 355
  newborn, 45
Wheat germ, 306
Whiteheads on face, 68
Whole grains
  diets, 538
  in infant diet, 221
  in postpartum/
    breastfeeding diets, 538

in protein combinations,
  361
in toddler diet, 362
serving exclusively, 305
starting baby on, 258
Whole-wheat bread
  starting baby on, 259
Whooping cough, 642
  immunization against, 149
Words, first, 281
Work
  returning to, 12, 587
  taking baby to, 199
Working mother
  baby forgetting, 581
  time with baby for, 581

Y

Yeast infection
  in diaper area, 179
  in mouth, 69
Yellow fruits and vegetables
  in infant diet, 221
  in postpartum diet, 537
  in toddler diet, 361
Yellow vegetables in infant
  diet, 221
Yogurt, as a first food, 219
Yogurt, peachy frozen, 626